Self Assessment and Review of Anatomy

Second Edition

Rajesh K Kaushal

MD Anatomy (AIIMS, Delhi)
Director, Human Anat Academia
New Delhi

The Health Sciences Publisher
New Delhi | London | Panama

Jaypee Brothers Medical Publishers (P) Ltd

Headquarters

Jaypee Brothers Medical Publishers (P) Ltd.
4838/24, Ansari Road, Daryaganj
New Delhi 110 002, India
Phone: +91-11-43574357
Fax: +91-11-43574314
E-mail: jaypee@jaypeebrothers.com

Overseas Offices

JP Medical Ltd.
83, Victoria Street, London
SW1H 0HW (UK)
Phone: +44-20 3170 8910
Fax: +44(0)20 3008 6180
E-mail: info@jpmedpub.com

Jaypee Brothers Medical Publishers (P) Ltd.
17/1-B, Babar Road, Block-B, Shyamoli
Mohammadpur, Dhaka-1207
Bangladesh
Mobile: +08801912003485
E-mail: jaypeedhaka@gmail.com

Jaypee-Highlights Medical Publishers Inc.
City of Knowledge, Bld. 235, 2nd Floor, Clayton
Panama City, Panama
Phone: +1 507-301-0496
Fax: +1 507-301-0499
E-mail: cservice@jphmedical.com

Jaypee Brothers Medical Publishers (P) Ltd.
Bhotahity, Kathmandu, Nepal
Phone: +977-9741283608
E-mail: kathmandu@jaypeebrothers.com

Website: www.jaypeebrothers.com
Website: www.jaypeedigital.com

Self Assessment and Review of Anatomy

First Edition: 2017
Second Edition: 2018

ISBN: 978-93-5270-441-5

Printed at: Ajanta Offset & Packagings Ltd., Faridabad, Haryana.

It all begins with one word
'Passion' !

Dedicated to

All those teachers and students,
who illuminate the world around by their honest work, sacrifices, and a purpose of duty !

PREFACE

Long ago I thought of a mission—Human Anatomy Made Simple. Then it was a dream, now realizing that dream into concrete reality is a profound matter of satisfaction and joy.

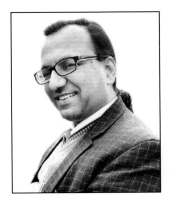

As Steve Maraboli mentioned: 'The best way to succeed is to have a specific **Intent,** a clear **Vision,** a plan of **Action,** and the ability to maintain **Clarity.**'

Anatomy is an integral component of PG Entrance exams at multiple levels. It is not an important individual subject in itself but, in terms of conceptual and clinical correlates, touches and fetches improved scoring in almost all the major and minor subjects, once mastered well.

The present book is a simplistic quintessential approach to master basic and conceptual Anatomy and its clinical application. Maximum possible content has been covered under various sub-sections of Anatomy, so that the student does not need to look into a plethora of books—in a sense it is 'all in one approach'. It is written in a simple lucid language with neatly labelled line diagrams, along with tables and flowcharts to improve memorization and recall of the vast content.

The latest edition of Gray's Anatomy has abundance of updated information, which is not in accordance with the traditional/conventional teaching. Such information has been included in the present book but its usage in the exams is not yet advisable, and depends upon the discretion of the teacher and the students.

Controversies arise when different authors follow different standard textbooks, for example, a particular question on pemphigus vulgaris may be asked by Anatomy department, but may also interest, Pathology, Dermatology and Medicine departments equally. Such questions have been dealt with profound and relentless research, referring to respective department standard textbooks and Journals to bring you the most appropriate answer possible.

Dear students, I was a medical student, and will remain so throughout my life. We all have been trained to work hard in the best interest of our patients and peers. I respect and honour your tenacity in keeping the fire and zeal alive in your heart and mind, and remain highly motivated despite tough scenarios in life keep presenting in front of you, every possible moment.

Wishing a great success to all the students, in all arenas of life !

Rajesh K Kaushal
MD Anatomy (AIIMS, Delhi)
February, 28, 2018

ACKNOWLEDGMENTS

I would like to thank Shri Jitendar P Vij (Group Chairman), Mr Ankit Vij (Group President) and Mrs Chetna Malhotra Vohra (Associate Director–Content Strategy) of Jaypee Brothers Medical Publishers (P) Ltd. New Delhi, India, for enabling me to publish this book. I would also like to thank Ms Payal Bharti (Sr Manager, Publishing), and the complete Production Team for helping me in the whole process.

CONTENTS

1. General Anatomy 1

2. Embryology 14

3. Histology 75

4. Neuroanatomy 126

5. Head and Neck 207

6. Back Region 324

7. Thorax 334

8. Upper Limb 392

9. Abdomen 451

10. Pelvis and Perineum 543

11. Lower Limb 588

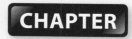
General Anatomy

▸ Skeleton

Bone is a calcified connective tissue consisting of **cells** (osteocytes) embedded in a **matrix** of ground substance and collagen fibers.

- ❑ It has a superficial thin layer of compact bone around a central mass of spongy bone, and contain internal soft tissue, the marrow, where blood cells are formed.
- ❑ It serve as a reservoir for calcium and phosphorus and act as biomechanical levers on which muscles act to produce the movements permitted by joints.

Long bones have a shaft (diaphysis) and two ends (epiphyses). The metaphysis is a part of the diaphysis adjacent to the epiphyses.

- ❑ **Diaphysis**
  - ➤ Forms the shaft (central region) and is composed of a thick tube of compact bone that encloses the marrow cavity.
- ❑ **Metaphysis**
  - ➤ Is a part of the diaphysis, the growth zone between the diaphysis and epiphysis during bone development.
- ❑ **Epiphyses**
  - ➤ Are expanded articular ends, separated from the shaft by the epiphyseal plate during bone growth and composed of a spongy bone surrounded by a thin layer of compact bone.

▸ Ossification

- ❑ **Ossification** is the process of laying down new bone material by cells called osteoblasts. It is of two types:
  - ➤ Membranous ossification is the direct laying down of bone into the mesenchyme (embryonic connective tissue).
  - ➤ Endochondral ossification involves osteogenesis in a precursor model of cartilage.
- ❑ **Membrane** (dermal) bones ossify in membrane (intramembranous ossification), and are thus derived from mesenchymal condensations. The flat bones of the skull and face, the mandible, and the clavicle develop by intramembranous ossification.
- ❑ **Cartilaginous** bones ossify in cartilage (endochondral ossification), and are thus derived from preformed cartilaginous models. The bones of the extremities (limbs) and those parts of the axial skeleton that bear weight (vertebral column and thoracic cage) develop by endochondral ossification.
- ❑ **Membrano-cartilaginous** bones are initially formed in membrane but later partly in cartilage. Examples: clavicle, mandible, occipital, temporal, sphenoid.
- ❑ Cartilaginous ossification involves primary and secondary centers of ossification:
- ❑ **Primary center of ossification**
  - ➤ In long bones, bone tissue first appears in the diaphysis **(middle of shaft)**.
  - ➤ Primary centers starts appearing at **week 6** of intrauterine life.
  - ➤ Chondrocytes multiply and form trabeculae and cartilage is progressively eroded and replaced by bone, extending towards the epiphysis.
  - ➤ A perichondrium layer surrounding the cartilage forms the periosteum, which generates osteogenic cells that make a collar to encircles the exterior of the bone and remodels the medullary cavity on the inside.
  - ➤ The **nutrient artery** enters via the nutrient foramen from a small opening in the diaphysis.
    - ▪ It invades the primary center of ossification, **bringing osteogenic cells** (osteoblasts on the outside, osteoclasts on the inside.)
    - ▪ The canal of the nutrient foramen is directed away from more active end of bone when one end grows more than the other.
    - ▪ When bone grows at same rate at both ends, the nutrient artery is perpendicular to the bone.
- ❑ **Secondary center of ossification**
  - ➤ The secondary centers generally appear at the ends **(epiphysis)** of long bones.

➢ Secondary ossification mostly occurs after birth **except** for secondary centers around knee joint (distal femur and proximal tibia), which appear during last weeks of fetal life (or immediately after birth).

➢ The epiphyseal arteries and osteogenic cells invade the epiphysis, depositing osteoblasts and osteoclasts which erode the cartilage and build bone. This occurs at both ends of long bones but only one end of digits and ribs.

Ossification centers which appear **prenatally** (ossified at birth) are: diaphysis of long bones, skull bones, vertebral column, ribs and sternum, few foot bones (talus, calcaneum, cuboid).

Primary center of all carpal and tarsal bones (**except** talus, calcaneum and cuboid) appear after birth.

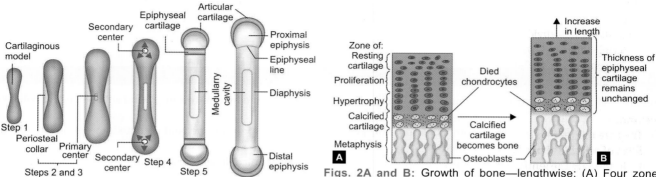

Fig. 1: Ossification of a long bone

Figs. 2A and B: Growth of bone—lengthwise: (A) Four zones of epiphyseal cartilage; (B) Conversion of calcified cartilage into bone

Time period	Bones affected
Second month of fetal development	Ossification in long bones beginning
Fourth month	Most primary ossification centers have appeared in the diaphyses of bone
Birth to 5 years	Secondary ossification centers appear in the epiphyses
5 years to 12 years in females, 5 to 14 years in males	Ossification is spreading rapidly from the ossification centers and various bones are becoming ossified
17 to 20 years	Bone of upper limbs and scapulae becoming completely ossified
18 to 23 years	Bone of the lower limbs and os coxae become completely ossified
23 to 25 years	Bone of the sternum, clavicles, and vertebrae become completely ossified
By 25 years	Nearly all bones are completely ossified

▶ Growing End

❑ The growing ends of bones in upper limb are **upper end** of humerus and **lower ends** of radius and ulna.

❑ In lower limb, the **lower end** of femur and **upper end** of tibia are the growing ends.

❑ The nutrient foramen is **directed away** from the growing end of the bone; their directions are indicated by a memory aid: 'Towards the elbow I go, from the knee I flee'.

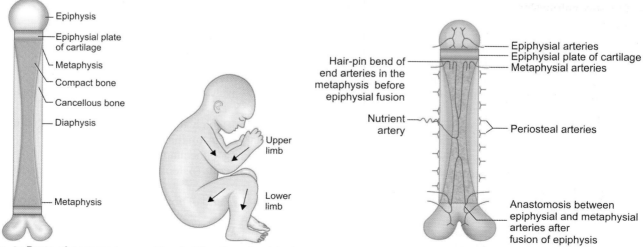

Fig. 3: Parts of a young long bone

Fig. 4: Direction of nutrient foramina in the limb bones

Fig. 5: Arterial supply of a long bone. The upper epiphysis (growing end) has not yet fused with the diaphysis

Blood Supply

Nutrient artery enters the diaphysis (shaft) through the nutrient foramen, runs obliquely through the cortex, and divides into ascending and descending branches in the medullary cavity.

- ❑ Each branch divides into a number of small parallel channels which **terminate in the adult metaphysis** by anastomosing with the epiphysial, metaphysial and periosteal arteries.
- ❑ It supplies medullary cavity, inner 2/3 of cortex and metaphysis.
- ❑ The nutrient foramen is **directed away** from the growing end of the bone. **Memory aid:** Towards the elbow I go, from the knee I flee.
- ❑ Bony skeleton is divided into two parts: the axial skeleton and the appendicular skeleton.
    - ➤ **Axial skeleton** is the central core unit, consisting of the skull, vertebrae, ribs, and sternum.
    - ➤ **Appendicular skeleton** comprises the bones of the extremities.

Sesamoid Bones

Sesamoid bones develop in certain **tendons** and reduce friction on the tendon, thus protecting it from excessive wear.

- ❑ They are commonly found where tendons cross the ends of long bones in the limbs.
- ❑ **Sites of sesamoid bones:**
    - ➤ In the ear: The lenticular process of incus is a sesamoid bone and therefore is considered the fourth ossicle of middle ear.
    - ➤ In the hand: Two sesamoid bones in the distal portions of the first metacarpal bone (within the tendons of adductor pollicis and flexor pollicis brevis).
    - ➤ In the wrist: The pisiform of the wrist is a sesamoid bone (within the tendon of **flexor carpi ulnaris**), develops at age 9–12.
    - ➤ In the knee: The patella (within the quadriceps tendon).
    - ➤ **Fabella** in the lateral head of gastrocnemius behind the knee joint.
    - ➤ Sesamoid bone in the tendon of peroneus longus where it binds around the cuboid bone.
    - ➤ In the foot: Two sesamoid bones in the distal portions of the first metatarsal bone (within the tendons of flexor hallucis brevis.

Pneumatic Bones

Note: **Pneumatic bones** are the **irregular** bones which contain air-filled cavities within them.

- ❑ They are generally produced during development by **excavation of bone** by pneumatic diverticula (air sacs) from an air-filled space such as the nasal cavity.
- ❑ E.g., maxilla, frontal, sphenoid, and ethmoid bones and a part of the mastoid part of the temporal bone.

Note: At birth, the mastoid is **not pneumatized**, but becomes aerated over the first year of life.

Epiphysis

There are **four types** of epiphysis:

- ❑ **Pressure epiphysis** are the parts of bone involved in weight transmission (and are intracapsular), e.g. head of humerus and femur and condyles of humerus, femur, tibia, etc.

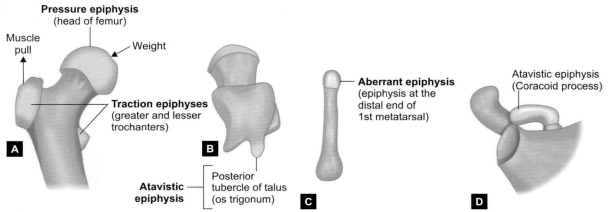

Figs. 6A to D: Types of epiphyses: (A) Pressure and traction epiphyses; (B) and (D) Atavistic epiphyses; (C) Aberrant epiphysis

❑ **Traction epiphysis** are present at the ends of bones and develop due to traction by the attached muscles (and are therefore extracapsular), e.g. greater (and lesser) tubercles in humerus and greater (and lesser) trochanter in femur.
  ➢ These epiphyses ossify later than pressure epiphyses.
  ➢ Examples of traction epiphyses are tubercles of the humerus (greater tubercle and lesser tubercle), and trochanters of the femur (greater and lesser). Mastoid process is also a traction epiphysis.
❑ **Atavistic epiphysis:** These types of fused bones are called atavistic, another example is the coracoid process of the scapula, **posterior tubercle** of talus (as trigonum), which has been fused in humans with the main bone, but is separate in lower animals.
❑ **Aberrant** (unusual) epiphysis are deviations from the norm and are **not always present.** E.g., Epiphyses at the **head of the first metacarpal** and at the **base of other metacarpals.**

QUESTIONS

1. Endochondral ossification is/are seen in: *(PGIC 2015)*
   a. Long bones   b. Clavicle
   c. Mandible   d. Nasal bones
   e. Flat bones of skull

2. Bones ossified at birth: *(PGIC 2015)*
   a. Upper end of humerus   b. Lower end of humerus
   c. Lower end of femur   d. Upper end of tibia
   e. Calcaneum

3. Nutrient artery runs: *(NEET Pattern 2012)*
   a. Towards metaphysis   b. Away from metaphysis
   c. Away from epiphysis   d. None

4. All of the following statements are true for metaphysis of bone EXCEPT: *(AIPG 2003)*
   a. It is the strongest part of bone
   b. It is the most vascular part of bone
   c. Growth activity is maximized here
   d. It is the region favouring hematogenous spread of infection

5. TRUE statement is: *(AIPG 2000)*
   a. Osteoblasts give rise to osteocytes
   b. Growth of bone occurs at diaphysis
   c. Epiphysis is present between metaphysis and diaphysis
   d. Interphalangeal joint is a saddle joint

6. Traction epiphysis is/are: *(PGIC)*
   a. Head of humerus   b. Lesser tubercle
   c. Deltoid tuberosity d. Coracoid process
   e. Greater trochanter

7. Which of the following is an aberrant epiphysis: *(NEET Pattern 2015)*
   a. Coracoid process
   b. Greater tubercle of humerus
   c. Base of 1st metacarpal   d. Base of 2nd metacarpal

8. Bones which is/are pneumatic: *(PGIC May 2015)*
   a. Maxillary   b. Parietal
   c. Temporal   d. Frontal
   e. Ethmoidal

ANSWERS

1. a. Long bones; b. Clavicle
   ❑ Long bones and medial end of clavicle bone develop by endochondral ossification.
   ❑ Flat bones of skull; facial skeleton; mandible and lateral end of clavicle develop by intramembranous ossification.

2. c. Lower end of femur; d. Upper end of tibia; e. Calcaneum
   ❑ **Secondary centers** around knee joint (**distal femur** and **proximal tibia**) appear during last weeks of intrauterine life (or immediately after birth).
   ❑ Primary center of all tarsal bones (except talus, calcaneum and cuboid) appear after birth.

3. a. Towards metaphysis
   ❑ **Nutrient artery** enters the shaft (diaphysis) of the bone, divides into ascending and descending branches, which run towards and terminate in the adult **metaphysis** by anastomosing with the epiphyseal, metaphyseal and periosteal arteries.

4. a. It is the strongest part of bone
   ❑ The strongest part of bone is diaphysis (**not metaphysis**).
   ❑ During growth of bone maximum activity occurs at growth plate (physis) and the adjacent section of the **metaphysis**.
   ❑ Metaphysis is richly supplied with arteries forming hairpin bends, hence becomes a common site of osteomyelitis in children, as infectious agents are easily trapped in **sluggish blood flow** in hairpin bends.

5. a. Osteoblasts give rise to osteocytes
   ❑ **Osteoblasts** that get trapped in Haversian lamellae **become osteocyte** and assume the function of bone maintenance. They are no longer involved in bone formation.
   ❑ Growth activity is **maximum at the growth plate** (physis) and adjacent metaphysis.
   ❑ Metaphysis is present **between** diaphysis and epiphysis.
   ❑ Interphalangeal joint is a **hinge variety** of synovial joint.

6. b. Lesser tubercle; e. Greater trochanter
   ❑ **Traction epiphysis** are usually present at the ends of bones and develop **due to traction** by the attached muscles (and are therefore extracapsular), e.g. Greater (and lesser) tubercles in humerus and greater (and lesser) trochanter in femur.
   ❑ **Pressure** epiphysis are involved in weight transmission (and are intracapsular) e.g. head of humerus and femur and condyles of humerus, femur, tibia, etc.
   ❑ **Coracoid process** in scapula is an example of **atavistic** epiphysis.
   ❑ Deltoid tuberosity is **not an epiphysis** (it is present on the shaft/diaphysis).

7. d. Base of 2nd metacarpal
   ❑ Aberrant epiphyses are **deviations from the normal** anatomy and are **not always present**. For example, the epiphysis at the head of the first metacarpal bone and at the bases of other metacarpals.

8. a. Maxillary; c. Temporal; d. Frontal; e. Ethmoidal
- ❑ Pneumatic bones have **air spaces** within them and are present around the nasal cavity.
- ❑ Temporal bone is morphologically classified as pneumatic bone because it has an **internal air sinus** and **mastoid air cells**.
- ❑ Parietal bone is **not a pneumatic bone**.

- ■ **Trochanter** of femur is an example of **traction** epiphysis *(NEET Pattern 2012)*
- ■ **Mastoid** process is **traction** epiphysis *(NEET Pattern 2015)*
- ■ **Mandible** is **not** a pneumatic bone *(AIPG 2011)*
- ■ **Metaphysis** is the epiphyseal end of the diaphysis.
- ■ Parietal bone is **not** a pneumatic bone *(AIIMS 2003)*
- ■ **Pisiform** is a sesamoid bone *(NEET Pattern 2015)*

▶ Joints

Union between bones can be in one of three types: by fibrous tissue; by cartilage; or by synovial joints.

Classification

The **structural** classification divides joints into **fibrous**, **cartilaginous**, and **synovial** joints depending on the material composing the joint and the presence or absence of a cavity in the joint. The **functional** classification divides joints into three categories: **synarthroses**, **amphiarthroses**, and **diarthroses**.

Synarthrosis (immovable)	Fibrous joints
Amphiarthrosis (slight mobile)	Cartilaginous joint
Diarthrosis (freely mobile)	Synovial joints

Fibrous joints occur where bones are separated only by connective tissue and movement between them is negligible. Examples of fibrous joints are the **sutures** that unite the bones of the vault of the skull and the **syndesmosis** between the lower ends of the tibia and fibula.

Types of fibrous joint	Examples
Suture	Spheno-vomerine joint (schindylesis)
Gomphosis	Tooth and socket joints
Syndesmosis	Middle radioulnar joint Inferior radioulnar joint

Cartilaginous joints are of two varieties, primary and secondary.
- ❑ Primary Cartilaginous Joints (synchondroses) are united by hyaline cartilage and permit no movement but growth in the length.
  - ➤ A primary cartilaginous joint **(synchondrosis)** is one where bone and hyaline cartilage meet. Thus, all epiphyses are primary cartilaginous joints, as are the junctions of ribs with their own costal cartilages.
  - ➤ All primary cartilaginous joints are **quite immobile** and are very strong. The adjacent bone may fracture, but the bone–cartilage interface will not separate.
  - ➤ They Includes epiphyseal cartilage plates (the union between the epiphysis and the diaphysis of a growing bone) and spheno-occipital and manubrio-sternal synchondroses.
- ❑ Secondary cartilaginous joints **(Symphysis)** have bones are united by hyaline plus fibrocartilage.
  - ➤ These joints are usually in the midline and are slightly mobile.
  - ➤ Include pubis symphysis, midline intervertebral joints.
    - ■ Symphysis is a union between bones whose articular surfaces are covered with a thin lamina of hyaline cartilage. The hyaline laminae are united by fibrocartilage.
    - ■ There may be a cavity in the fibrocartilage, but it is never lined with synovial membrane and it contains only tissue fluid.
    - ■ Examples are the **pubic symphysis** and the joint of the sternal angle (between the manubrium and the body of the sternum).
    - ■ An intervertebral disc is part of a secondary cartilaginous joint, but here the cavity in the fibrocartilage contains a gel.
    - ■ A limited amount of movement is possible in secondary cartilaginous joints, depending on the amount of fibrous tissue within them. All symphyses occur in the **midline** of the body.

Types of cartilaginous joint	Examples
Synchondrosis	Spheno-occipital joint Epiphysio-diaphyseal joint (growing bone)
Symphysis	Midline intervertebral joint Sacrococcygeal joint

- ❏ **Synovial joints** are freely mobile joints.
- ❏ Synovial joints are uniaxial: Plane, hinge and pivot; Biaxial: Condylar and ellipsoid; Multiaxial: Saddle, ball and socket.

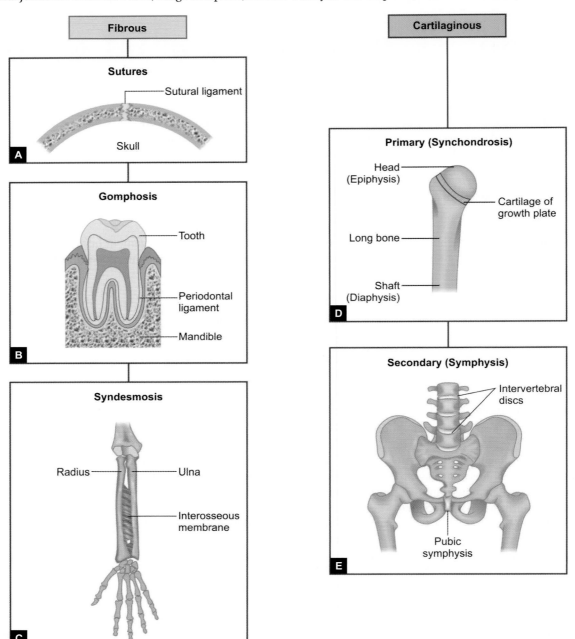

Figs. 7A to E: Fibrous joints (A to C) and Cartilaginous joints (D and E)

▶ Synovial Joints

Synovial joints are **freely mobile** joints. They are **uniaxial**: Plane, hinge and pivot; **Biaxial**: Condylar and ellipsoid and **Multiaxial**: Saddle, ball and socket.

Types of synovial joint	Examples
Plane	▪ Acromioclavicular ▪ Intercarpal ▪ Intertarsal
Hinge	▪ Elbow ▪ Interphalangeal
Pivot (Trochoid)	▪ Atlanto-axial ▪ Superior radio-ulnar ▪ Inferior radio-ulnar
Condylar	▪ Temporo-mandibular ▪ Knee joint

Types of synovial joint	Examples
Ellipsoid	▪ Atlanto-occipital ▪ Wrist (radio-carpal) ▪ Metacarpo-phalangeal (knuckle)
Saddle	▪ Malleus-incus joint ▪ Sternoclavicular ▪ First carpo-metacarpal ▪ Calcaneocuboid
Ball and socket	▪ Incus-stapes joint ▪ Shoulder ▪ Hip ▪ Talo-calcaneo-navicular

Some authors consider these joints condylar: Atlanto-occipital, wrist (radio-carpal), metacarpo-phalangeal (knuckle).

Some authors consider these joints as modified hinge: Temporo-mandibular, knee joint.

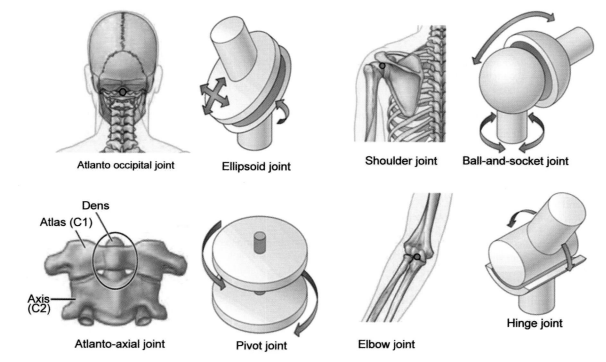

Fig. 8: Types of synovial joints

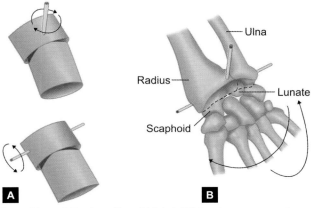

Figs. 9A and B: An ellipsoid joint (A) is shown as analogous to the radiocarpal joint (wrist) (B) The two axes of rotation are shown by the intersecting pins

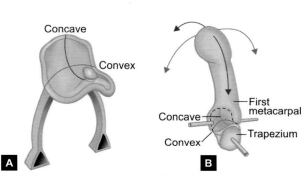

Figs. 10A and B: A saddle joint (A) is illustrated as analogous to the carpometacarpal joint of the thumb (B). The saddle in A. Represents the trapezium bone. The rider, if present, would represent the base of the thumb's metacarpal. The two axes of rotation are shown in (B)

❑ Knee joint is a **complex** joint (involving more than two bones).

❑ Femoro-tibial joint structurally resembles a hinge joint, but is considered as a condylar type of synovial joint between two condyles of the femur and tibia. In addition, it includes a saddle joint between the femur and the patella.

Hilton's law: A joint is **innervated** by articular branches of the nerves that supply the **muscles** acting on the joint and that also supply the **skin** covering the joint.

QUESTIONS

1. What type of joint is the growth plate? (AIPG 2010)
a. Fibrous　　　　　　　　b. Primary cartilaginous
c. Secondary cartilaginous　d. Plane joint

2. Atlanto-occipital joint is of synovial variety:
a. Trochoid　　　　b. Ellipsoid
c. Condylar　　　　d. Saddle

3. Which of the following is a compound condylar joint?
(NEET Pattern 2012)
a. Knee　　　　　　b. TM joint
c. Wrist　　　　　　d. Elbow

4. Metacarpophalangeal joint is:
a. Condylar　　　　b. Ellipsoid
c. Saddle　　　　　d. Hinge

5. Which of the following is a synovial joint of the condylar variety? (NEET Pattern 2012)
a. First carpometacarpal joint　b. Metacarpophalangeal joint
c. Interphalangeal joint　　　　d. Radiocarpal joint

6. Vomer ala and sphenoidal rostrum junction is:
(NEET Pattern 2013)
a. Syndesmosis　　b. Synostosis
c. Schindylesis　　d. Gomphosis

ANSWERS

1. b. Primary cartilaginous
❑ Growing bones have epiphyseal (growth) plate between the **epiphysis** and **diaphysis**, this epiphyseo-diaphyseal joint is primary cartilaginous (**synchondrosis**).
❑ It is found in the growing bone, where the growth plate (**hyaline** cartilage) connects the epiphysis with the diaphysis, creating a hyaline cartilaginous joint.
❑ At this site the **fate** of synchondrosis is **synostosis** (bony fusion) after the growth plate gets **removed** and **replaced** by the bone.

2. b. Ellipsoid > c. Condylar
❑ **Functionally** it is an **ellipsoid** synovial joint but **structurally** it is a **condylar** synovial joint.
❑ Head **flexion and extension** occurs at this joint for the **nodding (yes)** movement.

3. a. Knee
❑ Knee joint has **more than two** bones participating (hence **compound** joint). It is formed by the lateral and medial femorotibial and the femoropatellar joints.
❑ It is a compound synovial joint incorporating **two condylar joints** between the condyles of the femur and tibia and one **saddle joint** between the femur and the patella.
❑ TM joint is a **condylar joint** but it involves only 2 bones (not a compound joint).
❑ **Wrist** joint is an **ellipsoid** synovial joint and **elbow** is a **hinge** synovial joint.

4. b. Ellipsoid > a. Condylar
❑ Metacarpophalangeal joint has a condyle with elliptical articular surface.
❑ **Structurally** it is **condylar** but **functionally ellipsoid** synovial joint.

5. b. Metacarpophalangeal joint > d. Radiocarpal joint
❑ This a **wrong** Questions, since both the joints have condyles with ellipsoid articular surface - are structurally condylar but functionally ellipsoid synovial joints.
❑ Some authors mention metacarpophalangeal as condylar synovial joint only (**hence** the answer of first preference).

6. c. Schindylesis
❑ **Spheno-vomerine** joint is a **schindylesis** suture at the roof of the nasal cavity.

Rostrum of sphenoid
Ala of vomer
Vomer

Schindylesis

- **Innervated** structures of joints are **Synovium, Capsule** and **Ligaments** (NEET Pattern 2013)
  - **Articular cartilage** has **no** neurovascular bundle
- **Hilton's** law is related to **Nerve** innervation (NEET Pattern 2016)
- Knee is a **diarthrosis** type of joint.
- Joint between **epiphysis** and **diaphysis** of a long bone is a type of **Synchondrosis** (AIIMS 2004)
- **Ear ossicles** articulate with each other through **Synovial** type of joints (NEET Pattern 2012)
  - Malleus-incus joint is a **saddle** synovial joint and incus -stapes is **ball and socket** synovial joint.
- **Intracapsular** articular disc is present in Sternoclavicular joint (NEET Pattern 2012)
- **Vomerine** ala and **sphenoidal** rostrum junction is a **Schindylesis** (NEET Pattern 2013)
- **Pubic symphysis** is **Cartilaginous** type of joint (NEET Pattern 2015)

- Inferior tibio-fibular joint is a **Syndesmosis.**
- **Midline** intervertebral joint with intervertebral disc is **Secondary cartilagenous** *(NEET Pattern 2016)*
- The type of joint between the sacrum and the coccyx is a **Symphysis** *(AIPG 2005)*
- Atlantoaxial joint is a **Pivot** synovial joint *(NEET Pattern 2015, 16)*

Muscles

The orientation of individual skeletal muscle fibers is either **parallel or oblique** to the line of pull of the whole muscle. The range of contraction is long with the former arrangement, while the latter provides increased force of contraction. Sartorius is an example of a muscle with parallel fibers.

Muscles with an oblique disposition of fibers fall into several patterns:

- Muscles with **parallel fasciculi**: These are muscles in which the fasciculi are parallel to the line of pull and have greater degree of movement. These muscles may be:
  - Quadrilateral, e.g. thyrohyoid, Pronator quadratus
  - Strap-like, e.g. **sternohyoid** and **sartorius**
  - Strap-like, with tendinous intersections, e.g. **rectus abdominis**
  - Fusiform, e.g. biceps brachii, digastric
- Muscles with oblique fasciculi: When the fasciculi are oblique to the line of pull, the muscle may be triangular, or pennate (feather-like) in the construction. This arrangement makes the muscle more powerful, although the range of movement is reduced. Oblique arrangements are of the following types:
- **Convergent fasciculi:** The muscle fibers or fasciculi converge at the insertion point to maximize contraction. Such muscles may be: (a) Triangular, e.g. temporalis (b) Fan-shaped, e.g. temporalis.

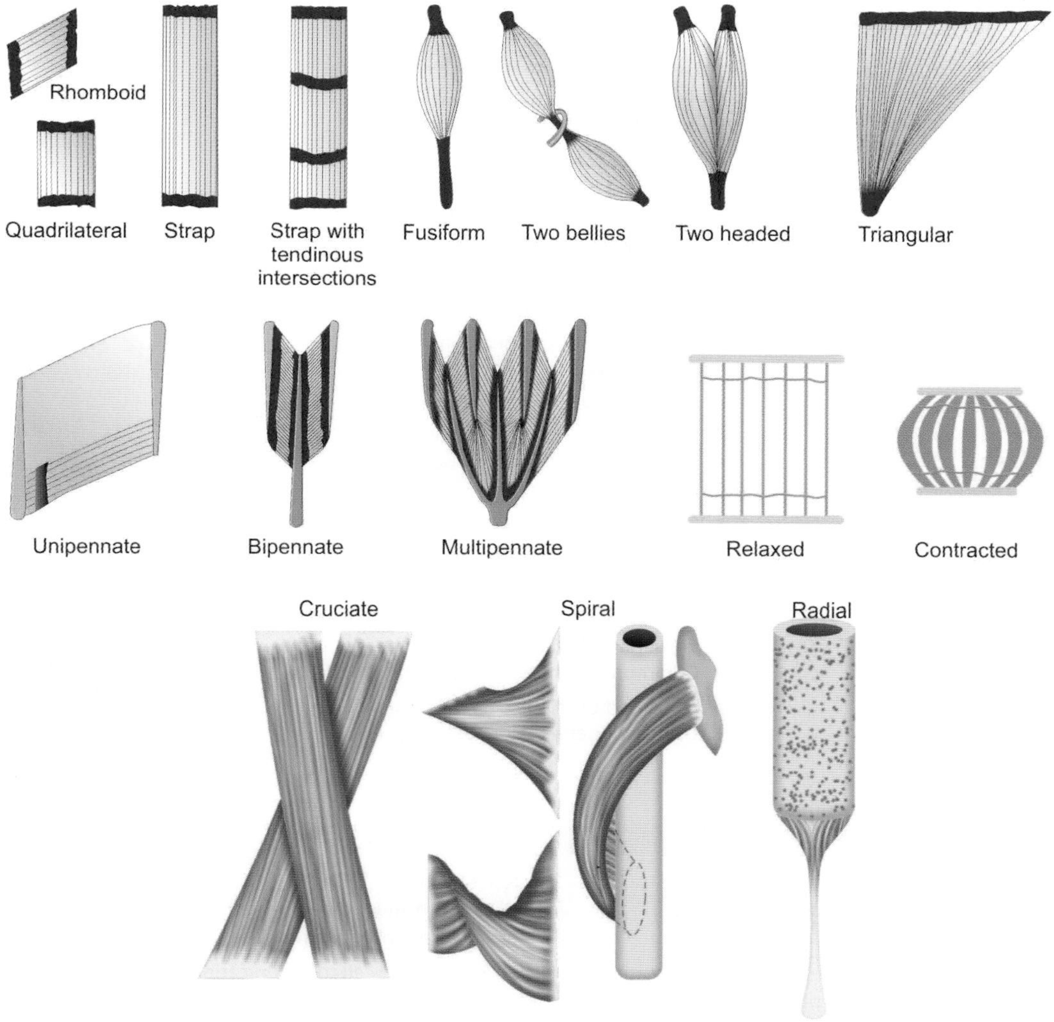

Fig. 11: Morphological 'types' of muscle based on their general form and fascicular architecture.

- ❑ **Spiral or twisted fasciculi:** In some muscles the fibers are twisted or spiraled, e.g. trapezius, latissimus dorsi, pectoralis major, supinator.
- ❑ **Cruciate muscles:** In some muscles, fibers or fasciculi are arranged in superficial and deep planes and crossed 'X', e.g. sterno-cleidomastoid, masseter, adductor magnus.
- ❑ **Sphincteric fasciculi:** In some muscles, the muscle fibers or fasciculi surround an opening or orifice, thus when they contract the opening is closed or constricted, e.g. orbicularis oculi around the eye and orbicularis oris surrounding the oral orifice.
- ❑ **Pennate fasciculi:** The pennate-fiber muscles resemble the feather, the fleshy fibers correspond to the bars of the feather and the tendon to the shaft, as they are all inserted by tendon. They may be:
  - ➢ **Uni pennate**, e.g. flexor pollicis longus, extensor digitorum longus
  - ➢ **Bipennate**, e.g. rectus femoris, flexor hallucis longus
  - ➢ **Multipennate**, e.g. tibialis anterior, subscapularis, deltoid (acromial fibers).
- ❑ Common sites of intramuscular injection

Upper arm (Deltoid)	▪ 5 cm distal to the acromion or ▪ 4 cm proximal to the insertion of deltoid ▪ This is to prevent injury to circumflex humeral nerve.
Gluteal region	▪ Upper outer (superolateral) quadrant ▪ This is to avoid damage to superior and inferior gluteal vessels and sciatic nerve. ▪ The muscle in which the injection is given is gluteus medius.
Thigh (lateral aspect)(vastus lateralis)	▪ Infant: Upper lateral quadrant of thigh below GT ▪ Adult: Middle third of lateral aspect.

Hybrid (composite) muscles have **more than one** set of muscles fibers and **more than one** nerve supply.

- ❑ They lie **at the boundaries** between muscle groups. Usually it incorporates fibers from two **adjoining groups** and is therefore **supplied by two nerves** usually.

Musle	Nerve supply (Part of muscle)
Trapezius	▪ Spinal accessory nerve (motor) ▪ Ventral rami of C3, C4 (proprioception)
Digastric	▪ Trigeminal nerve (anterior belly) ▪ Facial nerve (posterior belly)
Pectoralis major	▪ Medial pectoral nerve ▪ Lateral pectoral nerve
Subscapularis	▪ Upper subscapular nerve ▪ Lower subscapular nerve
Brachialis	▪ Musculocutaneous nerve (motor) ▪ Radial nerve (proprioceptive)
Flexor digitorum profundus	▪ Median nerve (lateral half) ▪ Ulnar nerve (medial half)
Opponens pollicis	▪ Median nerve (superficial part) ▪ Ulnar nerve (deep part)
Ilio-psoas	▪ Direct branches of the anterior rami of L1-L3 (psoas major) ▪ Femoral nerve (iliacus)
Pectineus	▪ Femoral nerve (anterior fibers) ▪ Obrurator nerve (posterior fibers)
Biceps femoris	▪ Tibial part of sciatic nerve (long head) ▪ Common peroneal nerve (short head)
Adductor magnus	▪ Tibial part of sciatic nerve (ischial part) ▪ Obturator nerve (adductor part)

Unit Concept of Muscle

Single-unit (unitary)	Multi-unit
Most of the smooth muscles	Few smooth muscles
Either the whole muscle contracts or whole of it relaxes	Smooth muscle cells in a in an organ all behave independently- each cell contract and relaxes on its own.
Gap junctions are present between the muscle cells (creating a syncytium), where an action potential can be progapated through neighboring muscle cells making them contract in a coordinated fashion.	Some cell to cell communication and activators/inhibitors produced locally leads to a somewhat coordinated response even in multiunit smooth muscle.

Single-unit (unitary)	Multi-unit
Myogenic: Muscle can contract regularly without input from a motor neuron	Neurogenic: Muscle contraction must be initiated by an autonomic nervous system neuron.
A few of the cells in a given single unit may behave as pacemaker cells, generating rhythmic action potentials due to their intrinsic electrical activity. Because of its myogenic nature, single-unit smooth muscle is usually active, even when it's not receiving any neural stimulation.	Requires neural stimulation
E.g., Digestive tract (including biliary ducts), urinary tract (including ureter, bladder), genital tract (including uterus), Blood vessels (except any neural)	E.g., Trachea & bronchi, large elastic arteries, iris muscles (sphincter and dilator pupillae), erector ductus, ductus deferens

Note: A series of axon-like swelling, called **varicosities** (boutons) from autonomic neurons form motor units through the smooth muscle.

QUESTIONS

1. **All are composite muscles EXCEPT:** (AIPG 2009)
   a. Pectineus
   b. Flexor carpi ulnaris
   c. Biceps femoris
   d. Flexor digitorum profundus

2. **Muscle having double nerve supply:** (PGIC 2015)
   a. Digastric muscle
   b. Omohyoid muscle
   c. Trapezius
   d. Thyrohyoid muscle
   e. Adductor magnus

3. **Digastric muscles are the following EXCEPT:** (AIPG 2008)
   a. Occipitofrontalis
   b. Sternocleidomastoid
   c. Omohyoid
   d. Muscular fibers in the ligament of Treitz

4. **Which of the following is multipennate muscle:** (NEET Pattern 2015)
   a. Flexor pollicis longus
   b. Extensor pollicis longus
   c. Deltoid
   d. Flexor hallucis longus

5. **Muscle with parallel fibers are all EXCEPT:** (AIIMS 2016)
   a. Sartorius
   b. Rectus abdominis
   c. Sternohyoid
   d. Tibialis anterior

6. **Multi-unit smooth muscle present at all EXCEPT:** (NEET Pattern 2012)
   a. Blood vessels
   b. Gut
   c. Iris
   d. Ductus deferens

7. **Single unit smooth muscles are seen in:** (NEET Pattern 2012)
   a. Iris
   b. Ductus deferens
   c. Ureter
   d. Trachea

8. **Which of the following muscle has intracapsular origin:** (PGIC 2012)
   a. Anconeus
   b. Coracobrachialis
   c. Long head of biceps femoris
   d. Popliteus
   e. Peroneus longus

9. **Identify the type of muscle shown in the image** (NEET Pattern 2018)
   a. Cruciate
   b. Spiral
   c. Multipennate
   d. Convergent

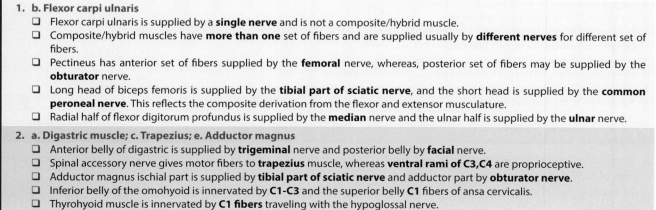

ANSWERS

1. **b. Flexor carpi ulnaris**
   - Flexor carpi ulnaris is supplied by a **single nerve** and is not a composite/hybrid muscle.
   - Composite/hybrid muscles have **more than one** set of fibers and are supplied usually by **different nerves** for different set of fibers.
   - Pectineus has anterior set of fibers supplied by the **femoral** nerve, whereas, posterior set of fibers may be supplied by the **obturator** nerve.
   - Long head of biceps femoris is supplied by the **tibial part of sciatic nerve**, and the short head is supplied by the **common peroneal nerve**. This reflects the composite derivation from the flexor and extensor musculature.
   - Radial half of flexor digitorum profundus is supplied by the **median** nerve and the ulnar half is supplied by the **ulnar** nerve.

2. **a. Digastric muscle; c. Trapezius; e. Adductor magnus**
   - Anterior belly of digastric is supplied by **trigeminal** nerve and posterior belly by **facial** nerve.
   - Spinal accessory nerve gives motor fibers to **trapezius** muscle, whereas **ventral rami of C3,C4** are proprioceptive.
   - Adductor magnus ischial part is supplied by **tibial part of sciatic nerve** and adductor part by **obturator nerve**.
   - Inferior belly of the omohyoid is innervated by **C1-C3** and the superior belly **C1** fibers of ansa cervicalis.
   - Thyrohyoid muscle is innervated by **C1 fibers** traveling with the hypoglossal nerve.

ANSWERS

3. b. Sternocleidomastoid
- ❑ Sternocleidomastoid is a muscle with two heads and **one belly**, like the biceps brachii.
- ❑ Digastric muscles have two bellies.
- ❑ Occipitofrontalis muscle has **two bellies:** Occipital belly and frontal belly.
- ❑ Omohyoid: Superior and inferior **belly**.
- ❑ Ligament of Treitz is a **digastric** muscle with a **skeletal muscle belly**, which arises from the left crus of diaphragm and a **smooth muscle belly** which arises from the duodeno-jejunal junction. It has an intermediate tendon attaching to the connective tissue around the celiac trunk of aorta.

4. c. Deltoid
- ❑ **Multipennate** muscle has the fiber bundles converge to several tendons.

5. d. Tibialis anterior
- ❑ The individual fibers of a muscle are arranged **either parallel** or **oblique** to the long axis of the muscle.
- ❑ Tibialis anterior muscle is a **multipennate** muscle with **oblique** fibers.
- ❑ Muscles with **parallel fasciculi**: These are muscles in which the fasciculi are parallel to the line of pull and have greater degree of movement. Few examples are:
  - ■ Strap-like, e.g. sternohyoid and sartorius
  - ■ Strap-like with tendinous intersections, e.g. rectus abdominis

6. b. Gut > a. Blood vessels
- ❑ **Gut** comes under **single-unit** smooth muscle, where the whole bundle or sheet contracts as a syncytium.
- ❑ Blood vessels are **also under single unit** smooth muscles but there are **few exceptions** like large elastic arteries (which are multi-unit).

7. c. Ureter
- ❑ In **single-unit** smooth muscle, either the whole muscle contracts or the whole muscle relaxes, as a **syncytium**.
- ❑ **Urinary tube** components, like **ureter** have the same arrangement.

8. d. Popliteus
- ❑ Long head of **biceps brachii** and the **popliteus** muscle has **intracapsular** origin.

9. Ans. b. Spiral> d. Convergent
- ❑ Muscles may exhibit a **spiral** or twisted arrangement (e.g. **sternocostal fibres of pectoralis major** or latissimus dorsi, which undergo a 180°-twist between their medial and lateral attachments).
- ❑ Some authors consider it as a muscle with **convergent** fibres as well. The muscle fibers or fasciculi converge at the insertion point to maximize contraction.
- ❑ Muscles may **spiral** around a bone (e.g. supinator, which winds obliquely around the proximal radial shaft), or contain two or more planes of fibres arranged in differing directions, a type of spiral sometimes referred to as **cruciate** (sternocleidomastoid, masseter and adductor magnus are all partially spiral and cruciate).

- ■ Smallest muscle in the body is **Stapedius** (NEET Pattern 2015)
  - – The smallest **skeletal** muscle in the body is **stapedius**.
  - – The **smallest muscle** in the body is **arrector pilorum**, a smooth muscle in the skin for erection of hair.
- ■ **Longest** muscle in the body is **Sartorius** (NEET Pattern 2012)
- ■ Flexor digitorum superficialis **does not** have dual nerve supply (NEET Pattern 2012)
- ■ Most common muscle to be congenitally absent is **Pectoralis major** (AIPG 2009)
- ■ Popliteus muscle has an **intra-articular** tendon (JIPMER 2016)
- ■ Rectus femoris is **not** a hybrid muscle (AIPG 2008)
- ■ Flexor carpi ulnaris is **not** a hybrid muscle.
- ■ All the muscles of body develop from mesenchyme **except** arrector pili, muscles of iris and myoepithelial cells, which develop from ectoderm.
- ■ Largest muscle in the body is gluteus maximus.
- ■ Functional unit of a muscle is **sarcomere**.
- ■ **Most variable** muscle in the body is palmaris longus.
- ■ **Longest tendon** in the body is **plantaris** in the leg.
- ■ **Largest tendon** in the body is tendo calcaneus (Achilles tendon).
- ■ Most commonly used muscle for intramuscular injection is **deltoid**.
- ■ Muscles with smallest motor unit are **extraocular muscles** and largest are lower limb muscles like gluteus maximus.
- ■ **Talus** bone in the foot and **Incus** bone in the middle ear cavity have **no muscle attachments**.

▼ Portal Venous Circulation

- ❑ Portal circulation is a **capillary network** that lies between two veins. Blood supplying the organ thus passes through **two sets** of capillaries before it returns to the heart.
- ❑ In **hepatic** portal system blood supplying the abdominal organs passes through two sets of capillaries before it returns to the heart.

- ❏ A portal circulation also connects the **median eminence** and infundibulum of the hypothalamus with the adenohypophysis.
- ❏ In the **renal glomeruli**. The glomerular capillary bed lies between afferent and efferent arterioles and may be considered as a portal circulation, but most of the authors do not mention so (including Gray's anatomy).

Shunt vessels are direct **arteriovenous** communication between smaller arteries and veins.

- ❏ Normal flow of blood: Artery → arterioles → capillaries → venules → veins.
- ❏ Shunt vessels **basically bypass the capillary circulation** and connect small arteries to the small veins in case of resting organ.
- ❏ **Sites of AV shunts**: Skin of the nose, lips, and ears, nasal and alimentary mucosa, erectile tissue, thyroid gland, sympathetic ganglia, etc.
- ❏ Shunt vessels are important for **temperature regulation** as evidenced in cold environment.
- ❏ To **conserve central (core) temperature** the shunt vessels open up in the peripheries (hand, feet, etc.) and the blood **bypasses** the capillary beds at the tip of the fingers. Hence, we feel our finger tips getting cold very quickly as relative to the central body.
- ❏ Shunt vessels are under the **vasoconstrictive** action of **sympathetic** nervous system.
- ❏ Under sympathetic control the shunt vessel is able to close completely, **diverting blood** into the normal pathway.

Heat lost by radiation   Skin surface
More blood flow through dilated capillaries
Shunt vessel constricted diverting blood to capillaries
Arteriole
Venule

QUESTION

1. **NOT true about shunt vessel is:**   (AIPG 2009)
   a. It controls temperature regulation
   b. It is direct communication between artery and vein
   c. It is under control of local mediators
   d. It is not under autonomic control

ANSWERS

1. **d. It is not under autonomic control**
   - ❏ **Shunt** vessels are under the **vasoconstrictive** action of **sympathetic** nervous system.
   - ❏ Under **sympathetic control** the shunt vessel is able to close completely, **diverting blood** into the normal pathway.

▶ Miscellaneous

QUESTIONS

1. **Embalming solution constituents are all EXCEPT:**
                                                       (AIIMS 2008)
   a. Ethanol   b. Phenol
   c. Glycerine   d. Formalin

2. **In the following nutrient arteries to bones, choose the WRONG pair:**
   a. Humerus: Profunda brachii   b. Radius: Anterior interosseous
   c. Fibula: Peroneal   d. Tibia: Anterior tibial

3. **All are Valveless EXCEPT:**
   a. Dural venous sinus   b. Hepatic veins   c. Inferior vena cava   d. Femoral vein

ANSWERS

1. **a. Ethanol**
   - ❏ Ethanol is a preservative and **can be used** for embalming **but is not** the usual content of embalming fluid/solution. **In its place methanol** is used, which is cheaper and more toxic to bacteria than ethanol. Methanol also holds the formaldehyde in solution.
   - ❏ **Embalming** is the process of treatment of the dead body with antiseptics and preservatives to **prevent putrefaction**.
   - ❏ Typically, embalming fluid contains a mixture of formaldehyde, glutaraldehyde, methanol, and other solvents. The formaldehyde content generally ranges from 5 to 37 percent and the methanol content may range from 9 to 56 percent.
   - ❏ **Preservative** is the substance added to destroy or inhibit the growth of **microorganisms**. It alters enzymes and lysins of the body and arrest decomposition — fixing the specimen in such a way that it retains its original structure with minimal alteration.
   - ❏ Formalin is the **most commonly** used fixative/ preservative and less commonly used are – Ethanol/ Phenol.
   - ❏ Phenol is a powerful **Fungicide**.
   - ❏ Glycerine is used in the embalming fluid as a **hygroscopic**/humectant/wetting agent and decreases the loss of water of the preserved structures (maintains hydration). But it is **not the actual preservative by definition**.
   - ❏ Wetting agents lower the **surface tension** of water and facilitate penetration and distribution of embalming fluids through the vascular beds into the tissues.

2. **d. Tibia: Anterior tibial**
   - ❏ Nutrient artery to tibia is a branch of **posterior tibial** artery.

3. **d. Femoral vein**
   - ❏ Femoral veins contain between **one and six valves**, and popliteal veins contain between zero and four valves.
   - ❏ Deep vein valves are **consistently** located in the common femoral vein (**within 5 cm of the inguinal ligament**), the femoral vein (within 3 cm of the deep femoral vein tributary) and in the popliteal vein near the adductor hiatus.

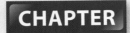

CHAPTER
2

Embryology

Prenatal period is divided into three parts: Pre-embryonic, embryonic and fetal period.
- ❏ **Pre-embryonic** period extends from fertilization to the end of second week of intrauterine life.
- ❏ **Embryonic period** extends from beginning of the third week to the end of eighth week of intrauterine life.
- ❏ **Fetal** stage extends from beginning of the ninth week to birth.

Note: Some authors consider the embryonic period from fertilization to the end of eight week.

Flowchart 1: Subdivision of prenatal period and events occurring in these periods.

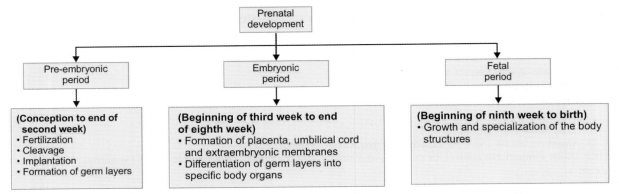

Table 1: Key developmental events during the embryonic period	
Developmental events	**Day/days of gestation**
Fertilization	Day 1
Blastocyst	Day 4
Bilaminar embryonic disc	Days 8
Implantation	Day 10
Primary streak appears	Day 15
Primitive heart tube	Day 17
Neurulation, first pair of somite	Day 21
Limb buds	Days 26–28
Primitive gut	Day 31
Physiological herniation	Day 36
Face appears	Day 37
External genitalia	Day 53
Miniature human form	Day 56

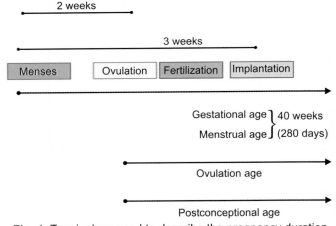

Fig. 1: Terminology used to describe the pregnancy duration

1. **At the end of 5th week of gestation, how many number of somites can be seen?** *(NEET Pattern)*
   - a. 24
   - b. 26
   - c. 38
   - d. 44

2. **Embryonic period of development is:** *(NEET Pattern 2012)*
   - a. Up to 16 weeks
   - b. Up to 12 weeks
   - c. Up to 10 weeks
   - d. Up to 8 weeks

3. **Identify the CORRECT pair:** *(NEET Pattern 2013)*
   - a. Embryonic period: 9–20 weeks
   - b. Fertilization to implantation: 0–4 weeks
   - c. Embryonic period: 4–8 weeks
   - d. None

1. **d. 44**
   - ❑ The first pair of somites arises in the occipital region of the embryo at approximately the 20th day of development.
   - ❑ From here, new somites appear in craniocaudal sequence at a rate of approximately three pairs per day until, at the end of the fifth week, 42 to 44 pairs are present.
   - ❑ The first occipital and the last five to seven coccygeal somites later disappear (now the total is 37), these remaining somites form the axial skeleton.
   - ❑ The age of an embryo can be accurately determined by counting number of somites

2. **d. Up to 8 weeks**
   - ❑ Embryonic period extends from beginning of the third week to the end of eighth week of intrauterine life.
   - ❑ Some authors consider the embryonic period from fertilization to the end of eight week.

3. **c. Embryonic period: 4–8 weeks**
   - ❑ Embryonic period extends from beginning of the third week to the end of eighth week of intrauterine life.
   - ❑ There is no correct answer, the most appropriate option has been chosen as the answer.
   - ❑ **Total number** of somites developing in fetus are **42 pair** (NEET Pattern 2016)

▶ Cell Division

Table 2: Distinguishing features between mitosis and meiosis

Mitosis	Meiosis
▪ Takes place in somatic cells	▪ Takes place in germ cells
▪ Completes in one sequence	▪ Completes in two sequences, i.e., there are two successive divisions, viz., meiosis I and meiosis II
▪ Crossing over of chromatids does not take place	▪ Crossing over of chromatids takes place
▪ Daughter cells have the same number of chromosomes as parent cells	▪ Daughter cells have half the number of chromosomes as parent cells
▪ Daughter cells are identical to each other and to the parent cell	▪ Daughter cells are not identical to each other and to the parent cell
▪ Equational division	▪ Reductional division

Table 3: Events during mitotic and meiotic cell divisions in the germ line

Stage	Events	Name of cell	Condition of Genome
Resting interval between mitotic cell divisions	Normal cellular metabolism occurs	F Oogonium M Spermatogonium	Diploid, 2N
Mitosis			
Preparatory phase	DNA replication yields double-stranded chromosomes	F Oogonium M Spermatogonium	Diploid, 4N
Prophase	Double stranded chromosomes condense		
Metaphase	Chromosomes align along the equator; centromeres replicate		
Anaphase and telophase	Each double stranded chromosome splits into two single stranded chromosomes, one of which is distributed to each daughter nucleus		
Cytokinesis	Cell divides	F Oogonium M Spermatogonium	Diploid, 2N
Meiosis I			
Preparatory phase	DNA replication yields double-stranded chromosomes	F Primary oocyte M Primary spermatocyte	Diploid, 4N
Prophase	Double stranded chromosomes condense two chromosomes of each homologous pair align at the centromeres to form a four imbed chiasma; recombination by crossing over occurs		
Metaphase	Chromosomes align along the equator; centromeres do not rep/kale		
Anaphase and telophase	One double-stranded chromosome of each homologous pair is distributed to each daughter cell		

Stage	Events	Name of cell	Condition of Genome
Cytokinesis	Cell divides	F One secondary oocyte and the first polar body M Two secondary spermatocytes	Haploid, 2N
Meiosis II			
Prophase	No DNA replication takes place during the second meiotic division; double stranded chromosomes condense		
Metaphase	Chromosomes align along the equator; centromeres replicate		
Anaphase and telophase	Each chromosome splits into two single stranded chromosomes, one of which is distributed to each daughter nucleus		
Cytokinesis	Cell divides	F One definitive oocyte and three polar bodies M Four spermatids	Haploid, 1N

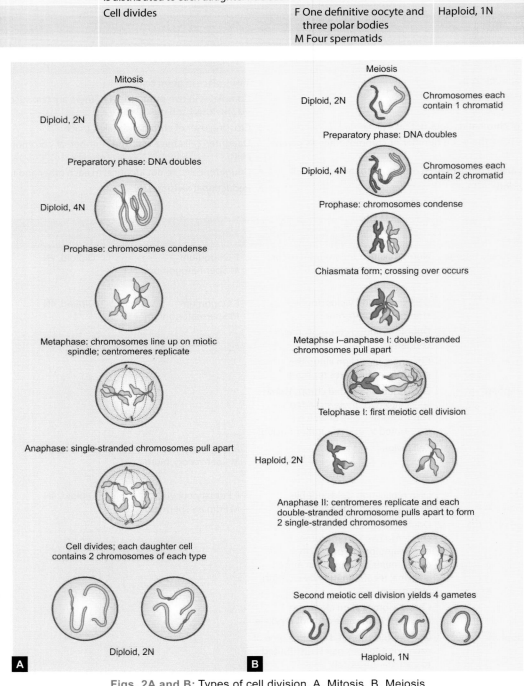

Figs. 2A and B: Types of cell division. A, Mitosis. B, Meiosis

1. Prophase of meiosis-I, TRUE statement is/are:
a. Chromosomes separate
c. Resultant cell is haploid
e. Sister chromatids separate
b. Resultant cell is diploid
d. Sister chromatids replicate

(PGIC 2017)

1. b. Resultant cell is diploid
- During prophase of meiosis-I, pairing of maternal and paternal (homologous) chromosomes (**synapsis**) occurs, followed by **chiasma** (site for genetic exchange) formation and crossover of genetic material between non-sister chromatids. There is **no change of ploidy status**, i.e., the diploid cell remains diploid. Maternal and paternal (homologous) chromosomes separate during Anaphase I of Meiosis I.
- During the **synthesis (S) phase** of interphase, **chromosomes** in a cell are **replicated** and sister chromatids are **created**.
- A sister chromatid is 'one-half' of the duplicated chromosome. Sister chromatids separate during **anaphase II** of meiosis II.

◤ Gametogenesis

- Gametogenesis is formation of gamete from primordial germ cells and involves cell division mitosis and meiosis.
- Primordial germ cells (PGCs) are derived from the epiblast, they migrate to the endodermal wall of the yolk sac (fourth week) and then reach the indeterminate gonad by the end of the fifth week, to differentiate into gametes (gametogenesis).
- Aberrant migration may lead to germ cell tumors (for e.g., teratoma).
- **Teratomas** may arise from PGCs (or from epiblast cells), which are pluripotent cells.
- Therefore, within teratomas are present derivatives of all three germ layers and may include skin, bone, teeth, gut tissue.

◤ Spermatogenesis

- **Spermatogenesis** is the process in which spermatozoa are produced from spermatogonial stem cells by way of mitosis and meiosis
- The primordial germ cells form spermatogonia, which yield primary spermatocytes by **mitosis**.
- The primary spermatocyte divides meiotically **(Meiosis I)** into two secondary spermatocytes; each secondary spermatocyte divides into two spermatids by Meiosis II. These later develop into mature spermatids.
- Thus, the primary spermatocyte gives rise to two cells, the secondary spermatocytes, and the two secondary spermatocytes by their subdivision produce four spermatids.
- Meiosis has two stages, Meiosis I is the actual meiotic **reduction division**, whereas meiosis II is just like mitosis (**equational** division).
- The **spermatid is the haploid** male gamete that results from division of secondary spermatocytes. As a result of meiosis, each spermatid contains only half of the genetic material present in the original primary spermatocyte. Early round spermatids undergo further maturational event (spermiogenesis) to develop into spermatozoa.
- Initial stages of spermatogenesis takes place within the testes **(seminiferous tubules)** and progress to the epididymis where the developing gametes mature, gain progressive motility and are stored until ejaculation.
- Spermatogenesis takes **74 days** to complete. If the transport through ductal system is included, it takes 3 months.
- The transit of sperm through the epididymis is thought to take up to **12 days**. Though sperms can be stored in the epididymis for several weeks (? 3 month). *(Campbell Walsh Urology - 10th ed)*
- There are **three subtypes** of spermatogonia in humans:
- Type A (dark) cells, with dark nuclei.
  ➢ These cells are reserve spermatogonial stem cells which do not usually undergo active mitosis.
- Type A (pale) cells, with pale nuclei.
  ➢ These are the spermatogonial stem cells that undergo active mitosis.
  ➢ These cells divide to produce Type B cells.
- Type B cells, which divide (mitosis) to give rise to primary spermatocytes.

Cell type	Chromosomes in human	DNA copy number/ chromatids in human	Process entered by cell
Spermatogonium (types Ad, Ap and B)	Diploid (2N)/46	2C/46	Spermatocytogenesis (mitosis)
Primary spermatocyte	Diploid (2N)/46	4C/2 x 46	Spermatogenesis (meiosis I)
Two secondary spermatocytes	Haploid (N)/23	2C/2 x 23	Spermatogenesis (meiosis 11)
Four spermatids	Haploid (N)/23	C I 23	Spermiogenesis
Four functional spermatozoids	Haploid (N)/23	C I 23	Spermiation

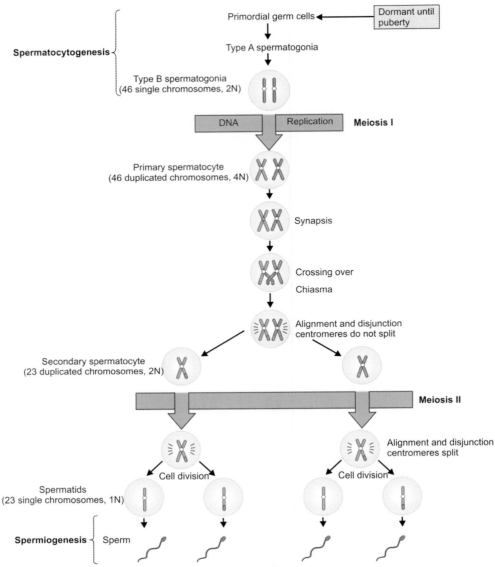

Fig. 3: Spermatogenesis. Only one pair of homologous chromosomes has been shown (red, maternal origin; blue, paternal origin). Synapsis is the process of pairing of homologous chromosomes. The point at which the DNA molecule crosses over is called the chiasma and is where exchange of small segments of maternal and paternal DNA occurs. Note that synapsis and crossing over occur only during meiosis I.

QUESTIONS

1. Spermatogonia divides by which cell division?

(NEET Pattern 2014)

a. Meiosis
b. Mitosis
c. Both Meiosis and Mitosis
d. Maturation

2. TRUE about spermatid: *(NEET Pattern 2015)*

a. Derived from primary spermatocyte
b. Derived from secondary spermatocyte
c. Undergoes mitotic division
d. Undergoes meiotic division

3. Haploid number of chromosomes is seen in:

(NEET Pattern 2012)

a. Spermatogonia
b. Primary spermatocytes
c. Secondary spermatocyte
d. None

4. Spermatogenesis is completed in:

a. 60 days
b. 64 days
c. 70 days
d. 74 days

5. Independent assortment of chromosome occurs at which level? *(AIIMS 2015)*

a. Primordial germ cells to spermatogonia
b. Spermatogonia to primary spermatocyte
c. Primary spermatocyte to secondary spermatocyte
d. Secondary spermatocyte to spermatids

ANSWERS

1. b. Mitosis
  ❑ There are **three subtypes** of spermatogonia in humans:
    ■ Type A (dark) cells, which are **reserve** spermatogonial stem cells which do not usually undergo active mitosis.
    ■ Type A (pale) cells, which are the spermatogonial stem cells that **undergo active mitosis** to produce Type B cells.
      – Type B cells, which divide (mitosis) to give rise to primary spermatocytes.
  ❑ Primary spermatocyte **subsequently enters meiosis** cell division.

2. b. Derived from secondary spermatocyte
- ❏ Spermatid is the **haploid male gamete** that results from division of **secondary spermatocytes**.
- ❏ As a result of meiosis, each spermatid contains **only half** of the genetic material present in the original primary spermatocyte.
- ❏ Spermatids **spermiogenesis** to form the spermatozoa. They undergo **no cell division** (mitosis or meiosis).

3. c. Secondary spermatocyte
- ❏ Spermatogonia are diploid (2n) cells containing 46 chromosomes, which divide (mitosis) to give rise to primary spermatocytes.
- ❏ Primary spermatocytes are diploid (2n) cells, which undergo meiosis I, to give two secondary spermatocytes.
- ❏ Secondary spermatocytes are haploid (n) cells that contain 23 chromosomes.

4. d. 74 days > b. 64 days.
- ❏ Spermatogenesis is the process in which spermatozoa are produced from spermatogonial stem cells by way of mitosis and meiosis and takes **74 days to complete**.
- ❏ Earlier editions of standard textbooks used to mention it as 64 days (2 months).

5. c. Primary spermatocyte to secondary spermatocyte
- ❏ **Primary** spermatocyte changes to **secondary** spermatocyte during **meiosis I.**
- ❏ **Maternal** and **paternal** chromosomes **separate during Meiosis - I** by **independent assortment**.
- ❏ During meiosis, the pairs of homologous chromosome are divided in half to form haploid cells, and this **separation, or assortment**, of homologous chromosomes is 'random'.
- ❏ This means that all of the maternal chromosomes **will not** be separated into one cell, while the all paternal chromosomes are separated into another. **Instead**, after meiosis occurs, each haploid cell contains a 'mixture' of genes from the individual's mother and father, and that too at **random** levels, i.e. its **not predetermined**.

- ▪ **Meiosis** occurs in **Seminiferous tubules** (AIIMS 2004)
  - – Sperms reach **epididymis** where they **mature**, gain **progressive motility** and are **stored until ejaculation**.
- ▪ Spermatogenesis begins **at Puberty** (NEET Pattern 2016)
  - – Primordial germ cells **remain dormant until** puberty.
- ▪ Development of spermatozoa (sperm) from spermatogonium takes **70–75 days** (NEET Pattern 2014)
- ▪ **Spermatogenesis** occurs at temperature **lower** than core body temperature (AIPG 2008)
- ▪ **Meiosis** occurs at transformation of **primary** spermatocyte to **secondary** spermatocyte (AIIMS 2007)
- ▪ Primary spermatocytes are **diploid** (2n) cells containing **46 chromosomes** (46-XY) (NEET Pattern 2014)

Oogenesis

- ❏ **Primordial germ cells** (46, 2N) derived from the epiblast cells, reach the **endodermal wall of the yolk sac** and differentiate into oogonia (46, 2N), which populate the ovary through mitotic division.
- ❏ Oogonium is unique in that it is only female cell in which both 'X' chromosomes are active.
- ❏ The majority of oogonia continue to divide by **mitosis**, but some of them arrest their cell division in prophase of meiosis I and undergo DNA replication to form primary oocytes (46, 4N).
- ❏ All primary oocytes are formed by month 5 of fetal life. At birth there are no primordial germ cells or oogonia in the ovary.
- ❏ Primary oocytes enter prophase I (of meiosis I), but get **arrested** there, due to OMI **(Oocyte Maturation Inhibitor)**, which alters the levels of cyclic AMP.
- ❏ Primary oocytes remain arrested in prophase (diplotene) of meiosis I from month 5 of fetal life **until exposed to LH surge**, which starts happening after puberty.
- ❏ After puberty, 5 to 15 primary oocytes begin maturation with each ovarian cycle, but only 1 reaches full maturity to undergo ovulation.
- ❏ During the ovarian cycle and triggered by the luteinizing hormone (LH) surge, a primary oocyte completes meiosis I to form two daughter cells: the secondary oocyte (23, 2N) and the first polar body, which degenerates.
- ❏ LH surge occurs approximately **34–36 hours** (wider range: 24-48 hours) before ovulation and **LH peak** occurs at 10–12 hours before ovulation. First polar body is released at about LH peak (10-20 hours before ovulation).
- ❏ The secondary oocyte promptly begins meiosis II but is **arrested in metaphase of meiosis II** about 3 hours before ovulation. The secondary oocyte remains arrested in metaphase of meiosis II until fertilization occurs.
- ❏ Secondary oocyte is **degenerated after 24 hours** of ovulation, hence fertilization must take place within a few hours, and no more than a day after ovulation. Almost all pregnancies result when intercourse occurs during the 2 days preceding or on the day of ovulation.
- ❏ At fertilization, the secondary oocyte completes meiosis II to form a mature oocyte (23, 1N) and a second polar body.
- ❏ Approximate number of primary oocytes at 5th month of intrauterine life is **7 million**, most of them get degenerated by birth and the count comes down to **600,000 to 2 million**. The degeneration continues and at puberty, only 40,000 are present, out of which **400–500 undergo ovulation** in the female reproductive life.
- ❏ Twelve secondary oocytes are ovulated per year, up to 480 over the entire reproductive life of the woman (40 years × 12 secondary oocytes per year = 480).
- ❏ Meiosis consists of two cell divisions (meiosis I and meiosis II) and results in the formation of gametes containing 23 chromosomes and 1N amount of DNA (1n, 1N), where n is the number of chromosomes and N is the unit (amount) of DNA.

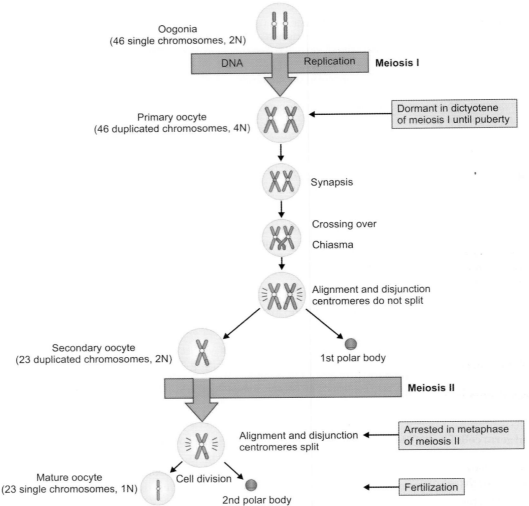

Fig. 4: Oogenesis. Only one pair of homologous chromosomes is shown (red, maternal origin; blue, paternal origin). Synapsis is the process of pairing of homologous chromosomes. The point at which the DNA molecule crosses over is called the chiasma and is where exchange of small segments of maternal and paternal DNA occurs. Note that synapsis and crossing over occur only during meiosis I. The polar bodies are storage bodies for DNA unnecessary for the further function of the cell and probably degenerate. There is no evidence that polar bodies divide or undergo any other activity.

- ❑ Meiosis I is a **reduction division** and reduces the chromosome number to half in gamete.
- ❑ Meiosis II is an **equational division** (chromosome numbers remain the same).
- ❑ During oogenesis, primordial germ cells differentiate into oogonia (46, 2N), which enter meiosis I and undergo DNA replication to form primary oocytes (46, 4N).
- ❑ All primary oocytes are formed by the fifth month of fetal life (about 7 million), and remain dormant in prophase (diplotene/dictyotene stage) of meiosis I until the beginning of LH surge (puberty).
- ❑ Primary oocyte completes meiosis I to form a secondary oocyte (23, 2N) and a first polar body (which later degenerates).
- ❑ The secondary oocyte enters meiosis II, remains arrested in metaphase of meiosis II until fertilization occurs.
- ❑ At fertilization, the secondary oocyte completes meiosis II to form a mature oocyte (23, 1N) and a second polar body.

Cell type	Ploidy/chromosomes	Chromatids	Process	Time of completion
Oogonium	Diploid/46(2N)	2C	Oocytogenesis (mitosis)	Third trimester
Primary Oocyte	Diploid/46(2N)	4C	Ootidogenesis (meiosis I) (Folliculogenesis)	Dictyate in prophase I for up to 50 years
Secondary Oocyte	Haploid/23(1N)	2C	Ootidogenesis (meiosis II)	Halted in metaphase II until fertilization
Ootid	Haploid/23(1N)	1C	Ootidogenesis (meiosis II)	Minutes after fertilization
Ovum	Haploid/23(1N)	1C		

QUESTIONS

1. **All is true regarding events related to oogenesis EXCEPT:**
   a. Primary oocyte is arrested at prophase – I at birth
   b. LH surge occurs 24–48 hrs. prior to ovulation
   c. First polar body is released before ovulation
   d. Meiosis-II is a reduction division

2. **Secondary oocyte is:** *(NEET Pattern 2013)*
   a. Haploid (n) and N
   b. Haploid (n) and 2N
   c. Diploid (2n) and N
   d. Diploid (2n) and 2N

3. **Germ cells are derivative of:** *(NEET Pattern 2012)*
   a. Epiblast
   b. Endodermal sinus
   c. Mesoderm
   d. Ectoderm

4. **Primordial germ cell is derived from:** *(AIPG 2007)*
   a. Ectoderm
   b. Mesoderm
   c. Endoderm
   d. Mesodermal sinus

5. **Cells which surround the oocyte in Graafian follicle are called:** *(NEET Pattern 2014)*
   a. Discus proligerus
   b. Cumulus oophorus
   c. Luteal cells
   d. Villus cells

6. **Fertilization is complete when:** *(NEET Pattern 2015)*
   a. 1st polar body is formed
   b. 2nd polar body is formed
   c. Primary oocyte is formed
   d. Secondary oocyte is formed

7. **Fertilization takes place after how much time of ovulation?**
   a. 1–2 days
   b. 5–6 days *(NEET Pattern 2014)*
   c. 8–12 days
   d. 12 days

8. **Primary oocyte is formed after:** *(NEET Pattern 2013)*
   a. First meiotic division
   b. Second meiotic division
   c. Mitotic division
   d. None of the above

9. **CORRECT statement(s) about meiosis:** *(PGIC 2016)*
   a. Meiosis is needed to produce large number of eggs and sperms
   b. Germ cell undergoes division to form diploid cell and increase their number
   c. Occur in germ cell which result in haploid cells
   d. One spermatocyte produces one sperm and one oocyte produces one ovum
   e. Somatic cells not divide by meiosis because number of chromosomes reduces to half

ANSWERS

1. **d. Meiosis II is a reduction division**
   - ❑ Chromosome number gets reduced to half during meiosis- I (**reduction division**).
   - ❑ Maternal and paternal chromosomes **separate** during meiosis- I.
   - Meiosis- II **doesn't reduce** the number of chromosomes (hence, it is **not** a reduction- division).

2. **b. Haploid (n) and 2N**
   - ❑ Secondary oocyte is a haploid cell (n) with two units of DNA (2N).
   - ❑ Key: n- number of chromosomes and N- amount of DNA.

3. **a. Epiblast > b. Endodermal sinus**
   - ❑ Primordial germ cell is a derivative of **epiblast**, earlier they were believed to arise from **endoderm of yolk sac** (endodermal sinus) *Gray's Anatomy (Ed. 41)*
   - ❑ They are derivatives of epiblast cells, developing in **primitive streak** and later **migrate** to the endodermal yolk sac and pass through the **dorsal mesentery** of hindgut to **finally reach** the genital ridge.

4. **c. Endoderm**
   - ❑ Primordial germ cell is a derivative of **epiblast**, earlier they were believed to arise from endoderm of yolk sac (endodermal sinus) *Gray's Anatomy (Ed. 41)*
   - ❑ They become evident at the distal end of primitive streak by the **2nd week** of development.
   - ❑ These cells are migratory cells and reach the **endodermal** wall of yolk sac (fourth week).
   - ❑ They reach the indeterminate gonad by the end of the fifth week, to differentiate into gametes (gametogenesis).
   - ❑ Note: Aberrant migration may lead to germ cell tumours (for example, **teratoma**).

5. **b. Cumulus oophorus**
   - ❑ Oocyte lies eccentrically in the ovarian (Graafian) follicle surrounded by some granulosa cells called **cumulus oophorus**.
   - ❑ **Discus proligerus** is the attachment point of the cumulus oophorus to the most peripheral granulosa cells of an antral follicle.

6. **b. 2nd polar body is formed**
   - ❑ At fertilization, the secondary oocyte completes meiosis II to form a mature oocyte (23, 1N) and a **second polar body**.

7. **a. 1–2 days**
   - ❑ After ovulation has occurred, the oocyte (ovum) remains **fertilizable for 48 hours**, although the chance is mostly lost by 18–24 hours.
   - ❑ If no fertilization occurs, the oocyte will degenerate between **12 and 24 hours** after ovulation.
   - ❑ Sperm is capable of fertilization **for 48 hours**, once ejaculated in the female genital tract.

8. **c. Mitotic division**
   - ❑ The majority of oogonia continue to divide by mitosis, but some of them arrest their cell division in prophase of meiosis I and form primary oocytes.
   - ❑ After **first** meiotic division secondary oocyte is formed and after **second** meiosis mature oocyte (ovum) is formed.

9. **a. Meiosis is needed to produce large number of eggs and sperms; c. Occur in germ cell which result in haploid cells; e) Somatic cells not divide by meiosis because number of chromosomes reduces to half**
   - ❑ Meiosis is a **reduction** division, since it reduces the chromosome number to half. Primary gametocyte (diploid) undergoes meiosis-I to become secondary gametocyte (haploid).
   - ❑ Male produces **four functional sperm** for each spermatocyte that enters meiosis, but the female produces only **one functional ovum** for each oocyte that completes meiosis.

- **Polar bodies** are formed during **Oogenesis** *(AIPG 2006)*
- **First polar body** is formed after **First meiosis** *(NEET Pattern 2014)*
  - **Primary oocyte** completes meiosis I to form **two daughter cells**: the secondary oocyte (23, 2N) and the first polar body.
- **Diplotene** and **zygotene** stages are seen in **Prophase** *(NEET Pattern 2015)*
  - Prophase I (of meiosis I) is divided into 4 stages: Leptotene, Zygotene, Pachytene and Diplotene, followed by Diakinesis.
- **At birth** the ovary contains **primary oocyte** in **Prophase-I** of meiosis *(AIIMS 2015)*
  - In the ovaries, primary oocytes reach **diplotene** stage of prophase I (meiosis I), by the **fifth month** in utero and each remains at this stage **until the period before ovulation** (may be as long as up to 50 years).
- After first meiotic division, the primary oocyte **remains arrested in Diplotene** stage *(NEET Pattern 2012)*
  - Primary oocytes enter prophase I (of meiosis I) and **remains arrested** in prophase (diplotene) of meiosis I **until exposed to LH surge,** which starts happening **after puberty**.
- **One** primary oocyte forms **one** ovum *(NEET Pattern 2013)*
- Abnormal persistence of **Primordial germ cells** in **primitive streak** result in **sacrococcygeal teratoma**.
  - Teratomas may arise from PGCs (or from **epiblast** cells), both being **pluripotent** cells.
  - Therefore, within teratomas are present derivatives of **all three germ layers** and may include skin, bone, teeth, gut tissue.

▼ Menstrual cycle

- ❑ Luteinizing hormone is produced by gonadotropic cells in the anterior pituitary gland.
- ❑ In females, an acute rise of LH triggers ovulation and development of the corpus luteum.
  - ➢ LH surge occurs 34–36 hours before ovulation. Some authors mention a wider range: Range: 24-48 hours before ovulation.
- ❑ After ovulation has occurred, the oocyte (ovum) remains fertilizable for 48 hours, although the chance is mostly lost by **18–24 hours**. If no fertilization occurs, the oocyte will degenerate between 12 and 24 hours after ovulation.

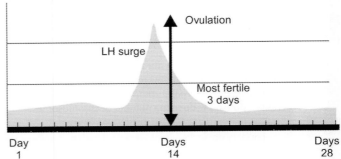

Fig. 5: Menstrual cycle (28 days), showing LH hormonal variation, period of ovulation (mid-cycle, day 14) and most fertile period (two days before ovulation and the day of ovulation)

- ❑ After coitus, semen containing mature and immature spermatozoa is discharged into the upper vagina and near the external os.
- ❑ Some active sperms enter the cervical canal within a few minutes and invade the mucous alkaline cervical plug which, at the time of ovulation, is softened to allow easier penetration.
- ❑ Once they are through the cervix, spermatozoa ascend quickly in 1 to 1 1/2 hours to the tubes and may meet the mature ovum.
- ❑ All sperms remaining in the vagina for 2 hours or longer are killed by vaginal acidic discharge.
- ❑ Although **sperms** remain alive and motile in the cervical canal and uterus for 5–7 days and in the fallopian tubes for 85 hours, they usually do not retain their power of fertilization after **24-48 hours of coitus**.
- ❑ Recently, donor **insemination** has indicated that sperms can retain their fertilizing capacity up to 4 days.
- ❑ Conception is therefore extremely unlikely unless coitus takes place 1 or 2 days before, or immediately after ovulation (**fertile period - 3 days**); the latter takes place around the 14th day of the 28-day-cycle and is related to the next menstrual period.
- ❑ However, pregnancy can occur following coitus on any day of the cycle due to irregularity in the time of ovulation.

▼ Ovulation and Fertilization

- ❑ Fertilization, which normally occurs in the oviduct, must take place within a few hours, and no more than a day after ovulation. Because of this narrow opportunity window, spermatozoa must be present in the fallopian tube at the time of oocyte arrival.
- ❑ Almost all pregnancies result when intercourse occurs during the 2 days preceding or on the day of ovulation.
- ❑ *****Fertilization** occurs in the ampulla of fallopian tube. Zona pellucida is a glycoprotein membrane, which attracts sperms for fertilization.
- ❑ Once a single sperm has fertilized the oocyte, the membrane prevents polyspermy. a. Zona pellucida attracts sperm → b. Sperm binds to the membrane → c. **Acrosome reaction** with release of enzymes → d.
- ❑ Penetration of sperm into the zona pellucida → e. Fusion of sperm membrane with oocyte membrane → f. **Cortical reaction** (release of cortical granules) → g. **Zona reaction**: Change in the permeability of zona pellucida, preventing polyspermy.

- *Acrosome reaction:* As the sperm is attracted by zona pellucida (a glycoprotein membrane) it releases enzymes (like acrosin) which allows sperm to penetrate the zona, thereby coming in contact with the plasma membrane of the oocyte.
- *Cortical reaction:* As the head of the sperm comes in contact with the oocyte surface, it results in release of lysosomal enzymes from cortical granules lining the plasma membrane of the oocyte. The trigger for the cortical granules to exocytose is the release of calcium ions from cortical smooth endoplasmic reticulum in response to sperm binding to the egg.
- *Zona reaction:* In turn, these enzymes alter properties of the zona pellucida to prevent another sperm penetration (polyspermy) and inactivate species-specific receptor sites for spermatozoa on the zona surface.
- The sequence of reactions is: Acrosome reaction → Cortical reaction → Zona reaction.

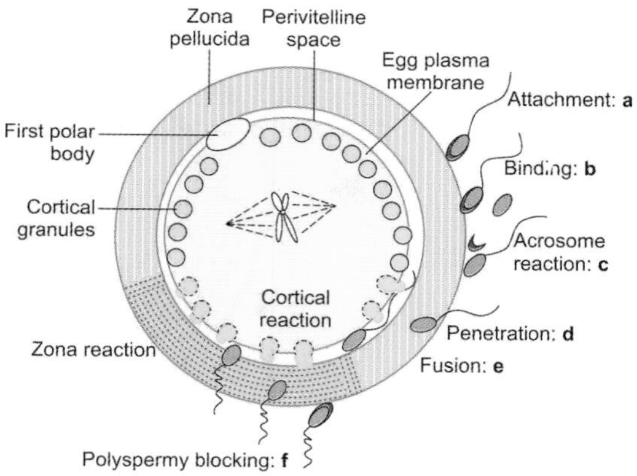

Fig. 6: Stages of sperm attachment (to zona pellucida), acrosome reaction, penetration, fusion, cortical reaction and zona reaction. (a-f)

QUESTIONS

1. Sperm remains fertile for how many hours in female genital tract? *(NEET Pattern 2013)*
   a. 6-8 hrs
   b. 12-24 hrs
   c. 24-48 hrs
   d. 72-96 hrs

2. Average reproductive life span of ovum is: *(NEET Pattern 2013)*
   a. 6-12 hrs
   b. 12-24 hrs
   c. 24-26 hrs
   d. 3 days

3. After how many hours of LH surge does ovulation occur?
   a. 12-24
   b. 24-48
   c. 24-36
   d. 36-48

ANSWERS

1. **c. 24-48 hrs**
   - Although sperms remain alive and motile in the cervical canal and uterus for **5-7 days** and in the fallopian tubes for 85 hours, they **usually do not retain** their power of fertilization **after 24-48 hours** of coitus.

2. **b. 12–24 hrs**
   - After ovulation has occurred, the oocyte (ovum) remains fertilizable for 48 hours, although the **chance is mostly lost by 18-24 hours**.
   - If no fertilization occurs, the oocyte will **degenerate between 12 and 24 hours** after ovulation.

3. **c. 24–36**
   - The most appropriate option has been taken as the answer.
   - An **acute rise of LH** triggers ovulation and development of the corpus luteum.
   - LH surge occurs **34-36 hours before ovulation**. Some authors mention a **wider** range: 24-48 hours before ovulation.
   - **Ion** responsible to **prevent polyspermy** at the time of fertilization is **Ca** (Calcium) *(NEET Pattern 2015)*
   - **Correct** sequence of the embryonic events is **Acrosome** reaction → **Cortical** reaction → **Zona** reaction *(NEET Pattern 2013)*

▶ First Week of Development

- Advanced morula (**16-64 celled**) enters the uterine cavity at **day 4** to become **blastocyst**. Blastocyst has an inner cell mass (**embryoblast**) and outer cell mass trophoblast. Embryoblast forms the embryo chiefly and **trophoblast** contributes to extraembryonic tissue majorly.
- At **day 6** trophoblast forms two type of cells: **cytotrophoblast** (inner layer) and **syncytiotrophoblast** (outer layer). Syncytiotrophoblast help in endometrial attachment of blastocyst at **day 6** itself (implantation in progress).
- Inner cell mass (embryoblast) of the blastocyst forms a bilayered embryonic disc having two type of cells: dorsal **epiblast** and ventral **hypoblast**. **Amniotic cavity** develops on the dorsal side and epiblast cell layer lies at the floor of amniotic cavity, whereas hypoblast cell layer is at the roof of **blastocyst cavity** (now called exocoelomic cavity).

Amnioblasts cells separate from the epiblast and organize to form a thin membrane, the **amnion**, which encloses the amniotic cavity. Epiblast cells are continuous peripherally with the amnion. Some cells migrate from hypoblast to surround the exocoelomic cavity and form **exocoelomic membrane**, which lines the internal surface of the cytotrophoblast.

The exocoelomic membrane and cavity soon become modified to form the **primary umbilical vesicle** (primary yolk sac). The embryonic disc then lies between the amniotic cavity and primary umbilical vesicle. The outer layer of cells from the umbilical vesicle forms a layer of loosely arranged connective tissue, the **extraembryonic mesoderm**.

- At first the walls of the amniotic cavity and yolk sac are in contact with trophoblast. They are soon separated from the latter by extraembryonic mesoderm.
- A cavity, the extraembryonic coelom appears and splits the extraembryonic mesoderm into a somatopleuric layer (in contact with trophoblast) and a splanchnopleuric layer (in contact with yolk sac).
- The trophoblast and underlying somatopleuric mesoderm form a membrane called the **chorion**.
- The cells forming the wall of the amniotic cavity form the **amnion**.

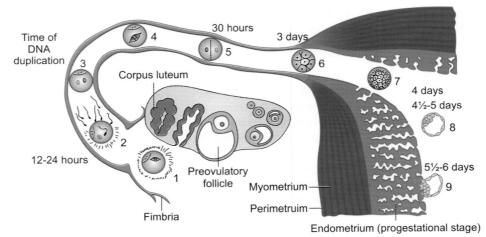

Fig. 7: Events during the first week of human development. 1, oocyte immediately after ovulation; 2, fertilization, approximately 12 to 24 hours after ovulation; 3, stage of the male and female pronuclei; 4, spindle of the first mitotic division; 5, two-cell stage [approximately 30 hours of age]; 6, morula containing 12 to 16 blastomeres [approximately 3 days of age]; 7, advanced morula stage reaching the uterine lumen [approximately 4 days of age]; 8, early blastocyst stage [approximately 4.5 days of age; the zona pellucida has disappeared]; 9, early phase of implantation [blastocyst approximately 6 days of age]. The ovary shows stages of transformation between a primary follicle and a preovulatory follicle as well as a corpus luteum. The uterine endometrium is shown in the progestational stage.

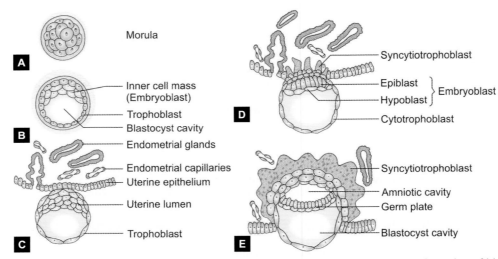

Figs. 8A to E: First week of development: Formation of morula and blastocyst and implantation of blastocyst

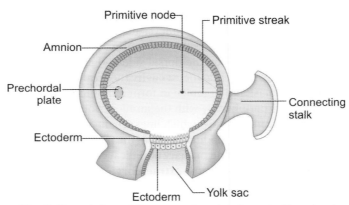

Fig. 9: Dorsal view of the conceptus showing primitive streak.

❏ The amniotic cavity is now attached to trophoblast by some mesoderm into which the extraembryonic coelom has not extended. This mesoderm forms the connecting stalk.

- The embryonic disc viewed from the ectodermal side near one edge shows a rounded area called the **prochordal plate**. Here ectoderm and endoderm are **not** separated by mesoderm.
- An elevation, the **primitive streak**, is also seen on the embryonic disc. A line drawn through the prochordal plate and the primitive streak divides the embryonic disc into right and left halves.
- Cells multiplying in the primitive streak move into the interval between epiblast and hypoblast form the **mesoderm** (Gray's anatomy mentions it as **mesoblast**) (third germ layer).
- Caudal to the primitive disc a round area called the **cloacal membrane** is present.
  - ➤ **Cloacal membrane** (plate) is formed at the caudal end of the embryo from adhesion between epiblast and hypoblast cells.
  - ➤ Later, it covers the cloaca and eventually breaks down to form openings into the urogenital sinus and anus.

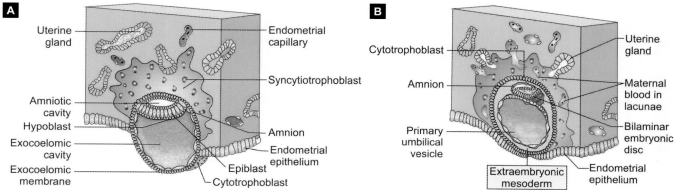

Figs. 10A and B: Implantation of blastocyst. A. Illustration of a section of a partially implanted blastocyst (approximately 8 days after fertilization). B, Illustration of a section through a blastocyst at approximately 9 days.

▼ Blast Cells

Embryoblast

- The embryoblast differentiates into two distinct cell layers: the **dorsal epiblast** and the **ventral hypoblast**. The epiblast and hypoblast together form a flat, ovoid-shaped disk known as the bilaminar embryonic disk.
- Within the epiblast, clefts develop and eventually coalesce to form the amniotic cavity.
- Hypoblast cells migrate and line the inner surface of the cytotrophoblast and eventually delimit a space called the definitive yolk sac.
- The epiblast and hypoblast fuse to form the **prochordal plate**, which marks the future site of the mouth.

Trophoblast

- The **syncytiotrophoblast** continues its growth into the endometrium to make contact with endometrial blood vessels and glands.
- The syncytiotrophoblast does not divide mitotically. The cytotrophoblast does divide mitotically, adding to the growth of the syncytiotrophoblast.
- The syncytiotrophoblast produces human chorionic gonadotropin (**hCG**).
- Primary chorionic villi formed by the cytotrophoblast protrude into the syncytiotrophoblast.

Extraembryonic Mesoderm

- Is a new layer of cells derived from the primary yolk sac.
- Extraembryonic somatic mesoderm (somatopleuric mesoderm) lines the cytotrophoblast, forms the connecting stalk, and covers the amnion.
- The conceptus is suspended by the connecting stalk within the chorionic cavity.
- The wall of the chorionic cavity is called the **chorion** and consists of three components: extraembryonic somatic mesoderm, cytotrophoblast, and syncytiotrophoblast.
- Extraembryonic visceral mesoderm (splanchnopleuric mesoderm) covers the yolk sac.

▼ Implantation

Implantation is the process by which the conceptus (blastocyst) is embedded within the endometrium of the uterus.

- Blastocyst usually implants within the **posterior superior wall** of the uterus in the functional layer of the endometrium during the progestational (**secretory**) phase of the menstrual cycle.
- On average, it occurs during the **20th to the 23rd day** after the last menstrual period.

- ❑ It is a **week long process**, beginning at day 5 (post-ovulation, or post fertilization) and is completed at day 12.
- ❑ It begins at day 5 when blastocyst is hatching out of zona pellucida.
- ❑ At day 6 it **attaches to the endometrium**. On the same day 6, the cells of trophoblast divide mitotically into **cytotrophoblast** and **syncytiotrophoblast**.
- ❑ The syncytiotrophoblast **invade** the endometrium with the help of proteolytic enzymes secreted by its cells.
- ❑ The blastocyst implants deep and completely lies within the endometrium (**interstitial implantation**).

QUESTIONS

1. Trophoblast differentiates into cyto and syncytiotrophoblast at post fertilization day:
   - a. 6-8
   - b. 8-12
   - c. 12-14
   - d. 16-18

2. Fertilized ovum reaches the uterus: *(NEET Pattern 2012)*
   - a. 3-4 days
   - b. 6- 8 days
   - c. 10- 12 days
   - d. 12-14 days

3. Conceptus enters uterine cavity in which cell stage? *(NEET Pattern 2014)*
   - a. 4 cells
   - b. 8 cells
   - c. 16 cells
   - d. 32 cells

4. Implantation occurs at: *(NEET Pattern 2012)*
   - a. 2-3 days
   - b. 5-7 days
   - c. 7-9 days
   - d. 20-25 days

5. Extra embryonic mesoderm is derived from: *(AIIMS 2016)*
   - a. Primary yolk sac
   - b. Secondary yolk sac
   - c. Epiblast
   - d. Hypoblast

ANSWERS

1. **a. 6-8**
   - ❑ Trophoblast differentiates into **cytotrophoblast** and **syncytiotrophoblast** at **6th day post-ovulation** (or post-fertilization).

2. **a. 3-4 days**
   - ❑ Fertilized ovum forms the morula, which enters uterine cavity on day 4, post ovulation (or post-fertilization).

3. **d. 32 cells**
   - ❑ Conceptus enters the uterine cavity at **advanced morula** stage (more than 16 cells) at **day 4**.
   - ❑ It gets converted into blastocyst **same day** and later attaches to endometrium on **day 6** (implantation).

4. **b. 5-7 days > c. 7-9 days**
   - ❑ Implantation is a **week-long** process, **beginning at day 5** (post-ovulation, or post-fertilization) and is **completed at day 12**.
   - ❑ It is **20th to the 23rd day** after the **last menstrual period**.

5. **a. Primary yolk sac**
   - ❑ **Extra-embryonic mesoderm** is formed by the cell lining of **primary yolk sac** (most appropriate option).
   - ❑ The origin of the extraembryonic mesoderm is **by no means clear**; it may arise from **several sources**, including the **caudal region of the epiblast**, the **parietal hypoblast**; **trophoblast** or a new germinal population which is **yet to be established** *(Gray's Anatomy Ed 41)*
   - ❑ Blastocyst **comes out of zona pellucida** on day 4-7, after fertilization *(NEET Pattern 2014)*
   - ❑ The **outer** layer of the blastocyst forms **trophoblast** *(NEET Pattern 2012)*
     - ■ **Inner** cell mass (**embryoblast**) forms embryo proper and **outer** layer of cells (**trophoblast**) contribute to **placenta**.
   - ❑ **Morula** is **16 cells** stage *(NEET Pattern 2014)*
     - ■ The conceptus is called a morula stage when it has **more than 12 cells** (blastomeres). The stage ends **when the blastocyst forms**, which occurs when there are **50 to 60 blastomeres present**.

▼ Primitive streak

- ❑ It starts developing by the **end of the second week** (day 14-15) and continues into the third week.
- ❑ It appears on the dorsum (back) of the developing embryo, **at the caudal** (or posterior) end and proceeds towards the cephalic (anterior) end.
- ❑ It originates from the anterior epiblast, and appears as an elongating groove (primitive groove) on the dorsal midsagittal surface of the epiblast, along the anterior-posterior axis of the embryo.
- ❑ The rostrocaudal and medial-lateral axis of the embryo are defined by the primitive streak.
- ❑ The rounded primitive (**Hensen's**) node is situated at the cranial tip of the primitive streak, and contains a depression called the **primitive pit**. The primitive pit is continuous with the primitive groove.
- ❑ The presence of the primitive streak determine the site of gastrulation and initiate germ layer formation.

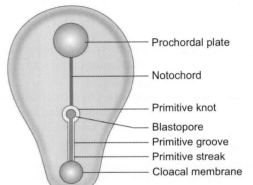

Fig. 11: Dorsal view of embryonic disc showing notochord

- Prochordal plate
- Notochord
- Primitive knot
- Blastopore
- Primitive groove
- Primitive streak
- Cloacal membrane

Primitive streak is the groove formed in the epiblast at the caudal end of the bilaminar germ disc stage embryo through which epiblast cells migrate to form endoderm and mesoderm during gastrulation.

Primitive node is the elevated region around the cranial end of the primitive streak that is known as the 'organizer' because it regulates important processes such as laterality and formation of the notochord.

Primitive pit is the depression in the primitive node.

Notochord

- ❑ Notochord (chordamesoderm) arises from epiblast cells of the medial part of the primitive node.
- ❑ It is also called axial mesoderm), is an early forming midline structure in the trilaminar embryo mesoderm layer initially ventral to the ectoderm, then neural plate and finally neural tube.
- ❑ It is a transient embryonic anatomy structure, not existing in the adult, defines the axis of embryo and is required for induction and Patterning the surrounding tissues. The Patterning signal secreted by notochord cells is sonic hedgehog (SHH).
- ❑ It forms in week 3, is eventually lost from vertebral regions and contributes to the nucleus pulposus of the intervertebral disc during the formation of the vertebral column.
- ❑ It forms during gastrulation and soon after induces the formation of the neural plate (neurulation), synchronizing the development of the neural tube.
- ❑ Notochord formation:
  - ➢ Epiblast cells at the floor of the amnion cavity in the blastopore region, form a notochordal process, which later becomes notochordal canal and fuses with the endoderm to form notochordal plate.
  - ➢ This occurs on the ventral aspect of the neural groove, where an axial thickening of the endoderm takes place next. This thickening appears as a furrow, the margins of which anastomose (come into contact), and so convert it into a solid rod of polygonal-shaped cells (the definitive notochord) which is then separated from the endoderm.
  - ➢ Notochord extends throughout the entire length of the future vertebral column, and reaches as far as the anterior end of the midbrain, where it ends in a hook-like extremity in the region of the future dorsum sellae of the sphenoid bone.
  - ➢ Initially it exists between the neural tube and the endoderm of the yolk-sac, but soon becomes separated from them by the mesoderm, which grows medially and surrounds it.
  - ➢ From the mesoderm surrounding the neural tube and notochord, the skull, vertebral column, and the membranes of the brain and spinal cord are developed.

QUESTIONS

1. True about notochord are all EXCEPT: *(NEET Pattern 2015)*
  a. Defines axis of embryo   b. Serves as primary inductor
  c. Derived from hypoblast   d. Remains as nucleus
     pulposus

2. All is true about notochord EXCEPT:
  a. Endodermal
  b. Appears at week 3
  c. Becomes nucleus pulposus
  d. Embryonic notochordal remnant may result in chordoma

ANSWERS

1. c. Derived from hypoblast
  ❑ Epiblast (not hypoblast) cells at the floor of the amnion cavity, form a notochordal process, which later evolve into definitive notochord.

2. a. Endodermal
  ❑ Notochord is the axial mesoderm forming the axis of the embryo.
  ❑ It appears at week 3 and later becomes nucleus pulposus of the intervertebral disc.
  ❑ Occasionally it may form a tumour- chordoma.
  ❑ Primitive streak initiation and maintenance is by Nodal gene a member of the transforming growth factor β (TGF-β) family *(AIIMS 2007)*
  Primitive streak is derived from epiblast, appear at caudal end and is 1st sign of gastrulation *(NEET Pattern 2015)*

Gastrulation

- ❑ During gastrulation epiblast cells (in primitive streak) undergo ingression and form three germ layers: endoderm, mesoderm and ectoderm.

Gastrulation
- ❑ The first germ layer to form is endoderm.
- ❑ Cells settling between the epiblast and endoderm were termed mesoderm and, more recently, it is being called as mesenchyme.
- ❑ The remaining epiblast cells then form the ectoderm.
- ❑ Later the fourth germ layer develops named as neural crest cells.
- ❑ The terms primary and secondary mesenchyme have been used to distinguish between those cells that arise from ingression through the primitive streak and those that arise from neural crest ingression, respectively.
- ❑ Head & neck mesenchyme is chiefly derived from neural crest cells.

This process is first indicated by the formation of the **primitive streak** in the midline of the epiblast. As early as the bilaminar and trilaminar stages of embryogenesis, left side/right side (L/R) axis determination begins with the asymmetric activity sonic hedgehog protein (SHH) only on the future left side since SHH activity is suppressed on the future right side by Activin. In addition, the neurotransmitter serotonin (5HT) plays an important role in L/R axis determination. After L/R axis determination, the L/R asymmetry of a number of organs (e.g., heart, liver, stomach) can be Patterned by the embryo.

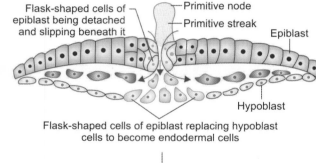

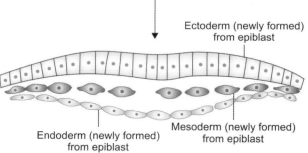

Fig. 13: Gastrulation

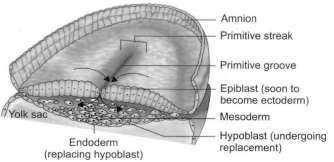

Fig. 12: Gastrulation: Formation of three germ layers from epiblast cells, in the third week of development.

1. **All the following statements are true concerning the early embryological development EXCEPT:**
   a. Zona pellucida is a glycoprotein membrane preventing implantation
   b. Blastocyst attaches to endometrium on day 6
   c. Primordial germ cells are derivative of epiblast
   d. The first germ layer to form is ectoderm

2. **Indicator of start of gastrulation is the formation of:**
   (NEET Pattern 2013)
   a. Neural groove
   b. Neural pit
   c. Primitive streak
   d. Formation of notochord

3. **Which of the following is FALSE regarding gastrulation?**
   a. Establishes all the three germ layers   *(AIPG 2002)*
   b. Occurs at the cephalic end of the embryo prior to its caudal end
   c. Involves the hypoblast cells of inner cells mass
   d. Occurs at 3 rd week

4. **Which of the following is present at the beginning of third week?**
   a. Notochord
   b. Primitive streak
   c. Mesoderm
   d. Neural crest cells

1. **d. The first germ layer to form is ectoderm.**
   ❑ **Endoderm** is the first germ layer to develop from the epiblast, followed by mesoderm and **lastly ectoderm**.

2. **c. Primitive streak**
   ❑ The **primitive streak** leads the way for development of the **primitive groove** and primitive fold. The primitive groove deepens into a **primitive pit**, an enlargement exists (the **primitive knot**) at the cephalic end of the primitive streak.

3. **c. Involves the hypoblast cells of inner cells mass**
   ❑ Gastrulation is the process by which the epiblast cells (**not hypoblast**) undergo ingression and establish three germ layers: endoderm, mesoderm and ectoderm.
   ❑ It occurs in the **third week** of development.
   ❑ Gastrulation has a **cephalocaudal direction**: It begins at the cephalic end and proceeds towards the caudal end. Hence, the three germ layers are first seen near the head region and consequently towards the tail region.

4. **b. Primitive streak**
   ❑ Primitive streak appears at the **end of second week** and beginning of third week (**day 14-15**).
   ❑ **Epiblast cells** in the primitive streak forms the **notochord, mesoderm** and **neural crest cells** later in the third week.
   ❑ **Disc** with **three** germ layers are formed at **3rd** week of gestation *(NEET Pattern 2012)*
   ❑ The **first epiblast cells** to ingress through the primitive streak form the **endoderm** and **notochord**, and initially occupy a midline position.
   ❑ The **earliest population** of endodermal cells rostral to the notochordal plate is termed the **prechordal plate**.

❑ The embryonic period, which extends from the **third to the eighth** weeks of development, is the period during which each of the three germ layers, ectoderm, mesoderm, and endoderm, gives rise to its own tissues and organ systems. As a result of organ formation, major features of body form are established.

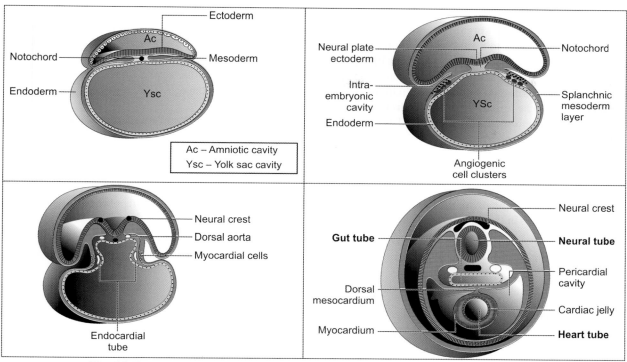

Fig. 14: Three germ layers forming three tubes: Neural tube, Gut tube and Heart tube

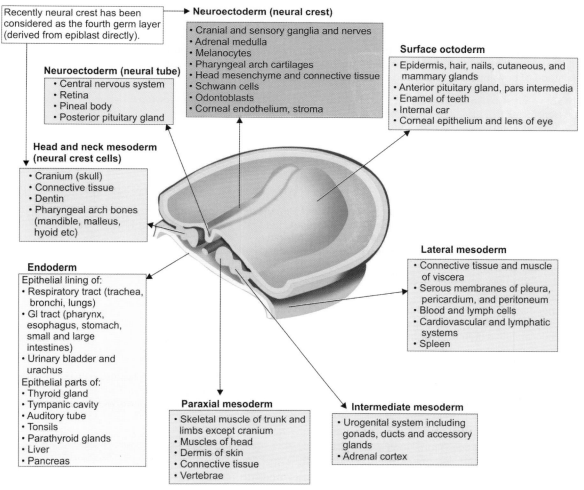

Recently neural crest has been considered as the fourth germ layer (derived from epiblast directly).

Neuroectoderm (neural crest)
- Cranial and sensory ganglia and nerves
- Adrenal medulla
- Melanocytes
- Pharyngeal arch cartilages
- Head mesenchyme and connective tissue
- Schwann cells
- Odontoblasts
- Corneal endothelium, stroma

Surface octoderm
- Epidermis, hair, nails, cutaneous, and mammary glands
- Anterior pituitary gland, pars intermedia
- Enamel of teeth
- Internal car
- Corneal epithelium and lens of eye

Neuroectoderm (neural tube)
- Central nervous system
- Retina
- Pineal body
- Posterior pituitary gland

Head and neck mesoderm (neural crest cells)
- Cranium (skull)
- Connective tissue
- Dentin
- Pharyngeal arch bones (mandible, malleus, hyoid etc)

Endoderm
Epithelial lining of:
- Respiratory tract (trachea, bronchi, lungs)
- GI tract (pharynx, esophagus, stomach, small and large intestines)
- Urinary bladder and urachus
Epithelial parts of:
- Thyroid gland
- Tympanic cavity
- Auditory tube
- Tonsils
- Parathyroid glands
- Liver
- Pancreas

Lateral mesoderm
- Connective tissue and muscle of viscera
- Serous membranes of pleura, pericardium, and peritoneum
- Blood and lymph cells
- Cardiovascular and lymphatic systems
- Spleen

Paraxial mesoderm
- Skeletal muscle of trunk and limbs except cranium
- Muscles of head
- Dermis of skin
- Connective tissue
- Vertebrae

Intermediate mesoderm
- Urogenital system including gonads, ducts and accessory glands
- Adrenal cortex

Fig. 15: Germ layer derivatives

❑ Craniocaudal Patterning of the embryonic axis is controlled by **homeobox genes**.
❑ As a result of formation of organ systems and rapid growth of the central nervous system, the initial flat embryonic disc begins to lengthen and to form head and tail regions (folds) that cause the embryo to curve into the fetal position. The embryo also forms two lateral body wall folds that grow ventrally and close the ventral body wall. As a result of this growth and folding, the amnion is pulled ventrally and the embryo lies within the amniotic cavity. Connection with the yolk sac and placenta is maintained through the vitelline duct and umbilical cord, respectively.
❑ **Earliest** system to be function in fetus is **Circulatory** (*NEET Pattern 2013*)
  ➢ Uteroplacental circulation is established as early as **12th day** of life, embryoplacental circulation at **day 17**.
  ➢ **Heart beat** begins as early as **day 22** of life.

▶ Endoderm

The endodermal germ layer provides the epithelial lining of the gastrointestinal tract, respiratory tract, and urinary bladder. It also forms the parenchyma of the thyroid, parathyroids, liver, and pancreas. The epithelial lining of the tympanic cavity and auditory tube originates in the endodermal germ layer.

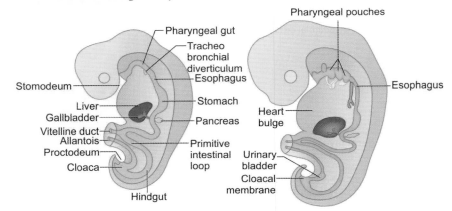

Figs. 16A and B: Sagittal sections through embryos showing derivatives of the endoderm germ layer. A. Pharyngeal pouches, epithelial lining of the lung buds and trachea, liver, gallbladder, and pancreas. B. The urinary bladder is derived from the cloaca and, at this stage of development, is in open connection with the allantois.

QUESTIONS

1. All are endodermal in origin EXCEPT:
  a. Hepatocyte   b. Odontoblast
  c. Alveolar lining cells   d. Urinary bladder

2. Which of the following is derived from endoderm?
  a. Gallbladder   b. Lens
  c. Spleen   d. Lymph nodes

3. Endoderm gives all EXCEPT:
  a. Urethra   b. Endocardium
  c. Lungs   d. Vagina

4. Rectum develops from: (*NEET Pattern 2012*)
  a. Cloaca   b. Hind gut
  c. Allantoic remnants d. Urogenital sinus

ANSWERS

1. b. Odontoblast
  ❑ **Odontoblasts** develop from the **neural crest cells** and form the **dentine** of teeth.
  ❑ **Hepatocytes** (liver) are endodermal derivative of **foregut**.
  ❑ Alveolar cells (**lung**) are derivative of the endoderm of **foregut**.
  ❑ Urinary bladder develops from **endoderm of urogenital sinus**.

2. a. Gallbladder
  ❑ Gallbladder develops from an **endodermal** outpouching of the embryonic **gut tube.**

3. b. Endocardium
  ❑ Endoderm of the urogenital sinus forms the **urethra** and **vagina epithelium**.
  ❑ Lung develops from the **endoderm** of anterior part of **foregut**.
  ❑ Endocardium is present in the heart tube (**mesodermal** origin).

4. a. Cloaca > b. Hind gut
  ❑ Rectum develops in the **cloaca** region of **hind gut**.
  ❑ The terminal end of the **hindgut** is an endoderm-lined pouch called the **cloaca**, which is partitioned by the **urorectal septum**.
  ❑ **Anterior** to the septum develops **urogenital sinus**, whereas **rectum** develops **posteriorly**.
  ❑ **Buccopharyngeal** membrane and **Cloacal** membrane have ectoderm **fused** with endoderm, with **no intervening mesoderm**
  (*AIIMS 2014*)

▶ Mesoderm

Components of the mesodermal germ layer are **paraxial, intermediate,** and **lateral plate** mesoderm
  ❑ Paraxial mesoderm give rise to somites, which further subdivide into the sclerotomes, myotomes and dermatomes.

- ❑ Somites give rise to the vertebrae of the vertebral column, rib cage, and part of the occipital bone; skeletal muscle, cartilage, tendons, and skin dermis (of the back).
- ❑ Somites are differentiated into:
  - ➢ Dermomyotome: Form skeletal muscles and dermis.
  - ➢ Sclerotomes: Surround notochord and project posteriorly to surround neural tube and divide into three parts:
  - ➢ Ventral sclerotomes: Forms vertebral body and annulus fibrosus.
    - ▪ Lateral sclerotomes: Forms vertebral arch (pedicle and lamina).
    - ▪ Dorsal sclerotomes: Forms the spinous process.
- ❑ Each lateral plate splits horizontally into the dorsal somatic (parietal) mesoderm, which underlies the ectoderm, and the ventral splanchnic (visceral) mesoderm, which overlies the endoderm.

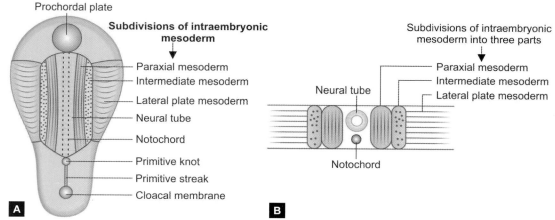

Figs. 17A and B: Subdivisions of intraembryonic mesoderm. A. As seen in embryonic disc. B. As seen in the horizontal section of the embryonic disc

- ❑ The space between these layers becomes the body cavity—the coelom—which stretches from the future neck region to the posterior of the body.
- ❑ During later development, the right- and left-side coeloms fuse, and folds of tissue extend from the somatic mesoderm, dividing the coelom into separate cavities.
- ❑ The coelom is subdivided into the pleural, pericardial, and peritoneal cavities, enveloping the thorax, heart, and abdomen, respectively.
- ❑ Parietal layers of pleura, pericardium and peritoneum develop from the dorsal somatic lateral plate mesoderm, whereas visceral layers of pleura, pericardium and peritoneum develop from the ventral visceral lateral plate mesoderm.

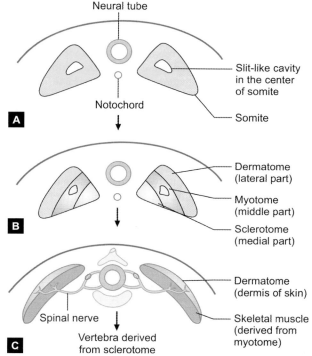

Figs. 19A to C: Subdivisions of the somites

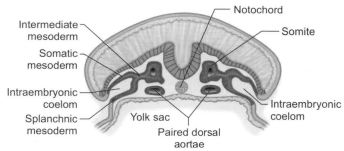

Fig. 18: Development of mesoderm into various subdivisions.

1. **All develop form mesoderm EXCEPT:** *(NEET Pattern 2012)*
   a. Skeletal muscle
   b. Testes
   c. Enamel
   d. Ureter

2. **Paraxial mesoderm contribution to development of:**
   (NEET Pattern 2013)
   a. Parietal peritoneum
   b. Visceral peritoneum
   c. Skeletal muscles
   d. Peritoneal cavity

QUESTIONS

3. Which of the following gives rise to the muscular component of dorsal aorta? *(AIPG 2011)*
   a. Intermediate mesoderm   b. Lateral plate mesoderm
   c. Axial mesoderm   d. Para-axial mesoderm

4. Which of the following marked structure forms nucleus pulposus embryologically? *(AIIMS 2017)*
   a. A   b. B
   c. C   d. D

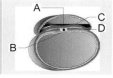

ANSWERS

1. **c. Enamel**
   ❑ **Enamel** of teeth develops from the **surface ectoderm**.

2. **c. Skeletal muscles**
   ❑ Paraxial mesoderm give rise to **somites**, whose myotome component forms the **skeletal muscles**.
   ❑ Each lateral plate splits horizontally into the dorsal somatic (parietal) mesoderm and the ventral splanchnic (visceral) mesoderm by a **space** called **coelomic cavity**
   ❑ The cavity is subdivided into the **pleural**, **pericardial**, and **peritoneal** cavities.
   ❑ **Parietal layers** of pleura, pericardium and peritoneum develop from the **dorsal somatic lateral plate mesoderm**, whereas **visceral layers** of pleura, pericardium and peritoneum develop from the **ventral visceral** lateral plate mesoderm.

3. **d. Para-axial mesoderm**
   ❑ Muscular component of the **dorsal aorta** is derived from **para-axial mesoderm**.
   ❑ Smooth muscles of most of the blood vessels are derived from **lateral plate mesoderm** (splanchnic layer), with few exceptions:
   ❑ Tunica media of
      ■ Proximal vessels of heart and head & neck, develop from **neural crest cells**.
      ■ Dorsal aorta develops from **para-axial mesoderm** *(AIPG 2011)*

4. **a. A**
   ❑ **Nucleus pulposus** is the adult remnant of **notochord** (marker A).
   Key: Marker B: Endoderm; C: Ectoderm; D: Mesoderm

- **Remnant** of notochord is **Nucleus pulposus** *(NEET Pattern 2013)*
- **Somites** develop from **paraxial** mesoderm *(NEET Pattern 2014)*
- **Pupillary muscles** do **not** develop from mesoderm *(AIIMS 2014)*
- Development of **peritoneal** cavity is from **Intraembryonic** coelom *(NEET Pattern 2012)*
  – Intraembryonic **coelom** forms the cavities like pericardial, pleural and peritoneal **cavities**.
- **Pericardial** cavity is an **intraembryonic** coelomic cavity *(NEET Pattern 2014)*
- **First pair** of somites arises in the occipital/**cervical** region of the embryo at approximately the **20th day** of development *(NEET Pattern 2014)*
- Mesoderm refers to cells derived from the **epiblast** and **extraembryonic tissues**.
- **Mesenchyme** refers to loosely organized embryonic connective tissue **regardless of origin**.
- **Sclerotome** forms the **vertebrae** and the **ribs** and **part of the occipital bone**
- **Myotome** forms the musculature of the back, the ribs and the limbs
- **Syndetome** forms the tendons and the **dermatome** forms the **skin dermis on the back**.
- Majority of the **skeletal** muscle in the body develops from **paraxial mesenchyme** and its segmental derivatives, the **somites**.
- **Smooth muscles** develop from the **splanchnopleuric mesenchyme** in the walls of the viscera and around the endothelium of blood vessels.

▶ Ectoderm

The ectodermal germ layer gives rise to the organs and structures that maintain contact with the outside world: Central and Peripheral nervous system, Sensory epithelium of ear, nose, and eye, skin, including hair and nails, pituitary, mammary, and sweat glands and enamel of the teeth.

QUESTIONS

1. All are derived from ectoderm EXCEPT: *(NEET Pattern 2012)*
   a. Lens   b. Eustachian tube
   c. Brain   d. Retina

2. All are derived from ectoderm EXCEPT: *(NEET Pattern 2012)*
   a. Hypophysis   b. Retina
   c. Spinal cord   d. Adrenal cortex

3. Ameloblasts in teeth are derived from: *(NEET Pattern 2012)*
   a. Mesoderm   b. Endoderm
   c. Neural crest cells   d. Ectoderm

4. All are derived from ectoderm EXCEPT: *(AIIMS 2014)*
   a. Hair follicle   b. Sebaceous gland
   c. Arrector pilorum   d. Mammary gland

ANSWERS

1. **b. Eustachian tube**
   ❑ Eustachian tube is a derivative of the **first pharyngeal pouch** and is lined by **endodermal** epithelium.

2. **d. Adrenal cortex**
   ❑ The suprarenal (adrenal) cortex is formed during the second month by a **proliferation of the coelomic epithelium**. (Some authors mention its origin from **intermediate mesoderm**).
   ❑ Adrenal medulla receives **neural crest cell** derived neurone bodies.

3. **d. Ectoderm**
   ❑ Ameloblasts develop from the **surface ectoderm** and form the **enamel of teeth**.

4. c. Arrector pilorum
- ❑ **Arrector pilorum** muscle is a smooth muscle in the skin derived from the **mesenchyme**.
- ❑ Ectoderm forms skin epithelium (**epidermis**) and the associated appendages (hair) and glands (sebaceous and sweat).
- ❑ Mammary gland is a **modified sweat gland**.
- ❑ Sphincter **and** dilator pupillae muscles of iris develop from the **neural plate ectoderm** (*NEET Pattern 2013*)

▶ Neural Crest Cell Derivatives

- ❑ Neural crest cells have been considered to arise from the embryonic ectoderm cell layer.
- ❑ After gastrulation, neural crest cells are located at the border of the neural plate and the non-neural ectoderm.
- ❑ During neurulation, the borders of the neural plate (neural folds) converge to form the neural tube.
- ❑ Subsequently, neural crest cells from the roof plate of the neural tube undergo an epithelial to mesenchymal transition, separating from the neuroepithelium and migrating through the periphery where they differentiate into varied cell types.
- ❑ Recently neural crest cells are called as fourth germ layer.
- ❑ The neural crest cells (NCCs) have multipotency and long range migration through embryo and its capacity to generate a prodigious number of differentiated cell types.
- ❑ For these reasons, although derived from the ectoderm, the neural crest (NC) has been called the fourth germ layer (in addition to the ectoderm, mesoderm and endoderm).
- ❑ The neural crest meets all the criteria used to define and identify a germ layer.
- ❑ As the fourth germ layer, the neural crest is confined to vertebrates, which are therefore tetrablastic not triploblastic.

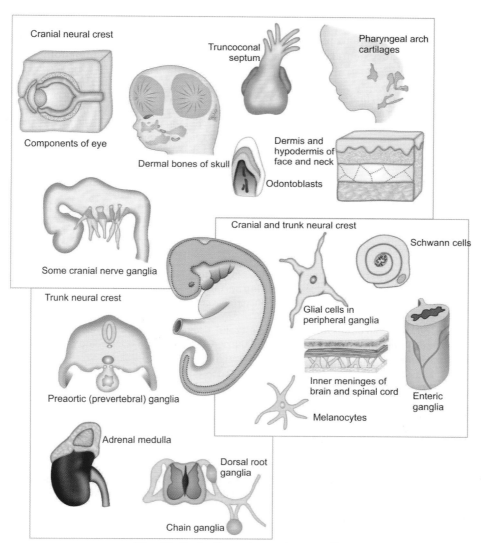

Fig. 20: Derivatives of neural crest cells

❑ Derivatives
❑ Neural crest cells originating from different positions along the anterior-posterior axis are divided into four regions: Cranial neural crest, trunk neural crest, vagal and sacral neural crest and cardiac neural crest.
❑ Neural crest cells give rise to secondary mesenchyme (also called mesoectoderm) and contributes to most of the skeletal and connective tissue components of the head and neck region:
  ➢ Odontoblasts, dental papillae, the chondrocranium (nasal capsule, Meckel's cartilage, scleral ossicles, hyoid), tracheal and laryngeal cartilage, the dermato-cranium (membranous bones), pericytes and smooth muscle of branchial arteries and veins, tendons of ocular and masticatory muscles, connective tissue of head and neck glands (pituitary, salivary, lacrymal, thymus, thyroid) dermis and adipose tissue of calvaria, ventral neck and face.
❑ Neural crest cells form one of the three pigment cell types - **melanocytes**, which develop from a subpopulation of neural crest cells derived from both the head and the trunk.
❑ The others pigment cells: Retinal pigment epithelium and pigment cells of the pineal organ, both originate from the neuroectoderm (diencephalon).
❑ Glomus cell type I are very similar structurally to neurons, and they are derived from the **neural crest**, while the glomus cells of type II are similar in function to neuroglia (derived from **neuroectoderm**).
❑ Glomus cell (type I) is a peripheral chemoreceptor, mainly located in the carotid bodies and aortic bodies, that helps the body regulate breathing. A decrease in the blood's pH, a decrease in oxygen (pO_2), or an increase in carbon dioxide (pCO_2), leads to the carotid bodies and the aortic bodies sending signal to the medulla oblongata (dorsal inspiratory center) to increase the volume and rate of breathing.
❑ Autonomic ganglia innervate the glomus cells, and some presynaptic sympathetic ganglia synapse with glomus cells.
❑ Clusters of glomus cells, of which the carotid bodies and aortic bodies are the most important, are called non-chromaffin or parasympathetic paraganglia. They are also present along the vagus nerve, in the inner ears, in the lungs, and at other sites.
❑ Neoplasms of glomus cells are known as paraganglioma, among other names, they are generally nonmalignant.
❑ Placodes: Cells within the rostral porencephalic neural fold and smaller populations of cells in bilateral sites lateral to the early brain do not form migratory neural crest cells but remain within the surface epithelium are called as ectodermal placodes.

QUESTIONS

1. Enumerate the derivatives of neural crest cells: *(PGIC 2016)*
  a. Tunica media of ascending aorta
  b. Connective tissue of thymus gland
  c. Enamel of teeth
  d. Choroid and sclera of eye
  e. Mandible bone

2. Derivatives of neural crest is/are *(PGIC 2003)*
  a. Para follicular cells of thyroid   b. Adrenal cortex
  c. Adrenal medulla   d. Dorsal root ganglia
  e. Autonomic ganglia

3. Structures derived from neural crest cells are all EXCEPT:
  a. Ganglia (PGIC)
  b. Mesenchyme of brain
  c. Astrocyte and oligodendrocyte
  d. AP septum of heart
  e. Enamel

4. Glomus cells are derived from: *(NEET Pattern 2015)*
  a. Surface ectoderm   b. Neuroectoderm
  c. Mesoderm   d. Endoderm

ANSWERS

1. a. Tunica media of ascending aorta; b. Connective tissue of thymus gland; d. Choroid & sclera of eye; e. Mandible bone
  ❑ Tunica media of proximal vessels of heart like **ascending aorta**, develop from **neural crest cells**.
  ❑ Few glands like **thymus** develop from endoderm of pharyngeal pouches, **but connective tissue** is derived from neural crest cell derived **secondary mesenchyme**.
  ❑ Dentine of teeth develop from **odontoblast** (neural crest cells), whereas the enamel develops from surface ectoderm.
  ❑ Most of the **eyeball** develop from neural crest cells and the derived mesenchyme, including **choroid** and **sclera** of eyeball.
  ❑ **Pharyngeal arch bones** like mandible develop from neural crest cells.

2. a. Para follicular cells of thyroid; c. Adrenal medulla; d. Dorsal root ganglia; e. Autonomic ganglia
  ❑ **Parafollicular** 'C' cells of thyroid are derived from neural crest cells.
  ❑ Adrenal **medulla** is a derivative of neural crest cells, whereas adrenal **cortex** develops from intermediate mesoderm.
  ❑ Most of the ganglia have contributions from neural crest cells, **including** autonomic and dorsal root ganglia.

3. c. Astrocytes and oligodendrocyte; e. Enamel
  ❑ Astrocyte and oligodendrocyte develop from the **neural plate ectoderm**.
  ❑ **Enamel** develops from ameloblasts (**surface ectoderm**).
  ❑ Most of the **ganglia**, head & neck **mesenchyme** and **AP septum** of heart develop from **neural crest cells**.
  ❑ Teeth develop from neural crest cells (**odontoblast** forms dentine) and are covered by surface ectoderm (**ameloblast** forms enamel).

4. b. Neuroectoderm
  ❑ Glomus **cell type I** are very similar structurally to **neurons**, and they are derived from the **neural crest**, while the glomus cells of **type II** are similar in function to **neuroglia** (derived from neuroectoderm).

- A **glomus cell** (type I) is a peripheral **chemoreceptor**, mainly located in the **carotid** bodies and **aortic** bodies, that helps the body regulate breathing.
- **Neural crest cells** are the **fourth germ layer**, derived from **epiblast**. Some authors consider neural crest cells are derived from **neuroectoderm**.
- Sympathetic **ganglion** develops from **Neural crest cells** (NEET Pattern 2015)
- Auerbach's plexus and Meissner's **ganglion** cell are derived from **Neural crest cells** (AIIMS 2009)
- **Melanoblasts** precursors of melanocytes) are derived from **Neural crest cells**
- **Leptomeninges** (pia-arachnoid) are contributed by **neural crest cells**.
- Skeletal and connective tissue components of the pharyngeal arches are chiefly derived from **secondary mesenchyme** (neural crest cells derived).

Yolk Sac (Umbilical Vesicle)

- Yolk sac (umbilical vesicle) is a membranous sac attached to an embryo, formed by cells of the hypoblast adjacent to the embryonic disk.
- It is important in early embryonic blood supply, and much of it is incorporated into the primordial gut during the fourth week of development.
- It is the first element seen within the gestational sac during pregnancy, usually at 3 days gestation.
- It is situated on the ventral aspect of the embryo; it is lined by extra-embryonic endoderm, outside of which is a layer of extra-embryonic mesenchyme.
- **Yolk sac** develops from the cavity of blastocyst and passes through **three** stages:
- **Primary** yolk sac is the vesicle which develops in the second week.
  - The blastocyst cavity gets converted into primary yolk sac, as it gets lined by flattened cells derived from extraembryonic endoderm (which themselves are derived from hypoblast).
  - This lining formed of flattened cells is called **Heuser's membrane**, which is attached to the undersurface of the hypoblast in the embryonic disc.
  - It is also known as the **exocoelomic cavity**.
- **Secondary** yolk sac is formed when the extraembryonic coelom develops in the extraembryonic mesoderm.
  - It is the remnant of primary yolk sac, has become smaller and lined by cuboidal cells.
- **Definitive** yolk sac is seen during the fourth week of development.
  - Part of the yolk sac gets surrounded by endoderm and incorporated into the embryo as the gut and the remaining part of the yolk sac is called as the final (definitive) yolk sac.
  - It communicates with the midgut via vitellointestinal duct.
- The **vitellointestinal duct** undergoes complete obliteration during the **seventh week**, but in about two percent of cases its proximal part persists as a diverticulum from the small intestine, **Meckel's diverticulum**.
- **Vitelline circulation** functions for absorption of nutritive material from the yolk sac to the embryo. Primitive aorta convey the blood to the wall of the yolk sac, which circulate through a wide-meshed capillary plexus and is carried by the vitelline veins to the tubular heart of the embryo.

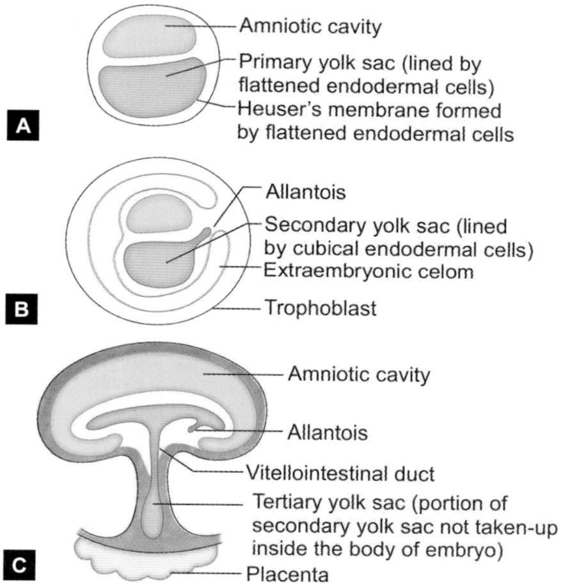

Figs. 21A to C: Yolk sac. A. Primary yolk sac (lined by Heuser's membrane made of flattened cells derived from endoderm B. Secondary yolk sac (becomes smaller due to the formation of extraembryonic celom and cells lining it becomes cuboidal) C. Tertiary yolk sac (part of secondary yolk sac which is not taken up inside the embryonic disc)

Amnion and Chorion

- **Amnion** is a thin extraembryonic membrane that is derived from the **epiblast** and surrounds the fluid-filled amniotic cavity around the embryo and fetus.
- It loosely envelops the embryo forming an amniotic sac that is filled with the amniotic fluid.
- It consists of two layers: an outer layer made up of somatopleuric layer of extraembryonic membrane and an inner layer made up of amniogenic cells.
- **Chorion** is the multilayered structure consisting of the somatic layer of **extraembryonic mesoderm**, **cytotrophoblast**, and **syncytiotrophoblast**.
- It contributes the fetal portion of the placenta, including the villi and villus lakes.
- Numerous small finger like projections arise from its surface called villi.

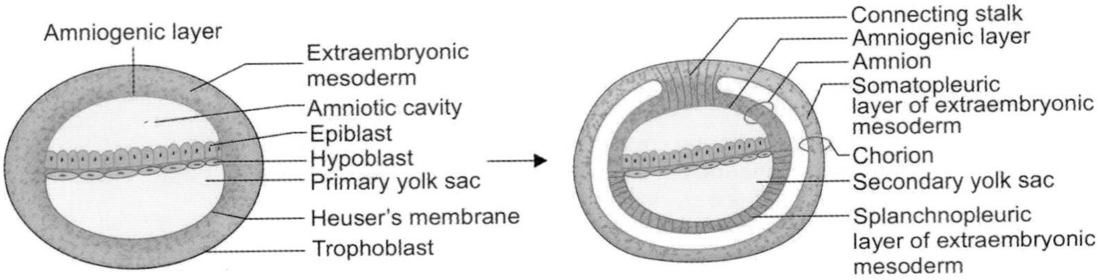

Fig. 22: Formation of amnion

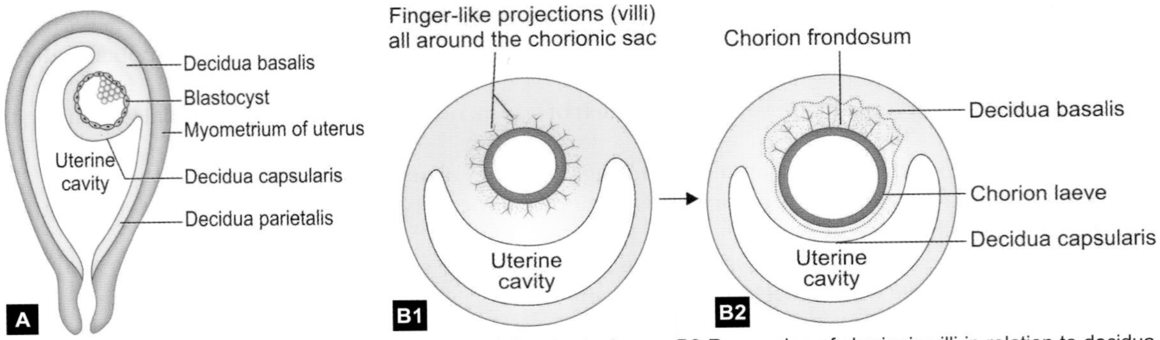

A-Parts (subdivisions) of decidua. B1-Formation of villi all around the chorionic sac. B2-Regression of chorionic villi in relation to decidua capsularis

Figs. 23A and B: Formation of chorion frondosum and chorion laeve. A. Formation of villi all around the chorionic sac. B. Regression of chorionic villi in relation to decidua capsularis.

- Decidua capsularis: Chorionic villi regress leaving a smooth surface called chorion laeve.
- Decidua basalis: Chorionic villi are well developed (chorion frondosum) and contribute the fetal portion of the placenta.

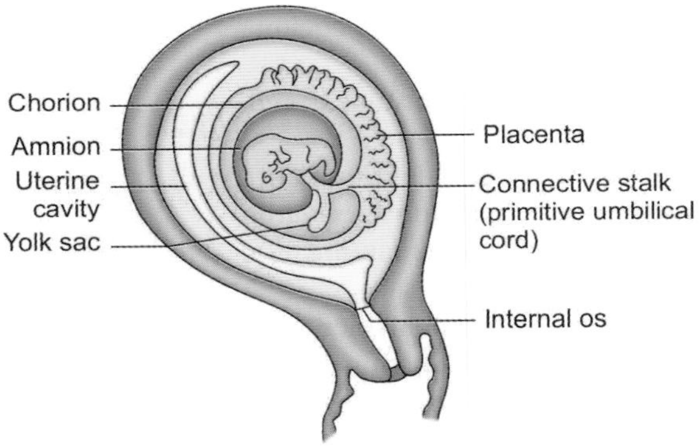

Fig. 24: Fetal membranes

Placenta, Fetal Membranes and Umbilical Cord

- The placenta consists of two components: (1) a fetal portion, derived from the chorion frondosum or villous chorion, and (2) a maternal portion, derived from the decidua basalis. The space between the chorionic and decidual plates is filled with intervillous lakes of maternal blood. Villous trees (fetal tissue) grow into the maternal blood lakes and are bathed in them. The fetal circulation is at all times separated from the maternal circulation by:
  - A syncytial membrane (a chorion derivative) and
  - Endothelial cells from fetal capillaries. Hence, the human placenta is of the hemochorial type.

Villus stage	Primary villus	Secondary villus	Tertiary villus
Time of appearance (post fertilization)	Day 12	Day 13-15	Day 17-21 (week 3)
Structure	A core of cytotrophoblast cells covered by a layer of syncytium (syncytiotrophoblast)	Cytotrophoblast core invaded by extraembryonic mesoderm	Fetal blood invade the mesoderm

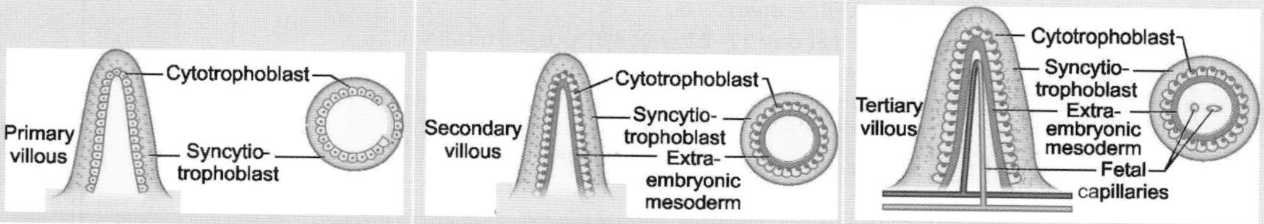

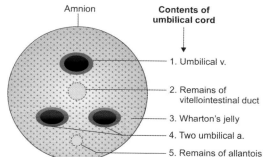

Fig. 25: Three stages of development of villi. Figures on the right side are the sectional views of three types of villi

During week 2 of development, the embryoblast receives its nutrients from endometrial blood vessels, endometrial glands, and decidual cells via diffusion.

Uteroplacental circulation is established at day 9–12 (week 2), yet no blood vessels are formed in the extraembryonic mesoderm to carry nutrients directly to the embryoblast. That fetoplacental circulation is established at day 17–22.

▶ Umbilical cord

❏ A patent opening called the primitive umbilical ring exists on the ventral surface of the developing embryo through which three structures pass: the yolk sac (vitelline duct), connecting stalk, and allantois. The allantois is not functional in humans and degenerates to form the median umbilical ligament in the adult.

❏ As the amnion expands, it pushes the vitelline duct, connecting stalk, and allantois together to form the primitive umbilical cord.

❏ The definitive umbilical cord at term is pearl-white, 1–2 cm in diameter, 50–60 cm long, eccentrically positioned, and contains the right and left umbilical arteries, left umbilical vein, and mucus connective tissue (Wharton's jelly).

❏ The right and left umbilical arteries carry deoxygenated blood from the fetus to the placenta. The left umbilical vein carries oxygenated blood from the placenta to the fetus.

Amnion

Contents of umbilical cord

1. Umbilical v.
2. Remains of vitellointestinal duct
3. Wharton's jelly
4. Two umbilical a.
5. Remains of allantois

Fig. 26: Cross-section of the umbilical cord

QUESTIONS

1. **Placenta develops from:**   *(NEET Pattern 2014)*
   a. Decidua capsularis and Chorion frondosum
   b. Decidua capsularis and Decidua basalis
   c. Decidua basalis and Chorion frondosum
   d. Decidua parietalis and Chorion frondosum

2. **Amnion is present on:**
   a. Decidua basalis   b. Fetal surface
   c. Maternal surface   d. All of the above

3. **TRUE about umbilical cord:**   *(NEET Pattern 2015)*
   a. Contains two umbilical veins
   b. Contains one umbilical artery
   c. Right umbilical vein disappears
   d. Length is 25-30 cm

4. **Cytotrophoblasts invades:**   *(NEET Pattern 2012)*
   a. Decidua basalis   b. Decidua parietalis
   c. Decidua capsularis   d. None

5. **Before formation of head and tail folds, the most cranial part of embryo**   *(NEET Pattern 2014)*
   a. Septum transversum   b. Neural plate
   c. Notochord   d. Primitive streak

ANSWERS

1. **c. Decidua basalis and Chorion frondosum**
   ❏ Placenta develops from decidua basalis (**maternal** component) and chorion frondosum (**fetal** component).

2. **b. Fetal surface**
   ❏ Amnion is the **inner most** layer facing fetus.

3. **c. Right umbilical vein disappears**
   ❏ Right umbilical vein Regresses (**R-R**) and Left umbilical vein is Left (**L-L**).
   ❏ Umbilical cord has **two** umbilical arteries and the **left umbilical vein**.
   ❏ An average umbilical cord is **55 cm long**, with a diameter of 1-2 cm and 11 helices.

4. **a. Decidua basalis**
   ❏ The cytotrophoblast within the villi continues to grow through the invading syncytiotrophoblast and makes direct contact with the **decidua basalis**, forming anchoring villi.

5. **a. Septum transversum**
   ❏ Before formation of head and tail folds, **septum transversum** is the **most cranial** structure in embryonic disc.
   ❏ Umbilical vesicle (yolk sac) is fully developed at **week four** and is called as **definitive** (final) yolk sac.

- Yolk sac is derived from **Hypoblast** (*NEET Pattern 2016*)
- Fetoplacental circulation is established at **day 17–22** (week 3), post fertilization.
- Tertiary villi develop by the **end of week 3** (day 17–21).
- Two **umbilical arteries** are normally joined at the chorionic plate, by **transverse anastomosis** called Hyrtl's anastomosis (*NEET Pattern 2015*)
- **Wharton jelly** is the connective tissue of the cord (*NEET Pattern 2018*)

▼ Cardiovascular system

Arteries

The arterial system develops from the **aortic arches** and branches of the **dorsal aorta**.

Aortic arch branch from the aortic sac to the dorsal aorta traveling in the center of each pharyngeal arch.

- ❏ Initially, there are five pairs, but these undergo considerable remodelling to form definitive vascular Patterns for the head and neck, aorta, and pulmonary circulation.
- ❏ In the rest of the body, the arterial Patterns develop mainly from the right and left dorsal aortae.
- ❏ The right and left dorsal aortae fuse to form the dorsal aorta, which then sprouts posterolateral arteries, lateral arteries, and ventral arteries (vitelline and umbilical).

Aortic arch artery	Adult derivative
1.	Maxillary artery (portion of)
2.	Stapedial and hyoid arteries (portion of)
3.	Right and left common carotid artery (portion of) Right and left internal carotid artery (portion of)
4.	Right side: Proximal part of right subclavian artery Left side: Arch of aorta (portion of)
5.	Regresses
6.	Right and left pulmonary arteries (portion of) Ductus arteriosus**

External carotid artery is a de-novo branch: Right regresses; left is left.

- ❏ Early in development, the recurrent laryngeal nerves hook around aortic arch 6. Later on the right side, the distal part of aortic arch 6 regresses, and the right recurrent laryngeal nerve moves up to hook around the right subclavian artery. On the left side, aortic arch 6 persists as the ductus arteriosus (or ligamentum arteriosus in the adult); the left recurrent laryngeal nerve remains hooked around the ductus arteriosus.

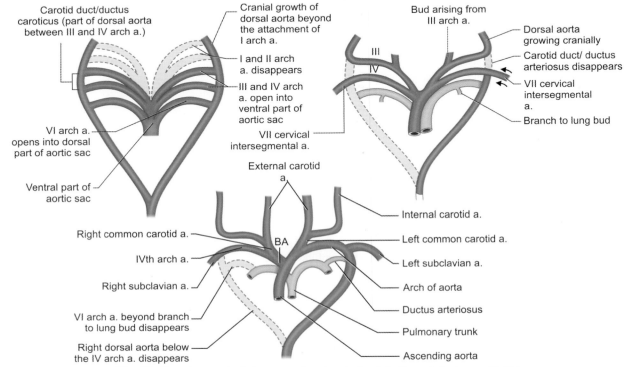

Fig. 27: Development of pharyngeal arch arteries into the adult stage arteries

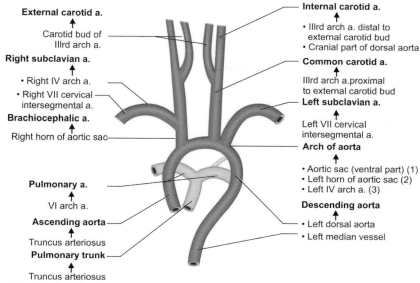

Fig. 28: Development of pharyngeal arch arteries into the adult stage arteries

Table 4: Source of development of main arteries	
Arteries	**Source of development**
Arch of aorta	(a) Aortic sac (ventral part), (b) left horn of aortic sac, and (c) left fourth arch artery
Brachiocephalic artery	Right horn of aortic sac
Right subclavian artery	(a) Proximal part from right fourth arch artery and (b) distal part from right seventh cervical intersegmental artery
Left subclavian artery	Left seventh cervical intersegmental artery
Common carotid artery	Third arch artery proximal to the external carotid artery bud
Internal carotid artery	Third arch artery distal to the external carotid bud and cranial part of dorsal aorta distal to the attachment of third arch artery
External carotid artery	Bud from third arch artery
Pulmonary arteries	Part of the sixth arch artery between pulmonary trunk and branch to lung bud on each side
Descending aorta	(a) Proximal part from left dorsal aorta distal to attachment of fourth arch artery and (b) distal part from fused dorsal aortae forming single median artery

* Arch of aorta also gets contributions from left dorsal aorta (between the attachment of the fourth aortic arch (artery) and 7th cervical intersegmental artery

◤ Applied anatomy

❑ Abnormal origin of the right subclavian artery. It happens due to disappearance of Right fourth aortic arch and proximal portion of right dorsal aorta. In this case the right subclavian artery is formed by distal portion of right dorsal aorta and right intersegmental subclavian artery (A). Abnormal subclavian artery crosses the midline behind esophagus and trachea creating a vascular ring around them (B).

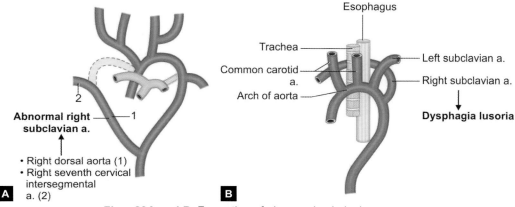

Figs. 29A and B: Formation of abnormal subclavian artery

❏ Double aortic arch results due to abnormal persistence of distal portion of right dorsal aorta (A). It leads to formation of double aortic arch, which forms vascular ring around trachea and esophagus and may cause compression.

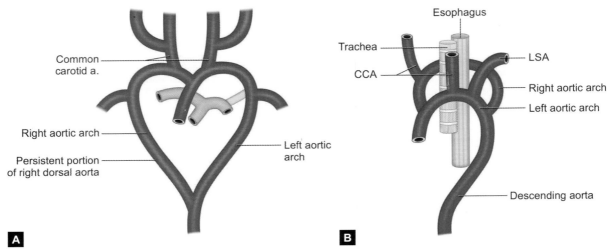

Figs. 30A and B: Formation of right aortic arch leading to double aortic arch

Derivatives of dorsal aorta

Embryonic artery	Adult derivative
Posterolateral (somatic intersegmental) branches	Arteries of upper and lower limbs Intercostal, lumbar and lateral sacral arteries
Lateral splanchnic arteries	Phrenic arteries Renal and suprarenal arteries Gonadal arteries
Ventral splanchnic arteries (a) Vitelline arteries (b) Umbilical arteries	(a) Coeliac, superior mesenteric and inferior mesenteric arteries (b) Internal iliac arteries (portion of), superior vesical arteries, medial umbilical ligaments

1. **Embryological dorsal aorta forms:** *(NEET Pattern 2016)*
   a. Ascending aorta   b. Descending aorta
   c. Common carotid artery   d. Pulmonary trunk

2. **Arch of aorta is derived from all EXCEPT:** *(NEET Pattern 2016)*
   a. Left horn of aortic sac   b. Left 2nd arch artery
   c. Left 4th arch artery   d. Left dorsal aorta

3. **Aberrant subclavian artery formed due to:** *(AIIMS 2016)*
   a. Persistent A
   b. Persistent B
   c. Obliterated A and persistent B
   d. Persistent A and obliterated B

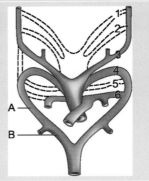

4. **Double aortic arch occurs due to:**
   a. Nondevelopment of right 4th aortic arch
   c. Non-division of truncus arteriosus
   b. Nondevelopment of left 4th aortic arch
   d. Persistent distal portion of right dorsal aorta

(NEET Pattern 2012)

1. **b. Descending aorta**
   ❏ Proximal part of descending aorta develops from 1) left **dorsal aorta** distal to attachment of fourth arch artery and (2) distal part from fused **dorsal aortae** forming single median artery.

2. **b. Left 2nd arch artery**
   ❏ Arch of aorta develops from 1. **Aortic sac** (ventral part). 2. **Left horn** of aortic sac and 3. **Left 4th** arch artery.

ANSWERS

3. c. Obliterated A and persistent B

❑ **Aberrant** subclavian artery: Right fourth aortic arch and **proximal portion** of right dorsal aorta ('A') **disappears** and distal portion of right dorsal aorta ('B') persists. In this case, the right subclavian artery is formed by **distal portion of right dorsal aorta** ('B') and **right seventh intersegmental** artery.

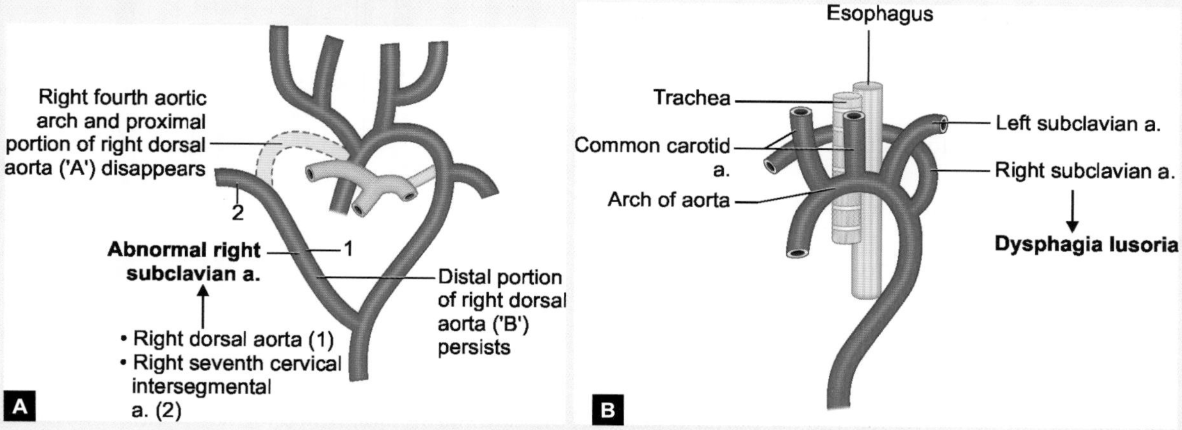

Figs. 31A and B: Formation of abnormal subclavian artery

❑ Since this abnormal artery crosses the **midline behind** esophagus and trachea, a **vascular ring** is formed by right subclavian artery and aortic arch, which may **compress** the two visceral tubes.

4. d. Persistent distal portion of right dorsal aorta

❑ Double aortic arch occurs when an abnormal **right aortic arch develops** in addition to a left aortic arch due to **persistence of the distal portion of the right dorsal aorta**.

❑ This forms a **vascular ring** around the trachea and esophagus, which may cause difficulties in **breathing** and **swallowing**.

- **2nd arch** artery does NOT take part in formation of **right subclavian** artery *(NEET Pattern 2015)*
- Artery of **2nd** pharyngeal arch is **stapedial** artery *(NEET Pattern 2012)*
- Artery **of 3rd arch** is **common** carotid artery *(NEET Pattern 2015)*
- **Right fourth** arch artery gives rise to **right subclavian** artery *(NEET Pattern 2014)*
- **External** carotid artery arises as a **sprout** from the **common** carotid artery.
- 6th aortic arch forms ductus arteriosus *(JIPMER 2017)*
  - **Proximal** part of 6th aortic arch forms **pulmonary arteries** on both sides.
  - The **distal** portion of 6th arch forms ductus arteriosus, which later **Regresses on Right** (RR) and Left is Left (LL).

Veins

The venous system develops from the vitelline, umbilical, and cardinal veins, which drain into the sinus venosus.

A. Vitelline veins

❑ Return poorly oxygenated blood from the yolk sac.

❑ Right vein forms the hepatic veins and sinusoids, ductus venosus, hepatic portal, superior mesenteric, inferior mesenteric, and splenic veins and part of the IVC.

❑ Left vein forms the hepatic veins and sinusoids and ductus venosus.

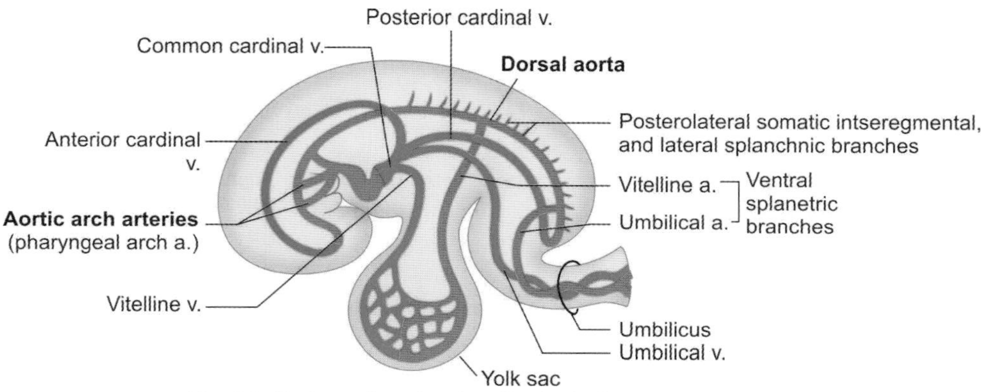

Fig. 32: Embryonic veins (cardinal, vitelline and umbilical).

B. Umbilical veins

- ❑ Carry welloxygenated blood from the placenta.
- ❑ Right vein degenerates during early development.
- ❑ Left vein forms the ligamentum teres hepatis.

Cardinal Veins

- ❑ Return poorly oxygenated blood from the body of the embryo.
- ❑ Anterior cardinal vein forms the internal jugular veins and SVC.
- ❑ Posterior cardinal vein forms a part of the IVC and common iliac veins.
- ❑ Subcardinal vein forms a part of the IVC, renal veins, and gonadal veins.
- ❑ Supracardinal vein forms a part of the IVC, intercostal, azygos, and hemiazygos veins.

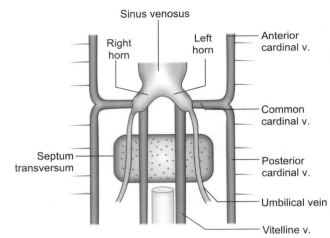

Fig. 33: Three sets of primitive veins

Venous System. Three systems can be recognized: (1) the vitelline system, which develops into the portal system; (2) the cardinal system, which forms the caval system; and (3) the umbilical system, which degenerates after birth.

Table 5: Embryonic veins and their future derivatives	
Embryonic	**Adult**
Vitelline veins	
Right and left	Portion of the IVC/hepatic veins and sinusoids, ductus venosus, portal vein, inferior mesenteric vein, superior mesenteric vein, splenic vein
Umbilical veins	
Right	Degenerates early in fetal life
Left	Ligamentum teres
Cardinal veins	
Anterior	SVC, internal jugular veins
Posterior	Portion of IVC, common iliac veins
Subcardinal	Portion of IVC, renal veins, gonadal veins
Supracardinal	Portion of IVC, intercostal veins, hemiazygos vein, azygos vein

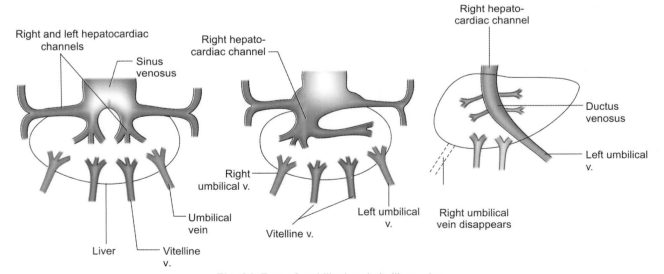

Fig. 34: Fate of umbilical and vitelline veins

In the majority of persistent left superior venae cavae, blood drains into the right atrium via the coronary sinus. When this does not happen, the coronary sinus is absent, and the persistent left superior vena cava drains directly into the atrium.

▼ Veins in the upper body

Cardinal veins are system of anterior, posterior, and common cardinal veins that drain the head and body of the embryo in the late third and early fourth weeks.

The major veins of the upper part of the body, viz., internal jugular veins, subclavian veins, right and left brachiocephalic vein, and superior vena cava are derived as follows:

1. **Internal jugular vein:** It develops from anterior cardinal vein cephalic to the opening of the subclavian vein.
2. **Subclavian vein:** It develops in the region of the upper limb bud by enlargement of the intersegmental veins in this region.
3. **Right brachiocephalic vein:** It develops from right anterior cardinal vein above the opening of oblique communicating channel and below the opening of the right subclavian vein.
4. **Left brachiocephalic vein:** It develops from oblique channel connecting left and right anterior cardinal veins, and left anterior cardinal vein between the opening of communicating channel (vide supra) and left subclavian vein.
5. **Superior vena cava:** Developmentally it consists of two parts: first and second.
   The first part develops from the right anterior cardinal vein caudal to the oblique transverse anastomosis. The second part develops from the right common cardinal vein. As the right common cardinal vein opens into the right horn of sinus venosus, the superior vena cava at first opens into the right horn of sinus venosus. As and when the right horn of sinus venosus is absorbed into the right atrium, the superior vena cava finally opens into the right atrium.
6. Other veins: As most of the blood is shunted from left to right the following changes occur:
   a. Part of the left anterior cardinal vein below the transverse anastomosis obliterates.
   b. The most of left posterior cardinal vein also regresses. The small cranial part of left posterior cardinal vein along with regressed part of the left anterior cardinal vein caudal to transverse anastomosis forms left superior intercostal vein.
   c. The left horn of sinus venosus regresses and forms coronary sinus. The left common cardinal vein obliterates in its lateral part and forms oblique vein of the left atrium (oblique vein of Marshall) while its medial part contributes to the formation of coronary sinus.

External jugular veins develop as separate channels.

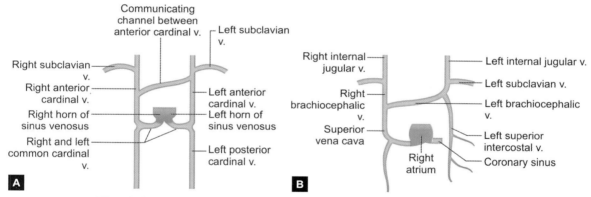

Figs. 35A and B: Development of major veins of the upper parts of the body

Clinical Correlation

Anomalies of superior vena cava

- **Double superior vena cava:** It occurs when the anastomosis between the two anterior cardinal veins fails to form and left anterior cardinal vein persists. Thus, anterior cardinal vein on both sides develops into the superior vena cava. The left superior vena cava opens into the coronary sinus, which in turn opens into the right atrium.

- **Left superior vena cava:** It occurs when the anastomosis does develop between the two anterior cardinal veins, but the blood is shunted from right to left through brachiocephalic vein. As a result, the right anterior cardinal vein below the oblique transverse anastomosis regresses and the left anterior cardinal vein develops into the superior vena cava. The left superior vena cava opens into the coronary sinus.

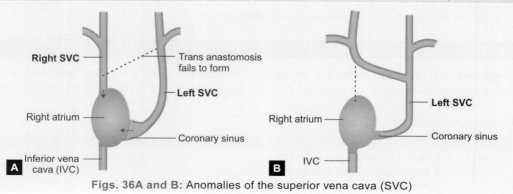

Figs. 36A and B: Anomalies of the superior vena cava (SVC)

Portal vein formation

The two vitelline veins lie one on either side of developing duodenum. They soon get interconnected by three anastomotic channels: two ventral and one dorsal.

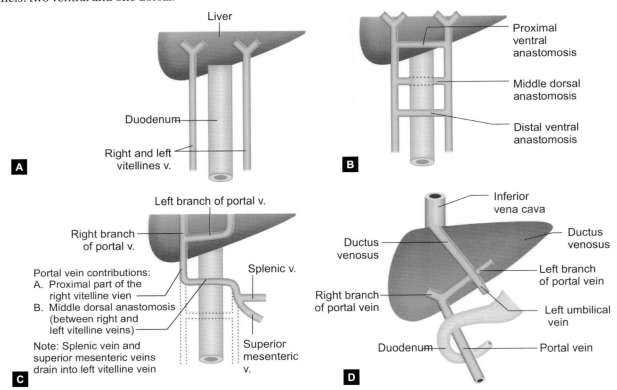

Figs. 37A to D: Development of portal vein

These anastomotic channels are:
- ❏ Proximal ventral anastomosis
- ❏ Middle dorsal anastomosis
- ❏ Distal ventral anastomosis

The superior mesenteric and splenic veins that develop independently unite with the left vitelline vein just below dorsal anastomosis.

The portal vein develops from three components:
1. Caudal part of left vitelline vein between point at which superior mesenteric and splenic vein open, and the point where dorsal anastomosis joins the left vitelline vein.
2. Middle dorsal anastomosis.
3. Part of right vitelline vein between the dorsal and proximal ventral anastomosis.

The right branch of portal vein develops from the part of right vitelline vein distal to proximal ventral anastomosis.

The left branch of portal vein develops from proximal ventral anastomosis and left vitelline vein distal to proximal ventral anastomosis. Remaining parts of vitelline veins and distal ventral anastomosis disappear along with left hepatocardiac channel.

Note: The development of portal vein explains that it is formed by union of superior mesenteric and splenic veins; it passes dorsally to the duodenum and divides into right and left branches that enter the liver.

IVC formation

Initially, three systems of veins are present: The umbilical veins from the chorion, vitelline veins from the umbilical vesicle, and cardinal veins from the body of the embryos. Next the subcardinal veins appear, and finally the supracardinal veins develop.

Inferior vena cava develops from six components.

Component	Contributions
Post renal (Sacrocardinal) segment	▪ Right posterior cardinal vein (1) ▪ Right supracardinal vein (2) ▪ Anastomosis between right supracardinal and subcardinal vein (3)

Component	Contributions
Renal segment	▪ Right subcardinal vein (4)
Hepatic segment	▪ Anastomotic channel between subcardinal vein and right hepatocardiac channel (5) ▪ Right hepatocardiac channel (6)

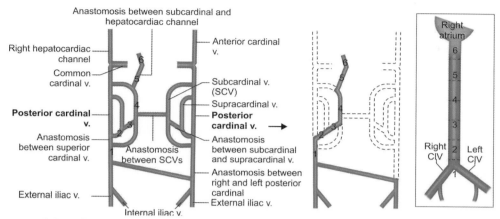

Fig. 38: Development of the inferior vena cava. Figure in the inset on the right shows 1 = Right posterior cardinal vein (sacrocardinal segment). 2 = Supracardinal vein. 3 = Supracardinal-subcardinal anastomosis. 4 = Right subcardinal vein (renal segment). 5 = Anastomotic channel between subcardinal vein and right hepatocardiac channel. 6 = Right hepatocardiac channel (hepatic segment). CIV = Common iliac vein.

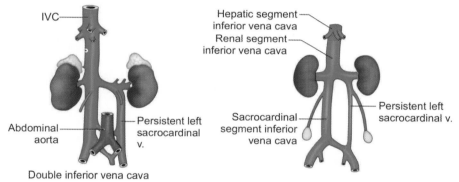

Fig. 39: Formation of double inferior vena cava

❑ Right hepatocardiac channel forms terminal segment (hepatic segment) of the inferior vena cava that first opens into right horn of sinus venosus, and, after the right horn is absorbed in the right atrium, in the right atrium directly.

❑ Double inferior vena cava may result from due to absence of the anastomosis between two posterior cardinal veins. The left posterior cardinal vein below the level of the renal vein develops into left inferior vena cava while normal inferior vena cava develops on the right side. As a result, inferior vena cava is duplicated below the renal veins. The left inferior vena cava into left renal vein. Double inferior vena cava may result due to persistence of left supracardinal vein is mentioned by most of the authors. Double inferior vena cava may also arise due to persistence of left sacrocardinal vein is mentioned by Langman's embryology. Some authors mention it is due to persistence of both (right and left) subcardinal and supracardinal veins. .

❑ Absence of inferior vena cava may result due to absence of the anastomosing channel between right subcardinal vein and right hepatocardiac channel. The cranial part of right subcardinal vein which normally disappears, persists and carries the blood from the inferior vena cava to the superior vena cava. The hepatic veins directly open into the right atrium at the site of the inferior vena cava.

▶ Veins In The Lower Body

❑ The anastomosis between the subcardinal veins forms the **left renal vein**. When this communication has been established, the left subcardinal vein disappears, and only its distal portion remains as the **left gonadal vein**.

❑ Hence, the **right subcardinal vein** becomes the main drainage channel and develops into **the renal segment of the inferior vena cava**.

❑ With **obliteration** of the major portion of the **posterior cardinal veins**, the supracardinal veins assume a greater role in draining the body wall. The 4th to 11th right intercostal veins empty into the right supracardinal vein, which together with a portion of the posterior cardinal vein forms the **azygos vein**.

❑ On the left, the 4th to 7th intercostal veins enter into the left supracardinal vein, and the left supracardinal vein, then known as the **hemiazygos vein**, empties into the azygos vein

❑ Right **common iliac** vein: It develops from the caudal part of **right posterior cardinal** vein below the **transverse anastomosis** between the two posterior cardinal veins.

❑ Left **common iliac** vein: It develops from the **transverse anastomosis** between the two posterior cardinal veins and part of **left posterior cardinal** vein below the anastomosis.

QUESTIONS

1. All of the following veins are formed from vitelline vein EXCEPT:
a. Hepatic vein
b. Superior vena cava
c. Inferior vena cava
d. Superior mesenteric vein

2. Derivative of vitelline vein is: *(NEET Pattern 2015)*
a. IVC
b. SVC
c. Ligamentum venosum
d. Ligamentum teres

3. Superior vena cava develops from: *(NEET Pattern 2016)*
a. Right anterior cardinal vein
b. Left anterior cardinal vein
c. Left common cardinal vein
d. Right subcardinal vein

4. Left sided SVC drains into: *(AIPG 2010)*
a. Right atrium
b. Left atrium
c. Coronary sinus
d. Pericardial space

5. The most important structure involved in development of inferior vena cava is: *(AIIMS)*
a. Supracardinal vein and subcardinal vein
b. Umbilical vein
c. Anterior cardinal vein
d. Posterior cardinal vein

6. Double inferior vena cava is formed due to persistence of: *(JIPMER)*
a. Sacrocardinal vein
b. Supracardinal vein
c. Subcardinal vein
d. Posterior cardinal vein

7. Double inferior vena cava is formed due to: *(NEET Pattern 2013)*
a. Persistence of sacrocardinal veins
b. Persistence of supracardinal veins
c. Persistence of subcardinal veins
d. Persistence of both supracardinal and subcardinal veins

8. Posterior cardinal vein develops into: *(NEET Pattern 2016)*
a. Superior vena cava
b. Internal jugular vein
c. External jugular vein
d. Common iliac vein

9. Portal vein develops from which of the following marked structures? *(AIIMS 2016)*
a. A
b. B
c. C
d. D

ANSWERS

1. b. Superior vena cava
❑ Vitelline vein forms portion of the **IVC, hepatic veins** and sinusoids, ductus venosus, portal vein, inferior mesenteric vein, **superior mesenteric vein**, splenic vein, etc.
❑ Superior vena cava is basically contributed by **anterior cardinal vein**.

2. a. IVC > c. Ligamentum venosum
❑ Vitelline vein forms **hepatic portion** of the **IVC**.
❑ Within the substance of the liver, the vitelline system also forms the **ductus venosus**, a channel shunting blood from the left umbilical vein directly to the inferior caval vein during gestation.

3. a. Right anterior cardinal vein
❑ Superior vena cava develops from:
 ▪ **Right anterior cardinal** vein (caudal to the oblique transverse anastomosis)
 ▪ **Right common cardinal** vein

4. c. Coronary sinus > a. Right atrium
❑ Left sided superior vena cava drains into the **coronary sinus** and thence into the **right atrium** (occasionally directly into the right atrium).
❑ The aetiology is **failure of regression** of left anterior and common cardinal veins and left sinus horn.
❑ In this case the **right** brachiocephalic vein becomes **longer, oblique and crosses** the midline to reach the superior vena cava.

5. a. Supracardinal vein and subcardinal vein
❑ Inferior vena cava develops from several sources, **subcardinal vein** having significant contribution, especially the renal segment and the postrenal segment (anastomosis between right **supracardinal** and **subcardinal** vein).
❑ Right posterior cardinal vein contributes to the inferiormost component of IVC (sacrocardinal segment).

6. b. > a. > c. > d.
❑ Double inferior vena cava may result due to **persistence** of left **supracardinal** vein is mentioned by most of the authors.
❑ Double inferior vena cava **may also** arise due to persistence of **left sacrocardinal vein i**s mentioned by Langman's embryology.
❑ Some authors mention it is due to persistence of **both** (right and left) subcardinal and supracardinal veins. It involves the **posterior cardinal vein** as well.

7. **b. > a. > c. > d.**
  ❏ Double inferior vena cava may result due to persistence of **left supracardinal vein** is mentioned by most of the authors.

8. **d. Common iliac vein**
  ❏ Posterior cardinal veins contribute to **inferior vena cava** and **common iliac veins**.
  ❏ Superior vena cava and jugular veins develop from anterior cardinal veins.

9. **a. A**
  ❏ Portal vein develops from the right vitelline vein.
  ❏ Portal vein is contributed by **middle dorsal anastomosis** (between right and left vitelline veins) and **proximal part of the right vitelline vein.**
  Key: A - Right vitelline vein; B - Right umbilical vein; C - Left vitelline vein; D - Left umbilical vein.

Diaphragm is contributed by the septum transversum mesenchyme (ventrally); the dorsal mesoesophagus and paired pleuroperitoneal membranes (posteriorly) and excavated body wall (posteriorly and laterally).

❏ Skeletal muscles of diaphragm develop from **cervical somites** (myotomes), hence it is supplied by phrenic nerve (C: 3,4,5).

❏ **Septum transversum** is the primordium of the central tendon of the diaphragm.

❏ Paired **pleuroperitoneal membranes** are sheets of somatic mesoderm that appear to develop from the dorsal and dorsolateral body wall.

❏ **Dorsal mesentery of the esophagus** is invaded by myoblasts and forms the crura of the diaphragm in the adult.

❏ **Body wall** contributes muscle to the peripheral portions of the definitive diaphragm.

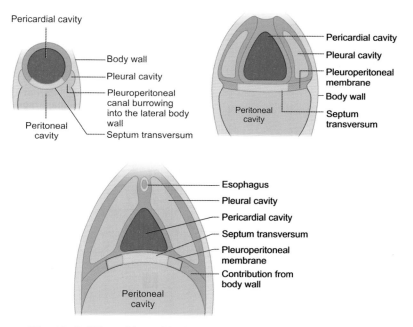

Fig. 40: Splitting of lateral body wall by developing pleural cavities

Embryonic structure	Adult derivative
Cervical somites (myotomes)	Skeletal muscle of diaphragm
Septum transversum	Central tendon of diaphragm
Pleuroperitoneal membrane	Posterior and peripheral part of diaphragm
Dorsal mesentery of esophagus (dorsal meso-esophagus)	Crura of diaphragm
Body wall mesoderm	Peripheral posterolateral portion

Positional Changes of the Diaphragm

❏ During week 4 of development, the developing diaphragm becomes innervated by the **phrenic nerves**, which originate from C3, C4, and C5 and pass through the pleuropericardial membranes.

❏ By week 8, there is an apparent **descent of the diaphragm** to L1 because of the rapid growth of the neural tube.

❏ The phrenic nerves are **carried along with** the 'descending diaphragm', while they remain associated with the fibrous pericardium.

Bochdalek Hernia

Deficiency in the pleuroperitoneal membrane or its failure to fuse with the other parts of the diaphragm leads to **Bochdalek** hernia (congenital diaphragmatic hernia), presenting as neonatal emergency.

❑ Abdominal contents are herniate into the **left pleural cavity**, usually the stomach and/or the small bowel, colon, liver and spleen.

    There is associated **left lung hypoplasia** and right mediastinal shift (and resulting cyanosis).

❑ Mother presents with polyhydramnios and baby has scaphoid (flattened) abdomen, **cyanosis**, and difficulty in breathing.

❑ Immediate nasogastric intubation is performed, and the surgery is postponed by few days till the patient is stabilized.

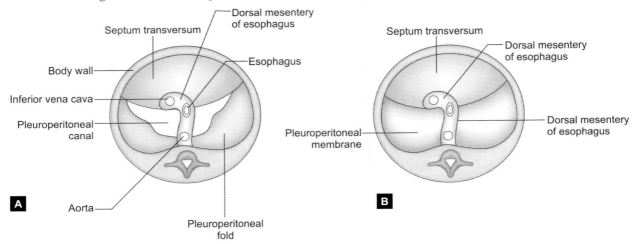

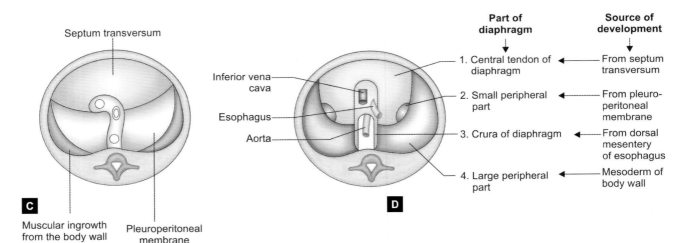

Figs. 41A to D: Successive stages (A, B, C, and D) of the development of the diaphragm

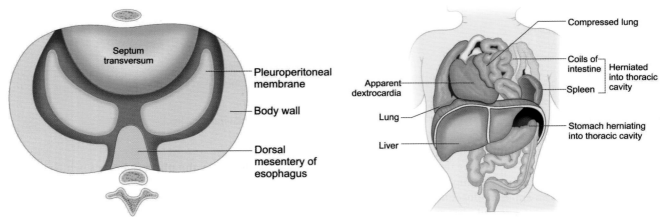

Fig. 42: Developmental components of the diaphragm   Fig. 43: Posterolateral hernia of diaphragm

QUESTIONS

1. **All are derivatives of septum transversum EXCEPT:**
   (AIIMS 2010)
   a. Falciform ligament   b. Ligamentum teres
   c. Coronary ligament   d. Lesser omentum

2. **Most common site of Morgagni Hernia is:** *(AIPG)*
   a. Left anterior   b. Right posterior
   c. Right anterior   d. Left posterior

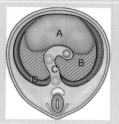

3. **In the following diagram for diaphragm development, congenital diaphragmatic hernia occurs usually due to defect in:**
   a. A   b. B
   c. C   d. D

ANSWERS

1. **b. Ligamentum teres**
   - ❑ **Ligamentum teres** is the adult remnant of **left umbilical vein** (and is not derived from septum transversum).
   - ❑ Septum transversum gives rise to **central tendon** of diaphragm and the **ventral mesentery** of the foregut.
   - ❑ Ventral mesentery itself gives derivatives: **Falciform** ligament, **Lesser omentum**, **Coronary** ligament.

2. **c. Right anterior**
   - ❑ Morgagni's hernia is a **congenital** diaphragmatic hernia, which is a rare entity (Bochdalek hernia is more common).
   - ❑ Morgagni's hernia is commonly seen on the **right anteromedial** aspect of diaphragm.

3. **b. B**
   - ❑ The most common congenital diaphragmatic hernia is **Bochdalek hernia**. It occurs due to deficiency in the **pleuroperitoneal** membrane (B), usually on the left side.
   - ❑ Bochdalek hernia presents with **left postero lateral defect** in the diaphragm, leading to intestinal herniation into the thorax.
   - **Key:** A - Septum transversum; B - Pleuroperitoneal membrane; C - Dorsal mesentery of esophagus; D - Body wall mesoderm.

- ▪ **Septum transversum** develops from mesoderm *(NEET Pattern 2016)*
  - Septum transversum is a plate of **cranial mesoderm**, descending down to reach the **junction** of thorax and abdomen and contributing to **central tendon** of diaphragm.
- ▪ Diaphragm **does not** develop from pleuropericardial membrane *(AIIMS 2015)*
- ▪ Diaphragm **doesn't** develop form dorsal mesocardium *(AIPG 2011, NEET Pattern 2016)*
- ▪ **Crus** of diaphragm develops from **dorsal mesentery of esophagus** *(NEET Pattern 2016)*
- ▪ **Myoblasts** of diaphragm develops from **cervical 3-5 somites** *(NEET Pattern 2012)*

▶ GIT - Embryology

- ❑ Primitive gut tube is formed from the incorporation of the dorsal part of the yolk sac into the embryo due to the craniocaudal folding and lateral folding of the embryo.
- ❑ The **epithelium** of the digestive system and the parenchyma of its derivatives originate in the **endoderm**; whereas, connective tissue, muscular components, and peritoneal components originate in the **mesoderm**.
- ❑ **HOX genes** in the mesoderm are induced by SHH secreted by gut endoderm and regulate the craniocaudal organization of the gut and its derivatives.
- ❑ The primitive gut tube extends from the oropharyngeal membrane to the cloacal membrane and is divided into the foregut, midgut, and hindgut.
- ❑ Early in development, the epithelial lining of the gut tube proliferates rapidly and obliterates the lumen, which later is reacquired by recanalization.

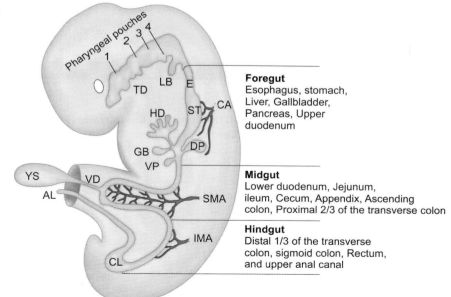

Foregut
Esophagus, stomach, Liver, Gallbladder, Pancreas, Upper duodenum

Midgut
Lower duodenum, Jejunum, ileum, Cecum, Appendix, Ascending colon, Proximal 2/3 of the transverse colon

Hindgut
Distal 1/3 of the transverse colon, sigmoid colon, Rectum, and upper anal canal

Fig. 44: Derivatives of the three parts of gut tube

- ❑ The **pharyngeal** gut gives rise to the pharynx and related glands.
- ❑ The **foregut** gives rise to the esophagus, the trachea and lung buds, the stomach, and the duodenum proximal to the entrance of the bile duct.
  - ➢ In addition, the liver, pancreas, and biliary apparatus develop as outgrowths of the endodermal epithelium of the upper part of the duodenum.
  - ➢ The epithelial **liver** cords and biliary system growing out into the septum transversum differentiate into parenchyma.
  - ➢ Hematopoietic cells (present in the liver in greater numbers before birth than afterward), the Kupffer cells, and connective tissue cells originate in the mesoderm.
  - ➢ The **pancreas** develops from a ventral bud and a dorsal bud that later fuse to form the definitive pancreas.
- ❑ The **midgut** forms the primary intestinal loop, gives rise to the duodenum distal to the entrance of the bile duct, and continues to the junction of the proximal two-thirds of the transverse colon with the distal third.
  - ➢ At its apex, the primary loop remains temporarily in open connection with the yolk sac through the vitelline duct.
  - ➢ During the sixth week, the loop grows so rapidly that it protrudes into the umbilical cord (physiological herniation).
  - ➢ During the 10th week, it returns into the abdominal cavity.
  - ➢ While these processes are occurring, the midgut loop rotates 270° counterclockwise.
- ❑ **Hindgut** gives rise to the region from the distal third of the transverse colon to the upper part of the anal canal.
  - ➢ The distal part of the anal canal originates from ectoderm.
  - ➢ The hindgut enters the posterior region of the cloaca (future anorectal canal), and the allantois enters the anterior region (future urogenital sinus).
- ❑ The **urorectal septum** will divide the two regions and breakdown of the cloacal membrane covering this area will provide communication to the exterior for the anus and urogenital sinus.
- ❑ The **anal canal** itself is derived from endoderm (cranial part) and ectoderm (caudal part).
- ❑ The caudal part is formed by invaginating ectoderm around the proctodeum.

Structures	Foregut	Midgut	Hindgut
Organs	Esophagus, stomach, liver, gallbladder, pancreas, 1/2 of duodenum	1/2 of duodenum, jejunum, ileum, cecum, ascending colon, 2/3 of transverse colon	1/3 of transverse colon, descending and sigmoid colon, rectum, and 2/3 of anal canal
Arteries and branches	**Celiac** splenic, left gastric, short gastric, common hepatic, right gastric, gastroduodenal	**Superior Mesenteric** inferior pancreaticoduodenal, intestinal middle colic, right colic, ileocolic	**Inferior Mesenteric** left colic, superior rectal
Veins	Portal vein	Portal vein	Portal vein
Lymph	Celiac nodes (supracolic compartment)	Superior mesenteric nodes (infracolic compartment)	Inferior mesenteric nodes (infracolic compartment)
Nerves: Parasympathetic	Vagus	Vagus	Pelvic splanchnic (S2-S4)
Sympathetic	Greater thoracic splanchnic (T5-T9)	Lesser thoracic splanchnic (T10, T11)	Least thoracic splanchnic (T12), upper lumbar splanchnic (L1, L2)
Pain refers to:	Epigastric region	Umbilical region	Suprapubic region

▼ Clinical Correlations

Tracheoesophageal Fistula

The upper part of the foregut is divided by a septum (the tracheoesophageal septum) into the esophagus posteriorly and the trachea and lung buds anteriorly, deviation of the septum may result in abnormal openings between the trachea and esophagus.

Hirschsprung's Disease

- ❑ Hirschsprung disease occurs due to **nonmigration of neural crest cells** into the distal part of the gut tube colon/rectum.
- ❑ It is usually characterized by an **aganglionic** portion of gut that does not display peristalsis, and a dilated segment of structurally normal colon (mega) proximal to this site.
- ❑ Histologically, there is either an absence or a reduction in the number of ganglia and

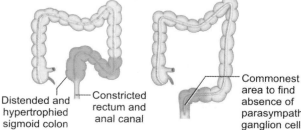

Distended and hypertrophied sigmoid colon — Constricted rectum and anal canal — Commonest area to find absence of parasympathetic ganglion cells

Fig. 45: Main characteristics of primary megacolon (Hirschsprung's disease)

postganglionic neurons in the **Auerbach's** myenteric plexus of the affected segment of gut; postganglionic innervation of the muscle layers is also often defective.

❏ **Midrectum** are the most common sites but, in severe cases, the rectum, sigmoid, descending and even proximal colon can be aganglionic. **Rectal biopsy is a-ganglionic**.

❏ Infants with Hirschsprung's disease show delay in the passage of meconium, constipation, vomiting and abdominal distension.

Meckel's Diverticulum

❏ A congenital ileal diverticulum (of Meckel); found in **2–3% of individuals** and represents the remnant of the proximal part of the **vitellointestinal duct**.

❏ It projects from the **antimesenteric border** of the terminal ileum and is commonly located between **50 and 100 cm** (2 feet) from the ileocaecal junction.

❏ It is variable in length (usually **2 inches** in adults) and often possesses a short 'mesentery'.

❏ The lumen of the diverticulum usually has a calibre similar to that of the ileum.

❏ Small heterotopic areas of gastric body type epithelium, pancreatic, colonic or other tissues may also occur in the wall of a diverticulum.

❏ Heterotopic gastric tissue may lead to ulceration and bleeding in the adjacent normal ileal mucosa.

❏ Diverticular inflammation may mimic acute appendicitis; pain is referred to the periumbilical region.

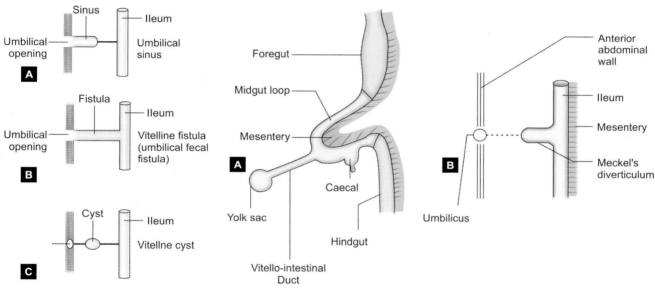

Figs. 46A to C: A. Umbilical sinus. B. Umbilical fistula. C. Vitelline cyst

Figs. 47A and B: Meckel's anomalies arise from the abnormal persistence of vitellointestinal duct

▼ Peritoneal fold (embryology) and mesentery

Peritoneum

❏ Parietal layer is derived from somatopleuric layer (lateral plate mesoderm)
  ➢ Innervated by somatic nerves (sensitive to prick and cut).

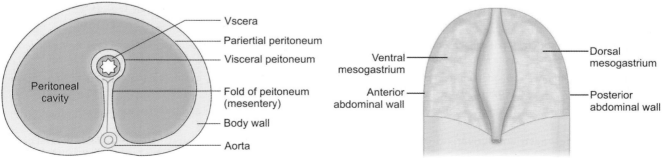

Fig. 48: Schematic transverse section of the abdomen showing arrangement of the peritoneum

Fig. 49: Side view of stomach showing dorsal and ventral mesogastrium

❑ Visceral layer is derived from splanchnopleuric layer (lateral plate mesoderm)
  ➤ Innervated by ANS (insensitive to prick and cut).

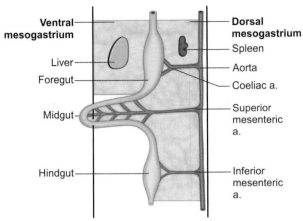

Fig. 50: Schematic diagram showing three parts of the primitive gut with their arteries and mesenteries

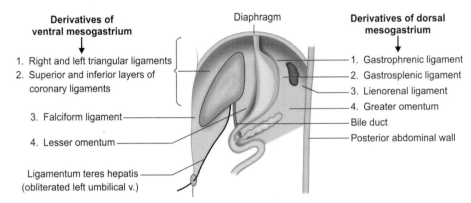

Fig. 51: Derivatives of ventral and dorsal mesogastrium

Mesenteries

The primitive gut tube is suspended within the peritoneal cavity of the embryo by a ventral and dorsal mesentery from which all adult mesenteries are derived.

Table 6: Derivation of adult mesenteries	
Embryonic mesentery	**Adult mesentery**
Ventral	Lesser omentum (hepatoduodenal and hepatogastric ligaments), falciform ligament of liver coronary ligament of liver, triangular ligament of liver
Dorsal	Greater omentum (gastrorenal, gastrosplenic, gastrocolic, and splenorenal ligaments), mesentery of small intestine, mesoappendix, transverse mesocolon, sigmoid mesocolon

Table 7: Characterization of abdominal structures by location and support	
Characterization	**Organ**
Intraperitoneal (supported by mesentery)	Abdominal esophagus, stomach, first 2 cm of superior part of duodenum (duodenal cap), liver, gallbladder, pancreatic tail, spleen, jejunum, ileum, caecum (variable), appendix, transverse colon, sigmoid colon
Secondarily retroperitoneal (adherent)	Duodenum (except initial 2 cm), pancreas (except tail), caecum, ascending and descending colon, rectum (upper 2/3)
Extra/ retroperitoneal	Thoracic esophagus, rectum, kidneys, ureters, adrenals, abdominal aorta, Inferior vena cava

QUESTIONS

1. **Ventral mesogastrium derivatives include all EXCEPT:**
   (JIPMER 2001)
   a. Falciform ligament   b. Coronary ligament
   c. Lesser omentum   d. Gastrosplenic ligament

2. **Which of the following structure develop in ventral part of ventral mesentery of stomach?**
   a. Falciform ligament   b. Hepatogastric ligament
   c. Lesser omentum   d. Splenogastric ligament

1. **d. Gastrosplenic ligament**
   ❏ **Gastrosplenic** ligament develops in **dorsal mesogastrium**.

2. **a. Falciform ligament**
   ❏ Falciform ligament develops in the **ventral** part of the **ventral** mesentery and lesser omentum (hepatogastric ligament) in the dorsal part of ventral mesentery.

- Kidney **doesn't** develop in **mesentery** of stomach *(AIIMS 2010)*
  – It lies on the posterior abdominal wall and develops behind peritoneum (is **retroperitoneal**).
- **Ascending** colon has **no mesentery** *(NEET Pattern 2015)*
- **Gastrosplenic** ligament contains **short gastric** artery *(NEET Pattern 2015)*
- **Splenic artery** is carried by **splenorenal** ligament *(NEET Pattern 2014)*
- **Spleen** develops from cephalic part of **dorsal mesogastrium** *(NEET Pattern 2015)*
- During development spleen **lobulation** is related to **superior** border *(NEET Pattern 2015)*
- Greater omentum develops from **dorsal mesentery** *(NEET Pattern 2018)*

▶ Gut rotation

❏ Midgut forms a U-shaped loop (**midgut loop**) that herniates through the **primitive umbilical ring** into the extraembryonic coelom (i.e. physiological umbilical herniation) beginning at **week 6.**

❏ The midgut loop consists of a cranial limb and a caudal limb.

❏ The cranial limb forms the jejunum and upper part of the ileum.

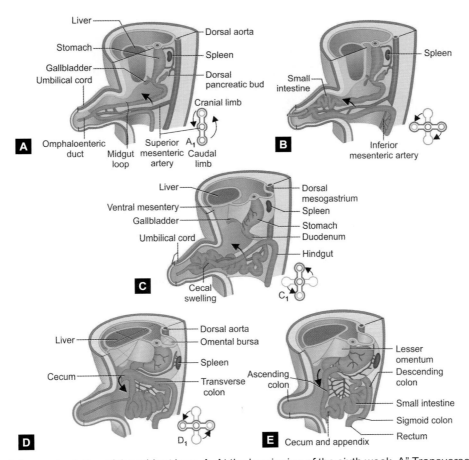

Figs. 52A to E: Herniation and rotation of the midgut loop. A, At the beg inning of the sixth week. A" Transverse section through the midgut loop, illustrating the initial relationship of the limbs of the midgut loop to the superior mesenteric artery. Note that the midgut loop is in the proximal part of the umbilical cord. B, Later stage showing the beginning of midgut rotation. B1, Illustration of the 90-degree counterclockwise rotation that carries the cranial limb of the midgut to the right. C. At approximately 10 weeks, showing the intestines returning to the abdomen. C_1, Illustration of a further rotation of 90 degrees. D, At approximately 11 weeks, showing the location of the viscera (internal organs) after contraction of intestines. D1, Illustrations of a further rotation of 90-degrees rotation of the viscera, for a total of 270 degrees. E, Later in the fetal period, showing the cecum rotating to its normal position in the lower right quadrant of the abdomen

❑ The caudal limb forms the **caecal diverticulum**, from which the cecum and appendix develop; the rest of the caudal limb forms the lower part of the ileum, ascending colon, and proximal 2/3 of the transverse colon.

❑ The midgut loop rotates a total of **270° anticlockwise** around the superior mesenteric artery as it returns to the abdominal cavity, thus reducing the physiological herniation, around week 10–11.

Omphalocele is a ventral body wall defect caused by failure of physiologically herniated loops of bowel to return to the body cavity in the 10-11th week.

❑ Omphalocele occurs when abdominal contents herniate through the umbilical ring and persist outside the body covered variably by a translucent peritoneal membrane sac (a light-gray, shiny sac) protruding from the base of the umbilical cord.

❑ Large omphaloceles may contain stomach, liver, and intestines.

❑ Omphaloceles are usually associated with multiple congenital anomalies like chromosomal defects, cardiovascular and neural tube defects.

Gastroschisis occurs when there is a defect in the ventral abdominal wall usually to the **right of the umbilical ring** through which there is a massive evisceration of intestines (other organs may also be involved).

❑ The intestines are **not covered by a peritoneal membrane**, are directly exposed to amniotic fluid, and are thickened and covered with adhesions.

❑ It is seen on the right side of the umbilicus (unlike omphalocele, which is a midline defect).

❑ Operative correction is possible, but volvulus remains a problem, due to presence of a long mesentery.

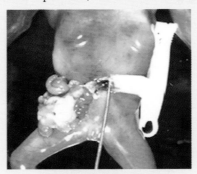
Fig. 53: Gastroschisis

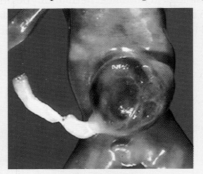
Fig. 54: Omphalocele

Rotation anomalies (**Malrotations**) are defects of gut rotation and commonly classifies as **three** variants:

▼ Rectum and Anal Canal

❑ The terminal end of the hindgut is an endoderm-lined pouch called the **cloaca**, which contacts the surface ectoderm of the proctodeum to form the **cloacal membrane**.

❑ **Cloaca** is partitioned by the **urorectal septum** into the rectum and upper anal canal and the urogenital sinus.

❑ The cloacal membrane is partitioned by the urorectal septum into anal membrane and urogenital membrane.

❑ The urorectal septum fuses with the cloacal membrane at the future site of the **perineal body**.

❑ The **upper anal canal** develops from the hindgut and the **lower anal canal** develops from the proctodeum, which is an invagination of surface ectoderm caused by a proliferation of mesoderm surrounding the anal membrane.

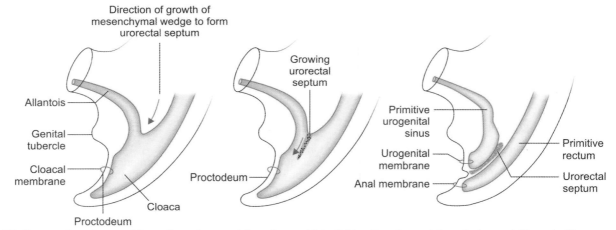
Fig. 55: Successive stages of formation of urorectal septum, which divides the cloaca into anterior part (the primitive urogenital sinus) and posterior part (the primitive rectum)

❑ The junction between the upper and lower anal canals is indicated by the **pectinate line**, which also marks the site of the former anal membrane.

❑ Pectinate line lies at the lower border of the anal columns.

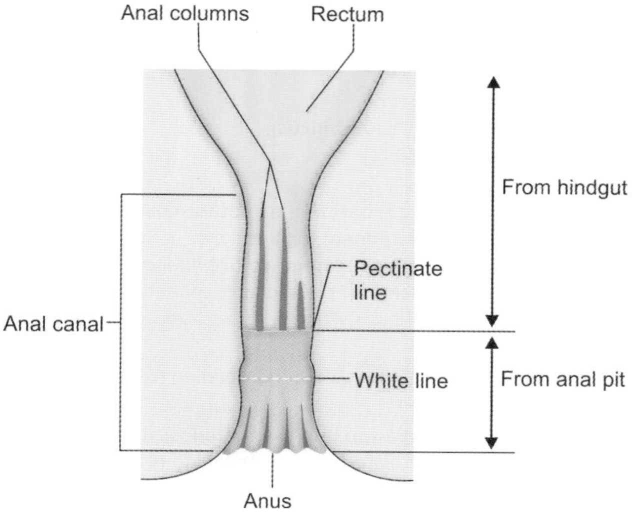

Fig. 56: The rectum and anal canal, showing their developmental origins. Note that the superior two-thirds of the anal canal are derived form the hindgut, whereas the inferior one-third of the anal canal is derived form the anal pit. Because of their different embryologic origins, the superior and inferior parts of the anal canal are supplied by different arteries and nerves and have different venous and lymphatic drainages

QUESTIONS

1. **Regarding Meckel's diverticulum all are true EXCEPT:**
   a. At anti-mesenteric border   *(AIIMS 2015)*
   b. Vitello-intestinal duct remnant
   c. 3" long
   d. Pain at umbilicus

2. **Remnant of omphalomesenteric duct is /are:**   *(PGIC 2013)*
   a. Umbilical fistula   b. Umbilical sinus
   c. Meckel's diverticulum   d. Median umbilical fold
   e. Omphalocele

3. **TRUE regarding Meckel's diverticulum is:**   *(JIPMER 2016)*
   a. Present in mesenteric border
   b. All 3 layers of gut wall are present
   c. Presents commonly with lower abdominal pain
   d. Second commonest congenial anomaly of GI tract

4. **Hirschsprung's disease is specifically known as:**   *(AIIMS)*
   a. Congenital megacolon
   b. Aganglionic megacolon
   c. Congenital aganglionic megacolon
   d. Congenital atretic aganglionic megacolon

5. **The caecum is found to be placed below the stomach and in midline. Which of the following abnormalities would have taken place in the rotation of gut?**   *(AIIMS Pattern 2010)*
   a. Malrotation   b. Non-rotation
   c. Mixed rotation   d. Reverse rotation

6. **An infant present with an omphalocele at birth. Which of the following applies to this condition?**
   a. It is also seen in patients with congenital aganglionic megacolon
   b. It results from herniation at the site of regression of the right umbilical vein
   c. It is caused by a failure of recanalization of the midgut part of the duodenum
   d. It is caused by failure of the midgut to return to the abdominal cavity after herniation into the umbilical stalk

7. **Regarding Gastroschisis and omphalocele, which one is FALSE?**
   a. Intestinal obstruction is common in gastroschisis
   b. Liver is the content of omphalocele
   c. Gastroschisis is associated with multiple anomalies
   d. Umbilical cord is attached in normal position in gastroschisis

8. **Rectum develops from:**   *(NEET Pattern 2012)*
   a. Cloaca   b. Hind gut
   c. Allantoic remnants d. Urogenital sinus

9. **TRUE about anal membrane:**   *(NEET Pattern 2013)*
   a. Perforates at 6 weeks
   b. Develops from anterior part of cloacal membrane
   c. Lies at proximal part of proctodaeum
   d. Covers urogenital sinus

10. **All develop from endodermal cloaca EXCEPT:**
    (NEET Pattern 2012)
    a. Rectum   b. Anal canal
    c. Sigmoid colon   d. Primitive urogenital sinus

11. **Endodermal cloaca gives rise to all of the following EXCEPT:**   *(NEET Pattern 2012)*
    a. Rectum   b. Lower 1/2 of anal canal
    c. Upper 1/2 of anal canal   d. Urinary bladder

ANSWERS

1. **c. 3" long**
   ❑ Meckel's diverticulum is usually mentioned to be **2 inches long**.
   ❑ Meckel's diverticulum is an outpouching (finger like pouch) of the ileum, derived from an unobliterated **vitelline duct** and located 2 feet proximal to the ileocecal junction on the **antimesenteric** side.
   ❑ Patient may present with discomfort (and pain) in epigastrium and **umbilical** region (**midgut pain**).

2. **a. Umbilical fistula; b. Umbilical sinus; c. Meckel's diverticulum**
   - ❑ **Omphalomesenteric** (vitello-intestinal) duct is an embryonic structure which connects the yolk sac to the midgut.
   - ❑ It gets obliterated between the 5th and 9th week of gestation, failure of which result in remnants like Meckel's **diverticulum/ cyst/fistula**.
   - ❑ Median umbilical fold is a **peritoneal fold** raised by allantoic remnant called **urachus**.
   - ❑ Omphalocele occurs due to **non-regression** of the physiological umbilical hernia.

3. **b. All 3 layers of gut wall are present**
   - ❑ Meckel's diverticulum is called a **true diverticulum**, since it has all the layers of gut tube.
   - ❑ It is located at the **antimesenteric** border and is a **midgut** derivative (pain around the **umbilicus**).
   - ❑ It is the **most common** congenital anomaly of gastrointestinal tract.

4. **c. Congenital aganglionic megacolon**
   - ❑ Hirschsprung disease occurs due to **non-migration** of neural crest cells into the **distal part** of the gut tube colon/rectum.
   - ❑ There is **absence** of myenteric (Auerbach's) **ganglia**, which is a parasympathetic component for faecal evacuation.
   - ❑ The **diseased** segment gets **narrowed** down and the normal proximal segment is **dilated (mega-colon)** due to faecal retention.
   - ❑ Rectal biopsy is **a-ganglionic**. The presenting complaint is chronic constipation and on per rectal examination, there occurs sudden gush of the retained faeces.

5. **c. Mixed rotation**
   - ❑ In mixed rotation the intestine **doesn't rotate as it re-enter**s the abdomen after physiological hernia leading to **caecum located just inferior to the pylorus** of the stomach in the midline.

6. **d. It is caused by failure of the midgut to return to the abdominal cavity after herniation into the umbilical stalk**
   - ❑ **Omphalocele** is a ventral body wall defect caused by **failure** of physiologically herniated loops of bowel to **return** to the body cavity in the 10th week.
   - ❑ Congenital aganglionic megacolon is **Hirschsprung** disease.
   - ❑ **Gastroschisis** is a ventral **body wall defect** resulting from a lack of closure of the lateral body wall folds in the abdominal region resulting in protrusion of intestines and sometimes other organs through the defect. It results from herniation **at the site of regression of the right umbilical vein**.
   - ❑ Failure of **recanalization** of the midgut part of the duodenum leads to **duodenal atresia**.

7. **c. Gastroschisis is associated with multiple anomalies**
   - ❑ It is omphalocele (**not gastroschisis**) which is associated with multiple anomalies.

8. **a. Cloaca > b. Hindgut**
   - ❑ Rectum develops from the **distal** part of the **hind** gut - the **cloaca**.

9. **c. Lies at proximal part of proctodaeum**
   - ❑ Distal end of cloaca is covered by **cloacal membrane** which has two parts.
   - ❑ Urogenital membrane is the ventral (**anterior**) part of cloacal membrane and covers primitive urogenital sinus.
   - ❑ **Anal membrane** is the dorsal (**posterior**) part of cloacal membrane and covers primitive rectum.
   - ❑ Anal membrane lies between these two and line of junction of these two parts is represented in later life by anal valves (**pectinate line**).
   - ❑ Anal membrane **perforates at 9th week** to let open the gut tube to the exterior at proctodaeum.

10. **c. Sigmoid**
    - ❑ **Sigmoid** colon develops from the **hind gut**.

11. **b. Lower 1/2 of anal canal**
    - ❑ **Lower** part of anal canal below the pectinate line develops from **ectodermal** invagination i.e., **proctodeum**
    - ❑ Physiological hernia reduces at **3rd month**.
      - ◼ At **week 6,** the gut tube connected to the yolk sac herniates into the region of umbilical cord and returns back at **week 10-11** (3rd month).

- ▪ Meckel's diverticulum is a remnant of **vitellointestinal** duct (*AIIMS 2005; NEET Pattern 2013*)
- ▪ **Mesenteric cyst** is NOT an anomaly of **vitello-intestinal** duct.
- ▪ **Proximal** half of duodenum is derived from **foregut** and distal half from the midgut (*NEET Pattern 2013*)
- ▪ **Descending** colon is supplied by **Inferior** mesenteric artery (*JIPMER 2016*)
- ▪ **Vermiform appendix** is a derivative of **midgut** (*NEET Pattern 2015*)
- ▪ **Primitive gut** develops from the endoderm of **yolk sac** (*NEET Pattern 2014*)
- ▪ Inferior mesenteric artery supplies the derivatives of the hind gut (*NEET Pattern 2013*)

▶ Liver and Hepatobiliary Tree

- ❑ The **endodermal** lining of the foregut forms an outgrowth (called the **hepatic diverticulum**) into the surrounding mesoderm of the septum transversum.
- ❑ Cords of **hepatoblasts** (called hepatic cords) from the hepatic diverticulum grow into the **mesoderm of the septum transversum**.
- ❑ The hepatic cords arrange themselves around the vitelline veins and umbilical veins, which course through the septum transversum and form the hepatic sinusoids.

Table 8: Source of development of various components of the liver	
Embryonic structure	**Adult derivatives**
▪ Hepatic bud	Liver parenchyma
	Bile canaliculi and bile ductules
▪ Vitelline and umbilical veins within septum transversum	Liver sinusoids
▪ Septum transversum (mesodermal in origin)	▪ Connective tissue stroma of the liver including Glisson's capsule (fibrous capsule of the liver)
	▪ Peritoneal coverings of liver
	▪ Kupffer cells
	▪ Hemopoietic cells
	▪ Blood vessels of liver

▶ Pancreas

❑ Pancreas develops from the two pancreatic buds. The ventral pancreatic bud and dorsal pancreatic bud are direct outgrowths of foregut endoderm.

❑ Within both pancreatic buds, endodermal tubules surrounded by mesoderm branch repeatedly to form acinar cells and ducts (i.e., exocrine pancreas).

❑ Isolated clumps of endodermal cells bud from the tubules and accumulate within the mesoderm to form islet cells (i.e., endocrine pancreas).

❑ Due to the 90° clockwise rotation of the duodenum, the ventral bud rotates dorsally and fuses with the dorsal bud to form the definitive adult pancreas.

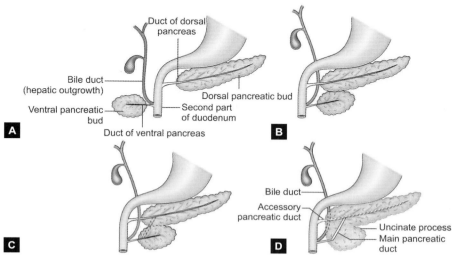

Figs. 57A to D: Schematic diagrams showing stages (A, B, C, and D) of formation of the adult pancreas and its ducts (main and accessory) by the fusion of the dorsal and ventral pancreatic buds

❑ The ventral bud forms the **uncinate** process and a portion of the head of the pancreas.

❑ The dorsal bud forms the remaining portion of the head, body, and tail of the pancreas.

❑ The **main pancreatic duct** is formed by the anastomosis of the distal two-thirds of the dorsal pancreatic duct (the proximal one-third regresses) and the entire ventral pancreatic duct.

❑ The proximal portion of the dorsal pancreatic bud gives rise to the **accessory pancreatic duct**

❑ **Pancreatic divisum** is the most common anomaly of pancreatic develop documented clinically (3–10%).
  ➢ The ducts of the pancreas are not fused to form a full pancreas, but instead it remains as a distinct dorsal and ventral duct.
  ➢ Without the proper fusion of both ducts the majority of the pancreas drainage is mainly through the accessory papilla.

❑ Pancreas develops from a ventral bud and a dorsal bud that later fuse to form the definitive pancreas. Sometimes, the two parts surround the duodenum **(annular pancreas)**, causing constriction of the gut.

1. **TRUE statement regarding development of pancreas:**
   a. Uncinate process from ventral bud   *(PGIC 2015)*
   b. Lower part of head from dorsal bud
   c. Body is formed from dorsal bud
   d. Duct of Wirsung develop from dorsal bud only
   e. Pancreatic divisum is due to abnormal development of duct of pancreas

2. **Pancreas divisum indicates which of the following:**
   (NEET Pattern 2012)
   a. Duplication of the pancreas
   b. Failure of fusion of dorsal and ventral pancreatic buds
   c. Formation of more than two pancreatic buds
   d. Formation of only one pancreatic bud

3. **FALSE about gastrointestinal development is:**
   (PGIC 2015)
   a. Lower respiratory system develops from foregut
   b. Stomach rotates 90° clock wise and its posterior wall grows faster
   c. Duodenum rotates to right and is retroperitoneal
   d. Dorsal bud form uncinate process
   e. Dorsal duct forms Santorini duct

1. **a. Uncinate process from ventral bud; c. Body is formed from dorsal bud; e. Pancreatic divisum is due to abnormal development of duct of pancreas**
   - ❑ Pancreas develops from the two **pancreatic buds**, which are direct outgrowths of foregut endoderm.
   - ❑ Ventral bud rotates dorsally and fuses with the dorsal bud to form the definitive adult pancreas.
   - ❑ Ventral (**not dorsal**) bud forms **lower part of head** of the pancreas & the **uncinate** process.
   - ❑ The **dorsal** bud forms the remaining portion of the head, **body**, and tail of the pancreas.
   - ❑ The main pancreatic duct (of **Wirsung**) is formed by the anastomosis of the **distal** two-thirds of the **dorsal** pancreatic duct and the entire ventral pancreatic duct.
   - ❑ In pancreatic **divisum** the ducts of the pancreas are **not fused** to form a full pancreas, but instead it remains as a distinct dorsal and ventral duct.

2. **b. Failure of fusion of dorsal and ventral pancreatic buds**
   - ❑ In Pancreatic divisum the ducts of the pancreas are **not fused** to form a full pancreas, but instead it remains as a distinct dorsal and ventral duct.

3. **d. Dorsal bud form uncinate process**
   - ❑ Foregut is subdivided into two parts: Prelaryngeal or cephalic part (pharyngeal gut)- which gives rise to floor of mouth, pharynx and lower respiratory tract.
   - ❑ Post-laryngeal (caudal part) gives rise to esophagus, stomach, proximal part of duodenum (up to opening of hepatopancreatic ampulla), liver and extrahepatic biliary system, and pancreas.
   - ❑ **Stomach** rotates by 90 degrees **clockwise** around its longitudinal axis and original **posterior** wall grows **faster** than anterior forming greater and lesser curvatures, respectively.
   - ❑ Duodenum grows rapidly forming a C- shaped loop that projects ventrally, rotates to the right and becomes retroperitoneal.
   - ❑ **Uncinate** process is formed by **ventral** pancreatic bud.
   - ❑ Proximal part of duct of **dorsal** bud forms accessory pancreatic duct (Duct of **Santorini**).
   - ❑ Liver **parenchyma** of the liver is derived from **endodermal** hepatic bud of **foregut**.
   - ❑ Liver **sinusoids** of liver develop from absorbed and broken **vitelline** and **umbilical** veins within the septum transversum.
   - ❑ **Fibrous stroma** of liver is derived from **septum transversum** (NEET Pattern 2016)
   - ❑ Most common site of ectopic pancreatic tissue is **Stomach** (AIIMS 2007)
     - ■ It is most frequently seen in the stomach, Meckel's diverticulum, duodenum & jejunum and rarely it may be seen in the wall of spleen
   - ❑ **Ventral** pancreatic duct give rise to **uncinate** process (NEET Pattern 2015)
   - ❑ **Most common** congenital anomaly of the pancreas is **Pancreas divisum** (NEET Pattern 2012)
   - ❑ If two buds of pancreas **do not fuse**, the anomaly is **Pancreatic divisum** (NEET Pattern 2012)

▼ Renal System

Major portion of genitourinary system develops from **intermediate mesoderm**. **Endoderm** of the hind gut contributes to the **terminal portion** of the tubes.

- ❑ **Intermediate mesoderm** forms a longitudinal elevation along the dorsal body wall called the **urogenital ridge**.
- ❑ A portion of the urogenital ridge forms the **nephrogenic cord**, which gives rise to the urinary system.
- ❑ The nephrogenic cord develops into three sets of nephric structures (from cranial to caudal segments): the pronephros, mesonephros, and the metanephros.
- ❑ **Pronephros**
  - ➤ Develops by the differentiation of mesoderm within the nephrogenic cord to form pronephric tubules and the pronephric duct.
  - ➤ It is the cranial-most nephric structure, develops in cervical region and is a transitory structure that regresses completely by week
- ❑ **Mesonephros**
  - ➤ Develops by the differentiation of mesoderm within the nephrogenic cord to form mesonephric tubules and the mesonephric duct (Wolffian duct).
  - ➤ It is the middle nephric structure, develops in thoracic and lumbar region and is a partially transitory structure.
  - ➤ Most of the mesonephric tubules regress, but the mesonephric/Wolffian duct persists and opens into the urogenital sinus.
  - ➤ Ducts and tubules from the mesonephros form the conduit for sperm from the testes to the urethra. Wolffian duct in females is mostly vestigial.
- ❑ **Metanephros**
  - ➤ Develops from an outgrowth of the mesonephric duct (called the ureteric bud) and from a condensation of mesoderm within the nephrogenic cord called the metanephric mesoderm.
  - ➤ It is the caudal-most nephric structure.
  - ➤ It begins to form at week 5 and is functional in the fetus at about week 10.
  - ➤ The fetal kidney is divided into lobes, in contrast to the definitive adult kidney, which has a smooth contour.

The **metanephros** forms the permanent kidney, having two portions: excretory & collecting system.

❑ Excretory system is constituted by the nephrons, collecting system originates from the ureteric bud, an outgrowth of the mesonephric duct.

❑ Ureteric bud gives rise to the ureter, renal pelvis, major & minor calyces, and the entire collecting system.

❑ Connection between the collecting and excretory tubule systems is essential for normal development.

Early division of the ureteric bud may lead to bifid or supernumerary kidneys with ectopic ureters.

Kidneys develop in the pelvic region and later ascend into the abdomen (lumbar area), abnormal ascent of the kidney, may result in anomalies like horseshoe kidney.

Urinary bladder develops from cloaca, which is a common collecting region for the primitive kidneys and gut system. Urorectal septum in cloaca region subdivides it into the urogenital sinus (anteriorly) and the rectum/anal canal (posteriorly).

Urogenital sinus gives us several derivatives like urinary bladder, **urethra** in the female and male (prostatic & membranous portions).

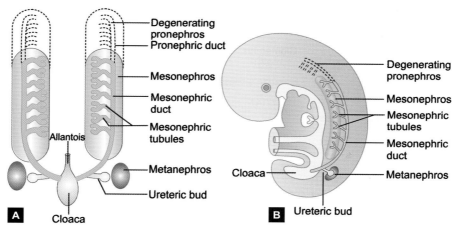

Figs. 58A and B: Formation of three successive kidneys in embryo. A. Ventral view. B. Lateral view.

Ascent of the Kidneys

Fetal metanephros is located at vertebral levels S1-S2, whereas the definitive adult kidney is located at vertebral level T12-L3.

❑ The change in location results from a disproportionate growth of the embryo caudal to the metanephros.

❑ During the relative ascent, the kidneys rotate 90°, causing the hilum, which initially faces ventrally, to finally face medially.

❑ Vascular buds from the kidneys grow toward and invade the common iliac arteries, while in pelvis.

❑ Growth of the embryo in length causes the kidneys to 'ascend' to their final position in the lumbar region.

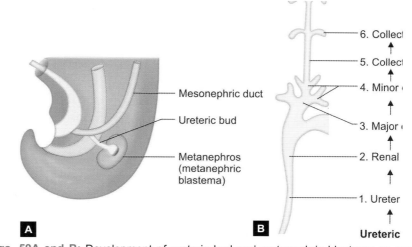

Figs. 59A and B: Development of ureteric bud and metanephric blastema as seen in lateral view of embryo. Figure in the insert shows structures derived from the ureteric bud.

❑ Rather than 'drag' their blood supply with them as they ascend, the kidneys send out new and slightly more cranial branches and then induce the regression of the more caudal branches.

❑ Eventually the renal arteries are branches of the abdominal aorta.

❑ Arteries formed during the ascent may persist and are called supernumerary arteries. Supernumerary arteries are end arteries. Therefore, any damage to them will result in necrosis of kidney parenchyma.

Development of Collecting System

❑ **Ureteric bud** is an outgrowth of the mesonephric duct.

❑ It initially penetrates the metanephric mesoderm and then undergoes repeated branching to form the ureters, renal pelvis, major calyces, minor calyces, and collecting ducts.

Development of Nephron

The inductive influence of the collecting ducts causes the metanephric mesoderm to differentiate into metanephric vesicles, which later give rise to primitive S-shaped renal tubules that are critical to nephron formation.

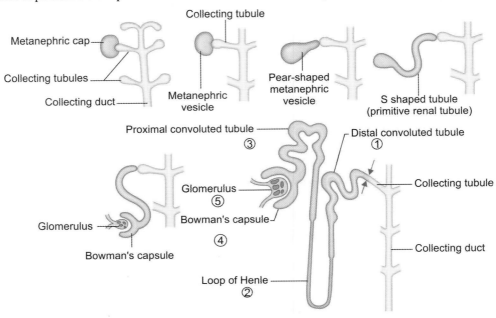

Fig. 60: Stages of development of nephron (excretory system of the kidney consisting of 3 million nephrons). Note each nephron consists of distal convoluted tubule (1), loop of Henle (2), proximal convoluted tubule (3), Bowman's capsule (4), and glomerulus (5). Arrows (red) indicate the place where excretory unit (blue) establishes a communication with the collecting system (yellow).

- ❏ The renal tubules differentiate into the connecting tubule, the distal convoluted tubule, the loop of Henle, the proximal convoluted tubule, and the Bowman's capsule.
- ❏ Tufts of capillaries called glomeruli protrude into Bowman's capsule.
- ❏ Nephron formation is complete at birth, but functional maturation of nephrons continues throughout infancy.

Development of excretory and collecting parts of kidney

Embryo	Adult Derivative
Metanephric mesoderm Metanephric vesicles S-shaped renal tubules	Connecting tubule Distal convoluted tubule Loop of Henle Proximal convoluted tubule Renal (Bowman's) capsule Renal glomerulus
Ureteric bud	Ureter Renal pelvis Major calyx Minor calyx Collecting duct

▶ Urinary bladder and urethra

Urinary bladder is formed from the upper portion of the urogenital sinus, which is continuous with the allantois.

- ❏ The **allantois** becomes a fibrous cord called the urachus (or median umbilical ligament) in the adult.
- ❏ The lower ends of the mesonephric ducts become incorporated into the posterior wall of the bladder to form the **trigone** of the bladder.

    Allantois is an **endodermal** diverticulum that extends from the ventral region of the urogenital sinus to the umbilicus.

- ❏ Later, its distal portion, called the **urachus**, becomes a fibrous cord and forms the **median umbilical ligament**.
- ❏ If it remains patent, then it may form a **urachal fistula** or **cyst** in this region.

Flowchart 2: Subdivision of cloaca

```
                    Cloaca
                      |  Urorectal septum
         ┌────────────┴────────────┐
   Primitive                   Primitive
 urogenital sinus               rectum
         │                         │
   ┌─────┴──────┐            ┌──────┴──────┐
Vesicourethral              Definitive
    canal                 urogenital sinus
   ┌──┴───┐                 ┌──────┴──────┐
Urinary  Primitive      Pelvic part   Phallic part
bladder  urethra
```

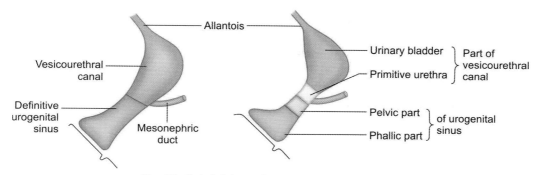

Fig. 61: Subdivisions of primitive urogenital sinus

Table 9: Development of the urinary blader	
Embryonic structure	Adult derivatives
Cranial dilated part of vesicourethral canal	Endodermal epithelial lining of the whole urinary bladder except in the region of trigone
Absorption of mesonephric ducts in the dorsal wall of the vesicourethral canal	Mesodermal epithelial lining in the region of trigone of urinary bladder
Splanchnopleuric intraembryonic mesoderm surrounding vesicourethral canal	Muscular and serous coats of the urinary bladder
Allantois	Urachus (median umbilical ligament) and apex of urinary bladder

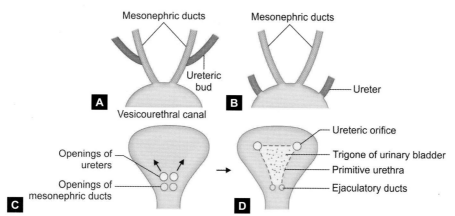

Figs. 62A to D: Formation of trigone of the urinary bladder. A. Opening of mesonephric ducts into the vesicourethral canal. B. Absorption of mesonephric ducts into the vesicourethral canal. C. At first, openings of ureters and mesonephric ducts are close together. D. Further absorption of ureters causes ureteric openings to shift laterally and upward.

In both sexes, the mesonephric (or Wolffian) duct gives origin on each side to the ureteric bud, which forms the ureter, the pelvis of the ureter, the major and minor calyces and the collecting tubules of the kidney. Its inferior end is absorbed into the developing bladder and forms the trigone and pat of the urethra.

The terminal portion of mesonephric duct gets absorbed into the posterior wall of urinary bladder to form the trigone (mesodermal).

Note: Proximal part of mesonephric duct (**Wolffian duct**) form the conduit for sperm from the testes to the urethra and give rise to **epididymis, ductus deferens, seminal vesicle, common ejaculatory duct**. In the female, these ducts regress.

❑ **Renal agenesis** occurs when the ureteric bud fails to develop, thereby eliminating the induction of metanephric vesicles and nephron formation.
❑ **Congenital polycystic kidney:** Luminal continuity between the nephrons and collecting tubules has failed to establish.
  ➢ The glomeruli continue to excrete urine which accumulates in the tubules due to lack of outlet.
  ➢ As a result tubules undergo cystic enlargements (retention cysts).
❑ **Pelvic kidney** is an ectopic kidney that occurs when kidneys fail to ascend and thus remain in the pelvis.
  ➢ Two pelvic kidneys may fuse to form a solid lobed organ called a cake (rosette) kidney.
❑ **Horseshoe kidney** develops as a result of fusion of the lower poles of two kidneys.
  ➢ The ureters pass anterior to the isthmus and may get obstructed due to impingement.

➤ The **inferior mesenteric artery** also passes anterior to the isthmus and the horseshoe kidney gets trapped behind the **inferior mesenteric artery** as it attempts to ascend toward the normal adult location

❑ **Bladder exstrophy** is a ventral body wall defect caused by lack of closure of the lateral body wall folds in the pelvic region resulting in protrusion of the bladder through the defect.

❑ **Urachal fistula or cyst** occurs when a remnant of the allantois persists, thereby forming fistula or cyst.

❑ It is found along the midline on a path from the umbilicus to the apex of the urinary bladder.

❑ A urachal fistula forms a direct connection between the urinary bladder and the outside of the body at the umbilicus, causing urine drainage from the umbilicus.

Urethra	Embryonic source of development
Female urethra	▪ Caudal part of vesicourethral canal ▪ Pelvic part of definitive urogenital sinus

Male urethra
1. Prostatic part
  a. Above the level of opening of ejaculatory ducts (colliculus seminalis)
  b. Below the level of openings of ejaculatory ducts
2. Membranous part
3. Penile part
4. Terminal part (which occupies the glans penis)
	▪ Caudal part of vesicourethral canal
	▪ Pelvic part of definitive urogenital sinus
	▪ Pelvic part of definitive urogenital sinus
	▪ Phallic part of definitive urogenital sinus
	▪ Surface ectoderm

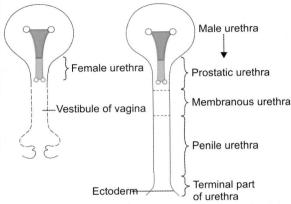

Figs. 63A and B: Development of urethra. A. Female urethra. B. Male urethra

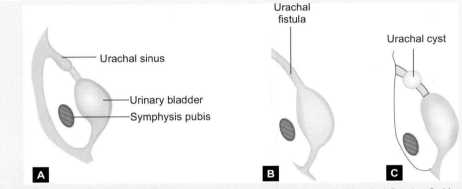

Figs. 64A to C: Congenital anomalies of urachus. A. Urachal sinus. B. Urachul fistula. C. Urachal cyst

Questions

1. WRONG statement regarding kidney development is: *(NEET Pattern 2015)*
   a. Glomerulus develops from metanephros
   b. Ureter develops from metanephric diverticulum
   c. Connecting tubule is a derivative of ureteric bud
   d. Terminal portion of mesonephric duct forms trigone

2. Initially renal arteries are branches of: *(NEET Pattern 2015)*
   a. Internal pudendal artery   b. External iliac artery
   c. Common iliac artery   d. Aorta

3. A child complains of fluid coming out of umbilicus on straining. The diagnosis is:
   a. Patent vitellointestinal duct   b. Gastroschisis
   c. Umbilical hernia   d. Urachal fistula

4. Kidney develops from: *(NEET Pattern 2015)*
   a. Metanephros   b. Mesonephros
   c. Blastema   d. All of the above

5. Epithelium of ureter develops from: *(AIIMS 2007)*
   a. Mesonephros
   b. Metanephros
   c. Pronephros
   d. Paramesonephric duct

6. Trigone of urinary bladder develops from: *(NEET Pattern 2015)*
   a. Urogenital sinus   b. Vesicourethral canal
   c. Mesonephric duct   d. Endoderm

Answers

1. c. Connecting tubule is a derivative of ureteric bud
   ❑ **Connecting tubule** is a part of nephron and develops from **metanephric blastema**.
   Note: Ureter develops from ureteric bud, which is also called as **metanephric diverticulum** by some authors.

ANSWERS

2. c. Common iliac artery
- ❑ Kidney start developing in the **pelvic** region and are supplied by branches of **common iliac** arteries.
- ❑ Subsequently as kidneys begin to ascend into the abdomen they receive their blood supply from the **distal end of the aorta**.
- ❑ Eventually they receive their most cranial arterial branches, which become the **renal arteries**, from the abdominal aorta.
- ❑ Normally, the caudal primordial branches undergo involution and disappear.

3. d. Urachal fistula
- ❑ Non-obliteration of allantois (hindgut diverticulum) may result in patent allantoic (**urachal**) **fistula**, which leads to leakage of urine from the urinary bladder towards the umbilicus, especially on straining.

4. d. All of the above
- ❑ Kidney has two parts: The **excretory** system (true kidney) develops from the **metanephric blastema**.
- ❑ The **collecting** system develops from **Mesonephric duct (**ureteric bud).
- ❑ Ureteric bud **penetrates** metanephros to convert it into metanephric blastema, which later develops into true kidney.

5. a. Mesonephros
- ❑ Epithelium of ureter develops from the **mesonephric** duct, as the ureteric bud.

6. c. Mesonephric duct
- ❑ The **terminal** portion of mesonephric duct (mesodermal) gets absorbed into the posterior wall of urogenital sinus and forms the **trigone** of urinary bladder.
- ❑ Urinary bladder (except trigone) develops from **endodermal** vesicourethral canal (cranial part of urogenital sinus).

- ▪ Ureter develops **from mesonephric duct** (AIIMS 2007; NEET Pattern 2018)
- ▪ **Most common** aberration in renal vessel development is **supernumerary arteries** (AIPG 2010)
- ▪ Urinary bladder, liver, pancreas are **endodermal** derivatives, but kidney is **mesodermal** (JIPMER 2006)
- ▪ Urinary bladder develops from **endoderm** (NEET Pattern 2012)
  - – It develops from the **cranial** vesicourethral canal, which is continuous above with the **allantoic** duct.
- ▪ **Ureteric bud** arises from Mesonephric duct (NEET Pattern 2013)
  - – Hence called **mesonephric diverticulum**.
  - – As it stimulates metanephros, it is also known as the **metanephrogenic diverticulum.**
- ▪ Ascending kidney receives its blood supply sequentially from arteries in its immediate neighbourhood, i.e. the **middle sacral** and **common iliac** arteries.
- ▪ Epithelium of urinary **bladder**, **urethra** and **vagina** develop from **endoderm of urogenital sinus**.
- ▪ **Ascent** of horseshoe-shaped kidney is prevented by **Inferior mesenteric** artery (NEET Pattern 2016)
- ▪ **Collecting tubules** of kidney develop from **Ureteric duct**/bud (NEET Pattern 2013)
- ▪ Proximal convoluted tubules develop from **Metanephric tubules.**
- ▪ Uro-rectal septum separates the **cloaca** into rectum and urogenital sinus.
- ▪ **Urachus** fistula is patent **allantois** (PGIC 2004)

◤ Genital system

- ❑ Genital system consists of (a) gonads or primitive sex glands, (b) genital ducts, and (c) external genitalia.
- ❑ The sex of the individual is not established till week 7 **(indeterminate embryo)**.
- ❑ Indeterminate embryo
  - ➢ The genotype of the embryo (46,XX or 46,XY) is established at fertilization.
  - ➢ During week 1–6, the embryo remains in a sexually indifferent or **undifferentiated stage**. The genetically female and male embryos are **phenotypically indistinguishable**.
  - ➢ During week 7, the indifferent embryo begins phenotypic sexual differentiation.
  - ➢ By **week 12**, female or male characteristics of the external genitalia can be recognized.
  - ➢ By week 20, phenotypic differentiation is complete.
  - ➢ Phenotypic sexual differentiation is determined by the **SRY gene** located on the short arm of the **Y chromosome** and may result in individuals with a female phenotype, an intersex phenotype, or a male phenotype. The SRY gene encodes for a protein called testes-determining factor (TDF).
- ❑ The SRY gene on the Y chromosome produces **testes determining factor** (TDF) and regulates male sexual development.
  - ➢ **Sertoli** and **Leydig** cells start developing in the testes.
  - ➢ Expression of the SRY gene causes (a) development of the medullary (testis) cords, (2) formation of the tunica albuginea, and (c) failure of the cortical (ovarian) cords to develop.
- ❑ Ovarian development occurs in the absence of the SRY gene and in the presence of **WNT4**, the master gene for this differentiation process.
  - ➢ It leads to formation of ovaries with (1) typical cortical cords, (2) disappearance of the medullary (testis) cords, and (3) failure of the tunica albuginea to develop.
- ❑ **Primordial germ cells** originate in the epiblast cells (primitive streak), migrate to the endodermal wall of yolk sac and thence to the genital ridge (during the 4th to 6th weeks).

- ❑ During the indifferent stage, there are two duct systems: the mesonephric duct and paramesonephric duct.
- ❑ **Testosterone**, produced by Leydig cells in the testes, stimulates development of the mesonephric ducts to form the efferent ducts, epididymis, vas deferens, seminal vesicle and ejaculatory duct.
- ❑ **Müllerian inhibiting** substance (Anti Mullerian hormone), produced by Sertoli cells in the testes, causes regression of the paramesonephric (Mullerian) ducts.
- ❑ Dihydrotestosterone stimulates development of the external genitalia, including the penis and scrotum.
- ❑ Estrogens (together with the absence of testosterone) regulate development of the paramesonephric ducts, which leads to genesis of the uterus, uterine tube and upper 1/3 of the vagina.
- ❑ Estrogens also stimulate differentiation of the external genitalia, including the clitoris, labia, and lower portion of the vagina.

Table 10: Embryonic structures and their homologous adult derivatives in male and female		
	Adult derivatives	
Embryonic structure	**In male**	**In female**
1. Indifferent gonad	Testis	Ovary
a. Primordial germ cells	Spermatogonia	Oogonia
b. Surface epithelium of gonad	Sertoli cells/supporting cells	Follicular cells
c. Mesenchyme	Leydig cells (interstitial cells)	Theca cells (forming theca interna and externa)
2. Gubernaculum	Gubernaculum testis	a. Round ligament of ovary b. Round ligament of uterus

3. Mesonephric tubules
  a. Cranial tubules
  b. Caudal tubules
	
	Efferent ductules
	Paradidymis
		
		Epoophoron
		Paroophoron

4. Mesonephric duct	Duct of epididymis Vas deferens Seminal vesicle Ejaculatory duct	Gartner's duct
5. Paramesonephric duct	Appendix of testis Prostatic utricle	Uterine tubes Uterus Cervix Upper part of vagina
6. Urogenital sinus	Urinary bladder Urethra (prostatic membranous and penile) Prostate gland Bulbourethral glands	Urinary bladder Urethra (membranous) and vestibule of vagina Paraurethral glands (of Skene) Greater vestibular glands
7. Mullerian tubercle	Seminal colliculus (verumontanum)	Hymen
8. Genital tubercle	Penis	Clitoris
9. Urethral folds	Penile urethra	Labia minora
10. Genital swellings	Scrotum	Labia majora

The **urogenital sinus** is considered in three parts: (1) the cephalad or vesicle portion, which will form the urinary bladder; (2) the middle or pelvic portion, which creates the female urethra; and (3) the caudal or phallic part, which will give rise to the distal vagina and to the greater vestibular (Bartholin) and paraurethral (Skene) glands.

Gubernaculum is the embryonic structures which begin as undifferentiated mesenchyme attaching to the caudal end of the gonads (testes and ovaries).

- ❑ As the **scrotum** and **labia majora** form in males and females, respectively, the gubernaculum aids in the descent of the gonads (both testes and ovaries).
- ❑ The testes descend to a greater degree than the ovaries and ultimately pass through the inguinal canal.

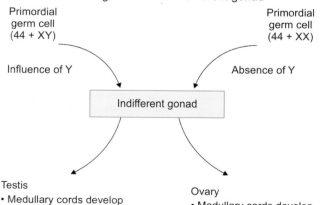

Flowchart 3: Influence of chromosome complement of primordial germ cells on indifferent gonad

Primordial germ cell (44 + XY) → Influence of Y → Indifferent gonad → Testis
- Medullary cords develop and persist
- No cortical cords
- Tunica albuginea develops

Primordial germ cell (44 + XX) → Absence of Y → Indifferent gonad → Ovary
- Medullary cords develop and degenerate
- Cortical cords develop
- Tunica albuginea does not develop

Table 11: Differences in development of testis and ovary	
Testis	**Ovary**
▪ Formation of only one generation of sex cords (medullary cords) that produce seminiferous tubules and rete testis	Formation of two generations of sex cords: a. First generation of sex cords (medullary cords) form stroma of ovarian medulla b. Second generation of sex cords (cortical cords) form primordial follicles (ovarian follicles)
▪ Formation of tunica albuginea separating seminiferous tubules from surface epithelium	▪ No formation of tunica albuginea. Hence ovarian follicles are not separated from surface epithelium

Flowchart 4: Influence of gonads on further sex differentiation

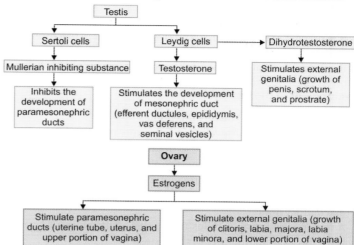

- In males the upper part of the gubernaculum degenerates and lower part persists as the gubernaculum testis (scrotal ligament), which secures the testis to the most inferior portion of the scrotum, tethering it in place and limiting the degree to which the testis can move within the scrotum.
- In females the gubernaculum has two vestigial remnants in females, the ovarian ligament and the round ligament of the uterus (ligamentum teres uteri) which respectively serve to support the ovaries and uterus in the pelvis.

Male Reproductive System

Testis

Intermediate mesoderm forms a longitudinal elevation along the dorsal body wall called the **urogenital ridge**, which later forms the **gonadal ridge**.

- Primary sex cords develop from the gonadal ridge and incorporate primordial germ cells (XY genotype), which migrate into the gonad from the wall of the yolk sac.
- The primary sex cords extend into the medulla of the gonad and lose their connection with the surface epithelium as the thick tunica albuginea forms.
- The primary sex cords form the seminiferous cords, tubuli recti, and rete testes.
- Seminiferous cords consist of primordial germ cells and sustentacular (Sertoli) cells, which secrete MIF.
- Mesoderm between the seminiferous cords gives rise to the interstitial (Leydig) cells, which secrete testosterone.
- Seminiferous cords remain as solid cords until puberty, when they acquire a lumen and are then called seminiferous tubules.

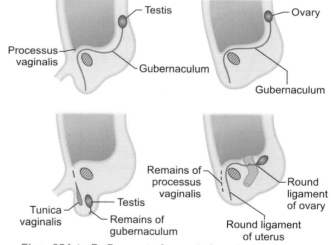

Figs. 65A to D: Descent of gonads from the abdomen region, pulled by gubernaculum

Descent of Testis

Testis starts developing in the **abdomen** (lumbar region) and later descends down to the **pelvis** and reach the **scrotum** eventually, as a result of disproportionate growth of the upper abdominal region away from the pelvic region.

- Gubernaculum pulls the caudal pole of testis to the scrotum and eventually anchor the testes within the scrotum.

Position of testis	Month (week) of Intrauterine life
Abdomen	2nd month (7th week)
Pelvis (Iliac fossa)	During 3rd month (12th week)
Deep inguinal ring	At the end of 6th month (24th week)
Pass inguinal canal	During 7th month (25–28 week)
At superficial inguinal ring	Eight month (29–32 week)
Enters scrotum	Beginning of ninth month (33 week)
At the base of scrotum	Before birth (End of 9th month/36th week)

- ❏ The peritoneum enaginates alongside the gubernaculum to form the **processus vaginalis**. Later in development, most of the processus vaginalis is obliterated except at its distal end, which remains as a peritoneal sac called the tunica vaginalis of the testes.
- ❏ Testis is present in the abdomen at **2nd month** (7th week), descends down to pelvis (iliac fossa) during **third month.**
- ❏ It is present at the deep inguinal ring at the **end of 6th month**, and starts passing through inguinal canal at **7th month**.
- ❏ It lies at superficial ring at **eighth month** and enters the scrotum at the **beginning of ninth month**.
- ❏ It reaches its final position in the scrotum just before birth (**end of ninth month**) and after birth (in few babies).

Development of the Genital Ducts

Mesonephric (Wolffian) ducts and tubules

- ❏ Mesonephric ducts develop in the male as part of the urinary system because these ducts are critical in the formation of the definitive metanephric kidney.
- ❏ Mesonephric ducts then proceed to additionally form the epididymis, ductus deferens, seminal vesicle, and ejaculatory duct.
- ❏ A few mesonephric tubules in the region of the testes form the efferent ductules of the testes.
- ❏ Vestigial remnants of the mesonephric duct (appendix epididymis) and mesonephric tubules (paradidymis) may be found in the adult male.

Paramesonephric (Mullerian ducts)

- ❏ Under the influence of MIF, the cranial portions of the paramesonephric ducts and the uterovaginal primordium regress.
- ❏ Vestigial remnants of the paramesonephric duct (called the appendix testis) is present in the adult male.

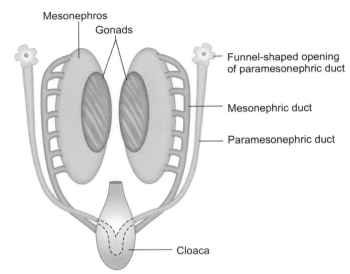

Fig. 66: Two pairs of genital ducts during the indifferent stage of development of gonads.

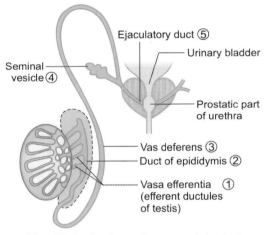

Fig. 67: Derivatives of mesonephric duct

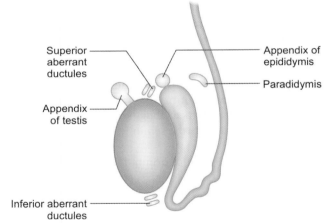

Fig. 68: Vestigeal remnants of mesonephric and paramesonephric ducts in males

1. **Testis lies at deep inguinal ring up to:**   *(NEET Pattern 2013)*
   - a. 4 months
   - b. 5 months
   - c. 7 months
   - d. 9 months

2. **Position of testis at 24–28 weeks of intrauterine life:**
   (NEET Pattern 2015)
   - a. Inguinal region
   - b. Lumbar region
   - c. Superficial inguinal ring
   - d. Deep inguinal ring

3. **Testes completely descend in the scrotum by the age of:**
   - a. End of 7th month of intrauterine life
   - b. End of 8 month of intrauterine life
   - c. End of 9 month of intrauterine life
   - d. After birth

1. **c. 7 months**
   - ❏ The most appropriate option has been chosen as the answer.
   - ❏ Testis is present at the deep inguinal ring at the end of **6th month** and starts passing through inguinal canal at 7th month.

2. **a. Inguinal region**
   - ❑ Testis passes through the inguinal canal during **25 – 28th week (7th month)** of intrauterine life.

3. **c. End of 9th month of intrauterine life**
   - ❑ Testis lies at **superficial ring** at **eighth** month and enters the scrotum at the **beginning of ninth month**.
   - ❑ It reaches its final position in the scrotum **just before birth** (end of ninth month) and after birth (in few babies).

▼ Female reproductive system

Ovary

Intermediate mesoderm forms a longitudinal elevation along the dorsal body wall called the urogenital ridge, which later forms the **gonadal ridge**.
- ❑ Primary sex cords develop from the gonadal ridge and incorporate primordial germ cells (XX genotype), which migrate into the gonad from the wall of the yolk sac.
- ❑ Primary sex cords extend into the medulla and develop into the rete ovarii, which eventually degenerates.
- ❑ Secondary sex cords develop and incorporate primordial germ cells as a thin tunica albuginea forms.
- ❑ The secondary sex cords break apart and form isolated cell clusters called primordial follicles, which contain primary oocytes surrounded by a layer of simple squamous cells.

Development of Genital Ducts

Paramesonephric (Mullerian ducts)
- ❑ Cranial (unfused) portions of the paramesonephric ducts develop into the uterine tubes.

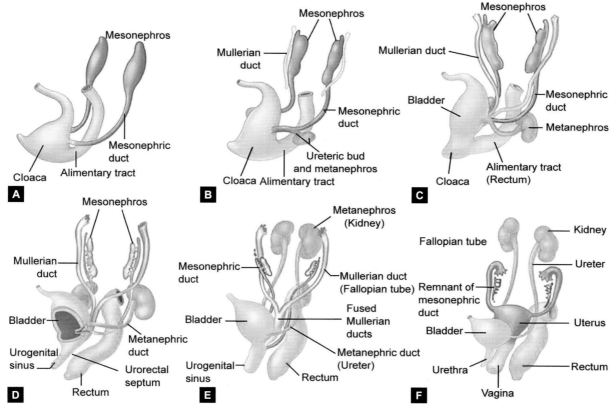

Figs. 69A to F: Development of reproductive system in female. Mullerian (paramesonephric) duct (mesodermal) gives: Uterus, uterine tube and upper third of vagina. Lower third of vagina, urinary bladder and urethra develop from urogenital sinus (endoderm). Kidney develops from metanephric blastema after it is stumulated by the ureteric bud (formed in mesonephric duct)

- ❑ **Caudal portions** of the paramesonephric ducts fuse in the midline to form the uterovaginal primordium and thereby bring together two peritoneal folds called the broad ligament.
- ❑ Uterovaginal primordium develops into the uterus, cervix, and superior 1/3 of the vagina.
- ❑ **Paramesonephric ducts** project into the dorsal wall of the cloaca and induce the formation of the sinovaginal bulbs. The sinovaginal bulbs fuse to form the solid vaginal plate, which canalizes and develops into the inferior two-thirds of the vagina.

❑ Vestigial remnants of the paramesonephric duct may be found in the adult female and are called the **hydatid of Morgagni**.

Mesonephric (Wolffian) ducts and tubules

❑ Mesonephric ducts develop in the female as part of the urinary system because these ducts are critical in the formation of the definitive metanephric kidney. However, they degenerate in the female after formation of the metanephric kidney.

❑ Vestigial remnants of the mesonephric ducts may be found in the adult female called the **appendix vesiculosa** and **Gartner's** duct.

❑ Vestigial remnants of the mesonephric tubules are called the epoophoron and the paroophoron.

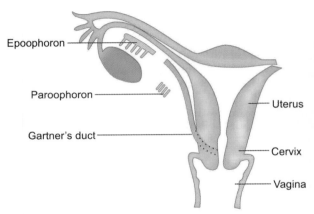

Fig. 70: Vestigeal remnants of mesonephric duct in females

Development of Vagina

❑ **Upper 1/3rd** of vagina develops from Mullerian (paramesonephric) duct **(mesoderm)** and lower 2/3 is derived from the endoderm of urogenital sinus.

❑ The caudal portions of the Mullerian ducts fuse in the midline to form the uterovaginal primordium, which contributes to upper 1/3 of vagina.

❑ The paramesonephric ducts project into the dorsal wall of the cloaca (urogenital sinus) and induce the formation of the **sinovaginal bulbs**.

❑ The sinovaginal bulbs fuse to form the solid vaginal plate, which canalizes and develops into the lower two-thirds of the vagina.

Table 12: Development of vagina and its associated structures	
Embryonic structures	**Adult derivatives**
▪ Mesodermal upper part of vaginal plate (derived from uterovaginal canal)	▪ Upper part of vagina including fornices of vagina
▪ Endodermal lower part of vaginal plate (derived from sinovaginal bulbs)	▪ Lower part of vagina
▪ Thin plate of tissue separating vagina and phallic part of urogenital sinus	▪ Hymen
▪ Phallic part of definitive urogenital sinus	▪ Vestibule of vagina

Structure	Origin
Epithelium	Urogenital sinus (Endoderm)
Smooth muscles	Lateral plate mesoderm (Splanchnic)
Skeletal muscles	Para-axial mesoderm
Hymen	Endoderm

❑ Human chorionic gonadotrophin (hCG) is a glycoprotein hormone produced by the syncytiotrophoblast; it stimulates the production of progesterone by the corpus luteum (i.e., maintains corpus luteum function).

❑ hCG can be assayed in maternal blood at day 8 or maternal urine at **day 10 using RIA (radioimmunoassay)** with antibodies directed against the β-subunit of hCG.

❑ Hydatid cyst of Morgagni arises from the hydatid of Morgagni, which is a remnant of the paramesonephric duct.

❑ Kobelt's cyst arises from the appendix vesiculosa, which is a remnant of the mesonephric duct.

❑ Mullerian agenesis involves the paramesonephric ducts can result in vaginal, cervical, uterine, uterine tube, or combined anomalies. For e.g., Lower vagina agenesis, cervix agenesis, uterus and cervix hypoplasia, and uterine tube agenesis.

❑ Uterus anomalies may occur when
  ➢ One paramesonephric duct fails to develop or incompletely develops–Unicornuate uterus.
  ➢ There is a complete lack of fusion of the paramesonephric ducts–Didelphys (double uterus).
  ➢ There is partial fusion of the paramesonephric ducts–Bicornuate uterus.
  ➢ The medial walls of the caudal portion of the paramesonephric ducts partially or completely fail to resorb- Septate uterus.

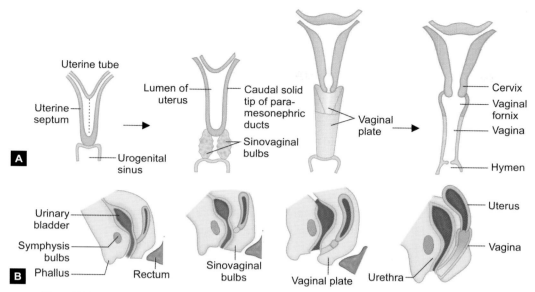

Figs. 71A and B: Development of the uterus and vagina. A. Frontal view. B. Side view

1. **Gartner's duct is present in:**
   a. Vaginal wall
   b. Broad ligament of uterus
   c. Transverse cervical ligament
   d. Perineal body

2. **Vaginal epithelium is derived from:** *(AIIMS 2013)*
   a. Endoderm of genital ridge
   b. Endoderm of urogenital sinus
   c. Mesoderm of genital ridge
   d. Mesoderm of urogenital sinus

3. **NOT true about development of ovary:** *(NEET Pattern 2015)*
   a. Develops in genital ridge
   b. Sex cords are derived from coelomic epithelium
   c. Oocytes are mesodermal in origin
   d. At birth ovary contains 2 million follicles

1. **a. Vaginal wall > b. Broad ligament of uterus**
   ❑ Gartner's duct is present in the anterolateral wall of the **vagina**. It may persist between the layer of the **broad ligament** of the uterus as well.

2. **b. Endoderm of urogenital sinus > Mesoderm of genital ridge**
   ❑ Vaginal epithelium is derived from **endoderm of the urogenital sinus** as per standard textbooks on embryology, though the topic is **controversial**.
   ❑ Upper 1/3 of vagina develops from the **Mullerian duct (mesoderm)** and 2/3 portion from endoderm of urogenital sinus.
   ❑ Later the endodermal epithelium of lower vagina **encroaches** upon the upper 1/3rd vagina, so that the epithelial lining of the **entire** vagina **eventually** gets lined by **endodermal epithelium**.
   ❑ **Recently** this concept has been challenged and there is a **new school of thought** expressing that vaginal origin (including epithelium) is entirely **mesodermal** (Few Journals mention, but no textbook yet).

3. **c. Oocytes are mesodermal in origin**
   ❑ Oocytes develop from the primordial germ cells, which themselves are derivatives of epiblast (**not mesoderm**).

- Total number of oocytes at birth are **1-2 million** *(NEET Pattern 2013)*
- **Upper 3/4th** of vagina develops from Mullerian duct *(NEET Pattern 2012)*
- **Vaginal** wall is derived from endoderm and mesoderm *(NEET Pattern 2013)*
- **Ovary is present** in Mullerian duct anomaly *(AIPG 2008)*
- Organ of Rosenmüller (epoophoron/parovarium) is a remnant of the **mesonephric tubules** *(NEET Pattern 2012)*
  - It can be found next to the ovary and fallopian tube.
- **Gartner's duct:** The paravaginal duct; a mesonephric duct remnant.
  - **Gartner's cyst** is the vaginal remnant of Gartner's duct, usually a benign cyst in the **anterolateral** wall of vagina.
- Round ligament of uterus are derivatives of **Gubernaculum** *(NEET Pattern 2014)*
- **Prostate** analogue in female is **Skene gland** *(NEET Pattern 2016)*

◤ External Genitalia

Proliferation of mesoderm (dorsal somatic, lateral plate mesoderm) around the cloacal membrane causes the overlying ectoderm to rise up so that three structures are visible externally, which include the phallus, urogenital folds, and labioscrotal swellings.

Male

- ❑ Phallus forms the penis (glans penis, corpora cavernosa penis, and corpus spongiosum penis).
- ❑ Urogenital folds form the ventral aspect of the penis (i.e., penile raphe).
- ❑ Labioscrotal swellings form the scrotum.

Female

- ❑ Phallus forms the clitoris (glans clitoris, corpora cavernosa clitoris, and vestibular bulbs).
- ❑ Urogenital folds form the labia minora.
- ❑ Labioscrotal swellings form the labia majora and mons pubis.
- ❑ Clitoris is embryologically derived from Genital tubercle *(NEET Pattern 2015)*
- ❑ Labia majora develops from the genital swelling *(NEET Pattern 2012)*
- ❑ **External genitalia** develop from **somatopleuric** lateral plate mesoderm *(NEET Pattern 2015)*

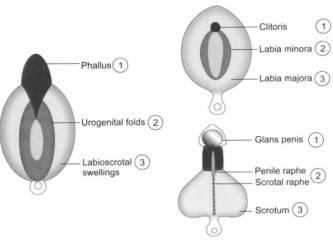

Fig. 72: Development of external genitalia

1. **INCORRECT statement about genital system development is:**
   a. Develop from mesoderm
   b. Genital ridge forms at week 5
   c. Testes develops earlier to ovary
   d. External genitalia are fully differentiated at week 10

2. **Male and female differentiation of fetus occurs at:**
   (NEET Pattern 2016)
   a. 2-4 weeks
   b. 10-12 weeks
   c. 16-18 weeks
   d. 24-26 weeks

3. **Faster sperm is with which sex chromosome:**
   (NEET Pattern 2012)
   a. X chromosome
   b. Y chromosome
   c. Both same
   d. None

4. **Mesonephric derivatives are all EXCEPT:** *(AIIMS 2015)*
   a. Glomerulus
   b. Para-oophoron
   c. Vas deferens
   d. Epididymis

5. **Derivative(s) of mesonephric duct includes:** *(PGIC 2014)*
   a. Some part of prostatic urethra
   b. Seminal vesicle
   c. Round ligament of uterus
   d. Vas deferens
   e. Common ejaculatory duct

6. **Sertoli cells are derived from:** *(NEET Pattern 2016)*
   a. Genital tubercle
   b. Genital swelling
   c. Primordial germ cells
   d. Sex cords

7. **Which of the following is derived from Wolffian duct?**
   (NEET Pattern 2012)
   a. Appendix of testis
   b. Uterus
   c. Appendix of epididymis
   d. Hydatid of Morgagni

8. **Which of the following is a derivative of paramesonephric duct in males:** *(NEET Pattern 2015)*
   a. Trigone of bladder
   b. Paroophoron
   c. Prostatic utricle
   d. Gartner's duct

1. **d. External genitalia are fully differentiated at week 10**
   - ❑ External genitalia become well differentiated, **after 12-13 weeks** age. Beyond 12-13-week sex determination is possible by **ultrasonographic** examination of external genitalia.
   - ❑ Genitourinary system develops from **intermediate mesoderm** and the genital ridge is first identified at **32 days (Week 5)** after ovulation and is **indistinguishable** between males and females.
   - ❑ Genetic sex is determined at fertilization by the presence or absence of the Y chromosome.
   - ❑ The testes, however, do not form **until the seventh week** of development.
   - ❑ Sex determination is **not possible before** an age of 7 weeks. During the 7th week, the gonad begins to assume the characteristics of a testis or ovary.
   - ❑ The ovary closely resembles the testis early in development, except that its characteristically female features are **slower to differentiate** (Testes develops earlier to ovary).

2. b. 10-12 weeks
- ❑ Genotype of the embryo is established at fertilization, but male and female embryos are phenotypically indistinguishable till week 6.
- ❑ Testis starts developing at week 7, whereas ovarian development begins at week 8-10.
- ❑ Male and female characteristics of the external genitalia can be recognized by week 12-13.
- ❑ Phenotypic differentiation is completed by week 20.

3. c. Both same
- ❑ Recent data confirms that Y sperm **do not** swim faster than X sperm, as mentioned in earlier literature by the scientist Shettles.

4. a. Glomerulus.
- ❑ Glomerulus (excretory system) is derived from 'metanephric' blastema (**not mesonephros**).
- ❑ Mesonephric duct gives ureteric bud to form the collecting system of kidney (**not excretory system**).
- ❑ Wolffian system (developing from Mesonephric duct) gives male reproductive tubes (and becomes **vestigial** in females).
- ❑ Wolffian system in males forms: Epididymis, Vas deferens, Seminal vesicle, Common ejaculatory ducts, etc.
- ❑ Vestigial remnant of **Wolffian** (mesonephric) system in females are: Epi-oophoron, Para-oophoron, Gartner's duct etc.

5. a. Some part of prostatic Urethra; b. Seminal vesicle; d. Vas deferens; e. Common ejaculatory duct
- ❑ In **both sexes**, the mesonephric duct gives origin to the **ureteric bud**, which forms the ureter, renal pelvis, major and minor calyces and the collecting tubules of the kidney.
- ❑ Its inferior (caudal) end is **absorbed** into the developing urinary bladder and forms the **trigone** and posterior wall of the proximal (prostatic) urethra.
- ❑ In males mesonephric duct becomes Wolffian duct and its superior (**cranial**) end is joined to the developing testis by the **efferent ductules** of the testis.
- ❑ **Its** derivatives are: Epididymis, vas (ductus) deferens, seminal vesicle, common ejaculatory duct etc.
- ❑ Round ligament of the uterus develops from the part of **gubernaculum** lying between uterus and the labium majus.

6. d. Sex cords
- ❑ **Sertoli** cells are the epithelial supporting cells of the seminiferous tubules. They develop from the **surface epithelium of early gonad**.
- ❑ **Few** authors mention them to be derived from the epithelial sex cords of the developing gonads.

7. c. Appendix of epididymis > d. Hydatid of Morgagni
- ❑ The appendix of the epididymis (or pedunculated hydatid) is a small stalked appendage (sometimes duplicated) on the head of the epididymis. It is usually regarded as a detached efferent duct.
- ❑ This structure is derived from the **Wolffian duct** (Mesonephric Duct) as opposed to the appendix testis which is derived from the Mullerian duct (Paramesonephric Duct) remnant.
- ❑ **The** Hydatid of Morgagni can refer to one of two closely related structures:
  - ▪ Para-tubal cyst (in the **female**)
  - ▪ Appendix testis (in the **male**)
- ❑ **Para**-tubal cysts originate from the mesothelium and are presumed to be remnants of the Mullerian duct and Wolffian ducts.
- ❑ **The** appendix testis (or hydatid of Morgagni) is a vestigial remnant of the **Mullerian** duct, present on the upper pole of the testis and attached to the tunica vaginalis

8. c. Prostatic utricle
- ❑ Prostatic utricle is a vestigial remnant of **Mullerian** (paramesonephric) duct.
- ❑ **Trigone** of bladder develop from the mesonephric duct **terminal portion**.
- ❑ **Para**-oophoron, and Gartner's duct are vestigial remnants of Wolffian (mesonephric) duct.

- ▪ **Differentiation** of genital ridge takes place at 2 months (*NEET Pattern 2013*)
- ▪ Male and female differentiation of fetus occurs at 7th week (*NEET Pattern 2016*)
- ▪ Y chromosome is a short acro-centric without the satellite (*NEET Pattern 2012*)
- ▪ **Gubernaculum** is attached to **caudal** pole of testis.
- ▪ **Appendix of testis** is derived from **cranial** end of paramesonephric duct (*NEET Pattern 2015*)

▶ Skeletal System

Vertebra

- ❑ Paraxial mesoderm give rise to somites, which have a component called sclerotome.
- ❑ Sclerotomes surround the notochord and project posteriorly to surround neural tube and divide into three parts:
  - ➢ Ventral sclerotomes: Forms vertebral body and annulus fibrosus.
  - ➢ Lateral sclerotomes : Forms vertebral arch (pedicle and lamina).
  - ➢ Dorsal sclerotomes : Forms the spinous process.
- ❑ **Ribs** are derived from the **sclerotome** portion of the **somite** (paraxial mesoderm) which form the costal process of the thoracic vertebrae.
- ❑ Primary ossification centers appear in the body of the ribs and mostly become cartilaginous during weeks 13-14 of development.

ANSWERS

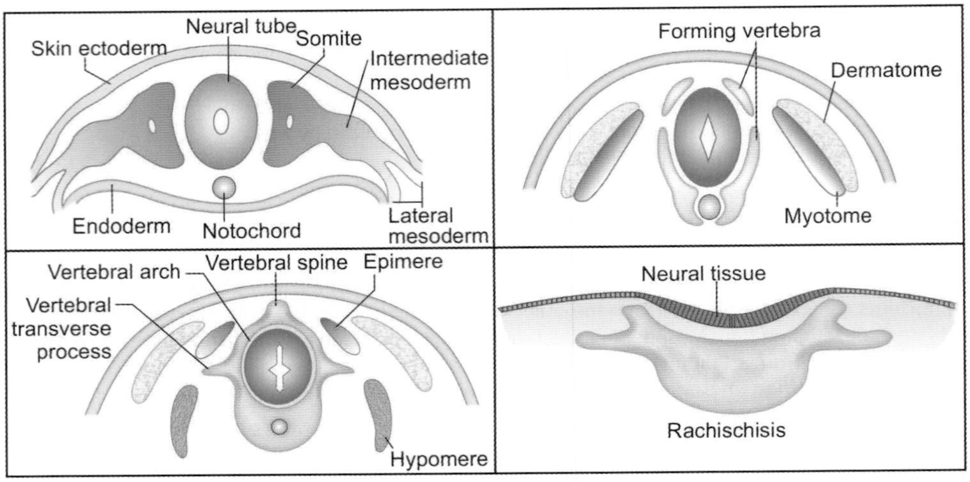

Neural tube Somite
Skin ectoderm
Intermediate mesoderm
Endoderm Notochord
Lateral mesoderm

Forming vertebra
Dermatome
Myotome

Vertebral arch Vertebral spine Epimere
Vertebral transverse process
Hypomere

Neural tissue
Rachischisis

Fig. 73: Formation of vertebra from sclerotomes. Spina bifida occurs in a case of open neural tube defect (rachischisis).

QUESTIONS

1. **Which of the following is TRUE about vertebral develop-ment?** *(NEET Pattern 2013)*
   a. The notochord forms the annulus fibrosus
   b. The sclerotome forms the nucleus pulposus
   c. The sclerotome surrounds the notochord only
   d. The sclerotome surrounds the notochord and the neural tube

2. **Lumbar hemivertebra results due to the abnormal development of:** *(AIIMS 2006)*
   a. Dorsal sclerotome
   b. Intermediate cell mass
   c. Notochord
   d. Ventral sclerotome

ANSWERS

1. **d. The sclerotome surrounds the notochord and the neural tube**
   ❑ Sclerotomes surround the **notochord** and project posteriorly to surround **neural tube** and divide into three parts:
   - **Ventral** sclerotomes: Forms vertebral **body** and annulus fibrosus.
   - **Lateral** sclerotomes : Forms vertebral arch (**pedicle and lamina**).
   - **Dorsal** sclerotomes : Forms the **spinous process**.

2. **d. Ventral sclerotome**
   ❑ Absence of **one half of the body** of the vertebra results in **hemivertebra** and is due to abnormal development of the **ventral** sclerotome.
   ❑ Ventral sclerotome forms the body of the vertebra, and absence of one half of the body (hemivertebra) may result in **scoliosis** (lateral bending of spine).
   ❑ **Dorsal** sclerotome forms the dorsal part of vertebral arch including the **spine**. Defective development of dorsal sclerotome may result in non-union of posterior vertebral arch results in **spina bifida**.
   ❑ **Notochord** forms the basis of **axial** skeleton and causes **induction** of the development of the vertebra. The adult remnant of notochord forms the **nucleus pulposus** of intervertebral disc.

▶ **Endocrine System**

Adrenal gland

Embryology

Suprarenal (adrenal) Gland
❑ Cortex is formed during the second month by a proliferation of the **coelomic epithelium** in the intermediate mesoderm. Cells pass into the underlying mesenchyme between the root of the dorsal mesogastrium and the mesonephros.
❑ The cortex is enveloped ventrally, and later dorsally, by a mesenchymal capsule that is derived from the mesonephros.
❑ **Medulla** forms from **neural crest cells**, which differentiate into chromaffin cells.

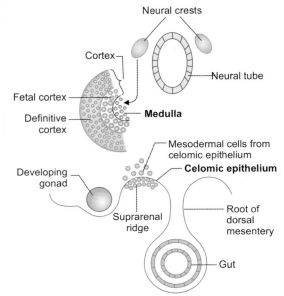

Fig. 74: Development of the adrenal gland

QUESTIONS

1. Adrenal cortex develops from:
   a. Para-axial mesoderm
   b. Intermediate mesoderm
   c. Lateral plate mesoderm
   d. Neural crest cells

2. Suprarenal gland develops from: *(NEET Pattern 2015)*
   a. Metanephros
   b. Ureteric bud
   c. Neural crest
   d. Endoderm

ANSWERS

1. b. Intermediate mesoderm
   ❑ The suprarenal (adrenal) cortex is formed during the second month by a proliferation of the coelomic epithelium. (Some authors mention its origin from intermediate mesoderm).
   ❑ Neural crest cells form the neurone bodies in adrenal medulla.

2. c. Neural crest
   ❑ Adrenal **medulla** develops from **neural crest** cells, which differentiate into **chromaffin cells**.
   ❑ **Cortex** is formed by a proliferation of the **coelomic epithelium** (in the vicinity of intermediate mesoderm).
   ❑ The cortex is enveloped ventrally, and later dorsally, by a mesenchymal **capsule** that is derived from the **mesonephros**.
   ❑ Metanephros forms the excretory portion of kidney system and ureteric bud forms the collecting system.
   ❑ Adrenal gland develops in mesoderm (**not endoderm**).

▼ Upper Limb and Lower Limb

❑ Limbs develop at the end of the fourth week as buds along the body wall adjacent to specific spinal segments determined by **HOX genes** (upper limb, C5-T2; lower limb, L2-S2).
❑ Development of the lower limb is approximately **1 to 2 days behind** that of the upper limb.

▼ Upper Limb and Lower Limb arteries

❑ The axis artery of the upper limb is derived from **seventh cervical intersegmental artery**. The axis artery runs on the **anterior** aspect of the lower limb and terminates in a palmar capillary plexus in hand. Main trunk of axis artery forms **axillary artery**, **brachial artery**, **anterior interosseous artery**, and **deep palmar arch**. The digital arteries of the hand arise from the **palmar capillary plexus**.

❑ The median artery develops from the anterior interosseous artery and communicate distally with the palmar capillary plexus. Radial and ulnar arteries develop from the axis artery close to bend of the elbow.

Axis artery	Adult derivatives
Axial artery of upper limb	• Axillary artery • Brachial artery • Anterior interosseous artery • Deep palmar arch
Axial artery of lower limb	• Inferior gluteal artery • Arteria nervi ischiadici • Popliteal artery above popliteus • Lower part of peroneal artery • Some parts of plantar arch

❑ The aortic arch 4 forms the proximal part of the **right subclavian artery**.
❑ The seventh intersegmental artery (ISA-7) contributes to the axial artery of upper limb and forms the distal part of the right subclavian artery and the entire left subclavian artery.
❑ The subclavian artery (right and left) continues into the limb bud as the axis artery, which ends in a terminal plexus near the tip of the limb bud.
❑ The axis artery persists in the adult as the **axillary artery, brachial artery, anterior interosseous artery, and deep palmar arch**.
❑ Developmentally, radial artery is pre-axial and ulnar is a post-axial artery.
   Axis Artery of the Lower Limb is derived from **fifth lumbar intersegmental artery**.
❑ The axis artery runs on the posterior aspect of the lower limb. It forms **inferior gluteal artery**, a small artery accompanying the sciatic nerve (ischiadic artery), part of popliteal artery (above the popliteus muscle), lower part of peroneal artery and part of plantar arch. The femoral artery is an entirely new (de novo) vessel formed on the ventral aspect of thigh. It develops a connection with the external iliac artery above and popliteal artery below. The external iliac artery is an offshoot of the axial artery.

QUESTIONS

1. Mis-expression of which of the following homeobox genes alters the position of the forelimbs during development? *(AIIMS)*
   a. HOX A7
   b. HOX B8
   c. HOX C9
   d. HOX D10

2. Melanoblast cells appear in basal layer of epidermis during:
   a. 3rd month of intrauterine life
   b. 5th month of intrauterine life
   c. 7th month of intrauterine life
   d. 8th month of intrauterine life

3. Merkel cells are derivatives of: *(NEET Pattern 2016)*
   a. Surface ectoderm
   b. Neural crest cell origin
   c. Endodermal origin
   d. Monocyte/Phagocyte origin

1. **b. HOX B8**
   - ❑ The **cranial limit** of expression of **HOX B8** is at the cranial border of the forelimb, and **mis-expression** of this gene **alters the position** of these limbs.
   - ❑ Positioning of the limbs along the **craniocaudal axis** in the flank regions of the embryo is regulated by the **HOX genes** expressed along this axis.
   - ❑ Specification of the **forelimb** is regulated by the transcription factor TBX5; specification of the **hind limb** is regulated by TBX4.
   - ❑ **Preaxial** border of limb is **radial** border of forearm *(NEET Pattern 2015)*
     - ■ For lower limb it is the tibial border.
   - ❑ Persistent remnant of **axial artery** of upper limb is **anterior interosseus artery** *(NEET Pattern 2015)*
     - ■ Radial and ulnar arteries develop later as **sprouts** of the axis artery close to bend of the elbow.
   - ❑ **Axis artery** of lower limb is derived from **5th lumbar intersegmental** artery *(NEET Pattern 2015)*
     - ■ The axis artery runs on the **posterior aspect** of the lower limb.
     - ■ It contributes to **inferior gluteal artery** and parts of **popliteal** artery, **peroneal** artery and **plantar** arch.

2. **a. 3rd month of intrauterine life**
   - ❑ During the first 3 months of development (as early as the **sixth to seventh weeks**), the epidermis is invaded by cells arising from the neural crest which synthesize melanin pigment in **melanosomes**.
   - ❑ Melanosomes are transported down **dendritic processes** of melanocytes and are transferred intercellularly to **keratinocytes** of the skin and hair bulb to **acquire pigmentation** of the skin and hair.

3. **a. Surface ectoderm > b. Neural crest cell origin**
   - ❑ **Earlier** Merkel cells were considered to be derived from **neural crest cells** *(Gray's Anatomy - 40th Edition)*, but more recent studies have indicated that they are in fact **epithelial** *(Gray's Anatomy - 41st Edition)* in origin.
   - ❑ Since skin epithelium is derived from **surface ectoderm**, the merkel cells are derivative of surface ectoderm.
   - ❑ **Langerhans** cells are derived from **monocyte**/phagocyte series, they capture antigens **from skin** and carry **to the lymph nodes** for further immune activity.

▶ Miscellaneous Questions

1. **If there is absence of precursor cell of an organ with the subsequent non development of the organ, the condition is called as:** *(NEET Pattern 2012)*
   - a. Agenesis
   - b. Aplasia
   - c. Atresia
   - d. Atrophy

2. **A person showing two cell lines derived from two different zygotes is known as:** *(AIIMS 2006)*
   - a. Chimerism
   - b. Mosaicism
   - c. Segregation
   - d. Pseudo dominance

3. **Which of the following marked structure is the heart primordium?** *(AIIMS 2017)*
   - a. A
   - b. B
   - c. C
   - d. D

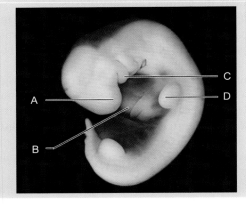

1. **a. Agenesis**
   - ❑ **Agenesis** is the **complete failure** of an organ to develop during embryonic growth due to the **absence** of primordial tissue.
   - ❑ **Aplasia** is the failure of organ to develop with only **rudiment** of organ present. It occurs, when precursor cells are present, but they do not differentiate into the organ.
   - ❑ **Atresia** is the **absence or closure** of an orifice, tube, duct.
   - ❑ **Atrophy** is the partial or **complete wasting away** of a part of the body due to a decrease in cell size and number.

2. **a. Chimerism**
   - ❑ A **chimera** is a single organism composed of **cells from different zygotes**. It may occur by organ transplantation, giving one individual tissues that developed from two genomes. For example, a bone marrow transplant can change someone's blood type.
   - ❑ **Mosaicism** describes the presence of two or more populations of cells with **different genotypes in one** individual, who has developed from a single fertilized egg.
   - ❑ Mosaics and chimera have **more than one genetically distinct population of cells**. But all genetically different cell lines arise form **single zygote in mosaics** and form **more than one zygote in chimeras**.

3. **b. B**
   Key: A: Nasal placode; B: Heart primordium; C: First pharyngeal arch; D: Upper limb bud.

Histology

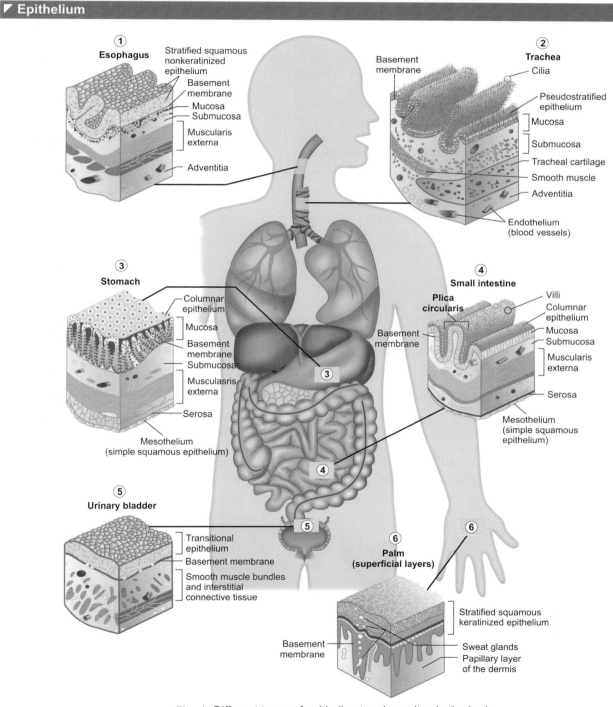

Fig. 1: Different types of epithelia at various sites in the body

▼ Types of Epithelia

❏ **Epithelium** is the layer of cells that cover the body surfaces or line the body cavities that open on to it. Epithelial lining at important sites is given in the following table:

Lining	Site
Simple squamous	▪ Pericardium, pleura and peritoneum ▪ Type – I pneumocytes (alveoli) ▪ Bowman capsule and Loop of Henle (major part)
Stratified squamous*	▪ External ear canal (including external surface of tympanic membrane) ▪ Cornea, conjunctiva ▪ Nasal vestibule ▪ Oral cavity: Lips, tongue, palate, tonsils, epiglottis (oral part) ▪ Terminal anal canal (below dentate/pectinate line) ▪ Terminal urethra
Simple cuboidal	▪ Thyroid follicles ▪ Germinal epithelium of ovary ▪ PCT, DCT and some parts of Henle's loop
Stratified cuboidal	▪ **Exocrine ducts**, like lacrimal, salivary, sweat
Simple columnar	▪ Stomach and intestine ▪ Gallbladder ▪ **Collecting tubules** of kidney
Stratified columnar	▪ Male urethra
Pseudostratified columnar	▪ Male urethra ▪ Olfactory epithelium ▪ Respiratory tract, e.g. trachea ▪ Eustachean tube ▪ Epididymis, ductus deferens ▪ Urethra
Ciliated columnar	▪ Respiratory tract ▪ Eustachian tube ▪ Uterine tube and uterus ▪ Central canal of spinal cord and ventricles of brain
Columnar with microvilli	▪ Small intestine (striated border) ▪ **Gallbladder (brush border)**
Neuroepithelium	▪ Ear, nose, tongue and eye (retina)

* **Rule**: Epithelium which can be **touched by fingers** is usually lined by **stratified squamous** epithelium and is a **derivative of ectoderm**.

❏ **Transitional epithelium** is a specialized stratified epithelium with large dome-shaped (umbrella) cells that bulge into the lumen.
  ➤ The dome-shaped cells have a **modified apical membrane** containing plaques and fusiform vesicles that accommodate the invaginated excess of the plasma membrane which is needed for the extension of the apical surface when the organ is **stretched**.

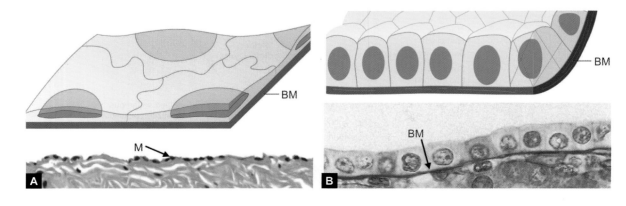

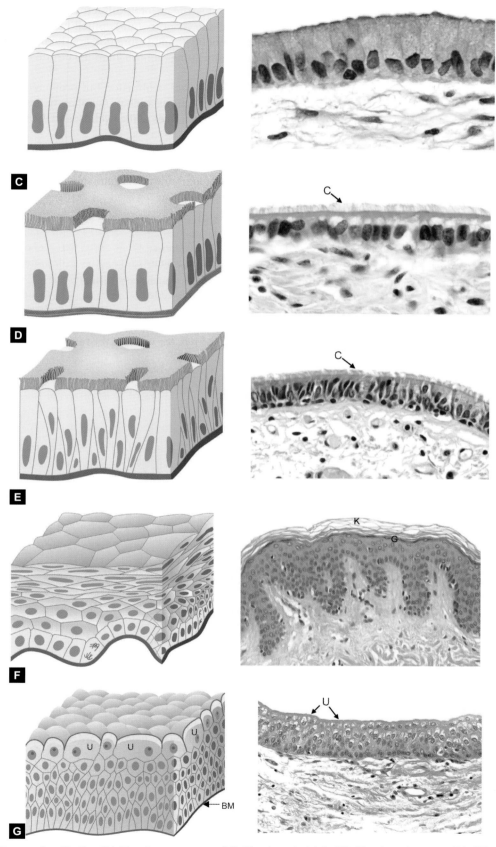

Figs. 2A to G: Types of epithelia: (A) Simple squamous; (B) Simple cuboidal; (C) Simple columnar; (D) Ciliated columnar; (E) Pseudostratified ciliated columnar; (F) Stratified squamous (keratinized); (G) Transitional. (BM - Basement membrane, C - Cilia, K - Keratin, U - Umbrella shaped cell).

- ❑ Sensory epithelium **(neuroepithelium)** is present in the special sense organs of the **olfactory (nose), gustatory (tongue)** and **vestibulocochlear (ear)** receptor systems. Some authors include **visual(retina)** epithelium under this category.
- ❑ **Keratinized epithelium** lies in the entire epidermis and the mucocutaneous junctions of the lips, nostrils, distal anal canal, outer surface of the tympanic membrane and parts of the oral lining (gingiva, hard palate and filiform papilla on the anterior part of the dorsal surface of the tongue).
- ❑ **Non-keratinized epithelium** is present at the surfaces that are subject to abrasion but protected from drying. These include: the buccal cavity (EXCEPT: for the areas noted above); oropharynx and laryngopharynx; esophagus; part of the anal canal; vagina; distal uterine cervix; distal urethra; cornea; inner surfaces of the eyelids; and the vestibule of the nasal cavities.

Myoepithelial cells (basket cells) are fusiform or stellate in shape contain actin and myosin filaments, and contract when stimulated by nervous or endocrine signals.

- ❑ They **surround** the secretory portions and ducts of some glands, e.g. mammary, lacrimal, salivary and sweat glands, and lie between the basal lamina and the glandular or ductal epithelium.

QUESTIONS

1. **Microvilli are absent in:** *(AIIMS 2015)*
   a. Proximal convoluted tube   b. Collecting duct
   c. Gallbladder   d. Duodenum

2. **Secreting active thyroid follicles are lined by which type of epithelium:** *(NEET Pattern 2013)*
   a. Columnar   b. Cuboidal
   c. Squamous   d. Pseudostratified squamous

3. **The ducts of all the following glands consist of stratified cuboidal epithelium EXCEPT:** *(AIIMS 2005)*
   a. Sweat glands   b. Sebaceous glands
   c. Salivary glands   d. Pancreas

4. **Simple squamous cells line:** *(PGIC)*
   a. Gallbladder   b. Blood vessels
   c. Pleura   d. Ependyma
   e. Male urethra

5. **Basal layer of cell in stratified squamous epithelium is:** *(PGIC 2014)*
   a. Squamous   b. Cuboidal
   c. Cuboidal-columnar   d. Pseudostratified
   e. Transitional

6. **Identify the organ in the following histology slide:** *(AIIMS 2016)*
   a. Urinary bladder   b. Gallbladder
   c. Bile duct   d. Skin

(NEET Pattern 2018)

7. **Hard palate lining contains:**
   a. Keratinized mucosa, absent submucosal layer, minor salivary glands
   b. Keratinized mucosa, submucosal layer, minor salivary glands
   c. Non-keratinized mucosa, submucosal layer, minor salivary glands
   d. Non-keratinized mucosa, absent submucosal layer, minor salivary glands

ANSWERS

1. **b. Collecting duct**
   - ❑ All of the given structures are lined by microvilli. Collecting duct has been taken as an answer of first preference.
   - ❑ The **proximal convoluted tubule** is lined by cuboidal (or low columnar) epithelium with a brush border of **tall microvilli** on its luminal surface.
   - ❑ **Collecting ducts** are lined by simple cuboidal or columnar epithelium. The **pale-staining** principal cells have occasional **microvilli**. A second cell type, intercalated or **dark cells** have longer **microvilli**.
   - ❑ **Gallbladder** epithelium is a single layer of columnar cells with apical microvilli (**brush border**) to actively absorb water and solutes from the bile and concentrate it up to ten-fold.
   - ❑ **Duodenum** has enterocytes which are columnar absorptive cells. Their surfaces bear numerous microvilli (**striated border**), which greatly increase the surface area for absorption.

2. **a. Columnar**
   - ❑ Thyroid follicles are **normally** lined by **simple cuboidal** epithelium, but **actively secreting** thyroid follicles (with abundant endoplasmic reticulum) are lined by simple **columnar** epithelium.

3. **b. Sebaceous glands**
   - ❑ The ducts of all exocrine glands are generally lined by **stratified** cuboidal/columnar epithelium with few **EXCEPT:ions** (sebaceous duct) which carries the same lining as that of skin (stratified **squamous** epithelium).

ANSWERS

4. b. Blood vessels; c. Pleura
- ❑ **Endothelium** (blood vessels) and **mesothelium** (pleura, pericardium, peritoneum) are lined by **simple squamous** epithelium.
- ❑ Gallbladder is lined by simple columnar epithelium with microvilli (**brush border**).
- ❑ **Ependyma** lies the ventricles of brain and has simple **cuboidal** (to **columnar**) cells with **cilia and microvilli**.
- ❑ Male urethra is lined by **stratified columnar** epithelium in entire length **EXCEPT:** the beginning (**transitional** epithelium) and the tip (**stratified squamous** epithelium).

5. c. Cuboidal-columnar
- ❑ The basal layers in stratified squamous epithelium are **columnar** give rise to layers of cells that change to acquire **cuboidal** and eventually **squamous** nature, as they migrate from **base towards the surface**.

6. a. Urinary bladder
- ❑ The slide shows **transitional epithelium** which is present in urinary tube; hence called **urothelium** as well.
- ❑ The most superficial cells have a **thickened plasma membrane** as a result of the presence of intramembranous **plaques** which give an **eosinophilic appearance** to the luminal surface.
- ❑ Large dome-shaped (umbrella) cells that **bulge into** the lumen may be evident.
- ❑ **Identification:** At first glance, it looks like a stratified cuboidal epithelium. Several rows of nuclei appear to be topped by a layer of dome-shaped cells which bulge into the lumen of the viscus.
  - ■ Cells of the basal layer are **cuboidal or columnar**, while the cells of the superficial layer vary in appearance depending on the degree of distension (may appear squamous, if stretched).

7. b. Keratinized mucosa, submucosal layer, minor salivary glands
- ❑ **Mucosa** of the hard palate is covered by **keratinized stratified squamous** epithelium which shows regional variations and may be **ortho-** or **parakeratinized**.
- ❑ Mucosa is bound **tightly** to the underlying periosteum. In its more lateral regions, it also possesses a **submucosa** containing the main neurovascular bundle.
- ❑ The submucosa in the posterior half of the hard palate contains **minor mucus-type salivary glands**.

- ▪ **Mesothelium** of serous cavities (pleura, pericardium and peritoneum) is lined by **simple squamous** epithelium.
- ▪ Thyroid follicles are lined by **cuboidal** epithelium (*NEET Pattern 2013*)
  - – **Actively secreting** thyroid follicles are lined by **simple columnar** epithelium.
  - – **Resting** follicles are lined by **simple squamous** epithelium.
- ▪ Cells in **transitional** epithelium are provided with **extra reserve of cell membrane** (*AIPG 2003*)
  - – Gets used up while **stretching**, helps in **increased storage**.
- ▪ **Cornea** is lined by squamous non-keratinized epithelium (*NEET Pattern 2012*)
- ▪ Lining epithelium of ventricles of brain is **columnar** epithelium (*NEET Pattern 2013*)
- ▪ Ventricles of brain and central canal of spinal cord are lined by **ciliated** simple columnar epithelium with **microvilli**.

▼ Surface Projections

- ❑ **Gallbladder** is lined by columnar cells with irregular microvilli- **brush border** (*AIIMS 2007*)
- ❑ **Small intestine** is lined by microvilli arranged in regular fashion—**striated border**.
- ❑ **Brush border** is also present in the proximal convoluted tubule (**PCT**) of kidney.
- ❑ **Stereocilia** are present in the hair cells of **internal ear** and **epididymis**.

▼ Cell Junctions

Cell junctions consist of multiprotein complexes that provide contact between neighboring cells or between a cell and the extracellular matrix.
- ❑ **Tight junctions** (zonula occludens) between two cells form a barrier **virtually impermeable** to fluid with almost **negligible intercellular gap**. It lies towards the **apical surface** of the cells.
- ❑ **Zona adheres** have an intercellular gap of **20 nm**.
- ❑ **Desmosomes** (macula adherens) are specialized for **cell-to-cell adhesion**, use **cadherins** as the cell adhesion molecule, have **25 nm** of intercellular gap and are damaged in **pemphigus vulgaris**.
- ❑ **Hemidesmosomes** use **integrins** and anchoring filaments (laminin 5) as their adhesion molecules anchored to the basal lamina, whereas **desmosomes** use **cadherins**.
- ❑ **Gap junctions** (communicating junctions) resemble tight junctions in transverse section, but the two apposed lipid bilayers are separated by an apparent gap of 3 nm which is bridged by a cluster of transmembrane channels (**connexons**).
  - ➢ Each connexon is formed by a ring of six connexin proteins whose external surfaces meet those of the adjacent cell in the middle. A minute central pore links one cell to the next. Larger assemblies of many thousands of channels are often packed in hexagonal arrays.
  - ➢ Gap junctions occur between numerous cells, including hepatocytes and **cardiac myocytes**.

- Gap junctions form **metabolic coupling** between cells and allow **free exchange of molecules** between cells (passive diffusion according to concentration gradient).
- They also work like an **electrical synapse** helping in **conducting impulses** between cells like **cardiac** and **smooth** muscle cells.

Pemphigus vulgaris is the most common and severe form of pemphigus seen usually in persons 40 to 60 years old, characterized by chronic, flaccid, easily ruptured **blisters** on the **skin and mucus** membranes.

❑ It begins focally but then becomes generalized, leaving large, weeping, denuded surfaces that partially crust over but do not heal and enlarge by confluence.

❑ **Autoantibodies** are detected against the **cadherins** of desmosomes. **Nikolsky sign** becomes **positive**.

Bullous pemphigoid is a usually mild, self-limited, **subepidermal** blistering skin disease, sometimes with **oral involvement**, predominantly affecting the elderly.

❑ It's characteristics include large, **tense bulla** that rupture to leave denuded areas and have a tendency to heal spontaneously, and cleft formation and deposition of complement usually with the IgG class of immunoglobulins at the **dermoepidermal junction**.

❑ **Autoantibodies** are detected against the **hemidesmosomes**.

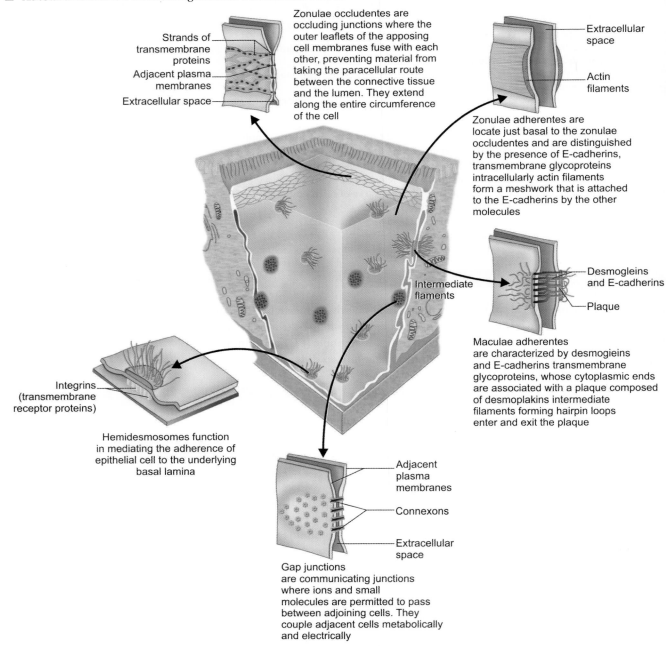

Fig. 3: Cell junctions and their characteristic features

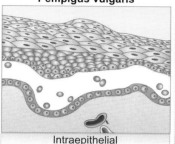

Pempigus vulgaris

Intraepithelial

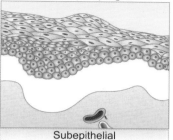

Bullous pemphigoid

Subepithelial

QUESTIONS

1. **In the electron micrograph below, the structure labeled 'D' primarily does which of the following**
   a. Forms a spot-weld between cells
   b. Facilitates communication between adjacent cells
   c. Seals membranes between cells
   d. Moves microvilli

2. **Intraepidermal blistering of skin is observed in**
   a. Erythema
   b. Bullous pemphigoid
   c. Pemphigus vulgaris
   d. SLE

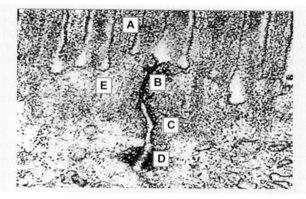

ANSWERS

1. **a. Forms a spot-weld between cells**
   - ❑ The present diagram is an Electron Microscopic (EM) picture showing microvilli, basal body and various cell junctions.
   - ❑ Marker A - **Microvilli** (apical surface projections), B - **Zona occludens** (tight junction) - identified by the apical location and narrow intercellular gap, C - **Zona adherens** - located below tight junction and has widened intercellular gap (20 nm), D - **Macula adherens** (desmosomes or spot weldings) have still lower location and more widened intercellular gap (25 nm) and E - **Basal body** (with centriole mechanism), located at the base and functions in the moving of microvilli.

2. **c. Pemphigus vulgaris**
   - ❑ Intraepidermal blistering is a sign of intraepithelial separation as observed in pemphigus vulgaris.
   - ❑ In bullous pemphigoid, there is a separation of epithelium from the basement membrane (subepidermal lesion).

- ❑ In **pemphigus vulgaris**, autoantibodies are formed against **cadherin**.
- ❑ Gap junction functions in **metabolic coupling** between adjacent cells.
- ❑ 20 nm of intercellular gap is found in the **zona adherens**.
- ❑ **Microvilli** are finger-like projections of epithelia that extend into a lumen and **increase** the cell's **surface area.**
- ❑ Microvilli constitute the **brush border** of kidney, proximal tubule cells and the **striated border** of intestinal absorptive cells.

▶ Glands

Table 1: Exocrine gland characteristics	
Cellular composition	**Example**
Unicellular (single cell)	Goblet cell
Multicellular (more than one cell)	Submandibular gland
Duct form	**Example**
Simple (unbranched)	Sweat gland
Compound (branched)	Mammary gland
Type of secretion	**Example**
Serous (watery)	Parotid gland
Mucus (viscous)	Palatal gland
Mixed (serous and mucus)	Sublingual gland
Mode of secretion	**Example**
Merocrine (only secretory product released)	Parotid gland
Apocrine (secretory product along with a portion of cell cytoplasm)	Lactating mammary gland (according to some authors)
Holocrine (cell dies and becomes the secretion)	Sebaceous gland

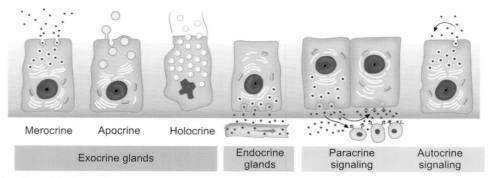

Fig. 4: Types of glands and their mechanism of secretion. Two types of glands (exocrine and endocrine) are shown and two types of signaling mechanisms (paracrine and autocrine) are visualized. Three basic types of secretions are shown in the cells of the exocrine glands. Merocrine secretion (most common) involves exocytosis of the vesicle content at the apical cell membrane. Apocrine secretion (like in mammary gland cells) the apical portion of the membrane covers the secretion and leaves the cell. Holocrine secretion cause disintegration of secretory cells is seen (as seen in sebaceous glands of hair follicles)

☐ Based upon the mode of secretion, there are three types of glands: Merocrine (eccrine), apocrine and holocrine.

1. **Merocrine**: The secretions are excreted via exocytosis from secretory cells into an epithelial-walled duct into the lumen or body surface.
   - It is the most common manner of secretion.
   - The gland releases its product and no part of the gland is lost.
   - Example, most of the sweat glands are of merocrine variety.

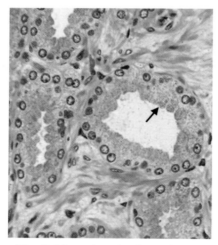

Fig. 5: Merocrine gland—entire cell remains intact.

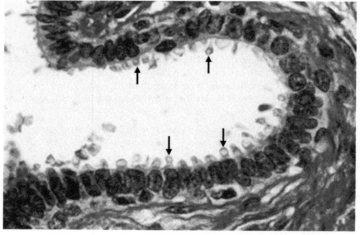

Fig. 6: Apocrine gland—cells are intact EXCEPT: the upper portions being detached as secretions (blebs).

2. **Apocrine**: The secretions of the cell take off a part of plasma membrane producing membrane-bound vesicles in the lumen.
   - The apical portion of the secretory cell of the gland pinches off and enters the lumen.
   - It loses part of its cytoplasm in their secretions.
   - Few sweat glands belong to apocrine variety, e.g. ceruminous gland and mammary glands are modified sweat glands of apocrine variety.

3. **Holocrine**: The secretions are produced in the cytoplasm of the cell and released by the rupture of the plasma membrane, which destroys the cell and results in the secretion of the product into the lumen.
   - Examples: Sebaceous gland (skin), meibomian glands (eyelid).

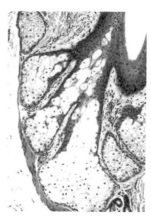

Fig. 7: A sebaceous gland (holocrine) showing a group of secretory acini opening into a hair follicle (top right). The distended sebocytes are filled with their oily secretion (sebum), which is discharged into the hair follicle by the holocrine disintegration of secretory cells.

Table 2: Difference between eccrine and apocrine sweat glands	
Eccrine sweat gland	**Apocrine sweat gland**
Found over most parts of the body	Confined to axilla, pubic and perineal regions, and areola of the nipples
Develops before birth	Develops after birth at puberty
Develops directly from surface epithelium	Develops from epidermal bud that produces hair follicle
Pours its secretion directly on the skin surface	Pours its secretion in the hair follicles just above the opening of sebaceous gland
Secretes by merocrine mechanism (exocytosis)	Secretes by apocrine mechanism (a portion of secretory cells is shed/pinched off and incorporated into the secretion)
Secretion is watery and involved in temperature control	Secretion is thick and produces an odor that acts as a sexual attractant

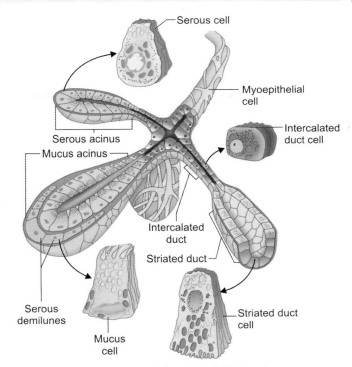

Fig. 8: Types of glands and duct system.

❑ Based upon the type of secretion, there are three types of glands: Serous, mucus and mixed.
   1. **Serous glands:** They contain serous acini (cuboidal cells), secreting fluid which is thin, watery in nature and isotonic with blood plasma, e.g. alpha-amylase.
      ▪ E.g. Parotid salivary gland, lacrimal gland.
   2. **Mucus glands:** They contain mucus acini (columnar cells), secreting fluid which is thick and viscous.
      ▪ E.g. Sublingual salivary gland.
   3. **Mixed glands:** Sero-mucous nature e.g. Submandibular salivary gland.

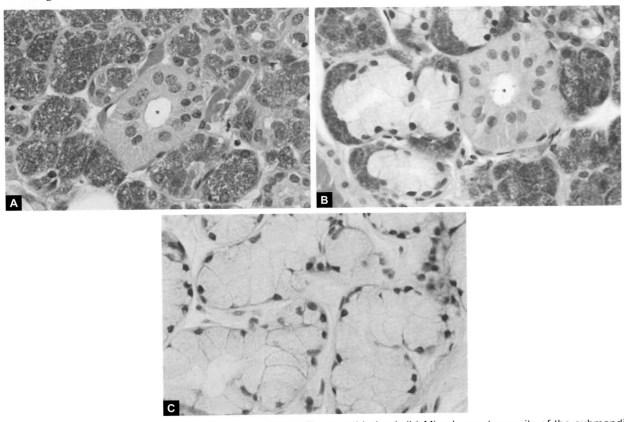

Figs. 9A to C: The microstructure of the salivary glands. (A) The parotid gland. (b) Mixed secretory units of the submandibular gland. (C) Mucus acini in the sublingual gland.

QUESTIONS

1. Which of the following is a holocrine gland:
(NEET Pattern 2012)
a. Sweat gland
b. Breast
c. Pancreas
d. Sebaceous gland

3. Sweat glands are which types of gland: *(NEET Pattern 2015)*
a. Simple tubular
b. Simple coiled tubular
c. Compound tubular
d. Compound acinar

2. Serous demilunes are present in the large number in which gland:
(AIIMS)
a. Parotid
b. Submandibular
c. Sublingual
d. Pituitary

4. Histology slide of a gland is given figure, identify the type of gland:
(AIIMS 2016)
a. Apocrine
b. Merocrine
c. Holocrine
d. Endocrine

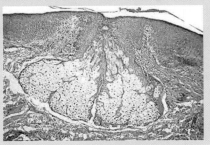

5. Which marker shows the holocrine gland: *(AIIMS 2017)*
a. A
b. B
c. C
d. D

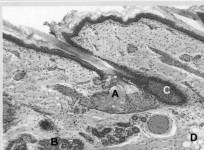

ANSWERS

1. d. Sebaceous gland
- Sebaceous gland is a **holocrine** gland since the discharged **secretion contains entire secreting cells.**
- Sweat glands are of two types: **Eccrine** (merocrine) is more common in occurrence as compared to **apocrine** variety.
- Breast (mammary gland) is **modified sweat** gland of **apocrine** variety. Another example for similar type is **ceruminous** (wax) gland in the ear.
- Pancreas is a mixed (exocrine and endocrine) gland. Exocrine secretory units are of **merocrine** type.

2. b. Submandibular
- **Parotid gland** is predominantly a **serous** gland and **sublingual** gland is **mucus** type.
- Submandibular gland is **mixed** (serous and mucus) type and shows large number of **serous demilunes** (a cap of serous gland appearing on mucus gland).

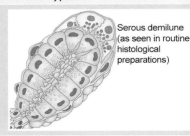

Serous demilune (as seen in routine histological preparations)

3. b. Simple coiled tubular
- Sweat glands are lined by the simple **coiled tubular** epithelium.

4. c. Holocrine
- The given slide in the figure appears to be taken from a **section of skin** showing sebaceous glands.
- In **holocrine** glands, the secretions are produced in the cytoplasm of the cell and released by the rupture of the plasma membrane which **destroys the cell** and results in the secretion of the product into the lumen.
- Examples: Sebaceous gland (skin), meibomian glands (eyelid).

5. a. A
- This is a figure of histological section of **skin**. **Sebaceous** gland (marker A) is a **holocrine** gland.
- In holocrine secretion, secretory product is released through the **total deterioration** of the cell. In this instance, as the lipid droplets accumulate, the cytoplasm is choked and disrupted, and the cell undergoes necrosis. Finally, total cell deterioration leads to release of the **sebum** as well as cellular debris into the duct.
- **Key**: A: Sebaceous gland (holocrine); B: Sweat gland (Eccrine); C: Hair follicle; D: Adipose tissue.

- **Ceruminous** glands present in the ear are modified **apocrine** glands. *(AIIMS 2005)*
- **Vagina** has **no glands** are seen in the mucosa, its surface receives the secretions of glands in the cervix.
- Mammary gland is a type of **modified sweat gland**. *(NEET Pattern 2015)*

Connective Tissue

Table 3: Review of supporting/connective tissue

Category	Component/nature	Details	Function
Matrix fibers	Collagen fibers	Type I collagen, type III collagen, etc.	Strength and structure
	Elastin	Elastin and fibrillin	Stretch and elasticity; elastin is formed on fibrillin microfibers
Ground substances	Glycosaminoglycans (GAGs)	Hyaluronate; proteoglycans	Water-binding gel provides volume, structure and interacts with supporting cells, epithelial cells, blood vessels and immune cells
	Structural glycoproteins	Fibronectin	Structural glycoprotein; binds and interacts with many connective tissue, molecular components
Basement membrane	Interface of cells with connective tissue	Type IV collagen, nidogen, integrins, heparan sulfate, etc.	Specialized structures formed where epithelia and other cells meet connective tissue matrix. Binds the epithelial cells to the connective tissue. Connective tissue and epithelial cells contribute to its formation and maintenance

Table 4: Classification of connective or supporting tissues

	General organization	Major functions	Examples
Connective tissue proper			
Loose (areolar) connective tissue	Much ground substance; many cells and little collagen, randomly distributed	Supports microvasculature, nerves, and immune defense cells	Lamina propria beneath epithelial lining of digestive tract
Dense irregular connective tissue	Little ground substance; few cells (mostly fibroblasts); much collagen in randomly arranged fibers	Protects and supports organs; resists tearing	Dermis of skin, organ capsules, submucosa layer of digestive tract
Dense regular connective tissue	Almost completely filled with parallel bundles of collagen; few fibroblasts, aligned with collagen	Provides strong connections within musculoskeletal system; strong resistance to force	Ligaments, tendons, aponeuroses, corneal stroma
Embryonic connective tissues			
Mesenchyme	Sparse, undifferentiated cells, uniformly distributed in matrix with sparse collagen fibers	Contains stem/progenitor cells for all adult connective tissue cells	Mesodermal layer of early embryo
Mucoid (mucus) connective tissue	Random fibroblasts and collagen fibers in viscous matrix	Supports and cushions large blood vessels	Matrix of the fetal umbilical cord
Specialized connective tissues			
Reticular connective tissue	Delicate network of reticulin/collagen III with attached fibroblasts (reticular cells)	Supports blood forming cells, many secretory cells, and lymphocytes in most lymphoid organs	Bone marrow, liver, pancreas, adrenal glands, all lymphoid organs EXCEPT: the thymus

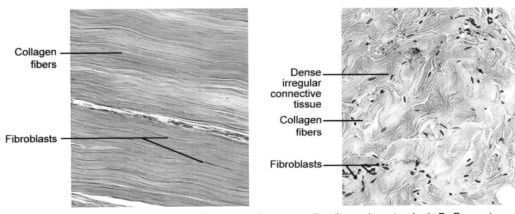

Figs. 10A and B: Arrangement of collagen fibres in A. Dense regular connective tissue (e.g. tendon); B. Dense irregular connective tissue (e.g. periosteum)

▶ Collagen Fibers

Table 5: Characteristics of some of the best known collagen types			
Molecular type	Cells synthesizing	Major locations in the body	Functions
I	Fibroblasts	Dermis of skin, tendons, ligaments, fibrocartilage, capsules of some organs	Resists tension
	Osteoblasts	Bone matrix	The arrangement of collagen fibers in compact bone reduces the presence of cleavage planes
	Odontoblasts	Dentin matrix	Structural support and provides a degree of elasticity to dentin
II	Chondroblasts	Hyaline and elastic cartilages	Resists intermittent pressure
III	Fibroblasts	Dermis of skin and capsules of some organs	Forms structural framework
	Reticular cells	Lymph nodes, spleen	
	Smooth muscle cells	Smooth muscle	Forms external lamina
	Schwann cells	Nerve fibers	
	Hepatocyte	Liver	Forms reticular fibers
IV	Endothelial cells	Blood vessels	Forms lamina densa of the basal lamina
	Epithelial cells	Epidermis and lining of body cavities	
	Muscle cells	Skeletal muscles, smooth muscles, heart	Forms external lamina
	Schwann cells	Nerve fibers	

QUESTIONS

1. The type of collagen fibres in hyaline cartilage are:
(NEET Pattern 2015)
- a. Type I
- b. Type II
- c. Type IV
- d. Type V

2. Reticular fibers of collagen tissues are present in all EXCEPT:
(AIIMS 2015)
- a. Thymus
- b. Bone marrow
- c. Spleen
- d. Lymph node

3. Following are given the collagen types and the sites of location. Choose the INCORRECT pair: *(PGIC)*
- a. Skin: Type – I
- b. Lens capsule: Type – I
- c. Blood vessel: Type – III
- d. Spleen: Type – III
- e. Hyaline cartilage: Type – I

4. Dense and regular arrangement of collagen fibers is seen in all EXCEPT: *(AIIMS 2014)*
- a. Tendon
- b. Ligament
- c. Aponeurosis
- d. Periosteum

5. Dense irregular connective tissue is found in:
(AIIMS 2017)
- a. Dermis
- b. Lamina propria
- c. Tendon
- d. Ligament

ANSWERS

1. b. Type II
- ❏ Hyaline and elastic cartilage have **type II** collagen fibers.
- ❏ Fibrocartilage has predominantly **type I** collagen fibers.

2. a. Thymus
- ❏ Reticular fibers/collagen type III are **absent in thymus**.

3. b. Lens capsule: Type i.e. Hyaline cartilage: Type I
- ❏ Generally, capsules have type – I collagen fibers; lens capsule/filtration membrane have **type IV** collagen fibers.
- ❏ Hyaline cartilage has **type II** collagen fibers.

4. d. Periosteum
- ❏ Periosteum has **dense but** no definite orientation (**irregular**) of collagen fibers.
- ❏ Tendon, aponeurosis and ligaments have collagen fiber bundles which are arranged in a **uniform parallel (regular)** fashion.

5. a. Dermis
- ❏ In **dense irregular** connective tissue, the collagen fibres are densely packed but are **not arranged in parallel** bundles (irregular).
- ❏ The **papillary** region of dermis is composed of **loose areolar** connective tissue, but the **reticular dermis** found under the papillary dermis is composed of **densely packed** collagen fibers but randomly arranged (**not parallel**).
- ❏ **Lamina propria** is a thin layer of **loose areolar** connective tissue (not dense) which lies beneath the epithelium in the mucosa.
- ❏ Tendon and aponeurosis have **dense** collagen fiber bundles, arranged in a uniform parallel (**regular**) fashion.

- ▪ In **hyaline** cartilage, type of collagen present is **type II**. *(AIIMS 2007)*
- ▪ **Basement membrane** has **type IV** collagen fibers. *(AIIMS 2015, 17)*
- ▪ The **papillary** region of dermis is composed of **loose areolar** connective tissue.
- ▪ The **reticular** dermis found under the papillary dermis is composed of **dense irregular** connective tissue featuring densely packed collagen fibers.
- ▪ **Muscle** is NOT a connective tissue. *(NEET Pattern 2012)*

Adipose Tissue

❏ The adipose organ is a complex endocrine system composed of white and brown fat. **White adipose tissue** serves as the primary site of energy storage, storing triglycerides within individual adipocytes, whereas **brown adipose tissue** stores little fat, burning it instead to produce heat and regulate body temperature.

Table 6: Summary of adipose tissue features		
Features	White adipose tissue	Brown adipose tissue
Location	Subcutaneous layer, mammary gland, greater omentum, mesenteries, retroperitoneal space, visceral pericardium, orbits (eye sockets), bone marrow cavity	Large amounts in newborns. Remnants in adults at the retroperitoneal space, deep cervical and supraclavicular regions of the neck, interscapular, paravertebral regions of the back, mediastinum
Function	Metabolic energy storage, insulation, cushioning, hormone production, source of metabolic water	Heat production (thermogenesis)

QUESTION

1. **Brown adipose tissue is present in all of the following sites EXCEPT:**   *(AIIMS 2015)*
   a. Subcutaneous tissue
   b. Around blood vessels
   c. Scapula
   d. Adrenal cortex

ANSWER

1. **c. Scapula**
   ❏ **Brown** adipose tissue is present in interscapular (**not scapular**) region.
   ❏ It is present in large amounts in the **new born** which helps offset the extensive heat loss, **later it disappears** from most sites **EXCEPT:** for regions around the kidney, adrenal glands, large vessels (i.e. aorta), and regions of the neck (deep cervical and supraclavicular), regions of the back (**interscapular** and paravertebral), and thorax (mediastinum).

Hemopoiesis

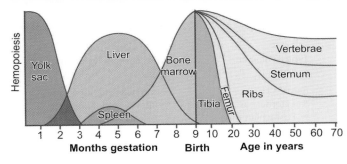

Fig. 11: Three major organs involved in hemopoiesis: Yolk sac (early stages), liver (second trimester), and bone marrow (third trimester). Spleen participates to a very limited time-period. Hemopoiesis occurs in the red bone marrow of all bones including long bones such as the femur and tibia. In adults, hemopoiesis is maintained primarily in flat bones (e.g. pelvic bones, sacrum, ribs, sternum, cranium) and vertebrae.

Cartilage and Bone

❏ **Osteoblasts** synthesize type I collagen and bone matrix proteins to form an unmineralized osteoid. Calcium and phosphate are deposited on the cartilaginous matrix to form mineralized bone. Blood supply within the haversian canals supply osteoblasts. Later, osteoblasts become surrounded by bone matrix to become **osteocytes**.

❏ **Osteocytes** are present in the space called lacuna and communicate with other osteocytes via cytoplasmic extensions called **canaliculi**. They are not directly involved in bone resorption but under the influence of parathyroid hormone (PTH) they stimulate osteoclastic bone resorption which allows calcium to be transferred rapidly into the blood.

❏ **Osteoclasts** are multinucleated cells (formed from monocytes) contain acid phosphatase and under the influence of PTH cause bone resorption.
   1. Bone formation occurs in two ways: During **endochondral ossification**, a cartilage model first forms and is eventually replaced with bone, EXCEPT: at epiphyseal plates and articular

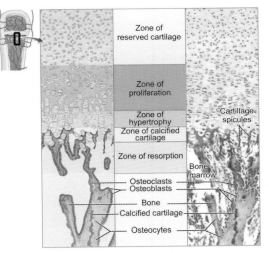

Fig. 12: Active bone formation on the diaphyseal side of the epiphyseal growth plate. Various zones are apparent: Chondrocytes undergo divisions, hypertrophy, and eventual apoptosis. Calcified cartilage (blue) is seen in the bone spicules

cartilages. This type of ossification underlie formation of the axial (vertebral column and ribs) and appendicular (limb) skeletons with the EXCEPT:ion of part of the clavicles.

2. During **intramembranous** ossification, bone forms directly from mesenchymal cells without the prior formation of cartilage. This type of ossification underlies the formation of the majority of bones of the face and skull.

❑ **Cancellous** bone is metabolically more active than the cortical bone. **Endosteum** is metabolically more active than periosteum.

❑ During endochondral ossification, **five** distinct zones can be seen at the light-microscope level.

1. Zone of **resting** cartilage: This zone contains normal, resting hyaline cartilage.
2. Zone of **proliferation:** In this zone, chondrocytes undergo rapid mitosis, forming distinctive looking stacks.
3. Zone of **maturation/hypertrophy**: It is during this zone that the chondrocytes undergo hypertrophy (become enlarged). Chondrocytes contain large amounts of glycogen and begin to secrete alkaline phosphatase.
4. Zone of **calcification**: In this zone, chondrocytes are either dying or dead, leaving cavities that will later become invaded by bone-forming cells. Chondrocytes here die when they can no longer receive nutrients or eliminate wastes via diffusion. This is because the calcified matrix is much less hydrated than hyaline cartilage.
5. Zone of **ossification**: The osteoprogenitor cells (OPCs) are available to continue the process of bone formation.

❑ Growth plate is made up of hyaline cartilage and is avascular.
❑ It starts getting vascularized by the formation of new blood vessels—vasculogenesis in the zone of calcification, and as it gets vascularized, erosion starts there.
❑ Then as the chondrocytes are eroded, new cells appear—the bone cells creating zone of ossification.
❑ It is evident that at epiphyseal growth plate, the cartilage gets destroyed and replaced by bone in a gradual manner.

Note: As the growth plate is ossified, it receives vascular buds and vasculogenesis occurs, the new blood vessels helping the metaphyseal artery to anastomose with the epiphyseal artery.

❑ Thus, metaphyseal arteries are no more termed as end-artery in an adult.
❑ Erosion of bone keep happening by the osteoclast cells which help in enlarging the marrow cavity.

▶ Cartilage

Table 7: Cartilage features

Types	Hyaline cartilage	Elastic cartilage	Fibrocartilage
Identifying characteristics	Type II collagen	Type II collagen	Type I collagen (predominantly)
Perichondrium	Present (EXCEPT: at articular cartilage)	Present	Absent
Location	Most common type ▪ Fetal cartilage ▪ Growth plate ▪ Articular cartilage ▪ Respiratory tube (with few EXCEPT:ions) ▪ Costal cartilage	Rare (E³ T³ C²) ▪ External ear ▪ Eustachian tube ▪ Epiglottis ▪ Tip of nose ▪ Tip of arytenoid ▪ Tritiate cartilage ▪ Corniculate ▪ Cuneiform	Found near the bone/joint ▪ Intervertebral disc ▪ Articular disc ▪ Knee meniscus ▪ Glenoid/acetabular labrum ▪ Insertion of tendons

❑ **Respiratory tube** cartilages-Nasal cartilage, thyroid, cricoid, arytenoid cartilage (**EXCEPT: tip**) are **hyaline** variety.
❑ **Hyaline** cartilage is the **articular** cartilage in **most** of the synovial joints **EXCEPT:** few joints. For e.g. articular cartilage in temporomandibular, sternoclavicular, acromioclavicular joints is **fibrocartilage** (**and not** of hyaline variety).

Table 8: Summary of cartilage features

Features	Hyaline cartilage	Elastic cartilage	Fibrocartilage
	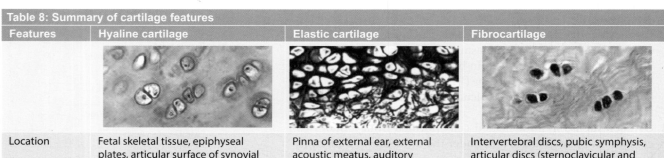		
Location	Fetal skeletal tissue, epiphyseal plates, articular surface of synovial joints, costal cartilages of rib cage, cartilages, of nasal cavity, larynx (thyroid, cricoid, and arytenoids), rings of trachea, and plates in bronchi	Pinna of external ear, external acoustic meatus, auditory (Eustachian) tube, and cartilages of larynx (epiglottis, corniculate, and cuneiform cartilages)	Intervertebral discs, pubic symphysis, articular discs (sternoclavicular and temporomandibular joints). menisci (knee joint), triangular fibrocartilage complex (wrist joint), and insertion of tendons

Features	Hyaline cartilage	Elastic cartilage	Fibrocartilage
Function	Resists compression provides cushioning. smooth and low-friction surface for joints provides structural support in respiratory system (larynx, trachea, and bronchi). Forms foundation for development of fetal skeleton and further endochondral bone formation and bone growth	Provides flexible support for soft tissues	Resists deformation under stress
Presence of perichondrium	Yes (EXCEPT: articular cartilage and epiphyseal plates)	Yes	No
Undergoes calcification	Yes (i.e. during endochondral bone formation, during aging process)	No	Yes (i.e. calcification of fibrocartilaginous callus during bone repair
Main cell types present	Chondroblasts and chondrocytes	Chondroblasts and condrocytes	Chondrocytes
Characteristic features of extracellular matrix	Type II collagen fibrils and aggrecan monomers (the most important proteoglycan)	Type II collagen fibrils, elastic fibers, and aggrecan monomers	Types I and II fibers, Proteoglycan monomers: Aggrecan-monomers (secreted by chondrocytes) and sersican (secreted by fibroblasts)
Growth	Interstitially and appositionally, very limited in adults		
Repair	Very limited capability, commonly forms scar, resulting in fibrocartilage formation		

QUESTIONS

1. All of the following cartilage types are covered by perichondrium EXCEPT: *(NEET Pattern 2012)*
   a. Articular cartilage
   b. Hyaline
   c. Elastic
   d. Fibrocartilage

2. TRUE about hyaline cartilage: *(AIPG 2000)*
   a. Hyaline cartilage covers the articular surface of synovial joints
   b. Hyaline cartilage is present in all synovial joints
   c. Articular cartilage may undergo ossification with ageing
   d. Articular cartilage limits the mobility of the joint

3. The articular cartilage is characterized by all of the following features EXCEPT: *(AIPG 2004)*
   a. It is devoid of perichondrium
   b. It has a rich nerve supply
   c. It is avascular
   d. It lacks the capacity to regenerate

4. Fibrocartilage is found in:
   a. Costal cartilage
   b. Nasal septum
   c. Intervertebral disc
   d. Auditory tube

5. The type of structure shown in the figure following slide is found in: *(AIIMS 2016)*
   a. Intervertebral disc
   b. Articular disc
   c. Epiphyseal plate
   d. Pinna

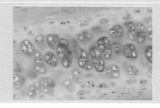

ANSWERS

1. **d. Fibrocartilage > a. Articular cartilage**
   ❏ Fibrocartilage and articular hyaline cartilage **do not have a perichondrium**.

2. **a. Hyaline cartilage covers the articular surface of synovial joints**
   ❏ Hyaline cartilage is the articular cartilage to cover the articular surfaces of **most** of the synovial joints **EXCEPT:** few joints. For example, articular cartilage in **temporomandibular** joint and **sternoclavicular** joints is fibrocartilage (**and not** of hyaline variety).
   ❏ Hyaline cartilage has **high tendency to get ossified** with few EXCEPT:ions, e.g. articular cartilage never gets ossified.
   ❏ Articular cartilage **smoothens** the articular surfaces and increase (**not limit**) the joint mobility.

3. **b. It has a rich nerve supply**
   ❏ Articular cartilage of typical synovial joints is **devoid** of nerves and blood vessels.
   ❏ It is **devoid** of perichondrium and has a **very low potential** for regeneration.

4. **c. Intervertebral disc**
   ❏ **Costal** cartilage and **nasal septum** contain hyaline cartilage. **Auditory tube** has elastic cartilage.

5. **c. Epiphyseal plate**
   ❏ This is a slide of **hyaline cartilage** which is found in growth (**epiphyseal**) plate.
   ❏ Identification points:
      ■ Islands of chondrocytes, scattered in the **hyalos matrix**.
      ■ Collagen fibers have the **same refractive index** as the matrix and are invisible. **So** the matrix appears glass-like (hyalos).
      ■ Intervertebral disc and articular disc has **fibrocartilage**.
      ■ Fibrocartilage has relatively **few chondrocytes**, and they are present among the visible bundles of collagen fibers running in a **wavy fashion**.
      ■ Pinna is made up of **elastic** cartilage.
      ■ Elastic cartilage slide shows numerous chondrocytes scattered among the **irregularly arranged** elastic fibers.

- Temporomandibular joint has fibrocartilage (**not hyaline**). *(NEET Pattern 2012)*
  - **Usually** synovial joints have **hyaline** cartilage.
- **Meniscus** is NOT a hyaline cartilage. *(NEET Pattern 2012)*
- **Elastic** cartilage is seen in **epiglottis**. *(NEET Pattern 2012)*

▶ Bone

Osteon is the fundamental functional unit of compact bone which contains **haversian system.**

❑ Each osteon consists of concentric layers, or **lamella**, of compact bone tissue that surround a central canal, the **haversian canal**.

❑ Haversian canal carries the **neurovascular** bundles to the bone.

❑ Osteons are connected to each other and the periosteum by oblique channels called **Volkmann's canals** or perforating canals.

Table 9: Summary of bone types and their organization

Types of bone	Histological features	Major locations	Synonyms
Woven bone, newly calcified	Irregular and random arrangement of cells and collagen; lightly calcified	Developing and growing bones; hard callus of bone fractures	Immature bone; primary bone
Lamellar bone, remodeled from woven bone	Parallel bundles of collagen in thin layers (lamella), with regularly spaced cells between; heavily calcified.	All normal regions of adult bone	Mature bone; secondary bone
Compact bone, ~80% of all lamellar bone	Parallel lamella or densely packed osteons, with interstitial lamella	Thick, outer region (beneath periosteum) of bones	Cortical bone
Cancellous bone, ~20% of all lamellar bone	Interconnected thin spicules or trabecula covered by endosteum	Inner region of bones adjacent to marrow cavities	Spongy bone; trabecular bone; medullary bone

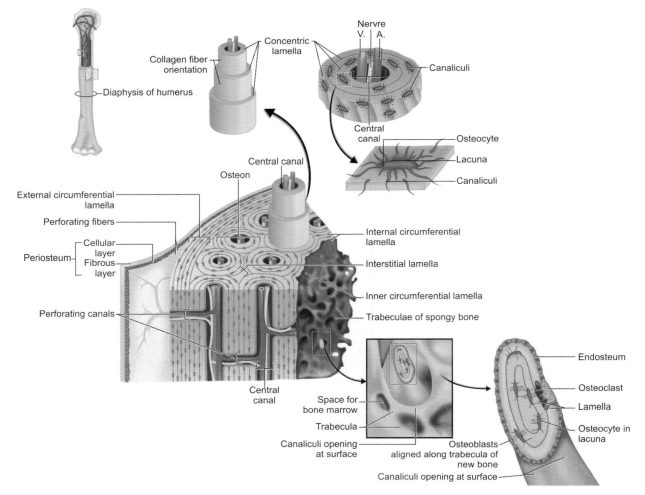

Fig. 13: Structural details of a bone with osteon arrangement and Haversian system.

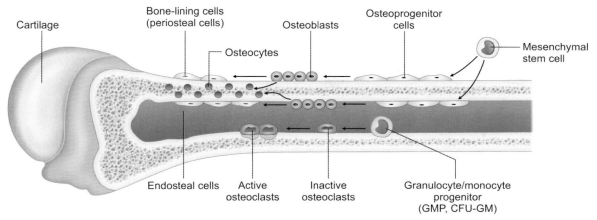

Fig. 14: Cells associated with bone. All cells EXCEPT: osteoclasts originate from the mesenchymal stem cells which differentiate into osteoprogenitor cells, osteoblasts, and finally osteocytes and bone lining cells. Bone-lining cells on external bone surfaces are the part of the periosteum, hence the term periosteal cells. Bone-lining cells on internal bone surfaces are frequently called endosteal cells. Osteoclasts originate from hemopoietic progenitor cells which differentiate into bone-resorbing cells

Table 10: Cells associated with bone

Features	Osteoblast	Osteocyte	Osteoclast
Location	Bone surface; closing cone of resorption canals	Lacunae and canaliculi of bone matrix	Bone surface; cutting cone of resorption canals
Percentage of all cells in the bone	>5%	~95%	>1%
Function	Deposits bone matrix; initiates mineralization by releasing matrix vesicles	Maintains bone matrix; senses mechanical stress; regulates calcium and phosphate hemostasis	Resorbs bone by enzymatic hydrolysis of the mineralized bone matrix
Cell morphology	Cuboidal or polygonal, mononuclear cells; basophilic cytoplasm; negative Golgi	Small, oval, mononuclear cell; pale cytoplasm; long cell processes	Large, multinuclear cell; acidophilic cytoplasm; rffled border; underlying Howship's lacuna
Precursor cells	Osteoprogenitor cell	Osteoblast	Hemopoietic cells (GMP, CFU-GM)
Lifespan	Weeks (~12 days)	Years (~10-20 years)	Days (~3 days)

- ❑ **Periosteum** is a membrane that covers the outer surface of all bones EXCEPT: at the joints of long bones.
- ❑ It consists of **dense irregular connective tissue** divided into an outer 'fibrous layer' and inner 'osteogenic layer'.
  - ➢ The fibrous layer contains fibroblasts, while the osteogenic layer contains progenitor cells that develop into osteoblasts.
  - ➢ The osteoblasts are responsible for increasing the width of a long bone and the overall size of the other bone types.
  - ➢ After a bone fracture the progenitor cells develop into osteoblasts and chondroblasts which are essential to the healing process.
- ❑ As opposed to osseous tissue, the periosteum has **nociceptive nerve endings** making it very sensitive to manipulation. It also provides nourishment by providing the blood supply to the body from the marrow.
- ❑ Periosteum is attached to the bone by strong collagenous fibers called **Sharpey's fibers** which extend to the outer circumferential and interstitial lamella. It also provides an attachment for muscles and tendons.
- ❑ **Endosteum** is a thin vascular membrane of connective tissue that lines the surface of the medullary cavity of long bones.
- ❑ The osteoblasts and osteoprogenitor cells within the endosteum play an important role in remodeling and repair
- ❑ To prevent the bone from becoming unnecessarily thick, osteoclasts resorb the bone from the endosteal side.
- ❑ Endosteal surface is resorbed during long periods of malnutrition, resulting in less cortical thickness.
- ❑ **Endosteum** is metabolically **more active** than periosteum. The periosteum is highly active during fetal development, when it generates osteoblasts for the appositional growth of bone. The population of osteogenic layer of the periosteum is markedly diminished with age and remodelling of bone is in adult life is a very slow process, but osteoblasts below the endosteum are **more active** than those below the periosteum.

Red Bone Marrow

- ❑ It is vascular and appears red in color due to presence of red blood cells.
- ❑ It consists of network of fine **reticular fibers** containing blood forming cells showing all the stages of development.

❑ At birth it is present in all the bones at all sites, and is an important site of hemopoiesis, but as the age advances the marrow in the medullary cavity of long bones is gradually replaced by yellow marrow.

In adults, the **red marrow** is found in the cancellous bone. e.g. ends of long bones, sternum, ribs, skull bones, iliac crests of hip bones, vertebrae.

QUESTIONS

1. All physiological processes occur during the growth at the epiphyseal plate EXCEPT: *(AIPG 2005)*
   a. Proliferation and hypertrophy
   b. Calcification and ossification
   c. Vasculogenesis and erosion
   d. Replacement of red bone marrow with yellow marrow

2. Most metabolically active layer in bone is: *(AIIMS 2015)*
   a. Periosteum
   b. Endosteum
   c. Cancellous bone
   d. Cortical bone

ANSWERS

1. **d. Replacement of red bone marrow with yellow marrow**
   ❑ Replacement of red bone marrow with yellow bone marrow occurs **mainly at the diaphysis**.
   ❑ During endochondral ossification, **five distinct zones** can be seen at the light-microscope level.

2. **b. Endosteum**
   ❑ This question has **confusing options** and the most appropriately appearing option has been taken as the answer.
   ❑ **Cancellous** bone is metabolically **more active** than the cortical bone. **Endosteum** is metabolically **more active** than periosteum.
   ❑ The periosteum is highly active during **fetal** development, when it generates osteoblasts for the appositional growth of bone.
   ❑ The population of osteogenic layer of the periosteum is **markedly diminished with age** and remodelling of bone is in adult life is a very slow process, but **osteoblasts below the endosteum are more active** than those below the periosteum.

▪ **Haversian** system is found in **diaphysis** of long bones. *(AIPG 2000)*

▼ Muscular System

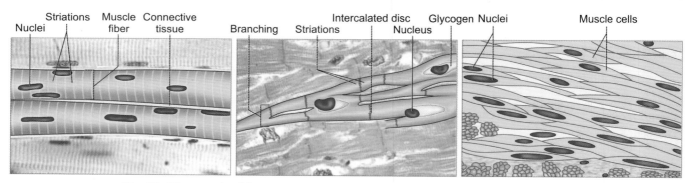

Fig. 15: Microscopic slide and corresponding details shown for three type of muscles.

Table 11: Important comparisons of the three types of muscles			
	Skeletal muscle	**Cardiac muscle**	**Smooth muscle**
Fibers	Single multinucleated cells	Aligned cells in branching arrangement	Single small, closely packed fusiform cells
Cell/fiber shape and size	Cylindrical 10–100 μm diameter, many cm long	Cylindrical 10-20 μm diameter, 50–100 μm long	Fusiform, diameter 0.2–10 μm, length 50–200 μm
Striations	Present	Present	Absent
Locations of nuclei	Peripheral, adjacent to sarcolemma	Central	Central, at widest part of cell
T tubules	Center of triads at A-I junctions	In diads at Z discs	Absent; caveola may be functionally similar
Sarcoplasmic reticulum (SR)	Well-developed with two terminal cisterns per sarcomere in triads with T tubule	Less well-developed, one small terminal cistern per sarcomere in diad with T tubule	Irregular smooth ER without distinctive organization
Special structural features	Very well-organized sarcomeres, SR, and transverse tubule system	Intercalated discs, joining cell with many adherent and gap junctions	Gap junctions, caveola, dense bodies

▼ Skeletal Muscle

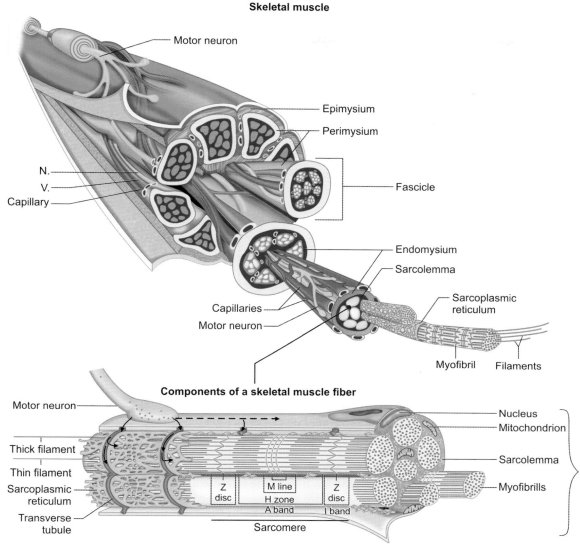

Fig. 16: Microscopic structure of a skeletal muscle, with reference to sarcomere.

❏ A **sarcomere** is defined as the segment between two neighboring Z-lines (or Z-discs, or Z bodies). In electron micrographs of cross-striated muscle, the Z-line (from the German 'Zwischenscheibe', the disc in between the I-bands) appears as a series of dark lines.

❏ Surrounding the Z-line is the region of the **I-band** (for **isotropic**). I-band is the zone of thin filaments that is not superimposed by thick filaments.

❏ Following the I-band is the **A-band** (for **anisotropic**). Named for their properties under a polarizing microscope. An A-band contains the entire length of a single thick filament.

❏ Within the A-band is a paler region called the **H-zone** (from the German 'heller', brighter). Named for their lighter appearance under a polarization microscope. H-band is the zone of the thick filaments that is not superimposed by the thin filaments.

❏ Within the H-zone is a thin **M-line** (from the German 'Mittelscheibe', the disc in the middle of the sarcomere) formed of cross-connecting elements of the cytoskeleton.

❏ The relationship between the proteins and the regions of the sarcomere are as follows:
  ➢ **Actin filaments,** the thin filaments are the major components of the I-band and extend into the A-band.
  ➢ **Myosin filaments,** the thick filaments are bipolar and extend throughout the A-band. They are cross-linked at the center by the M-band.
  ➢ The giant protein titin (connectin) extends from the Z-line of the sarcomere where it binds to the thick filament (myosin) system to the **M-band**, where it is thought to interact with the thick filaments. **Titin** (and its splice isoforms) is the biggest

single highly elasticated protein found in nature. It provides binding sites for numerous proteins and is thought to play an important role as sarcomeric ruler and as blueprint for the assembly of the sarcomere.

➤ Another giant protein, **nebulin**, is hypothesized to extend along the thin filaments and the entire I-Band. Similar to titin, it is thought to act as a molecular ruler along for thin filament assembly.

➤ Several proteins important for the stability of the sarcomeric structure are found in the Z-line as well as in the M-band of the sarcomere.

➤ Actin filaments and titin molecules are cross-linked in the Z-disc via the Z-line protein alpha-actinin.

➤ The M-band proteins **myomesin** as well as C-protein cross-link the thick filament system (myosins) and the M-band part of titin (the elastic filaments).

➤ The interaction between actin and myosin filaments in the A-band of the sarcomere is responsible for the muscle contraction (sliding filament model).

Table 12: Effects of contraction on skeletal muscle cross-bands

Bands	Myofilament component	Change in bands during contraction
I	Thin only	Shorten
H	Thick only	Shorten
A	Thick and thin	N change in length
Z discs	Thin only (attached by α-actinin)	Move closer together

◤ Cardiac Muscles

❑ **Intercalated discs** are microscopic identifying features of cardiac muscle. Cardiac muscle consists of individual heart muscle cells (cardiomyocytes) connected by intercalated discs to work as a single functional organ or **syncytium**. By contrast, skeletal muscle consists of multinucleated muscle fibers and exhibit no intercalated discs. Intercalated discs support synchronized contraction of cardiac tissue. They occur at the Z-line of the sarcomere and can be visualized easily when observing a longitudinal section of the tissue.

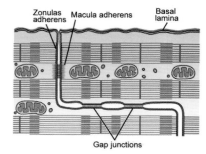

❑ **Three types** of cell junction make up an intercalated disc—fascia adherens, desmosomes and gap junctions.
1. **Fascia adherens** are anchoring sites for actin, and connect to the closest sarcomere.
2. **Desmosomes** stop separation during contraction by binding intermediate filaments joining the cells together. Desmosomes are also known as macula adherens.
3. **Gap junctions** allow action potentials to spread between cardiac cells by permitting the passage of ions between cells, producing depolarization of the heart muscle.

Fig. 17: Cardiac muscles showing various types of cell junctions.

QUESTIONS

1. In the following figure, the structure marked with arrow has all of the following cell junctions EXCEPT: *(AIIMS 2016, 17)*

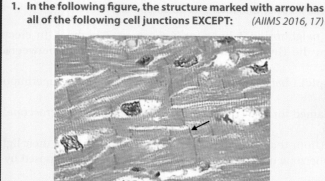

a. Zonula occludens   b. Zonula adherens
c. Macula adherens   d. Gap junction

2. In the given EM picture of a sarcomere, identify the structure at marker 'A'. *(AIIMS 2016)*

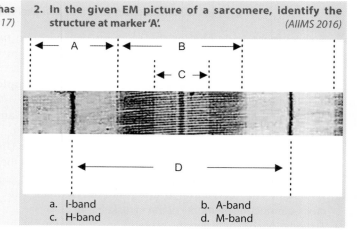

a. I-band   b. A-band
c. H-band   d. M-band

ANSWERS

1. a. Zonula occludens
❑ This is a diagram of **cardiac muscle** and the marker is pointing towards the **intercalated disc** which does not have **zonula occludens** present in the structure.
❑ **Three** types of cell junction make up an intercalated disc — fascia adherens, desmosomes and gap junctions.

2. a. I-band
- ❏ This figure is an **electron microscopic** picture of sarcomere showing various zones including **isotropic** I (marker 'A') band.
- ❏ Key: A – I (Isotropic) band; B – A (Anisotropic) band; C – H (Heller) band; D – Sarcomere.
- ❏ A sarcomere ('D') is defined as the segment **between two neighboring Z-lines** (dark lines).
- ❏ Surrounding the Z-line is the region of the I (Marker 'A') band having thin filaments that are **not superimposed** by thick filaments.
- ❏ An A-band (marker 'B') contains the entire length of **a single thick filament**.
- ❏ Within the A-band is a paler region called the **H-band** (marker 'C') which is the zone of the thick filaments that are **not** superimposed by the thin filaments.

▶ Nervous System

A **nerve** is an enclosed, bundle of axons in the peripheral nervous system (PNS). It carries electrochemical nerve **impulses** transmitted along each of the axons.

- ❏ Within a nerve, each axon is surrounded by a layer of connective tissue called the **endoneurium**. The axons are bundled together into groups called **fascicles**.
- ❏ Each fascicle is wrapped in a layer of connective tissue called the **perineurium**.
- ❏ Finally, the entire nerve is wrapped in a layer of connective tissue called the **epineurium.**

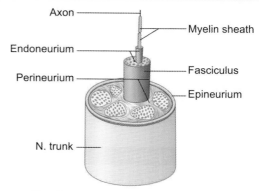

Fig. 18: Microscopic details of a nerve.

Cerebellum

- ❏ **Identification point:** Cerebellar cortex forms a series of deeply convoluted folds or folia supported by a branching central white matter.

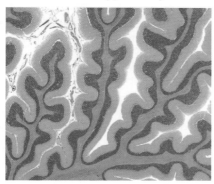

Fig. 19: Cerebellum (low magification).

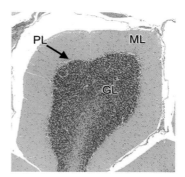

Fig. 20: Cerebellum (Higher magification), showing three layers in cerebellar cortex.

- ❏ Triple layered cortex
- ❏ Cerebellar outer **molecular layer** (ML) contains relatively few neurons and large numbers of unmyelinated fibers.
- ❏ The inner **granular cell layer** (GL) is extremely cellular.
- ❏ Between the two is a single layer of huge neurons called **Purkinje cells** (PL).

▶ Circulatory System

Table 13: Characteristics of different types of capillaries			
Characteristics	**Continuous capillaries**	**Fenestrated capillaries**	**Sinusoidal capillaries**
Location	CT, muscle, nerve tissue; modified in brain tissue	Endocrine glands, pancreas, intestines	Bone marrow, spleen, liver, lymph nodes, certain endocrine glands
Diameter	Smallest diameter	Intermediate diameter	Largest diameter
Endothelium	Forms tight junctions at marginal fold with itself or adjacent cells	Forms tight junction at marginal fold with itself or adjacent cells	Frequently the endothelium and basal lamina are discontinuous
Fenestra	Not present	Present	Present in addition to gaps

▶ Veins

Sinusoids are **expanded** capillaries. They have **true discontinuities** in their walls allowing intimate contact between blood and the parenchyma.

- ❏ The discontinuities are formed by gaps between **fenestrated endothelial** cells such that the sinusoidal lining, and sometimes also the basal lamina, is incomplete.
- ❏ Sinusoids are found in the **liver**, lymphoid tissue (spleen, lymph node), **endocrine** organs (like adenohypophysis, adrenal medulla, parathyroids), and **hematopoietic organs** such as the bone marrow, carotid body, etc.

QUESTIONS

1. Sinusoids are seen in all of the following EXCEPT:

   (NEET Pattern 2012)

   a. Liver   b. Kidney
   c. Lymph nodes   d. Spleen

2. Vasa vasorum includes: *(NEET Pattern 2012)*

   a. Small blood vessels supplying walls of large blood vessels
   b. Small blood vessels supplying nerves
   c. Vessels accompanying artery
   d. Vessels accompanying nerves

ANSWERS

1. **b. Kidney**
   - ❏ Sinusoids are **expanded capillaries** with discontinuous walls.
   - ❏ Sinusoids are found in the liver, lymphoid tissue (lymph nodes, spleen), endocrine organs, hematopoietic organs (bone marrow), etc.
   - ❏ **Non-sinusoidal** fenestrated blood capillaries with open fenestra are only known to be present in the **kidney** glomerulus.

2. **a. Small blood vessels supplying walls of large blood vessels**
   - ❏ Vasa vasorum is a network of small blood vessels that **supply the walls of large blood vessels**. These are found in large arteries and veins, e.g. **aorta**, **vena cavae**
   - ❏ These vessels supply blood and nutrition for tunica adventitia and outer part of tunica media of large vessels.
   - ❏ Vasa **nervorum**: These are small arteries that provide blood supply to nerves and their coverings

▶ Lymphoid System

- ❏ Lymphoid system consists of capsulated lymphoid tissues (thymus, spleen, tonsils, and lymph nodes); diffuse lymphoid tissue; and lymphoid cells, primarily T lymphocytes (T cells), B lymphocytes (B cells), and macrophages.

Table 14: Review of the immune system

Organ/tissue	Basic structural components	Component functions
Bone marrow	Red marrow	Production of all circulating and tissue resident blood cells including immature T and B lymphocytes. Site of B lymphocytes maturation
	Yellow marrow	Resting bone marrow with little hematopoietic activity
Thymus	Cortex	Maturation of immature T lymphocytes
	Medulla	Development of self-tolerance by deletion of self-reactive clones of T cells
Lymph node	Cortex	B cell activation and clonal expansion to produce large numbers of B lymphocytes reactive to specific antigens. Production of memory T lymphocytes
	Paracortex	T cell activation and clonal expansion to produce large numbers of T lymphocytes reactive to specific antigens. Production of memory T lymphocytes.
	Medulla	Plasma cell maturation and secretion of antibody
Mucosal-associated lymphoid tissue (MALT)	Tonsils Bronchial-associated lymphoid tissue (BALT) Gut-associated lymphoid tissue (GALT)	All components of MALT function in the same fashion as lymph nodes to protect the body from infective organisms presenting at mucosal surfaces.
Spleen	White pulp	Mounts an adaptive immune response against blood borne infective agents
	Red pulp	Filtering the blood to remove particulate matter. Removing damaged and aged erythrocytes. Recycling of iron to the bone marrow.

Table 15: Comparison of the major lymphatic organs

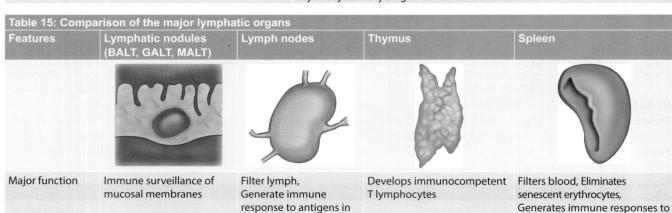

Features	Lymphatic nodules (BALT, GALT, MALT)	Lymph nodes	Thymus	Spleen
Major function	Immune surveillance of mucosal membranes	Filter lymph, Generate immune response to antigens in the lymph	Develops immunocompetent T lymphocytes	Filters blood, Eliminates senescent erythrocytes, Generates immune responses to circulating antigens

Features	Lymphatic nodules (BALT, GALT, MALT)	Lymph nodes	Thymus	Spleen
Connective tissue capsule	No	Yes	Yes	Yes; contains myofibroblasts
Cortex	No	Yes	Yes	No
Medulla	No	Yes	Yes	No
Lymph nodules	Yes	Yes; in the superficial cortex only	No	Yes; in white pulp only
Afferent lymphatic vessels	No	Yes; passing through the capsule	No	No
Efferent lymphatic vessels	Yes	Yes; leaving the node at the hilum	Yes (few); originate in connective tissue septa and capsule	Yes; inconspicuous, originate in white pulp near trabeculae
High endothelial venules (HEVs)	Yes; in well-established lymph nodules (i.e. tonsils, appendix, Peyer's patches)	Yes; associated with deep cortex	No	No
Characteristic features	Diffuse lymphatic tissue with randomly distributed lymphatic nodules underlying epithelial surface	Presence of lymphatic sinuses (subcapsular, trabecular and medullary) Reticular meshwork	Thymic lobules Meshwork of epithelioreticular cells, Hassall's corpuscles in medulla only	White pulp with PALS splenic noduling central artery

BALT: Bronchus-associated lymphatic tisse; GALT: Gut-associated lymphatic tissue; MALT: Mucosa-associated lymphatic tissue; PALS: Periarterial.

Primary lymphoid organs: Lymphocytes differentiate and acquire immunocompetency in the primary (central) lymphatic organs which for B lymphocytes is the **bone marrow** and gut-associated lymphatic tissue (GALT), and for T lymphocytes is the **thymus**.

Secondary lymphoid organs: Lymphocytes enter into the blood or lymphatic vessels to colonize secondary (peripheral) lymphatic tissues, where they undergo the final stages of antigen-dependent activation.

❑ Secondary lymphatic tissues consist of various groups of **lymph nodes** and aggregations of lymphatic nodules, such as **tonsils**, bronchus-associated lymphatic tissue (BALT) in lungs, and mucosa-associated lymphatic tissue (**MALT**) throughout the genitourinary system, **spleen**.

▶ Lymph Node

Lymph nodes contain aggregates of lymphocytes organized into an **outer cortex** (majorly B lymphocytes), a **paracortex** (majorly T lymphocytes), and an **inner medulla**.

❑ The darkly stained 'cortex' just **under the capsule** consists of **lymphoid nodules** (B lymphocytes). These lymphatic nodules contain pale staining **'Germinal centers'** which are major sites of B lymphocyte proliferation.

❑ The subcapsular sinus is the space between the capsule and the cortex which receives the incoming **lymph**.

❑ Lymph → subcapsular sinus → trabecular sinuses → medullary sinuses.

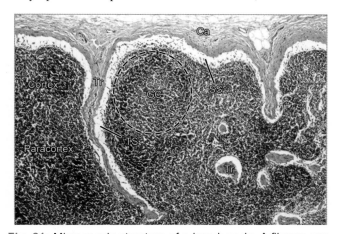

Fig. 21: Microscopic structure of a lymph node. A fibrous connective tissue capsule (Ca) sends in trabecula (Tr) that extend deeply into the node. A prominent subcapsular sinus (SS) is continuous with trabecular sinuses (TS). The outer cortex consists mostly of B lymphocytes. Deeper parts of the cortex—the paracortex—contain mostly T lymphocytes. A lymphoid nodule (broken line) in the cortex contains a germinal center (GC).

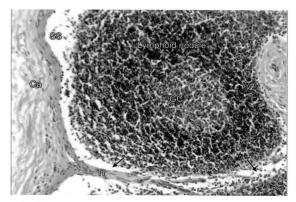

Fig. 22: **Microscopic structure of a lymph node** (Higher magnification). Collagen fibers of the capsule (Ca) and trabecula (Tr) are seen clearly. A broad subcapsular sinus (SS) drains lymph into smaller trabecular sinuses (arrows). Aside from lymph and lymphocytes, sinuses contain reticular fibers and macrophages which cannot be seen at this magnification. The lymphoid nodule has a peripheral rim of closely packed lymphocytes around a pale central zone—a germinal center (GC) —that contains mainly activated B lymphocytes.

▾ Thymus

❑ Precursors of both B cells and T cells are produced in the bone marrow. T lymphocyte precursors migrate to the thymus where they develop into T lymphocytes. After the thymus undergoes involution, T lymphocytes (thymocytes) migrate out of the thymus to the peripheral lymphoid organs such as spleen, tonsils, and lymph nodes where they further differentiate into mature immunologically competent cells which are responsible for cell-mediated immunity. (However, B lymphocyte precursors remain in the bone marrow to develop into B lymphocytes which migrate to the peripheral lymphoid organs where they become mature immunocompetent B cells which are responsible for the humoral immunity. Also, B cells differentiate into plasma cells that synthesize antibodies [immunoglobulins].)

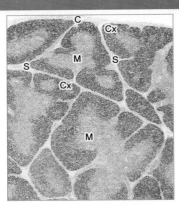

Fig. 23: Thymus is a lobulated organ invested by a loose collagenous *capsule C* from which interlobular *septa S* containing blood vessels radiate into the substance of the organ. The thymic tissue is divided into two distinct zones, a deeply basophilic outer cortex Cx and an inner eosinophilic medulla **M**.

▾ Spleen

Splenic parenchyma is divided into two principal regions – **white pulp** and **red pulp.**

    White pulp accounts for between 5 - 20% of the splenic tissue. It consists of **lymphoid follicles** and **PALS** (Peri Arteriolar Lymphatic Sheath.

❑ It has lymphoid follicles with B lymphocytes at the **germinal centers**, whereas T cell lie in the **periphery**.

❑ The **eccentric arterioles** in lymphoid follicles are surrounded by peripheral T lymphocytes forming PALS.

Red pulp

❑ Constitutes up to ~ 90% of the total splenic volume. It consists of **venous sinusoids** and **splenic cords** (of Billroth).

❑ **Venous sinusoids** that ultimately drain into tributaries of the splenic vein.

❑ Sinusoids show **discontinuous endothelium** that is unique to the spleen.

❑ **Stave** (Littoral) cells are the long, narrow endothelial cells are aligned with the long axis of the sinusoid. The cells arrangement shows **intermittent intercellular slits** that allow blood cells to squeeze into the lumen of the sinusoid from the surrounding splenic cords.

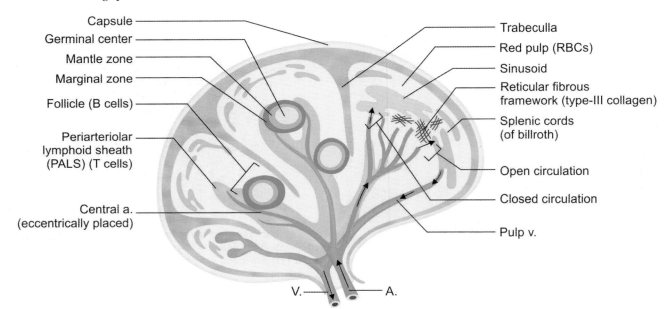

Fig. 24: Structure and blood circulation of spleen. **Note:** Spleen has both open and closed circulation, the blood is exposed to macrophages for filtering and removing abnormal cells and foreign antigens. (Note: direction of blood is shown by the arrows)

- ❑ **Splenic cords** (of Billroth) are present in the intersinusoidal regions contain type III (reticular) collagen fibres alongwith **fibroblasts** and splenic **macrophages**.
  - ➢ These contain half of the human body's **monocytes** as a reserve so that after tissue injury these monocytes can move in and aid locally sourced monocytes in wound healing.
- ❑ **Capsule** sends **trabecula** which extend into the splenic tissue.

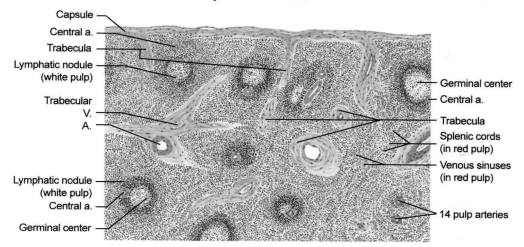

Fig. 25: Spleen (panoramic view). Stain: hematoxylin and eosin. Low magnification Note: **White pulp** is present as ovoid areas of basophilic tissue, alongwith eccentrically placed central artery and surrounding PALS. Red pulp lies between white pulp tissue and consists of splenic sinusoids and intervening cellular cords (of Billroth).

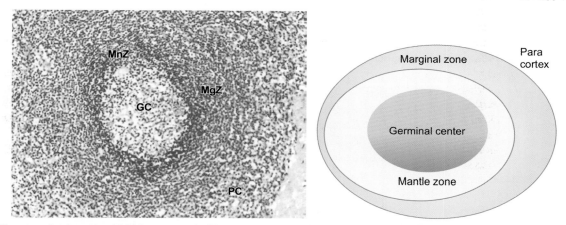

Fig. 26: The **germinal center** (GC) is surrounded by a narrow ring of deep-stained. **Mantle zone** (MnZ) which contains densely packed small lymphocytes (resting B-cells). Still peripheral is the broader. **Marginal zone** (MgZ) which contains less densely packed B lymphocytes. Marginal (perifollicular) zone lies at the interface between the white and red pulp; it contains macrophages and specialized B cells and is where antigen presenting cells (APCs) capture blood borne antigens for recognition by lymphocytes. The Paracortex (PC) is a T-cell zone which lies still peripheral and between lymphatic nodules.

▶ Tonsil

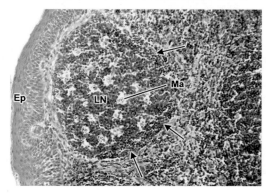

Fig. 27: Lymphoid nodule in the palatine tonsil. Under the stratified squamous epithelium (Ep) that covers the tonsil surface is a profusion of dark-staining, closely packed lymphocytes.

▶ Lymphatics

Lymph capillaries are present in **most tissues** of the body.

   Absent in:
- ❑ Avascular tissues (e.g. the cornea, epidermis, hair, nails, cartilage)
- ❑ Bone and bone marrow
- ❑ Placenta
- ❑ Eyeball, inner ear
- ❑ Striated muscles and tendons.
- ❑ Thymus, spleen
- ❑ Teeth
- ❑ Central or peripheral nervous system

Note: Unlike lymph nodes, the palatine tonsils do not possess afferent lymphatics or lymph sinuses.

QUESTIONS

1. **All of the following are categorized as secondary lymphoid organs EXCEPT:** *(PGIC)*
   - a. Lymph nodes
   - b. Spleen
   - c. Thymus
   - d. Subepithelial collections of lymphocytes
   - e. Bone marrow

2. **Which of the following is the most common site of mucosa associated lymphoid tissue:** *(AIIMS 2014)*
   - a. Stomach
   - b. Duodenum
   - c. Jejunum
   - d. Ileum

3. **Intestinal epithelium has which cell type:** *(AIIMS 2012)*
   - a. T lymphocytes
   - b. B lymphocytes
   - c. Macrophages
   - d. Plasma cells

4. **Follicles are present in which part of lymph nodes:** *(NEET Pattern 2013)*
   - a. Red pulp
   - b. White pulp
   - c. Cortex
   - d. Medulla

5. **GALT (Gut Associated Lymphoid tissue) is present in:** *(AIPG 2009)*
   - a. Submucosa
   - b. Lamina propria
   - c. Muscularis mucosa
   - d. Serosa

6. **All of the following are the components of the white pulp of spleen EXCEPT:** *(AIPG 2006)*
   - a. Periarteriolar lymphoid sheath
   - b. Vascular sinus
   - c. B cells
   - d. Antigen presenting cells

7. **Marked area in the following lymphoid tissue refers to:** *(AIIMS 2017)*

   - a. Marginal zone
   - b. Mantle zone
   - c. Germinal center
   - d. Para-cortical zone

8. **Identify the lymphatic structure shown in the figure** *(AIIMS 2016)*

   - a. Tonsil
   - b. Spleen
   - c. Thymus
   - d. Lymph node

9. **Absence of lymphatics is characteristic of** *(NEET Pattern 2012)*
   - a. Liver
   - b. Brain
   - c. Lung
   - d. Placenta

10. **Organ which have no lymphatic supply** *(PGIC 2016)*
   - a. Eyeball
   - b. Liver
   - c. Spinal cord
   - d. Brain
   - e. Kidney

ANSWERS

1. **c. Thymus; e. Bone marrow**
   - ❑ Primary (central) lymphoid organs have **stem cells** for lymphopoiesis (**bone marrow** and **thymus**). They are involved in **providing immunocompetence** to the lymphocytes.
   - ❑ Secondary (peripheral) lymphoid organs are in the periphery where the lymphocytes **execute** their immunocompetence, e.g. lymph node, tonsil, spleen, MALT (subepithelial collection of lymphocytes, etc.

2. **d. Ileum**
   - ❑ The mucosa-associated lymphoid tissue is a diffuse system of small concentrations of lymphoid tissue in the **lamina propria** of mucosa layer in gastrointestinal tract.
   - ❑ Terminal ileum has large concentrations of MALT arranged in the form of **Peyer patches**.
   - ❑ MALT is populated by lymphocytes such as **T cells** and **B cells**, as well as **plasma cells** and **macrophages** to encounter antigens passing through the mucosal epithelium.

3. **a. T lymphocytes**
   - ❑ Intestinal epithelium has many **scattered migratory immune cells**, predominantly Intra Epithelial Lymphocytes (IEL) for tackling with the antigens in the food (bacteria, protozoa).
   - ❑ IEL display many characteristics of **effector T lymphocyte** cells, hence the answer.

4. **c. Cortex**
   - ❑ Lymphoid follicles are present in the **cortex** region of lymph node.
   - ❑ The **medulla** has cords of lymphatic tissue and sinusoids.
   - ❑ Red and white pulp are features of spleen (**not lymph node**).

5. **b. Lamina propria > a. Submucosa**
   - ❑ GALT is present in the **lamina propria** (mucosa) of the body tubes, though it may also be found in the **submucosa occasionally** (e.g. vermiform appendix).
   - ❑ In vermiform appendix the smooth muscle layer of muscularis mucosa is **interrupted** at places and MALT is present **both** in mucosa and submucosa.
   - ❑ **Peyer's patches** of ileum are under GALT and are mainly present in the **lamina propria** but may also extend into the Submucosa.
   - ❑ GALT and BALT (Bronchus Associated Lymphoid Tissue) come under a common term – MALT (Mucosa Associated Lymphoid Tissue).
   - ❑ Lymphocytes are educated to **recognize and destroy** specific antigens in the MALT.
   - ❑ MALT components are observed at other sites also like Mucosa of reproductive tract.

6. **b. Vascular sinus**
   - ❑ Vascular sinus is included **under red pulp** in spleen.
   - ❑ Spleen is composed of red pulp (~ 90%) having **venous sinusoids** and **splenic cords** (of Billroth).
   - ❑ White pulp (~ 10%) of spleen has **lymphoid follicles** with B lymphocytes at the germinal centers, whereas T cell lie in the periphery. The eccentrically placed arterioles in lymphoid follicles are surrounded by peripheral T lymphocytes forming PALS (**Peri Arteriolar Lymphatic Sheath**).
   - ❑ Antigen presenting cells (APCs) are present in the **marginal zone** of lymphoid follicles.

7. **a. Marginal zone**
   - ❑ This is a histological picture of a **lymphoid organ** showing various **zones around** the lymphatic nodules. The marker represents the area of **Marginal zone**.
   - ❑ The germinal center is surrounded by a narrow ring of deep-stained. **Mantle zone** which contains densely packed small lymphocytes (resting B-cells). Still peripheral is the broader **Marginal** (perifollicular) zone which contains less densely packed B lymphocytes; lying at the interface between the white and red pulp.

8. **a. Tonsil**
   - ❑ This is a slide of **lymphatic tissue**, showing abundance of **lymphocytes** (blue dots), one **lymphoid follicle** is also evident and so is the lining **stratified squamous epithelium** (characteristic finding in **tonsil**). None of the other lymphoid organ show any such epithelium EXCEPT: tonsil, though the other findings may be evident.
   - ❑ Lymphoid tissue can be easily recognized by the presence of aggregation of dark-staining nuclei (lymphocytes), e.g. tonsil, lymph node, spleen, thymus, etc.
   - ❑ Identification point for **spleen** is the **lymphoid nodule** (with pale germinal center and **eccentrically placed** arteriole).
   - ❑ **Thymus** is identified by multiple **Hassall's corpuscles** in the central light staining area surrounded by dense/dark lymphatic tissue in periphery.
   - ❑ **Lymph node** has an outer capsule with a prominent **broad subcapsular sinus**. Lymphatic nodules are present with pale staining germinal center and dark, staining periphery.

9. **b. Brain**
   - ❑ Lymphatic capillaries are **absent from avascular** structures (e.g. epidermis, cornea, cartilage), from the CNS and meninges, choroid, internal ear; Eyeball (EXCEPT: conjunctiva); bone marrow; striated muscle and tendons etc.

10. **a. Eyeball; c. Spinal cord; d. Brain**

- ▪ Subcapsular sinuses are seen in the **lymph node**. *(NEET Pattern 2012)*
- ▪ Cords of Billroth are present in the **red pulp** of the spleen. *(NEET Pattern 2013)*
- ▪ **Stave cells** are seen in the spleen. *(NEET Pattern 2012)*

▰ Integumentary System

- ❑ **Skin** consists of two components: epidermis and dermis.
- ❑ The surface epithelium (epidermis) is of the keratinized stratified squamous variety.
- ❑ The deeper dermis consists mainly of bundles of collagen fibers together with some elastic tissue, blood vessels, lymphatics and nerve fibers.
- ❑ Color of skin is determined by the degree of pigmentation produced by melanocytes in the basal layer of the epidermis.
- ❑ Hair and nails are a hard type of keratin; the keratin of the skin surface is soft keratin. Each hair is formed from the hair matrix, a region of epidermal cells at the base of the hair follicle, which extends
- ❑ **Sweat glands** are exocrine glands with a small tubular structures of the skin that secrete sweat onto an epithelial surface by way of a duct.

- ❏ They are distributed all over the skin **EXCEPT:** on the tympanic membranes, lip margins, nipples, inner surface of prepuce, glans penis and labia minora.
- ❏ The greatest concentration is in the thick skin of the **palms** and **soles**, and on the face.
- ❏ They are two types: Eccrine and apocrine
  1. **Eccrine** sweat glands are distributed almost all over the human body and has water-based secretion meant primary form of cooling the body.
  ➤ Eccrine glands are innervated by the **sympathetic cholinergic** fibers.
  2. **Apocrine** sweat glands are rare to find and are mostly limited to axilla, areola, periumbilical, genital and perianal. regions
  ➤ **Ceruminous** glands (ear wax), **mammary** glands (milk), and **ciliary** glands in the eyelids are modified apocrine sweat glands.
  ➤ Their ducts open into hair follicles or directly on to the skin surface.
  ➤ Apocrine glands are innervated by the **sympathetic adrenergic** fibers.

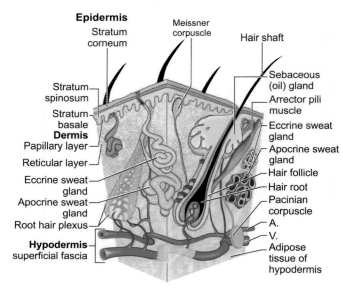

Fig. 28: Skin and its derivatives.

- ❏ **Sebaceous glands** are **holocrine** glands, small saccular structures in the dermis and open into the side of hair follicles.
- ❏ They also open directly on to the surface of the hairless skin of the lips, nipples, areolae, inner surface of prepuce, glans penis and labia minora.
- ❏ They are in large concentration on the face but **none** on the palms or soles.
- ❏ Androgens act on these glands which have no motor innervation.
- ❏ The epidermis of thick skin consists of **five layers** of cells (keratinocytes): stratum **corneum** (characterized by dead and dying cells with compacted keratin), stratum **lucidum** (a translucent layer not obvious in thin skin), stratum **granulosum** (characterized by keratohyalin granules), stratum **spinosum** (characterized by tonofibrils and associated desmosomes) and stratum **basale** (proliferative layer).

Table 16: Characteristics of thick and thin skin		
Cellular strata (Superficial to deepest)	**Thick skin**	**Thin skin**
Epidermis	Is a stratified squamous keratinized epithelium derived from ectoderm. Cells of the epidermis consist of four cell types: keratinocytes, melanocytes, Langerhans cells and Merkel cells.	
Stratum corneum (Cornified cell layer)	Composed of several layers of dead, anucleated, flattened keratinocytes (squames) that are being sloughed from the surface. As many as 50 layers of keratinocytes are located in the thickest skin (e.g. sole of the foot).	Only about five or so layers of keratinocytes (squames) comprise this layer in the thinnest skin (e.g. eyelids).
Stratum lucidum (Clear cell layer)	Poorly stained keratinocytes filled with keratin compose this thin, well-defined layer. Organelles and nuclei are absent.	Layer is absent but individual cells of the layer are probably present.
Stratum granulosum (Granular cell layer)	Only three to five layers thick with polygonal-shaped nucleated keratinocytes with a normal complement of organelles as well as keratohyalin and membrane-coating granules.	Layer is absent but individual cells of the layer are probably present.
Stratum spinosum (Prickle cell layer)	This thickest layer is composed of mitotically active and maturing polygonal keratinocytes (prickle cells) that interdigitate with one another via projections (intercellular bridges) that are attached to each other by desmosomes. The cytoplasm is rich in tonofilaments, organelles, and membrane-coating granules, Langerhans cells are present in this layer.	The stratum is the same as in thick skin but the number of layers is reduced.
Stratum basale (Stratum germinativum)	This deepest stratum is composed of a single layer of mitotically active tall cuboidal keratinocytes that are in contact with the basal lamina. Keratinocytes of the more superficial strata originate from this layer and eventually migrate to the surface where they are sloughed. Melanocytes and Merkel cells are also present in this layer.	This layer is the same in thin skin as in thick skin.

Cellular strata (Superficial to deepest)	Thick skin	Thin skin
Dermis	Located deep to the epidermis and separated from it by a basement membrane, the dermis is derived from mesoderm and is composed mostly of dense irregular collagenous connective tissue. It contains capillaries, nerves, sensory organs, hair follicles, seat and sebaceous glands, as well as arrector pilli muscles. It is divided into two layers: a superficial papillary layer and a deeper reticular layer.	
Papillary layer	Is composed of loose connective tissue containing capillary loops and terminals of mechanoreceptors. These dermal papillae interdigitate with the epidermal ridges of the epidermis. These interdiginations are very prominent in thick skin.	The papillary layer is comprised of the same loose connective tissue as in thick skin. However, its volume is much reduced. The depth of the dermal/epidermal interdiginations is also greatly reduced.
Reticular layer	Is composed of dense irregular collagenous connective tissue containing the usual array of connective tissue elements, including cells, blood and lymphatic vessels. Sweat glands and cutaneous nerves are also present and their branches extend into the papillary layer and into the epidermis.	Same as in thick skin. Sebaceous glands and hair follicles along with their arrector pilli muscles are observed.

Table 17: Nonkeratinocytes of the epidermis				
Nonepithelial cells	Origin	Location	Features	Function
Melanocytes	Derived from neural crest	Migrate into stratum basale during embryonic development. Some remain undifferentiated even in adulthood (reserved to maintain melanocyte population). Do not form desmosomal contact with keratinocytes but some may form hemidesmosomes with basal lamina.	Form long processes (dendrites) that pass into the stratum spinosum. Melanocytes possess melanosomes within their cytoplasm where melanin is manufactured. Melanocytes form associations with several keratinocytes (epidermal-melanin unit). Population = to about 3% of epidermal population.	Manufacture melanin pigment. Melanosomes located in the cytoplasm are activated to produce melanin (eumelanin in dark hair and pheomelanin in red and blond hair). Once melanosomes are filled with melanin, they travel up the dendrites and are released into the extracellular space. Keratinocytes of the stratum spinosum phagocytose these melanin-laden melanosomes. The melanosomes migrate to the nuclear region of the keratinocyte and form a protective umbrella, shielding the nucleus (and its chromosomes) from the ultraviolet rays of the sun. Soon, the melanosomes are destroyed by keratinocyte lysosomes.
				UV rays increase melanin production, its dark-skinned individuals. They are larger and dispersed throughout the cytoplasm. Melanosome destructions at a slower pace in darker skin.
Langerhans cells	Derived from bone marrow	Mostly located in the stratum spinosum	Possess long processes; thus they are known as dendritic cells. Nucleus possesses many indentations. Cytoplasm contains Birbeck granules, elongated vesicles exhibiting a ballooned-out terminus. Do not form desmosomal contact with keratinocytes.	Are antigen-presenting cells. These cells possess surface markers and receptors as well as langerin a transmembrane protein associated with Birbeck granules. Some of these elements facilitate an immune response against the organism responsible for leprosy. Additionally, Langerhans cells phagocytose antigens that enter the epidermis and migrate to lymph vessels located in the dermis and form there into the paracortex of a lymph node to present these antigens to T cells, thereby activating a delayed-type hypersensitivity response.
Merkel cells	Believed to be a modified keratinocyte, although origin is uncertain	Interspersed with keratinocytes of the stratum basale. They are most abundant in the fingertips	Merkel cells form complexes, known as Merkel discs with terminals of afferent nerves.	Merkel cells function as mechanoreceptors (touch receptor). There is some evidence that Merkel cells may also function as neurosecretory cells.

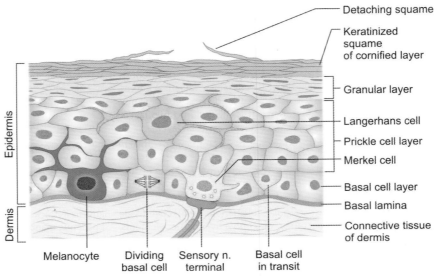

Fig. 29: Layers of skin and the various cells associated with its different layers.

Hypodermis

- **Hypodermis** the layer of loose connective tissue immediately deep to the dermis of the skin. It contains: loosely arranged elastic fibers fibrous bands anchoring skin to deep fascia; fat (**panniculus adiposus**); blood vessels and lymphatics on route to dermis, hair follicle roots; the glandular part of some sweat glands; nerves: free endings; Pacinian corpuscles; bursae: only in the space overlying joints in order to facilitate smooth passage of overlying skin; sheets of muscle: **panniculus carnosus**.

- **Panniculus** (a thin layer) **adiposus** is a layer of adipose connective tissue subjacent to the reticular layer of the dermis. It's distribution defines secondary sexual characteristic: it forms the breasts of females and accentuates the contour of female hips. It functions as an insulating compartment and as a storage site for energy. It is absent in eyelid, external ear, scrotum, penis, nipple and areola, e.g. superficial cervical fascia, Camper fascia (superficial fatty layer of the subcutaneous tissue of the abdomen, external to the membranous layer).

- The **panniculus carnosus** is a thin layer of skeletal muscle within the superficial fascia, deep to the panniculus adiposus. One end of each muscle fiber is attached to the skin, the other end being usually attached to deep fascia or bone. For example, some of the muscles of facial expression, platysma muscle of the neck, palmaris brevis in the hand, subareolar muscle of the nipple, dartos muscle in the scrotum, corrugator cutis ani, etc.

Receptors

- Sensory receptors are of three types :
    1. Exteroceptors—receive information from the outside environment.
    2. Proprioceptors—receive information from muscles, tendons, and joint structures.
    3. Interoceptors—receive information from within the internal environment.
- **Merkel cells** are surface ectoderm derivatives located at the basal layers of epidermis. They are slowly adapting receptors to detect light touch. They are the most capable cells detecting the braille characters (as compared with Meissner corpuscles).
- **Meissner corpuscles** are rapidly adapting, encapsulated receptors in the dermal papillae (dermoepidermo junction). They are distributed in eyelids, lips, nipples, fingertips. They carry fine touch perception, which is essential for tactile discrimination, and reading Braille.
- **Pacinian corpuscles** are rapidly adapting encapsulated receptors in the deep dermis and in the connective tissue of the mesenteries and joints. They carry the information of pressure, touch, and vibration.
- **Ruffini receptors** are slowly adapting encapsulated structure in the dermis and joints. They perceive dermal stretch and pressure.
- **Free nerve endings** are un-encapsulated, nonmyelinated terminations in the skin to carry pain, temperature, etc.
- **Golgi tendon organs** are encapsulated mechanoreceptors sensitive to stretch and tension in tendons and carry proprioceptive information.
- **Muscle spindle** receptors are also encapsulated and carry proprioception. They have intrafusal muscle fibers called flower spray endings and annulospiral endings that sense differences in muscle length and tension.

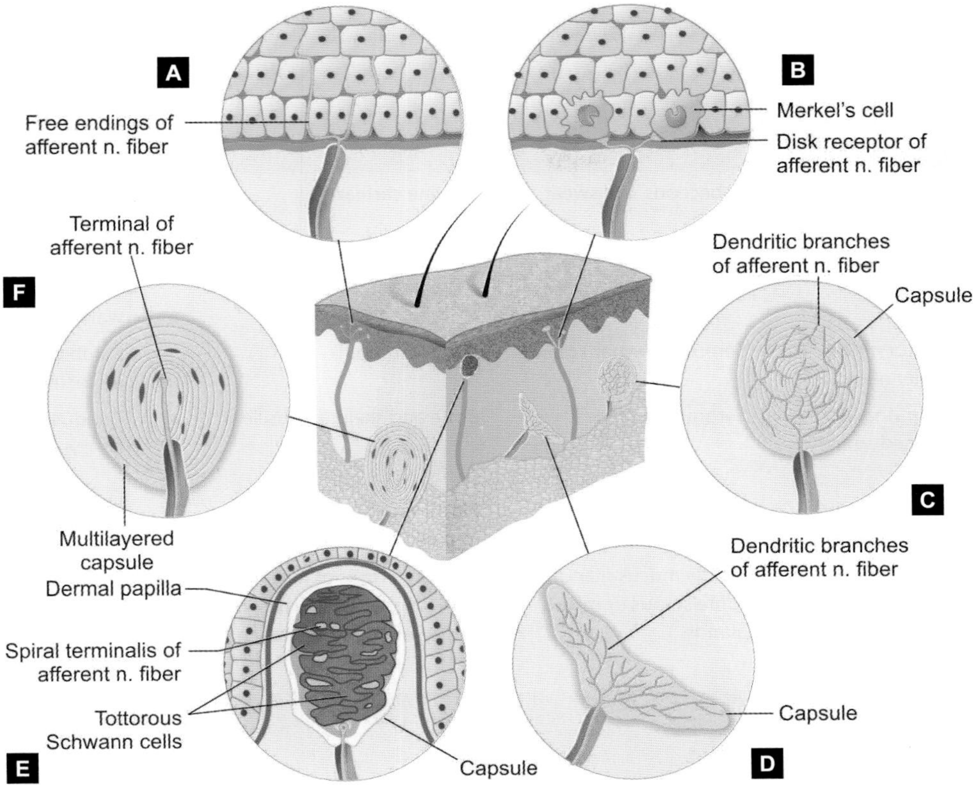

Figs. 30A to F: Various type of sensory receptors in skin. (A) Epidermal free endings. (B) Merkel's corpuscles containing merkel's cells and disc receptors of afferent myelinated nerve fibere. (C) Krause's end bulb serves as cold receptor. (D) Ruffini's corpuscle in deep layers of the dermis. (E) Meissner's corpuscle in dermal papilla. (F) Pacinian corpuscle located in the deep layer of deep dermis and hypodermis. Sensory nerve fibers in receptors c-f are encapsulated.

QUESTIONS

1. **Panniculus adiposus is seen in:** *(AIIMS 2014)*
   a. Scrotum   b. Orbit
   c. Eyelid   d. Penis

2. **Which of the following faithfully represents the Braille characters:** *(NEET Pattern 2015)*
   a. Meissner's corpuscle   b. Merkel cell
   c. Pacinian corpuscle   d. Ruffini receptor

3. **TRUE about Merkel cell:** *(PGIC)*
   a. Neural crest cell derivative
   b. Rapidly adapting receptor
   c. Dermal stretch receptor
   d. Neural basis for reading Braille text
   e. Detect pain and temperature

4. **What constitutes Malpighian layer:** *(NEET Pattern 2018)*
   a. Stratum lucidum
   b. Stratum spinosum
   c. Stratum granulosum
   d. Stratum spinosum and basale

ANSWERS

1. **b. Orbit**
   ❑ Panniculus adiposus is the **subcutaneous fat**, a layer of adipose tissue underlying the dermis.
   ❑ It is **absent** in eyelid, external ear, scrotum, penis, nipple and areola.

2. **b. Merkel cell > a. Meissner's corpuscle**
   ❑ Merkel fibers **faithfully** represent the pattern of Braille dots. Meissner's fibers produced a **blurry image**, while the deep sensors (the Pacinian and Ruffini) encode the Braille dots **poorly**.

3. **d. Neural basis for reading Braille text**
   ❑ Neural basis for reading Braille is **Merkel cell** > Meissner's corpuscle (**detection capability**).
   ❑ Merkel cell is a **slowly adapting** receptor at the basal layer of epidermis for detection of **light touch sensations**. It is derived from **surface ectoderm** (some authorities believe it is a **neural crest cell** derivative).
   ❑ Free nerve endings detect **pain and temperature** form the skin.
   ❑ Ruffini receptor perceives **dermal stretch**.

4. **d. Stratum spinosum and basale**
   ❑ Malpighian layer of the skin is generally defined as both the **stratum spinosum** and **stratum basale** as a unit.

❑ The **panniculus adiposus** is the fatty layer of the subcutaneous tissues, superficial to a deeper vestigial layer of muscle, the **panniculus carnosus**.

▶ Respiratory System

Table 18: Histologic features of the upper respiratory tract, larynx, and trachea.

Region	Epithelium	Glands	Musculoskeletal support	Other features and major functions
Vestibules of nasal cavities	Stratified squamous, keratinized to nonkeratinized	Sebaceous and sweat glands	Hyaline cartilage	Vibrissae (stiff hairs) and moisture both filter and humidify air
Most areas of nasal cavities	Respiratory	Seromucus glands	Bone and hyaline cartilage	Rich vasculature and glands warm. humidify, and clean air
Superior areas of nasal cavities	Olfactory, with bipolar neurons	Serous (Bowman) glands	Bone (ethmoid)	Soluble and detect odorant molecules in air
Nasopharynx and posterior oropharynx	Respiratory and stratified squamous	Seromucus glands	Bone and skeletal muscle	Conduct air to larynx; pharyngeal and palatine tonsils
Larynx	Respiratory and stratified squamous	Mucus glands, smaller seromucus glands	Elastic and hyaline cartilage, ligaments, skeletal muscle	Site for phonation; epiglottis closes while swallowing
Trachea	Respiratory	Mainly mucus glands, some serous or mixed glands	C-shaped rings of hyaline cartilage, with smooth (trachealis) muscle in posterior opening of each	Conduct air to primary bronchi entering lungs; some MALT

Table 19: Features of airways within the lungs.

Region of airway	Epithelium	Muscle and skeletal support	Other features and major functions
Bronchi	Respiratory	Prominent spiral bands of smooth muscle: irregular hyaline cartilage plates	Repeated branching; conduct air deeper into lungs
Bronchioles	Simple ciliated cuboidal to columnar with Clara cells	Prominent circular layer of smooth muscle: no cartilage	Conduct air; important in bronchoconstriction and bronchodilation
Terminal bronchioles	Simple cuboidal, ciliated and Clara cells	Thin. incomplete circular layer of smooth muscle; no cartilage	Conduct air to respiratory portions of lungs; Clara cells with several protective functions
Respiratory bronchioles	Simple cuboidal, ciliated and Clara cells, with scattered alveoli	Fewer smooth muscle fibers, mostly around alveolar openings	Conduct air deeper with some gas exchange and protective Clara cells
Alveolar ducts and sacs	Simple cuboidal between many alveoli	Bands of smooth muscle around alveolar openings	Conduct air, with much gas exchange
Alveoli	Types I and II alveolar cells (pneumocytes)	None (but with network of elastic and reticular fibers)	Sites of all gas exchange; surfactant from type II pneumocytes; dust cells

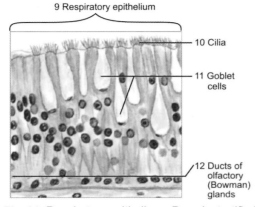

Fig. 31: Respiratory epithelium - Pseudostratified ciliated columnar epithelium with goblet cells.

9 Respiratory epithelium
10 Cilia
11 Goblet cells
12 Ducts of olfactory (Bowman) glands

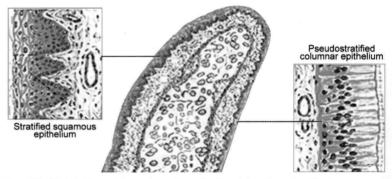

Stratified squamous epithelium

Pseudostratified columnar epithelium

Fig. 32: Epiglottis - Lingual surface is lined by the stratified squamous epithelium; Laryngeal surface is lined by respiratory epithelium and the core has elastic cartilage.

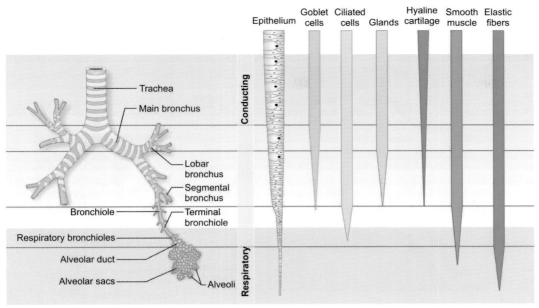

Fig. 33: Tracheobronchial tree and its characteristic microscopic features. Respiratory epithelium changes from columnar to cuboidal to squamous proximo-distally. The number of goblet cells, and hylaine cartilage are almost non-existent beyond the level of bronchus.

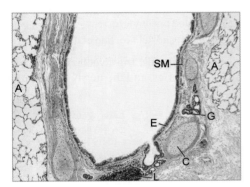

Fig. 34: Intrapulmonary bronchus (cross section) - Lumen is lined by pseudostratified ciliated columnar epithelium with goblet cells (E). Beneath the epithelium in the lamina propria of loose, fibroelastic connective tissue are bundle of smooth muscle cells (SM) wrapped in a spiraling arrangement around the lumen. In the submucosal connective tissue outside of the smooth muscle are irregular plates of cartilage (C), seromucus glands (G), and lymphoid tissue (L). Alveoli (A) are evident in the nearby respiratory tissue.

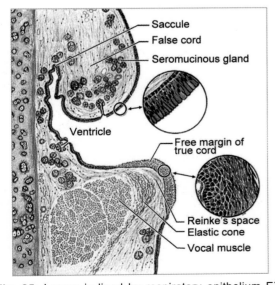

Fig. 35: Larynx is lined by respiratory epithelium EXCEPT: at the vocal cords (which are lined by stratified squamous epithelium). The core cartilage is hyaline in nature.

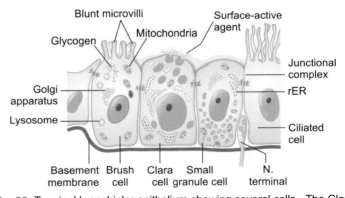

Fig. 36: Terminal bronchiolar epithelium showing several cells - The Clara cell in interposted between the brush cell and the small granule cell. The Clara cell is a nonciliated cell that has rounded apical surface, well-developed basal eER and Golgi apparatus and contains secretory vesicles filled with a surface-active agent containing blunt microvilli, which are distinctive features of this cell. Cytoplasm of the brush cell shows a Golgi apparatus and glycogen inclusions. A small granule cell is shown located between the Clara cell and ciliated cell. This cell contains small secretory vesicles, most of which are in the basal portion of the cell. In addition to the vesicles, the most conspicuous organelles of this cell are rER, a Golgi apparatus, and mitochondria. A nerve terminal is shown within the epithelium.

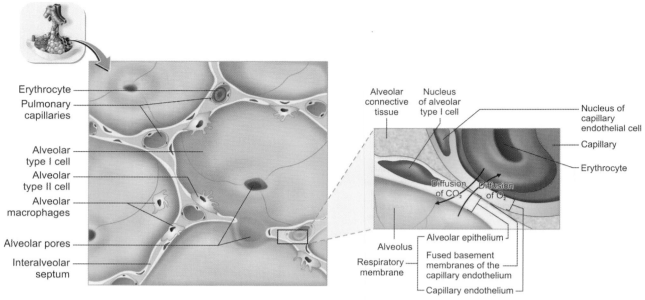

Fig. 37: Microscopic picture of an alveolus, showing respiratory membrane and the respiratory gas exchange.

Table 20: Components of the blood-air barrier		
Endothelial component	**Epithelial and pneumocyte component**	**Pneumocyte component**
Attenuated endothelial cell	Combined basal laminae	Attenuated penumocyte I
		Surfactant and fluid coating of the alveolous

❑ The air–blood barrier consists of alveolar **type I cells,** basal lamina, and capillary endothelial cells. The alveolar **type II** cells secrete surfactant. Gas exchange occurs between the walls of alveoli and pulmonary capillaries, and the newly oxygenated blood enters venules and then pulmonary veins.

QUESTIONS

1. Epithelium lining of lingual surface of epiglottis is:
   a. Simple columnar
   b. Pseudostratified ciliated columnar
   c. Simple cuboidal
   d. Stratified squamous epithelium

2. Hyaline cartilage of respiratory tree extends up to:
   (NEET Pattern 2012)
   a. Tertiary bronchiole
   b. Secondary bronchiole
   c. Terminal bronchiole
   d. Bronchus

3. The structure lying distal to respiratory bronchiole is:
   (NEET Pattern 2015)
   a. Bronchi
   b. Tertiary bronchiole
   c. Terminal bronchiole
   d. Alveolar duct

4. All of the following cells are found in lung EXCEPT:
   (AIPG 2008)
   a. Kulchitsky cells
   b. Clara cells
   c. Brush cells
   d. Langerhans cells

5. Trachea is lined by: *(NEET Pattern 2012)*
   a. Stratified squamous epithelium
   b. Ciliated columnar epithelium
   c. Simple columnar epithelium
   d. Pseudostratified columnar epithelium

6. Which of the following is lined by an epithelium containing ciliated cells and Clara cells:
   a. Nasopharynx
   b. Trachea
   c. Respiratory bronchiole
   d. Intrapulmonary bronchi

ANSWERS

1. d. Stratified squamous epithelium
   ❑ Epiglottis has **two surfaces,** the lingual surface is lined by oral epithelium, which is **stratified squamous** epithelium.
   ❑ The **laryngeal** surface has **respiratory** epithelium—**pseudostratified ciliated columnar** epithelium with goblet cells.
   ❑ **Larynx** is lined by respiratory epithelium (pseudostratified ciliated columnar epithelium with goblet cells) **EXCEPT:** at the vocal cords, which are lined by **stratified squamous** epithelium.

2. d. Bronchus
   ❑ Hyaline cartilage extends **till the bronchi** and are absent (or scatteredly present) distally in the bronchioles.
   ❑ Bronchioles have **smaller lumen** and are lined by **more of smooth muscles** in place of cartilage.
   ❑ Goblet cells also **extend till bronchus** level; beyond that they are present scatteredly.

3. d. Alveolar duct
   ❑ Bronchioles have a diameter **smaller than 1 mm** and lack **cartilage** and **glands** within their walls. Goblet cells (and cilia) decrease in number and **almost negligible** at the levels of bronchioles (small lumen). **Hyaline cartilage** also is almost non-existent at the levels of bronchioles. **Epithelium gradually changes** from pseudostratified columnar to simple columnar to cuboidal to squamous.
   ❑ Alveolus is lined by **type-I pneumocyte** (simple squamous epithelium) for respiratory gas exchange. **Type- II pneumocyte** is a cuboidal cell for surfactant secretion.

ANSWERS

4. d. Langerhans cells

- **Langerhans** cells are **antigen presenting cells** located in the **skin** and migrate towards **lymphoid tissue.** In abnormal conditions like **histiocytosis**, there they invade the lung in large numbers.
- **Kulchitsky** cells are the **neuro-endocrine cells** found in the lining epithelium of lung and belong to the APUD system. They secrete hormones like **serotonin**.
- **Clara** cells are the non-ciliated cuboidal/columnar cells in the wall of **terminal** / respiratory **bronchioles**. They function as **stem cells for repair** of epithelium and also **secrete the surfactant** lipoproteins like the type- II pneumocytes.
- **Brush cells have microvilli** at their surface and are innervated by nerve fibers, and function as **receptor cells**.

5. d. Pseudostratified columnar epithelium > b. Ciliated columnar epithelium

- Trachea is lined by **respiratory** epithelium - Pseudostratified ciliated columnar epithelium **with goblet cells**.

6. c. Respiratory bronchiole

- Clara (club) cells are predominantly present in the **terminal bronchiole** and also in respiratory bronchiole.

- **Clara cells** are dome-shaped cells with **short microvilli**, found in the **terminal bronchioles** and extend into respiratory bronchioles as well in (*NEET Pattern 2012*)

▶ Digestive System

Table 21: Summary of distinguishing digesting tract features, by region and layers

Region and subdivisions	Mucosa (epithelium, lamina propria, muscularis mucosae)	Submucosa (with submucosal plexuses)	Muscularis (inner circular and outer longitudinal layers, with myenteric plexuses between them)	Adventitia/serosa
Esophagus (upper, middle, lower)	Nonkeratinized stratified squamous epithelium; cardiac glands at lower end	Small esophageal glands (mainly mucus)	Both layers striated muscle in upper region; both layers smooth muscle in lower region; smooth and striated muscle fascicles mingled in middle region	Adventitia, EXCEPT: at lower end with serosa
Stomach (cardia, fundus, body, pylorus)	Surface mucus cells and gastric pits leading to gastric glands with parietal and chief cells, (in the fundus and body) or to mucus cardiac glands and pyloric glands	No distinguishing features	Three indistint layers of smooth muscle (inner oblique, middle circular, and outer longitudinal	Serosa
Small intestine (duodenum, jejunum, ileum)	Plicae circulares; villi, with enterocytes and goblet cells, and crypts/glands with Paneth cells and stem cells; Peyer patches in ileum	Duodenal (Brunner) glands (entirely mucus); possible extensions of Peyer patches in ileum	No distinguishing features	Mainly serosa
Large intestine (cecum, colon, rectum)	Intestinal glands with goblet cells and absorptive cells	No distinguishing features	Outer longitudinal layer separated into three bands, the teniae coli	Mainly serosa, with adventitia at rectum
Anal canal	Stratified squamous epithelium; longitudinal anal columns	Venous sinuses	Inner circular layer thickened as internal sphincter	Adventitia

- **Gut tube has 4 layers:** Mucosa, submucosa, muscularis externa and adventitia/serosa.
- Lamina propria is a part of mucosa and contains glands, blood vessels and components of immune system-GALT.
- **Muscularis mucosa** is also a part of mucosa and mainly composed of smooth muscles. Its contraction moves the mucosa to facilitate secretion and absorption.
- **Submucosa** consists of mainly dense irregular connective tissue. It has neurovascular branches and some lymphatics also. The Meissner's plexus is mainly a collection of parasympathetic neurons observed in submucosa only.
- **Adventitia/Serosa** are the outermost covering of GI tube. Adventitia is chiefly made up of connective tissue, whereas, serosa has the serous membrane made up of squamous epithelium.

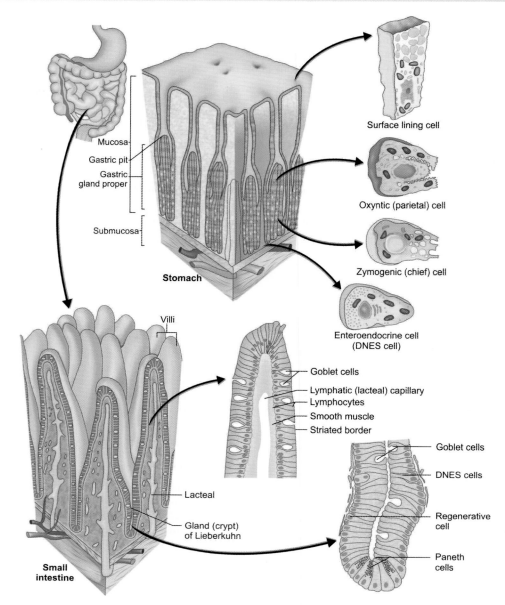

Fig. 38: Mucosa of stomach and intestine showing various type of cells.

▶ Oral Cavity

Table 22: Review of oral tissues	
Structure	**Details**
Oral mucosa	Stratified squamous epithelium with variable site-dependent keratinization
Teeth	Enamel: Surface layer of closely packed calcium hydroxyapatite crystals formed by an external ameloblast layer; destroyed with tooth eruption
	Dentine: Deeper zone of calcified tissue containing numerous fine parallel tubules radiating from odontoblasts which line the pulp cavity and form dentine
	Pulp: Central core of loose tissue with nerves and vessels supplying odontoblasts
Tongue	Muscular organ with layers of skeletal muscle fibers oriented perpendicular to each other; numerous minor salivary glands and surface stratified squamous eprthelium with filiform, fungiform and circumvallate papillae
Taste buds	Sensory organs of taste situated in tongue mucosa
Salivary glands	Serous and/or mucinous glands; found as large glands (parotid, submandibular and sublingual) and innumerable small (minor) glands
Tonsils and lingual tonsils	Lymphoid organs near posterior tongue and extension of similar structures onto posterior tongue

□ Oral cavity has non-keratinized stratified squamous epithelium. **Para-keratinization:** persistence of the nuclei of the keratinocytes into the stratum corneum; this is normal only in the epithelium of true mucus membranes of the mouth and vagina.

▶ Esophagus

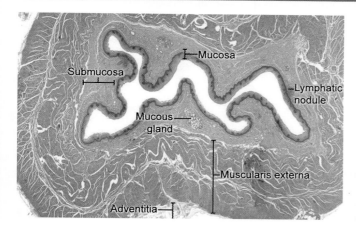

Fig. 39: Esophagus with its characteristically folded wall, giving the lumen an irregular appearance. The mucosa consists of a relatively thick stratified squamous epithelium, a thin layer of lamina propria containing occasional lymphatic nodules, and muscularis mucosae. Mucus glands are present in the submucosa, their ducts, which empty into the lumen of the esophagus, are not evident in this section. External to the submucosa in this part of the esophagus is a thick muscularis externa made up of an inner layer of circularly arranged smooth muscle and an outer layer of longitudinally arranged smooth muscle. The adventitia is seen just external to the muscularis externa.

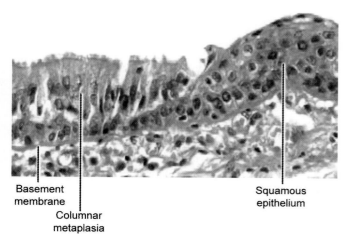

Fig. 40: Intestinal metaplasia in Barret's esophagus (Replacement of the normal stratified squamous epithelium by the columnar epithelium with goblet cells).

QUESTIONS

1. **All are true about esophagus EXCEPT:** (NEET Pattern 2013)
   a. Lined by stratified squamous epithelium
   b. Mucosa is thick
   c. Middle third contains both skeletal and smooth muscles
   d. Lower third contains only skeletal muscle

2. **Strongest layer of esophagus is:** (AIPG)
   a. Mucosa
   b. Submucosa
   c. Muscular externa
   d. Serosa

ANSWERS

1. **d. Lower third contains only skeletal muscle**
   □ In the **upper third** of the esophagus, the muscularis externa is formed by **skeletal** muscle; in the **middle third**, smooth muscle fascicles **intermingle** with striated muscle; and this increases distally such that the **lower third** contains **only smooth muscle**.
   □ Oesophagus is lined by a **thick mucosa** with the **stratified squamous** epithelium.

2. **b. Submucosa**
   □ The **submucosa** consists of a layer of fibroelastic connective tissue containing blood vessels and nerves. It is the **strongest component** of the esophagus and intestinal wall and therefore should be included in **anastomotic sutures**.

- Esophagus does not have **serosa** (NEET Pattern 2016)
- Barrett's esophagus is diagnosed by **intestinal metaplasia** (AIIMS)

▶ Stomach

Table 23: Principal secretions of the epithelial cells of the stomach		
Gastric glands of the stomach	Approximate life span of the cells	Secretions
Surface lining cells	3–5 days	Visible mucus
Mucus neck cells	6 days	Soluble mucus

Gastric glands of the stomach	Approximate life span of the cells	Secretions
Parietal cells	200 days	Hydrochloric acid, gastric intrinsic factor
Chief cells	60–90 days	Pepsin, rennin, lipase precursors
Diffuse neuroendocrine system cells	60–90 days	Gastrin, somatostatin, secretin, cholecystokinin
Regenerative cells	Function to replace epithelial lining of stomach and cells of glands	

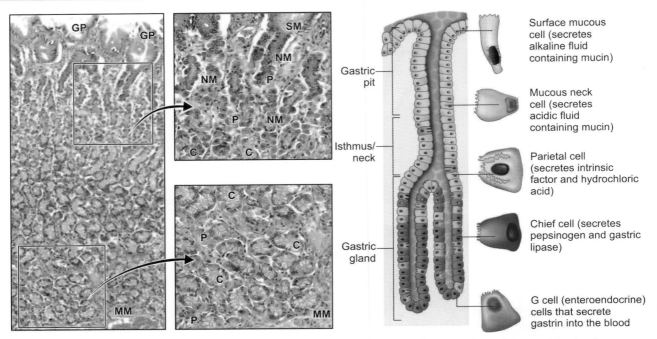

Fig. 41: Microscopic features of the various types of cells present in different regions of the gastric glands.

Table 24: Various type of cells present in the gastric mucosa

Cell type	Predominant location in stomach (gross anatomy)	Predominant location in gastric gland (histology)
Mucus	Cardia and pylorus	Neck
Parietal	Body	Body
Chief	Fundus	Fundus
NEC	Pylorus	Fundus
Stem	Omnipresent	Isthmus

❑ **Mucous** cells are small, dark stained, columnar cell
❑ Located close to gastric pit (neck region of gastric gland)
❑ **Parietal** (Oxyntic) cells are lightly eosinophilic (clear cytoplasm) large cuboidal cell, with central spherical nucleus (fried egg appearance).
❑ Predominantly present in the upper half of the gland, more so in the body region of the gastric gland.
❑ They secrete hydrochloric acid and intrinsic factor.
❑ Gastric intrinsic factor is essential for absorption of **vitamin B12** (and erythropoiesis).
   ➤ In pernicious anemia, autoantibodies destroy the parietal cells leading to deficiency of intrinsic factor and resultant Vit. B12 absorption, which further leads to megaloblastic anemia.
❑ **Chief cells** are small, basophilic columnar cells, more numerous in the lower half of the gland—more so at the base (fundus) of the gastric gland.
❑ Contain zymogen granules/pepsinogen.
❑ **Neuroendocrine cells** are small cells, found at the deeper areas—base (fundus) of the gastric gland, along with chief cells.
❑ **Stem cells** are pluripotent cell, located at the isthmus region of gastric gland.
❑ They help in repair of gastric epithelium.
❑ The secretory activities of the chief and parietal cells are controlled by the autonomic nervous system and the hormone gastrin, secreted by the enteroendocrine cells of the pyloric region of the stomach.
❑ The **enteroendocrine cells** are also called APUD (amine precursor uptake and decarboxylation) cells.

1. Chief Cells are found in which part of the gastric gland:
   a. Fundus   b. Pit   *(AIPG 2009)*
   c. Neck   d. Body

2. Oxyntic cells are present in: *(NEET Pattern 2016)*
   a. Pylorus   b. Cardiac notch
   c. Body   d. Fundus

3. All are correct about stomach EXCEPT: *(NEET Pattern 2016)*
   a. Pylorus has more acid secreting cells
   b. Lots of mucus secreting cells in pylorus
   c. Chief cells secrete pepsinogen
   d. Parietal cells secrete intrinsic factor

4. Which of the following marked cells in the slide secrete hydrochloric acid: *(AIIMS 2016)*

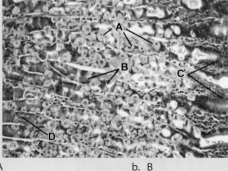

   a. A   b. B
   c. C   d. D

1. a. Fundus
   ❑ Chief cells are usually **basal (fundal)** in location.
   ❑ Neuroendocrine cells are also situated mainly in the **deeper/basal** parts of the glands, **along with the chief cells**.

2. c. Body
   ❑ Oxyntic cells are predominantly seen in the **body part** of the stomach. They are present in the **fundus part** as well.
   ❑ In the **cardiac** and **pylorus** portion of stomach, these cells are **present but sparse**. Their mucous cells are in predominance.

3. a. Pylorus has more acid secreting cells.
   ❑ **Cardia** and **pylorus** of stomach has **more mucus producing cells**, which help to **neutralize** the acid in the stomach and **prevent ulcer** in distal esophagus and proximal duodenum.
   ❑ **Chief cells** are the source of **digestive enzymes** like pepsin and lipase.
   ❑ **Parietal cells** produce **hydrochloric** acid and the **intrinsic factor**.

4. a. A
   ❑ HCl is secreted by **parietal** cells, shown at marker 'A'.
      ▪ They are identified by a **large** size, **eosinophilic** cytoplasm and **fried egg appearance**.
      ▪ They are located in the **upper half** of the gastric gland, more so in the **body region** of the gland.
   ❑ Key: A: Parietal cell, B: Mucous neck cell, C: Surface mucous cell, D: Chief cell
   ❑ **Mucous cells** are darker staining, **columnar cells** located close to gastric pit (neck region of gastric gland).
   ❑ **Chief cells are small**, **basophilic** columnar cells, more numerous in the **lower half** of the gland - more so at the base (fundus) of the gastric gland.

▶ Intestine

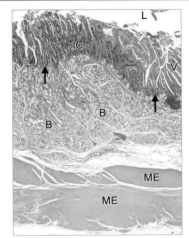

Fig. 42: Duodenum, with villi (V) projecting into the lumen (L); intestinal crypts (IC) of Lieberkuhn in the mucosa, seen mainly in transverse section; muscularis mucosae (arrows); submucosal seromucus (Brunner's) glands (B); and muscularis externa (ME).

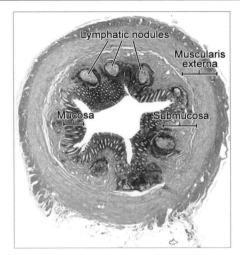

Fig. 43: Microscopic picture of vermiform appendix, showing presence of MALT in mucosa as well as submucosa, along-with disruption of the muscularis mucosa.

Intestinal Epithelium	
1.	Enterocyte (absorption)
2.	Goblet cell (mucus)
3.	Paneth cell (maintain intestinal flora/cytokines)
4.	Enteroendocrine cell (hormones)
5.	M (micro-fold) cell (immunity)
6.	Stem cell

▶ Anal Canal

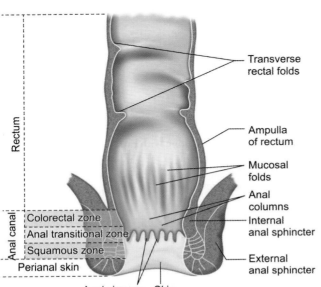

Labels: Transverse rectal folds, Ampulla of rectum, Mucosal folds, Anal columns, Internal anal sphincter, External anal sphincter, Skin, Anal sinuses, Perianal skin, Squamous zone, Anal transitional zone, Colorectal zone, Anal canal, Rectum

Fig. 44: Rectum and anal canal are the terminal portions of the large intestine, lined by the colorectal mucosa that possesses a simple columnar epithelium containing mostly goblet cells and numerous anal glands. In the anal canal, the simple columnar epithelium undergoes transition into a stratified columnar (or cuboidal) epithelium and then to a stratified squamous epithelium. This transition occurs in the area referred to as the anal transitional zone, which occupies the middle third of the anal canal between the colorectal zone and the squamous zone of the perianal skin.

QUESTIONS

1. All is true about Brunner's gland EXCEPT:
  a. Sub-mucosal glands
  b. Secrete urogastrone, which inhibit gastric HCl production
  c. Secrete human epidermal growth factor
  d. Present in the lower duodenum

2. Goblet cells are present in all EXCEPT:
  a. Small intestine
  b. Large intestine
  c. Esophagus
  d. Stomach

3. Cell which does not migrate from the base of the crypt to ends of villi is: *(AIIMS 2007)*
  a. Enterocyte
  b. Endocrine cell
  c. Paneth cell
  d. Goblet cell

4. Paneth cells are identified by:
  a. High zinc content
  b. Numerous lysozyme granules
  c. Rich rough endoplasmic reticulum
  d. Foamy appearance

5. All of these cells are found in small intestine EXCEPT: *(NEET Pattern 2014)*
  a. Stem cells
  b. Goblet cells
  c. Neck cells
  d. Paneth cells

6. Colon contains *(NEET Pattern 2012)*
  a. Parietal cells
  b. Chief cells
  c. Goblet cells
  d. Brunner's gland

7. Stem cells are seen in: *(NEET Pattern 2015)*
  a. Retina
  b. Endometrium
  c. Base of intestinal crypts
  d. None of the above

8. Lining epithelium of anal canal below pectinate line is:
  a. Columnar epithelium
  b. Transitional epithelium
  c. Non-keratinized stratified squamous epithelium
  d. Keratinized stratified squamous epithelium

ANSWERS

1. d. Present in the lower duodenum.
  ❑ **Brunner's glands** are present in the sub-mucosa of the **proximal** (**upper** duodenum).
  ❑ They secrete **urogastrone**, which **inhibit parietal** cell and acid secretion to **reduce the incidence** of duodenal ulcer.
  ❑ **Urogastrone** is also known as HEGF (human **epidermal growth factor**) and **increases the mitotic activity** of the region and helps **healing** the duodenal ulcer faster, if any.

2. d. Stomach > c. Esophagus
  ❑ Goblet cells are **absent** in the stomach and esophagus, **though** esophagus may have goblet cells in Barrett's metaplasia (pathology).

3. **c. Paneth cell**
   - ❑ **Most** of the cells in the mucosa of small intestine are derived from the **stem cells** located in the basal region of the crypts and this progeny **migrate** out along the wall of the crypts **towards the villi** (Paneth cell being an **EXCEPT:ion** migrate **towards the base**).
   - ❑ Paneth cells are present in the **deeper** parts of the intestinal crypts and **not at the ends of villi**. The villus has mainly the enterocytes and the goblet cells.
   - ❑ Endocrine cells are numerous in the intestinal **crypts** but few of them lie over the villi as well.

4. **b. Numerous lysozyme granules**
   - ❑ Paneth cells is distinguished by the **apical eosinophilia** in HandE staining. The apical region has large number of **lysozymes**, which takes **eosin**, making the paneth cell appear **dark pink at the apex**.
   - ❑ Paneth cells are **rich in zinc** and have large amount of endoplasmic reticulum as well but are **not** the answers of first preference.
   - ❑ **Mucus** in the cells like goblet cells give the **foamy appearance** and is **not** a feature of Paneth cells.

5. **c. Neck cells**
   - ❑ At least six types of cells are found in intestinal mucosal epithelium: 1. Columnar cell (**Enterocytes**): For absorption 2. **Goblet** cell: Mucus production, 3. **Paneth** cell: Maintain intestinal flora by secreting antimicrobial substances. 4. **Enteroendocrine** cell: Secrete paracrine and endocrine hormones 5. M cells (**microfold** cells), modified enterocytes that cover enlarged lymphatic nodules in the lamina propria. 6. **Stem** cell: for repair of epithelium.

6. **c. Goblet cells**
   - ❑ **Parietal** and **chief** cells are present in gastric glands.
   - ❑ **Brunner's** glands are present in the **proximal** duodenum.
   - ❑ **Goblet** cells are present in all parts of GIT and **increase towards the distal** segments - most abundant in the rectum and anal canal.

7. **c. Base of intestinal crypts**
   - ❑ Stem cells are located near the base (**lower half**) of crypts of Lieberkuhn, in the intestine.
   - ❑ Stem cells form the multiple layers of new epithelial cells, which **migrate upwards** and reach the tips of the villi.

8. **c. Non-keratinized stratified squamous epithelium.**
   - ❑ Uppermost (colorectal zone) anal canal is lined by the **columnar** epithelium.
   - ❑ Anal transition zone (above dentate line) is lined by the **transitional** epithelium (columnar changing to cuboidal to squamous epithelia).
   - ❑ Squamous zone (below dentate line) is lined by **non-keratinized** stratified squamous epithelium
   - ❑ The terminal most anal canal is lined by **keratinized** stratified squamous epithelium, where it merges with the anal skin.

▼ Hepatobiliary and Pancreatic System

Liver is covered by **Glisson's capsule** and is divided into **hexagonal lobules** oriented around the terminal tributaries of the **hepatic vein**. (Terminal hepatic veins), i.e. Terminal hepatic vein is in the center of the lobule and area around the hepatic vein is called centrilobular zone.

Name	Model	Shape	Centered on	Structure at peripheral angles/poles
Classical lobule	Anatomical	Hexagonal; divided into concentric centrilobular, midzonal, periportal parts	Terminal hepatic venule (central vein)	Portal triads*
Portal lobule	Bile secretion	Triangular; centerd on a portal triad	Portal triads	Terminal hepatic venules (central veins)
Liver acinus	Blood flow and metabolic	Diamond or ovoid-shaped; divided into zone I (periportal), zone II (transition zone), and zone III (pericentral)**	Terminal branches of hepatic arterioles and portal vein at equator	Terminal hepatic venules (central veins)

*Portal triads include branches of the hepatic portal vein, hepatic artery and bile duct.
**Most nutrient-oxygenated is zone I and least so is zone III.

❑ At periphery of lobule, lies the **portal tract** containing hepatic **artery**, bile **duct** and portal **vein**. Area around portal tract is called periportal zone.

❑ Area between periportal zone and centrilobular zone is called **midzonal area**. All around the central vein are the major parenchymal cells, i.e. hepatocytes.

Liver blood flow: Branches of **hepatic artery** and **portal vein** → hepatic sinusoids → **central veins** → hepatic veins → **inferior vena cava**.

The structural unit of the liver is the **lobule**: a roughly **hexagonal** arrangement of plates of **hepatocytes**, separated by intervening **sinusoids** that radiate outwards from a central vein, with portal triads at the vertices of each hexagon.

Hepatic (portal) **acinus** is an approximately ovoid mass of tissue, orientated around a terminal branch of a hepatic arteriole and portal venule, and with its **long axis** defined by two adjacent central veins. It includes the hepatic tissue served by these afferent vessels and is bounded by adjacent acini.

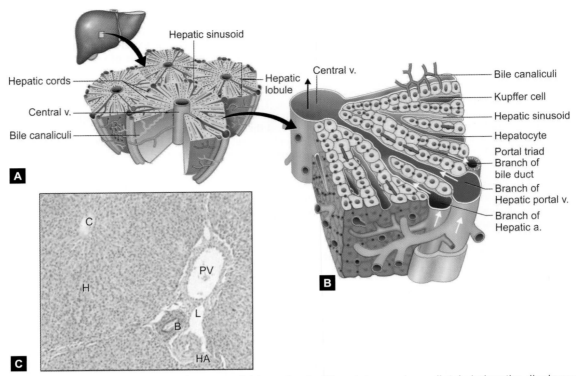

Figs. 45A to C: The liver, a large organ in the upper right quadrant of the abdomen, immediately below the diaphragm, is composed of thousands of polygonal structures called **hepatic lobules**, which are the basic functional units of the organ. **(a)** Diagram showing a small **central vein** in the center of a hepatic lobule and several sets of blood vessels at its periphery. The peripheral vessels are grouped in connective tissue of the **portal tracts** and include a branch of the portal vein, a branch of the hepatic artery, and a branch of the bile duct (the **portal triad**). **(b)** Both blood vessels in this triad branch as **sinusoids**, which run between plates of **hepatocytes** and drain into the central vein. **(c)** Micrograph of a lobule shows the central vein (C), plates of hepatocytes (H), and in an adjacent portal area a small lymphatic (L) and components of the portal triad: a portal venule **(PV)**, hepatic arteriole **(HA)**, and bile ductule **(B)**. X220, H&E

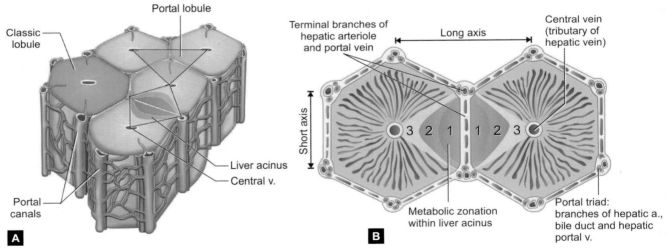

Figs. 46A and B: **Comparison of three models of liver organization and function.** (A) The outlines of a classic hepatic lobule, portal lobule, and liver acinus are visible on this section of the liver tissue. Note that the hexagonal-shaped classic lobule (red) has the terminal hepatic venule (central vein) at the center of the lobule and the portal canals containing portal triads at the peripheral angles of the lobule. The triangular portal lobule (green) has a portal canal at the center of the lobule and terminal hepatic venules (central veins) at the peripheral angles of the lobule. A diamond-shaped liver acinus (multicolor) has distributing vessels at the equator and terminal hepatic venules (central veins) at each pole. (B) The liver acinus is a functional interpretation of liver organization. It consists of adjacent sectors of neighboring hexagonal fields of classic lobules partially separated by distributing blood vessels. The zones, marked 1, 2, and 3, are supplied with blood that is richest and most nutrient-oxygenated in zone 1 and least so in zone 3. The terminal hepatic venules (central veins) in this interpretation are at the pointed edges of the acinus instead of in the center, as in the classic lobule. The portal triads (terminal branches of the portal vein and hepatic artery) and the smallest bile ducts are shown at the corners of the hexagon that outlines the cross-sectioned profile of the classic lobule

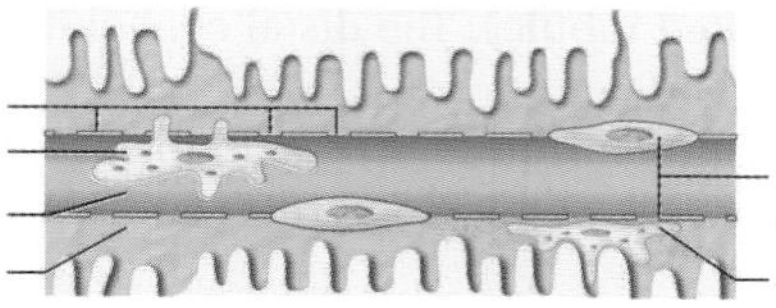

Fig. 47: A schematic illustration of a hepatocyte and adjacent sinusoids

The **endothelium** of the sinusoids is **fenestrated** and lacks a basal lamina, which enables it to act as a dynamic blood filter. The **sinusoids** are separated from the plates of hepatocytes by the **space of Disse**.

- Perisinusoidal space of **Disse** is a small area between the sinusoids and hepatocytes, containing blood plasma, the microvilli of adjacent hepatocytes, **hepatic stellate cells of Ito** etc.
  - It may be obliterated in liver disease, leading to decreased uptake by hepatocytes of nutrients and wastes such as bilirubin.
- **Kupffer cells** are hepatic **macrophages** derived from circulating blood **monocytes** and originate in the bone marrow. They lie within the sinusoidal lumen attached to the endothelial surface.
- **Hepatic stellate cells (HSC) of Ito** are **mesenchymal pericytes** found in the **peri-sinusoidal space (of Disse),** which secrete collagen type III (**reticular**) fibers and **store fat or fat-soluble vitamins** including vitamin A. These cells can transform into **myofibroblasts**, resulting in collagen production, fibrosis, and cirrhosis.

QUESTIONS

1. **Functional unit of liver is:** *(NEET Pattern 2016)*
   a. Hepatocytes
   b. Portal tracts
   c. Liver acinus
   d. Hepatic lobule
2. **Space of Disse contains all EXCEPT:** *(NEET Pattern 2015)*
   a. Microvilli
   b. Blood plasma
   c. Kupffer cell
   d. Hepatic stellate cell
3. **Gallbladder epithelium is:** *(AIIMS 2007)*
   a. Simple squamous
   b. Simple cuboidal with stereocilia
   c. Simple columnar
   d. Simple columnar with brush border
4. **Cell lining of common bile duct is:** *(NEET Pattern 2015)*
   a. Stratified columnar
   b. Stratified squamous
   c. Simple cuboidal
   d. Simple columnar
5. **Centroacinar cells are present in:** *(NEET Pattern 2013)*
   a. Pancreas
   b. Parotid gland
   c. Prostate
   d. None

ANSWERS

1. **c. Liver acinus > d. Hepatic lobule**
   - Functionally, the liver microarchitecture is better understood in terms of **liver acinus**, as compared with hepatic lobule (which has more of an anatomical description).
2. **c. Kupffer cell**
   - Kupffer cell lies **within the sinusoidal lumen** attached to the endothelial surface (**not in space of Disse**).
   - The peri-sinusoidal space (of Disse) is a location in the liver **between** a hepatocyte and a sinusoid. Microvilli of hepatocytes **extend into this space**. It contains the **blood plasma** and **hepatic stellate cells of Ito** as well.
3. **d. Simple columnar with brush border**
   - Gallbladder is lined by the **columnar epithelium with brush** border (irregularly placed microvilli).
   - Small intestine is lined by microvilli arranged in regular fashion-**striated** border.
   - **Brush border** is also present in the proximal convoluted tubule (**PCT**) of kidney.
   - **Stereo-cilia** are present in the hair cells of **internal ear** and **epididymis**.
4. **d. Simple columnar > c. Simple cuboidal**
   - The intrahepatic ducts, cystic duct, and the common bile duct are lined by a **tall columnar** epithelium.
   - Bile ducts are lined by a single layer of columnar/cuboidal-shaped cholangiocytes which display **numerous short microvilli** as well as a single, **long primary cilium** that monitors bile flow and bile composition within the bile duct.
5. **a. Pancreas**
   - **Centroacinar cells** are an extension of the **intercalated duct** cells into each **pancreatic acinus**. The intercalated ducts continue as intralobular ducts which eventually become lobular ducts. These lobular ducts finally converge to form the main pancreatic duct.

- Hepatic vein NOT the component of portal triad in liver *(NEET Pattern 2015)*
- **Stellate cells of von Kupffer** are seen in the sinusoids of liver.
- **Stellate cells of Ito** are present in liver *(NEET Pattern 2016)*
  - These are also called **hepatic stellate cells** and are present in liver for storage of fat or fat-soluble vitamins including vitamin A.
- Space of Disse is seen in liver *(NEET Pattern 2012, 14)*

Urinary System

- The **nephron** is the structural and functional unit of the kidney.
- The nephron consists of the **renal corpuscle** and a long tubular part that includes a proximal thick segment (proximal convoluted tubule and proximal straight tubule), thin segment (thin part of the loop of Henle), and distal thick segment

(distal straight tubule and distal convoluted tubule). The distal convoluted tubule connects to the collecting tubule that opens at the renal papilla.

❑ The renal corpuscle contains the **glomerulus** surrounded by a double layer of **Bowman's capsule**.

❑ The filtration apparatus of the kidney consists of the glomerular endothelium, glomerular basement membrane (GBM), and the Bowman's capsule podocytes.

❑ **Podocytes** extend their processes around the capillaries and develop numerous secondary processes called pedicels (foot processes), which interdigitate with other foot processes of the neighboring podocytes. The spaces between the interdigitating foot processes form filtration slits that are covered by the filtration slit diaphragm.

❑ **Mesangial cells** are involved in phagocytosis and endocytosis of residues trapped in the filtration slits, secretion of paracrine substances, structural support for podocytes, and modulation of glomerular distention.

Table 25: Important structural and functional characteristics of the uriniferous tubule

Region	Epithelium	Major functions	Summary
Renal corpuscle	Simple squamous epithelium lining Bowman capsule: podocytes (visceral layer), outer (parietal layer)	Filters blood	Filteration barrier of fenestrated endothelial cells, fused basal laminate, filtration slits between podocyte secondary processes (pedicels)
Proximal convoluted tubule	Simple cuboidal epithelium with brush border, many compartmentalised mitochondria	Resorbs all glucose, amino acids, filtered proteins; at least 80% Na, Cl, H_2O	The activity of Na pumps in basolateral membranes, transporting Na out of tubule, reduces volume of ultrafiltrate, maintains its isotonicity with blood
Loop of Henle, descending thick limb	Lined by simple cuboidal epithelium with brush border	Same as for proximal convoluted tubule	Same as for proximal convoluted tubule
Loop of Henle, descending thin limb	Simple squamous epithelium	Somewhat permeable to H_2O which enters ultrafiltrate; Na, exist ultrafiltrate	Ultrafiltrate becomes hypotonic with respect to blood: Cl pump in basolateral membranes is primarily responsible for establishing osmotic gradients in interstitium of outer medulla
Loop of Henle, ascending thick limb	Simple cuboidal epithelium; compartmentalized mitochondra	Impermeable to H_2O; Cl actively transported out of trouble into interstitium; Na follows	Ultrafiltrate becomes hypotonic with respect to blood; Cl pump in basolateral membranes is primarily responsible for establishing osmotic gradients in interstitium of outer medulla
JG apparatus macula densa	Simple cuboidal epithelium	Monitors level of Na (or decrease of fluid volume) in ultrafiltrate of distal tubule	Macula densa cells communicate with JG cells in afferent arteriole via gap junctions
JG cells in afferent arteriole	Modified smooth muscle cells containing renin granules	Cells synthesis renin, release it into bloodstream	Renin acts on plasma protein, to trigger events leading to formation of angiotensin II, release of aldosterone from adrenal gland
Distal convoluted tubule	Simple cuboidal cells; compartmentalised mitochondria	Cells respond to aldosterone by removing Na from ultrafiltrate	Ultrafilterate more hypotonic in presence of adolosterone; K^+, NH^+, H^+ enter ultrafiltrate
Collecting tubules	Simple cuboidal epithelium; simple columnar epithelium	In absence of ADH, tubule impermeable to H_2O; hypotonic urine excreted	In presence of ADH, tubule permeable to H_2O, which is removed from filtrate, producing hypertonic urine

Table 26: Features of excretory passages

Region	Epithelium	Lamina propria	Muscularis	Comments
Calyces, minor, major	Transitional epithelim	Reticular, elastic fibers	A few inner longitudinal and outer circular smooth muscle fibers	Urine from collecting tubules (ducts of Bellini) empty into minor calyces.
Renal pelvis	Transitional epithelim	Reticular, elastic fibers	Inner longitudinal, outer circular layer of smooth muscle	Expanded upper portion of ureter receives urine from the major calyces.
Ureters	Transitional epithelium lines steliate lumen	Collagen, elastic fibers	Inner longitudinal, outer circular layer of smooth muscle; lower third has additional outermost longitudinal layer	Peristaltic waves propel urine, so it enters bladder in sports.

Region	Epithelium	Lamina propria	Muscularis	Comments
Urinary bladder	Transitional epithelium: 5 or 6 cell layers in empty bladder; 3 or 4 cell layers in distended bladder. Trigone; triangular region; apices are openings of ureters and urethra	Fibroelastic connective tissue rich in blood vessels	Three poorly defined layers of smooth muscle; inner longitudinal, middle circular, outer longitudinal	Plasmalemma of dome-shaped cells in epithelium has unique plaques, elliptical vesicles underlying remarkable (empty vs. full) transition. Trigone, unlike most of bladder mucosa, always presents smooth surface.
Urethra female	Transitional epithelim near bladder; remainder stratified squamous	Fibroelastic vascular connective tissue; mucus-secreting glands of Littre	Inner longitudinal, outer circular layer of smooth muscle; skeletal muscle sphincter surrounds urethra at urogenital diaphragm	Female urethra is conduit for urine. External sphincter of skeletal muscle permits voluntary control of micturition.
Urethra male prostatic	Transitional epithelium near bladder; pseudostratified or stratified columnar	Fibromuscular stroma of prostate gland; a few glands of Littre	Inner longitudinal, outer circular layer of smooth muscle	Conduit for urine and semen. Receives secretions from prostate glands, paired ejaculatory ducts.
Urethra male membranous	Pseudostratified or stratified columnar	Fibroelastic stroma; a few glands of Littre	Striated muscle fibers of urogenital diaphragm form external sphincter	Conduit for urine and semen. External shpincter of skeletal muscle permits voluntary control of micturition.
Urethra male cavernous	Pseudostratified or stratified columnar; at fossa navicularis stratified squamous	Replaced by erectile tissue of corpus spongiosum; many glands of Littre	Replaced by sparse smooth muscle, many elastic fibers in septa lining vascular spaces in erectile tissue	Conduit for urine and semen. Receives secretions of bulbourethral glands present in urogenital diaphragm.

- ❏ PCT (Proximal convoluted tubules) lined with cuboidal brush border
- ❏ DCT: Shorter than proximal convoluted tubules, less frequent in cortex, and lack brush border

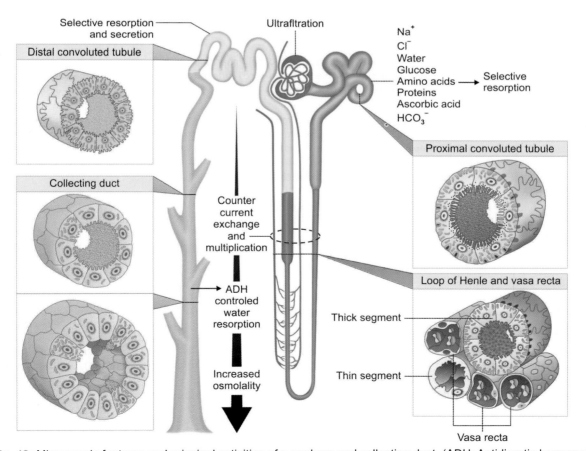

Fig. 48: Microscopic features and principal activities of a nephron and collecting duct. (ADH: Antidiuretic hormone).

Epithelium

- ❑ **Urothelium** (transitional epithelium) begin to appear at the tip of collecting ducts and continues into the minor calyx region and lines major calyx, pelvis, ureter, urinary bladder and the proximal 2 cm of prostatic urethra.
- ❑ Male urethra: **Proximal half** of prostatic urethra (till the opening of common ejaculatory ducts) is lined by the continuation of bladder epithelium – Urothelium. Distally, **major length** of the male urethra is lined by pseudo-stratified or stratified columnar epithelium. **Terminal urethra** is lined by stratified squamous epithelium. The terminal most urethra becomes keratinized.

Site	Lining
Proximal	Transitional (Urothelium)
Major lining	Pseudo-stratified or stratified columnar epithelium
Terminal	Stratified squamous (non- keratinized) epithelium

Female Urethra

Site	Lining
Proximal	Transitional (Urothelium)
Main lining	Stratified squamous (non- keratinized) epithelium

QUESTIONS

1. **Urothelium lines all EXCEPT:** (AIIMS 2009)
   a. Minor calyx b. Ureter
   c. Urinary bladder d. Membranous urethra

2. **Transitional epithelium is present in:** (NEET Pattern 2012)
   a. Renal pelvis b. Loop of Henle
   c. Terminal part of urethra d. PCT

3. **Urothelium does NOT line:** (AIIMS 2007)
   a. Collecting ducts b. Minor calyx
   c. Ureter d. Urinary bladder

4. **Which cells line the collecting ducts:** (NEET Pattern 2013)
   a. Simple cuboidal b. Simple squamous
   c. Simple columnar d. Transitional

5. **Ansa nephroni is lined by:** (JIPMER)
   a. Columnar b. Squamous epithelium
   c. Cuboidal squamous epithelium d. Cuboidal and squamous

ANSWERS

1. **d. Membranous urethra:**
   - ❑ **Membranous** urethra is lined by **stratified** (or pseudostratified) columnar epithelium.
   - ❑ **Urothelium** (transitional epithelium) is present at **terminal lining of collecting tubules**, minor and major calyces, renal pelvis, ureter, urinary bladder and **proximal urethra**.

2. **a. Renal pelvis**
   - ❑ **Transitional epithelium** begins to appear at the **terminal portion of collecting ducts** and further continue to line minor calyx, major calyx, renal pelvis, ureter, urinary bladder and **proximal half of prostatic urethra**.
   - ❑ Loop of Henle is lined by **simple cuboidal** epithelium/ simple **squamous** epithelium (thin segment).
   - ❑ Terminal part of urethra is lined by **stratified squamous** epithelium.
   - ❑ PCT is lined by **simple cuboidal** epithelium with microvilli (**brush border**).

3. **a. Collecting ducts**
   - ❑ Collecting ducts are majorly lined by **columnar epithelium**, though the **tip** of collecting ducts are lined by **urothelium** (or transitional) epithelium.

4. **c. Simple columnar**
   - ❑ Collecting tubules are lined by **simple cuboidal** epithelium which gradually change to **simple columnar** in collecting ducts as the duct system passes from the cortex to the renal papilla.

5. **d. Cuboidal and squamous**
   - ❑ Ansa nephroni (loop of Henle) is lined by **simple squamous** epithelium.
   - ❑ The **thick** descending and ascending limbs are lined by simple **cuboidal** epithelia.

- ❑ **Duct of Bellini** are present in kidney (NEET Pattern 2015)
- ❑ Collecting duct of kidney is also called as papillary duct or **duct of Bellini**.
  - ➢ They are the **largest straight** excretory ducts in the kidney medulla and the papillae of which openings form the area cribrosa that open into a minor calyx.
- ❑ Renal filtrate (urine) flow: Collecting tubule → Collecting ducts of Bellini → minor calyx

▶ Genital System

- ❑ **Squamo-columnar junction** is present at the endocervix and ectocervix junction. **Uterus** is lined by columnar epithelium and **vagina** has stratified squamous epithelium.

Male

Table 27: Review of male genital tract			
Organ	**Main components**	**Cell types**	**Functions**
Testis	Seminiferous tubules	Spermatogenic series cells Sertoli cells	Production of male gametes, spermatozoa Support cells for spermatogenesis
	Interstitium	Leydig cells	Synthesis of androgenic hormones, principally testosterone
	Rete testis	Cuboidal epithelium with cilia and smooth muscle coat	Convey spermatozoa to ductules efferentes and thence to epididymis
Epididymis		Columnar epithelium with stereocilia and smooth muscle coat	Store and mature spermatozoa
Vas deferens		Columnar epithelium and smooth muscle coat, three layers	Carry sperm to urethra during ejaculation
Prostate	Central, transition and peripheral zones and anterior fibromuscular stroma	Epithelium with two cell layers, luminal tall columnar layer and basal cell layer	Produces secretions that mix with seminal fluid
Seminal vesicle		Cuboidal to columnar epithelium with muscular wall	Produce seminal fluid
Penis	Corpus spongiosum and corpora cavernosa	Spongy fibrous tissue containing anastomosing vascular sinuses	Erectile tissue
	Urethra	Lined by urothelium proximally Pseudostratified columnar epithelium distally	Duct for ejaculation (and micturition)

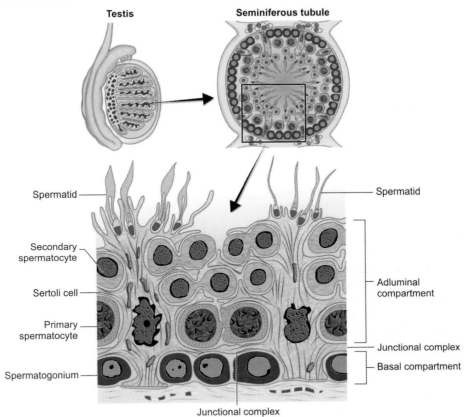

Fig. 49: Seminiferous tubules epithelium. Intercellular bridges are present between spermatocytes and the junctional complexes near the bases of adjacent Sertoli cells. These junctional complexes of the Sertoli cells divide the epithelium into an adluminal and a basal compartment.

Table 28: Summary of histology and functions of male genital ducts				
Duct	**Location**	**Epithelium**	**Support tissues**	**Function(s)**
Seminiferous tubules	Testicular lobules	Spermatogenic, with sertoli cells and germ cells	Myoid cells and loose connective tissue	Produce sperm

Duct	Location	Epithelium	Support tissues	Function(s)
Straight tubules (tubuli recti)	Periphery of the mediastinum testis	Sertoli cells in proximal portions, simple cuboidal in distal portions	Connective tissue	Convey sperm into the rete testis
Rete testis	In mediastinum testis	Simple cuboidal	Dense irregular connective tissue	Channels with sperm from all seminiferous tubules
Efferent ductules	From rete testis to head of epididymis	Alternating patches of simple cuboidal nonciliated and simple columnar ciliated	Thin circular layer of smooth muscle and vascular loose connective tissue	Absorb most fluid from seminiferous tubules; convey sperm into the epididymis
Epididymal duct	Head, body, and tail of the epididymis	Pseudostratified columnar, with small basal cells and tall principal cells bearing long stereocilia	Circular smooth muscle initially, with inner and outer longitudinal layers in the tail	Site for sperm maturation and short-term storage; expels sperm at ejaculation
Ductus (vas) deferens	Extends from epididymis to ejaculatory ducts in prostate gland	Pseudostratified columnar, with fewer stereocilia	Fibroelastic lamina propria and three very thick layers of smooth muscle	Carries sperm by rapid peristalsis from the epididymis to the ejaculatory ducts
Ejaculatory ducts	In prostate, formed by union of ductus deferens and ducts of the seminal vesicles	Pseudostratified and simple columnar	Fibroelastic tissue and smooth muscle of the prostate stroma	Mix sperm and seminal fluid; deliver semen to urethra, where prostatic secretion is added

Table 29: Functions of Sertoli cells	
During gestation	**After puberty**
Synthesize and release antimullerian hormone to suppress the formation of the female genital system and support the development of the male genital system	Physical and nutritional support of developing germ cells
	Synthesize and release testicular transferrin to transfer iron from seum transferrin to developing germ cells
	Synthesize and release ABP
	Establish blood-testis barrier
	Phagocytose cytoplasm shed during spermiogenesis
	Synthesize and release inhibin
	Secrete fructose-rich medium to provide nutrients for spermatozoa released into the male genital ducts

*ABP: Androgen binding protein

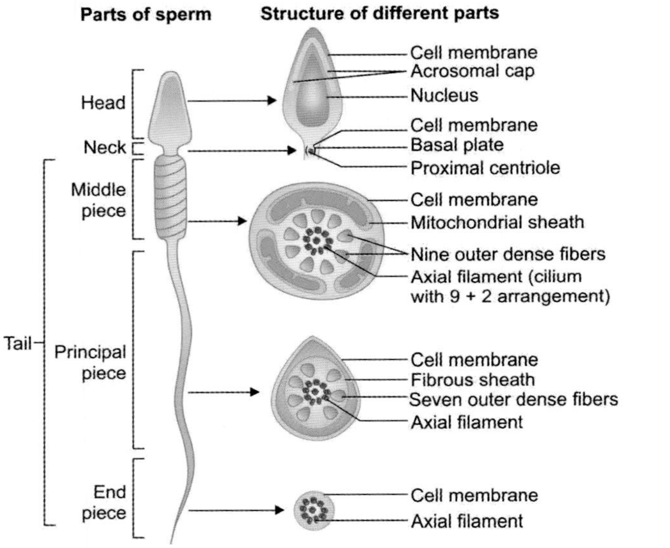

Fig. 50: Parts of the mature sperm are shown on the left side and the sections through the head, neck, middle piece, principal piece, and end piece along with their composition are shown onto the right side.

Sperm consist of **four key functional components**:

- [ ] **Acrosome** which contains enzymes that aid in digesting and penetrating the cumulus oophorus.
- [ ] **Nucleus** which contains highly compacted DNA.
- [ ] **Midpiece**, which includes the centrosome that is key in human embryogenesis, as well as mitochondria which provide the energy source for sperm.
- [ ] **Tail**, which contains the axoneme and the dynein motor proteins.
- [ ] To maximize transport efficiency, the sperm has **no ribosomes**, endoplasmic reticulum, or **Golgi apparatus**. However, small ribonucleic acids (**RNAs**) are transported within the sperm and may have a role in embryogenesis.
- [ ] **Blood testis barrier:** The adjacent cytoplasm of **Sertoli** cells are joined by occluding tight junctions, producing a blood–testis barrier that subdivides each seminiferous tubule into a basal compartment and an adluminal compartment. This important barrier segregates the spermatogonia from all successive stages of spermatogenesis in the adluminal compartment and excludes plasma proteins and **bloodborne antibodies** from the lumen of seminiferous tubules. The more advanced spermatogenic cells can be recognized by the body as foreign and cause an immune response.
- [ ] The blood–testis barrier protects developing cells from the immune system by restricting the passage of membrane antigens from developing sperm into the bloodstream. Thus, the blood–testis barrier prevents an autoimmune response to the individual's own sperm, antibody formation, and eventual destruction of spermatogenesis and **induction of sterility**. The blood–testis barrier also keeps harmful substances in the blood from entering the developing germinal epithelium.

Table 30: Comparison of structural components of the spermatid and the spermatozoon

Spermatid (round cell)	Spermatozoon (elongated cell)
▪ Nucleus	▪ Head
▪ Golgi apparatus	▪ Acrosomal cap
▪ One centrosome	▪ Two centrioles – One lies in the neck and forms axial filament – Other forms annulus at the distal end of middle piece
▪ Mitochondria	▪ Spirally surround the axial filament between the neck and annulus to form the middle piece; the remaining axial filament forms the tail
▪ Cell membrane	▪ Cell membrane

QUESTIONS

1. Sertoli cells in the testis have receptors for: *(AIIMS 2007)*

a. FSH
b. LH
c. Inhibin
d. GnRH

2. Sperm doesn't contain: *(NEET Pattern 2016)*

a. Golgi apparatus
b. Mitochondria
c. Endoplasmic reticulum
d. Lysosome

ANSWERS

1. a. FSH
- ❑ Sertoli cell (a kind of **sustentacular** cell) is a **'nurse'** cell of the testes which is part of a seminiferous tubule.
- ❑ It is activated by follicle-stimulating hormone and has **FSH-receptor** on its membranes. FSH binds to sertoli cells stimulate **testicular fluid production** and synthesis of intracellular **androgen receptor proteins.** Sertoli cells secrete **anti-Mullerian hormone** and activins also.
- ❑ LH binds to receptors on interstitial cells of Leydig and stimulate **testosterone production**, which in turn binds to Sertoli cells to promote spermatogenesis.
- ❑ **Inhibin** is a hormone that **inhibits FSH production**. It is secreted from the **Sertoli** cells, located in the seminiferous tubule inside the testes.

2. c. Endoplasmic reticulum > a. Golgi apparatus
- ❑ To maximize transport efficiency, the sperm has **no ribosomes**, **endoplasmic reticulum**, or **Golgi apparatus**.
- ❑ **Golgi apparatus** forms a cap-like structure, **acrosome** over the anterior half of the head.

- ▪ Blood testis barrier lies between **Sertoli – Sertoli** cells.
- ▪ Acrosome cap of sperm is derived from **Golgi body** *(NEET Pattern 2014)*
- ▪ Middle piece of sperm contains **mitochondria** *(NEET Pattern 2015)*
- ▪ Corpora amylacea is seen in **prostate** *(NEET Pattern 2012)*

Female

Table 31: Review of the female reproductive system

Part of the female genital tract	Key features
Ovary	Primordial and developing follicles embedded in ovarian stroma Surface covering of epithelium (mesothelium) Corpora lutea and corpora albicantes
Fallopian tube	Muscular wall Folded mucosa Ciliated columnar epithelium
Uterus	Muscular wall—the myometrium Lining endometrium consisting of glands and stroma, varies with the menstrual cycle
Endocervix	Bulk consists of a dense fibromuscular stroma Surface has deep cletts lined by simple columnar mucus-secreting epithelium
Ectocervix	Stroma same as for endocervix Stratified squamous non-keratinising surface epithelium
Vagina	Fibromuscular wall Stratified squamous non-keratinising surface epithelium
Vulva	Stratified squamous epithelium/modified skin
Placenta	Chorionic villi with core of mesenchyme and double surface layer of trophoblast
Breast	Stroma consists of adipose tissue with fibrous septa Branching tubulo-acinar glands Glandular epithelium consists of luminal epithelial cells and underlying myoepithelial cells

Uterine tube

❑ The mucosa is lined by a single-layered, tall, **columnar epithelium**, which contains mainly **ciliated** cells and **secretory** (peg) cells (so called because they project into the lumen further than their ciliated neighbors), and occasional intraepithelial lymphocytes. In the tube, ciliated cells predominate distally and secretory cells proximally

> ➤ Uterus: Single-layered columnar epithelium.
> ➤ (**Before puberty**, the epithelium is ciliated and cuboidal).

Ovary

❑ An **ovarian follicle** is a rounded structure that contains a developing **ovum** surrounded by **follicular cells** and a fluid filled **antral cavity**.

❑ Ovarian follicles have a cellular covering called the **theca interna** whose cells produce estrogen.

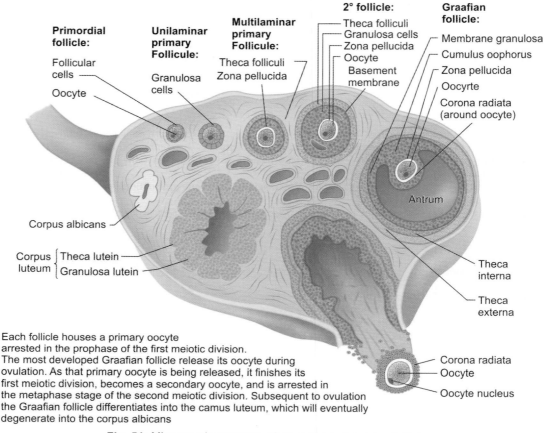

Each follicle houses a primary oocyte arrested in the prophase of the first meiotic division. The most developed Graafian follicle release its oocyte during ovulation. As that primary oocyte is being released, it finishes its first meiotic division, becomes a secondary oocyte, and is arrested in the metaphase stage of the second meiotic division. Subsequent to ovulation the Graafian follicle differentiates into the camus luteum, which will eventually degenerate into the corpus albicans

Fig. 51: Microscopic structure of an ovary and ovarian follicles.

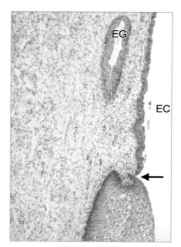

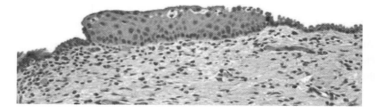

Fig. 52: Uterine cervix showing the transformation zone. The single-layered columnar epithelium lining the endocervical canal (EC) and its endocervical glands (EG) changes abruptly (arrow) to the stratified squamous non-keratinizing epithelium of the external os and ectocervix (below arrow).

Fig. 53: Squamous metaplasia of the uterine cervix. The center of the image is occupied by an island containing squamous stratified epithelium. This metaplastic epithelium is surrounded on both sides by simple columnar epithelium. Since metaplasia is triggered by reprogramming of stem cells, metaplastic squamous cells have the same characteristics as normal stratified suqamous epithelium.

QUESTIONS

1. **Lining epithelium of fallopian tube is:** *(NEET Pattern 2012)*
   a. Simple columnar
   b. Pseudostratified columnar
   c. Ciliated columnar
   d. Simple cuboidal

2. **Lining epithelium of uterus is:** *(NEET Pattern 2012)*
   a. Simple columnar
   b. Simple cuboidal
   c. Ciliated columnar
   d. Ciliated cuboidal

3. **Lining epithelium of vagina is:** *(NEET Pattern 2012)*
   a. Pseudostratified columnar epithelium
   b. Keratinized stratified squamous epithelium
   c. Non-keratinized stratified squamous epithelium
   d. Ciliated columnar epithelium

4. **Mucus glands are absent in:** *(NEET Pattern 2012)*
   a. Cervix
   b. Esophagus
   c. Vagina
   d. Duodenum

5. **Ratio of connective tissue: smooth muscle in cervix:** *(NEET Pattern 2013)*
   a. 2:1
   b. 5:1
   c. 7:1
   d. 8:1

ANSWERS

1. **c. Ciliated columnar**
   ❑ The mucosa of fallopian tube is lined by a single-layered, tall, **columnar** epithelium, which contains mainly **ciliated** cells and secretory (**peg**) cells.
   ❑ Uterine cavity is also lined by the **columnar** epithelium.

2. **a. Simple columnar**
   ❑ Uterus has a single-layered tall **columnar** epithelium.
   ❑ Some of the cells bear cilia, the remainder having surface **microvilli**.
   Note: **Before puberty**, the epithelium is ciliated and cuboidal (G-41).

3. **c. Non-keratinized stratified squamous epithelium**
   ❑ Vagina and ectocervix are lined by **non-keratinized** stratified squamous epithelium.
   ❑ Vagina has **no glands** though cervix has glandular epithelium.
   ❑ Squamo-columnar junction is present at the **endocervix** and **ectocervix** junction.
   ❑ Uterus is lined by **columnar epithelium** (some of the cells bear cilia) and vagina has stratified squamous epithelium.

4. **c. Vagina**
   ❑ Vaginal mucosa has **no glands**.
   ❑ Vaginal secretions are primarily from the uterus, cervix, and vaginal epithelium in addition to minuscule vaginal lubrication from the **Bartholin's glands** upon sexual arousal.
   ❑ The significant majority of vaginal lubrication is provided by **plasma seepage** from the vaginal walls (vaginal transudation).

5. **d. 8:1**
   ❑ Cervix consists of **fibroelastic** connective tissue and contains **relatively little** (10%) **smooth** muscle.
   ❑ The **elastin** component of the cervical stroma is essential to the **stretching** capacity of the cervix during childbirth.
   ❑ The amount of smooth muscle varies between the upper (25%), middle (16%) and lower (6%) portions of the cervix.

- Epithelium of ovarian follicle is **stratified cuboidal** while that of ovary is **simple cuboidal**.
- Corpora **arenacea** (or brain sand) are calcified structures in the pineal gland which become increasingly visible on X-rays over time *(NEET Pattern 2012)*

Neuroanatomy

- ❑ Nervous system has two major divisions, the **central nervous system** (CNS) and the **peripheral nervous system** (PNS).
- ❑ **CNS** consists of the brain, spinal cord, optic nerve and retina, and contains the majority of neuronal cell bodies.
- ❑ **PNS** includes all nervous tissue outside the CNS and consists of the cranial and spinal nerves, peripheral autonomic nervous system (ANS) and the special senses (taste, olfaction, vision, hearing and balance).
  - ➤ It is composed mainly of the axons of sensory and motor neurons that pass between the CNS and the body.
  - ➤ ANS is subdivided into **sympathetic** and **parasympathetic** components. It consists of neurones that innervate secretory **glands** and **cardiac** and **smooth** muscle, and is concerned primarily with control of the internal environment.
  - ➤ Neurons in the wall of the gastrointestinal tract form the **enteric nervous system** (ENS) and are capable of sustaining local reflex activity that is independent of the CNS.
  - ➤ **ENS** contains as many intrinsic neurons in its ganglia as the entire spinal cord is often considered as a third division of the nervous system.

▶ Brain

- ❑ Brain **(encephalon)** has 12 pairs of cranial nerves through which it communicates with structures of the head and neck and through connections with the spinal cord, it controls the activities of the trunk and limbs.
- ❑ The brain is divided into major regions on the basis of ontogenetic growth and phylogenetic principles: **Forebrain** (prosencephalon), **midbrain** (mesencephalon) **hindbrain** (rhombencephalon).

Primary vesicles	Secondary vesicles	Adult derivatives
Prosencephalon	Telencephalon	Cerebral hemispheres, caudate, putamen, amygdaloid claustrum, lamina terminalis, olfactory bulbs, hippocampus
	Diencephalon	Epithalamus, subthalamus, thalamus, hypothalamus, mammillary bodies, neurohypophysis, pineal gland, retina, iris, ciliary body, optic nerve (CN II), optic chiasm, optic tract
Mesencephalon	Mesencephalon	Midbrain
Rhombencephalon	Metencephalon	Pons, cerebellum
	Myelencephalon	Medulla

- ❑ **Prosencephalon** is subdivided into the **telencephalon** and the **diencephalon**.
  - ➤ **Telencephalon** is mainly composed of the two **cerebral hemispheres** or cerebrum. Each hemisphere has an outer layer of gray matter, the cerebral cortex, beneath which lies a thick mass of white matter.
  - ➤ **Internal capsule** contains nerve fibers that pass to and from the cerebral cortex and lower levels of brain.
  - ➤ **Basal ganglia** gray matter nuclei partly embedded in the subcortical white matter.
  - ➤ **Corpus callosum** is the nerve fiber connection between corresponding areas on either side of the brain, which cross the midline within commissures.
  - ➤ **Diencephalon** equates mostly to the thalamus and hypothalamus, but also includes the smaller epithalamus and subthalamus.
- ❑ **Mesencephalon** (midbrain) comprises of the tectum, tegmentum, the cerebral aqueduct, cerebral peduncles, and certain nuclei and fasciculi.
  - ➤ Caudally the midbrain adjoins the metencephalon and rostrally the diencephalon.
- ❑ **Rhombencephalon** is subdivided into **metencephalon** (pons and the cerebellum) and **myelencephalon** (medulla oblongata).
  - ➤ **Pons** lies between the midbrain and the medulla oblongata and in front of the cerebellum. It has two parts: the basilar part ventrally, and pontine tegmentum, dorsally.
  - ➤ **Cerebellum** consists of paired hemispheres united by a median vermis and lies within the posterior cranial fossa, dorsal to the brainstem (midbrain, pons and medulla) and connected with cerebellar peduncles.

> **Medulla oblongata** is the most caudal part of the brainstem and is continuous with the spinal cord below the level of the foramen magnum.
❑ **Brainstem** is the collective term which includes midbrain, pons and medulla oblongata. It lies upon the basal portions of the occipital and sphenoid bones (**clivus**).

▶ Basic Neuroanatomy

Table 1: Glial cells in the central nervous system and peripheral nervous system	
Cell type	**Functions**
Central nervous system	
Astrocytes	Maintain blood-brain barrier, regulate ion, nutrient, and dissolved gas concentrations. Form scar tissue after injury
Oligodendrocytes	Form myelin around CNS axons
Microglia	Remove cellular debris, and pathogens in CNS by phagocytosis
Ependymal cells	Line ventricles of the brain and central canal of the spinal cord. Assist in production, circulation and monitoring of cerebrospinal fluid
Peripheral nervous system	
Satellite cells	Surround nerve cell bodies in peripheral ganglia
Schwann cells	Surround all axons in PNS. Responsible for myelination of axons in PNS. Participate in repair process after injury

▶ White Matter

❑ **White matter** is constituted by the bundles of **myelinated axons**, which connect various gray matter areas and carry nerve impulses between neurons.
❑ Collection of axons are categorized on the basis of their course and connection into **association** fibers, **projection** fibers, and **commissural** fibers.
> **Association fibers** connect cortical regions within the same cerebral hemisphere of the brain.
> **Projection fibers** project from higher to lower centers (or vice versa) in CNS.
> **Commissural fibers** are transverse fibers that interconnect similar regions in the left and right sides of CNS (cerebral hemisphere, brainstem, cerebellum, spinal cord).

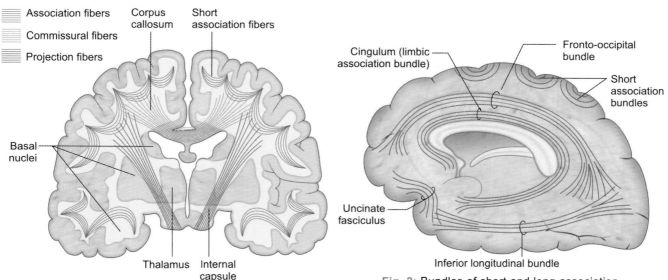

Fig. 1: Types of white matter fibers

Fig. 2: Bundles of short and long association fibers within the cerebral hemisphere

❑ **Association** fibers:

Name	From	To
Uncinate fasciculus	Frontal lobe	Temporal lobe
Cingulum	Cingulate gyrus	Entorhinal cortex
Superior longitudinal fasciculus	Frontal lobe	Occipital lobe
Inferior longitudinal fasciculus	Occipital lobe	Temporal lobe
Fornix	Hippocampus	Mammillary bodies
Arcuate fasciculus	Frontal lobe	Temporal lobe

❑ **Projection** fibers: Corona radiata, internal capsule, fimbria
❑ **Commissural** fibers: Corpus callosum, hippocampal commissure, anterior and posterior commissure, habenular commissure.

Corpus Callosum

❑ The anterior is called the **genu** and posterior part is **splenium**; between the two is the **body** of the corpus callosum.
❑ The part between the body and the splenium is the **isthmus** and **rostrum**, the part that projects posteriorly and inferiorly from the anterior most genu.
❑ The fibers curving forward from the genu into the frontal lobe constitute the **forceps minor**, and those curving backward into the occipital lobe, the **forceps major**. Between these two parts is the main body of the fibers which constitute the **tapetum** and extend laterally on either side into the temporal lobe, and cover in the central part of the lateral ventricle.

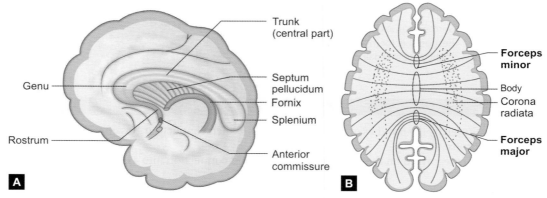

Figs. 3A and B: Parts of corpus callosum. (A) Median sagittal section of the cerebrum showing shape and different parts of corpus callosum, (B) Horizontal section of the cerebrum showing components of the fires of corpus callosum

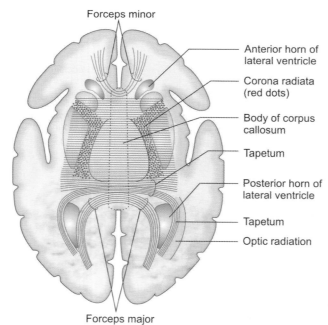

Fig. 4: Horizontal section of the cerebrum (schematic) to show the course and components of the fibres of corpus callosum. Fibres of coronal radiata are seen cut at right angle to their course

1. Association fibers are all EXCEPT: *(AIIMS 2014)*
   a. Uncinate
   b. Cingulum
   c. Forceps major
   d. Longitudinal fasciculus

2. All are parts of corpus callosum EXCEPT:
   a. Forceps minor
   b. Forceps major
   c. Tapetum
   d. Indusium griseum

3. In the given image, the marked structure connects which of the following: *(AIIMS 2017)*
   a. Striate cortex
   b. Orbital cortex
   c. Dentate nucleus
   d. Hippocampus

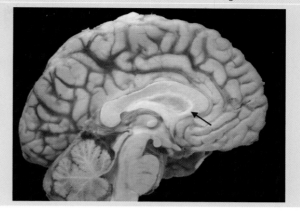

1. c. Forceps major
   ❑ **Forceps major** is the collection of **commissural** fibers in the splenium part of the corpus callosum, communicates somatosensory information between the two halves of the parietal lobe and the visual cortex at the occipital lobe.
   ❑ Uncinate fasciculus connects parts of the **limbic system** (hippocampus and amygdala in the temporal lobe) with frontal lobe structures such as the orbitofrontal cortex.
   ❑ **Cingulum** fibers project from the cingulate gyrus to the entorhinal cortex, allowing for communication between components of the **limbic system**.
   ❑ Superior longitudinal fasciculus connects the frontal, occipital, parietal, and temporal lobes on the **same** cerebral hemisphere.

2. d. Indusium griseum
   ❑ Indusium griseum is a thin layer of **gray matter** in contact with the **dorsal surface** of the corpus callosum and continuous laterally with the gray matter of the cingulate gyrus.

3. b. Orbital cortex
   ❑ This is a **sagittal section** of brain, the marker showing **rostrum part of corpus callosum** (a commissural fibers system connecting left and right cerebral hemispheres). The **orbital** regions of the **frontal lobes** are connected via the rostral fibers of corpus callosum.

❑ Corpus callosum is **commissural** type of fibers *(NEET Pattern 2012)*
   ➢ It connects the left and right cerebral hemispheres and facilitates **interhemispheric** communication.
❑ **Largest** commissural fibers are seen in **corpus callosum** *(NEET Pattern 2016)*

Development of Nervous System

Nervous system and special sense organs are derivatives of the neuroectoderm and develop from **three sources**:
❑ **Neural plate**, which forms the CNS (including the preganglionic autonomic nerves).
❑ **Neural crest** cells appear at the junction of neural plate and peripheral ectoderm, undergo epithelial to mesenchymal transition and migrate away just prior to its fusion of neural plate to form neural tube.
   ➢ Neural crest cells form majority of the neurons and glia outside the CNS.
   ➢ Most of the ganglia (somatic and autonomic) develop from neural crest cells.
   ➢ Neural crest cells also form neurons in adrenal medulla and chromaffin cells.
❑ **Ectodermal placodes** develop from a common panplacodal ectoderm (PPE) a horseshoe-shaped region of ectoderm surrounding the anterior neural plate and neural crest.

Flowchart 1: Development of nervous system and special sense organs

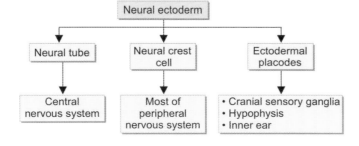

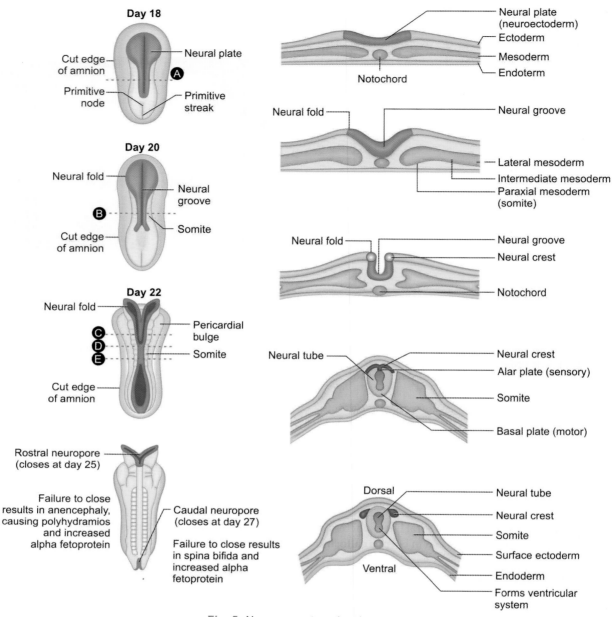

Fig. 5: Nervous system development

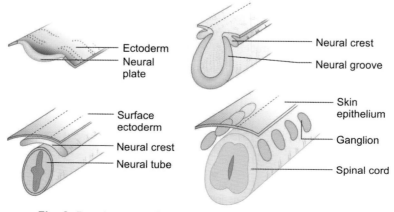

Fig. 6: Development of neural tube (CNS) and ganglia (PNS)

- **Macroglial** cells are derived from neuroectoderm and include: Astrocytes, oligodendrocytes, ependymal cells, Schwann cells.
- During hematopoiesis, some of the stem cells differentiate into monocytes and travel from the bone marrow to the brain, where they settle and further differentiate into **microglia**.
- **Neurulation** begins in the **third week** of development.
  - As the primitive streak regresses caudally, the **notochord** develops in the axial line of the embryo (between the buccopharyngeal membrane and cloacal membrane).
  - Notochord **induces** the overlying ectoderm to form the **neural plate**.
  - By the end of the third week, the lateral margins of the neural plate thicken and become elevated to form the **neural folds** with the neural groove located centrally between the two folds.
  - The neural folds then grow over the midline and begin to fuse to form the **neural tube** which later separate from the surface ectoderm.
  - Closure of the neural tube begins in the **cervical** region and continues cranially and caudally (The recent literature mentions **multiple levels of fusion**).
  - Neural tube has a cavity **neural canal**, which is in continuity with amniotic cavity in the beginning. The cavity gives rise to the central canal of the spinal cord and ventricles of the brain.
  - When neural tube starts closing in the cervical region, the neural canal is still open at the cranial end (anterior neuropore) and caudal end (posterior neuropore).

Table 2: Congenital defects of the nervous system

Condition	Clinical features
Spina bifida	<ul><li>Improper closure of posterior neuropore</li><li>Several forms:</li></ul> A. *Spina bifida occulta* (mildest form): Failure of vertebrae to close around spinal cord (tufts of hair often evident). No ↑ AFP B. *Spinal meningocele* (spina bifida cystica): Meninges extend out of defective spinal canal, ↑ AFP C. *Meningomyelocele*: Meninges and spinal cord extend out of spinal canal. ↑ AFP D. *Myeloschisis* (most severe form): Neural tissue is visible externally. ↑ AFP
Anencephaly	<ul><li>Failure of brain and cranium to develop</li><li>Caused by lack of closure of anterior neuropore</li><li>Associated with increased maternal α– fetoprotein (AFP) and polyhydramnios</li><li>Severe cranial nerve defects</li></ul>
Hydrocephaly	<ul><li>Accumulation of cerebrospinal fluid (CSF) in ventricles and subarachnoid space</li><li>Caused by congenital blockage of cerebral aqueducts</li><li>Increased head circumference in neonates</li></ul>
Dandy-Walker malformation	<ul><li>Dilation of fourth ventricle leading to hypoplasia of cerebellum</li><li>Failure of formaina of Luschka and Magendie to open</li></ul>
Arnold-Chiari malformation Type II	<ul><li>Herniation of the *cerebellar vermis* through the foramen magnum</li><li>Hydrocephaly</li><li>Myelomeningocele and syringomyelia</li><li>Newborn</li></ul>
Fetal alcohol syndrome	<ul><li>*Most common cause of intellectual disability*</li><li>*Cardiac septal defects*</li><li>Facial malformations including widely spaced eyes and long philtrum</li><li>Growth retardation</li></ul>

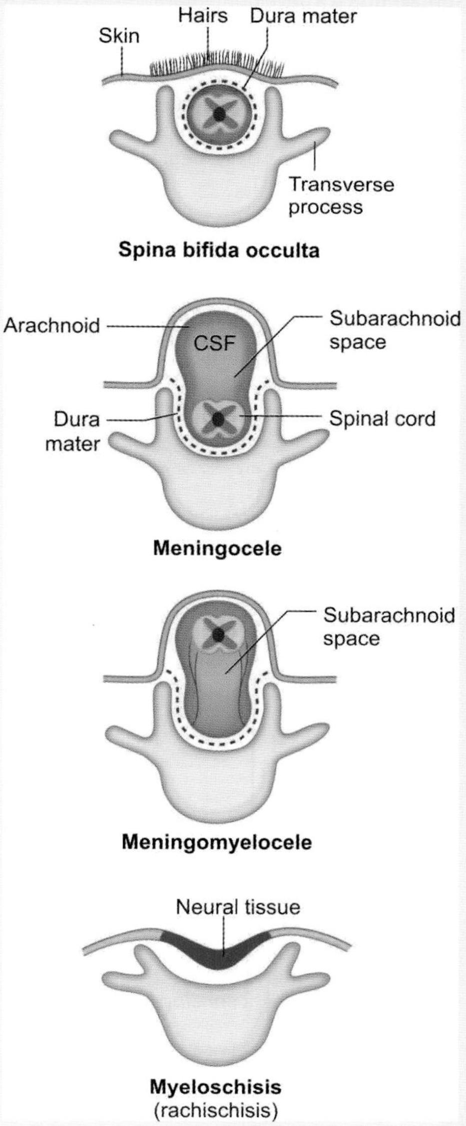

Fig. 7: Spina bifida

- ➢ These neuropores gradually shut close the neural canal from the amniotic cavity. The anterior (cranial) neuropore closes earlier (Day 25) than the posterior (caudal) neuropore (day 28).
- ➢ Failure of closure of the neuropores results in **open neural tube defects.** Non-closure anterior neuropore leads to anencephaly and non-closure of posterior neuropore leads to spina bifida. These conditions present with **elevated** levels of alpha-fetoprotein levels (and acetylcholine-esterase).
- ➢ Neural crest cells are the **fourth germ layer** cells, which appear at the margins of the neural folds during closure of the neural tube. (Some authorities consider neural crest cells are derived from **neuro-ectoderm**).
- ➢ **Neural crest cells** contribute to the peripheral nervous system and most of the ganglia are derived from these cells.
- ❏ Neural tube closure begins in the **cervical** region and proceeds **bidirectionally** towards cranial and caudal region (Langman's embryology).
- ❏ Moore embryology: Fusion of the neural tube starts in embryos with 4–6 somites, at the level of somites 1 and 2, forming the future rhombencephalon.
  - ➢ The tube closes caudally and rostrally, forming sequentially cervical and thoracic cord regions, then mesencephalic and prosencephalic brain regions.
  - ➢ Rostrally, two sites of fusion can be seen. The initial fusion, termed α, or the dorsal lip of the rostral neuropore, proceeds caudorostrally. A second site, termed β, or the terminal lip of the rostral neuropore, closes from the rostral end of the neural plate and proceeds rostrocaudally.
  - ➢ Closure of these lips of the rostral neuropore is completed when 19–20 pairs of somites are present.

Spina bifida is a developmental anomaly characterized by defective closure of the vertebral arch associated with maternal folic acid deficiency and is classified as various types.
- **Alpha fetoprotein** (AFP) is found in the amniotic fluid and maternal serum. It is an indicator of neural tube defects (e.g. spina bifida, anencephaly). AFP levels are reduced in mothers of fetuses with Down syndrome.
- Neural tube defect **Prophylaxis**: Women who may become pregnant are advised to get 400 micrograms of folic acid daily. Women who are pregnant should receive 1.0 mg (1000 mcg), and women who have previously given birth to a child with a neural tube defect should get 4.0 mg/5.0 mg daily, beginning one month before they start trying to get pregnant and continuing through the first three months of pregnancy.

1. **Remnant of rostral neuropore is:**   (NEET Pattern 2016)
   - a. Septum pellucidum
   - b. Crista terminalis
   - c. Lamina terminalis
   - d. Cerebellum

2. **Identify the anomaly:**   (AIIMS 2014)
   - a. Anencephaly
   - b. Rachischisis
   - c. Craniorachischisis
   - d. Meningoencephalocele

3. **Identify the congenital anomaly:**   (AIIMS 2015)
   - a. Rachischisis
   - b. Meningocele
   - c. Meningomyelocele
   - d. Meningoencephalocele

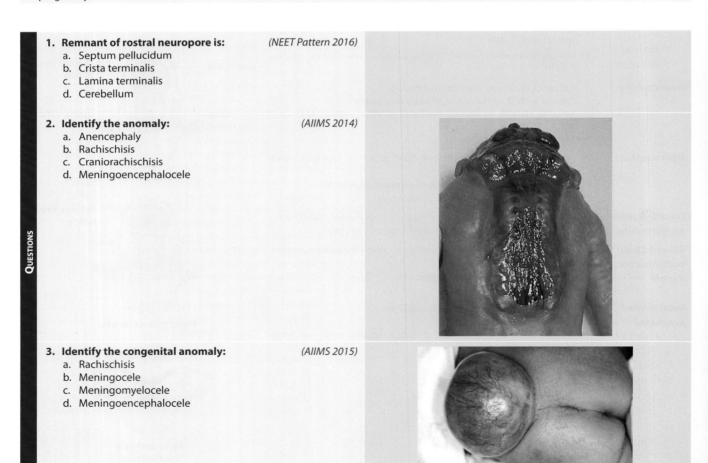

QUESTIONS

1. c. **Lamina terminalis**
   - ❑ **Lamina terminalis** represents the **cephalic end** of the primitive neural tube and corresponds with the **site of closure** of rostral (anterior) neuropore. It lies at the **anterior boundary** of third ventricle.

2. c. **Craniorachischisis**
   - ❑ This clinical case is craniorachischisis, which is the most severe form of dysraphism. It occurs due to total failure of neural tube closure.
   - ❑ Brain and spinal cord are exposed to the surrounding amniotic fluid, resulting in necrosis, degeneration or angioma-like formations.
   - ❑ Entire neural tube remains open.

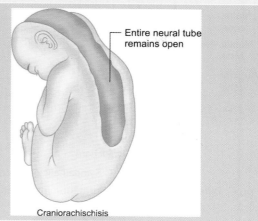

Craniorachischisis

3. c. **Meningomyelocele**
   - ❑ The present case shows a cystic swelling in the lumbosacral region, filled with fluid and has visible neural tissue as well, indicative of meningomyelocele.
   - ❑ In Myelomeningocele, the skin is intact, and the placode-containing remnants of nervous tissue is observed in the center of the lesion, which is filled with cerebrospinal fluid.

▶ Neural Tube

Layers of the neural tube wall:
- ❑ **Neuroepithelial** (ventricular) layer is the innermost layer having ependymal cells that lines the central canal and developing brain ventricles.
- ❑ **Mantle** (intermediate) layer is the middle layer consisting of neurons and glial cells, gets organized into a pair of anterior (**basal**) plates and posterior (**alar**) plates.
- ❑ **Marginal** layer is the outermost layer containing nerve fibers of neuroblasts of the mantle layer and glial cells. It forms the white matter of the spinal cord through the myelination of axons growing into this layer.

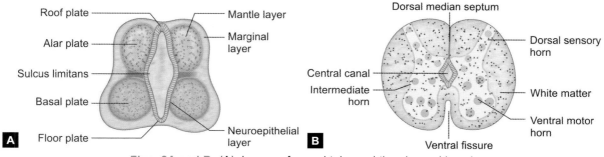

Figs. 8A and B: (A). Layers of neural tube and the alar and basal plates giving origin to ventral horn cells and dorsal horn cells (B)

- ❑ **Alar plate** is the posterolateral thickening of the mantle layer of the neural tube which give rise to second-order **sensory** neuroblasts of the posterior horn (general somatic afferent and general visceral afferent) cell regions.
  - ➤ It becomes the dorsal horn of the spinal cord and receives axons from the spinal ganglion which form the dorsal roots.
- ❑ **Basal plate** is the anterolateral thickening of the mantle layer of the neural tube giving rise to the **motor** neuroblasts of the anterior horn (general somatic efferent) and lateral horns (general visceral efferent) cell regions.
  - ➤ It becomes the anterior horn of the spinal cord and the axons from motor neuroblasts exiting the spinal cord form the anterior roots.
- ❑ **Sulcus limitans** is the longitudinal groove in the lateral wall of the neural tube that appears during the fourth week and **separates** the alar (sensory) and the basal (motor) plates.
  - ➤ It extends from rostral midbrain to the spinal cord, disappears in the adult spinal cord but is retained in the rhomboid fossa of the brainstem.
  - ➤ **Sulcus limitans** is present between the two plates; dorsally and ventrally, they are connected by non-neurogenic structures (**roof plate** and **floor plate**).
  - ➤ Floor plate contains the anterior white commissure.

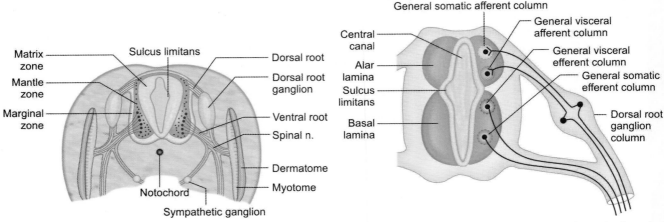

Fig. 9: Differentiation of the neural tube into three distinct layers, zones, and associated structures

Fig. 10: Transverse section of the developing spinal cord showing four longitudinal cell columns

Myelination begins in the fourth month (intrauterine life) in the spinal cord motor roots.

> Myelination of the corticospinal tracts is not complete until the end of the second postnatal year.
> Myelination of the association neocortex extends into the third decade.

Brain Development

❑ **Three primary** brain vesicles and associated flexures develop during the fourth week.
> **Prosencephalon** (forebrain) further divides into telencephalon and diencephalon.
> **Mesencephalon** (midbrain).
> **Rhombencephalon** (hindbrain) gives rise to metencephalon (pons and cerebellum) and myelencephalon (medulla oblongata).

❑ **Cephalic** flexure (midbrain flexure) is located between the prosencephalon and the rhombencephalon and **cervical** flexure is located between the rhombencephalon and the future spinal cord.

❑ **Five secondary** brain vesicles (with four ventricles) appear in the sixth week, which form the five major divisions of brain
> **Telencephalon** develops an out pocketing that form the **cerebral hemispheres** and olfactory bulbs. its ventricles are called as **lateral ventricles**.
> **Diencephalon** has the **thalamus** and the related thalami, with **third ventricle**. Its extensions form the optic nerves, neurohypophysis, etc.

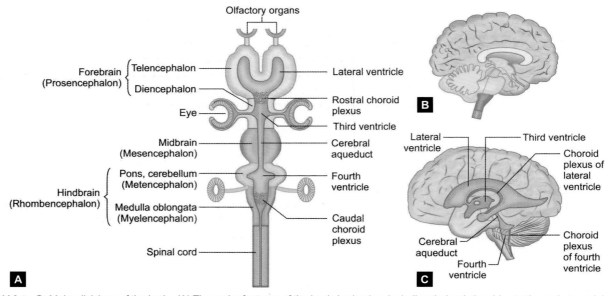

Figs. 11A to C: Major divisions of the brain. (A) The major features of the basic brain plan, including their relationships to the major special sensory organs of the head; (B) The corresponding regions in the adult brain, seen in sagittal section; (C) The organization of the ventricular system in the brain

➢ **Mesencephalon** presents with the cerebral **aqueduct** of Sylvius.
➢ **Metencephalon** is separated from the mesencephalon by the **rhombencephalic isthmus** and from the myelencephalon by the **pontine flexure**.
  ▪ It forms the **pons** and has rhombic lips on the dorsal surface that give rise to the **cerebellum**.
  ▪ Rostral half of the **fourth ventricle** is present in metencephalon.
➢ **Myelencephalon** is present between the pontine and cervical flexures and forms the **medulla oblongata**.
  ▪ Upper half of the medulla oblongata has **fourth ventricle** and lower half has **central canal**.

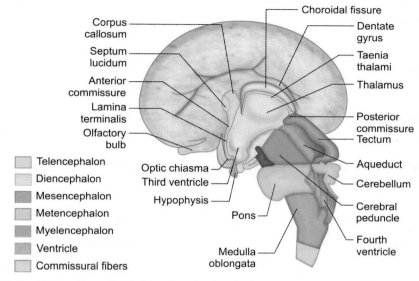

Fig. 12: Sagittal section of brain showing the developing anterior and posterior commissures

Cerebral hemispheres develop further into frontal, parietal, occipital, and temporal lobes.
❑ The temporal lobes overlie the insula and posterior brainstem.
❑ Telencephalon gives rise to commissural tracts that integrate the activities of the left and right cerebral hemispheres: the corpus callosum, anterior commissure, and hippocampal commissure.
  ➢ **Anterior commissure** is the first commissure to appear and interconnects the olfactory structures and the middle and inferior temporal gyri.
  ➢ **Hippocampal commissure** (fornix) is the second commissure to appear which interconnects the two hippocampi.
  ➢ **Corpus callosum** is the third commissure to appear interconnects the corresponding neocortical areas of the two cerebral hemispheres.
❑ The small posterior and habenular commissures develop from the epithalamus.

Corpus striatum appears as a bulging eminence on the floor of the lateral **telencephalic** vesicle.
❑ It forms the **caudate** nucleus, **putamen**, **amygdaloid** nucleus, and **claustrum**.
❑ The neurons of the **globus pallidus** originate in the subthalamus; they migrate into the telencephalic white matter and become the medial segments of the lentiform nucleus.
❑ **Corpus striatum** is divided into the **caudate** nucleus (medially) and the **lentiform** nucleus (laterally) by some projection fibers which make up the **internal capsule**.

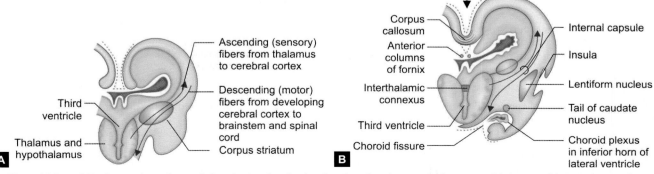

Figs. 13A and B: Coronal sections of developing forebrain showing development of corpus striatum and internal capsule

Hippocampus which is initially dorsal to the thalamus migrates **into the temporal lobe** and several brain components gradually assume **'C' curvature** with thalamus at the center: the cerebrum, corpus callosum, choroid plexus, fornix, caudate nucleus. Caudate nucleus has a head, body and tail eventually.

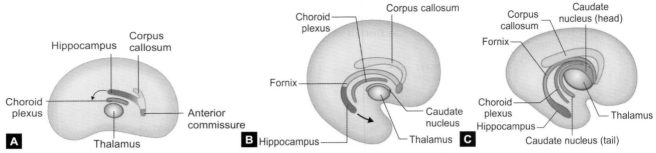

Figs. 14A to C: Coronal section of the developing brain components, showing the 'C' curvature assumed by the cerebrum, corpus callosum, choroid plexus, fornix, caudate nucleus, with thalamus at the center

▼ Neural Crest Cells

Ectodermal Placodes

❏ Before the neural tube closes, the elevating neural folds contain two distinctive neuronal populations. The larger population, **neural crest cells**, migrates from the neural epithelium prior to the fusion of neural tube and the smaller population, **neuroepithelial cells**, becomes incorporated into the surface ectoderm after neural tube closure.

❏ These areas of **neuroepithelium** within the surface ectoderm have been termed **ectodermal placodes**. Majority of the ectodermal placodes form nervous tissue and few of them are non-neurogenic placodes.

❏ After an appropriate inductive stimulus, placodes present as **localized thickenings** of the cephalic surface ectoderm and either they generate **migratory neuronal cells** that will contribute to the cranial sensory ganglia, or the whole placodal region invaginates to form a **vesicle** beneath the remaining surface ectoderm.

❏ **Otic placodes** are the first placodes visible on the surface of the embryo and forms the otic pit and the otic vesicle, giving rise eventually to inner ear (hearing and equilibrium).

❏ **Olfactory** (Nasal) placodes have 2 components (medial and lateral) and form the nose olfactory epithelium.

❏ **Optic** (Lens) placodes which form the lens, lie on the surface adjacent to the out pocketing of the diencephalon (which forms retina).

❏ **Trigeminal** placode gives rise to the cells of the trigeminal ganglion.

❏ **Adenohypophyseal** placode forms the anterior lobe of the pituitary gland.

1. Mesodermal in origin: (NEET Pattern 2012)
  a. Astrocytes
  b. Oligodendrocytes
  c. Ependymal cells
  d. Microglial cells

2. All of these arises from neuroepithelial cells EXCEPT: (NEET Pattern 2013)
  a. Neuron
  b. Oligodendrocyte
  c. Microglial cells
  d. Ependymal cells

3. Spinal cord develops from: (NEET Pattern 2014)
  a. Neural tube
  b. Mesencephalon
  c. Rhombencephalon
  d. Prosencephalon

4. Brainstem nucleus NOT derived from alar plate: (AIIMS 2008)
  a. Dentate
  b. Inferior olivary
  c. Hypoglossal
  d. Substantia nigra

5. Part of neural tube from which corpus callosum develops: (NEET Pattern 2016)
  a. Lamina terminalis
  b. Basal lamina
  c. Alar lamina
  d. Roof plate

6. Which of the following part of corpus callosum develops first: (NEET Pattern 2016)
  a. Dorsal part of genu
  b. Ventral part of genu
  c. Rostrum
  d. Splenium

7. All are disorders due to non-migration of neural crest cells EXCEPT: (AIIMS 2011)
  a. Porencephaly
  b. Lissencephaly
  c. Microgyria with ballooning
  d. Schizencephaly

1. d. Microglial cells
❏ **Microglia** are specialized macrophages (**mesodermal** in origin) capable of **phagocytosis** that protect neurons of the central nervous system.
  ■ They are derived from the earliest wave of **mononuclear** cells that originate in blood islands early in development and colonize the brain shortly after the neural precursors begin to differentiate.
  ■ They are **self-renewing** population and are distinct from macrophages and monocytes.
❏ **Macroglia** cells are derived from **neuroectoderm** and include: Astrocytes, oligodendrocytes, ependymal cells, Schwann cells.

2. c. Microglial cells
- ❑ **Neuroepithelial** cells are **neuroectodermal** in origin and are found in the ventricular zone of the neural tube. These are the **'stem cells'** which differentiate further into neurons, astrocytes and other glial cells.
- ❑ Most glia are derived from **ectodermal** tissue (neural tube and crest). The **exception** is microglia, which are derived from hemopoietic stem cells (**mesenchymal** in origin).

3. a. Neural tube
- ❑ **Neural tube** develops into brain and spinal cord.
- ❑ Brain: Forebrain (Prosencephalon); Midbrain (Mesencephalon); Hindbrain (Rhombencephalon)

4. c. Hypoglossal
- ❑ Hypoglossal nucleus is a **pure motor** nucleus derived from the **anterior basal plate** of neural tube.
- ❑ Posterior alar plate gives **sensory** (not motor) nuclei.

5. a. Lamina terminalis
- ❑ Initially, corpus callosum forms a small bundle in the **lamina terminalis** and later extends first anteriorly and then posteriorly, **arching over** the thin roof of the diencephalon. It connects the **nonolfactory** areas of the right and the left cerebral cortices.

6. a. Dorsal part of genu
- ❑ During the development of the corpus callosum, the **dorsal part of the genu** and the corpus form **first**. Subsequently, the anterior part of the genu and then the splenium arise. The **rostrum** is the **last** part to be formed.

7. a. Porencephaly
- ❑ Neuronal migration disorders (NMDs) **do not include porencephaly**.
- ❑ Under neuronal migration disorders are Lissencephaly, Microgyria, Schizencephaly.
- ❑ **Lissencephaly**, which literally means smooth brain, is a rare brain formation disorder caused by defective neuronal migration during the 12th to 24th weeks of gestation, resulting in a lack of development of brain folds (gyri) and grooves (sulci).
- ❑ Terms such as 'agyria' (no gyri) or 'pachygyria' (broad gyri) are used to describe the appearance of the surface of the brain.
- ❑ **Microgyria** is a neuronal migration disorder, a developmental anomaly of the brain characterized by development of numerous small convolutions (microgyri), presenting with mental retardation. It is present in a number of specific neurological diseases, notably multiple sclerosis and Fukuyama congenital muscular dystrophy, a specific disease cause by mutation in the Fukutin gene.
- ❑ Alternate names for the condition are polygyria and micropolygyria.
- ❑ **Schizencephaly** is a neuron migration disorder leading to clefts in the brain, which extend from the CSF cavity (ventricles) and reach till the surface of brain. It is characterized by abnormal continuity of gray matter tissue extending from the ependyma lining of the cerebral ventricles to the pial surface of the cerebral hemisphere surface.

- ❑ Neural tube begin to close from **cervical** region *(AIPG 2009)*
  - ➢ Neural tube closure begins in the cervical region and proceeds **bidirectionally** towards cranial and caudal region.
- ❑ Caudal (posterior) neuropore closes at **day 28** (three days later (25+3) to cranial (anterior) neuropore.
- ❑ Alpha-fetoprotein levels are **elevated** in Anencephaly, Myeloschisis, Omphalocele (but in Down syndrome the levels are **down**).
- ❑ The **retina** is an outgrowth of the **Diencephalon** *(NEET Pattern 2014)*
  - ➢ Diencephalon extends into the eyeball to become **retina** and **optic nerve**.
- ❑ **Myelination** of optic nerve begins at **7 months** of gestational age *(NEET Pattern 2016)* terminates shortly after birth at the level of the lamina cribrosa.
- ❑ **First commissure** to develop is **anterior** commissure *(NEET Pattern 2013)*

▼ CSF and Ventricles

- ❑ CSF (Cerebrospinal Fluid) is the ultrafiltrate of blood produced in the choroid (capillary) plexuses of the ventricles of the brain.
- ❑ The first CSF (cerebrospinal fluid) is formed of amniotic fluid, and is later secreted by the choroid (capillary) plexus in the lateral ventricles (chiefly) and partly in third and fourth ventricles.
- ❑ It escapes from the lateral ventricle into third ventricle via **foramen of Monro**, passes through **aqueduct of Sylvius** into the fourth ventricle, then it enters **central canal** eventually.
- ❑ It escapes the ventricular space at the roof of fourth ventricles at three foramina (midline Magendie and two lateral Luschka) into the subarachnoid space. (Sub – under).
- ❑ CSF absorption from the subarachnoid space occurs by the arachnoid villi (granulations) projecting into the dural venous sinuses (e.g. superior sagittal sinus).
- ❑ **Dural venous sinus** is the intradural space (between two layers of dura mater), contains venous blood from several tributaries including veins of brain.
- ❑ The most important lymphatic CSF absorption pathway is along the **olfactory** nerve route but there are other nerves that may conduct CSF extracranially. Tracers injected into the CSF system appear to exit the cranium along almost all of the cranial nerves including the **optic**, trigeminal, **vestibulo-cochlear**, vagus and hypoglossal nerves.

❏ The total volume of CSF in the adult ranges from 140–270 mL. The volume of the ventricles is about 25 mL. CSF is produced at a rate of 0.2–0.7 mL per minute (600–700 mL per day), which means that the entire CSF volume is replaced approximately 4 times per day.

Circulation and absorption of CSF:

CSF in **lateral ventricles** → Interventricular **foramen of Monro** → **Third** Ventricle (midline) → Cerebral **aqueduct of Sylvius** → **Fourth** ventricle →

Foramina in the roof of fourth ventricle (**Magendie** and **Luschka**) → **Sub-arachnoid space** (Cerebellomedullary and pontine cistern) → Tentorial notch → Inferior and superolateral surface of cerebrum → **Arachnoid villi** and granulations → Dural venous sinus (**Superior sagittal sinus**).

Choroid plexus develops by the close apposition of vascular pia mater and ependyma without intervening nervous tissue.

❏ The vascular layer is infolded into the ventricular cavity and develops a series of small villous projections, each covered by a cuboidal epithelium derived from the ependyma.

❏ The cuboidal cells display numerous microvilli on their ventricular surfaces.

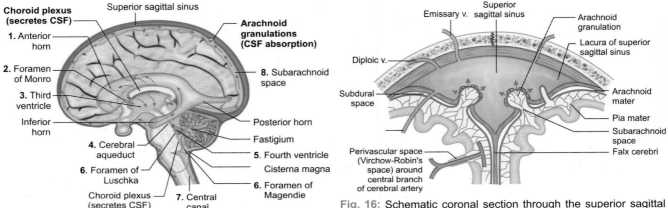

Fig. 15: Circulation of cerebrospinal fluid

Fig. 16: Schematic coronal section through the superior sagittal sinus showing arachnoid granulations and absorption of the cerebrospinal fluid

Hydrocephalus is the dilation of the ventricles due to an excess of CSF. It may result from blockage of CSF circulation or overproduction of CSF.

❏ **Non-communicating** hydrocephalus may result from obstruction within the ventricles (e.g. congenital aqueductal stenosis).

❏ **Communicating** hydrocephalus results from blockage distal to the ventricles (e.g. adhesions after tuberculous meningitis).

CSF Cisterns of the Brain

Table 3: Location and vascular contents of various cisterns of the brain		
Cistern	**Location**	**Contents**
Cerebellomedullary cistern/cisterna magna	In the interval between medulla oblongata and inferior surface of cerebellum	–
Pontine cistern/cisterna pontis	On the ventral surface of pons	Basilar artery and its branches
Interpeduncular cistern/basal cistern	At the base of brain in the interval between two temporal lobes	Circle of Willis (circulus arteriosus)
Cistern of lateral sulcus/sylvian cistern	In the stem of lateral sulcus in front of temporal pole	Middle cerebral artery
Cistern of great cerebral vein of Galen/cisterna ambiens	In the interval between splenium of corpus callosum and superior surface of cerebellum	Great cerebral vein of Galen

- ❑ **Lateral ventricles**, one in each cerebral hemi-sphere, is a C-shaped cavity lined with **ependyma** and communicate with the 3rd ventricle through the interventricular foramen (of **Monro**).
- ❑ Parts: It has a **central** part (body) and three horns (**Anterior**, **Posterior** and **Inferior**).
  - ➢ **Central** part (body) is located in the medial portion of the frontal and parietal lobes.
    - ▪ **Floor** (lateral to medial): Body of caudate nucleus, stria terminalis, thalamostriate vein, and thalamus.
    - ▪ **Roof**: **Corpus callosum**
    - ▪ **Medial wall**: Septum pellucidum
  - ➢ **Frontal** (anterior) horn is located in the **frontal** lobe; lies **in front of** interventricular foramen.
    - ▪ Roof: **Body** of corpus callosum
    - ▪ Floor: **Rostrum** of corpus callosum
    - ▪ Anterior wall: **Genu** of corpus callosum
    - ▪ Medial wall: Septum pellucidum
    - ▪ Lateral wall: Head of the caudate nucleus
  - ➢ **Occipital** (posterior) horn is located in the parietal and occipital lobes.
    - ▪ Medial wall: Upper- **Bulb** of posterior horn (formed by the forceps major of corpus callosum) and Lower- **Calcar avis** (formed by calcarine sulcus).
    - ▪ Roof, lateral wall, and floor: **Tapetum** of the corpus callosum.
  - ➢ **Temporal** (inferior) horn is located in the medial part of the temporal lobe and is **the largest** horn.
    - ▪ Floor: **Hippocampus** (medially) and collateral eminence (laterally)
    - ▪ Roof (medially): Tail of caudate nucleus & stria terminalis and (laterally): **Tapetum** of corpus callosum
  - ➢ **Trigone** (atrium) is present at the junction of the body, occipital horn, and temporal horn of the lateral ventricle.
- **Third ventricle** is the ventricle of diencephalon and presents as a median cleft between the two thalami.
- ❑ **Thalamus and hypothalamus** are at the **lateral** wall of third ventricle.
- ❑ **Lamina terminalis** is at the **anterior** wall of third ventricle.
- ❑ The anterior part of the **floor** of the third ventricle is formed mainly by **hypothalamic** structures.
  - ➢ Immediately behind the **optic chiasma** lies the thin **infundibular recess**, which extends into the pituitary stalk.
  - ➢ Behind this recess, the **tuber cinereum** and the **mammillary bodies** form the floor of the ventricle.
- ❑ **Pineal gland** is at the **posterior** wall of third ventricle.
- ❑ **Roof** is formed by the **ependyma**, lining the undersurface of the tela choroidea of the third ventricle.
- ❑ Certain regions of the lining of the third ventricle become highly specialized, and develop concentrations of tanycytes or other modified cells that are collectively termed the **circumventricular organs**, e.g. the subfornical organ, the organum vasculosum (intercolumnar tubercle) of the lamina terminalis, the subcommissural organ, and the linings of the pineal, suprapineal and infundibular recesses.

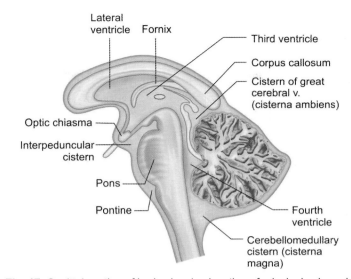

Fig. 17: Sagittal section of brain showing location of principal subarach-noid cisterns

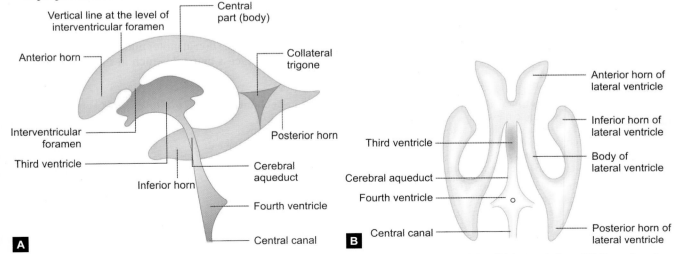

Figs. 18A and B: Ventricular system of the brain showing different parts of lateral ventricle: (A) Lateral view; (B) Superior view

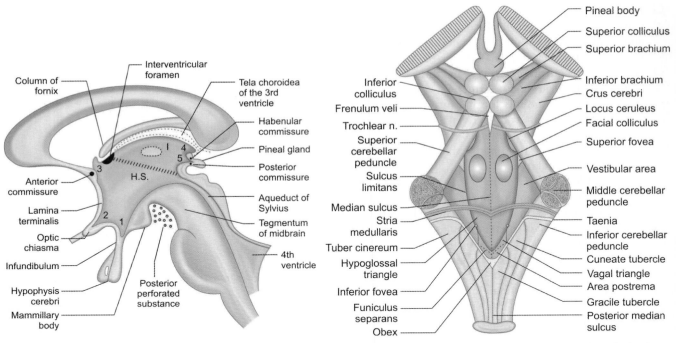

Fig. 19: Boundaries and recesses of the 3rd ventricle as seen in sagittal section (HS - hypothalmic sulcus, I - interthalamic adhesion, 1 - infundibular recess, 2 - optic recess, 3 - anterior recess, 4 - suprapineal recess, 5 - pineal recess)

Fourth ventricle is located within the pons and the upper part of the medulla.

❑ **Roof** of the fourth ventricle is formed by the **cerebellum** (superior and inferior medullary vela).

❑ **Floor** of the fourth ventricle is formed by the rhomboid fossa. Structures present at the floor of the fourth ventricle are:

➢ **Facial colliculus** is the rounded elevation formed by the axons of facial nerve as they loop around (internal genu) the abducens nucleus in the lower pons.

➢ Lesion to the facial colliculus results in ipsilateral facial paralysis and ipsilateral unopposed eye medial deviation.

➢ **Obex** represents the caudal tip of the fourth ventricle. It is a marker for the level of the foramen magnum of the skull and the imaginary dividing line between the medulla and spinal cord.

➢ **Median sulcus** divides the floor into right and left halves. It extends from cerebral aqueduct of the midbrain to central canal of the spinal cord.

➢ **Stria medullaris** are the fibers derived from arcuate nuclei, which emerge from the median sulcus and run transversely across the floor to enter into the inferior cerebellar peduncle.

➢ **Medial eminence** are the elevations on either side of the median sulcus and are laterally bounded by sulcus limitans.

➢ **Sulcus limitans** represents the border between the alar plate and the basal plate of the developing neural tube.

➢ The upper end of the sulcus limitans widens into a triangular depression **superior fovea**. Above the superior fovea sulcus limitans presents a flattened gray area called **locus ceruleus**.

➢ The lower end of the sulcus limitans widens into a triangular depression **inferior fovea**.

➢ **Vestibular area** is over the vestibular nuclei and lies lateral to sulcus limitans.

➢ **Vagal trigone** is the prominence in the floor of the inferior fovea that overlies the dorsal motor nucleus of the vagus.

➢ **Hypoglossal trigone** is the slight elevation in the floor of the inferior recess beneath which lies the nucleus of the hypoglossal nerve.

QUESTIONS

1. **TRUE about cerebrospinal fluid is:**   *(PGIC 2000)*
   a. Produced by choroid plexus
   b. Travels from subarachnoid space to the fourth ventricle
   c. Absorbed by arachnoid villi
   d. Drains into the dural venous sinuses
   e. Aqueductal stenosis dilates 4th ventricle

3. **Posterior limit of lateral ventricle is:**   *(NEET Pattern 2016)*
   a. Corpus callosum
   b. Occipital lobe
   c. Septum pellucidum
   d. Calcar avis

2. **Anterior horn of lateral ventricle is closed anteriorly by:**   *(NEET Pattern 2015)*
   a. Thalamus   b. Septum pellucidum
   c. Lamina terminalis   d. Corpus callosum

4. **Floor of third ventricle is formed by all EXCEPT:**   *(NEET Pattern 2015)*
   a. Tuber cinereum
   b. Posterior perforated substance
   c. Tegmentum
   d. Anterior pituitary

QUESTIONS

5. All are seen in the floor of 3rd ventricles EXCEPT:
(AIIMS 2014)
- a. Infundibulum
- b. Oculomotor nerve
- c. Mammillary body
- d. Optic chiasma

7. Floor of fourth ventricle contains all EXCEPT: *(JIPMER 2011)*
- a. Abducent nucleus
- b. Facial nucleus
- c. Dorsal vagal nucleus
- d. Hypoglossal nucleus

9. Which cranial nerve nucleus lies under the facial colliculus:
(AIIMS 2014,15, NEET Pattern 2016)
- a. Fifth
- b. Sixth
- c. Seventh
- d. Eighth

6. Floor of 4th ventricle has: *(NEET Pattern 2015)*
- a. Infundibulum
- b. Vagal triangle
- c. Mammillary body
- d. Tuber cinerium

8. Substantia ferruginea is present in: *(NEET Pattern 2016)*
- a. Gray matter
- b. White matter
- c. Hypothalamus
- d. Pituitary gland

10. Damage to the structure producing the elevation marked leads to paralysis of which of the following muscle:
(AIIMS 2016)
- a. Lateral rectus
- b. Risorius
- c. Levator palpebrae superioris
- d. Superior oblique

ANSWERS

1. a. Produced by choroid plexus; c. Absorbed by arachnoid villi; d. Drains into dural venous sinuses.
- ❏ CSF moves out of fourth ventricle into the subarachnoid space (not the other way around).
- ❏ Aqueductal stenosis dilates the proximal ventricles 1, 2 and 3 (not 4th).

2. d. Corpus callosum
- ❏ The anterior horn of the lateral ventricle lies anterior to its central part, the two being separated by an imaginary vertical line drawn at the level of the interventricular foramen.
- ❏ Anterior horn is closed anteriorly by the genu and rostrum of the corpus callosum.

3. b. Occipital lobe
- ❏ Occipital (posterior) horn of lateral ventricle reaches posterior extent of the occipital lobe.

4. d. Anterior pituitary
- ❏ Floor of third ventricle has infundibular recess, which extends into the pituitary stalk (not anterior pituitary).

5. b. Oculomotor nerve
- ❏ Oculomotor nerve is not in the floor of 3rd ventricle, it passes under the floor, within the interpeduncular fossa.
- ❏ The anterior part of the floor of the third ventricle is formed mainly by hypothalamic structures.
- ❏ Immediately behind the optic chiasma lies the thin infundibular recess, which extends into the pituitary stalk.
- ❏ Behind this recess, the tuber cinereum and the mammillary bodies form the floor of the ventricle.

6. b. Vagal triangle
- ❏ Vagal triangle is seen at the floor of the fourth ventricle raised by vagal nucleus underneath.
- ❏ Floor of 4th ventricle has areas related to Abducent (6), vestibular (8), vagus (10), hypoglossal (12) nuclei.

7. b. Facial nucleus
- ❏ Facial nucleus is not present in the floor of the fourth ventricle.
- ❏ Facial colliculus is raised due to the axons of facial nerve winding around the abducent nucleus.

8. a. Gray matter
- ❏ A group of nerve cells (gray matter) containing melanin pigment constitute the substantia ferruginea, at the floor of fourth ventricle.

9. b. Sixth
- ❏ Facial colliculus is raised due to the axons of facial nerve winding around the abducent nucleus.
- ❏ It is the facial nerve axons (not the abducent nucleus) that raises the elevation called facial colliculus.

10. b. Risorius > a. Lateral rectus
- ❏ The diagram shows the floor of the fourth ventricle, with the arrow showing the facial colliculus.
- ❏ Facial colliculus is a rounded elevation formed by the axons of facial nerve winding around the abducent nucleus.
- ❏ Damage to the facial nerve axons paralyzes muscles of facial expression like risorius.
- ❏ In facial colliculus syndrome, even the deeper abducent nucleus may be damaged, leading to paralysis of lateral rectus muscle.

❑ The color in locus ceruleus is imparted by the underlying group of nerve cells containing melanin pigment which constitute the substantia ferruginea.
  ➤ The neurons of locus ceruleus contain large quantities of norepinephrine (noradrenaline).
❑ CSF escapes the fourth ventricle into the subarachnoid space via three foramina: One midline Magendie and two lateral Luschka *(PGIC 2000)*
❑ Arachnoid villi responsible for cerebrospinal fluid absorption protrude mainly in the superior sagittal sinus *(AIIMS 2002)*
❑ Third ventricle is the midline ventricle located in diencephalon *(NEET Pattern 2012)*
❑ Cerebral aqueduct of Sylvius is a cavity within the mesencephalon *(NEET Pattern 2013)*
❑ Ventricles of brain are lined by ependymocytes *(NEET Pattern 2015)*
  ➤ These are cuboidal or columnar in shape with tuft of cilia.
❑ Lateral ventricle is connected in third ventricle by foramen of Monro *(NEET Pattern 2013)*
❑ Pineal gland forms Posterior boundary of third ventricle *(NEET Pattern 2013)*
❑ Foramen of Magendie is the central opening of 4th ventricle *(NEET Pattern 2013)*
❑ Facial colliculus is located at pons *(AIPG 2008)*

▶ Cerebrum

Cerebrum is the highest and largest part of brain to control and modulate emotions, personality, hearing, vision, and voluntary activities.

It is made up of the two cerebral hemispheres having the outer layers of cortex (gray matter) and the underlying regions of axons (white matter).

❑ Cerebral cortex is folded into ridges (gyri) and furrows (sulci) to increase the surface area.
❑ The two cerebral hemispheres are separated from each other by a deep fissure called the **longitudinal fissure**.
❑ Cerebral hemisphere is divided into **six lobes**: frontal, parietal, occipital, temporal, insular and limbic lobes.
❑ Frontal, parietal, temporal, and occipital lobes named upon their overlying neurocranial bones.
❑ Dominant hemisphere is responsible for propositional language consisting of grammar, speech and calculations.
  ➤ The left hemisphere is dominant in 95% of cases.
  ➤ Nondominant hemisphere is primarily responsible for three-dimensional or spatial perception and nonverbal ideation (music and poetry).

Cerebral cortex consists of the **neocortex** (90%) and the **allocortex** (10%).

❑ Neocortex has six layers and allocortex three.
❑ Allocortex itself is two types:
  ➤ Archicortex which includes the hippocampus and the dentate gyrus.
  ➤ Paleocortex which includes the olfactory cortex.

The **six layers** in the neocortex:

❑ Layers II and IV of the neocortex are mainly afferent and Layers V and VI are mainly efferent.
❑ Layer I is the molecular and layer II is the external granular.
❑ Layer III is the external pyramidal layer which gives rise to association and commissural fibers and is the major source of corticocortical fibers.
❑ Layer IV is the internal granular layer which receives thalamocortical fibers from the thalamic nuclei of the ventral tier (i.e., ventral posterolateral and ventral posteromedial).
  ➤ In the visual cortex (Brodmann's area 17), layer IV receives input from the lateral geniculate body.
❑ Layer V is the internal **pyramidal layer** and gives rise to corticobulbar, corticospinal, and corticostriatal fibers.
  ➤ It contains the giant **pyramidal cells of Betz**, which are found only in the motor cortex (Brodmann's area 4).
❑ Layer VI is the multiform layer and is the major source of corticothalamic fibers.
  ➤ It gives rise to projection, commissural, and association fibers.

Sulci in Cerebrum

Central sulcus (of Rolando) begins by cutting the superomedial border of the hemisphere about 1 cm behind the midpoint between the frontal and occipital poles.

❑ It runs sinuously downwards and forwards at an angle of 70° and ends just above the lateral sulcus.
❑ Its upper end extends onto the medial surface.
❑ It is the boundary between the frontal motor area and the parietal sensory area posteriorly.

Lateral sulcus (of Sylvius) begins as a deep cleft on the inferior surface of the cerebral hemisphere at the anterior perforated substance.

❑ It extends laterally between the temporal pole and the posterior part of the orbital surface of the hemisphere.
❑ It continues posteriorly and slightly upwards across the lateral surface and ends in the inferior parietal lobule by an upturned posterior end.

Calcarine sulcus develops on the medial surface of the cerebral hemisphere.
- ❏ It begins below the posterior end of the splenium part of corpus callosum and follows an arched course with a convexity upwards to the occipital pole and extends upon the superolateral surface.

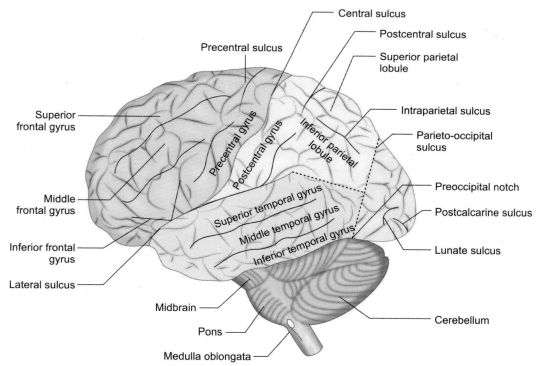

Fig. 20: Lateral aspect of the left side of the brain. Note the four lobes on the superolateral surface of the cerebral hemisphere

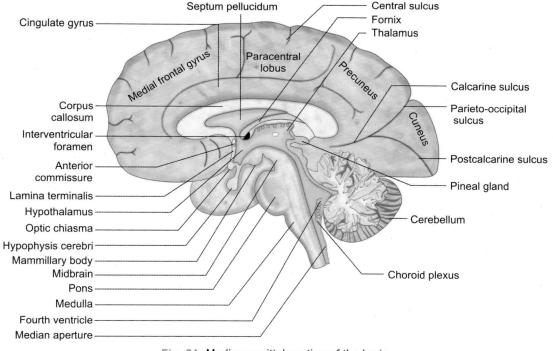

Fig. 21: Median sagittal section of the brain

Types of sulci: **Axial, limiting, operculated,** and **ctomplete**.
- ❏ **Axial sulci** develop along the long axis of rapidly growing homogeneous areas. They are longitudinally infolded (as seen in the **posterior part of calcarine sulcus** of the visual cortex).
- ❏ **Limiting sulci** develop along planes separating cortical areas, which differ in the functions. **Central sulcus** limiting frontal motor cortex from the parietal sensory cortex.

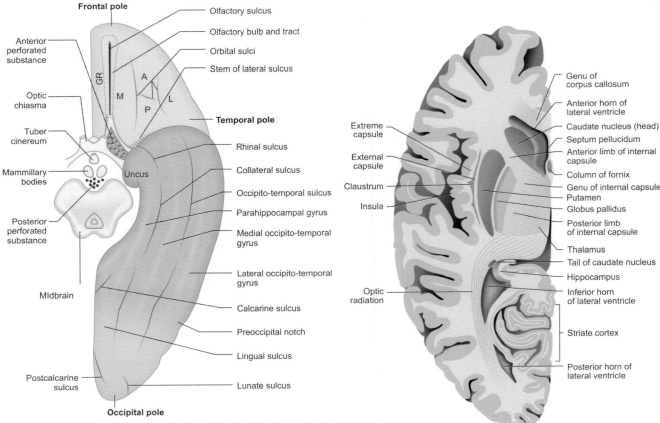

Fig. 22: Inferior surface of the cerebral hemisphere is divided into small anterior part, the orbital surface and large posterior part, the tentorial surface. Midbrain is seen in a transverse section

Fig. 23: The superior view of a horizontal section through the left cerebral hemisphere

- ❑ **Operculated sulcus** is similar to a limiting sulcus in that it separates structurally and functionally different areas but the transition occurs at the lip and not the floor. Often a third area of function is present in the floor and walls of the sulcus. An example is the **lunate sulcus** (separating the striate and peristriate areas at the surface) which contains the peristriate area within its walls.
- ❑ **Complete sulcus** is deep enough to produce an elevation in the wall of a ventricle. For example, the **collateral sulcus** produces collateral eminence in the inferior horn of the lateral ventricle and the **anterior part of the calcarine sulcus** produces calcar avis in the medial wall of the occipital horn of the lateral ventricle.
- ❑ **Insula** is a portion of the cerebral cortex folded deep within the floor of the lateral sulcus.
  - ➤ During development insula becomes hidden due to the overgrowth of the surrounding cortical areas and may be seen by pulling the lips of the lateral sulcus wide apart.
  - ➤ It is triangular in shape and surrounded entirely by the circular sulcus except anteroinferiorly at its apex (limen insulae).

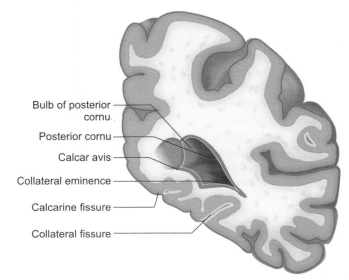

Fig. 24: Cut-section of cerebrum to show calcarine fissure (raising calcar avis) and collateral fissure (raising collateral eminence) into the depths of the cavity of lateral ventricle. These two sulci are thence called complete sulci

QUESTIONS

1. Which of the following is a complete sulcus:
(NEET Pattern 2012)

- a. Lunate sulcus
- b. Lateral sulcus
- c. Collateral sulcus
- d. Calcarine sulcus

2. Identify Insula in the coronal section of brain: *(AIIMS 2016)*

- a. A
- b. B
- c. C
- d. D

ANSWERS

1. c. Collateral sulcus > d. Calcarine sulcus
- ❏ Complete sulcus is the one which is **deep enough** to reach the wall of the **ventricle** and **raise an elevation** on the interior wall.
- ❏ Inside the lateral ventricle, **collateral sulcus** invaginates to produces an elevation called collateral eminence and **anterior part of calcarine** sulcus (pre-calcarine sulcus) raises the elevation known as calcar avis.

2. c. C
- ❏ Insula (marker 'C') is the lobe of cerebrum which lies **deep to the lateral sulcus** of brain.
- ❏ Key: A: Frontal cortex (in the vicinity of superior longitudinal fissure); B: **Basal ganglia**; C: **Insular cortex**; D: **Thalamus**

- ❏ **Hippocampus** is concerned with **recent memory traces** and is related to the inferior **(temporal)** horn of **lateral** ventricle.
- ❏ **Lunate** sulcus is an **operculated** sulcus *(NEET Pattern 2012)*

▼ Brodmann Areas

Brodmann area is a region of the cerebral cortex defined by its cytoarchitecture, or histological structure and organization of cells correlated closely to specific cortical functions. There are a total of 52 areas grouped into 11 histological areas.

- ❏ Brodmann areas 1, 2 and 3 (postcentral gyrus) are the primary somatosensory cortex and area 5 is the somatosensory association cortex.
- ❏ Area 4 (precentral gyrus) is the primary **motor** cortex and 6 is the **premotor** cortex and **supplementary** motor cortex (secondary motor cortex).
- ❏ Area 17 (occipital cortex) is the **primary** visual area (V1). Area 18 is the **secondary** visual cortex (V2) and Area 19 is **associative** visual cortex (V3, V4, V5).
- ❏ Auditory cortex (41 and 42) is located at the anterior part of the superior temporal gyrus (transverse temporal gyri of Heschl's).
- ❏ **Wernicke's sensory speech area** (22) is present at the **posterior** part of the **superior temporal gyrus**.
  - ➤ There is **uncertainty** about the precise extent of Wernicke's area. Some authorities consider it as a large parietotemporal area that includes areas 22 and 37 to be visuo-auditory areas associated with speech and language respectively.
  - ➤ There is a mention of areas 39 (angular gyrus) and 40 (supramarginal gyrus) by few other authors.
  - ➤ It is responsible for the **comprehension of language** but its stimulation causes speech arrest.
- ❏ **Broca's motor speech area** is part of the inferior frontal gyrus on the left Brodmann areas 44 (pars opercularis), and 45 (pars triangularis).
  - ➤ It works for the planning of movement of speech muscles and is involved in production of language.
- ❏ **Frontal eye field** (8) is present in the middle frontal gyrus.
  - ➤ Frontal eye field is the center for contralateral horizontal gaze. A lesion results in an inability to make voluntary eye movements toward the contralateral side. Since the activity of the intact frontal eye field in the opposite cortex is unopposed in such a lesion, the result is conjugate slow deviation of the eyes toward the side of the lesion.
- ❏ Area 43 is the primary gustatory (taste) cortex.
- ❏ Area 13 and Area 14 are insular cortex.

Para-central lobule is present near the midline encroaching upon the medial surface of the hemisphere and is the continuation of the precentral and postcentral gyri.

❑ The paracentral lobule controls motor and sensory innervations of the contralateral **lower limb** and **perineal region**.

❑ It is also responsible for control of **bladder and bowel** (defecation and urination).

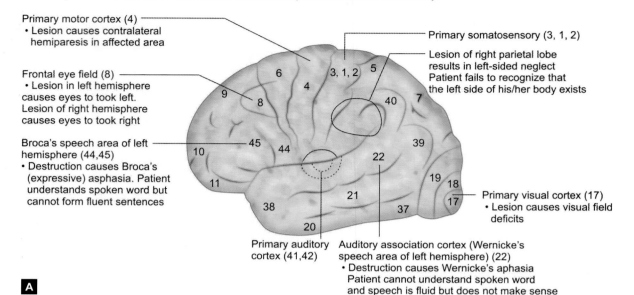

A

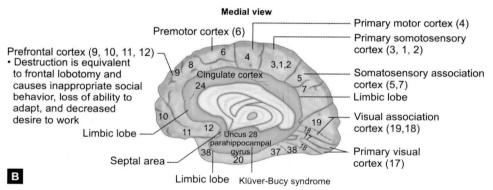

B

Figs. 25A and B: Brodmann areas on lateral (A) and medial (B) surfaces of cerebrum

1. **All of the following pairs for Brodmann area are correct EXCEPT:**
   a. Superior temporal gyrus: Auditory cortex (41,42)
   b. Superior temporal gyrus: Wernicke's sensory speech area (22)
   c. Inferior frontal gyrus: Broca's motor speech area (44)
   d. Superior frontal gyrus: Frontal eye field (8)

2. **Wernicke's Brodmann area is:**   *(NEET Pattern 2013)*
   a. 22
   b. 37
   c. 39
   d. 40

3. **Broca's area is located at**   *(NEET Pattern 2018)*
   a. Inferior frontal gyrus
   b. Inferior temporal gyrus
   c. Superior temporal gyrus
   d. Parietal lobe

1. **d. Superior frontal gyrus: Frontal eye field (8)**
   ❑ Frontal eye field (8) is located at the middle frontal gyrus.

2. **a. 22**
   ❑ Wernicke's Brodmann area is number 22 and is present at the **posterior part** of the **superior temporal gyrus**.
   ❑ There is **uncertainty** about the precise extent of Wernicke's area. Some authorities consider it as a large **parietotemporal area** that includes areas 22 **and 37** to be visuo-auditory areas associated with speech and language respectively.
   ❑ There is a mention of **areas 39** (angular gyrus) and 40 (supramarginal gyrus) by few other authors.

3. **a. Inferior frontal gyrus**
   ❑ **Broca's** motor speech area (44, 45) is located at **inferior frontal gyrus**.

- ❑ Primary **visual** area is located in the walls of **posterior part** of calcarine sulcus.
  - ➢ It shows lines (stria) of Gennari and is also called as **striate cortex**.
- ❑ Primary **auditory** area (41, 42) is present in the **superior temporal gyrus** (*NEET Pattern 2015*)
- ❑ **Broca's** area is present in **Inferior frontal** gyrus (*NEET Pattern 2012*)
- ❑ **Heschl's** gyrus in brain is located in Primary auditory cortex (*JIPMER 2016*)
  - ➢ It is the **transverse temporal gyrus** in the area of primary auditory cortex **buried within** the lateral sulcus.

▸ Homunculus

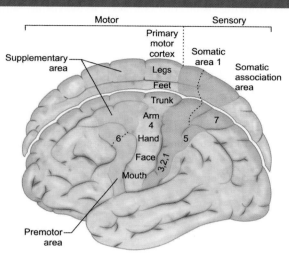

Fig. 26: Motor and somatosensory functional areas of the cerebral cortex (with Brodmann numbers)

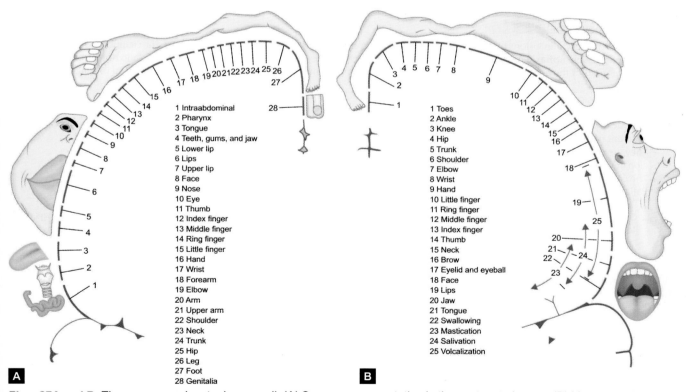

A

| 1 Intraabdominal |
| 2 Pharynx |
| 3 Tongue |
| 4 Teeth, gums, and jaw |
| 5 Lower lip |
| 6 Lips |
| 7 Upper lip |
| 8 Face |
| 9 Nose |
| 10 Eye |
| 11 Thumb |
| 12 Index finger |
| 13 Middle finger |
| 14 Ring finger |
| 15 Little finger |
| 16 Hand |
| 17 Wrist |
| 18 Forearm |
| 19 Elbow |
| 20 Arm |
| 21 Upper arm |
| 22 Shoulder |
| 23 Neck |
| 24 Trunk |
| 25 Hip |
| 26 Leg |
| 27 Foot |
| 28 Genitalia |

B

| 1 Toes |
| 2 Ankle |
| 3 Knee |
| 4 Hip |
| 5 Trunk |
| 6 Shoulder |
| 7 Elbow |
| 8 Wrist |
| 9 Hand |
| 10 Little finger |
| 11 Ring finger |
| 12 Middle finger |
| 13 Index finger |
| 14 Thumb |
| 15 Neck |
| 16 Brow |
| 17 Eyelid and eyeball |
| 18 Face |
| 19 Lips |
| 20 Jaw |
| 21 Tongue |
| 22 Swallowing |
| 23 Mastication |
| 24 Salivation |
| 25 Volcalization |

Figs. 27A and B: The sensory and motor homunculi. (A) Sensory representation in the postcentral gyrus. (B) Motor representation in the precentral gyrus

QUESTIONS

1. While doing surgery for meningioma on cerebral hemisphere, there occurred injury to left paracentral lobule, it will lead to paresis of:
   - a. Left face
   - b. Right neck and scapular region
   - c. Right leg and perineum
   - d. Right shoulder and trunk

Answers

1. **c. Right leg and perineum**
   - **Para-central lobule** is present near the midline encroaching upon the **medial surface** of the hemisphere and is the continuation of the precentral and postcentral gyri.
   - The paracentral lobule controls **motor and sensory** innervations of the **contralateral lower limb** and part of perineal region. It is also responsible for control of **bladder and bowel** (defecation and urination).

Language Pathway

- Visual image of a word is projected from the visual cortex (area 17) to the visual association cortices (areas 18 and 19) and next to the angular gyrus (area 39).
- Further processing occurs in Wernicke speech area (area 22), where the auditory form of the word is recalled.
- Arcuate fasciculus carries this information to Broca's speech area (areas 44 and 45), which has motor speech programs to control the vocalization mechanisms of the precentral gyrus (4).

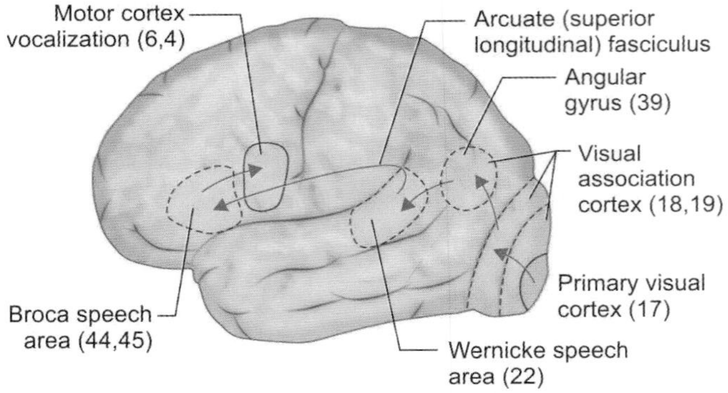

Fig. 28: Cortical areas involved in language production

Clinical Correlations

- **Dysphasia** may occur in lesions of Broca's motor speech area, Wernicke sensory speech area, or the arcuate fasciculus.
- **Broca's expressive aphasia** patient presents with hesitant speech (fluency is decreased), speaks in few words (and not in sentences).
  - The planning of movement of speech muscles is compromised and muscles are unable to articulate properly to produce meaningful voice.
  - Comprehension of language is good.
  - They are aware of their language disorder and may get frustrated by the deficit.
- In **Wernicke's receptive aphasia**, comprehension (understanding) of the language is compromised and the patient incessantly speaks in incoherent (irrelevant) sentences, making little sense.
  - They are often unaware of their mistakes.
- Lesion in the arcuate fasciculus result in **conduction aphasia**, with poor naming and problems in repetition of speech.
  - The comprehension of language and fluency of speech is intact.
  - Patients are aware of their errors but have significant difficulty correcting them.

Questions

1. **Speech in words and not in sentence occurs due to the lesion of:**
   a. Wernicke's sensory speech area
   b. Broca's motor speech area
   c. Arcuate fasciculus
   d. Primary auditory area

2. **A man comes with aphasia, is unable to name things and repetition is poor. However, comprehension, fluency and articulation are unaffected. He is probably suffering from:** *(AIIMS 2015)*
   a. Anomic aphasia
   b. Transcortical sensory aphasia
   c. Conduction aphasia
   d. Broca's aphasia

Answers

1. **b. Broca's motor speech area**
   - Speech in words **and not in sentences** is a feature suggesting **hesitant speech**, which occurs **Broca's motor aphasia**.
   - The **fluency** of speech is affected due to problem of **planning the speech movements**.
2. **c. Conduction aphasia**
   - A patient with **conduction aphasia** presents with inability to **name things** and **poor repetition** of language.
   - These features are evident in other conditions as well but since the comprehension is good, its **not a case of Wernicke's** and on the other hand intact fluency **rules out Broca's aphasia**.

Basal Ganglia

Brain components involved in **control of voluntary movements**

- Idea of voluntary movement originate in **cerebral** cortical association areas.
- The cerebral cortex, **basal ganglia**, and **cerebellum** work cooperatively to plan movements.

❑ Movement executed by the cortex is relayed via the **pyramidal tract** (corticospinal and corticobulbar tracts) to the motor neurons.

❑ Cerebellum provides feedback to adjust and smoothen movement.

Basal ganglia is involved in starting (initiation), and stopping of the voluntary motor activity and inhibiting unwanted movements.

❑ It consists of numerous nuclei, generally mentioned are three structural nuclei deep in the cerebrum (caudate nucleus, putamen, and globus pallidus) and two functional nuclei: Substantia nigra (midbrain) and the subthalamic nucleus (diencephalon).

❑ Amygdaloid nucleus and claustrum are also considered a part of basal ganglia.

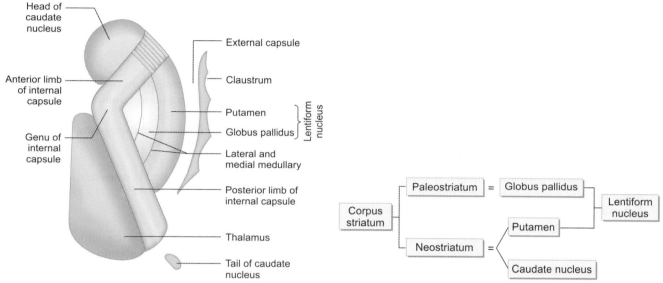

Fig. 29: Basal ganglia components (horizontal section of brain)

Fig. 30: Components of basal ganglia

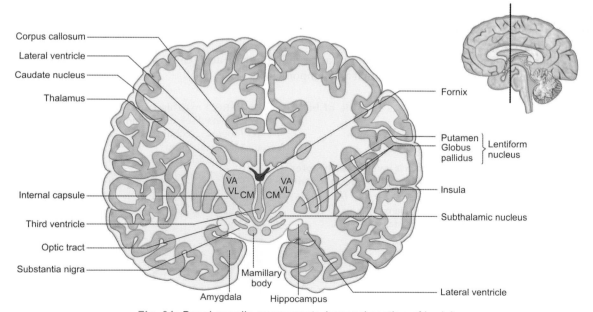

Fig. 31: Basal ganglia components (coronal section of brain)

Basal Ganglia Connections

❑ The **striatum** receives major input from three sources: the **thalamus**, **neocortex**, and **substantia nigra**.

❑ The striatum projects to the **globus pallidus** and **substantia nigra**.

❑ The globus pallidus is the **effector nucleus** of the striatal system; it projects to the **thalamus** and **subthalamic** nucleus.

❏ The substantia nigra also projects to the thalamus.
❏ The striatal motor system is expressed through the pyramidal system (corticobulbar and corticospinal tracts).

Basal Ganglia Functions

❏ **Planning** and **programming** of movement or, more broadly, in the processes by which an abstract thought is converted into voluntary action.
❏ Plays a role in the **initiation** and **execution** of voluntary motor activity, especially willed movement.
❏ It is also involved in **automatic stereotyped** postural and reflex motor activity (e.g. normal subjects swing their arms when they walk).
❏ Regulate the **muscle tone** and thus helps in smoothening the voluntary motor activities of the body. Decrease muscle tone to inhibit unwanted muscular activity.
❏ Determine how rapidly a movement is to be performed and how large the movement must be.
❏ Control group of movements for **emotional expression**.
❏ Control reflex muscular activity.

Lesions

❏ **Parkinson's disease** is a degenerative disease that affects the **substantia nigra** and its projections to the striatum resulting in depletion of dopamine in the substantia nigra and striatum as well as a loss of melanin-containing dopaminergic neurons in the substantia nigra.
❏ Patient presents with tremors (pill rolling), rigidity (cogwheel/lead pipe) and hypokinesia. Stooped posture, shuffling gait and masked facies.
❏ Lewy bodies are found in the melanin containing neurons of the substantia nigra.
❏ **Wilson's disease** (hepato-lenticular degeneration) is an autosomal recessive disorder that is caused by a defect in the metabolism of copper, in pediatric patients.
❏ Deposition of copper in the **lentiform** nucleus and liver (multilobar cirrhosis).
❏ Clinical signs include choreiform or athetotic movements, rigidity, and wing beating tremor.
❏ Copper deposition in the limbus of the cornea gives rise to the corneal Kayser-Fleischer ring (pathognomonic sign).
❏ **Hemiballismus** is a movement disorder that usually results from a vascular lesion of the **subthalamic nucleus**.
❏ Clinical signs include violent contralateral flinging (ballistic) movements of an entire limb.
❏ Lesions in the **globus pallidus** frequently lead to spontaneous and often continuous writhing movements of a hand, an arm, the neck, or the face-movements called **athetosis**.
❏ Multiple small lesions in the **putamen** (of striatum) lead to flicking movements in the hands, face, and other parts of the body, called **chorea**.
❏ **Huntington's** disease (chorea) is an inherited autosomal dominant movement disorder that is traced to a single gene defect on chromosome 4.
❏ It is associated with degeneration of the cholinergic and γ-aminobutyric acid (GABA)-ergic neurons of the **striatum**.
❏ It is accompanied by gyral atrophy in the frontal and temporal lobes.

QUESTIONS

1. **Which of the following clearly states the role of basal ganglia in motor function?**
   a. Planning
   b. Skilled function
   c. Coordinate function
   d. Balance

3. **The marked structure in the diagram is involved with motor activities. It receives afferents from all of the following EXCEPT:** *(AIIMS 2016)*
   a. Spinal cord
   b. Thalamus
   c. Cerebral cortex
   d. Substantia nigra

2. **INCORRECT matching pair about basal ganglia lesion is:**
   a. Wilson's disease: Lentiform nucleus
   b. Athetosis: Globus pallidus
   c. Chorea: Striatum
   d. Hemiballismus: Substantia nigra

1. a. Planning
- ❑ Basal ganglia are involved in the planning and programming of voluntary motor activity, especially in the processes by which an abstract thought is converted into voluntary action.

2. d. Hemiballismus: Substantia nigra
- ❑ A lesion in the subthalamus often leads to sudden flailing movements of an entire limb, a condition called hemiballismus.
- ❑ Lesions of the substantia nigra lead to the common and extremely severe disease of rigidity, akinesia, and tremors known as Parkinson's disease.

3. a. Spinal cord
- ❑ The structure marked in the diagram is **caudate nucleus** (part of basal ganglia).
- ❑ Caudate and putamen nucleus constitute striatum part of basal ganglia, which has three major inputs: Thalamus, neocortex, and substantia nigra.

  Note: Caudate nucleus do **not** receive any afferent from spinal cord.

❑ **Globus pallidus** and **putamen** are present in Basal ganglia *(NEET Pattern 2012)*
❑ **Amygdaloid** nucleus is a part of **basal ganglia.**

Internal Capsule

Internal capsule is the structure composed of collection of axons (**white matter**) in the inferomedial part of cerebral hemisphere.
- ❑ It has projection fibers (both **ascending** and **descending**) connecting higher brain centers with the lower and vice versa.
- ❑ It **separates** the caudate nucleus and the thalamus from the lentiform nucleus (putamen and globus pallidus).
- ❑ In a transverse section, it appears **V shaped**, with an anterior and posterior limb and the bend called as the genu.
- ❑ **Anterior limb** lies between the head of the caudate nucleus and lentiform nucleus and the **posterior limb** between the thalamus and lentiform nucleus.
- ❑ **Anterior limb** of internal capsule carries fibers connecting the **cerebral cortex** with the **thalamus** and **basal ganglia**.
- ❑ **Sensory** and **motor** fibers of the **head region** pass through the **genu.**
- ❑ **Sensory** and **motor fibers** of the **body** (neck, trunk and limb regions) pass through the anterior 2/3 of **posterior limb** of internal capsule (upper body fibers are arranged more anterior and lower body fibers more posterior).
- ❑ Posterior 1/3 of **posterior limb** carries sensory fibers (including audio-visual pathways).
- ❑ **Retrolenticular** portion is caudal to the lentiform nucleus and carries the **optic radiation** (geniculo-calcarine tract) from the lateral geniculate body to the occipital visual cortex (calcarine fissure).
- ❑ **Sublentiform** portion is beneath the lentiform nucleus and carries the **auditory pathway** from the medial geniculate nucleus to the primary auditory cortex (superior temporal gyrus).

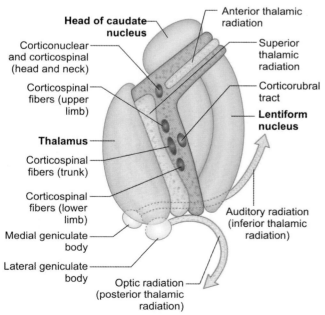

Fig. 32: Main components of internal capsule and their constituent fibers (yellow = thalamocortical, green = corticopontine fibers)

Table 4: Constituent motor and sensory fibers in different parts of the internal capsule		
Part	**Motor fibers**	**Sensory fibers**
Anterior limb	Corticopontine fibers	Anterior thalamic radiation
Genu	Corticopontine fibers Corticonuclear and corticospinal fibers for head and neck	Superior thalamic radiation (anterior part only)
Posterior limb	Corticopontine fibers Corticospinal (pyramidal) fibers for upper limb, trunk and lower limb Corticorubral (extrapyramidal) fibers	Superior thalamic radiation
Retrolentiform part	Corticopontine fibers	Posterior thalamic radiation (optic radiation)
Sublentiform part	Corticopontine fibers	Inferior thalamic radiation (auditory radiation)

- ❑ **Pyramidal tract** (corticospinal and corticonuclear tracts) constitutes a significant proportion of the internal capsule, carrying information from the upper motor neurones (in cerebral cortex) to the lower motor neurons (in brainstem and spinal cord) to modulate the **skeletal muscle** activity in the body.
  - ➤ Above the basal nuclei the pyramidal tract is a part of the **corona radiata**, below the basal nuclei the tract is called **crus cerebri** (a part of the cerebral peduncle).
  - ➤ In **genu** part of internal capsule lies the **corticonuclear tracts**, which carry the upper motor neurone fibers for the skeletal muscles of head region. These fibers undergo decussation and end in the motor nuclei of the cranial nerves of the opposite side.
  - ➤ In **posterior limb** runs the **corticospinal tract**, which carry the upper motor neurone fibers for the skeletal muscles of lower body (neck, trunk and limb regions).
- ❑ **Sensory** fibers are carried by **trigeminal** system from the **head** region and fibers pass through the **genu** of internal capsule.
- ❑ **Sensory** fibers from the **lower body** are carried by various tracts (e.g. dorsal column and spinothalamic tract) and the fibers pass through the **posterior limb** of internal capsule.

Arterial Supply

- ❑ Internal capsule is supplied by arteries that arise from the circle of Willis and its associated vessels. Lateral and medial **striate arteries** from the **middle** and **anterior cerebral arteries** supply major part of internal capsule.
- ❑ The arteries supplying internal capsule are:
  - ➤ Middle cerebral artery (major supply)
  - ➤ Anterior cerebral artery (including recurrent branch of Heubner)
  - ➤ Anterior choroidal artery (branch of internal carotid artery)

Note: Internal capsule also receives additional branches from internal carotid artery, posterior communicating artery, and posterior cerebral artery.

- ❑ Arterial supply to internal capsule is discussed in two parts: superior (dorsal) and inferior (ventral) part.
  - ➤ Superior (dorsal) part of the anterior limb, genu and the posterior limb are supplied by the **lenticulo-striate branches of middle cerebral artery**.
  - ➤ Inferior (ventral) part of internal capsule:
    - ▪ Anterior limb: Anterior cerebral artery (including recurrent branch of Heubner)
    - ▪ Genu: Internal carotid artery
    - ▪ Posterior limb: Anterior choroidal artery
    - ▪ Sublentiform and retrolentiform parts are chiefly supplied by anterior choroidal artery.
- ❑ One of the larger striate branches of the middle cerebral artery is known as 'Charcot's artery of cerebral hemorrhage'.

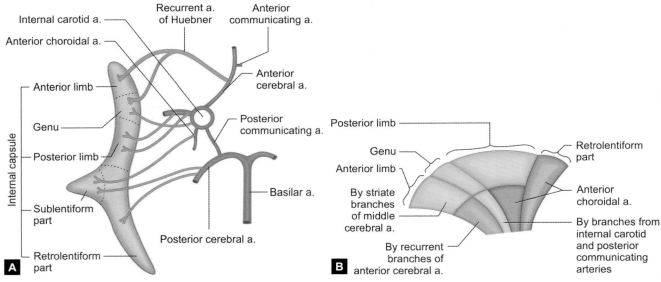

Figs. 33A and B: Arteries supplying the internal capsule

- ❑ Ischemic injury to internal capsule result in sensory and motor loss (hypesthesia and hemiparesis with the Babinski sign) on the contralateral side of the body.
- ❑ Lesion at
  - ➤ **Genu** results in sensory and motor loss on the **head** region.
  - ➤ **Posterior limb** (anterior 2/3) results in sensory and motor loss in **body** (neck, trunk and limb) region.
  - ➤ **Posterior limb** (posterior 1/3) results in audio-visual disturbances (e.g. homonymous hemianopia)

QUESTIONS

1. **Relations of internal capsule are:**
   a. Thalamus medially, caudate and lentiform nuclei laterally
   b. Thalamus laterally, caudate and lentiform nuclei medially
   c. Thalamus and caudate nucleus medially and lentiform nucleus laterally
   d. Thalamus and caudate nucleus laterally and lentiform nucleus medially

2. **Corticospinal fibers pass through which part of internal capsule:**
   a. Posterior one-third of anterior limb
   b. Anterior two-third of posterior limb
   c. Posterior two-third of anterior limb
   d. Anterior two-third of anterior limb

3. **Regarding anterior choroidal artery syndrome, all are true EXCEPT:**
   a. Hemiparesis
   b. Hemi-sensory loss
   c. Predominant involvement of anterior limb of internal capsule
   d. Homonymous hemianopia

4. **All of the following pairs are correct for the artery supply to the lower parts of internal capsule EXCEPT:**
   a. Anterior limb: Recurrent branch of anterior cerebral artery
   b. Genu: Internal carotid artery
   c. Posterior limb: Anterior choroidal artery
   d. Sublentiform part: Heubner's artery

5. **Blood supply of posterior limb of internal capsule includes all EXCEPT:**
   a. Middle cerebral artery   b. Anterior cerebral artery
   c. Anterior choroidal artery   d. Posterior cerebral artery

ANSWERS

1. **c. Thalamus and caudate nucleus medially and lentiform nucleus laterally**
   - Internal capsule **separates** the caudate nucleus and the thalamus from the lentiform nucleus (putamen and globus pallidus).
   - In a transverse section, it appears **V shaped**, with an anterior and posterior limb and the bend called as the genu.
   - **Anterior limb** lies between the head of the caudate nucleus and lentiform nucleus and the **posterior limb** between the thalamus and lentiform nucleus.

2. **b. Anterior two-third of posterior limb**
   - **Corticospinal** fibers pass through the **anterior two-third** of the posterior limb of internal capsule.
   - Posterior 1/3 of **posterior limb** carries sensory fibers (including **audio-visual** pathways).

3. **c. Predominant Involvement of anterior limb of internal capsule**
   - Anterior choroidal artery (branch of internal carotid artery) does not supply the anterior limb of internal capsule.
   - It supplies inferior (ventral) part of posterior limb of internal capsule.
   - Fibers passing through posterior limb of internal capsule are compromised in this syndrome, which include:
     - Sensory and motor fibers from the body
     - Auditory and visual pathway fibers

4. **d. Sublentiform part: Heubner's artery**
   - The sublentiform and retrolentiform parts are chiefly supplied by **anterior choroidal artery**.
   - **Heubner's artery** is a recurrent branch of anterior cerebral artery, which supplies the **anterior limb** of internal capsule.

5. **b. Anterior cerebral artery**
   - **Superior** (dorsal) part of the posterior limb of internal capsule is supplied by the striate branches of **middle cerebral artery**.
   - **Inferior** (ventral) part of posterior limb is supplied by : **anterior choroidal artery** (branch of internal carotid artery).
   - The sublentiform and retrolentiform parts are chiefly supplied by **anterior choroidal artery**.
   - Some authors mention **posterior cerebral artery** as well, as a source of blood supply to posterior limb of internal capsule.

- Neural pathway passing through **genu** of internal capsule is **corticonuclear tract** (NEET Pattern 2014)
- **Sublentiform** part of the internal capsule are associated with **acoustic radiation**.

Diencephalon

Diencephalon is the part of the prosencephalon (forebrain), which includes **thalamus** and the related thalami.
- It plays the important role in the **integration** of the sensory and motor systems.
- The ventricle of thalamus is the **third ventricle**, which lies in the midline between the two thalami.
- Components of diencephalon:
  - Thalamus
  - Hypothalamus (neurohypophysis included)
  - Epithalamus which consists of anterior and posterior Paraventricular nuclei, medial and lateral Habenular nuclei, Stria medullaris thalami, Posterior commissure, Pineal body
  - Subthalamus
  - Metathalamus (medial and lateral geniculate bodies).
- Embryonic diencephalon forms the optic cup, which later forms the retina and optic nerve.

▶ Thalamus

Thalamus is a division of the diencephalon and is a **relay** and **integration center** for the sensory and motor signals to the cerebral cortex.

❑ It is also involved in regulation of consciousness, sleep, and alertness.

❑ The two thalami form the **lateral wall of the third ventricle** and are interconnected by a flattened gray band (**interthalamic adhesion**), which passes through the ventricle.

Thalamic Nuclei

❑ It has a ventral posterior (VP) nucleus, which has two parts: medial and lateral.

    ➢ VPM **(Ventero-Posterior-Medial)** nucleus receive sensory input from 'head' region, whereas VPL **(Ventero-Postero-Lateral)** nucleus receive sensory information from the 'body'.

❑ Trigeminal nerve (first order neurone) carries information from the head region continues in the trigeminal lemniscus (second order neurone in brainstem) and synapses on **VPM nucleus** of thalamus.

❑ **Thalamus** has **third** order neurones, which in turn project on to the parietal sensory cortex (1,2,3).

❑ Spinothalamic tract—spinal lemniscal system (pain, temperature) and dorsal column—medial lemniscal system (tactile discrimination, vibration, etc.) carry information from the 'body' region to synapse on VPL nucleus of thalamus, which further project the information to area 1,2,3.

Connections

Thalamus receives input from all sensory systems **except** the olfactory system.

❑ It is connected to the **cerebral cortex** via the thalamocortical radiations and to the **hippocampus** via the mammillo-thalamic tract.

❑ It has important connections with **basal nuclei.**

❑ **Spinothalamic tract** in the spinal cord transmits information to the thalamus about crude touch, pressure, pain and temperature.

Table 5: Connections of the specific thalamic nuclei			
Nucleus	**Afferents**	**Efferents**	**Functions**
Ventral posterior (VP)			
Ventral posteromedial (VPM)	Trigeminal lemniscus Solitariothalamic tract	To postcentral gyrus (area 3, 1, and 2)	Relay station for impulses from face and head, and taste buds
Ventral posterolateral (VPL)	Medial lemniscus Spinal lemniscus	To postcentral gyrus (area 3, 1 and 2)	Relay station for exteroceptive (pain, touch, and temperature) and proprioceptive sensations from whole of body except face and head
Ventral anterior (VA)	From globus pallidus through subthalamic fasciculus	To premotor cortex (area 6 and 8)	Relay station for striatal impulses
Ventra lateral (VL) (also called ventral intermediate (VI))	From cerebellum (denta-tonubrothalamic fibers and dentatothalamic fibers)	To motor and premotor areas of cerebral cortex (area 4 and 6)	Relay station for cerebellar impulses
Medial geniculate body	Auditory fibers from inferior colliculus	To primary auditory area (area 41 and 42)	Relay station for auditory impulses
Lateral geniculate body	Optic tract	To primary visual cortex (area 17)	Relay station for visual impulses

Arterial Supply

❑ Posterior communicating artery

❑ Posterior cerebral artery

❑ Anterior choroidal artery

❑ **Thalamic syndrome** leads to contralateral hemiparesis and hemi-anesthesia; elevated pain threshold;

❑ Spontaneous agonizing, burning pain (hyperpathia); and thalamic hand (athetotic posturing of the hand).

❑ **Korsakoff's syndrome** may result from damage to the mammillary body or the mammillothalamic tract.

❑ **Fatal familial insomnia** is a hereditary prion disease in which degeneration of the thalamus occurs, causing the patient to gradually lose his ability to sleep and progressing to a state of total insomnia, and eventual death.

Metathalamus

Metathalamus includes the **medial** and **lateral geniculate bodies**.

❑ **Lateral geniculate body** is a part of **visual pathway** and serves as a relay nucleus.
  ➤ It receives retinal input through the optic tract and projects to the primary visual cortex (area 17).
  ➤ It has six layered structure.

❑ **Medial geniculate body** is a part of **auditory pathway** and serves as an auditory relay nucleus.
  ➤ It receives auditory input through the brachium of the inferior colliculus and projects to the primary auditory cortex (areas 41 and 42).

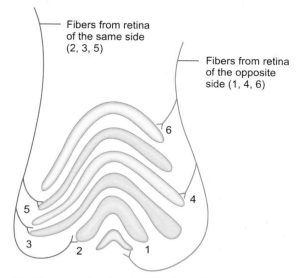

Fibers from retina of the same side (2, 3, 5)

Fibers from retina of the opposite side (1, 4, 6)

Fig. 34: Six layers (laminae) of the lateral geniculate body and their afferent connections

Table 6: Comparison between the medial and lateral geniculate bodies

Medial geniculate body	Lateral geniculate body
Oval-shaped collection of gray matter on the inferior aspect of the pulvinar	Bean-shaped collection of gray matter on the inferior aspect of inferior aspect of the pulvinar
Hilum absent	Hilum present
No lamination	Consists of 6 laminae, numbered 1 to 6 from ventral surface to dorsal surface
Destruction of medial geniculate on one side has little or no effect on hearing	Destruction of lateral geniculate body on one side produces blindness in the opposite half of the field of vision
Last relay station on the auditory pathway	Last relay station on the optic pathway
Sends auditory impulse through auditory radiation to the auditory area of temporal lobe	Sends visual impulses through optic radiation to the visual radiation to the cortex of the occipital lobe

Hypothalamus

❑ **Hypothalamus** is a division of the diencephalon which lies within the floor and ventral part of the walls of the third ventricle. It helps to maintain homeostasis by regulating the autonomic nervous system, endocrine system, and the limbic system.
❑ **Hypothalamic nuclei** and their functions.

Anterior	Medial	Posterior
Preoptic	Paraventricular	Posterior
Supraoptic	Dorsomedial	Mammillary
Suprachiasmatic	Lateral	Tuberomammillary
	Ventromedial	Dorsal
	Arcuate	

Table 7: Main hypothalamic nuclei and their functions

Region		Nucleus	Hormone secreted	Function
Chiasmatic	Medial	Median preoptic Periventricular	GnRH GnRH, somatostatin, CRH, TRH	
	Intermediate	Suprachiasmatic Supraoptic Paraventricular	Vasopressin Vasopressin, oxytocin	

Region		Nucleus	Hormone secreted	Function
Tuberal	Medial	Dorsomedial	TRH, ANP	Satiety center
		Ventromedial	TRH	Secrete to portal system
		Arcuate	GHRH, dopamine	
	Lateral	Lateral		Feeding center
Posterior	Medial	Mammillary body		Memory

(ANP, atrial natriuretic peptide; CRH: Corticotrophin-releasing hormone; GHRH: Growth hormone-releasing hormone; GnRH: Gonadotrophin-releasing hormone; TRH: Thyrotrophin-releasing hormone).

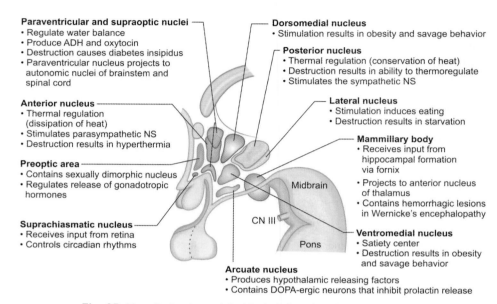

Fig. 35: Hypothalamic nuclei with their functional significance

Connections of Hypothalamus

❑ **Fornix** has five parts: the alveus, fimbria, crus, body, and columns.
❑ It projects from the hippocampal formation to the mammillary nucleus, anterior nucleus of the thalamus, and septal area.
❑ Bilateral transection results in an **acute amnestic syndrome**.
❑ **Stria terminalis** arises from the amygdaloid complex and interconnects the septal area, the hypothalamus, and the amygdaloid complex.
❑ It lies in the sulcus terminalis between the caudate nucleus and the thalamus.
❑ **Mammillothalamic tract** projects from the mammillary nuclei to the anterior nucleus of the thalamus.
❑ **Hypothalamospinal tract** contains descending autonomic fibers that influence preganglionic sympathetic neurons of the lateral horn cells and preganglionic neurons of the sacral parasympathetic nucleus in the spinal cord.
❑ The lesion of the tract may result in **Horner syndrome**.

▶ Subthalamus

Subthalamus is a part of diencephalon and is located lies beneath (sub) the thalamus, medial to the internal capsule and dorsolateral to the hypothalamus.

Connections

Subthalamus has efferent connections to:
❑ Striatum (caudate nucleus and putamen) in the telencephalon
❑ Dorsal thalamus (medial and lateral nuclear groups) in the diencephalon
❑ Red nucleus and substantia nigra in the mesencephalon.
❑ It has afferent connections from the substantia nigra and striatum.
❑ Its neurons contain glutamate and have excitatory effects over neurons of globus pallidus and substantia nigra.

▶ Reticular Nuclei

Reticular nucleus of the thalamus surrounds the thalamus as a thin layer of gamma-aminobutyric acid (GABA)-ergic neurons.
- ❏ It lies between the **external medullary lamina** and the **internal capsule** and receives excitatory collateral input from corticothalamic and thalamocortical fibers.
- ❏ It projects inhibitory (GABAergic) fibers to thalamic nuclei, from which it receives input.
- ❏ Reticular nuclei have intrathalamic connections and **do not** project to the cortex.

1. **Which of the following is/are projected to ventral posterior nucleus of thalamus?** *(PGIC)*
   a. Lateral lemniscus
   b. Medial lemniscus
   c. Corticospinal tract
   d. Spinal lemniscus
   e. Trigeminal lemniscus

2. **Which of the following thalamic nuclei does NOT project to neocortex?** *(AIIMS 2003)*
   a. Intralaminar nuclei
   b. Reticular nuclei
   c. Pulvinar nuclei
   d. Anterior thalamic nuclei

3. **Which of the following is NOT a part of epithalamus?**
   a. Pineal body
   b. Posterior commissure
   c. Trigonum habenula
   d. Geniculate bodies

4. **All of the following pairs are correct for nuclei of hypothalamus EXCEPT:**
   a. Ventero-medial: Hunger
   b. Supra-optic: Water conservation
   c. Posterior nucleus: Shivering center
   d. Supra-chiasmatic: Circadian rhythm

1. **b. Medial lemniscus; d. Spinal lemniscus; e. Trigeminal lemniscus**
   - ❏ Thalamus has a **ventral posterior** (VP) nucleus, which has two parts: **medial** and **lateral**.
   - ❏ VPM (Ventero-Posterior-**Medial**) nucleus receive sensory input from '**head**' region, whereas VPL (Ventero-Postero-**Lateral**) nucleus receive sensory information from the 'body'.
   - ❏ Trigeminal nerve (first order neurone) carries information from the head region continues in the **trigeminal lemniscus** (second order neurone in brainstem) and synapses on **VPM nucleus of thalamus**.
   - ❏ **Thalamus** has **third** order neurones, which in turn project on to the **parietal sensory cortex** (1,2,3).
   - ❏ Spinothalamic tract- spinal lemniscal system (pain, temperature) and dorsal column- medial lemniscal system (tactile discrimination, vibration, etc.) carry information from the '**body**' region to synapse on VPL nucleus of thalamus, which further project the information to area 1,2,3.
   - ❏ Lateral lemniscus carry **auditory** pathway and synapses with **medial geniculate** body (meta-thalamus).

2. **b. Reticular nuclei**
   - ❏ Reticular nuclei have **intrathalamic** connections and **do not project to the cortex**.
   - ❏ Reticular nuclei lie **between** the external medullary lamina and the internal capsule.
   - ❏ They use the neurotransmitter **GABA** and have **inhibitory** control over thalamic nuclei.
   - ❏ They play important role in normal EEG readings.
   - ❏ Most of the thalamic nuclei project to the neo-cortex, including intra-laminar, Pulvinar and anterior thalamus.

3. **d. Geniculate bodies**
   - ❏ The **epithalamus** is the dorsal (posterior) segment of the diencephalon.
   - ❏ It includes the **habenula** and their interconnecting fibers the habenular commissure, the **stria medullaris** and the pineal gland.
   - ❏ The medial and lateral **geniculate bodies** belong to **metathalamus**.

4. **a. Venteromedial: Hunger**
   - ❏ **Venteromedial** nucleus is the center for satiety (**not hunger**).
   - ❏ Anterior hypothalamus has osmoreceptors and centers like **supra-optic nucleus** secrete vasopressin (ADH) for **water conservation**.
   - ❏ **Posterior** nucleus works for heat conservation (**shivering** center).
   - ❏ Supra-chiasmatic regulates the circadian rhythm.

▶ Brainstem

Brainstem includes midbrain, pons and the medulla.
- ❏ It extends from the posterior commissure to the pyramidal decussation.
- ❏ It contains the nuclei for cranial nerve 3–12 and the nerves fibers exit from it.
- ❏ Various motor and sensory pathways (lemnisci) pass through the brainstem: Corticospinal tract (motor), dorsal column-medial lemniscal tract, spinothalamic tract—spinal lemniscal system, trigeminal lemniscus, lateral lemniscus (auditory pathway).
- ❏ It contains reticular formation at its central core.
- ❏ Brainstem has role in the regulation of cardiac and respiratory function (heart rate, breathing).
- ❏ It also regulates the central nervous system and maintains consciousness and regulating the sleep cycle.
   Arterial supply to brainstem is from the branches of vertebral arteries and the basilar arteries.

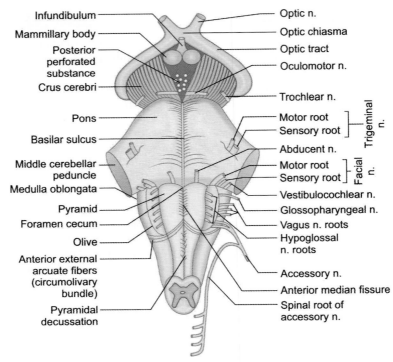

Fig. 36: External features on the anterior (ventral) aspect of the brainstem

Midbrain

- **Mesencephalon** (midbrain) comprises of three parts: the dorsal tectum, intermediate tegmentum, and the base.
- It extends from the posterior commissure to the superior medullary velum.
- It is connected to the cerebellum by the **superior cerebellar peduncle**.
- **Oculomotor** nucleus is present at the level of superior colliculus and **trochlear** nucleus at the level of inferior colliculus.
- It contains a center for vertical conjugate gaze in its rostral extent.
- Substantia nigra is the largest nucleus of the midbrain.
- Paramedian reticular formation is present along the midline.
- Has four lemnisci (medial to lateral): Medial, trigeminal, spinal and lateral.
- The **ventricle** of midbrain is called the **cerebral aqueduct of Sylvius, which lies** between the tectum and the tegmentum.
  A **transverse section** of midbrain shows following structures:
- **Dorsal structures:** Superior and inferior colliculi.

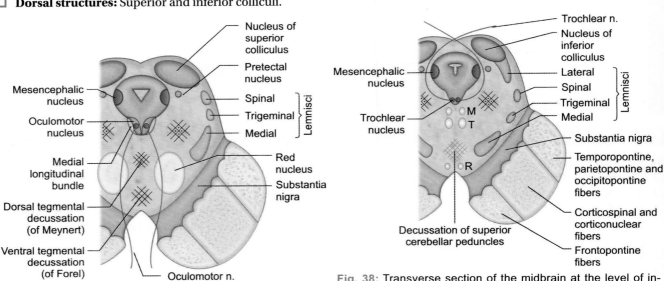

Fig. 37: Transverse section of the midbrain at the level of superior colliculi

Fig. 38: Transverse section of the midbrain at the level of inferior colliculi (M = medial longitudinal bundle, R = rubrospinal tract, T = tectospinal tract)

- **Tegmentum**: Oculomotor nucleus, Medial longitudinal fasciculus, Red nucleus, Substantia nigra, Dentatothalamic tract (crossed), Medial lemniscus, Lateral spinothalamic tract (in the spinal lemniscus).
- **Crus cerebri** (cerebral peduncle): Corticospinal tract lies in the middle three-fifths.
- **Weber (Medial midbrain) syndrome** (due to occlusion of paramedian branches of upper basilar and proximal posterior cerebral arteries)
- **Ipsilateral** sign and symptoms (structure involved)
  - ‘Down and out eye’ with dilated and unresponsive pupil and ptosis (Oculomotor nerve fibers)
    - Eye abduction and depression occur due to the unopposed action of the lateral rectus (CN 6) and the superior oblique (CN 4)
    - Severe ptosis (paralysis of the levator palpebrae)
    - Fixed and dilated pupil (complete internal ophthalmoplegia)
- **Contralateral** sign and symptoms (structure involved)
  - Weakness of lower face (CN 7), Palate (CN 10) and tongue (CN 12) (**Corticobulbar** tract in crus cerebri)
  - Hemiparesis of trunk and limbs (**Corticospinal** tract in crus cerebri)
  - ? Parkinsonism features (substantia nigra)

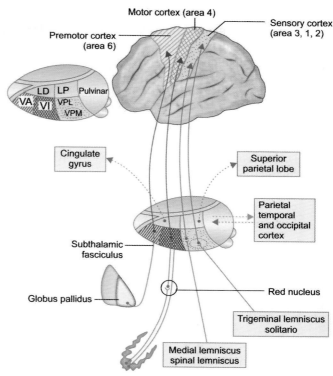

Fig. 39: Scheme to show connections of ventral and lateral groups of thalamic nuclei. The figure inset on left upper corner shows the dorsolateral view of thalamus and its major subdivisions. (LD = Lateral dorsal nucleus, LP = Lateral posterior nucleus, VA = Ventral anterior nucleus, VI = Ventral intermediate n, VPL = Ventral posterolateral n. VPM = Ventral posteromedial n.)

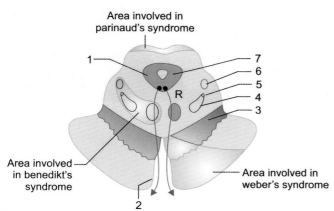

Fig. 40: Transverse section through the upper part of the midbrain. The Golden areas indicate the sites of lessions: 1. oculomotor nucleus, 2. oculomotor nerve, 3. substantia nigra, 4. medial lem-niscus, 5. trigeminal lemniscus, 6. spinal lemniscus, 7. cerebral aqueduct.

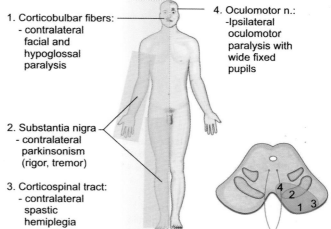

Fig. 41: Weber syndrome

- **Lateral** midbrain syndrome (occlusion of posterior cerebral artery branches)
- **Ipsilateral** sign and symptoms (structure involved)
  - ‘Down and out eye’ with dilated and unresponsive pupil and ptosis (Occulomotor nerve nucleus and fibers)
- **Contralateral** sign and symptoms (structure involved)
  - Hemiataxia, hyperkinesia, tremors (Red nucleus and dentato-rubro-thalamic tract)

- ❑ **Benedikt** (paramedian midbrain) syndrome (occlusion of paramedian branches of posterior cerebral artery)
- ❑ **Ipsilateral** sign and symptoms (structure involved)
  - ➤ 'Down and out eye' with dilated and unresponsive pupil and ptosis (Oculomotor nerve fibers)
    - ▪ Eye abduction and depression occurs due to the unopposed action of the lateral rectus (CN 6) and the superior oblique (CN 4)
    - ▪ Severe ptosis (paralysis of the levator palpebrae)
    - ▪ Fixed and dilated pupil (complete internal ophthalmoplegia)
- ❑ **Contralateral** sign and symptoms (structure involved)
  - ➤ Hemiataxia, hyperkinesia, tremors (Red nucleus and dentato-rubro-thalamic tract)
  - ➤ Loss of proprioception, discriminative touch and vibrations (medial lemniscus)
- ❑ **Parinaud** (posterior midbrain) syndrome may result due to a pineal tumour
  - ➤ Paralysis of upward and downward gaze, pupillary disturbances and absence of convergence (lesion in superior colliculus and pretectal area)
  - ➤ Non-communicating hydrocephalus (compression of aqueduct of Sylvius).

1. Red nucleus is situated at the level of:
a. Mid-brain; superior colliculus
b. Mid-brain; inferior colliculus
c. Pons
d. Medulla

2. Fibers passing through crus cerebri are:
a. Corticonuclear and corticospinal fibers
b. Medial lemniscus
c. Spinothalamic
d. All

3. Ventral tegmental decussation in cerebral peduncle is due to: *(NEET Pattern 2016)*
a. Tectospinal tract
b. Tectobulbar tract
c. Vestibulospinal tract
d. Rubrospinal tract

4. The marked structure is involved in which pathology: *(AIIMS 2017)*
a. Dementia
b. Alzheimer
c. Paralysis agitans
d. Chorea

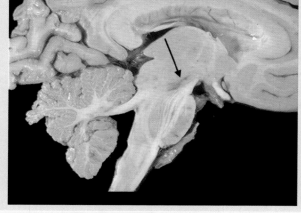

5. All of the following structures are involved in Weber syndrome EXCEPT *(NEET Pattern 2018)*
a. Oculomotor nerve roots
b. Corticobulbar tracts
c. Cerebellar peduncles
d. Corticospinal tract

1. a. Midbrain; superior colliculus
- ❑ A transverse section of midbrain, taken at the level of superior colliculus displays the red nucleus.
- ❑ At this level three syndrome may occur:
  - ▪ Weber syndrome: anterior midbrain lesion at this level involving crus cerebri and oculomotor nerve;
  - ▪ Benedict's syndrome: anterior and mid region is affected involving red nucleus.
  - ▪ Parinaud syndrome: Posterior midbrain lesion involving superior colliculi (upward gaze disturbances).

2. a. Corticonuclear and corticospinal fibers
- ❑ Crus cerebri is the anterior portion of the cerebral peduncle which contains the motor tracts: corticonuclear and corticospinal tracts.

3. d. Rubrospinal tract
- ❑ The ventral tegmental decussation is a decussation of the rubrospinal tract. The fibers from red nucleus before forming these tracts decussate forming 'ventral tegmental decussation of Forel'. The fibers of rubrospinal tract end in the anterior horn cells of the opposite side.

4. c. Paralysis agitans
- ❏ This is a sagittal section of the brain, showing substantia nigra in midbrain. Parts of the substantia nigra appear darker than neighboring areas due to high levels of neuromelanin in dopaminergic neurons.
- ❏ Paralysis agitans (parkinsonism) is characterized by the death of dopaminergic neurons in the substantia nigra pars compacta and abnormal pallor of the substantia nigra, correlating with loss of the pigment-containing nigral neurones.

5. b. Cerebellar peduncles
- ❏ In Weber syndrome there is lesion of cerebral (not cerebellar) peduncles.
- ❏ Cerebral peduncles carry corticospinal and corticobulbar tracts, whose lesion results in contralateral hemiplegia.
- ❏ Occulomotor nerve is lesions in Weber syndrome leading to ipsilateral eye involvement (down and out eye).

- ❏ Corpora quadrigemina is present in Midbrain
  - ➢ Corpora quadrigemina (four bodies) are the four colliculi (two superior and two inferior) located at the dorsal aspect of midbrain (tectum).
- ❏ Superior colliculus is related to visual reflexes, and inferior colliculus to auditory.
- ❏ In Parinaud (posterior midbrain) syndrome, superior colliculus is involved leading to disturbances in upward gaze.

▶ Pons

The **pons** is part of the brainstem lies between the midbrain (above) and the medulla oblongata (below) and in front of the cerebellum.

- ❏ It has two parts: The basilar part of the pons (ventrally) and the pontine tegmentum (dorsally).
  - ➢ Basilar part contains corticobulbar, corticospinal, and corticopontine tracts and pontine nuclei
  - ➢ Tegmentum contains cranial nerve nuclei, reticular nuclei, and the major ascending sensory pathways.
- ❏ Cranial nerve 5–7 nuclei (trigeminal, abducent and facial nerve) are present in pons. Vestibulocochlear nerve nuclei are present at the pontomedullary junction.
- ❏ Center for lateral gaze is present in pons.
- ❏ It is connected to the cerebellum by the **middle cerebellar peduncle**.

  A **transverse section** of pons shows following structures:
- ❏ **Medial structures**: Medial longitudinal fasciculus, internal genu of facial nerve producing facial colliculus, Abducent nucleus (underlies facial colliculus), Medial lemniscus, Corticospinal tract (in the base of the pons).
- ❏ **Lateral structures**: Facial nucleus, Descending (Spinal) sensory nucleus and tract of trigeminal nerve, Lateral spinothalamic tract—spinal lemniscus, Vestibular and cochlear nuclei.

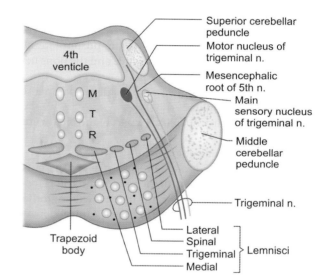

Fig. 42: Transverse section through the upper part of the pons (M = medial longitudinal bundle, R = rubrospinal tract, T = tectospinal tract)

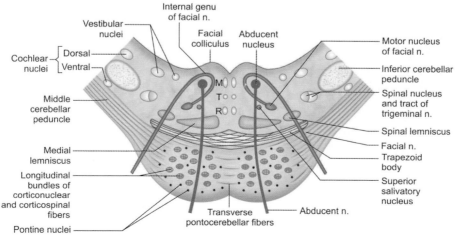

Fig. 43: Transverse section through the lower part of the pons (M = medial longitudinal bundle, T = tectospinal tract, R = rubrospinal tract)

	Lower part	Upper part
Gray matter	Contains: nuclei of VIth, VIIth and VIIIth cranial nerves; and nucleus of spinal tract of trigeminal nerve	Contains: motor and principal sensory nuclei of trigeminal nerve; and caudal part of nucleus ceruleus
White matter	Contains 2 lemnisci: medial and spinal Trapezoid body and nuclei present	Contains 4 lemnisci: medial, trigeminal, spinal and lateral Trapezoid body and nuclei absent

▼ Medulla Oblongata

Medulla oblongata is present in the lower part of the brainstem and is continuous with the spinal cord. Its upper part is continuous with the pons.
- ❏ It extends from inferior pontine sulcus to the pyramidal decussation.
- ❏ Cranial nerve **9–12 nuclei** (glossopharyngeal, vagus, cranial accessory nerve and hypoglossal nerve) are present in the medulla.
- ❏ Vestibulocochlear nerve nuclei are present at the **pontomedullary junction**.
- ❏ Medulla contains the cardiovascular, respiratory, vomiting and vasomotor centers dealing with heart rate, breathing and blood pressure.
- ❏ It is connected to the cerebellum by the **inferior cerebellar peduncle**.
  Olive (medulla oblongata)
- ❏ **Olives** are a pair of prominent oval structures in the medulla oblongata containing the olivary nuclei.
- ❏ Olive is present on the anterior surface of the medulla lateral to the pyramid, from which it is separated by the antero-lateral sulcus and the fibers of the hypoglossal nerve.
- ❏ Posteriorly it is separated from the posterolateral sulcus by the ventral spinocerebellar fasciculus. In the depression between the upper end of the olive and the pons lies the vestibulocochlear nerve.
- ❏ It has two parts:
  - ➢ Superior olivary nucleus is considered part of the pons and part of the auditory system, is a part of auditory pathway for sound perception.
  - ➢ Inferior olivary nucleus is a part of the olivo-cerebellar system and is mainly involved in cerebellar motor-learning and function.
  Pyramid (medulla oblongata)
- ❏ Medullary pyramids are paired ridge-like structures present on the ventral aspect of the medulla oblongata.
- ❏ It contains motor fibers of the **pyramidal tracts** (corticospinal and corticobulbar tracts).
- ❏ Pyramidal decussation occurs in the **lower medulla**. Approximately 90% of the fibers decussate and travel down the lateral corticospinal tract while the other 10% travel down the anterior corticospinal tract.

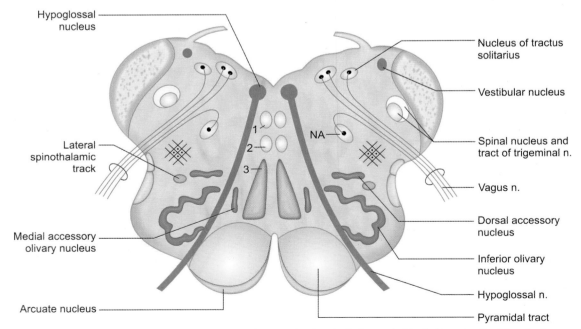

Fig. 44: Transverse section of medulla at the level of olives: 1. Medial longitudinal fasciculus, 2. tectospinal tract, 3. medial lemniscus. (NA = nucleus ambiguus)

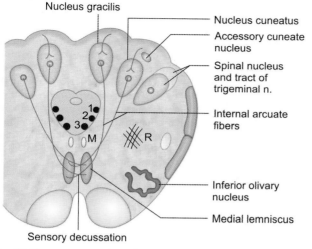

Fig. 45: Transverse section of medulla at the level of sensory decussation (1 = nucleus tractus solitarius, 2 = dorsal nucleus of vagus, 3 = hypoglossal nucleus; M = medial longitudinal fasciculus, R = reticular formation)

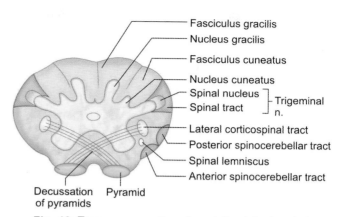

Fig. 46: Transverse section of medulla at the level of pyramidal decussation

- ❑ Anterior median fissure is present in the midline and separates the two pyramids.
- ❑ Anterolateral sulcus, which is present along their lateral borders, separates pyramid from olives.
- ❑ Hypoglossal nerve fibers emerge from anterolateral sulcus.

A **transverse section** of medulla shows following structures:
- ❑ **Medial** structures
  - ➢ Hypoglossal nucleus, medial lemniscus, pyramid (corticospinal fibers)
- ❑ **Lateral** structures
  - ➢ Nucleus ambiguus, vestibular nuclei, inferior cerebellar peduncle (carrying dorsal spinocerebellar, cuneocerebellar, and olivocerebellar tracts), lateral spinothalamic tract—spinal lemniscus, spinal nucleus and tract of trigeminal nerve

- ❑ **Medial medullary syndrome** (occlusion of vertebral artery or anterior spinal artery or a branch of basilar artery)
- ❑ **Ipsilateral** sign and symptoms (structure involved)
  - ➢ **Flaccid** (LMN) paralysis and atrophy of one half of tongue (Hypoglossal nerve)
- ❑ **Contralateral** sign and symptoms (structure involved)
  - ➢ **Spastic** (UMN) paralysis of trunk and limbs (contralateral corticospinal tract)
  - ➢ Impaired tactile, proprioceptive and vibration sense of trunk and limbs (contralateral medial lemniscus).

- ❑ **Wallenberg (Lateral medullary)** syndrome (occlusion of vertebral artery > posterior inferior cerebellar artery)
- ❑ **Ipsilateral** sign and symptoms (structure involved)
  - ➢ Loss of pain and temperature over half face (Descending tract and nucleus of trigeminal nerve)
  - ➢ Cerebellar ataxia of limbs, falling to side of lesion (? Spinocerebellar tract)
  - ➢ Nystagmus, vertigo, nausea (Vestibular nucleus)
  - ➢ Horner's syndrome—miosis, ptosis, anhydrosis (Descending sympathetic tract)
  - ➢ Paralysis of palate, pharynx and larynx muscles - difficulty in speech and swallowing (Nucleus ambiguus)
  - ➢ Loss of taste on half of tongue (nucleus tractus solitarius).
- ❑ **Contralateral** sign and symptoms (structure involved)
  - ➢ Loss of pain and temperature over half of the body (Lateral spinothalamic tract)
- ❑ Total unilateral medullary syndrome (occlusion of vertebral artery) presents with combination of medial and lateral syndromes.

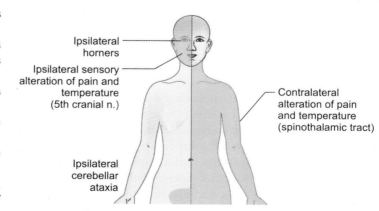

Fig. 47: Right sided Wallenberg syndrome: Clinical features.

QUESTIONS

1. Cross section through medulla at the level of mid-olivary section through floor of fourth ventricle contains which of the following structures: *(PGIC 2016)*
   a. Dorsal nucleus of vagus
   b. Trapezoid body
   c. Nucleus of tractus solitarius
   d. Superior vestibular nucleus
   e. Nucleus ambiguus

2. A 68-year-old woman presents in the emergency room with dizziness and nystagmus. Examination reveals a loss of pain and temperature sensation over the right side of the face and the left side of the body. The patient exhibits ataxia and intention tremor on the right in both the upper and lower extremities and is unable to perform either the finger-to-nose or heel to-shin tasks on the right. In addition, she is hoarse and demonstrates pupillary constriction and drooping of the eyelid on the right. Finally, the right side of her face is drier than the left. Which of the following artery block would explain the patient's condition: *(AIIMS 2016)*
   a. Right posterior inferior cerebellar artery
   b. Left posterior inferior cerebellar artery
   c. Right anterior inferior cerebellar artery
   d. Basilar artery

   (NEET Pattern 2018)

3. Wallenberg syndrome involves which artery
   a. Anterior inferior cerebellar artery
   b. Posterior inferior cerebellar artery
   c. Subclavian artery
   d. Posterior cerebral artery

ANSWERS

1. **a. Dorsal nucleus of vagus; c. Nucleus of tractus solitarius; e. Nucleus ambiguus**
   ❑ **Trapezoid body** and **superior vestibular nucleus** are seen in a section of **lower pons**.

2. **a. Right posterior inferior cerebellar artery**
   ❑ This is a case of right sided **Wallenberg syndrome** due to occlusion in the right **posterior inferior cerebellar artery**, leading to lateral medullary ischemia and lesion of certain nuclei and tracts.
   ❑ The patient has alternating hemi-anesthesia: ipsilateral loss of pain and temperature on face and contralateral loss of pain and temperature on the body. It occurs due to lesion of **lateral spinothalamic tract** and **spinal sensory nucleus of trigeminal**.
   ❑ Ataxia and intentions tremors indicate injury to **spinocerebellar tract** in the lateral medulla.
   ❑ There is hoarseness of voice which indicates lesion of **nucleus ambiguus** (which controls muscles of larynx).
   ❑ Patient also has features of right sided Horner syndrome due to lesion of the **hypothalamo-spinal pathway** in the lateral medulla.

3. **b. Posterior inferior cerebellar artery**
   ❑ **Wallenberg syndrome** usually occurs due to involvement of ipsilateral **vertebral artery**, but occasionally it is due to block in ipsilateral **posterior inferior cerebellar artery**.

❑ Nucleus **fasciculatus** (another name for cuneatus) is seen in **Medulla oblongata** *(NEET Pattern 2012)*
❑ **Nuclei** cuneatus and gracilis are present in **Medulla oblongata**.
❑ **Facial nerve** does NOT arise from the **medulla** *(NEET Pattern 2014)*
❑ Nucleus ambiguus is **postero-medial** to olive *(NEET Pattern 2014)*
❑ **Olive** is seen in Medulla oblongata *(NEET Pattern 2014)*
❑ **Internal arcuate fibers** of medulla comes from Nucleus gracilis and cuneatus *(NEET Pattern 2015)*
❑ These fibers cross to the opposite side to continue as the **medial lemniscus**.
❑ **Trochlear** nerve arises from **lower midbrain** and Abducent arises from pons.

▶ Interpeduncular Fossa

❑ **Interpeduncular fossa** is a rhomboidal space bounded on either side by crus cerebri of cerebral peduncles, anteriorly by optic chiasma and optic tracts; and posteriorly by the pons.
❑ It contains (anterior to posterior):
   ➢ A narrow stalk which connects the hypophysis cerebri with the tuber cinereum called **infundibulum**
   ➢ A raised area of gray matter lying anterior to the mammillary bodies called **tuber cinereum**
   ➢ Two small spherical bodies called **mammillary bodies**
   ➢ **Posterior perforated substance**, which is a layer of gray matter in the angle between the crus cerebri, and is pierced by central branches of the posterior cerebral arteries
   ➢ **Oculomotor nerve** which emerges immediately dorsomedial to the corresponding crus.
❑ **Contents** of interpeduncular fossa are Tuber cinerium, Infundibular stalk, Posterior perforated substance, Occulomotor nerve.
❑ Trochlear nerve is **not** a content of interpeduncular fossa.

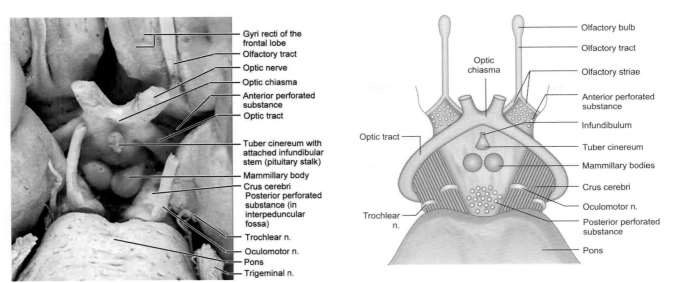

Fig. 48: Inferior aspect of hypothalamus and interpeduncular fossa

Fig. 49: Boundaries and contents of the interpeduncular fossa

CNS and Brain Stem Nuclei

❑ Neural tube forms the CNS (central nervous system) and is divided transversely into dorsal (sensory) and ventral (motor) parts by the **sulcus limitans**. It has a **dorsal alar plate** which gives origin to the **sensory** nuclei and a **ventral** plate separated forming the **motor** nuclei. The sensory and motor nuclei are separated from each other by the sulcus limitans.

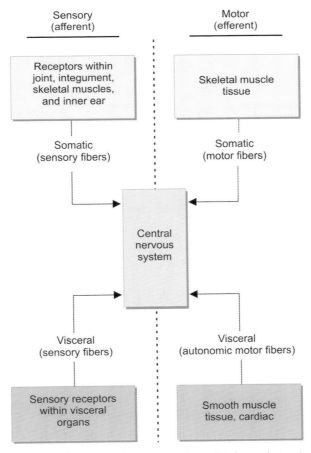

Fig. 50: Motor (efferent) and sensory (afferent) information categories

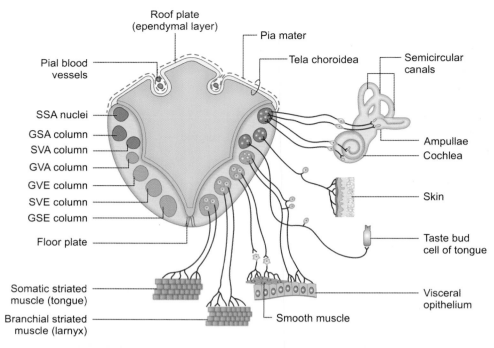

Fig. 51: Brainstem illustrating the cell columns derived from the alar and basal plates. The seven cranial nerve modalities are shown. (GSA: General somatic afferent, GVA: General visceral afferent, GVE: General visceral efferent; SSA: Special somatic afferent, SSE: Special somatic efferent; SVA: Special visceral afferent, SVE: Special visceral efferent)

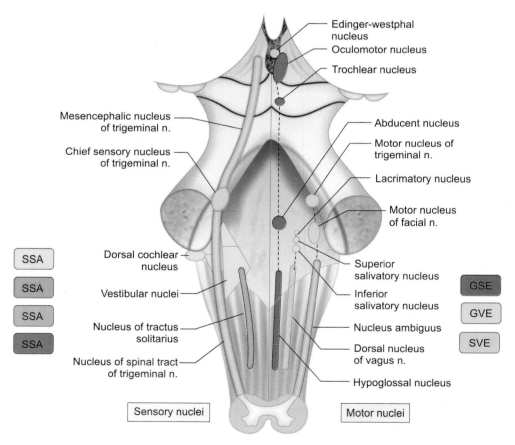

Fig. 52: Cranial nerve nuclei in brainstem and their related neural columns

GSE column	SVE column	GVE column	GVA/SVA column	GSA column	SSA column
▪ Oculomotor nucleus	▪ Motor nucleus of trigeminal nerve	▪ Edinger-Westphal nucleus	▪ Nucleus of solitary tract (nucleus tractus solitarius)	▪ Sensory nuclei of trigeminal nerve	▪ Vestibular nuclei
▪ Trochlear nucleus	▪ Motor nucleus of facial nerve	▪ Lacrimatory nucleus		– Chief	▪ Cochlear nuclei
▪ Abducens nucleus	▪ Nucleus ambiguus	▪ Superior salivatory nucleus		– Mesencephalic	
▪ Hypoglossal nucleus		▪ Inferior salivatory nucleus		– Spinal	
		▪ Dorsal nucleus of vagus nerve			

Table 8: Functional components, nuclei, distribution and functions of cranial nerves

Cranial nerve	Functional components	Nuclei	Distribution	Functions
I	SVA	–	Olfactory epithelium	Smell
II	SSA	–	Retina of eyeball	Sight (vision)
III	SE	Oculomotor nucleus	All extrinsic muscles of eyeball except lateral rectus and superior oblique	Movements of eyeball
	GVE	Edinger-Westphal nerve	Sphincter pupillae and ciliary muscle	Constriction of pupil and accomodation
IV	SE	Trochlear nucleus	Superior oblique muscle of eyeball	Movement of eyeball
V	SVE	Motor nucleus	Muscle of mastication	Movement of mandilble
	GSA	(a) Chief sensory nerve	Skin of face and mucous membrane of mouth and nose	Tourch
		(b) Spinal nucleus	Skin of face and mucous membrane of mouth and nose	Pain and temperature
		(c) Mesencephalic nucleus	Muscles of mastication	Proprioceptive sensations
VI	SE	Anducent nucleus	Lateral rectus of eyeball	Abduction of eyeball
VII	GVE SVE	Superior salivatory nucleus	Submandibular and sublingual salivary glands	Secretomotor
	SVA GSA	Motor nucleus	Muscles of facial expression stylohyoid, posterior belly of digastric, platysma and stapedius	Facial expression, elevation of hyoid, etc.
		Nucleus of tractus solitarius	Taste buds in the anterior 2/3rd of tongue except vallate papillae	Taste sensations from anterior 2/3rd of tongue except vallate papillae
		Spinal nucleus of Vth nerve	Part of skin of external ear	Exteroceptive sensations
VIII	SSA	Cochlear nuclei	Organ of Corti in the cochlea of internal ear	Equilibrium and balance
		Vestibular nuclei	Vestibular receptors in the semicircular ducts, utricle and saccule of internal ear	
IX	SVE	Nucleus ambiguus	Stylopharyngeus muscle	Elevation of larynx
	GVE	Inferior salivatory nucleus	Parotid gland	Secretomotor
	GVA	Nucleus tractus solitarius (lower part)	Pharynx, posterior 1/3rd of tongue	Touch, pain and temperature from pharynx and posterior 1/3rd of tongue
	SVA	Nucleus tractus solitarius (upper part)	Taste buds in posterior 1/3rd of tongue and vallate papillae	Taste sensations from posterior 1/3rd of tongue and vallate papillae
X	SVE	Nuclees ambiguus	Muscles of palate, pharynx and larynx	Movements of palate, pharynx and larynx
	GVE	Dorsal nucleus of vagus	Smooth muscles and glands of thoracic and abdominal viscera	Motor and secretomotor to bronchial tree and gut; Inhibitory to heart
	GVA	Nucleus tractus solitarius	Thoracic and abdominal viscera	General sensations from thoracic and abdominal viscera
	SVA	Nucleus tractus solitarius	Taste buds in posterior most par of tongue and epiglottis	Taste sensations from posterior-most part of tongue and epiglottis
	GSA	Spinal nucleus of Vth nerve	Part of skin of external ear	General sensations from skin of external ear

Cranial nerve	Functional components	Nuclei	Distribution	Functions
XI	SVE	Nucleus ambiguus	Muscles of palate, pharynx and larynx	Movements of palate, pharynx and larynx Movements of head and shoulder
	GSE	Spinal nucleus of accessory nerve (anterior gray column of upper 5 cervical spinal segments)	Trapezius and sternocleidomastoid muscles	
XII	SE	Hypoglossal nucleus	All intrinsic and extrinsic muscles of tongue except palatoglossus	Movements of tongue

(SE: Somatic efferent; SVE: Special visceral efferent; GVE: General visceral efferent; GVA: General visceral efferent; SVA: Special visceral efferent; GSA: General somatic afferent; SSA: Special somatic afferent).

Brainstem has three subdivisions: Midbrain, Pons and Medulla oblongata and has cranial nerve 3–12 nuclei. Nuclei for CN 3 and 4 (midbrain); CN 5–8 (pons); and 9–12 (medulla). Motor nuclei are located medially (and sensory nuclei are lateral).

❏ Motor nuclei of cranial nerve are **lower motor neurons** that innervate the skeletal muscles of the head. These lower motor neurons are under influence of upper motor neurons by corticobulbar fibers. The neuron bodies of corticobulbar fibers are located in the cerebrum (frontal motor cortex).
  ➢ Cranial nerve 1, 2 and 8 are pure sensory nerves.
  ➢ Cranial nerve 3, 4, 6 and 11, 12 are pure motor nerves.
  ➢ Mixed (sensory and motor) nerves are cranial nerve 5, 7, 9 and 10.
❏ **General somatic efferent** (GSE) fibers conduct motor impulses to the skeletal (somatic) muscles of the body.
❏ **Special visceral efferent** (SVE) fibers convey motor impulses to the muscles of the head and neck, which develop from pharyngeal arches such as muscles of mastication, muscles of facial expression, and muscles of palate, pharynx and larynx (speech and swallowing).
❏ **General visceral efferent** (GVE) fibers transmit motor impulses to smooth muscle, cardiac muscle, and glandular tissues (Autonomic nervous system).
❏ **General somatic afferent** (GSA) fibers transmit general sensations like touch, pain, temperature, proprioception from the body to the CNS.
❏ **Special visceral afferent** (SVA) fibers transmit taste sensations to the CNS.
❏ **General visceral afferent** (GVA) fibers carry sensory impulses from visceral organs to the CNS, e.g. carotid sinus pressure sensation.
❏ **Special somatic afferent** (SSA) fibers convey special sensory impulses of vision, hearing and balance to the CNS.
❏ SVE: Special (S) muscles (E) which develop around the pharynx viscera (V) – pharyngeal arch muscles:
  ➢ Arch – I (Muscles of mastication, 5th nerve)
  ➢ Arch – II (Muscles of facial expression, 7th nerve)
  ➢ Arch – III, IV and VI (Palate, pharynx and larynx muscles), Nucleus Ambiguus (9, 10, 11 nerves).
❏ GVE and GVA: General visceral efferent and afferent are under ANS (autonomic nervous system).
  ➢ Motor fibers control three effectors: cardiac, smooth muscles and glands.
  ➢ Sensory fibers receive visceral sensations like angina pain, colicky pain, etc.

Nucleus Tractus Solitarius (NTS)

❏ It is a **sensory** nucleus present in the medulla oblongata and through its center runs the solitary tract axons from the **facial, glossopharyngeal and vagus nerves**.
❏ It has both SVA and GVA neural columns.
❏ SVA (Special visceral afferent) is related to taste sensations which reach the **upper part** of the nucleus.
❏ GVA (General visceral afferent) is related to sensations like carotid sinus pressure sensations, carotid body chemoreception and information from cardio-respiratory and gastrointestinal processes etc., reach the **lower part** of the nucleus.
❏ NTS receives **taste sensation** from three nerves:
  ➢ Anterior two-thirds of the tongue via the chorda tympani nerve of the facial nerve (CN VII).
  ➢ Posterior third of the tongue via the glossopharyngeal nerve (CN IX).
  ➢ Posteriormost tongue (and epiglottic region of the pharynx) via the vagus nerve (CN X).
❏ Cranial nerve 9 and 10 carry the **general visceral sensations** (GVA) to lower part of the nucleus. The nucleus mediate the gag reflex, the carotid sinus reflex, the aortic reflex, the cough reflex, the baroreceptor and chemoreceptor reflexes, several respiratory reflexes and reflexes within the gastrointestinal system regulating motility and secretion.
❏ Information from NTS is projected the **paraventricular nucleus** of the hypothalamus and the central nucleus of the amygdala, as well as to other nuclei in the brainstem (such as the parabrachial area, the Locus coeruleus, the dorsal raphe nucleus, and other visceral motor or respiratory networks).

Nucleus Ambiguus

- ❏ It contains lower motor neurons belonging to cranial nerves **9, 10 and 11** (cranial part).
- ❏ It belongs to **special visceral efferent** (SVE) column and innervate the pharyngeal arch muscles of the **palate, pharynx, and larynx** involved in the movements of **speech** and **swallowing**. It also supplies the muscles of upper esophagus.
- ❏ Its 'external formation' contains cholinergic preganglionic parasympathetic neurons for the heart.
- ❏ It is located in the upper medulla oblongata, deep in the medullary reticular formation.
- ❏ It lies posterior to the inferior olivary nucleus and posteromedial to olive.
- ❏ It receives upper motor neuron innervation via the corticobulbar tract.
- ❏ Lesions of nucleus ambiguus results in:
  - ➤ Difficulty of speech and swallowing—nasal speech, dysphagia, and dysphonia.
  - ➤ Uvula deviate towards the contralateral side, due to prominent activity of contralateral (normal side) muscles.

QUESTIONS

1. Which of the following brainstem nuclei is not derived from alar plate? *(AIIMS 2008)*
- a. Dentate
- b. Inferior olivary
- c. Hypoglossal
- d. Substantia nigra

2. All of the following pairs regarding neural columns and associated nuclei are correct EXCEPT:
- a. Hypoglossal nucleus: GSE
- b. Nucleus ambiguus: SVE
- c. Dorsal nucleus of vagus: GVA
- d. Nucleus tractus solitarius: SVA

3. All of the following cranial nerves contains somatic efferents EXCEPT: *(NEET Pattern 2013)*
- a. VII nerve
- b. III nerve
- c. IV nerve
- d. VI nerve

4. Visceral efferent column in the lateral horns of spinal cord arises from which plate of the neural tube?
- a. Alar
- b. Basal
- c. Roof
- d. Floor

5. General visceral motor nuclei are present for all the following cranial nerves EXCEPT: *(NEET Pattern 2016)*
- a. Oculomotor
- b. Trigeminal
- c. Facial
- d. Glossopharyngeal

6. All of the following nerves have general visceral fibers EXCEPT: *(AIIMS 2015)*
- a. Olfactory
- b. Oculomotor
- c. Facial
- d. Glossopharyngeal

7. Nerves of branchial arch develop from *(NEET Pattern 2018)*
- a. Neuroectoderm
- b. Neural crest cells
- c. Mesoderm
- d. Endoderm

8. Special visceral efferent DOESN'T include *(NEET Pattern 2018)*
- a. Motor nucleus of fifth cranial nerve
- b. Motor nucleus of seventh cranial nerve
- c. Dorsal nucleus of tenth cranial nerve
- d. Nucleus ambiguus

ANSWERS

1. c. Hypoglossal
- ❏ **Alar plate** of neural tube gives sensory **(afferent)** neurons and basal plate forms motor (efferent) neurons.
- ❏ **Hypoglossal** nucleus is a **motor** nucleus developing from the **basal** plate (not alar plate).

2. c. Dorsal nucleus of vagus: GVA
- ❏ Dorsal nucleus of vagus is a **motor** nucleus to control cardiac and smooth muscles and glands, hence belongs to GVE **(not GVA)** neural column.

3. a. VII nerve
- ❏ GSE (General somatic efferent) neural column includes supply to **all the skeletal muscle, except** the pharyngeal arch muscles.
- ❏ Muscles of **eyeball** are supplied by cranial nerve 3, 4 and 6, which are under GSE neural column.
- ❏ **Pharyngeal arch muscles** are under the SVE (Special visceral efferent) neural column. **Facial** nerve supplies muscles of **facial expression**, which develop in **second pharyngeal arch**.

4. b. Basal
- ❏ Visceral efferent column in the **lateral horns** of spinal cord are sympathetic **and** parasympathetic motor neurons, which controls **cardiac** and **smooth** muscles and the **glands**.
- ❏ Since these are motor neurones they take origin from the anterior **basal** plate of neural tube.

5. b. Trigeminal
- ❏ General visceral motor nuclei send **parasympathetic** fibers, which are **not** carried by trigeminal nerve.

6. a. Olfactory
- ❏ **Olfactory** nerve carries sense of smell and belongs to SVA **(Special visceral afferent)** neural column.
- ❏ GVE (General visceral efferent) neural column belongs to **autonomic nervous system** and supplies the three effectors: Cardiac muscles, smooth muscles and glands. Oculomotor nerve, facial nerve and glossopharyngeal nerve carry fibers under this column.
- ❏ SSA (Special sensory afferent) neural column includes CN II **(optic)** and CN VIII **(vestibulo-cochlear)**.

7. a. Neuroectoderm
- ❏ Nerves of **branchial arch** (CN V, VII, IX, X and XI) carry **motor fibres** to supply muscles of **pharyngeal arches**.
- ❏ Their neurone bodies (nuclei) are located inside the brainstem **(part of CNS)**.
- ❏ All the nerves which are derived from Central nervous system develop from neural plate ectoderm **(neuroectoderm)**, hence the answer.
- ❏ Cranial nerves like CN V (trigeminal) have **mixed** nature, i.e., they have motor **and sensory** fibres. The sensory fibres have their neurone bodies in trigeminal ganglia **(part of PNS - peripheral nervous system)**, hence they are derived from **neural crest cells**.

Note: A mixed nerve is derived from both neuroectoderm and neural crest cells. **Neuroectoderm** give motor fibres and **neural crest cells** give sensory fibres.

8. c. Dorsal nucleus of tenth cranial nerve
- ❑ **Dorsal nucleus** of tenth cranial nerve belongs to **GVE** (General Visceral efferent) neural column.
- ❑ It supplies the **three effectors** under autonomic system: Cardiac Muscles, smooth muscles and glands.
- ❑ Special visceral efferent **(SVE)** neural column supplies skeletal **muscles** developing in **pharyngeal arches**.

- ❑ Facial nerve does NOT have fibers in **nucleus ambiguus** *(NEET Pattern 2012)*
- ❑ CN VIII is associated with **special somatic afferent** nuclei.
- ❑ Dorsal nucleus of vagus belongs to the **general visceral efferent** column *(AIIMS 2004)*
- ❑ CN V is **not** a somatic efferent nerve *(AIPG 2008)*

▼ Cerebellum

Cerebellum is embryologically derived from the rhombic lips, which are the thickened **alar plates** of the mantle layer (neural tube).
- ❑ The rostral part of the cerebellum is derived from the caudal mesencephalon.
- ❑ Cerebellum is a part of the **metencephalon** (hindbrain) and lies in the posterior cranial fossa.
- ❑ Fourth ventricle, pons and medulla lie anterior to the cerebellum.
- ❑ It is separated from the overlying cerebrum (occipital lobes) by a layer of dura mater (**tentorium cerebelli**)
- ❑ It has two hemispheres and a narrow midline zone (vermis).
- ❑ It has an outer cerebellar **cortex** having tightly folded layer of gray matter, producing gyri (**folia**) and sulci.
- ❑ Deep to the gray matter lies white matter, made up largely of myelinated nerve fibers running to and from the cortex. White matter gives the appearance of **arbor vitae** (tree of life) because of its branched, tree-like appearance in cross-section.
- ❑ Embedded within the white matter are **four deep cerebellar nuclei** (gray matter).

Structurally, three lobes are distinguished within the cerebellum: the **anterior** lobe (above the primary fissure), the **posterior** lobe (below the primary fissure), and the **flocculonodular** lobe (below the posterior fissure).
- ❑ These lobes divide the cerebellum from top to bottom.

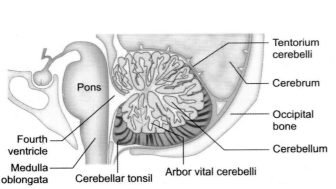

Fig. 53: Structure and relations of cerebellum

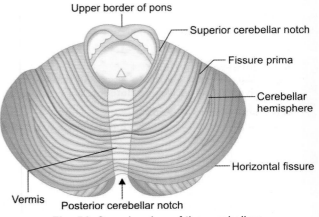

Fig. 54: Superior view of the cerebellum

Functionally the distinction is along the medial-to-lateral direction.
- ❑ Medial region : **Spinocerebellum** (paleocerebellum)
  - ➢ It includes the medial zone of the anterior and posterior lobes.
  - ➢ It works for fine tuning of body and limb movements.
  - ➢ It receives proprioceptive input from the dorsal columns of the spinal cord (including the spinocerebellar tract) and from the cranial trigeminal nerve, as well as from visual and auditory systems.
  - ➢ It sends fibers to deep cerebellar nuclei that, in turn, project to both the cerebral cortex and the brainstem, thus providing modulation of descending motor systems.
- ❑ Lateral region: **Cerebrocerebellum** (neocerebellum)
  - ➢ It receives input exclusively from the cerebral cortex (especially the parietal lobe) via the pontine nuclei (**cortico-ponto-cerebellar pathways**), and sends output mainly to the ventrolateral thalamus (in turn connected to motor areas of the premotor cortex and primary motor area of the cerebral cortex) and to the red nucleus.

Flowchart 2: Nuclear connection of the cerebellum

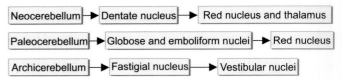

❏ Midline region: **Vermis** is a narrow strip of protruding tissue along the midline.
   Flocculonodular lobe (vestibulocerebellum) is the oldest part (archicerebellum), participating mainly in balance and spatial orientation.
❏ Its primary connections are with the **vestibular** nuclei, although it also receives **visual** and other sensory input.

Table 9: Various subdivisions (lobules) of vermis and cerebellar hemisphere

Lobes	Subdivisions of vermis	Subdivisions of cerebellar hemisphere

Anterior lobe	Lingula
	    Central lobule
	    Culmen
		No lateral projection
		    Alae
		    Quadrangular lobe

Posterior lobe	Declive
	    Follum
	    Tuber
	    Pyramid
	    Uvula
		Lobulus simplex
		    Superior semilunar lobule
		    Inferior semilunar lobule
		    Biventral lobule
		    Tonsil

Flocculonodular lobe	Nodule	Flocculus

Table 10: Components, nuclei, connections and functions of three morphological subdivisions of the cerebellum

Subdivisions	Components	Nucleus	Chief connections	Functions
Archicerebellum (oldest part)	Flocculonodular lobe + lingula	Nucleus fastigii	Vestibulocerebellar	Maintenance of equilibrium (responsible for maintaining the position of body in space)
Paleocerebellum (in between, i.e. neither oldest nor newest)	Whole of anterior lobe except lingula Pyramid Uvula	Nucleus interpositus consisting of nucleus globosus and nucleus emboliformis	Spinocerebellar	Controls crude movements of the limbs
Neocerebellum (most recent part)	Whole of posterior lobe except pyramid and uvula	Nucleus dentatus	Corticopontocerebellar	Smooth performance of high skilled voluntary movements of precision

❏ Two neurone types play dominant roles in the cerebellar circuit: **Purkinje** cells and **granule** cells.
❏ Three types of axons also play dominant roles: **mossy** fibers and **climbing** fibers (afferents to cerebellum), and **parallel** fibers (the axons of granule cells).
❏ There are two main pathways through the cerebellar circuit, originating from mossy fibers and climbing fibers, both eventually terminating in the deep cerebellar nuclei.
❏ Cerebellar cortex has **five cell types** arranged in **3 layers**:
  ➢ Outermost molecular layer has inhibitory (GABAergic) interneurons—2 cells (stellate and basket)
  ➢ Middle layer—Purkinje cells
  ➢ Inner (deeper/granular) layer—2 cells (granule and Golgi).
   Outermost **molecular** layer also contains the array of **parallel fibers** penetrating the **Purkinje cell dendritic trees** at right angles.
   Deep nuclei of the cerebellum are collections of gray matter lying within the white matter at the core of the cerebellum.
❏ Their arrangement is (lateral to medial): Dentate, emboliform, globose, and fastigial.
❏ Dentate nucleus is the latest in evolution, is the largest and the lateral most. It communicates exclusively with the lateral parts of the cerebellar cortex.
❏ Flocculonodular lobe is the only part of the cerebellar cortex that does not project to the deep nuclei, instead its efferent reach the vestibular nuclei.
❏ These nuclei receive collateral projections from mossy fibers and climbing fibers as well as inhibitory input from the Purkinje cells of the cerebellar cortex.
❏ These nuclei are (with the minor exception of the vestibular nuclei) the sole sources of output (efferents) from the cerebellum.

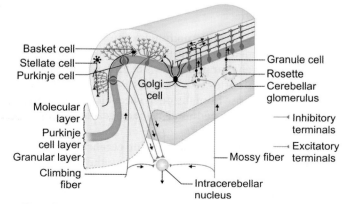

Fig. 55: Triple layers of cerebellar cortex and the triple fiber (mossy, climbing and parallel) neuronal circuitry

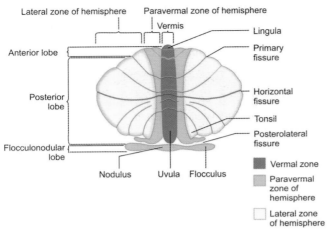

Fig. 56: Schematic diagram of the fissures, lobules, and lobes of the cerebellum. Functional longitudinal zones of the cerebellum are associated with cerebellar nuclei. The vermal (median) zone projects to the fastigial nucleus, the paravermal (paramedian) zone projects to the interposed nucleus, and the lateral zone projects to the dentate nucleus

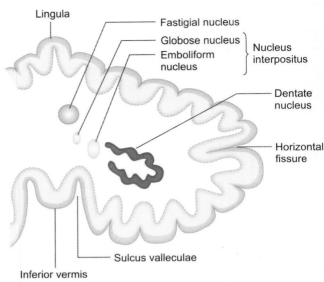

Fig. 57: Transverse section of the cerebellum showing intracerebellar nuclei

Climbing fibers (olivocerebellar fibers) originate from the inferior olivary nucleus on the contralateral side of the brainstem, pass through inferior cerebellar peduncle and project to Purkinje cells.

❑ Although the inferior olive lies in the medulla oblongata and receives input from the spinal cord, brainstem and cerebral cortex, its output goes entirely to the cerebellum.

❑ A climbing fiber gives off collaterals to the deep cerebellar nuclei before entering the cerebellar cortex, where it splits into about 10 terminal branches, each of which gives input to a single Purkinje cell.

Mossy fibers are the afferent fibers to cerebellum, arising from the pontine nuclei, spinal cord, vestibular nuclei etc.

❑ They form excitatory synapses with the granule cells and the cells of the deep cerebellar nuclei.

❑ Within the granular layer, a mossy fiber generates a series of enlargements called rosettes. The contacts between mossy fibers and granule cell dendrites take place within structures called glomeruli.

❑ Cerebellar glomerulus consists of a mossy fiber rosette, granule cell dendrites, and a Golgi cell axon.

Mossy fibers project directly to the deep nuclei, but also give rise to the following pathway:

Mossy fibers → granule cells → parallel fibers → Purkinje cells → deep nuclei.

Cerebellar Pathways

❑ Mossy fibers (and climbing fibers) are the afferent fibers reaching the cerebellum via the cerebellar peduncles. These are excitatory in nature and project directly (or indirectly via granule cells) to the Purkinje cells of the cerebellar cortex.

❑ The axons of the Purkinje cells are inhibitory (GABAergic) and are the only efferent (outflow) from the cerebellar cortex. They project to and inhibit the deep cerebellar nuclei (dentate, interposed, and fastigi) in the medulla.

❑ From the deep nuclei, efferents project through the superior cerebellar peduncle to the contralateral ventral lateral (and ventral anterior) nuclei of the thalamus, to reach the contralateral cerebrum (precentral gyrus).

❑ The upper motor neurons of the cerebrum thence influence the contralateral lower motor neurons of the spinal cord via corticospinal tract.

Three paired cerebellar peduncles connect the cerebellum to the brainstem (and different parts of the nervous system).

❑ These are named according to their position relative to the vermis as the superior, middle and inferior cerebellar peduncle.

❑ Superior cerebellar peduncle is mainly an output to the cerebral cortex, carrying efferent fibers to upper motor neurons in the cerebral cortex.

  ➢ The fibers arise from the deep cerebellar nuclei.

❑ Middle cerebellar peduncle is the largest and is connected to the pons. It receives all of its input from the pons mainly from the pontine nuclei.

  ➢ This input to the pons is from the cerebral cortex (Cortico-ponto-cerebellar tract).

❑ Inferior cerebellar peduncle receives input from afferent fibers from the spinal cord, vestibular nuclei and the tegmentum.

  ➢ Cerebellum receives entire modulatory input from the inferior olivary nucleus (via the climbing fibers passing through inferior cerebellar peduncle).

  ➢ Output (efferents) from the inferior peduncle is to the vestibular nuclei and the reticular formation.

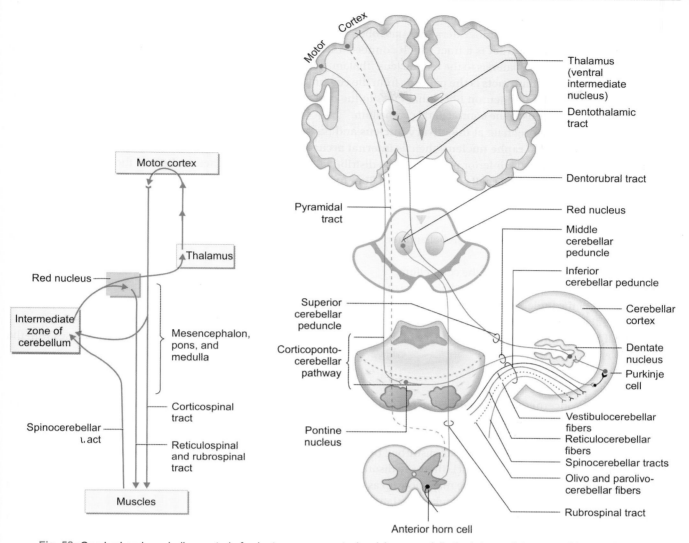

Fig. 58: Cerebral and cerebellar control of voluntary movements, involving especially the intermediate zone of the cerebellum

Cerebellar peduncle	Afferent tracts	Efferent tracts
Superior	Ventral spinocerebellar Tecto-cerebellar	Dentato-rubro-thalamic Dentato-olivary Fastigio-reticular
Middle	Pontocerebellar (cortico-ponto-cerebellar pathway)*	
Inferior	Dorsal spinocerebellar Olivo-cerebellar Parolivo-cerebellar Reticulo-cerebellar Vestibulo-cerebellar Anterior external arcuate fibers Cuneocerebellar (posterior external arcuate fibers) Stria medullaris Trigeminocerebellar	Cerebello-vestibular Cerebello-olivary Cerebello-reticular

*Middle cerebellar peduncle has only one tract: Incoming (afferent) fibers from the contralateral pons (pontocerebellar) fibers.

❑ **Spinocerebellar tract** originate in the spinal cord and terminate in the ipsilateral cerebellum.
  ➢ It conveys information to the cerebellum about length and tension of muscle fibers (i.e., unconscious proprioceptive sensation)

➤ Spinocerebellar tract conveys information from ipsilateral part of trunk and lower limb.

➤ Cuneocerebellar tract (posterior external arcuate fibers) carries information form the upper limbs and neck.

❑ **Dentato-rubro-thalamic tract** is a tract which connects the dentate nucleus and the thalamus (ventral intermediate nucleus) while sending collaterals to the red nucleus. Thalamus further project the information to the cerebral cortex.

❑ **Cortico-ponto-cerebellar tracts is the** pathway from the cerebral cortex to the contralateral cerebellum. Pontocerebellar fibers are the second order neuron fibers that cross to the other side of the pons and run within the middle cerebellar peduncles, from the pons to the contralateral cerebellum.

❑ **Olivocerebellar tract** originate at the **olivary nucleus** and pass out through the hilum and decussate with those from the opposite olive in the **raphe nucleus**, then as **internal arcuate fibers** they pass partly through and partly around the opposite olive and enter the inferior peduncle to be distributed to the **cerebellar hemisphere** of the opposite side. They terminate directly on **Purkinje cells** as the **climbing fiber** input system.

Arterial Supply

Three paired major arteries: **Superior** cerebellar artery (SCA), **Anterior inferior** cerebellar artery (AICA), and the **Posterior inferior** cerebellar artery (PICA).

❑ SCA supplies the upper region of the cerebellum.

❑ AICA supplies the front part of the undersurface of the cerebellum.

❑ PICA arrives at the undersurface, where it divides into a medial branch and a lateral branch.

➤ The medial branch continues backward to the cerebellar notch between the two hemispheres of the cerebellum.

➤ Lateral branch supplies the under surface of the cerebellum, as far as its lateral border, where it anastomoses with the AICA and the SCA.

Functions

❑ Cerebellum is concerned with **coordination of voluntary motor activity**, controls posture, equilibrium and muscle tone, and is involved learning of repeated motor functions.

❑ Cerebellum **does not** initiate movement, but contributes to coordination, precision, and accurate timing.

❑ Cerebellar lesion leads to abnormal gait, disturbed balance, and in-coordination of voluntary motor activity (no paralysis or inability to start or stop movement). There are disorders in fine movement, posture, and motor learning.

❑ Damage to the **flocculonodular lobe** may show up as a loss of equilibrium and in particular an altered, irregular walking gait, with a wide stance caused by difficulty in balancing.

❑ Damage to the **lateral zone** typically causes problems in skilled voluntary and planned motor movements which leads to errors in the force, direction, speed and amplitude of movements.

➤ Other manifestations include **hypotonia** (decreased muscle tone), **dysmetria** (problems judging distances or ranges of movement), **dysdiadochokinesia** (inability to perform rapid alternating movements such as walking), impaired check reflex or rebound phenomenon, **intention tremor** (involuntary movement caused by alternating contractions of opposing muscle groups) and **dysarthria** (problems with speech articulation).

❑ Damage to the **midline portion** may disrupt whole-body movements, whereas damage localized more laterally is more likely to disrupt fine movements of the hands or limbs.

❑ **Cerebellar ataxia**: Damage to the upper part of the cerebellum tends to cause gait impairments and other problems with leg coordination; damage to the lower part is more likely to cause uncoordinated or poorly aimed movements of the arms and hands, as well as difficulties in speed.

QUESTIONS

1. Function of spinocerebellar tract:
   a. Equilibrium
   b. Coordinates movement
   c. Learning induced by vestibular reflexes
   d. Planning and Programming

2. Structures NOT passing through inferior cerebellar peduncle: (PGIC 07, 08, 09)
   a. Pontocerebellar   b. Cuneocerebellar
   c. Anterior spinocerebellar   d. Posterior spinocerebellar
   e. Vestibulocerebellar

3. Efferents from cerebellum arise from:
   a. Purkinje cells
   b. Stellate neurons
   c. Deep nuclei
   d. Grade III fibers

4. Tract ABSENT in superior cerebellar peduncle:
   a. Tecto-cerebellar
   b. Dentato thalamic
   c. Dorsal spinocerebellar
   d. Ventral spinocerebellar

5. Pathology of the given structure will lead to which of the following speech disorder: *(AIIMS 2016)*
  a. Visual agnosia
  b. Sensory aphasia
  c. Dysarthria
  d. Verbal apraxia

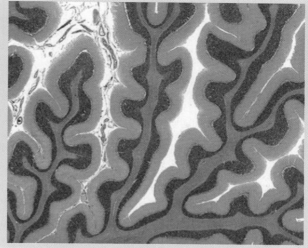

6. The marked cell inhibits which of the following structure: *(AIIMS 2017)*
  a. Golgi cell
  b. Basket cell
  c. Vestibular nuclei
  d. Deep cerebellar nuclei

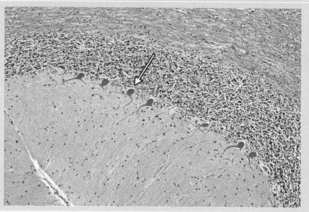

7. Cerebellar input is from which nucleus: *(JIPMER 2017)*
  a. Dentate nucleus
  b. Vestibular nucleus
  c. Inferior olivary nucleus
  d. Globose and emboliform nucleus

---

1. b. Coordinates movement
  ❑ Spinocerebellar tract carries the unconscious proprioception to the higher brain centers, for co-ordination of voluntary motor activity.

2. a. Pontocerebellar, c. Anterior spinocerebellar
  ❑ Pontocerebellar tract passes through the middle cerebellar peduncle and anterior spinocerebellar tract passes through the superior peduncle.

3. c. Deep nuclei
  ❑ Efferents from cerebellum arise from the deep cerebellar nuclei.
  ❑ Efferents from the cerebellar cortex arise from the purkinje cells.

4. c. Dorsal spinocerebellar
  ❑ Dorsal spinocerebellar fibers pass through inferior cerebellar peduncle.
  ❑ Ventral spinocerebellar tract sends fibers through superior cerebellar peduncle.
  ❑ Superior colliculus (visual reflexes) and inferior colliculus (auditory) are present in the tectum (midbrain).
  ❑ Tectocerebellar fibers in superior cerebellar peduncle carry visual and auditory information from the colliculi towards cerebellum.
  ❑ Dentatothalamic tract passes through the superior cerebellar peduncle to reach the contralateral thalamus.

5. c. Dysarthria
  ❑ It is the histology slide of cerebellum, lesion of which may lead to dysarthria. As speech production requires the coordinated and simultaneous contraction of a large number of muscle groups, cerebellar disorders could disrupt speech production and cause ataxic dysarthria.
  ❑ Identification point: Cerebellar cortex forms a series of deeply convoluted folds (folia) supported by a branching central white matter (Arbor vitae).
  ❑ Cerebellar outer molecular layer (ML) contains relatively few neurones and large numbers of unmyelinated fibers.
  ❑ The inner granular cell layer (GL) is extremely cellular.
  ❑ Between the two is a single layer of huge neurones called Purkinje cells (PL).

6. d. Deep cerebellar nuclei
- ❏ This slide shows the Purkinje cell in middle layer of cerebellar cortex. They are a class of GABAergic neurons with elaborate dendritic branching, characterized by a large number of dendritic spines.
- ❏ Purkinje cells send inhibitory projections to the deep cerebellar nuclei and constitute the sole output of all motor coordination in the cerebellar cortex.

7. c. Inferior olivary nucleus
- ❏ Inferior olivary nucleus sends climbing fibers (olivocerebellar tract) to reach the Purkinje cell in the cerebellum.

- ▪ Purkinje cells fibers from the cerebellum end in cerebellar nuclei *(NEET Pattern 2014)*
  - – The fibers are neuroinhibitory (neurotransmitter is GABA).
- ▪ Only tract present in middle cerebellar peduncle is Pontocerebellar *(NEET Pattern 2015)*
- ▪ In cerebellar lesion NOT seen is Resting tremors.
- ▪ Deep cerebellar nuclei are DEFG: Dentate, Emboliform, Fastigi and Globose.
- ▪ Superior cerebellar peduncle is attached to midbrain; middle to pons and inferior to medulla oblongata.
- ▪ Evolution wise, the latest and the lateral-most nucleus is dentate
  - – The oldest and medial most is Fastigi nucleus.
  - – Fastigi nucleus, as believed to be derived from fish (evolution-wise) is for maintenance of axial balance.
- ▪ Dentato-rubro-thalamic tract passes through the superior cerebellar peduncle to reach the contralateral thalamus.
- ▪ Cerebellar cortex has 3 layers: Outermost molecular layer – 2 cells (stellate and basket); middle layer – Purkinje cells and inner (deeper/ granular) layer– 2 cells (granule and Golgi).
- ▪ In adults the weight ratio of cerebellum to cerebrum is approximately 1:10 and in infants 1:20.

▶ SC - Vertebral Canal

- ❏ The number of **spinal segments** corresponds to the number of **vertebrae** in thoracic, lumbar and sacral regions,
- ❏ **But in cervical** region, **one segment is more** than the number of vertebrae,
- ❏ Whereas in **coccygeal** region there is **only one** segment for four coccygeal vertebrae.
- ❏ Thus, the spinal cord is made up of **31 spinal segments**: 8 cervical, 12 thoracic, 5 lumbar, 5 sacral, and one coccygeal.
- ❏ Since the cord is **shorter** than the vertebral column, **length and obliquity** of spinal nerve roots increase progressively from above downwards, so that spinal nerves may emerge through their **respective intervertebral foramina**.
- ❏ In **upper cervical** region the spinal nerve roots are **short and run almost horizontally** but the roots of the **lumbar and sacral** nerves are **long and run obliquely** (almost vertically).
- ❏ At thoracic, lumbar, sacral and coccygeal levels, the numbered nerve exits the vertebral canal by passing **below the corresponding vertebra**, e.g. L4 nerve exits the intervertebral foramen between L4 and L5.
- ❏ However, in the cervical region, nerves C1-7 pass **above their corresponding vertebrae**.
- ❏ **C1** leaves the vertebral canal **between** the occipital bone and atlas (termed suboccipital nerve).
- ❏ The **last pair of cervical nerves** does not have a correspondingly numbered vertebra and C8 passes **between** the 7th cervical and 1st thoracic vertebrae.
- ❏ First and second cervical spinal roots are short, running almost horizontally to their exits from the vertebral canal, and that from the third to the eighth cervical levels the roots slope obliquely down.
  - ➢ Lumbar, sacral and coccygeal roots descend with increasing obliquity to their exits.
  - ➢ Approximate vertebral levels of the spinal cord segments are shown in Table 13.
  - ➢ In the cervical region, the tip of a vertebral spinous process corresponds to the succeeding cord segment (i.e. the sixth cervical spine is opposite the seventh spinal segment).

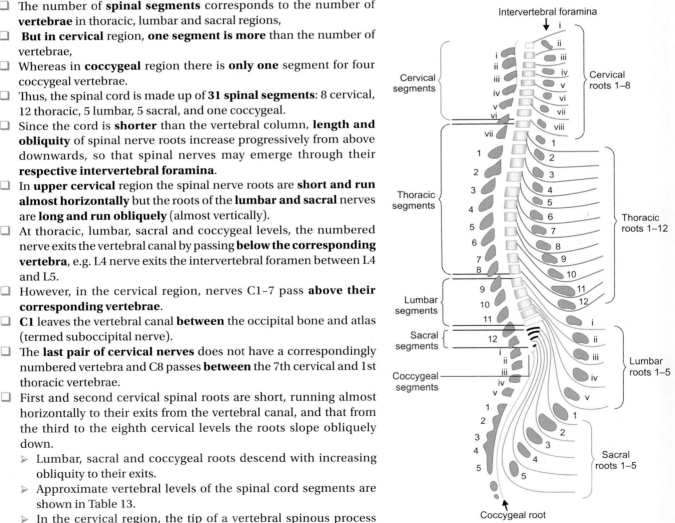

Fig. 59: Lateral view showing exit of emerging spinal nerves through the intervertebral foramina

➤ At upper thoracic levels, the tip of a vertebral spine corresponds to the cord two segments lower (i.e. the fourth spine is level with the sixth segment), and in the lower thoracic region, there is a difference of three segments (i.e. the tenth thoracic spine is level with the first lumbar segment).

➤ The eleventh thoracic spine overlies the third lumbar segment and the twelfth is opposite the first sacral segment.

Table 11: Approximate vertebral levels of the spinal cord segments

Regions	Spinal segments	Vertebral level	General rule
Upper cervical	C2	C2	Same level
Lower cervical	C6	C5	One vertebra above
Upper thoracic	T5	T3	Two vertebrae above
Lower thoracic	T10	T7	Three vertebrae above
Lumbar	L1-L5	T10-T11	Three to five vertebrae above
Sacral and coccygeal	S1-S5 and C × 1	T12-L1	Six to ten vertebrae above

❑ **Cervical** enlargement gives axons to the **brachial** plexus to supply the upper limbs.

❑ It **extends** from the C3-T2 segments.

❑ The maximum circumference is in the C6 segment.

❑ **Lumbar** enlargement gives axons to the lumbar and sacral plexus to supply the lower limbs.

❑ It **extends** from the L1-S3 segments.

❑ The equivalent vertebral levels are last four thoracic vertebra (T9-12).

❑ The maximum circumference is at the lower part of T12 vertebra.

❑ It is protected by the last four thoracic vertebrae (T9 – T12 vertebra).

❑ Upper 15 cm of filum terminale (**pial part**) is covered by dural and arachnoid meninges and reaches the caudal border of the **second sacral vertebra**.

❑ Lower 5 cm (**dural part**) fuses with the investing dura mater, and then **both descend** to the dorsum of the **first coccygeal** vertebral segment.

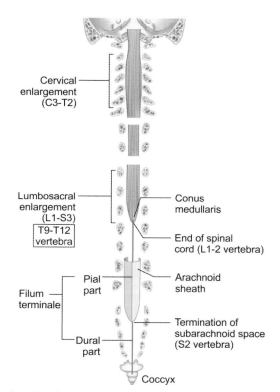

Fig. 60: Cervical and lumbosacral enlargements in the spinal cord. Terminal extent of various structures in relation to vertebral level is also evident

Table 12: Characteristic features of the spinal segments as seen in transverse sections at cervical, thoracic, and lumbar regions of the spinal cord

Features	Cervical	Thoracic	Lumbar
Gray matter	Large	Small	Large
Posterior horn	Slender and extends far posteriorly	Slender	Bulbous
Anterior horn	Massive	Slender	Bulbous
Lateral horn	Absent	Present	Present only in tL1 and L2 segments
Reticular formation	Well developed	Poorly developed	Absent
Amount of white matter	Massive + + + +	Large (less than in the cervical region)+++	Less (but slightly less than in the thoracic region) + + +

Table 13: Spaces associated with spinal meninges*		
Space	**Location**	**Contents**
Epidural	Space between periosteum lining bony wall of vertebral canal and spinal dura mater	Fat (loose connective tissue); internal vertebral venous plexuses; inferior to L2 vertebra, ensheathed roots of spinal nerves
Subarachnoid (leptomeningeal)	Naturally occurring space between arachnoid mater and pia mater	CSF; radicular, segmental, medullary, and spinal arteries; veins; arachnoid trabeculae

*Although it is common to refer to a "subdural space," there is no naturally occurring space at the arachnoid-dura junction (Haines, 2006).

❑ Epidural space lies between the spinal dura mater and the tissues that line the vertebral canal.
❑ It is closed above by fusion of the spinal dura with the edge of the foramen magnum, and below by the posterior sacrococcygeal ligament that closes the sacral hiatus.
❑ **Ligamenta denticulatum** is made up of piamater and attaches to duramater.
  ➢ It lies on each side between the dorsal and ventral nerve roots, forming narrow ribbon-like transparent bands.

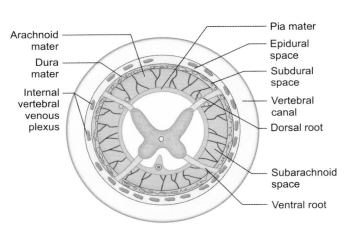

Fig. 61: Schematic transection of the vertebral canal showing its contents

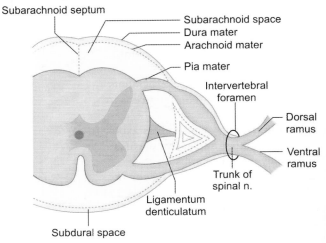

Fig. 62: Schematic transverse section of the spinal cord showing meninges and formation of meningeal sheaths onto the spinal nerve roots

➢ The lateral margin of each ligamentum denticulatum sends 21 teeth-like projections, which pass through subarachnoid space and arachnoid mater to gain attachment on the inner surface of the dural tube between the points of emergence of two adjacent spinal nerves.
➢ It helps to anchor the spinal cord in the middle of the subarachnoid space.
➢ The first tooth of ligamentum denticulatum is above the rim of the foramen magnum, while the last tooth lies between the exiting twelfth thoracic and first lumbar spinal nerves.

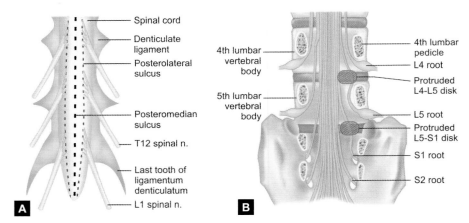

Figs. 63A and B: (A) Posterior view of part of the spinal cord showing ligamenta denticulata, (B) Posterolateral herniation of the nucleus pulposus in the lumbosacral region, doesn't affect the nerve root exiting at the same level, but the next subsequent nerve root

Herniated disc between	Compressed nerve root	Dermatome affected	Muscles affected	Movement weakness	Nerve and reflex involved
C4 and C5	C5	C5 Lateral surface of the arm	Deltoid	Abduction of arm	Axillary nerve ↓ biceps jerk
C5 and C6	C6	C6 Lateral surface of the forearm Thumb index finger	Biceps Brachialis Brachioradialis	Flexion of forearm Supination/pronation	Musculocutaneous nerve ↓ biceps reflex ↓ brachioradialis (supinator) reflex
C6 and C7	C7	C7 Middle finger	Triceps Wrist extensors	Extension of forearm Extension of wrist	Radial nerve ↓ triceps jerk
L3 and L4	L4	L4 Medial surface of the leg	Quadriceps	Extension of Knee	Femoral nerve ↓ knee jerk
L4 and L5	L5	L5 Lateral surface of leg Dorsum of foot Big toe	Tibialis anterior Extensor hallucis longus Extensor digitorum longus	Dorsiflexion of ankle (patient cannot stand on heels) Extension of toes	Common fibular Nerve No reflex loss
L5 and S1	S1	S1 Heel Little toe	Gastrocnemius Soleus	Plantar flexion of ankle (patient cannot stand on toes) Flexion of toes	Tibial nerve ↓ ankle jerk

Spinal Cord Termination

❏ Spinal cord occupies the upper two-thirds of the vertebral canal.
  ➤ It is continuous cranially with the medulla oblongata, just below the level of the foramen magnum, at the upper border of the atlas.
  ➤ It terminates caudally as the conus medullaris at lower border of L1 vertebra.
❏ During development, the vertebral column elongates more rapidly than the spinal cord, so that there is an increasing discrepancy between the anatomical level of spinal cord segments and their corresponding vertebrae.
  ➤ At week 8, the vertebral column and spinal cord are the same length and the cord ends at the last coccygeal vertebra.
  ➤ At birth, the conus medullaris extends to the upper border of third lumbar vertebra.
  ➤ With growth of the spine, the conus typically reaches the adult level (L1) by 2 years of age.
  ➤ In adults, the conus medullaris terminates at the lower border of L1 vertebra.

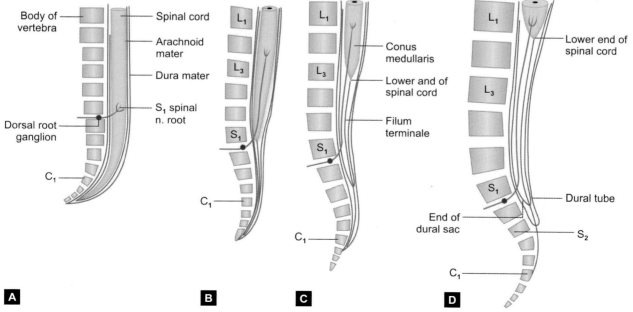

Figs. 64A to D: Termination of spinal cord in relation to vertebral canal at various stages of development. (A) At week 8. (B) At week 24. (C) At birth. (D) In adult.

❑ Disproportionate growth results in formation of the cauda equina, consisting of posterior and anterior roots (L3–Co) that descend inferior to the conus medullaris, and in formation of the filum terminale, which anchors the spinal cord to the dura mater and coccyx.

❑ Due to rostral shift of the spinal cord during development, the spinal nerve roots become progressively oblique from above downwards.

❑ In upper cervical region the spinal nerve roots are **short and run almost horizontally** but the roots of the lumbar and sacral nerves are long and run obliquely (**almost vertically**).

❑ The spinal cord and its blood vessels and nerve roots lie within a meningeal sheath (theca), which extends from the foramen magnum to the level of the second sacral vertebra in the adult.

❑ Distal to this level, the dura extends as a fine cord, the filum terminale externum, which fuses with the posterior periosteum of the first coccygeal segment.

❑ The filum terminale is a filament of connective tissue approximately 20 cm long, descends from the apex of the conus medullaris.
  ➢ The upper 15 cm, the filum terminale internum, is continued within extensions of the dural and arachnoid meninges and reaches the caudal border of the second sacral vertebra.
  ➢ The final 5 cm, the filum terminale externum, fuses with the investing dura mater, and then descends to the dorsum of the first coccygeal vertebral segment.
  ➢ The filum is continuous above with the spinal pia mater.

Structure/Space	Terminal extent
Spinal cord at birth	L3 vertebrae (upper border)
Spinal cord in 2 year infant	L1 vertebra (lower border)
Adult spinal cord	L1 vertebra (lower border) or L2 vertebra (upper border)
Filum terminale	Attached to first coccygeal segment
Filum terminale internum	S2 vertebra (lower border)
Filum terminale externum	Attached to first coccygeal segment
Piamater and duramater	Attached to first coccygeal segment
Subarachnoid sheath Subarachnoid space Subdural space	S2 vertebra (lower border)

QUESTIONS

1. Lowest projection of ligamentum denticulatum lies at which level of spinal nerves *(NEET Pattern 2016)*
   a. T9,10
   b. T12; L1
   c. S2,3
   d. S4,5

2. These ventral spinal rootlets are more prone to injury during decompressive operations because they are shorter and exit in a more horizontal direction *(AIIMS 2002)*
   a. C5
   b. C6
   c. C7
   d. T1

ANSWERS

1. **b. T12; L1**
   ❑ The first tooth of ligamentum denticulatum is at the level of the foramen magnum, while the last tooth lies between T12 and L1 spinal nerves *(NEET Pattern 2016)*

2. **a. C5**
   ❑ In upper cervical region the spinal nerve roots are short and run almost horizontally and are more prone to injury during decompressive operations.
   ❑ Roots of the lumbar and sacral nerves are long and run obliquely (almost vertically)

- In adults the spinal cord normally ends at the lower border of the L1 vertebra *(NEET Pattern 2015)*
- Spinal cord termination in a baby at birth is at upper border of L3 vertebra.
- Subarachnoid space ends at S2 vertebra *(NEET Pattern 2012)*
- Ligamentum denticulatum has 21 pair of teeth like projections *(NEET Pattern 2016)*
- There are 31 pairs of spinal nerves, one on each side of the vertebral column *(NEET Pattern 2013)*

Laminae and Reflex Arc

Table 14: Rexed laminae and nuclear groups

Laminae	Corresponding gray column nuclei
I	Posteromarginal nucleus
II	Substantia gelatinosa
III and IV	Nucleus proprius
V and VI	Base of dorsal column
VII	Nucleus dorsalis (Clarke's column) and intermediolateral nuclei of lateral horn
VIII and IX	Medial and lateral groups of nuclei of anterior gray column
X	Surrounds the central canal and composed of the gray commissure and substantia gelatinosa centralis

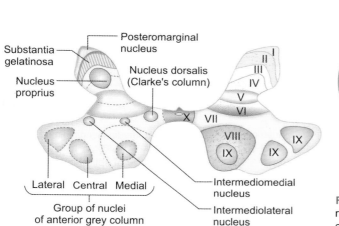

Fig. 65: The laminae of Rexed and related nuclear groups

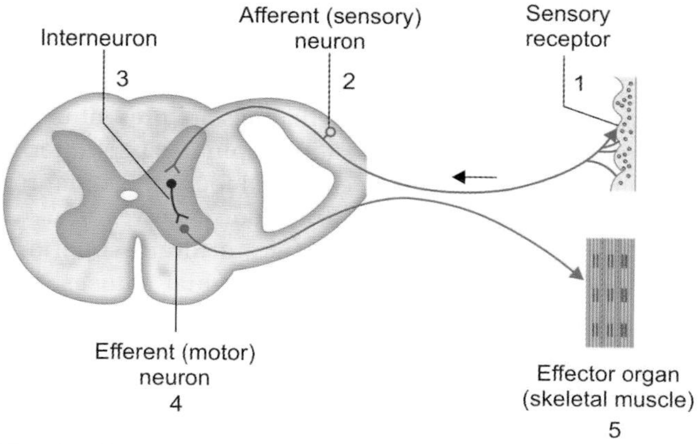

Fig. 66: Polysynaptic spinal reflex arc involved in withdrawal reflex. Note the five components: (1) a sensory receptor, (2) an afferent or sensory neuron, (3) an association neuron, (4) an efferent or motor neuron, and (5) an effector organ

Spinal Chord - Vascular Supply

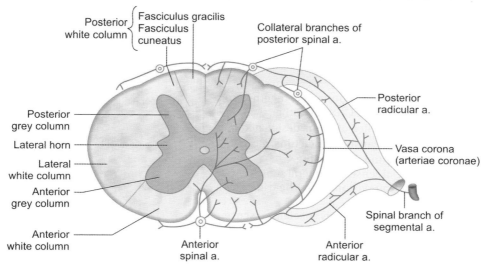

Fig. 67: Arterial supply of the interior part of spinal cord

- ❑ **Arterial supply**: Spinal cord is supplied by three major longitudinal vessels, a midline anterior and two posterior spinal arteries originating intracranially from the vertebral artery and terminating in a plexus around the conus medullaris.
  - ➢ The anterior spinal artery is a midline structure formed by the union of anterior spinal branches of the vertebral artery, and descends in the ventral median fissure of the cord.
  - ➢ Two posterior spinal arteries originates from the vertebral artery (or posterior inferior cerebellar artery) and descends in the posterolateral sulcus of the cord.

> The segmental arteries are derived in craniocaudal sequence from spinal branches of the vertebral, deep cervical, intercostal and lumbar arteries.
  - These vessels enter the vertebral canal through the intervertebral foramina and anastomose with branches of the longitudinal vessels to form a pial plexus on the surface of the cord.
> The great anterior radiculo-medullary artery (of Adamkiewicz) is the largest anterior medullary feeder.
  - It may arise from a spinal branch of either one of the lower posterior intercostal arteries (T9–11), or of the subcostal artery (T12), or less frequently of the upper lumbar arteries (L1 and L2).
  - It is mostly seen on the left side and may be the main supply to the lower two-thirds of the cord.

❏ **Venous drainage**: Intramedullary veins within the substance of the spinal cord drain into a circumferential plexus of surface veins, the coronal plexus (venous plexus of the pia mater).
  > Six tortuous longitudinal channels are present in this plexus: anterior and posterior spinal veins (anterior and posterior median veins) and four others that run on either side of the ventral and dorsal nerve roots.
  > These vessels connect freely and drain superiorly into the cerebellar veins and cranial sinuses, and segmentally into medullary veins mainly.
  > The segmental veins drain into the intervertebral veins and thence into the external vertebral venous plexuses, the caval and azygos systems.

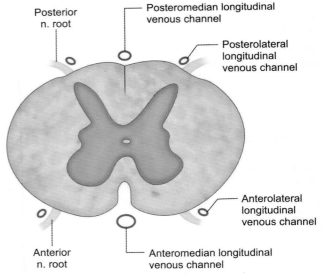

Fig. 68: Venous drainage of spinal cord

◤ Neural Pathways

Neural pathway is a series of neurons connected together to enable a signal to be sent from one part of CNS to another.
❏ It involves a single axon or a sequence of axons designated by terminologies: **Tract, lemniscus, capsule, fasciculus,** etc.
❏ They are classified as **ascending** and **descending**.
Sensory modalities are either special senses or general senses.
❏ The **special senses** are olfaction, vision, taste, hearing and vestibular function.
  > Afferent information is encoded by highly specialized sense organs and transmitted to the brain in cranial nerves I, II, VII, VIII and IX.
❏ The **general senses** include touch, pressure, vibration, pain, thermal sensation and proprioception (sense of posture and movement).
❏ Afferent impulses from the trunk and limbs are conveyed to the spinal cord in **spinal nerves**, while those from the head are carried to the brain in **cranial nerves**.
❏ **Generally** ascending sensory projections related to the general senses consist of a sequence of **three neurons** that extends from peripheral receptor to contralateral cerebral cortex.
  > These are referred to as first, second and third order neurons.

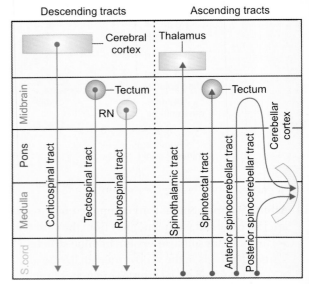

Fig. 69: Major ascending and descending tracts. (RN = Red nucleus)

- ❑ **First order neuron** afferents have peripherally located sensory endings and cell bodies that lie in dorsal root ganglia or the sensory ganglia associated with certain cranial nerves.
  - ➢ Their axons enter the CNS through spinal or cranial nerves and terminate by synapsing on the cell bodies of ipsilateral second-order neurons.
- ❑ Primary afferent fibers carrying **pain**, **temperature** and coarse **touch and pressure** information from the trunk and limbs are carried by **spinothalamic tract**.
  - ➢ Homologous fibers from the head terminate in the **trigeminal** sensory nucleus of the brainstem.
- ❑ Primary afferent fibers carrying **proprioceptive** information and **fine (discriminative) touch** from the trunk and limbs ascend ipsilaterally in the spinal cord as the **dorsal column - medial lemniscal system.**
  - ➢ A similar homologous projection exists for afferents derived from the head.

Tract	Location	Origin*	Termination	Functions
Lateral spinothalamic tract	Lateral white column	Posterior horn cells of spinal cord of opposite side	Ventral posterolateral (VPL) nucleus of thalamus	Carry pain and temperature from opposite side of the body
Anterior spinothalamic tract	Anterior white column	Posterior horn cells of spinal cord of opposite side	Ventral posterolateral (VPL) nucleus of thalamus	Carry light touch, pressure, tickle, and itch sensation from opposite side of the body
Spinotectal tract	Lateral white column	Posterior horn cells of spinal cord of opposite side	Superior colliculus of tectum of midbrain	Visuomotor reflexes, head and eye movements towards the source of stimulation
Spinocerebellar (anterior and posterior) tracts	Lateral white column (superficially)	Posterior horn cells of spinal cord of same side	Cerebellum	Unconscious kinesthesia (proprioception)
Fasciculus gracilis and fasciculus cuneatus (tracts of Gall and Burdach)	Posterior white column of spinal cord	Dorsal root ganglia of spinal nerves of the same side	Nucleus gracilis and nucleus cuneatus in medulla of the same side	Joint sense, vibration sense, two-point discrimination, stereognosis, conscious kinesthesia

Table 15: Major ascending tracts in the spinal cord

*Location of cell bodies of neurons from which the axons of tract arise

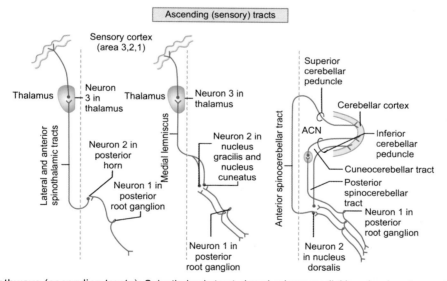

Fig. 70: Sensory pathways (ascending tracts): Spinothalamic tract, dorsal column-medial lemniscal system and spinocerebellar tract

▶ Dorsal Column–Medial Lemniscal System (DC-MLS)

- ❑ It carries the following sensory modalities - **fine (discriminative) touch**, pressure, vibration, conscious proprioception and stereognosis.
- ❑ **First order neurons** (dorsal root ganglion) carry the information ipsilaterally in the dorsal column (fasciculus cuneatus and gracilis) to synapse on **second order neurons** located in the gracile and cuneate nuclei of the caudal medulla.
- ❑ They give rise to axons (internal arcuate fibers) that **decussate** and form medial lemniscus.
- ❑ The **medial lemniscus** crosses midline and ascends through the **contralateral brainstem** and terminates in the **ventral posterolateral** (VPL) nucleus of the thalamus.
- ❑ **Third order neurons** are located in the VPL nucleus of the thalamus.

❑ They project through the posterior limb of the **internal capsule** to the **primary** somatosensory cortex—postcentral gyrus (Brodmann's areas 3, 1, and 2).

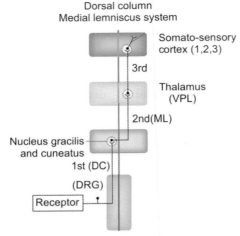

Fig. 71: Dorsal column- medial lemniscal system (overview)

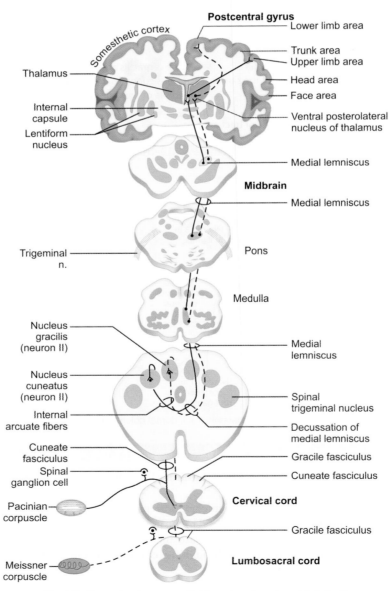

Fig. 72: Dorsal column-medial lemniscal system (detailed)

Spinothalamic Tract (STT)

❏ Primary afferent fibers carrying **pain** and **temperature** information from the trunk and limbs are carried by **lateral spinothalamic tract** and coarse **touch** and **pressure** information by **anterior spinothalamic tract**.

Lateral Spinothalamic Tract – Spinal Lemniscal System

❏ **First order neurons** (dorsal root ganglion) fibers **ascend up** by one or two spinal segments, before they terminate in the dorsal horn of the spinal gray matter.

❏ They synapse on the posterior horn cells (**second order neuron**), which further send the fibers decussating in the anterior white commissure and run as **lateral spinothalamic tract** (spinal cord) and further as **spinal lemniscus** (in the brainstem).

❏ **Third order neurons** are located in the **VPL nucleus of the thalamus**. They project through the **posterior limb** of the internal capsule to terminate in the postcentral gyrus of the parietal lobe, which is also known as the **primary somatosensory cortex** (Brodmann area 1,2,3).

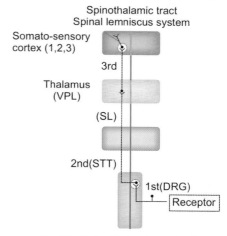

Fig. 73: Spinothalamic - spinal lemniscal system (overview)

Anterior spinothalamic tract has a minor role in carrying the touch and pressure of light and crude (coarse) nature. It carries the sensations of itch, tickling, etc.

❏ It has almost the same course as lateral spinothalamic tract and joins it in the brainstem at the level of **spinal lemniscus**, before it reaches the thalamus.

❏ Some of the axons carrying touch sensations may join **medial lemniscus**, before reaching the thalamus.

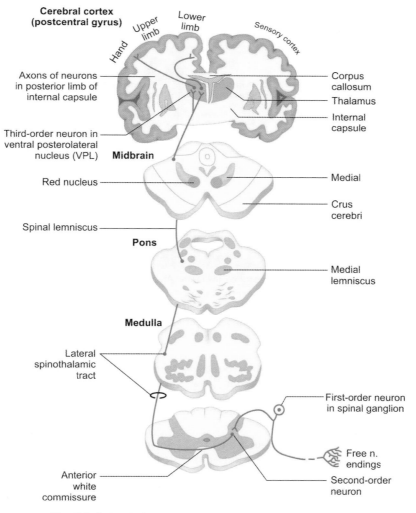

Fig. 74: Spinothalamic - spinal lemniscal system (detailed)

QUESTIONS

1. Which of the following is NOT carried by posterior column tract? *(AIIMS 2014)*
   a. Position sense
   b. Pain
   c. Touch
   d. Vibration

2. TRUE about medial lemniscus system *(PGIC)*
   a. Formed from fasciculus gracilis and cuneatus
   b. Carries discriminative touch and proprioception
   c. Convey pain and temperature
   d. Joins spinothalamic tract
   e. Decussates at lower medulla

ANSWERS

1. b. Pain
   ❑ **Posterior** (dorsal) column carries sensations like pressure, vibration, tactile discrimination, proprioception, stereognosis, conscious proprioception.
   ❑ **Pain and temperature** is carried by the **lateral spinothalamic tract**.

2. a. Formed from fasciculus gracilis and cuneatus; b. Carries discriminative touch and proprioception; e. Decussates at lower medulla
   ❑ Five sensations (pressure, **discriminative touch**, vibration, stereognosis and **proprioception**) are carried by **dorsal column (fasciculus gracilis and cuneatus)** of spinal cord and synapse in the respective nuclei in the lower medulla.
   ❑ **Second order** neurons begin as medial lemniscus and cross the midline (internal arcuate fibers) in the **lower medulla** and ascend up to synapse in thalamus (VPL nucleus).
   ❑ **Pain and temperature** is carried by **lateral spinothalamic tract** – spinal lemniscal system.

❑ **Ventral corticospinal tract** and medial descending brainstem pathways (tectospinal, reticulospinal, and vestibulospinal tracts) regulate **proximal muscles** and **posture**.

❑ **Lateral corticospinal** and rubrospinal tracts control **distal limb muscles** for fine motor control and **skilled voluntary movements**.

❑ Posterior column tract **does not** carry the temperature sensations, it is carried by the lateral spino-thalamic tract (AIPG 2008)

❑ Ability to recognise an unseen familiar object is known as **stereognosis** and is carried by the **dorsal column**.

❑ An **anterolateral cordotomy** relieving pain in left leg is effective because it interrupts the right **lateral spinothalamic tract**.

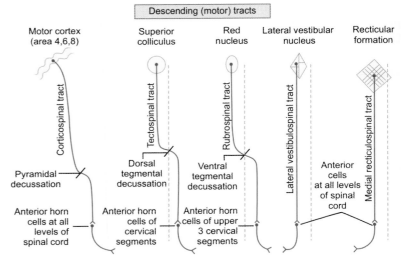

Fig. 75: Descending (motor) tracts

Table 16: Major descending tracts in the spinal cord

Tract	Location	Origin	Termination	Functions
Lateral corticospinal (crossed pyramidal) tract	Lateral white column of spinal cord	Primary motor cortex (area 4), premotor cortex (area 6) of the opposite cerebral hemisphere (upper motor neurons)	Anterior horn cells of the spinal cord (lower motor neurons)	Controls conscious skilled movements especially of hands (contraction of individual or small group of muscles particularly those which move hands, fingers, feet and toes)
Anterior corticospinal (uncrossed pyramidal) tract	Anterior white column	Primary motor cortex (area 4) premotor cortex (area 6) of the opposite cerebral hemisphere (upper motor neurons)	Anterior horn cells of the spinal cord (lower motor neurons)	Same as that of lateral corticospinal tracts
Rubrospinal tract	Lateral white column	Red nucleus of the opposite side located in midbrain	Anterior horn cells of the spinal cord	Unconscious coordination of movements (controls muscle tone and synergy)
Vestibulospinal tract	Anterior white column	Vestibular nucleus	Anterior horn cells of the spinal cord	Unconscious maintenance of posture and balance

Tract	Location	Origin*	Termination	Functions
Tectospinal tract	Anterior white column	Superior colliculus of the opposite side	Cranial nerve nuclei in medulla and anterior horn cells of the upper spinal segments	Controls movements of head, neck and arms in response to visual stimuli
Lateral reticulospinal tract	Lateral white column	Reticular formation in midbrain, pons and medulla	Anterior horn cells of the spinal cord	Mainly responsible for facilitatory influence on the motor neurons to the skeletal muscles
Medial reticulospinal tract	Anterior white column	Reticular formation in medulla	Anterior horn cells of the spinal cord	Mainly responsible for inhibitory influence on the motor neurons to the skeletal muscles

▼ Pyramidal System

Pyramidal tract: Fibers arise from pyramidal neurons in layer 5 of the precentral gyrus, premotor areas and somatic sensory cortex and descend through the posterior limb of internal capsule and basis pedunculi, cross at the spinomedullary junction and form the lateral corticospinal tract in the lateral funiculus of the spinal cord. They terminate on lower motor neurons in the ventral horn or on interneurons.

- ❑ Most muscles are represented in the contralateral motor cortex. However, some (such as the muscles of the upper face, the muscles of mastication, and muscles of the larynx) are represented bilaterally.

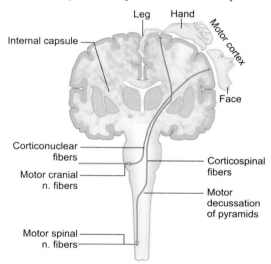

Fig. 76: The corticospinal and corticonuclear tracts

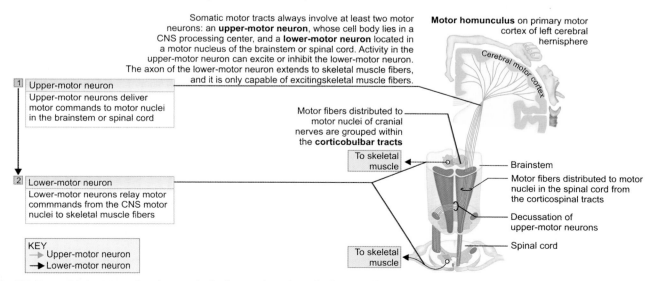

Fig. 77: Pyramidal system showing corticobulbar and corticospinal tracts. Upper motor neurons in the cerebrum modulate the lower motor neurons located in brainstem (cranial nerves) and spinal cord (spinal nerves), which themselves control the skeletal muscles

❑ With the noted bilateral exceptions, lesion of the pyramidal tract above the decussation results in spastic paralysis, loss of fine movements, and hyper-reflexia on the contralateral side.

❑ Lesion of the corticospinal tract in the spinal cord results in ipsilateral symptomology.

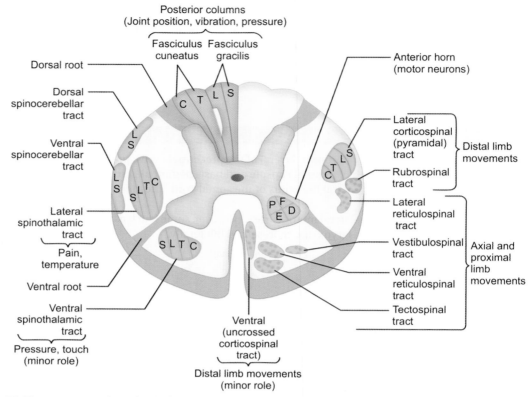

Fig. 78: Transverse section of spinal cord showing sensory tracts on left half and motor tracts on the right half

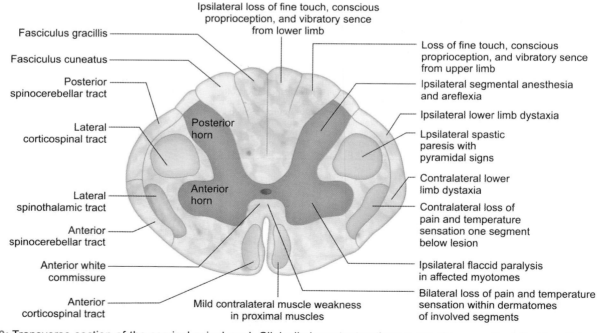

Fig. 79: Transverse section of the cervical spinal cord. Clinically important pathways are shown on the left side; clinical deficits resulting from the interruption of these pathways are shown on the right side. Destructive lesions of the posterior horns result in anesthesia and areflexia, and destructive lesions of the anterior horns result in LMN lesions and areflexia. Destruction of the anterior white commissure interrupts the central transmission of pain and temperature impulses bilaterally via the anterolateral system.

Table 17: Differences between conus medullaris syndrome and cauda equina syndrome

Features	Conus medullaris syndrome	Cauda equina syndrome
Part affected	Conus medullaris containing sacral segments of the cord and may be lumbar nerves	Sacral nerve roots
Presentation	Both upper motor neuron and lower motor neuron type paralysis	Only lower motor neuron type of paralysis
Onset	Sudden	Gradual
Laterality	Bilateral	May be unilateral
Low back pain	Severe	Not severe
Root pain	Not severe	Severe
Anesthesia	Perianal region	Saddle anesthesia
Paralysis	Bilateral upper motor neuron type with exaggerated tendon reflexes, increased tone below the level of lesion and lower motor neuron type paralysis at the level of lesion	Unilateral, lower motor neuron type paralysis with hypotonia, loss of reflexes and atrophy of muscles
Bladder and bowel involvement	Early, urinary retention with overflow urinary and bowel incontinence	Late, urinary and bowel retention
Sexual dysfunction	More frequent	Less frequent

❏ **Brown-Sequard syndrome** is characterized by a **Hemisection of spinal cord** which results in weakness or paralysis on same side (hemiplegia) of the body and a loss of sensation (hemianesthesia) on the opposite side.
➤ The patient presents with **contralateral** loss of crude touch sensations, since **anterior spinothalamic tract** carrying these sensations, crosses the midline and runs on the opposite half of spinal cord.

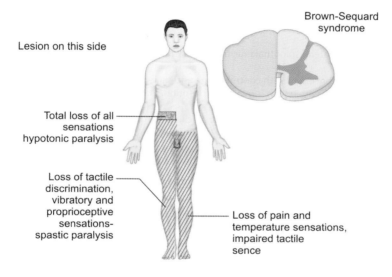

Fig. 80: Brown-Séquard syndrome with a spinal cord lesion at the right 10th thoracic level

Questions

1. **All true about conus syndrome EXCEPT:** *(AIPG 2008)*
   a. Begins at the level of lower 3 sacral and coccygeal segment
   b. Absent knee and ankle jerks
   c. Flexor plantar reflex
   d. Saddle anesthesia

2. **The final common pathway for horizontal gaze is nucleus:** *(AIPG 2008)*
   a. Abducent
   b. Oculomotor
   c. Trochlear
   d. Vestibular

3. **Most of the fibers in pyramidal tract originate from:**
   a. Primary motor cortex
   b. Pre-motor cortex
   c. Primary somato-sensory cortex
   d. Supplementary motor cortex

4. **All is true about Brown-Sequard syndrome EXCEPT:**
   a. Hemisection of spinal cord
   b. Ipsilateral loss of vibration sensations
   c. Ipsilateral loss of crude touch sensations
   d. Ipsilateral paralysis below the level of lesion

5. **About Brown-Sequard syndrome all are true EXCEPT** *(NEET Pattern 2018)*
   a. Ipsilateral hemiplegia
   b. Ipsilateral loss of position and vibration
   c. Ipsilateral loss of pain and temperature
   d. Contralateral loss of pain and temperature

ANSWERS

1. **b. Absent knee and ankle jerks**
   - ❑ Since the spinal segments involved in knee and ankle jerks are at higher level than the level of lesion, they are preserved, and not lost.
   - ❑ Root value of knee reflex is L-2, 3 and 4 and for the ankle reflex is S-1.
   - ❑ Conus medullary syndrome is a lower motor neuron lesion and involves the lower 3 sacral and coccygeal segments.
   - ❑ Plantar reflex remains flexor in this syndrome, since its spinal arc is also above the level of lesion and is unaffected.
   - ❑ Root value of plantar reflex is S-1, 2.
   - ❑ Conus medullary syndrome produces saddle anesthesia in the perineal region as per the dermatomal pattern.
2. **a. Abducent**
   - ❑ Subcortical center for horizontal conjugate gaze lies in the abducent nucleus in pons.
   - ❑ It receives input from the contralateral frontal eye field and controls ipsilateral lateral rectus and contralateral medial rectus muscle via projections of medial longitudinal fasciculus (MLF).
   - ❑ MLF connects the nuclei controlling eyeball muscles and mediates nystagmus and lateral conjugate gaze.
   - ❑ Its fibers originate in vestibular nucleus and terminate in abducent, trochlear and oculomotor nuclei.
   - ❑ It coordinates eyeball movements with the head. Trochlear nucleus is mainly concerned with vertical gaze movements.
3. **c. Primary somato-sensory cortex**
   - ❑ About 31% of the corticospinal tract neurons arise from the primary motor cortex.
   - ❑ The premotor cortex and supplementary motor cortex account for 29% of the corticospinal tract neurons.
   - ❑ The largest percentage of 40% originate in the parietal lobe and primary somatosensory area in the postcentral gyrus.
4. **c. Ipsilateral loss of crude touch sensations**
   - ❑ The patient presents with contralateral loss of crude touch sensations, since anterior spinothalamic tract carrying these sensations, crosses the midline and runs on the opposite half of spinal cord.
5. **c. Ipsilateral loss of pain and temperature**
   - ❑ **Brown-Sequard syndrome** presents with **contralateral** loss of pain and temperature, due to lesion of **lateral spinothalamic tract**.

High Yield

- Pain and temperature is carried by the lateral spinothalamic tract, whereas, anterior spinothalamic tract carries the crude touch and light touch.
- Pyramidal tract is a motor tract and is concerned with control of fine and skilled voluntary motor activity.
- Dorsal spinocerebellar tract is concerned with unconscious proprioception, mainly from the lower limbs.
- Upper limb proprioception is carried by the cuneocerebellar tract.
- Posterior column (dorsal column) of spinal cord has two fasciculi: gracilis and cuneatus.

Autonomic Nervous System

Autonomic nervous system (ANS) is responsible for the motor innervation of **three effectors**: Cardiac muscle, smooth muscle, and glands, and is divided into **three components**: Sympathetic, parasympathetic, and enteric divisions.

- ❑ It includes general visceral efferent (GVE) and general visceral afferent (GVA) fibers.
- ❑ Its motor (GVE) component is a ganglionated system involving **two neurons**: preganglionic and postganglionic.
- ❑ Preganglionic neurons with cell bodies are in the CNS (brainstem and in the lateral gray columns of the spinal cord). Their axons are usually finely **myelinated**, exit from the CNS in certain cranial and spinal nerves, and then pass to peripheral ganglia, where they synapse with postganglionic neurons.
- ❑ The axons of postganglionic neurons are usually **unmyelinated**. Postganglionic neurons are **more numerous** than preganglionic ones; one preganglionic neuron may synapse with 15–20 postganglionic neurons, which permits the wide distribution of many autonomic effects.

Location and Distribution

- ❑ Sympathetic flow is **thoracolumbar** outflow and **parasympathetic** is craniosacral outflow.
- ❑ Autonomic activity is not initiated or controlled solely by the reflex connections of general visceral afferent pathways; nor do impulses in these pathways necessarily activate general visceral efferents.
- ❑ Peripheral autonomic activity is integrated at higher levels in the **brainstem** and **cerebrum**, including various nuclei of the brainstem **reticular formation**, **thalamus** and **hypothalamus**, the **limbic lobe** and **prefrontal** neocortex, together with the ascending and descending pathways that interconnect these regions.
- ❑ The parasympathetic system is **restricted** in its distribution to the head, neck and body cavities (except for erectile tissues of genitalia), otherwise, parasympathetic fibers are **never** found in the body wall and limbs. Sympathetic fibers by comparison are distributed to all the vascularized portions of body.

Neurotransmitters

❏ Generally preganglionic neurons of both sympathetic and parasympathetic systems are **cholinergic** and postganglionic parasympathetic neurons are also **cholinergic** while those of the sympathetic nervous system are **noradrenergic** (with few exceptions).

❏ The principal co-transmitters in sympathetic nerves are **ATP** and **neuropeptide Y**; in parasympathetic nerves **vasoactive intestinal polypeptide (VIP)**; and in enteric nerves ATP, VIP and **substance P**.

❏ **Acetylcholine** (ACh) is the preganglionic neurotransmitter for both divisions of the ANS as well as the postganglionic neurotransmitter of the parasympathetic neurons; the preganglionic receptors are nicotinic, and the postganglionic are muscarinic in type.

❏ **Norepinephrine** (NE) is the neurotransmitter of the postganglionic sympathetic neurons, except for cholinergic neurons innervating the eccrine sweat glands.

Functions of Autonomic Nervous System (ANS)

❏ Sympathetic nervous system functions in **emergencies** (energy consumption), preparing for fight or flight, whereas the parasympathetic nerve functions in **homeostasis** (energy conservation), tending to promote quiet and orderly processes of the body.

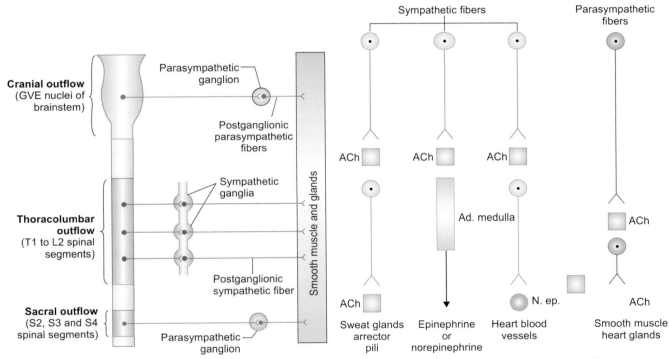

Fig. 81: ANS showing two components: sympathetic and parasympathetic

Fig. 82: ANS showing the various neurotransmitters at ganglion and effector levels

❏ Sympathetic activity, in general, results in the constriction of cutaneous arteries (increasing blood supply to the heart, muscles and brain), cardiac acceleration, an increase in blood pressure, contraction of sphincters and depression of peristalsis, all of which mobilize body energy stores for dealing with increased activity.

❏ Parasympathetic activity leads to cardiac slowing and an increase in intestinal glandular and peristaltic activities, which may be considered to conserve body energy stores.

❏ With the exception of coronary arteries, vasoconstriction is sympathetically stimulated; the effects of sympathetic stimulation on glands (other than sweat glands) are the indirect effect of vasoconstriction.

❏ **Sympathetic** nervous system works for bladder and bowel **storage** (decrease in peristalsis and sphincter constriction), whereas **parasympathetic** system is involved in bladder and bowel **evacuation** (increased peristalsis and relaxed sphincters).

❏ Pelvic viscera like urinary bladder and rectum are supplied by T10 - 12; L1-2 (sympathetic splanchnic nerves) supply which decrease the peristalsis of detrusor and constrict the urethral sphincters for **storage** of urine.

❏ Parasympathetic nervi erigentes (S2-4) increase the peristalsis of detrusor and relax the urethral sphincters for **evacuation** of urine.

❑ Somatic nervous system allows for the bladder and bowel continence by S-2-4 (somatic pudendal nerve) which constricts the external urethral sphincter (skeletal muscle) for voluntary holding of urine or fecal matter.

❑ Pain fibers from the bladder and proximal urethra (GVA) traverse both the **pelvic splanchnic nerves** and the inferior hypogastric plexus, hypogastric nerves, superior hypogastric plexus and lumbar splanchnic nerves to reach their cell bodies in ganglia on the **lower thoracic and upper lumbar dorsal spinal roots** (T10 - 12; L1-2).

▶ Parasympathetic Nervous System

Parasympathetic Nervous System is an energy conserving (**anabolic**) system, concerned with homeostasis and promoting quiet and orderly processes of the body.

❑ Preganglionic parasympathetic neuronal cell bodies are located in certain **cranial nerve nuclei** of the brainstem and in the **intermedio-lateral horn cells** of the second to fourth sacral segments of the spinal cord.

❑ Efferent fibers (GVE), which are **myelinated**, emerge from the CNS only in the **oculomotor**, **facial**, **glossopharyngeal** and **vagus** nerves, and in the **nervi erigentes** (S2-4) spinal nerves.

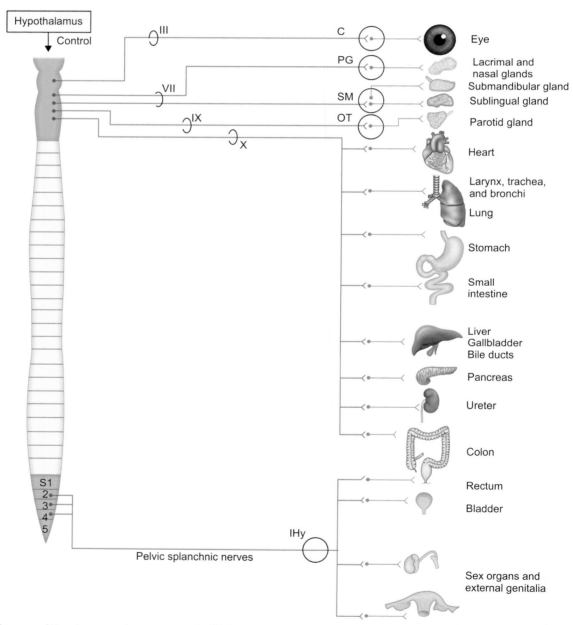

Fig. 83: Diagram of the visceromotor component of the parasympathetic nervous system. Preganglionic parasympathetic neurons (solid line; green), postganglionic parasympathetic neurons (solid line; red). C, ciliary ganglion; PG, pterygopalatine ganglion; SM, submandibular ganglion; OT, otic ganglion; IHy, inferior hypogastric plexus

- Both the preganglionic and postganglionic parasympathetic neurons are **cholinergic**.
- The cell bodies of postganglionic parasympathetic neurons are mostly located **distant** from the CNS, either in discrete ganglia located near the structures innervated, or dispersed in the walls of viscera.
- In the cranial part of the parasympathetic system there are **four** small peripheral ganglia: **ciliary**, **pterygopalatine**, **submandibular** and **otic**.
- These ganglia are **efferent** parasympathetic ganglia, **unlike** the trigeminal, facial, glossopharyngeal and vagal sensory ganglia, all of which are concerned exclusively with afferent impulses and contain the cell bodies of sensory neurons.
- The cranial parasympathetic ganglia are also traversed by afferent fibers, postganglionic sympathetic fibers and, in the case of the otic ganglion, by branchial efferent fibers; however, **none of these fibers synapse** in the ganglia.
- Postganglionic parasympathetic fibers are usually **unmyelinated** and **shorter** than their counterparts in the sympathetic system because the ganglia in which the parasympathetic fibers synapse are either in or near the viscera they supply.
- **Vagus** nerve has the **largest distribution** in the body and contains the parasympathetic preganglionic **GVE** fibers with cell bodies located in the medulla oblongata and the **GVA** fibers with cell bodies located in the inferior (nodose) ganglion.
- Parasympathetic fibers in the vagus nerve (CN X) that supply all of the thoracic and abdominal viscera, **except** the descending and sigmoid colons and other pelvic viscera (which are supplied by nervi erigentes).

▶ Sympathetic Nervous System

Sympathetic Nervous System is a catabolic (energy-consuming) system that enables the body to cope with emergencies, with a fight-or-flight reaction.

- It contains preganglionic cell bodies that are located in the intermediolateral horn cells of the spinal cord segments between T1 and L2 (thoracolumbar flow).

    Sympathetic trunks are two ganglionated nerve cords that extend on either side of the vertebral column from the cranial base to the coccyx.
- The trunk is composed primarily of ascending and descending **preganglionic** sympathetic fibers and **visceral afferent** fibers and contains the cell bodies of the postganglionic sympathetic fibers.
- The ganglia are joined to spinal nerves by short connecting nerves called **white** and **gray rami communicantes**.
- Preganglionic axons join the trunk through the white rami communicantes while postganglionic axons leave the trunk in the gray rami.
- In the neck, each sympathetic trunk lies **posterior to the carotid sheath** and anterior to the transverse processes of the cervical vertebrae.
- In the thorax, the trunks are **anterior to the heads of the ribs** and the posterior intercostal vessels and gives rise to cardiac, pulmonary, mediastinal, and splanchnic branches.
- Sympathetic trunks enter the abdomen **through the crus of the diaphragm** or behind the medial lumbocostal arch and in the abdomen they lie anterolateral to the bodies of the lumbar vertebrae.
- In the pelvis they are anterior to the sacrum and medial to the anterior sacral foramina.
- Anterior to the coccyx the two trunks meet in a single, median, terminal ganglion.
- **Cervical sympathetic** ganglia are usually reduced to **three** by fusion. The **internal carotid nerve**, a continuation of the sympathetic trunk arises from the cranial pole of the superior ganglion and accompanies the internal carotid artery through its canal into the cranial cavity.
- There are between 10 and 12 (usually 11) thoracic ganglia, 4 lumbar ganglia, and 4 or 5 ganglia in the sacral region.
- The cell bodies of preganglionic sympathetic neurons are located in the **lateral horn** of the spinal gray matter of all thoracic segments and the upper two or three lumbar segments.
- Their axons are **myelinated** and leave the cord in the corresponding ventral nerve roots and **pass into the spinal nerves**, but soon leave in white rami communicantes to join the sympathetic trunk.
- Neurons like those in the lateral gray column exist at other levels of the cord above and below the thoracolumbar outflow and small numbers of their fibers leave in other ventral roots.
- On reaching the sympathetic trunk, preganglionic fibers behave in one of several ways. They may synapse with neurons in the nearest ganglion, or traverse the nearest ganglion and ascend or descend in the sympathetic chain to end in another ganglion.
- A preganglionic fiber may terminate in a single ganglion or, through collateral branches, synapse with neurons in several ganglia.
- Preganglionic fibers may traverse the nearest ganglion, ascend or descend and, without synapsing, emerge in one of the medially directed branches of the sympathetic trunk to synapse in the ganglia of autonomic plexuses (mainly situated in the midline, e.g. around the coeliac and mesenteric arteries).
- More than one preganglionic fiber may synapse with a single postganglionic neurone.
- **Uniquely**, the suprarenal gland is innervated directly by preganglionic sympathetic neurons that traverse the sympathetic trunk and celiac ganglion **without synapse**.

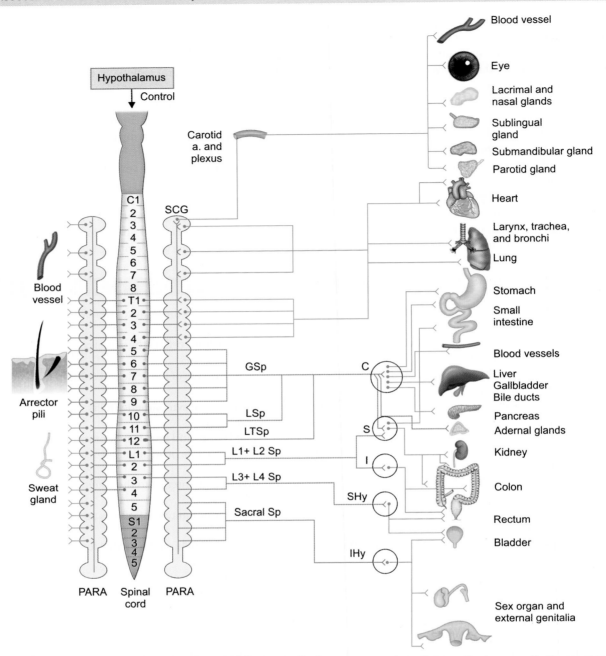

Fig. 84: Diagram of the visceromotor component of the sympathetic nervous system. Preganglionic sympathetic neurons (solid line; green), postganglionic sympathetic neurons (solid line; red). PARA, paravertebral chain ganglia; C, celiac ganglion; S, superior mesenteric ganglion; I, inferior mesenteric ganglion; SHy, superior hypogastric plexus; IHy, inferior hypogastric plexus; GSp, greater thoracic splanchnic nerve; LSp, lesser thoracic splanchnic nerve; LTSp, least thoracic splanchnic nerve; Sp, splanchnic nerve

❏ The neuron bodies of sympathetic postganglionic neurons are located mostly either in the ganglia of the sympathetic trunk or in ganglia in more peripheral plexuses.

❏ The axons of **postganglionic** neurons are, therefore, generally **longer than** those of preganglionic neurons, an exception being some of those that innervate pelvic viscera.

❏ The axons of ganglionic cells are **unmyelinated**. They are distributed to target organs in various ways.

❏ Those from a ganglion of the sympathetic trunk may return to the spinal nerve of preganglionic origin through a **gray ramus** communicans, which usually joins the nerve just proximal to the white ramus, and are then distributed through ventral and dorsal spinal rami to blood vessels (**vasomotor**), sweat glands (**sudomotor**), hair (**pilomotor**) in their zone of supply.

❏ **Alternatively**, postganglionic fibers may pass in a medial branch of a ganglion direct to particular viscera, or innervate adjacent blood vessels, or pass along them externally to their peripheral distribution. They may ascend or descend before leaving the sympathetic trunk as described above.

❏ Many fibers are distributed along arteries and ducts as plexuses to distant effectors.

- ❑ The sympathetic system has a much **wider distribution** than the parasympathetic. It innervates all sweat glands, the arrector pili muscles, the muscular walls of many blood vessels, the heart, lungs and respiratory tree, the abdominopelvic viscera, the esophagus, the muscles of the iris, and the non-striated muscle of the urogenital tract, eyelids, etc.
- ❑ Postganglionic sympathetic fibers that return to the spinal nerves are vasoconstrictor to blood vessels, secretomotor to sweat glands and motor to the arrector pili muscles within their dermatomes.
- ❑ Those that accompany the motor nerves to voluntary muscles are probably only dilatory.

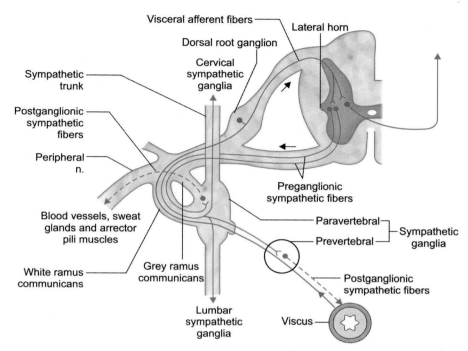

Fig. 85: Sympathetic nervous system showing efferent and afferent fibers. The preganglionic fibers are shown by solid red lines and postganglionic fibers by interrupted red lines. The afferent fibers are shown by green lines

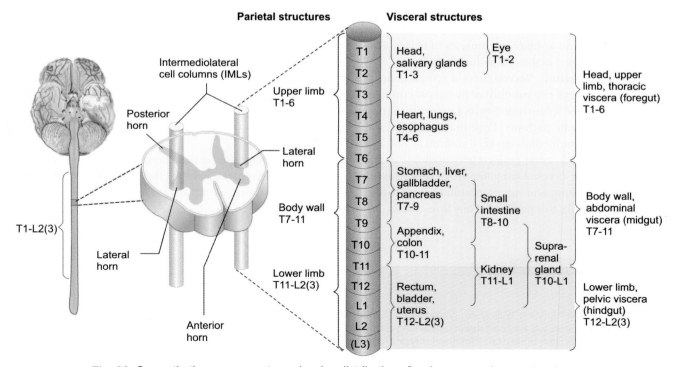

Fig. 86: Sympathetic nervous system, showing distribution of various root values to the viscera

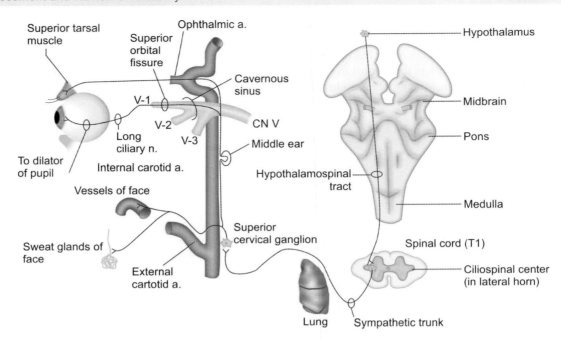

Fig. 87: Sympathetic pathway for controlling smooth muscles of eyeball, namely superior tarsal muscle and dilator pupillae muscle. It is three order neuron pathway and injury at any level leads to features of Horner syndrome

- Most, if not all, peripheral nerves contain postganglionic sympathetic fibers. Those reaching the viscera are concerned with general vasoconstriction, bronchial and bronchiolar dilation, modification of glandular secretion, pupillary dilation, inhibition of gastrointestinal muscle contraction, etc.

- Sympathetic fibers have a typical relation with the spinal nerves. The preganglionic sympathetic fibers may relay in their corresponding (or higher and lower) ganglion and pass to their corresponding spinal nerve for distribution or pass without synapse to a peripheral (prevertebral) ganglion for relay.

- **White Rami Communicantes** contain preganglionic sympathetic GVE (myelinated) fibers with cell bodies located in the lateral horn (intermediolateral cell column) of the spinal cord and GVA fibers with cell bodies located in the dorsal root ganglia. They are connected to the spinal nerves, limited to the spinal cord segments between T1 and L2.

- **Gray Rami Communicantes** contain postganglionic sympathetic GVE (unmyelinated) fibers that supply the blood vessels, sweat glands, and arrector pili muscles of hair follicles. They are connected to every spinal nerve and contain fibers with cell bodies located in the sympathetic trunk.

- **Thoracic Splanchnic Nerves** contain sympathetic preganglionic GVE fibers with cell bodies located in the lateral horn (intermediolateral cell column) of the spinal cord and GVA fibers with cell bodies located in the dorsal root ganglia. They include: **Greater** Splanchnic Nerve, **Lesser** Splanchnic Nerve and **Least** Splanchnic Nerves.

- Oculosympathetic pathway: Hypothalamus (first order neuron) send fibers which project to the ipsilateral ciliospinal center of the intermediolateral cell column at T1 (second order neurons).
  - ➢ The ciliospinal center projects preganglionic sympathetic fibers to the superior cervical ganglion (third order neuron).
  - ➢ The superior cervical ganglion projects perivascular postganglionic sympathetic fibers through the tympanic cavity, cavernous sinus, and superior orbital fissure to the dilator pupillae and superior tarsal muscle (part of Muller muscle).
  - ➢ Interruption of this pathway at any level results in **Horner syndrome**.

CLINICAL CORRELATIONS

Horner syndrome

Etiology

- **First order** neuron injury, e.g. Wallenberg syndrome. The hypothalamospinal pathway is lesioned in the lateral medullary ischemia.
- **Second order** neuron, e.g. Pancoast tumor (apical lung cancer like bronchial carcinomas) that invades the sympathetic trunk and is also a recognized complication of cervical sympathectomy or a radical neck dissection.
- **Third order** neuron, e.g. Carotid artery dissection

Clinical Features

❑ **Partial ptosis** (drooping eyelid) due to paralysis of *superior tarsal muscle* (part of Muller muscle) and unopposed (**over-activity) of orbicularis muscle**. Upside-down ptosis (slight elevation of the lower lid).

❑ **Enophthalmos** (sunken globe) due to paralysis of orbitalis muscle. Enophthalmos may be absent or patient may present with apparent enophthalmos (the impression that the eye is sunken, caused by a narrow palpebral aperture).

❑ **Miosis** (paralysed contracted pupil) occurs as the *dilator pupillae* is paralysed and sphincter pupillae is **unopposed**. If dilator pupillae is partly functional a pupillary dilatation lag is observed and pupil's light reflex may be elicited.

❑ **Vasodilation** occurs, since T-1 sympathetic vasoconstrictive fibers are lesioned—hyperemia and flushing on face, bloodshot conjunctiva and nasal congestion.

❑ **Anhydrosis** (lack of thermal sweating)

❑ **Loss of ciliospinal reflex** (The ciliospinal reflex is a pupillary-skin reflex, which consists of dilation of the ipsilateral pupil in response to pain applied to the neck, face, and upper limb).

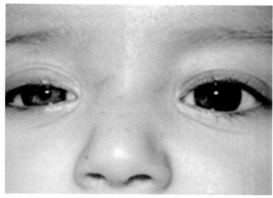

Fig. 88: Right sided Horner syndrome showing partial ptosis (paralysed superior tarsal muscle), miosis (paralysed dilator pupillae) and enophthalmos (paralysed orbitalis muscle). Also note blue green colur of right iris as compared to left normal brown iris (heterochromia iridis)

Congenital Horner syndrome: Difficult labor and hyper-abduction injury during birth may lead to avulsion of the first thoracic nerve from the spinal cord (**Klumpke's palsy**) presenting with heterochromia and unilateral straight hair.

Heterochromia iris is a difference in color between the two eyes that results from interference with melanocyte pigmentation of the iris by a lack of sympathetic stimulation during development.

❑ The affected iris color may remain blue while the other iris changes to brown.

❑ The color of iris at birth is deep blue and changes to green and brown eventually (decided by the sun exposure in various races).

❑ Iris pigmentation is under sympathetic control during development, which is completed by age 2 years.

❑ Heterochromia is uncommon in patients with Horner syndrome acquired later in life.

---

1. All of the following statements about the vagus nerve are true EXCEPT that it: *(AIIMS 2005)*
   a. Supplies heart and lung
   b. Carries postganglionic parasympathetic fibers
   c. Innervates right two third of transverse colon
   d. Stimulates peristalsis and relaxes sphincters

2. General visceral fibers do NOT supply: *(NEET Pattern 2013)*
   a. Smooth muscles
   b. Skeletal muscles
   c. Cardiac muscles
   d. Glands

3. All of the following nuclei belong to GVE (General Visceral Efferent) EXCEPT:
   a. Edinger-Westphal nucleus
   b. Lacrimatory nucleus
   c. Dorsal nucleus of vagus
   d. Abducent

4. Sweating is mediated by:
   a. Adrenal hormones
   b. Sympathetic adrenergic system
   c. Sympathetic cholinergic system
   d. Parasympathetic cholinergic system

5. Dilator pupillae is supplied by:
   a. Oculomotor nerve
   b. Sympathetic fibers from the fronto-orbital branch of trigeminal nerve
   c. Postganglionic sympathetic fibers from cervical sympathetic chain
   d. Postganglionic parasympathetic fibers

6. In a car accident the patient sustained crushed internal injury in the abdomen. The fibers in the vagus nerve are lesioned, which interferes with the functions of, which of the following structure:
   a. Urinary bladder   b. Splenic flexure of colon
   c. Kidney   d. Uterus

7. All are seen in Horner's syndrome EXCEPT: *(AIIMS 2008)*
   a. Heterochromia iridis   b. Ptosis
   c. Miosis   d. Apparent exophthalmos

8. Features of stellate ganglion lesions include: *(PGIC 2014)*
   a. Miosis
   b. Vasodilation in ipsilateral arm
   c. Mydriasis in contralateral eye
   d. Mydriasis in ipsilateral eye
   e. Nasal congestion

9. WRONG statement regarding gray rami communicantes is: *(AIIMS 2017)*
   a. Connected to spinal nerve
   b. Present medial to white rami communicantes
   c. Carries pre-ganglionic fibers
   d. Fibers are non-myelinated

QUESTIONS

1. b. Carries postganglionic parasympathetic fibers:
- ❏ **Vagus nerve carries preganglionic (and not post-ganglionic) fibers from the dorsal nucleus of vagus in the medulla oblongata.**
- ❏ Vagus nerve is the **longest** cranial nerve with **largest distribution** in the body. It supplies head and neck region, thorax, abdomen and some pelvic viscera as well.
- ❏ It causes bradycardia (heart) and bronchoconstriction (lung).
- ❏ It supplies **till the right 2/3 of transverse colon** (mid-gut). Splenic flexure is innervated by nervi erigentes.
- ❏ Vagus nerve is a parasympathetic nerve, which **increases peristalsis** and **relaxes the sphincters** for viscus evacuation.

2. b. Skeletal muscles
- ❏ General visceral efferent (GVE) includes the fibers under autonomic nervous system, which control three effectors: **Cardiac** muscle, **smooth** muscles and **glands**.
- ❏ General somatic efferent (GSE) neural column controls skeletal muscles.

3. d. Abducent
- ❏ General visceral efferent (GVE) includes the fibers under autonomic nervous system, which control three effectors: Cardiac muscle, smooth muscles and glands.
- ❏ Abducent nucleus is under general somatic efferent (GSE) neural column, which controls skeletal muscles, like lateral rectus.

4. c. Sympathetic cholinergic system > b. Sympathetic adrenergic system
- ❏ Sweat glands are two types: Eccrine and apocrine.
- ❏ Eccrine sweat glands are more common in occurrence and are supplied by sympathetic cholinergic fibers.
- ❏ Apocrine sweat glands (less common in occurrence) are supplied by adrenergic sympathetic fibers.

5. c. Postganglionic sympathetic fibers from cervical sympathetic chain
- ❏ Dilator pupillae is supplied by sympathetic fibers, which arise from the inter medio lateral horn of spinal cord segment T-1.
- ❏ These pre-ganglionic T-1 sympathetic fibers climb up the cervical sympathetic chain and synapse in the superior (highest) cervical ganglion.
- ❏ Post-ganglionic fibers make sympathetic plexus around the internal carotid artery and reach the dilator pupillae muscle.

6. c. Kidney
- ❏ Vagus nerve supplies till the kidney level. Pelvic viscera like urinary bladder and uterus are supplied by nervi erigentes.
- ❏ Splenic flexure of colon belongs to hind gut, supplied by nervi erigentes.

7. d. Apparent exophthalmos
- ❏ Horner syndrome presents with enophthalmos (and not exophthalmos).
- ❏ This is due to paralysis of **ciliaris** muscle which normally protrude the eyeball out of the socket. It's paralysis leads to eyeball staying back in the orbit, giving the appearance of **sunken eyeball** (enophthalmos).
- ❏ **Heterochromia iridis** may be present if the lesion occurred in a child younger than 2 years (congenital Horner syndrome).

8. a. Miosis; b. Vasodilation in ipsilateral arm
- ❏ Stellate ganglion lesions damage T1 sympathetic fibers and presents with the symptomology like Horner's syndrome.
- ❏ Miosis due to paralysis of dilator pupillae (and unopposed action of sphincter pupillae); Enophthalmos due to the paralysis of ciliaris muscle; loss of sympathetic vasoconstrictive tone resulting in dilated vessels- conjunctival redness, nasal congestion, vasodilatation in arm.

9. c. Carries pre-ganglionic fibers
- ❏ Each spinal nerve receives a branch called a **gray ramus communicans** from the adjacent paravertebral ganglion of the sympathetic trunk.
- ❏ The gray rami communicantes contain postganglionic **(not preganglionic)** nerve fibers of the sympathetic nervous system and are composed of largely unmyelinated (hence the name gray) neurons.
- ❏ It lies **medial** to white rami communicans, which also is connected to spinal nerve.

- ▪ Intraocular muscle supplied by Edinger-Westphal nucleus is Ciliary muscle *(NEET Pattern 2014)*
- ▪ Synaptic transmission in autonomic ganglia is Cholinergic.
  - – Synaptic transmission in autonomic ganglia (sympathetic and para-sympathetic) is cholinergic.
- ▪ Preganglionic parasympathetic neurons are located in brainstem and sacral spinal cord.
- ▪ Nerve carrying parasympathetic fibers are Cranial nerves 3, 7, 9, 10 and sacral nerves S2-4 *(AIIMS 2016)*
- ▪ Exophthalmos is NOT a sign of stellate ganglion block *(AIPG 2006)*
- ▪ Superior salivary nucleus controls Lacrimal, Palatine, Sublingual salivary glands.
- ▪ Pancoast tumor (superior pulmonary sulcus tumor) is a malignant neoplasm of the lung apex which may cause a lower trunk brachial plexopathy (which causes severe pain radiating toward the shoulder and along the medial aspect of the arm and atrophy of the muscles of the forearm and hand) and a lesion of cervical sympathetic chain ganglia with Horner syndrome (ptosis, enophthalmos, miosis, anhidrosis, and vasodilation).

▛ Enteric Nervous System

❏ Several peripheral **autonomic ganglia** contain neurons **derived from the neural crest** during embryonic development that are anatomically distinct from classical sympathetic and parasympathetic neurons.

❑ Enteric nervous system consists of neurons and enteric glial cells grouped into ganglionated plexuses lying in the wall of the gastrointestinal tract to form **myenteric** and **submucous** plexuses that extend from the esophagus to the anal sphincter.

❑ This intrinsic circuitry mediates numerous **reflex functions** including the **contractions** of the muscular coats of the gastrointestinal tract, **secretion** of gastric acid, intestinal transport of water and electrolytes, and the **regulation** of mucosal blood flow.

❑ Although complex interactions occur between the enteric and sympathetic and parasympathetic nervous systems, the enteric nervous system is capable of sustaining local reflex activity independent of the CNS and keeps working despite denervation of sympathetic and parasympathetic fibers.

❑ **Peristalsis** wave in ureter is generated in smooth muscle cells of the minor calyces (**pacemaker**). The sympathetic and parasympathetic nerves are not essential for the initiation and propagation of ureteric contraction waves, they are just **modulatory** in function.

▶ Arterial Supply

Brain is supplied by **two arterial systems**: Carotid and vertebrobasilar. Major arteries supplying the brain are given in Table.

Table 18: Arterial blood supply of cerebral hemispheres		
Artery	**Origin**	**Distribution**
Internal carotid:	Common carotid artery at superior border of thyroid cartilage	Gives branches to walls of cavernous sinus, pituitary gland, and trigeminal ganglion; provides primary supply to brain
Anterior cerebral	Internal carotid artery	Cerebral hemispheres, except for occipital lobes
Anterior communicating	Anterior cerebral artery	Cerebral arterial circle (of Willis)
Middle cerebral	Continuation of internal carotid artery distal to anterior cerebral artery	Most of lateral surface of cerebral hemispheres
Vertebral:	Subclavian artery	Cranial meninges and cerebellum
Basilar	Formed by union of vertebral arteries	Brainstem, cerebellum, and cerebrum
Posterior cerebral	Terminal branch of basilar artery	Inferior aspect of cerebral hemisphere and occipital lobe
Posterior communicating	Posterior cerebral artery	Optic tract, cerebral peduncle, internal capsule, and thalamus

Internal Carotid Artery is a branch of common carotid artery and enters the **carotid canal** in the petrous part of the temporal bone.

❑ It is separated from the tympanic cavity by a thin bony structure, lies within the cavernous sinus and gives branches to the pituitary (hypophysis) and trigeminal (semilunar) ganglion.

❑ Next it pierces the dural roof of the cavernous sinus between the anterior clinoid process and the middle clinoid process, which is a small projection posterolateral to the tuberculum sellae.

❑ The artery forms a carotid siphon (a bent tube with two arms of unequal length), which is the petrosal part just before it enters the cranial cavity.

❑ The four parts of internal carotid artery in its course and their branches are shown in the following table and Figure.

Part	Branches
Cervical	No branches
Petrous	Caroticotympanic Pterygoid
Cavernous	Cavernous Superior and inferior hypophyseal
Cerebral	Anterior cerebral Middle cerebral Ophthalmic Anterior choroidal Posterior communicating Mnemonic: AM-OCP

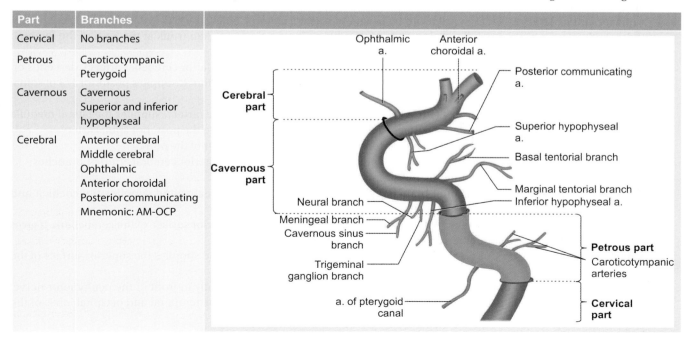

Five branches given in the cerebral part (AM-OCP): **Anterior Cerebral, Middle Cerebral, Ophthalmic, Choroidal and Posterior communicating arteries.**

- ❑ **Anterior Cerebral Artery** enters the longitudinal fissure of the cerebrum, supplies the optic chiasma and medial surface of the frontal and parietal lobes of the brain.
  - ➢ It is the major artery on the medial surface of cerebrum.
  - ➢ It supplies the lower body representation on the brain homunculus.
  - ➢ An occlusion/hemorrhage in the artery presents with sensory motor disturbances in lower limb and pelvis perineum area.
- ❑ **Middle Cerebral Artery** passes laterally in the lateral cerebral fissure and supplies the lateral convexity of the cerebral hemisphere.
  - ➢ It is the major artery on the supero lateral surface of cerebrum.
  - ➢ It supplies the upper body representation on the brain homunculus.
- ❑ **Ophthalmic Artery** enters the orbit via the optic canal with the optic nerve and supplies the eyeball and structures in the orbit and forehead.
  - ➢ Its occlusion results in monocular blindness.
- ❑ **Posterior Communicating Artery** arises from the carotid siphon and joins the posterior cerebral artery.
  - ➢ It connects the anterior circulation of the circle of Willis with the posterior circulation.
  - ➢ It runs backward below the optic tract and supplies the optic chiasma and tract and hypothalamus.
  - ➢ It is the second most common site of an aneurysm, which, if ruptured, will result in a subarachnoid hemorrhage and oculomotor nerve (CN III) paralysis.
- ❑ **Anterior Choroidal Artery** supplies the choroid plexus of the lateral ventricles, optic tract and radiations, lateral geniculate body and the posterior limb of internal capsule.
- ❑ **Circle of Willis** lies at the base of the brain, in the **interpeduncular fossa** (in sub-arachnoid space).
- ❑ It serves as a channel of collateral circulation in the events of arterial occlusions and is formed by the nine arteries:
  - ➢ Anteriorly: Anterior communicating artery
  - ➢ Anterolaterally: Paired anterior cerebral artery
  - ➢ Laterally: Proximal segments of both internal carotid arteries
  - ➢ Postero laterally: Paired posterior communicating arteries
  - ➢ Posteriorly: Proximal segments of both posterior cerebral arteries

Cerebral hemispheres are supplied by three cerebral arteries : anterior cerebral artery is a chief artery on medial surface, middle cerebral artery on superolateral surface and posterior cerebral artery on the inferior surface.

Vertebral Artery arise from the first part of the subclavian artery and ascend through the foramen transversium of upper six cervical vertebra (C1 to C6).

- ❑ Next it curve posteriorly winds around the superior articular process of the atlas, pierce the dura mater into the vertebral canal, and then enter the cranial cavity through the foramen magnum.
- ❑ The two vertebral arteries join to form the basilar artery.
- ❑ Branches:
  - ➢ **Anterior Spinal Artery** arises as two roots from the vertebral arteries shortly before the junction of the vertebral arteries. It descends in front of the medulla, and the two roots unite to form a single median trunk at the level of the foramen magnum. It supplies medial medulla and anterior 2/3 of spinal cord.
  - ➢ **Posterior Spinal Artery** is a branch given by vertebral artery (or the posterior inferior cerebellar artery), descends on the side of the medulla, and the right and left roots unite at the lower cervical region. It supplies posterior 1/3 of spinal cord.
  - ➢ **Posterior Inferior Cerebellar Artery (PICA)** is the largest branch of the vertebral artery, supplies the lateral medulla and distributes to the posterior–inferior surface of the cerebellum, and gives rise to the posterior spinal artery.

Basilar Artery is formed by the union of the two vertebral arteries at the lower border of the pons.

- ❑ It terminates near the upper border of the pons by dividing into the right and left posterior cerebral arteries. Branches:
  - ➢ **Pontine Arteries** are multiple in number and supply the pons.
  - ➢ **Labyrinthine Artery** is an occasional branch, enters the internal auditory meatus and supplies the cochlea and vestibular apparatus.
  - ➢ **Anterior Inferior Cerebellar Artery (AICA)** supplies the anterior part of the inferior surface of the cerebellum. It gives the labyrinthine artery in 85% of the population.
  - ➢ **Superior Cerebellar Artery** passes laterally just behind the oculomotor nerve and supplies the superior surface of the cerebellum.
  - ➢ Basilar artery bifurcates into two **Posterior Cerebral Arteries** which pass laterally in front of the oculomotor nerve, wind around the cerebral peduncle, and supplies the midbrain, thalamus and the temporal and occipital lobes of the cerebrum, with visual cortex.

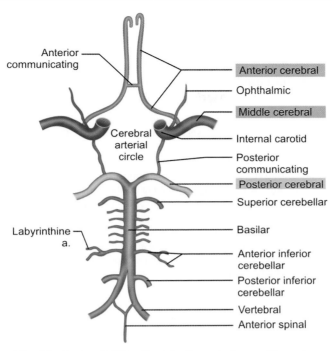

Fig. 89: Circle of Willis: Contributing arteries and branches

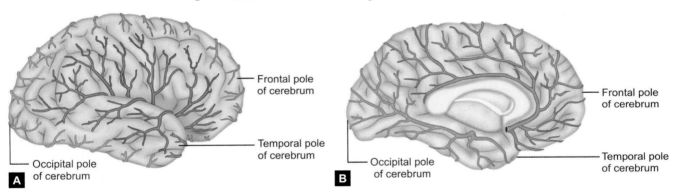

Figs. 90A and B: (A) Right lateral view of right hemisphere, (B) medial view of left hemisphere.
(Blue: Middle cerebral artery; Green: Anterior cerebral artery; Orange: Posterior cerebral artery)

Brief overview of arterial supply to various parts of brain:

❑ Cerebrum
  ➢ Cerebral hemispheres are supplied by three cerebral arteries : anterior cerebral artery is a chief artery on medial surface, middle cerebral artery on superolateral surface and posterior cerebral artery on the inferior surface.

❑ Basal ganglia
  ➢ The components are supplied by the striate (medial and lateral) arteries, which are branches from the roots of the anterior and middle cerebral arteries.
  ➢ The posteroinferior part of the lentiform complex is supplied by the thalamostriate branches of the posterior cerebral artery.
  ➢ Additional contributions are from anterior choroidal artery (branch of internal carotid artery).

❑ **Thalamus**
  ➢ Branches of the posterior communicating, posterior cerebral and basilar arteries.
  ➢ Some authors mention anterior choroidal artery as well.

❑ **Medulla oblongata**
  ➢ Branches of the vertebral, anterior and posterior spinal, posterior inferior cerebellar and basilar arteries.

❑ Pons
  ➢ Branches of basilar artery and the anterior inferior and superior cerebellar arteries.

❑ Mid brain
  ➢ Branches of posterior cerebral, superior cerebellar and basilar arteries

☐ Cerebellum
  ➢ Branches of posterior inferior, anterior inferior and superior cerebellar arteries.
☐ Choroid plexus
  ➢ In third and lateral ventricles is supplied by branches of the internal carotid and posterior cerebral arteries
  ➢ In fourth ventricle is supplied by the posterior inferior cerebellar arteries

CLINICAL CORRELATIONS

▪ **Berry aneurysms** are balloon (sac) like dilatations in the vessel wall and are common in the circle of Willis (at the base of the brain). These might rupture sometime and lead to subarachnoid hemorrhage.
▪ The most common sites for aneurysms include the anterior cerebral artery and anterior communicating artery (30–35%), the bifurcation, division of two branches, of the internal carotid and posterior communicating artery (20–25%), the bifurcation of the middle cerebral artery (20%), the bifurcation of the basilar artery, and the remaining posterior circulation arteries.
  – **Anterior communicating artery** is a short vessel connecting the two anterior cerebral arteries.
  – It is the most common site of an aneurysm (e.g., congenital berry aneurysm), which, if ruptured, will result in a subarachnoid hemorrhage and bitemporal lower quadrantanopia due to compression of optic chiasma.
  – **Posterior communicating artery** is the second most common site of an aneurysm (e.g., congenital berry aneurysm), which, if ruptured, will result in a subarachnoid hemorrhage and possibly oculomotor nerve (down and out eye with, fixed dilated pupil and ptosis).
▪ Aneurysms on the posterior communicating artery, superior cerebellar artery, or the tip of the basilar artery, can cause **oculomotor nerve** palsy by compression. Aneurysms on the internal carotid artery near its termination may compress the lateral aspect of the optic chiasma, and compromise axons derived from the temporal side of the ipsilateral retina, which causes a defect in the nasal visual field.

Cause	Abducens nerve (%) (n = 1918)	Trochlear nerve (%) (n = 578)	Oculomotor nerve (%) (n = 1130)
Undetermined	26	32	23
Neoplasm	22	5	12
Head trauma	15	29	14
Aneurysm	3	1	16
Vascular	13	18	20
Other	21	15	15

  – **Posterior cerebral artery** occlusion results in contralateral sensory loss of all modalities with concomitant severe pain (i.e., thalamic syndrome) due to damage to the thalamus and contralateral homonymous hemianopia with macular sparing.
  – **Middle cerebral artery** occlusion of leads to the following signs and symptoms:
▪ Contralateral paralysis and contralateral anesthesia of the face, neck, trunk and arm region along with and sensory impairment over the same area.
▪ Homonymous hemianopia and aphasia if the dominant hemisphere is involved.
  Lenticulostriate arteries (branches of middle cerebral artery) supply the basal ganglia and the internal capsule.
▪ Occlusion results in contralateral hemiplegia due to destruction of descending motor fibers in the posterior limb of the internal capsule
▪ Contralateral hemi-anesthesia due to lesion of ascending sensory thalamocortical fibers in the internal capsule.

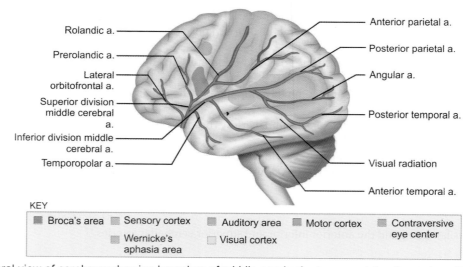

KEY
■ Broca's area   ■ Sensory cortex   ■ Auditory area   ■ Motor cortex   ■ Contraversive eye center
■ Wernicke's aphasia area   ☐ Visual cortex

Fig. 91: Lateral view of cerebrum showing branches of middle cerebral artery supplying the various Brodmann areas

1. **Primary motor area (Area no. 4) of brain is supplied by:**
   a. Anterior cerebral artery
   b. Middle cerebral artery
   c. Anterior and middle cerebral artery
   d. Anterior and posterior cerebral artery

2. **Which of the following is NOT a branch of the cavernous segment of internal carotid artery?** *(AIPG 2007; AIIMS 2008)*
   a. Inferior hypophyseal artery
   b. Branches to cavernous sinus
   c. Ophthalmic artery
   d. Meningeal artery

3. **Branch(es) of Internal carotid artery directly arising from it**
   a. Posterior cerebral artery *(PGIC 2016)*
   b. Posterior communicating artery
   c. Superior hypophyseal artery
   d. Inferior hypophyseal artery
   e. Recurrent artery of Heubner

4. **NOT affected in posterior cerebral artery infarct is:**
   a. Pons
   b. Midbrain
   c. Thalamus
   d. Striate cortex

5. **A block in the posterior cerebral artery supplying occipital lobe results in:**
   a. Ipsilateral homonymous hemianopia
   b. Contralateral homonymous hemianopia
   c. Ipsilateral homonymous hemianopia with macular sparing
   d. Contralateral homonymous hemianopia with macular sparing

6. **Most common site of berry aneurysm:**
   a. Internal carotid bifurcation
   b. Anterior cerebral circulation
   c. Middle cerebral circulation
   d. Anterior choroidal circulation

7. **Most commonly lesioned nerve in intracranial aneurysms is:**
   a. Optic *(AIPG 2007)*
   b. Oculomotor
   c. Trochlear
   d. Abducent

8. **Berry aneurysm of the posterior communicating artery causes compression of:** *(AIIMS 2008)*
   a. Optic nerve
   b. Oculomotor nerve
   c. Trochlear nerve
   d. Hypophysis cerebri

9. **All is true about branches of internal carotid artery EXCEPT:**
   a. Anterior choroidal artery is given in cerebral part
   b. Ophthalmic artery is given in cerebral part
   c. Posterior communicating artery is given in petrous part
   d. Caroticotympanic artery is given in petrous part

10. **Visual area of cortex is supplied by:** *(PGIC 2008)*
    a. Anterior cerebral artery
    b. Middle cerebral artery
    c. Posterior cerebral artery
    d. Posterior inferior cerebellar artery
    e. Posterior choroidal artery

11. **All of the following arteries supply medulla EXCEPT:**
    a. Anterior spinal artery
    b. Anterior inferior cerebellar artery
    c. Superior cerebellar
    d. Basilar

12. **Circle of Willis does not get contribution from:**
    a. Anterior cerebral artery
    b. Middle cerebral artery
    c. Posterior communicating artery
    d. Posterior cerebral artery

13. **Charcot's artery is** *(NEET Pattern 2016)*
    a. Medial striate branch of anterior cerebral artery
    b. Fronto parietal artery
    c. Striate branch of middle cerebral artery
    d. Calloso marginal artery

14. **Arterial supply to putamen includes all EXCEPT**
    a. Medial striate arteries *(NEET Pattern 2015)*
    b. Lateral striate arteries
    c. Anterior choroidal artery
    d. Posterior communicating artery

15. **Identify the marked artery in the diagram:** *(AIIMS 2016)*
    a. Anterior communicating artery
    b. Posterior communicating artery
    c. Superior cerebellar artery
    d. Anterior inferior cerebellar artery

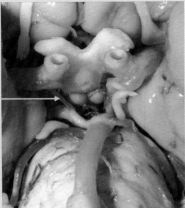

1. c. Anterior and middle cerebral artery
- ❏ Greater part of the lateral surface receives supply from middle cerebral artery, whereas medial surface of cerebrum is majorly supplied by anterior cerebral artery.
- ❏ The upper limb and head are represented on the lateral surface of the cortex in homunculus, whereas pelvis and lower limb are on the medial surface of the hemispheres.
- ❏ Therefore, the motor and sensory functions of the lower limb are supplied by the anterior cerebral artery while the motor and sensory functions of the upper limb and head are supplied by the middle cerebral artery.

◼ Anterior cerebral a.   ▭ Middle cerebral a.   ▨ Posterior cerebral a.

2. c. Ophthalmic branch
- ❏ Internal carotid artery gives ophthalmic branch in its cerebral part (**not** in cavernous segment).
- ❏ Cavernous branches supply the trigeminal ganglion, the walls of cavernous sinus and the nerves contained in it.
- ❏ The hypophyseal branches form pituitary portal system and meningeal branch supplies the bone and duramater of anterior cranial fossa.

3. b. Posterior communicating artery; c. Superior hypophyseal artery; d. Inferior hypophyseal artery
- ❏ Internal carotid artery gives ophthalmic branch in its cerebral part (**not** in cavernous segment).
- ❏ Cavernous branches supply the trigeminal ganglion, the walls of cavernous sinus and the nerves contained in it.
- ❏ The hypophyseal branches form pituitary portal system and meningeal branch supplies the bone and duramater of anterior cranial fossa.

4. b. Pons
- ❏ Posterior cerebral artery gives branches to only the midbrain part of brainstem (not pons or medulla oblongata).
- ❏ Pons are supplied by branches of basilar artery.
- ❏ Midbrain is supplied by branches of posterior cerebral artery and basilar artery.
- ❏ Thalamus is supplied by numerous arteries including posterior cerebral artery and posterior communicating artery.
- ❏ Posterior cerebral artery supplies the posterior cerebrum, including the occipital visual (striate) cortex.

5. d. Contralateral homonymous hemianopia with macular sparing
- ❏ Posterior cerebral artery supplies occipital visual (striate) cortex, and a block results in loss of visual field on the opposite side—contralateral homonymous hemianopia.
- ❏ Left half of each eye is blind in right posterior cerebral artery infarct.
- ❏ There is associated macular sparing, since the macular area on brain is additionally supplied by branch of middle cerebral artery.

6. b. Anterior cerebral circulation
- ❏ Berry aneurysms are more common at the site where anterior communicating artery is given by anterior cerebral artery (~30%)
- ❏ The incidence is ~25% at the origin of posterior communicating artery (from internal carotid artery).
- ❏ Bifurcation of middle cerebral artery presents with an incidence of ~20 %.

7. b. Oculomotor
- ❏ Intracranial aneurysms may involve oculomotor, abducent and optic nerve in descending order.
- ❏ Trochlear nerve is involvement is highest in head trauma.

8. b. Oculomotor nerve
- ❏ Berry aneurysm in the vicinity of posterior communicating artery can compress the third cranial nerve and cause oculomotor nerve palsy.
- ❏ Aneurysms of superior cerebellar artery or tip of the basilar artery can also compress the oculomotor nerve and produce its palsy.
- ❏ Berry aneurysm on the internal carotid artery (near its termination) compresses the lateral aspect of optic chiasma and hence damages the visual information from the ipsilateral nasal visual field.

9. c. Posterior communicating artery is given in petrous part:
- ❏ Posterior communicating artery is given in **cerebral part** of internal carotid artery.

10. b. Middle cerebral artery; c. Posterior cerebral artery
- ❏ The major artery to supply occipital visual cortex is posterior cerebral artery.
- ❏ An additional branch to the macular area on the brain is given by the middle cerebral artery.

ANSWERS

11. c. Superior cerebellar
- Medulla oblongata is supplied by numerous arteries (but **not** superior cerebellar).
- The arteries supplying medulla are: Vertebral, anterior spinal, posterior spinal, posterior inferior cerebellar, anterior inferior cerebellar, basilar etc.

12. b. Middle cerebral artery
- Circle of Willis is contributed by paired posterior cerebral arteries, posterior communicating arteries, internal carotid arteries, anterior cerebral arteries and one anterior communicating artery.

13. c. Striate branch of middle cerebral artery
- Charcot's artery is the lenticulostriate branch of the middle cerebral artery.
- Charcot–Bouchard aneurysms are located in the lenticulostriate vessels of the basal ganglia and are associated with chronic hypertension (common cause of cerebral hemorrhage.)

14. d. Posterior communicating artery
- Basal ganglia components (including putamen) are supplied by the striate (medial and lateral) arteries, which are branches from the roots of the anterior and middle cerebral arteries.
- The posteroinferior part of the lentiform complex is supplied by the thalamostriate branches of the posterior cerebral artery.
- Additional contributions are from anterior choroidal artery (branch of internal carotid artery).

15. b. Posterior communicating artery
- The marked artery is posterior communicating artery, branch of internal carotid artery, anastomosing with posterior cerebral artery, contributing to circle of Willis.
- This is inferior view of brain, showing the circle of Willis in the interpeduncular fossa at the base of the brain.

- Vertebral arteries of both sides unite to form Basilar artery *(NEET Pattern 2015)*
- Branches of basilar artery: Paramedian, Anterior inferior cerebellar artery, Labyrinthine artery, Superior cerebellar artery, Posterior cerebral artery *(PGIC 2002)*
- Major supply of medial surface of cerebral hemisphere is Anterior cerebral artery *(NEET Pattern 2012)*
- Chief artery of lateral surface of cerebral hemisphere is Middle cerebral artery *(NEET Pattern 2013)*
- Posterior communicating artery is a branch of Internal carotid artery.
- Posterior communicating artery connects Posterior cerebral artery with internal carotid artery *(NEET Pattern 2015)*
- Medulla oblongata is supplied by the branches of vertebral, anterior spinal and posterior spinal, posterior inferior cerebellar and basilar arteries.
- Labyrinthine artery is a branch of anterior inferior cerebellar artery, passes through internal auditory meatus (along with facial and vestibulo-cochlear nerve) and supply the inner ear.
- Occasionally labyrinthine artery is a direct branch of basilar artery.
- Branches of the vertebral artery are: Anterior spinal, Posterior spinal and Posterior inferior cerebellar artery.
- Anterior inferior cerebellar artery is a branch of basilar artery.

▼ Reflexes

Reflex	Afferent limb	Efferent limb
Corneal reflex	Ophthalmic nerve	Facial nerve
Conjunctival reflex	Ophthalmic nerve	Facial nerve
Lacrimation (tearing) reflex	Ophthalmic nerve	Facial nerve
Oculocardiac reflex	Ophthalmic nerve	Vagus nerve
Gag reflex	Glossopharyngeal nerve	Vagus nerve
Carotid sinus reflex	Glossopharyngeal nerve	Vagus nerve
Sneezing reflex	Ophthalmic/maxillary nerve	Vagus nerve
Jaw-jerk (masseteric) reflexes*	Mandibular nerve	Mandibular nerve
Papillary reflexes –Light reflex –Accommodation reflex		

*Jaw-jerk reflex is the only monosynptic reflexmediated by the cranial nerves.

Ankle jerk – Spinal segment **S-1**; Nerve: Tibial; Muscle: Gastrocnemius.

Knee jerk – Spinal segment **L- 2, 3, 4**; Nerve: Femoral; Muscle: Quadriceps.

Biceps jerk – Spinal segment **C-5, 6**; Nerve: Musculocutaneous; Muscle: Biceps.

Supinator reflex – Spinal segment **C-5, 6**; Nerve: Radial; Muscle: Brachioradialis.

Triceps reflex – Spinal segment **C-7, 8**; Nerve: Radial; Muscle: Triceps.

Memory aid: S-**1**; L-**2, 3, 4**; C-**5, 6**; C-**7, 8**.

Miscellaneous

1. **All are pain sensitive area of brain EXCEPT:** *(AIPG 2009)*
   a. Dural sheath surrounding vascular sinuses
   b. Middle meningeal artery
   c. Falx cerebri
   d. Choroid plexus

2. **Which structure is just lateral to anterior perforated substance?** *(AIPG 2009)*
   a. Uncus
   b. Limen insulae
   c. 3rd Ventricle
   d. Optic chiasma

1. **d. Choroid plexus**
   ❑ Choroid plexus is not a pain producing structure. Much of the brain parenchyma, Ventricular ependyma, pial veins and choroid plexus are not pain-producing structures.
   ❑ Few cranial structures are pain producing: The scalp, middle meningeal artery, dural sinuses, falx cerebri and proximal segments of large pial arteries.
   ❑ The structures involved in headache are few and the large intracranial vessels and dura mater innervated by the trigeminal nerve.

2. **b. Limen insulae**
   ❑ Limen insulae lies in the lateral relation of anterior perforated substance.
   ❑ It represents the level at the which the middle cerebral artery typically bifurcates/trifurcates.
   ❑ It is the **starting point of the insular cortex**. The limen insulae translates as the threshold to the insula and is the point at which the insular cortex is continuous with cortex over the amygdala and superior temporal gyrus.

Head and Neck

Landmarks and levels

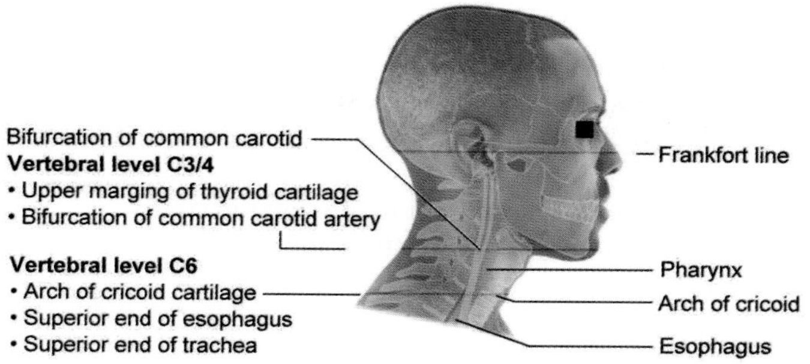

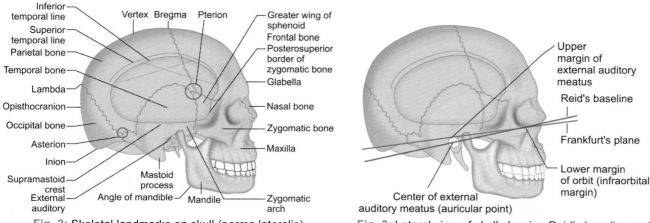

Bifurcation of common carotid
Vertebral level C3/4
• Upper marging of thyroid cartilage
• Bifurcation of common carotid artery

Vertebral level C6
• Arch of cricoid cartilage
• Superior end of esophagus
• Superior end of trachea

— Frankfort line

— Pharynx
— Arch of cricoid
— Esophagus

Fig. 1: Lateral view of head and neck to show structures at the C3/C4 and C6 vertebral levels

Vertebral level	Structures
C3	Level of greater cornu of hyoid bone
C3- C4 junction	Level of upper border (and notch) of thyroid cartilage and bifurcation of common carotid artery
C4-C5 Junction	Level of thyroid cartilage
C6	Level of cricoid cartilage

- **Upper border** of thyroid cartilage lies at C3-4 vertebral level. Common carotid artery **bifurcates** into two branches at this level (*NEET Pattern 2012*); (*AIIMS 2007*)
- **Cricoid cartilage** of larynx lies at the **C6 vertebra** level, which marks the **termination** of larynx and pharynx and **beginning** of trachea and oesophagus (*NEET Pattern 2012*)
- **Hyoid bone** is located at the level of C3 vertebra (*NEET Pattern 2013*)
- **Sylvian point** practically corresponds to the **pterion**, which is an H-shape suture, contributed by **four bones**, including the squamous part of temporal bone (*NEET Pattern 2015*)
- **Reid's base line** extends from infraorbital margin to center of external acoustic meatus (*NEET Pattern 2014*)
- The **anterior division** of the middle meningeal artery runs underneath the **pterion** (*NEET Pattern 2016*)

Inferior temporal line
Superior temporal line
Parietal bone
Temporal bone
Lambda
Opisthocranion
Occipital bone
Asterion
Inion
Supramastoid crest
External auditory

Vertex Bregma Pterion

Mastoid process
Angle of mandible Mandile

Greater wing of sphenoid
Frontal bone
Posterosuperior border of zygomatic bone
Glabella
Nasal bone
Zygomatic bone
Maxilla

Zygomatic arch

Upper margin of external auditory meatus

Reid's baseline

Frankfurt's plane

Lower margin of orbit (infraorbital margin)

Center of external auditory meatus (auricular point)

Fig. 2: Skeletal landmarks on skull (norma lateralis)

Fig. 3: Lateral view of skull showing Reid's baseline and Frankfurt's plane

- ❑ **Reid's baseline** extends from infraorbital margin to center of external acoustic meatus.
- ❑ **Frankfort's** horizontal plane extends from infraorbital margin to superior margin of external meatus.
- ❑ The lateral (**Sylvian**) fissure of the brain aligns with the anterior part of squamosal suture in a zone 2.5–4.0 cm anterior to the external acoustic meatus.
- ❑ **Coronal suture** lies between the frontal bone and the two parietal bones. Sagittal Suture is present between the two parietal bones.
- ❑ **Squamous** (squamoparietal) **suture** lies between the parietal bone and the squamous part of the temporal bone.

- ❏ **Lambdoid** suture is present between the two parietal bones and the occipital bone *(NEET Pattern 2014)*
- ❏ **Pterion** represents the junction of the four bones: the frontal, parietal, and temporal bones and the great wing of the sphenoid bone.
  - ➢ The central point of pterion is known as Sylvian point, the cranium is very thin at this point. Its immediate deep relations are **fontal branch of middle meningeal artery**, its accompanying vein and **stem of lateral sulcus of brain**.
  - ➢ Fracture at this point may injure middle meningeal artery and give rise to **extradural hemorrhage**.
  - ➢ Pterion helps in the positioning of **burr-holes** to evacuate extradural hematomas.

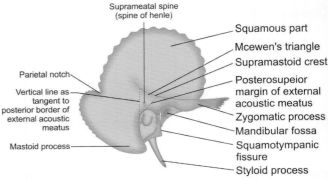

Fig. 4: Right temporal bone: External aspect

- ❏ Suprameatal triangle of McEwen is a small depression posterosuperior to the external auditory meatus on **squamous** part of the temporal bone.
- ❏ It is bounded
  - ➢ Superiorly by **supramastoid crest**, which is level with the floor of the middle cranial fossa
  - ➢ Anteroinferiorly, which forms the **posterosuperior margin of the external acoustic meatus**, indicates approximately the position of the descending part of the facial nerve canal.
  - ➢ Posteriorly by **a vertical tangent to the posterior margin of the meatus**, is anterior to the sigmoid sinus.
- ❏ The lateral wall of mastoid antrum corresponds to the **suprameatal triangle of McEwen** on the outer surface of the skull, palpable through the cymba conchae.
  - ➢ A small bony projection - suprameatal spine of Henle may be present in the anteroinferior part of this triangle.
  - ➢ It is an important landmark when performing a cortical mastoidectomy.
  - ➢ The **mastoid antrum** lies 1.25 cm deep to this triangle. The lateral wall of mastoid antrum is only 2 mm thick **at birth** but increases at an average rate of 1 mm a year, attaining a **final thickness of 12–15 mm**.
    - ▪ The adult capacity of the mastoid antrum is **1 mL**, with a general diameter of 10 mm.
    - ▪ Unlike the other air sinuses in the skull, it is present at birth, and **almost adult in size.**

▸ Embryology

- ❏ **Pharyngeal apparatus** consists of the pharyngeal arches, pouches, grooves, and membranes.
- ❏ Pharyngeal (Branchial) arches are composed majorly of **secondary mesenchyme** (neural crest origin) and **partly** primary mesenchyme.
- ❏ The mesenchymal core is covered externally by **ectoderm** and internally by **endoderm**.
- ❏ Pharyngeal arches develop in the **lateral wall of the primitive pharynx** and later extend ventrally and fuse with their counterparts of the opposite side in floor of the primitive pharynx to form **horseshoe-shaped cylindrical bars**.
- ❏ Initially there are six arches, but **fifth arch is rudimentary**.

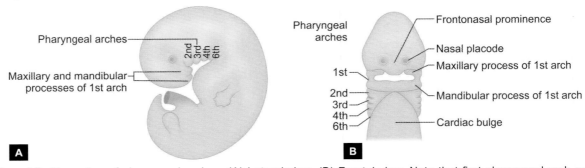

Figs. 5A and B: Formation of pharyngeal arches. (A) Lateral view. (B) Frontal view. Note that first pharyngeal arch consists of maxillary and mandibular processes

Table 1: Derivatives of the pharyngeal arches						
Arch No.	Nerve	Embryonic cartilage	NCCs/Mesoderm	Mesoderm (Muscles)	Misc	Artery
1.	CNV$_3$	Quadrate/ Meckel's	Maxilla Mandible (GT) Incus Malleus Anterior ligament of malleus Sphenomandibular ligament	Tensor tympani Tensor veli palatini Muscles of mastication Mylohyoid Anterior belly digastric	Anterior 2/3 of tongue	Maxillary (transitory)

Arch No.	Nerve	Embryonic cartilage	NCCs/Mesoderm	Mesoderm (Muscles)	Misc	Artery
2.	CN VII	Reichert's	Stapes Styloid process Stylohyoid ligament Lesser horn and upper part of body of hyoid bone	Stapedius Stylohyoid Facial muscles (incl. Buccinatory/Platysma, auricular, occipitofrontalis) Posterior belly digastric		Stapedial/Hyoid artery (transitory)
3.	CN IX		Greater horn and lower part of body of hyoid	Stylopharyngeus	Posterior 1/3 of tongue	Common caroitd artery Internal carotid artery (first part)
4.	CN X Pharyngeal branch superior laryngeal branch		NCSs: none Thyroid Cartilage Epiglottis	Palate (Levator, etc.) Pharynx Cricothyroid	Root of tongue	Right subclavian artery (proximal part) Arch of aorta (between origins of left common carotid and left subclavian arteries)
6	CN X Recurrent laryngeal branch		NCCs: none Cricoid Arytenoid cartilages	Larynx		Pulmonary arteries D arteriosus

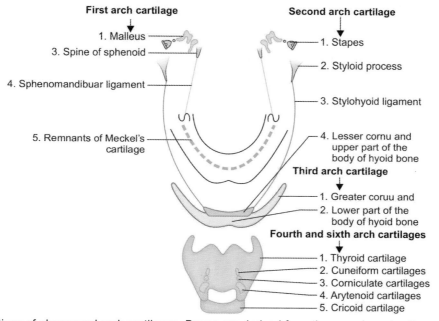

First arch cartilage
→
1. Malleus
3. Spine of sphenoid
4. Sphenomandibuar ligament
5. Remnants of Meckel's cartilage

Second arch cartilage
→
1. Stapes
2. Styloid process
3. Stylohyoid ligament
4. Lesser cornu and upper part of the body of hyoid bone

Third arch cartilage
→
1. Greater coruu and
2. Lower part of the body of hyoid bone

Fourth and sixth arch cartilages
→
1. Thyroid cartilage
2. Cuneiform cartilages
3. Corniculate cartilages
4. Arytenoid cartilages
5. Cricoid cartilage

Fig. 6: Skeletal derivatives of pharyngeal arch cartilages. Bones are derived from the neural crest cells and larynx cartilages are derived from lateral plate mesoderm

Pharyngeal Arch Muscles: Myoblasts from the pharyngeal arches, which originate from the unsegmented **paraxial mesoder** and prechordal plate form the muscles of mastication, facial expression, pharynx, and larynx.

❑ These muscles are innervated by pharyngeal arch nerves.

❑ Ocular Muscles: Extrinsic eye muscles are derived from mesenchymal cells near the prechordal plate. **Three preotic** myotomes, each supplied by its own nerve (cranial nerve Ill, IV and VI), form the extrinsic muscles of the eye.

❑ **Recurrent** laryngeal nerve (branch of vagus) is the nerve of **sixth** pharyngeal arch *(NEET Pattern 2013)*

❑ Both maxillary and mandibular processes develop in **first pharyngeal arch**. Frontonasal process is derived from the neural crest cells *(NEET Pattern 2015)*

❑ **Epiglottis** and upper part of thyroid cartilage develop in the **fourth** pharyngeal arch *(NEET Pattern 2013)*

❑ **Tensor tympani** muscle develops in the **first** pharyngeal arch and is hence, supplied by the **mandibular** branch of trigeminal nerve *(AIIMS 2010)*

❑ Most of the laryngeal muscles develop in sixth arch, with few **exceptions**. **Cricothyroid** muscle develops in fourth pharyngeal arch.

❑ Most of the pharyngeal muscles develop in fourth arch, with few **exceptions**. **Stylopharyngeus** muscle develops in third pharyngeal arch *(NEET Pattern 2015)*

QUESTIONS

1. Which of the following muscle is derivative of 1st arch:
(NEET Pattern 2015)

a. Stylopharyngeus
b. Tensor tympani
c. Platysma
d. Cricothyroid

2. WRONG match about the bone and cartilages in pharyngeal arches:

a. Meckel's cartilage: Mandible
b. Reichert's cartilage: Stapes
c. Second arch cartilage: Styloid process
d. Third arch: Lesser cornu of hyoid bone

3. Which of the following muscles develop from 6th pharyngeal arch:
(JIPMER 2017)

a. Cricothyroid
b. Thyrohyoid
c. Stylopharyngeus
d. Cricoarytenoid

4. Maxillary prominence develops in: *(JIPMER)*

a. 1st pharyngeal arch
b. 1st pharyngeal groove
c. 1st pharyngeal pouch
d. 1st pharyngeal membrane

ANSWERS

1. b. Tensor tympani
- ❑ Tensor tympani muscle develops in the first pharyngeal arch.
- ❑ Stylopharyngeus develops in 3rd arch, platysma in 2nd and cricothyroid in 4th arch, respectively.

2. d. Third arch: Lesser cornu of hyoid bone
- ❑ Third pharyngeal arch forms the lower body and greater (and not lesser) cornu of hyoid bone.

3. d. Cricoarytenoid
- ❑ Larynx muscles develop in 6th pharyngeal arch, cricoarytenoid is one among them.
- ❑ Cricothyroid is an exception in the sense that, despite being a larynx muscle it develops in fourth arch.

4. a. 1st pharyngeal arch
- ❑ Two prominences develop in 1st pharyngeal (mandibular) arch.
- ❑ Maxillary prominence, which forms maxilla, zygomatic bone, squamous part of temporal bone.
- ❑ Mandibular prominence, which has Meckel's cartilage and forms mandible.

▶ Pharyngeal Pouches and Clefts

Pouch	Adult derivatives
1.	Epithelium of middle ear cavity and Eustachian tube
2.	Epithelium of palatine tonsil crypts
3.	Thymus (ventral) Inferior parathyroid (dorsal)
4.	Superior parathyroid (dorsal) Ultimobranchial body (ventral) – Parafollicular C cells of thyroid

Groove	Adult derivatives
1	Epithelium of external auditory meatus
2–4	Obliterated

Membrane	Adult derivatives
1	Tympanic membrane
2–3	Obliterated

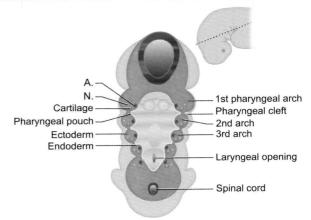

Fig. 7: Pharyngeal cleft, arch and pouches

❑ Cut section of pharyngeal arches. Each arch consists of a mesenchymal core derived from mesoderm and neural crest cells and each is lined internally by endoderm and externally by ectoderm. Each arch also contains an artery (one of the aortic arches) and a cranial nerve and each will contribute specific skeletal and muscular components to the head and neck. Between the arches are pouches on the inner surface and clefts externally.

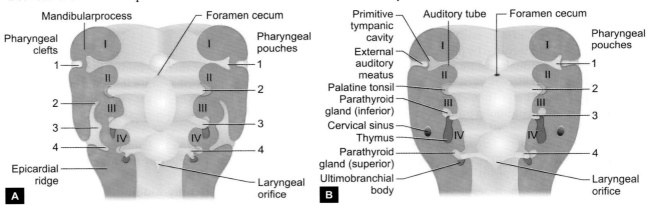

Figs. 8A and B: (A) Development of the pharyngeal clefts and pouches. The second arch grows over the third and fourth arches, burying the second, third, and fourth pharyngeal clefts. (B) Remnants of the second, third, and fourth pharyngeal clefts form the cervial sinus, which is normally obliterated

- ❑ Pharyngeal **pouches** are formed in the lateral wall of the pharynx and are lined by **endoderm**.
- ❑ Pharyngeal **clefts** (grooves) develop on the outer aspect and are lined by **ectoderm**.
- ❑ Pharyngeal **membranes** lie between the two.

Tonsil develops in the region of 2nd pharyngeal pouch.

- ❑ The endoderm of the second pouch proliferates and grows into the underlying secondary mesenchyme (neural crest cell derived).
- ❑ The central parts of these buds break down, forming tonsillar crypts (pit-like depressions).
- ❑ The pouch **endoderm** forms the **surface epithelium** and lining of the tonsillar crypts.
- ❑ At approximately 20 weeks, the mesenchyme around the crypts differentiates into lymphoid tissue, which soon organizes into the lymphatic nodules of the palatine tonsil.
- ❑ The **remnant** of 2nd pharyngeal pouch is seen as supratonsillar/**intratonsillar cleft**.

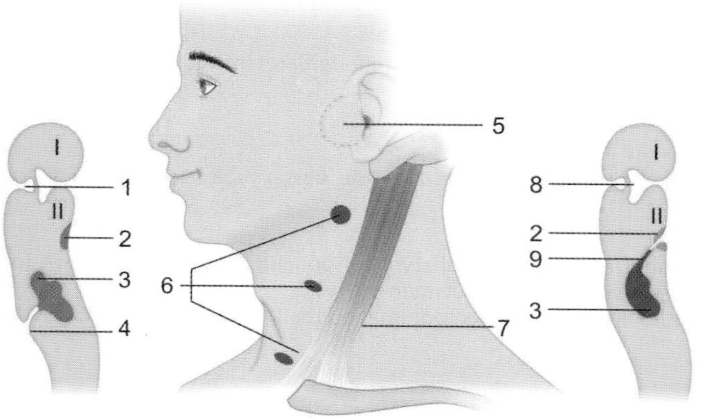

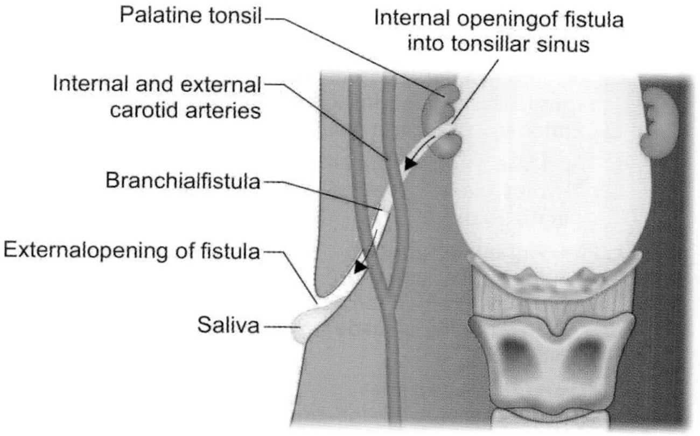

Fig. 9: 1. External auditory meatus; 2. Palatine tonsil; 3. Lateral cervical (branchial) cyst; 4. External branchial sinus; 5. Region of preauricular fistulae; 6. Region of lateral cervical cysts and fistulae; 7. Sternocleidomastoid muscle; 8. Tubotympanic recess; 9. Internal branchial sinus

The mesenchyme of second pharyngeal arch rapidly grows downward, overlaps the second, third, and fourth pharyngeal clefts (grooves), and fuses with the epicardial ridge.

- ❑ Thus, second, third, and fourth pharyngeal clefts get buried under the surface and form a slit-like cavity—the **cervical sinus** that is lined by ectoderm.
- ❑ The cervical sinus later disappears, if it fails to obliterate, it leads to the formation of **branchial cyst**.
- ❑ The branchial cyst is present at the **anterior border of the sternocleidomastoid** at the junction of its upper one-third and lower two-third, below and **behind the angle of mandible**.
- ❑ In some cases, branchial cyst may open externally on the surface of the neck forming **external branchial sinus**.
- ❑ Rarely the branchial cyst may communicate internally with tonsillar fossa, leading to **internal branchial sinus**.
- ❑ **Branchial fistula** may develop due to rupture of membrane between the second pharyngeal cleft and second pharyngeal pouch, which passes deep between the external and internal carotid arteries (carotid fork) and opens into the **tonsillar sinus**.
- ❑ **DiGeorge syndrome** presents with chromosome 22q11 deletion.
  - ➢ Neural crest cell migration is affected, and patients lack mature T cells (due to absence of thymus) *(JIPMER 2017)*
  - ➢ There is defective development of pharyngeal **pouch three** and four, leading to **thymic hypoplasia** and impaired function of T cell leading to **recurrent infections. Hypocalcaemic tetany/seizures** may be observed due to **(missing parathyroid gland).**
  - ➢ Other features observed is **mandibular hypoplasia**. Most common cause of death is cardiovascular defects.

QUESTIONS

1. **Which of these is CORRECT about the development of tonsil?**
   - a. Is a derivative of the first pharyngeal arch *(NEET Pattern 2012)*
   - b. Develops from the second pharyngeal pouch
   - c. Develops from the third pharyngeal pouch
   - d. Is a derivative of the neural crest cells

2. **Thymus develops from:**
   - a. Second pharyngeal pouch (ventral portion)
   - b. Third pharyngeal pouch (ventral portion)
   - c. Third pharyngeal pouch (dorsal portion)
   - d. Fourth pharyngeal pouch (ventral portion)

3. **During 4th week, endoderm and ectoderm approach each other in the head and neck region at:** *(AIIMS)*
   - a. Pharyngeal groove
   - b. Pharyngeal pouch
   - c. Pharyngeal membrane
   - d. Pharyngeal arch

4. **Which structure develops from all the 3 germ layers:**
   - a. Tympanic membrane
   - b. External acoustic meatus
   - c. Auditory tube
   - d. Middle ear

5. **TRUE statement regarding branchial anomalies:** *(AIIMS 2010)*
   - a. Most commonly second arch is involved
   - b. Cyst is more common than sinus
   - c. Sinus should always be excised
   - d. Cyst cause dysphagia and hoarseness

6. **A sinus is extending from the base of tongue to anterior border of sternomastoid, develop from which arch?**
   - a. I
   - b. II   *(JIPMER 2017)*
   - c. III
   - d. IV

7. A 5-year child presented with absence of thymus, hypoparathyroidism and thyroid hypoplasia. Identify the abnormality lies in which area?   (*AIIMS 2017*)
  a. A
  b. B
  c. C
  d. D

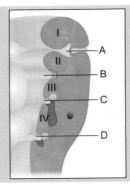

1. **d. Is a derivative of the neural crest cells > b. Develops from the second pharyngeal pouch**
  ❑ Neural crest derived (secondary) mesenchyme, in the region of second pharyngeal pouch differentiates into connective tissue of tonsil, which later is invaded by lymphocytes migrating from bone marrow and thymus.
  ❑ Endoderm of second pharyngeal pouch contributes to the tonsillar epithelium.

2. **b. Third pharyngeal pouch (ventral portion)**
  ❑ Thymus gland develops in the ventral portion of third pharyngeal pouch, whereas in the dorsal region develops inferior parathyroid.

3. **c. Pharyngeal membrane**
  ❑ During 4th week, at the lateral wall of primitive pharynx, inner endoderm (of pharyngeal pouch) and outer ectoderm (of pharyngeal cleft) approach each other and sandwich the pharyngeal membrane between the two.
  ❑ The membrane is made up of mesenchyme (connective tissue) lined by outer ectodermal epithelium and inner endodermal epithelium.

4. **a. Tympanic membrane**
  ❑ Tympanic membrane has an outer epithelial layer (ectodermal) and inner epithelial layer (endodermal) and sandwiched between the two is mesenchyme, forming the connective tissue.

5. **a. Most commonly second arch is involved**
  ❑ This is a **controversial QUESTIONS**, since all the statements can be proven correct. The most appropriate option has been chosen as the answer.
  ❑ Branchial arch anomalies are the most commonly associated with second arch, comprising more than 90% of the arch anomalies.
  ❑ Branchial cysts are more common than the branchial sinus statistically - nearly 74% of the branchial arch anomalies present as a branchial cyst (though in paediatric age group sinuses are more common than cysts).
  ❑ Branchial sinuses should always be excised (though some of the authors believe that excision should be done if they present with chronic inflammation, recurrent infections or have potential for malignant degeneration).
  ❑ Pressure symptoms like dysphagia and hoarseness are rarely seen with branchial cyst (though few cases have been documented in neonates).

6. **b. II**
  ❑ This is a case of second arch branchial fistula, with a cutaneous opening along the anterior border of the sternocleidomastoid, usually at the junction of the middle and lower thirds, and track up through the neck to run between the internal and external carotid arteries and end in the tonsillar fossa.

7. **c. C**
  ❑ This a variant of DiGeorge syndrome, presenting with absent thymus and parathyroid glands (with thyroid hypoplasia). It usually involves pharyngeal pouch 3 (Marker C) and pouch 4.
  ❑ Key: Marker A: Pharyngeal pouch 1; B: Pharyngeal pouch 2; C: Pharyngeal pouch 3; D: Pharyngeal pouch 4.

Thyroid Gland develops from the thyroid diverticulum, which forms from the **endoderm** at foramen cecum, in the floor of the foregut (pharynx) and divides into right and left lobes that are connected by the isthmus of the gland.
  ❑ It descends caudally into the neck, passing ventral to the hyoid bone and laryngeal cartilages.
  ❑ During migration, the developing gland remains connected to the tongue by the **thyroglossal duct**, which is an endodermal tube and extends between the thyroid primordium and posterior part of the tongue.
  ❑ This duct is later obliterated, and the site of the duct is marked by the foramen cecum.
  ❑ **Parafollicular C cells** of thyroid are derived from the **neural crest cells** via the ultimobranchial body in the fourth pharyngeal pouch and then migrate into the thyroid gland.
  ❑ **Ultimobranchial body** is a remnant of the fifth pharyngeal pouch (which regresses) and attaches to the fourth pharyngeal pouch later. It receives the neural crest cells, which get transformed into parafollicular C cells of thyroid.
  ❑ Later these cells migrate to the thyroid gland and secrete **thyrocalcitonin** hormone.

1. The parafollicular C cells of thyroid develops from:
    (*JIMPER 2016*)
  a. 1st and 2nd pharyngeal pouch
  b. 2nd and 3rd pharyngeal pouch
  c. 3rd and 4th pharyngeal pouch
  d. 4th and 5th pharyngeal pouch

2. Parafollicular C cells are derived from:
  a. Ultimobranchial body
  b. Pharyngeal pouch 4
  c. Pharyngeal pouch 5
  d. Neural crest cells

3. **True about development of pharyngeal arches are all EXCEPT:**   *(PGIC)*
   a. Parathyroid glands develop from 3rd and 4th pharyngeal pouch   b. Tongue muscles develop from occipital myotome
   c. Superior parathyroid gland develops from 4th pharyngeal pouch   d. Inferior parathyroid gland develops from 2nd pharyngeal pouch
   e. Thyroid develops from foramen cecum

1. **d. 4th and 5th pharyngeal pouch**
   - ❑ Parafollicular C cells of thyroid gland develop from the neural crest cells.
   - ❑ The fifth pharyngeal pouch is rudimentary and disappears, leaving behind ultimobranchial body, which attaches to the fourth pharyngeal pouch.
   - ❑ Neural crest cells reach the ultimobranchial body and get converted into parafollicular C cells of thyroid.

2. **d. Neural crest cells > a. Ultimobranchial body > b. Pharyngeal pouch 4 > c. Pharyngeal pouch 5**
   - ❑ Parafollicular C cells of thyroid gland develop from the neural crest cells.
   - ❑ The Fifth pharyngeal pouch is rudimentary and disappears, leaving behind ultimobranchial body, which subsequently attaches to the fourth pharyngeal pouch.
   - ❑ Neural crest cells reach the ultimobranchial body and get converted into parafollicular C cells of thyroid.

3. **d. Inferior parathyroid gland develops from 2nd pharyngeal pouch**
   - ❑ Inferior parathyroid gland develops from 3rd pharyngeal pouch.

▶ Development of Skull Bones

- ❑ **Neural crest cells** contribute to secondary mesenchyme which forms most of the skull bones.
- ❑ Additionally, there are two contributions from primary mesenchyme: **Cranial paraxial mesenchyme** and sclerotome (**paraxial mesenchyme**), which give parietal and occipital bone components.
- ❑ Skull has three types of bones developmentally: **Cartilagenous**, **membranous** and **membran ocartilaginous**.
- ❑ **Metopic suture** is the frontal suture between the two halves of frontal bone, runs through the midline across the frontal bone from the nasion to the bregma. It completely fuses between 3 and 9 months of age. Forensic books mention the closure between the age of 2–8 years.

Table 2: Types of skull bones according to their development (ossification)

Membranous bones (ossify in membrane)	Cartilaginous bones (ossify in cartilage)	Membranocartilaginous bones (ossify both in membrane and cartilage)
Frontal Parietal	Ethmoid Inferior nasal concha	Occipital (part above the superior nuchal line is membranous and the remaining part is cartilaginous)
Maxilla (Excluding premaxilla) Zygomatic Nasal		Sphenoid (lateral parts of greater wings and pterygoid processes are membranous and rest is cartilaginous)
Lacrimal		Temporal (squamous) and tympanic parts are membranous while petromastoid part and styloid process are cartilaginous
Vomer		Mandible (condylar and coronoid proesses are cartilaginous and the rest of the mandible is membranous)

▶ Skull at birth

Bones of the calvaria are unilaminar and lack diploe at birth. The fibrous membrane that forms the calvaria remains unossified at the six angles of the parietal bones, producing **six fontanelles**: two single midlines (anterior and posterior) and two lateral pairs: Sphenoidal (anterolateral) and mastoid (posterolateral).

- ❑ The anterior fontanelle is the **largest**, it occupies the junction between the sagittal, coronal and frontal sutures and is rhomboid in shape. The posterior fontanelle lies at the junction between the sagittal and lambdoid sutures and is triangular. The sphenoidal (anterolateral) and mastoid (posterolateral) fontanelles lie at the sphenoidal and mastoid angles of the parietal bones, respectively.

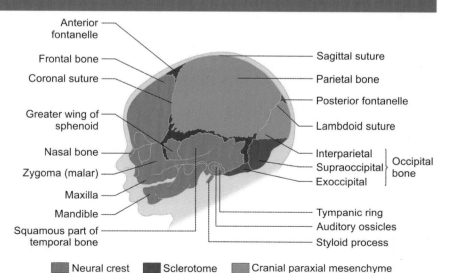

Fig. 10: The newborn skull, showing the tissue origins of the bones (based on combined mouse and human data). The darker green represents the sites of fontanelles.

❑ Posterior fontanelle closes **soon after birth**, lateral fontanelles close within a few weeks of birth and anterior fontanelle closes by **2 years of age**.

❑ At birth, the orbits are relatively large, the internal ear, tympanic cavity, auditory ossicles and mastoid antrum are all **almost adult in size**, and the mastoid process is **absent**.

❑ The external acoustic meatus is short, straight and wholly cartilaginous. The external aspect of the tympanic membrane faces more inferiorly than laterally.

❑ The styloid process has not yet commenced ossification, paranasal sinuses are rudimentary or absent and only the maxillary sinuses are usually identifiable.

❑ **Mandible** at birth is in **two halves**, united by the fibrous tissue at the **symphysis menti**.

❑ The inner ear and the petrous temporal bone around it grow very little after birth, so the increasing breadth of the skull draws the petrous temporal bone out laterally, creating the bony external acoustic meatus.

❑ Use of sternocleidomastoid to lift the head results in formation of the **mastoid process** of the temporal bone (during the later part of **2nd year**), which develops air-filled spaces (mastoid air cells) during 6th year.

❑ The paranasal sinuses begin to form in late fetal life as diverticula from the nasal cavity that gradually invade the maxilla, frontal, ethmoid and sphenoid bones.

❑ Paranasal sinuses are **rudimentary** at birth. The **maxillary** sinus is the **1st PNS to develop** and is identifiable at birth. Maxillary antrum enlarges with age.

❑ At birth, small ethmoidal sinuses are also present, but the **frontal sinus is nothing more than** an out-pouching from the nasal cavity, and there is no pneumatization of the sphenoid bone.

❑ Diploe (and diploic veins) are present in the skull at birth – they **appear by 4th year** of age.

Structures at adult size (at birth)	Structures not at adult size (at birth)
▪ Tympanic membrane ▪ Tympanic cavity ▪ Ear ossicles (malleus, incus and stapes) ▪ Tympanic (mastoid. antrum ▪ Internal ear: Cochlea, vestibule, semicircular canal	▪ Tegmen tympani ▪ Mastoid process ▪ External ear and external auditory canal ▪ Eustachian tube

QUESTIONS

1. **Facial skeleton develops form:**   *(NEET Pattern 2013)*
   a. Neural crest   b. Paraxial mesoderm
   c. Intermediate mesoderm   d. Lateral plate mesoderm

2. **All are of adult size at birth EXCEPT:**   *(AIIMS 2009)*
   a. Mastoid antrum   b. Ear ossicles
   c. Tympanic cavity   d. Maxillary antrum and orbit

3. **Which of the following attains adult size before birth:**   *(AIIMS 2010)*
   a. Ear ossicles   b. Maxilla
   c. Mastoid   d. Parietal bone

4. **Suture present between parietal and occipital bones is :**   *(NEET Pattern 2012)*
   a. Lambdoid suture   b. Coronal suture
   c. Sagittal suture   d. Metopic suture

ANSWERS

1. **a. Neural crest**
   ❑ The viscerocranium consists of the bones of the face that develop from the secondary mesenchyme, derived from neural crest cells in the 1st and 2nd pharyngeal arches.

2. **d. Maxillary antrum and orbit**
   ❑ Tympanic cavity, mastoid (tympanic) antrum, ear ossicles and the Internal ear are of adult size in the fetal skull.
   ❑ Mastoid process is absent at birth — appears during the later part of 2nd year and the mastoid air cells appear during 6th year.
   ❑ Paranasal sinuses are rudimentary at birth. The maxillary sinus is the 1st PNS to develop and is identifiable at birth. Maxillary antrum enlarges with age.
   ❑ At birth the orbits appear relatively large. Growth of the orbits is complete by 7th year.

3. **a. Ear ossicles**
   ❑ Ear ossicles are almost of adult size at birth. Maxilla, mastoid and parietal bones change their features significantly after birth.

4. **a. Lambdoid suture**
   ❑ Lambdoid suture is present between the two parietal bones and the occipital bone. It is continuous with the occipitomastoid suture.
   ❑ Coronal suture lies between the frontal bone and the two parietal bones.
   ❑ Sagittal Ssuture is present between the two parietal bones in the midline.
   ❑ Metopic suture lies in the median plane and separates the two halves of the frontal bone.
   ❑ Fontanel last to close is anterior fontanelle (NEET Pattern 2018)

▶ Skull bones

The skull is composed of 28 separate bones and is divided into two parts: The neurocranium and viscerocranium.

❑ **Neurocranium** consists of the flat bones of the skull (i.e. cranial vault) and the base of the skull, which include the 8 cranial bones for enclosing the brain (unpaired frontal, occipital, ethmoid, and sphenoid bones and paired parietal and temporal bones), which can be seen in the cranial cavity.

- **Viscerocranium**: The viscerocranium consists of the bones of the face that develop from the pharyngeal arches in embryologic development, which include the following 14 facial bones (paired lacrimal, nasal, palatine, inferior turbinate, maxillary, and zygomatic bones and unpaired vomer and mandible).
- **Cranium** is the skull without the mandible.
- **Calvaria** is the skullcap, which is the vault of the skull without the facial bones. It consists of the superior portions of the frontal, parietal, and occipital bones. Its highest point on the sagittal suture is the vertex.
- Frontal bone is a **pneumatic bone** which underlies the forehead and the superior margin and roof of the orbit and has a smooth median prominence called the **glabella**.
- Ethmoid is a **pneumatic** bone located between the orbits and consists of the cribriform plate, perpendicular plate, and two lateral masses enclosing ethmoid air cells. It is the **thinnest** skull bone (*NEET Pattern 2014*)
- Sphenoid is a **pneumatic** bone, consists of the body (with sphenoid air sinus), the greater and lesser wings, and the pterygoid process.
- Temporal bone consists of the squamous part, which is external to the lateral surface of the temporal lobe of the brain; the petrous part, which encloses the internal and middle ears; the mastoid part, which contains mastoid air cells (**pneumatic**); and the tympanic part, which houses the external auditory meatus and the tympanic cavity.
- **Styloid Process** extends downward and forward from the temporal bone and gives origin to **three** muscles (stylohyoid, styloglossus, and stylopharyngeus) and **two** ligaments (stylohyoid and stylomandibular).

▶ Cranial cavity and Skull foramina

Structures seen inside the cranial fossa:
- **Foramen cecum** is a small pit in front of the crista galli between the ethmoid and frontal bones.
- **Crista galli** is the triangular midline projection of the ethmoid bone extending upward from the cribriform plate, provides attachment for the dural fold falx cerebri.
- Anterior clinoid processes are two anterior processes of the lesser wing of the sphenoid bone, in the middle cranial fossa, provide attachment for the **free border of the tentorium cerebelli**.
- Posterior clinoid processes are two tubercles from each side of the dorsum sellae, provide attachment for the attached border of the tentorium cerebelli.

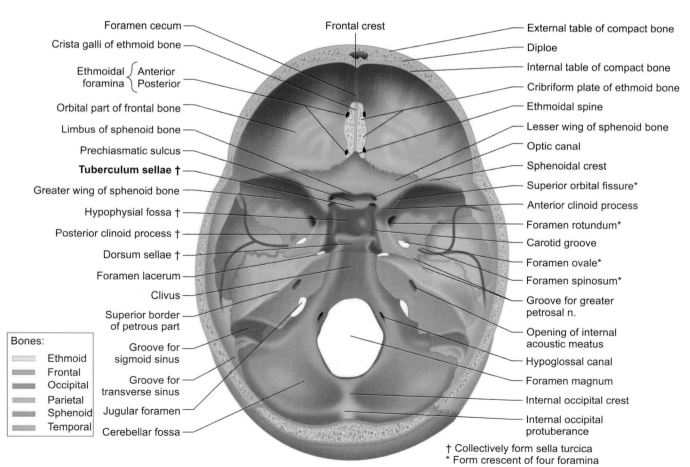

Fig. 11: Internal surface of cranial base (Superior view)

- ❑ **Lesser wing of the sphenoid** Bone forms the anterior boundary of the middle cranial fossa, forms the sphenoidal ridge separating the anterior from the middle cranial fossa, contributes to the boundary of the superior orbital fissure.
- ❑ **Superior orbital fissure** is a gap between the lesser wing of sphenoid and greater wing of sphenoid.
- ❑ **Greater wing of the sphenoid bone** forms the anterior wall and the floor of the middle cranial fossa. It has several openings: the foramen rotundum, foramen ovale, canaliculus innominatus and foramen spinosum.
- ❑ Jugum sphenoidale is a portion of the body of the sphenoid bone connecting the two lesser wings and forms the roof for the sphenoidal air sinus.
- ❑ **Turkish saddle** (sella turcica) is a saddle-shaped depression in the body of the sphenoid bone. The deepest part of the sella turcica known as the hypophyseal fossa, lodges the **pituitary gland** (hypophysis). It is bounded anteriorly by the tuberculum sellae and posteriorly by the dorsum sellae. It lies directly **above the sphenoid sinus** located within the body of the sphenoid bone; its dural roof is formed by the diaphragma sellae.
- ❑ **Clivus** is the downward sloping surface from the dorsum sellae to the foramen magnum. It is formed by a part of the body of the sphenoid and a portion of the basilar part of the occipital bone. The spheno-occipital joint is a **synchondrosis**. It is related to the anterior aspect of brainstem.

Anterior Cranial Fossa

Foramen	Contents
Cribriform plate	Olfactory nerve
Foramen cecum	Emissary vein from nasal mucosa to superior sagittal sinus
Anterior and posterior ethmoidal foramina	Anterior and posterior ethmoidal nerves, arteries, and veins

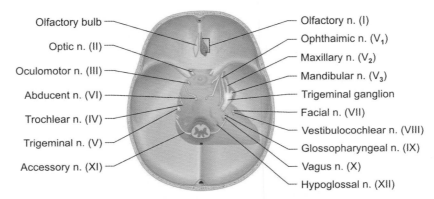

Fig. 12: Internal surface of cranial base (Superior view), showing cranial nerves and related foramina

Middle Cranial Fossa

Foramen	Contents
Optic canal	Optic nerve, ophthalmic artery, and central artery and vein of the retina
Superior orbital fissure (through CTRZ*)	Oculomotor nerve (superior and inferior division), abducent nerves and nasociliary nerve (branch of ophthalmic division of trigeminal nerve)
Superior orbital fissure (left outside the ring)	LFT* nerves: Lacrimal and frontal nerves (branches of ophthalmic division of trigeminal nerve), trochlear nerve and ophthalmic (superior and inferior) veins
Foramen rotundum	Maxillary division of trigeminal nerve
Foramen ovale	Mandibular division of trigeminal nerve, Accessory meningeal artery, Lesser petrosal nerve, Emissary vein. Mnemonic: MALE
Canaliculus innominatus	Lesser petrosal nerve (occasionally)
Foramen spinosum	Middle meningeal artery, nervus spinosus
Foramen lacerum	No structure passes through this foramen, but the upper part is traversed by the internal carotid artery (and sympathetic plexus around), deep petrosal nerves and greater petrosal nerves joining to form vidian nerve of pterygoid canal
Carotid canal	Internal carotid artery and sympathetic nerves (carotid plexus)
Hiatus of facial canal	Greater petrosal nerve

*CTRZ: Common tendinous ring of Zinn

Note: *LFT nerves are LeFT outside the common tendinous ring of Zinn.

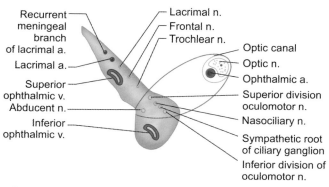

Fig. 13: Structures passing through superior orbital fissure

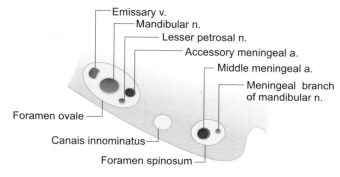

Fig. 14: Structures passing through foramen ovale and spinosum

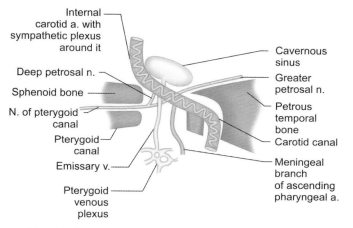

Fig. 15: Structures at the base and passing through the foramen lacerum

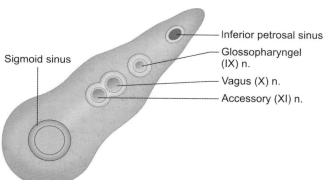

Fig. 16: Structures passing through the jugular foramen

Posterior Cranial Fossa

Foramen	Contents
Internal auditory meatus	Facial and vestibulocochlear nerves and labyrinthine artery
Jugular foramen (anterior part)	Inferior petrosal sinus
Jugular foramen (middle part)	Cranial nerves 9, 10, 11 (cranial and spinal)
Jugular foramen (posterior part)	Junction of sigmoid sinus and internal jugular vein Meningeal branch of occipital artery
Hypoglossal canal	Hypoglossal nerve and meningeal artery.
Foramen magnum (Anterior part)	Apical ligament of dens Membrana tectoria Vertical band of cruciate ligament
Foramen magnum (posterior part)	Lower part of medulla oblongata Meninges (dura, arachnoid and pia mater) In subarachnoid space: Spinal root of accessory nerves Vertebral arteries and sympathetic plexus Anterior and posterior spinal arteries Venous plexus of vertebral canal
Condyloid foramen	Condyloid emissary vein
Mastoid foramen	Branch of occipital artery to dura mater and mastoid emissary vein

- Major structures passing foramen magnum are: Medulla oblongata with the 3 meninges, Two vertebral arteries, Three spinal arteries (one anterior and two posterior), Spinal part of accessory nerve, few ligaments.
- **Membrana tectoria** is continuation of posterior longitudinal ligament on vertebral column and enters cranial cavity passing through foramen magnum.

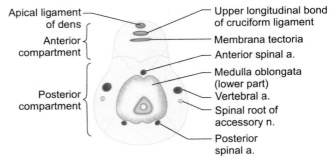

Fig. 17: Structures passing through the foramen magnum

Foramina in the Base of the Skull

Foramen	Contents
Petrotympanic fissure	Chorda tympani and often anterior tympanic artery
Stylomastoid foramen	Facial nerve
Incisive canal	Nasopalatine nerve and terminal part of the sphenopalatine or greater palatine vessels
Greater palatine foramen	Greater palatine nerve and vessels
Lesser palatine foramen	Lesser palatine nerve and vessels
Palatine canal	Descending palatine vessels and the greater and lesser palatine nerves
Pterygoid canal	Runs from the anterior wall of the foramen lacerum to the pterygopalatine fossa and transmits the nerve of the pterygoid canal (vidian nerve)
Sphenopalatine foramen	Sphenopalatine vessels and nasopalatine nerve

Foramina in the Front of the Skull

Foramen	Contents
Zygomaticofacial foramen	Zygomaticofacial nerve
Supraorbital notch or foramen	Supraorbital nerve and vessels
Infraorbital foramen	Infraorbital nerve and vessels
Mental foramen	Mental nerve and vessels

1. **All structures pass through foramen ovale EXCEPT:**
   a. Accessory meningeal artery   b. Middle meningeal artery
   c. Lesser petrosal nerve   d. Emissary vein

2. **Structure passing through the tendinous ring of Zinn:**
   a. Superior ophthalmic vein   b. Trochlear nerve
   c. Nasociliary nerve   d. Lacrimal nerve

3. **Mass in jugular foramen may result in all EXCEPT:**
   a. Difficulty in swallowing
   b. Hoarseness
   c. Difficulty in turning the neck to opposite side
   d. Tongue deviates to same side

4. **Incisive foramen transmits:**   (NEET Pattern 2015)
   a. Greater palatine artery and greater palatine nerve
   b. Greater palatine artery and lesser palatine nerve
   c. Greater palatine artery and sphenopalatine nerve
   d. Greater palatine artery and nasopalatine nerve

5. **Choose the INCORRECT pair regarding the skull foramina and the structures passing through:**   (PGIC)
   a. Maxillary nerve: Foramen rotundum
   b. Vestibulocochlear nerve: Internal acoustic meatus
   c. Anterior part of jugular foramen: Inferior petrosal sinus
   d. Foramen spinosum: Middle meningeal artery
   e. Superior orbital fissure: Optic nerve

6. **Structures which passes through the internal auditory meatus are all EXCEPT:**   (NEET Pattern 2014)
   a. Nerve of Wrisberg
   b. Anterior inferior cerebellar artery
   c. Superior vestibular nerve
   d. Cochlear nerve

7. **Cranial nerve related to apex of the petrous temporal bone:**   (PGIC 2005)
   a. IX   b. VIII
   c. VII   d. VI
   e. V

8. **Which structure passes through foramen magnum:**   (AIPG 2010)
   a. Vertebral artery   b. Internal carotid artery
   c. Hypoglossal nerve   d. Sympathetic chain

9. **Mandibular division of trigeminal nerve passes through, which of the following marked foramen:**   (AIIMS 2017)
   a. A
   b. B
   c. C
   d. D

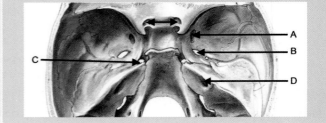

10. Which of the following structures do not pass through the marked foramen in the diagram? *(AIIMS 2014)*
   a. Maxillary nerve
   b. Sensory branch of mandibular nerve
   c. Lesser petrosal nerve
   d. Motor root of trigeminal nerve

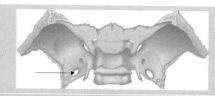

11. Maxilla doesn't articulate with: *(AIIMS 2015)*
   a. Lacrimal bone
   b. Plate of sphenoid bone
   c. Frontal bone
   d. Ethmoid bone

12. NOT a relation of sphenoid sinus: *(NEET Pattern 2015)*
   a. Optic nerve
   b. Mandibular nerve
   c. Maxillary nerve
   d. Vidian nerve

13. Identify the structure marked with arrow: *(AIIMS 2017)*
   a. Spinal accessory nerve
   b. Abducent nerve
   c. Vertebral artery
   d. Labyrinthine artery

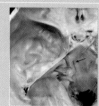

1. **b. Middle meningeal artery**
   ❑ 'MALE' structures pass through foramen ovale: Mandibular division of trigeminal nerve, Accessory meningeal artery, Lesser petrosal nerve, Emissary vein.
   ❑ Middle meningeal artery passes through foramen spinosum, along with nervus spinosus (branch of mandibular nerve).

2. **c. Nasociliary nerve**
   ❑ Nasociliary nerve passes inside (though) the common tendinous ring of Zinn.
   ❑ LFT nerves are left outside the ring (L - Lacrimal, F - Frontal, T - Trochlear).
   ❑ Superior and inferior ophthalmic veins usually remain outside the ring of Zinn, while passing through superior orbital fissure.

3. **d. Tongue deviates to same side**
   ❑ Hypoglossal nerve passes through hypoglossal canal (and not jugular foramen). Hence tongue doesn't show any deformity as such.
   ❑ Jugular foramen has cranial nerves 9, 10, and 11 passing through it, which supply the muscles of palate, pharynx and larynx (for speech and swallowing).
   ❑ A mass in the foramen leads to paralysis of these muscles and difficulty in speech and swallowing.
   ❑ Injury to spinal part of accessory nerve leads to paralysis of sternocleidomastoid muscle and difficulty in turning the neck to opposite side.

4. **d. Greater palatine artery and nasopalatine nerve**
   ❑ Incisive foramina are located behind the central incisor teeth in the incisive fossa of the maxilla (hard palate).
   ❑ It receives the nasopalatine nerves from the floor of the nasal cavity along with the greater palatine vessels supplying the mucous membrane covering the hard palate of the mouth.

5. **e. Superior orbital fissure: Optic nerve**
   ❑ Optic nerve passes through the optic canal.

6. **b. Anterior inferior cerebellar artery**
   ❑ Labyrinthine vessels passing through internal auditory meatus.
   ❑ Vestibulocochlear and facial nerves also pass through the meatus.
   ❑ Nerve of Wrisberg (nervus intermedius) is sensory component of facial nerve.

7. **d. VI; e. V**
   ❑ Apex of petrous temporal bone is related to cranial nerve V and VI.

8. **a. Vertebral artery**
   ❑ Foramen magnum has the two vertebral arteries and three spinal arteries passing through it.
   ❑ Internal carotid artery passes through the carotid canal in the petrous temporal bone at the base of the skull.
   ❑ Hypoglossal nerve passes the hypoglossal canal present in the occipital bone.
   ❑ Sympathetic chain begins at the foramen magnum and continues till the coccyx

9. **b. B**
   ❑ The diagram shows various foramina in the superior view of cranial cavity. Mandibular nerve (trigeminal) passes through the foramen ovale (Marker B).
   ❑ Key: Marker A: Foramen rotundum; C: Foramen lacerum; D: Internal auditory meatus

10. **a. Maxillary nerve**
   ❑ Maxillary nerve passes through foramen rotundum (not foramen ovale).
   ❑ The marked foramen in diagram is foramen ovale and structures passing through it are: Mandibular division of trigeminal nerve, Accessory meningeal artery, Lesser petrosal nerve, Emissary vein. (Mnemonic: MALE).

11. **b. Plate of sphenoid bone**
   ❑ Maxilla bone generally do not articulate with plate (pterygoid) of sphenoid bone, though sometimes it may form an articulation with the orbital surface or lateral pterygoid plate of the sphenoid bone.
   ❑ Maxilla articulates with nine bones: Frontal, ethmoid, nasal, lacrimal, zygomatic, inferior nasal concha, vomer, palatine, and the other maxilla.

12. b. Mandibular nerve
- ❏ Structures related to sphenoid sinus are foramen rotundum (maxillary nerve), optic canal (optic nerve and ophthalmic artery), vidian canal (with nerve), internal carotid artery.
- ❏ Mandibular nerve is not related to sphenoid sinus.

13. b. Abducent nerve
- ❏ This diagram shows the cranial cavity and the marker is put at abducent nerve, piercing duramater to enter the Dorello's canal. The nerve emerges from the brainstem and runs upward between the pons and the clivus, then pierces the dura mater to run through Dorello's canal, before it enters cavernous sinus.

- ❏ **Posterior cranial fossa** has the **brainstem** which gives cranial nerve **3–12**, hence these nerves are present in the fossa. The last six nerves (7–12) enter/exit through the foramina present in the posterior cranial fossa.
- ❏ Lesser petrosal nerve passes through the **foramen ovale** (and **canaliculus innominatus** in small percentage of population).
- ❏ **Sternberg's canal** is anteromedial to the foramen rotundum (not posterolateral). It connects middle cranial fossa with the nasopharynx. Infection may be carried from the nasopharynx towards the sphenoidal sinus via the canal *(AIPG 2009)*
- ❏ Tumors of anterior cranial fossa damage the olfactory bulb *(NEET Pattern 2015)*
- ❏ Maxillary nerve arises in the trigeminal ganglion (middle cranial fossa), passes through lateral wall of cavernous sinus and leaves the skull through foramen rotundum to enter the pterygopalatine fossa.
- ❏ **Dorello's Canal** is the bow-shaped enclosure surrounding the abducens nerve as it enters the cavernous sinus. It is present at the medial most end of the petrous ridge at the confluence of the inferior petrosal sinus and cavernous sinus *(NEET Pattern 2015)*
- ❏ Skull fracture of anterior cranial fossa causes anosmia, periorbital bruising (raccoon eyes). The cribriform plate of ethmoid bone may be involved, leading to **CSF rhinorrhea** and ethmoid air sinuses filled with CSF.
- ❏ Fracture of the petrous portion of the temporal bone may cause blood or cerebrospinal fluid (CSF) to escape from the ear (**otorrhea**), hearing loss, and facial nerve damage.

� Mandible

Mandible bone develops in **first pharyngeal arch**. It has **16 alveolar sockets** for teeth. It is the **most mobile bone of skull**.
- ❏ Ossification: Mandible is formed in relation to first pharyngeal arch (**Meckel's**) cartilage by **both** intramembranous and endochondral ossification. It is the **second bone to ossify in the body.**
- ❏ At birth, mandible consists of two halves connected at the symphysis menti by cartilaginous joint. The bony union starts from below upwards during the 1st year of the age and completed at the end of the 2nd year.
- ❏ Coronoid and condylar processes ossify from secondary cartilages not related to Meckel's cartilage.

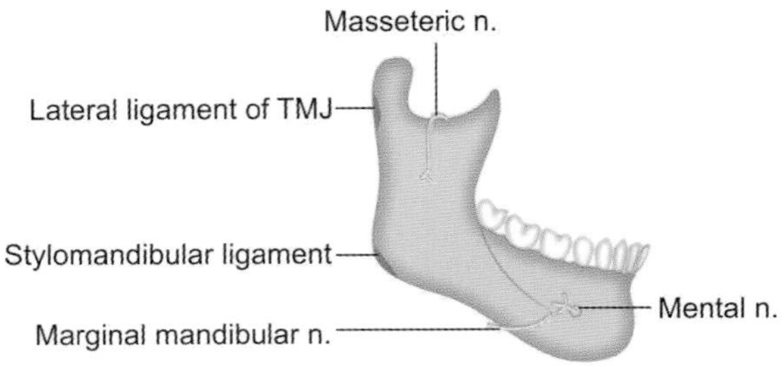

Fig. 18: Attachment of ligaments and nerves related to the mandible: Lateral surface of the right half of the mandible

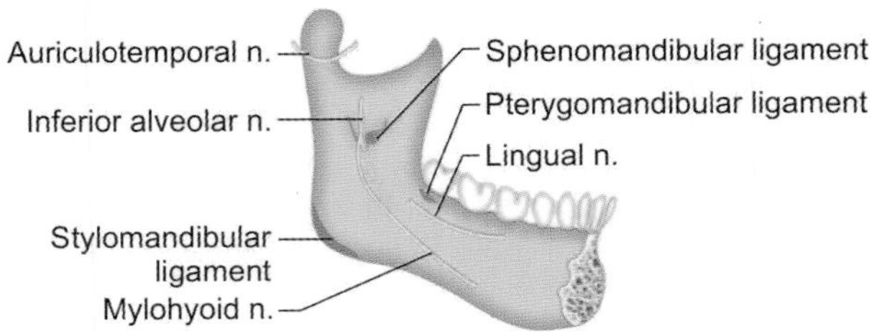

Fig. 19: Attachment of ligaments and nerves related to the mandible: Medial surface of the left half of the mandible

- ❏ **Lingual nerve** enters the submandibular region by passing just behind and inferior to the third molar tooth between medial surface of the mandible and the mucs membrane of the gum. In this position, it is accessible to local anesthetics and liable to be injured by the clumsy extraction of the adjacent tooth.
- ❏ **Inferior alveolar nerve** enters the mandibular foramen and passes through the mandibular canal; **mylohyoid nerve** runs in the mylohyoid groove; **masseteric nerve** runs through the mandibular notch; auriculotemporal nerve runs to the medial side of the neck; **marginal mandibular nerve** across the lower border of the mandible.
- ❏ Inferior to the **second premolar teeth** are the mental foramina for the **mental nerves and vessels**.

1. Mental foramen is located near: *(AIIMS 2002)*
- a. First premolar of mandible
- b. Second molar of mandible
- c. Canine of mandible
- d. Canine of maxilla

2. Which nerve is in close relation with root of the lower third molar? *(NEET pattern 2014)*
- a. Inferior alveolar nerve
- b. Chorda tympani nerve
- c. Lingual nerve
- d. Mylohyoid nerve

3. To give inferior alveolar nerve block the nerve is approached lateral to pterygomandibular raphe between the buccinator and:
- a. Temporalis
- b. Superior constrictor *(AIIMS 2002)*
- c. Middle constrictor
- d. Medial pterygoid

1. **a. First premolar of mandible**
    - ❑ The most frequent position (63%) of the mental foramen is in line with the longitudinal axis of the 2nd premolar tooth (not given in the choice).
    - ❑ On the medial surface of mandible is the mandibular foramen for inferior alveolar nerve and vessels.
    - ❑ The foramen leads into mandibular canal which opens on lateral surface of mandible at mental foramen, situated below the second premolar tooth.

2. **c. Lingual nerve**
    - ❑ Lingual nerve moves in a groove on the medial aspect of socket for lower third molar.

3. **b. Superior constrictor**
    - ❑ The coronoid notch is palpated with index finger and the needle is introduced 1 cm above the surface of last molar medial to finger (coronoid notch) but lateral to pterygomandibular raphe between the buccinator and superior constrictor muscle.

▶ Trigeminal nerve

Trigeminal nerve has **one motor** and **three sensory** nuclei.

❑ The **motor nucleus** is located in pons and send the motor fibers by mandibular nerve (branch of trigeminal) to control the eight muscles developing in the first pharyngeal arch, which include muscles of mastication.

❑ The **main sensory** nucleus is present in the pons, whereas midbrain has the **mesencephalic sensory** nucleus of trigeminal (for proprioception) and the **spinal sensory** nucleus of trigeminal has neurone bodies extending into the spinal cord (carry pain and temperature).

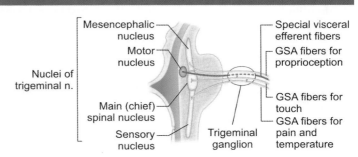

Fig. 20: Four nuclei and functional components of the trigeminal nerve

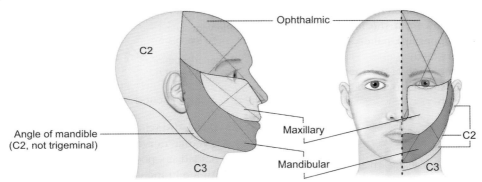

Fig. 21: Distribution of trigeminal & cervical plexus branches

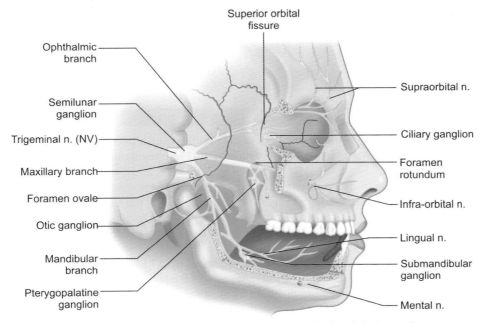

Fig. 22: Trigeminal nerve branches and anatomically related ganglia

❑ Sensations carried by trigeminal nerve fibers reach the corresponding nuclei in brainstem and synapse, second order neurone cross the midline as **trigeminal lemniscus** and synapse in VPM (Ventero-postero medial) nucleus of thalamus. Third order neurones in thalamus send fibers through the **genu of internal capsule** to the postcentral gyrus (parietal sensory cortex).

❑ Trigeminal (semilunar) **ganglion** consists of cell bodies of sensory fibers that distribute along three divisions: Ophthalmic
❑ (V1), maxillary (V2) and mandibular (V3). It creates an impression at the apex of the petrous portion of the temporal bone in the middle cranial fossa and is located in a pouch webbed with arachnoid between two layers of dura (**Meckel cave**).

❑ Artery supply to trigeminal ganglion is by cavernous part of internal carotid artery.

❑ **Ophthalmic** division innervates the area above the **upper eyelid** and **dorsum of the nose**. **Maxillary** division innervates the face below the level of the eyes and above the **upper lip**. **Mandibular** division innervates the face below the level of the **lower lip**.

❑ **Mandibular** nerve (branch of trigeminal) supply skin on the mandible (except the angle). Skin at the angle of jaw is supplied by the greater auricular nerve.

❑ Lesser occipital nerve supplies the skin in the lateral area of the head posterior to the ear.

❑ **Trigeminal** nerve has largest number of axons and is the **thickest** and **largest** (in size) neve *(NEET Pattern 2016)*

◢ Maxillary Nerve

Maxillary Division (V2) of trigeminal nerve is constituted by axons given by cell bodies in the trigeminal ganglion, pass through the lateral wall of the cavernous sinus in the middle cranial fossa and next the foramen rotundum to enter the pterygopalatine fossa (at the back of the orbit).

❑ It carries general somatic afferent (GSA) neural column, sensory fibers from the face (below the eyes and to the upper lip), palate, paranasal sinuses, and maxillary teeth.

❑ It mediates the afferent limb of the sneeze reflex (irritation of the nasal mucosa), vagus nerve being the efferent limb.

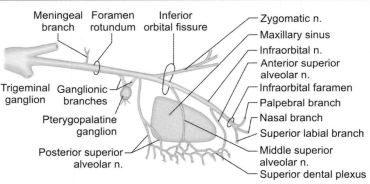

Fig. 23:Origin, course, and branches of the maxillary nerve

Table 3: Summary of branches of the maxillary nerve	
Region	**Branches**
In the middle cranial fossa	Meningeal branch
In the pterygopalatine fossa	▪ Ganglionic branches ▪ Posterior superior alveolar nerves ▪ Zygomatic nerve
In the infraorabital canal	▪ Middle superior alveolar nerve ▪ Anterior superior alveolar nerve
On the face	▪ Palpebral branch ▪ Nasal branch ▪ Labial branch

❑ Upper (Maxillary) teeth are supplied by the superior alveolar nerves which are three in number. They are named as—posterior, anterior and middle.

❑ All are branches of maxillary nerve—the nerve of upper jaw.

❑ **Posterior superior alveolar** nerve is a direct branch of maxillary nerve. It supplies mainly the molar teeth.

❑ Maxillary nerve continues as **inferior orbital nerve** and gives **middle** superior alveolar nerve (supplies premolars) and **anterior** superior alveolar nerve (supplies canine and incisors).

◢ Mandibular nerve

Mandibular nerve is given at trigeminal ganglion at the floor of the middle cranial fossa and passes through the foramen ovale to enter the infratemporal region. It provides sensory innervation to the lower teeth and gum and to the lower part of the face below the lower lip and the mouth.

❑ It supplies **8 muscles** developing in first pharyngeal arch: 2 tensors (tensor tympani and tensor palati), 3 elevators of mandible (MTM: Masseter, Temporalis, Medial pterygoid) and 3 depressors of mandible (Lateral pterygoid, mylohyoid and anterior belly of digastric).

❑ Muscles of mastication are supplied by anterior division of mandibular nerve **except medial pterygoid** being supplied by **main trunk** *(AIPG 2011)*

❑ Masseteric nerve is a branch from anterior division of mandibular nerve *(NEET Pattern 2012)*

❑ **Mandibular nerve** carries both the afferent and the efferent limbs of the **jaw jerk reflex**.

❑ Meningeal branch (**nervus spinosus**) arise from the main trunk of mandibular nerve *(NEET Pattern 2013)*
  ➤ Accompanies the middle meningeal artery, enters the cranium through the foramen spinosum, and supplies the meninges of the middle cranial fossa.

- **Buccal nerve** descends between the two heads of the lateral pterygoid muscle and innervates skin and fascia on the **buccinator** muscle and **penetrates this muscle** to supply the mucous membrane of the cheek and gums.
- **Auriculotemporal nerve** arises from two roots that encircle the middle meningeal artery. It carries postganglionic parasympathetic and sympathetic general visceral efferent (GVE) fibers to the parotid gland and sensory general somatic afferent (GSA) fibers to the temporomandibular joint and the skin of the auricle and the scalp.
- **Lingual nerve** is joined by the chorda tympani, passes deep to the mylohyoid muscle, and descends lateral to and loops under the submandibular duct. It carries general sensation from the anterior two-thirds of the tongue.

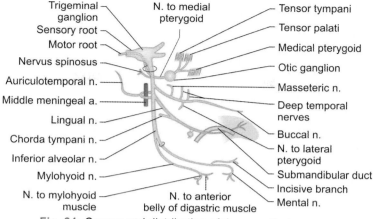

Fig. 24: Course and distribution of the mandibular nerve

  ➤ It also carries the postganglionic fibers from the submandibular ganglion to supply the submandibular and sublingual salivary gland. The preganglionic fibers are brought by the chorda tympani nerve.
  ➤ Lesion near the neck of the third molar causes loss of general sensation and taste to the anterior two-thirds of the tongue as well as salivary secretion from submandibular and sublingual glands.
- **Inferior alveolar nerve** passes deep to the lateral pterygoid muscle and then between the sphenomandibular ligament and the ramus of the mandible. It enters the mandibular canal through the mandibular foramen and supplies the tissues of the chin and lower teeth and gum.

Table 4: Branches of the mandibular nerve

From main trunk	From anterior division	From posterior division
Nerve spinosus (meningeal branch)	Masseteric nerve	Auriculotemporal nerve
Nerve to medial pterygoid	Deep temporal nerves	Lingual nerve
	Nerve to lateral pterygoid	Inferior alveolar nerve
	Nerve to lateral pterygoid	Inferior alveolar nerve
	Buccal nerve	

N.B. All the branches of posterior division of the mandibular nerve are sensory except nerve to mylohyoid, which is motor

- Posterior division of mandibular nerve gives ALI branches: A - Auriculotemporal nerve, L - Lingual nerve and I - Inferior alveolar nerve Mnemonic: P-ALI).

QUESTIONS

1. Post superior alveolar nerve is a branch of: *(AIPG 2009)*
   a. Mandibular
   b. Facial
   c. Lingual
   d. Maxillary

2. Middle superior alveolar nerve is: *(AIIMS 2010)*
   a. Palatal branch of maxillary nerve
   b. Nasal branch of maxillary nerve
   c. Branch of mandibular nerve
   d. Branch of inferior alveolar nerve

3. All are true for trigeminal nerve EXCEPT: *(NEET Pattern 2014)*
   a. Carries sensation from face
   b. Three sensory nuclei
   c. Two motor nuclei
   d. Maxillary nerve is a branch

4. Findings of trigeminal nerve injury include: *(PGIC 2013)*
   a. Pupillary dilation
   b. Loss of blinking reflex of eye
   c. Loss of jaw reflex
   d. Ptosis
   e. Weakness of muscle of mastication

ANSWERS

1. **d. Maxillary**
   - Posterior superior alveolar nerve is a direct branch of maxillary nerve. It supplies mainly the molar teeth. It also supplies the maxillary sinus, gingiva and inner cheek region.

2. **a. Palatal branch of maxillary nerve**
   - This questions doesn't have a proper answer and the most suitable option has been chosen.
   - Middle superior alveolar nerve supplies the palatal teeth on the maxilla and hence could be stated as the palatal branch of maxillary nerve.
   - It supplies teeth number 4, 5 (premolars) and 6 (first molar) and the lining of maxillary air sinus.
   - It is given by the infra-orbital nerve, while running in the infra-orbital groove.

3. **c. Two motor nuclei**
   - Trigeminal nerve has one motor nucleus and three sensory nuclei (total 4).
   - It carries sensation from the face by three branches, one of them being the maxillary nerve.

4. b. Loss of blinking reflex of eye; c. Loss of jaw reflex; e. Weakness of muscle of mastication
- ❑ Trigeminal nerve has 3 branches: ophthalmic, maxillary and mandibular, the lesions results in sensory loss on face.
- ❑ Injury to ophthalmic nerve injury leads to loss of corneal (blink) reflex; maxillary nerve injury results in loss of sneeze reflex and in mandibular nerve injury, there is loss of jaw jerk.
- ❑ Muscles of mastication are paralysed in mandibular nerve injury and manifests as a deviation of the mandible toward the side of the lesion.
- ❑ Partial deafness to low pitched sound due to paralysis of tensor tympani muscle is also observed.
- ❑ Mydriasis and ptosis are not clinical features of trigeminal nerve injury.

▼ Facial nerve

Facial nerve has two parts: **motor to facial expression** muscles and **nervus intermedius**. The motor part carries SVE component, while nervus intermedius carries GSA, SVA, and GVE fibers.

- ❑ SVE (Special visceral Efferent): Facial nerve supplies the muscles of facial expression (second pharyngeal arch).
  - ➤ The fibers arise from the motor nucleus of facial nerve (pons), loop around the abducent nucleus (internal genu), raising **facial colliculus** (at floor of fourth ventricle), exit the brainstem at the **ponto-medullary junction**.
  - ➤ Next the fibers enter the **internal auditory meatus**, pass through the facial canal in the middle ear cavity, give a branch to stapedius muscle, exit the skull through the **stylomastoid foramen**.
  - ➤ The nerve fibers innervate stylohyoid muscle, posterior belly of the digastric muscle, auricular muscles and enter

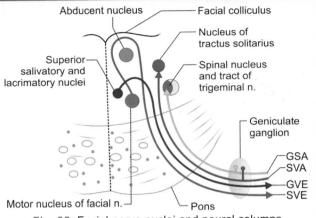

Fig. 25: Facial nerve nuclei and neural columns

the parotid gland to give rise to five terminal branches — the temporal, zygomatic, buccal, mandibular, and cervical branches that radiate forward in the face and supply muscles of facial expressions.
  - ➤ It supplies: Occipitofrontalis, **Risorius**, **Procerus**, **Zygomaticus**, **Auricular** muscles, Orbicularis oris etc.
- ❑ **Nervus intermedius** (nerve of Wrisberg) is the part of the facial nerve located between the motor component of the facial nerve and the vestibulocochlear nerve (cranial nerve VIII).
  - ➤ Upon reaching the facial canal, it joins with the motor root of the facial nerve at the geniculate ganglion.
  - ➤ It carries fibers for taste, salivation, lacrimation, and general sensation (from the external ear).
  - ➤ The first-order sensory neurons are found in the geniculate ganglion within the temporal bone.
- ❑ GSA (General Somatic Afferent) component brings general sensations from the posterior surface of the external ear through the posterior auricular branch.
- ❑ SVA (Special Visceral Afferent) component carries taste has from palate and the anterior two-thirds of the tongue to the **nucleus tractus solitarius**.
- ❑ GVE (General Visceral Efferent) component begins in the **superior salivatory nucleus** in the lower pons, carry preganglionic parasympathetic secretomotor fibers to glands.
- ❑ SVE (Special visceral Efferent): Supplies muscles of facial expression (second pharyngeal arch).
- ❑ **Superior salivatory nucleus** contains the cell bodies of parasympathetic axons within the nervus intermedius.
  - ➤ These secretomotor fibers reach the geniculate ganglion, pass through it without synapse and reach pterygopalatine ganglion to synapse, which further pass on the fibers to lacrimal, nasal and palatine glands.
- ❑ The sensory component of the nervus intermedius carries input about sensation from the skin of the external auditory meatus, mucous membranes of the nasopharynx and nose, and taste from the anterior two-thirds of the tongue, floor of the mouth, and the palate.
- ❑ The sensory information from the mucous membranes of the nasopharynx and palate is carried along the greater petrosal nerve, while the chorda tympani nerve (and lingual nerve) carries taste input from the anterior two thirds of the tongue, floor of mouth, and palate.
- ❑ GVE (General Visceral Efferent) component begins in the superior salivatory nucleus in the lower pons, carry preganglionic parasympathetic secretomotor fibers to glands by two pathways:
  - ➤ **Lacrimal pathway**—Secretomotor fibers pass through the nervus intermedius and greater petrosal nerves to the pterygopalatine (spheno-palatine. ganglion to supply LNP (**lacrimal, nasal, palatine**) glands.
  - ➤ **Submandibular pathway**—Secretomotor fibers pass through the nervus intermedius and chorda tympani to the submandibular ganglion to innervate the **submandibular and sublingual salivary glands**.
- ❑ **Greater petrosal nerve** is a branch of the facial nerve that arises distal to the geniculate ganglion, inside the facial canal, in middle ear cavity. It enters the middle cranial fossa through the hiatus for the greater (superficial) petrosal nerve (on the anterior surface of the petrous temporal bone).
  - ➤ It proceeds towards the foramen lacerum, where it joins the deep petrosal nerve (sympathetic) to form the vidian nerve of the pterygoid canal, which passes through the pterygoid canal to reach the pterygopalatine ganglion.

➤ The greater (superficial) petrosal nerve carries gustatory (taste) and parasympathetic fibers.

➤ Postganglionic parasympathetic fibers from pterygopalatine ganglion supply **lacrimal gland** and the mucosal glands of the **nose, palate, and pharynx**.

➤ The gustatory (**taste) fibers of palate** carried by this nerve, reach the geniculate ganglion and next run in facial nerve to reach eventually the nucleus tractus solitarius in medulla oblongata.

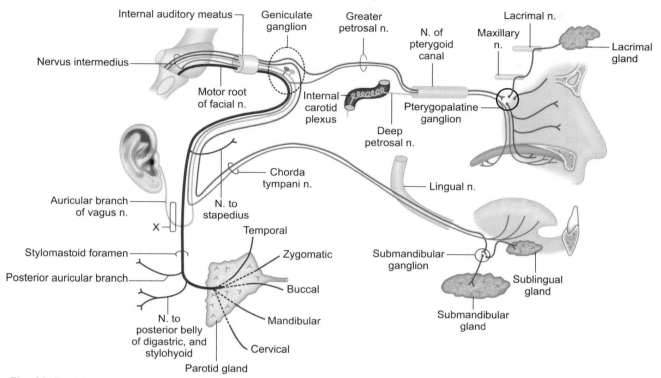

Fig. 26: Facial nerve: Origin, course and branches. Code for fibers: Black- Motor to muscles, Green- Secretomotor, Violet- Taste; Yellow- Sensory

❏ **Vidian nerve:** Sympathetic fibers around the internal carotid artery form the **deep petrosal nerve**, which joins **the greater petrosal nerve** (parasympathetic fibers) to form the **vidian nerve of pterygoid canal**.

➤ This nerve is formed at the floor of foramen lacerum and runs anteriorly in pterygoid canal to reach the pterygopalatine ganglion.

❏ **Chorda tympani nerve** is given in the middle ear cavity, runs medial to the tympanic membrane and malleus. It contains the SVA and GVE (parasympathetic) fibers.

➤ Taste sensations from anterior two third of tongue are carried by chorda tympani nerve towards the geniculate ganglion.

➤ Additionally, it carries pre-ganglionic fibers and is joined by lingual nerve (a branch of mandibular nerve), which carries post-ganglionic parasympathetic fibers to reach the submandibular and sublingual salivary glands.

❏ Facial nerve lesion causes **Bell's palsy**, which is marked by flaccid paralysis of the ipsilateral muscles of facial expression, typical distortion of the face such as no wrinkles on the forehead, drooping of the eyebrow, inability to close or blink the eye, sagging corner of the mouth, and inability to smile, whistle, or blow.

➤ The palsy also causes loss of taste in the anterior two-thirds of the tongue, decreased salivary secretion and lacrimation, painful sensitivity to sounds, and deviation of the lower jaw.

➤ MRI studies indicate that it may be caused by viral neuronitis either in the bony first part of the facial canal (labyrinthine segment) at the apex of the internal auditory canal, or in the adjacent brainstem. Depending upon the level of lesion the clinical features may differ.

Table 5: Facial nerve lesions at various levels and corresponding clinical features	
Level of injury	**Clinical features**
Stylomastoid foramen	Paralysis of muscles of facial expression
Proximal to chorda tympani branch	▪ Paralysis of muscles of facial expression ▪ Decreased salivation and loss of taste sensation on anterior 2/3 tongue
Proximal to nerve to stapedius	▪ Paralysis of muscles of facial expression ▪ Decreased salivation and loss of taste sensation on anterior 2/3 tongue ▪ Hyperacusis (loss of stapedial reflex)

Level of injury	Clinical features
Proximal to geniculate ganglion	▪ Paralysis of muscles of facial expression ▪ Decreased salivation and loss of taste sensation on anterior 2/3 tongue ▪ Hyperacusis (loss of stapedial reflex) ▪ Loss of lacrimation (later may present with crocodile syndrome)

❑ **Schirmer's test** evaluates the secretion of tears (function of lacrimal gland), which receives fibers through the greater petrosal nerve.

❑ **Crocodile tears syndrome** (Bogorad syndrome) is spontaneous lacrimation during eating caused by a lesion of the facial nerve proximal to the geniculate ganglion. It follows facial paralysis and is due to misdirection of regenerating parasympathetic fibers, which formerly innervated the salivary (submandibular and sublingual) glands, to the lacrimal glands.

❑ In **Bell's palsy** (lower motor neuron lesion of facial nerve), both the upper face and lower face muscles are paralysed on the same side (ipsilateral) of the lesion.

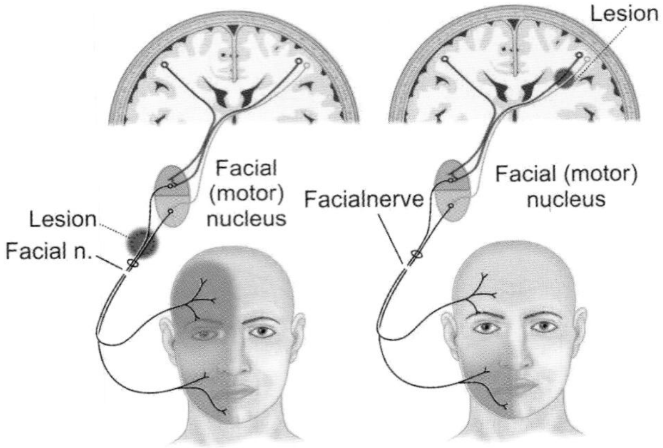

Fig. 27: Upper and lower motor neuron lesions of facial nerve

❑ Left sided **upper motor neuron** lesion result in contralateral (right sided) Facial palsy, where only lower face is involved, since the upper face has bilateral innervation.

  ➤ Lower face muscles like orbicularis oris have only contralateral innervation, as the left cortico-bulbar tract is lesioned, they get paralysed (dribbling of saliva).
  ➤ Upper face muscles like orbicularis oculi are functional, as they are additionally innervated by right cortico-bulbar tract (forehead wrinkles are not impaired.)

1. **All is true about facial colliculus EXCEPT:**
   a. Raised by axons of facial nerve internal genu
   b. Abducent nucleus lies deep to it
   c. Located at the floor of fourth ventricle
   d. Present on the dorsal aspect of upper pons

2. **Lacrimation is lost in lesion of:** (AIIMS May 2013)
   a. Nasociliary nerve
   b. Greater petrosal nerve
   c. Anterior ethmoidal nerve
   d. Supraorbital nerve

3. **Following statements concerning chorda tympani nerve are true EXCEPT:** (AIPG 2005)
   a. Is a branch of facial nerve
   b. Carries secretomotor fibers to submandibular gland
   c. Joins lingual nerve in the infratemporal fossa
   d. Carries post-ganglionic parasympathetic fibers

4. **Nerve to pterygoid canal is formed from:** (NEET Pattern 2012)
   a. Deep petrosal nerve joined by greater petrosal nerve
   b. Facial nerve
   c. Lesser superficial petrosal nerve
   d. Lesser petrosal nerve

5. **Loss of wrinkles on forehead on one side of face is due to:** (NEET Pattern 2016)
   a. Contralateral upper motor neuron facial paralysis
   b. Contralateral lower motor neuron facial paralysis
   c. Ipsilateral upper motor neuron facial paralysis
   d. Ipsilateral lower motor neuron facial paralysis

6. **A patient presents with hyperacusis, loss of lacrimation and loss of taste sensation in the anterior 2/3rd of the tongue. Inflammation extends up to which level of facial nerve:**
   a. Vertical part
   b. Vertical part proximal to nerve to stapedius
   c. Vertical part and beyond nerve to stapedius
   d. Proximal to geniculate ganglion

7. **Nerve of Wrisberg contain:** (PGIC 2013)
   a. Motor fibers
   b. Sensory fibers
   c. Secretory fibers
   d. Parasympathetic fibers
   e. Sympathetic fibers

8. **Arterial supply of facial nerve is/are:** (PGI 2015)
   a. Ascending pharyngeal artery
   b. Middle meningeal artery
   c. Greater palatine artery
   d. Stylomastoid branch of occipital artery
   e. Labyrinthine branch of ethmoidal artery

9. **Structure related to floor of sphenoidal sinus is:** (JIPMER 2017)
   a. Maxillary nerve   b. Mandibular nerve
   c. Vidian nerve   d. Greater petrosal nerve

10. **Greater petrosal nerve is formed from:** (NEET Pattern 2015)
    a. Geniculate ganglion
    b. Plexus around ICA
    c. Plexus around middle meningeal artery
    d. None of the above

1. **Present on the dorsal aspect of upper pons**
   ❑ Facial colliculus is present on the dorsal aspect of lower (not upper) pons.

2. **a. Greater petrosal nerve**
   ❑ Greater petrosal nerve carries the pre-ganglionic para-sympathetic secretomotor (GVE) fibers to the pterygo-palatine ganglion, which relays them to the lacrimal, nasal and palatine glands. Injury of greater petrosal nerve causes dryness in the eyes, nose and palate ipsilaterally.

3. **d. Carries post-ganglionic parasympathetic fibers**
   - ☐ Chorda tympani carries pre-ganglionic (not post-ganglionic) para-sympathetic fibers.
   - ☐ Chorda tympani nerve is a branch of facial nerve given in the facial canal (middle ear cavity) and carries secretomotor fibers to supply the sub-lingual and sub-mandibular salivary glands. It is joined by lingual nerve (branch of mandibular, trigeminal) in the infra-temporal fossa.
   - ☐ Lingual nerve carries the post-ganglionic fibers towards the salivary glands.

4. **a. Deep petrosal nerve joined by greater petrosal nerve**
   - ☐ Vidian nerve of pterygoid canal is formed by the union of greater petrosal nerve (parasympathetic fibers) and deep petrosal nerve (sympathetic fibers).
   - ☐ The nerve is formed at the floor of foramen lacerum and runs anteriorly in pterygoid canal to reach the pterygopalatine ganglion.

5. **d. Ipsilateral lower motor neuron facial paralysis**
   - ☐ Loss of wrinkles on forehead on one side of face is due to Ipsilateral lower motor neuron lesion of facial nerve (e.g., Bell's palsy), leading to frontalis muscle paralysis.
   - ☐ In Bell's palsy, both the upper face and lower face muscles are paralysed on the same side (ipsilateral) of the lesion.
   - ☐ In UMN lesion of facial nerve, contralateral lower face muscles are paralysed. Upper face muscles like frontalis are functional, as they have bilateral innervation.

6. **d. Proximal to geniculate ganglion**
   - ☐ If facial nerve inflammation extends proximal to geniculate ganglion, the clinical features are: Loss of lacrimation (later may present with crocodile syndrome); hyperacusis (loss of stapedial reflex); decreased salivation and loss of taste sensation on anterior 2/3 tongue; paralysis of muscles of facial expression.

7. **b. Sensory fibers; c. Secretory fibers; d. Parasympathetic fibers**
   - ☐ Facial nerve has two parts: motor to facial expression muscles and nervus intermedius.
   - ☐ The motor part carries SVE component, while nervus intermedius carries GSA, SVA, and GVE fibers.
   - ☐ Nervus intermedius (nerve of Wrisberg) carries fibers for taste, salivation, lacrimation, and general sensation (from the external ear).
   - ☐ The first-order sensory neurons are found in the geniculate ganglion within the temporal bone.

8. **a. Ascending pharyngeal artery; b. Middle meningeal artery; d. Stylomastoid branch of occipital artery**
   - ☐ Facial nerve in facial canal is supplied by: Superficial petrosal branch of middle meningeal artery, stylomastoid branch of posterior auricular or occipital arteries.
   - ☐ In extracranially course it is supplied by: Stylomastoid branches of posterior auricular or occipital arteries, superficial temporal, transverse facial and tympanic branch of ascending pharyngeal artery.

9. **c. Vidian nerve**
   - ☐ Vidian nerve lies in the vidian (pterygoid) canal, which is located at the floor of sphenoidal sinus. It is a passage connecting foramen lacerum (posteriorly) to the pterygopalatine fossa (anteriorly). If a fast-growing tumor erodes the floor of the sphenoidal sinus, the vidian nerve could be in danger.

10. **a. Geniculate ganglion**
    - ☐ Greater petrosal nerve is a branch of facial nerve, given at geniculate ganglion, carry a number of axons. Geniculate ganglion has sensory neurons, whose axons travel by greater petrosal nerve.
    - ☐ Sympathetic fibers from the superior cervical ganglion form plexus around the internal carotid artery to contribute to deep petrosal nerve and around middle meningeal artery to reach the otic ganglion.

▶ Glossopharyngeal nerve

- ☐ **Glossopharyngeal nerve** belongs to the third branchial arch and carries the fibers for neural columns SVE (pharyngeal arch muscles), SVA (taste), GVE (secretomotor), GVA (visceral sensations), and GSA (somatic sensations) fibers.
- ☐ Its nuclei are located in **medulla oblongata** and axons leave it at the postolivary sulcus to exit the cranial cavity through the **jugular foramen**.

Glossopharyngeal nerve gives the following branches:
- ☐ **Communicating branch** to join the auricular branch of the vagus nerve and provides general sensation and pain fibers to the ear.
- ☐ **Pharyngeal branch** to carry visceral sensory fibers to the posterior tongue and pharyngeal wall, including the tonsillar bed.

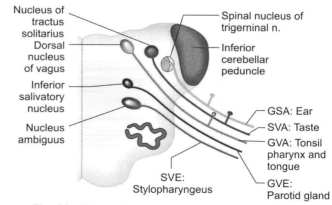

Fig. 28: Glossopharyngeal nerve and neural columns

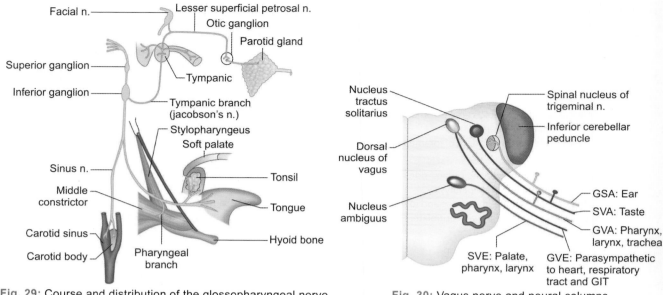

Fig. 29: Course and distribution of the glossopharyngeal nerve

Fig. 30: Vagus nerve and neural columns

> ➤ It joins with the pharyngeal branch of the vagus nerve and branches from the sympathetic trunk to form the **pharyngeal plexus** on the middle constrictor muscle.
> ➤ The sensory fibers mediate the afferent limb of the **gag reflex** (vagus nerve carry efferent limb).

❑ **Carotid sinus branch** to supply baroreceptive and chomoreceptive fibers (GVA) to the carotid sinus and the carotid body. It mediates the afferent limbs of the carotid sinus and body reflexes that can cause a drop in heart rate and blood pressure with carotid massage (vagus nerve carry efferent limb).

❑ Tonsillar branches carry sensory fibers to the **palatine tonsil** and the **soft palate**.

❑ Motor branch carry motor fibers (SVE) to the **stylopharyngeus**.

❑ Lingual branch carry taste and visceral afferent fibers to the **posterior one-third of the tongue** and the **circumvallate papillae**.

❑ **Tympanic Nerve** contributes to the tympanic plexus on the medial wall of the middle ear with sympathetic fibers from the internal carotid plexus (caroticotympanic nerves) and a branch from the geniculate ganglion of the facial nerve.
> ➤ It carries visceral sensory fibers from the tympanic cavity, the mastoid antrum and air cells, and the auditory tube.
> ➤ Its secretomotor axons continue beyond the tympanic plexus as the lesser petrosal nerve in the floor of the middle cranial fossa, which leaves through the foramen ovale to bring preganglionic parasympathetic fibers to the otic ganglion.
> ➤ Postganglionic parasympathetic fibers leave the otic ganglion to innervate the parotid gland.

▶ Vagus Nerve

Vagus Nerve is given by the **medulla oblongata**, comes out of the postolivary sulcus to exit the posterior cranial fossa through the **jugular foramen**.
> ➤ It mediates the afferent and efferent limbs of the **cough reflex** and the efferent limbs of the **gag** and **sneeze reflex**.

❑ **Auricular branch** of vagus nerve is joined by a branch from the glossopharyngeal nerve and the facial nerve and supplies general sensory fibers **(GSA)** to the external acoustic meatus.

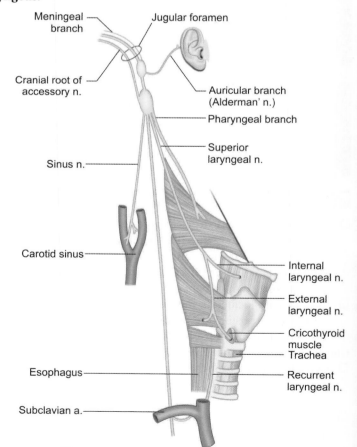

Fig. 31: Vagus nerve course and distribution

❑ The visceral afferent fibers (GVA) are carried from all mucous membranes in the lower pharynx, larynx, trachea, bronchus, esophagus, and thoracic and abdominal visceral organs (except for the descending colon, sigmoid colon, rectum, and other pelvic organs).

❑ It also carries parasympathetic preganglionic innervation (GVE) to **smooth muscles** and **glands** of the pharynx, esophagus, and gastrointestinal track (from the stomach to the transverse colon) as well as for the **cardiac muscle** of the heart.

❑ Vagus nerve contributes to vagus accessory complex and carries motor innervation (SVE) to all muscles of the **larynx**, **pharynx** (except stylopharyngeus), and **palate** (except tensor palati).

❑ **Taste sensations** (SVA) from posteriormost tongue and epiglottis are carried by superior laryngeal nerve (vagus).

❑ **Meningeal branch** arises from the superior ganglion and supplies the dura mater of the **posterior cranial fossa**.

❑ **Pharyngeal branch** supplies motor fibers to the skeletal muscles of the pharynx, by way of the pharyngeal plexus and all muscles of the palate.

❑ **Nerve to the carotid body**, which carry sensations from carotid body and the carotid sinus; superior, middle, and inferior cardiac branches which carry parasympathetic supply toward, and visceral afferent fibers back from, the cardiac plexuses.

❑ **Superior laryngeal nerve** which divides into internal and external branches.

❑ **Recurrent laryngeal nerve** which hooks around the **subclavian artery** on the right and around the **arch of the aorta** lateral to the ligamentum arteriosum on the left to ascends in the groove between the trachea and the esophagus. *(NEET Pattern 2016)*

❑ **Right vagus** nerve forms the **posterior vagal trunk** (or gastric nerves) and left vagus nerve forms the anterior vagal trunk at the lower part of the esophagus and both enter the abdomen through the esophageal hiatus.

QUESTIONS

1. Galen's anastomosis is between   *(NEET Pattern 2013)*
   a. Recurrent laryngeal nerve and external laryngeal nerve
   b. Recurrent laryngeal nerve and internal laryngeal nerve
   c. Internal laryngeal nerve and external laryngeal nerve
   d. None of the above

2. All of the following statements about the vagus nerve are true EXCEPT   *(AIIMS 2005)*
   a. Supplies heart and lung
   b. Carries postganglionic parasympathetic fibers
   c. Innervates right two third of transverse colon
   d. Stimulates peristalsis and relaxes sphincters

ANSWERS

1. **b. Recurrent laryngeal nerve and internal laryngeal nerve**
   ❑ **Galen's anastomosis** is the connecting branch between the inferior laryngeal nerve (a branch of the recurrent laryngeal nerve) and the internal laryngeal nerve (a branch of the superior laryngeal nerve).
   ❑ The internal laryngeal nerve is sensory down to the vocal cords, the recurrent laryngeal nerve is sensory below the vocal cords, and there is overlap between the territories innervated by the two nerves at the vocal cords themselves.

2. **b. Carries postganglionic parasympathetic fibers**
   ❑ Cranial nerve 3, 7, 9 and 10 (vagus) carry the preganglionic (and not post-ganglionic) parasympathetic fibers.
   ❑ It supplies the parasympathetic fibers to lungs and heart, and the GI system till the mid-gut.
   ❑ The right 2/3 of the transverse colon belongs to mid-gut and is supplied by the vagus nerve.
   ❑ Para-sympathetic system is generally evacuatory in nature and stimulates peristalsis and relaxes the sphincters, e.g. stomach empties into duodenum under vagal activity.

❑ Injury to vagus nerve leads to **loss of palate elevation** and the uvula deviates **toward the intact side** (away from the side of the lesion) during phonation.

❑ **Vagus** nerve has the **largest distribution in the body** and contributes about **75% to the parasympathetic** system *(NEET Pattern 2016)*

▶ Accessory Nerve

Accessory nerve has two parts: cranial and spinal.

❑ **Cranial roots** arise from the medulla oblongata below the roots of the vagus.

❑ **Spinal roots** arise from spinal cord C1-5, form a trunk that ascends in the vertebral canal, enter foramen magnum and join the cranial part.

❑ Both pass through the jugular foramen, cranial accessory fibers join the vagus nerve (vagus accessory complex) to innervate the muscles of palate, pharyngeal and larynx.

❑ The spinal accessory nerve supplies **sternocleidomastoid** muscle, lies on levator scapulae in the posterior cervical triangle, then reach and supply **trapezius**.

❑ Spinal accessory nerve may be damaged within the posterior (occipital) triangle due to surgery or a penetrating wound leading to paralysis of the trapezius muscle (resulting in drooping of shoulder and compromised overhead abduction).

▶ Vagus Accessory Complex

Nucleus ambiguus (in medulla oblongata) gives axons to form **cranial part of accessory nerve** which are carried by the vagus nerve (vagus accessory complex) to innervate the muscles of **palate, pharyngeal and larynx**.

❑ Vagus nerve gives pharyngeal branches to pharyngeal plexus (which carry axons of cranial accessory nerve and the plexus itself sends these axons to muscles of palate and pharynx.

❑ All the muscles of palate and pharynx are supplied by the **vagus accessory complex** and **pharyngeal plexus**, with few exceptions: **Tensor palati** (first pharyngeal arch muscle) is supplied by mandibular nerve (trigeminal) and **stylopharyngeus** (third pharyngeal arch muscle) is supplied by glossopharyngeal nerve (neuron bodies in nucleus ambiguus).

Vagus accessory complex:

❑ **Cranial accessory nerve** (neuron bodies in nucleus ambigus) fibers are carried by **vagal** branches to supply muscles of palate, pharynx and larynx.

❑ **Stylopharyngeus** muscle is supplied by the **glossopharyngeal nerve**, fibers arising from nucleus ambigus.

❑ Spinal accessory nerve roots arise from spinal cord, ascends in the vertebral canal, enter foramen magnum and join the cranial part.

❑ Both pass through the jugular foramen, **cranial accessory** fibers **join the vagus** nerve (vagus accessory complex) whereas, the spinal accessory nerve supplies sternocleidomastoid muscle and trapezius.

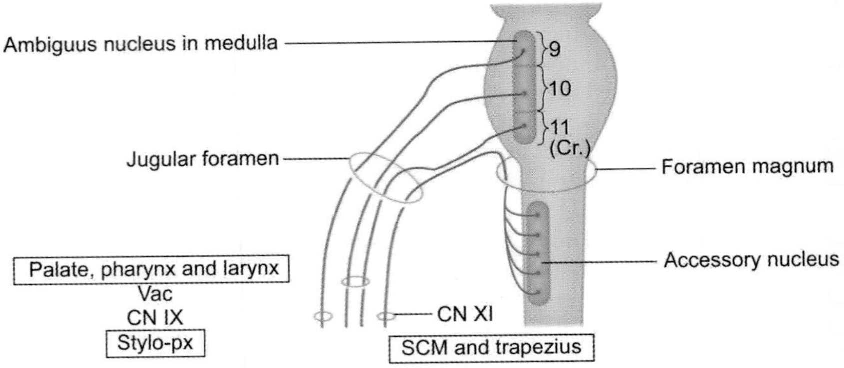

Fig. 32: Vagus - accessory complex

❑ Most of the muscles of the pharynx (including **palatopharyngeus**, **cricopharyngeus**, **salpingopharyngeus**) develop in the fourth pharyngeal arch and are supplied by the cranial part of accessory nerve, whose axons are carried by the vagus nerve through the pharyngeal plexus to the muscles. (vago – accessory complex) (AIIMS 2012)

QUESTIONS

1. Choose the INCORRECT statement concerning pharyngeal plexus:
   a. Receives contributions from vagus nerve carrying cranial accessory nerve component
   b. Supplies all pharyngeal muscles except stylopharyngeus
   c. Supplies tensor tympani
   d. Supply palatoglossus

2. Cranial part accessory nerve supplies all palatal muscles EXCEPT: *(NEET Pattern 2014)*
   a. Palatoglossus
   b. Palatopharyngeus
   c. Tensor veli palati
   d. Levator palati

ANSWERS

1. **c. Supplies tensor tympani**
   ❑ Tensor tympani muscle develops in first pharyngeal arch and is supplied by the mandibular nerve (trigeminal).
   ❑ Vagus nerve carry axons of cranial accessory nerve (vagus accessory complex) and gives pharyngeal branches to pharyngeal plexus. This plexus sends the axons to muscles of palate and pharynx.
   ❑ All the muscles of palate and pharynx are supplied by the vagus accessory complex and pharyngeal plexus, with few exceptions like stylopharyngeus (CN IX) and tensor tympani (CN V).
   ❑ Palatoglossus is a tongue muscle supplied by CN XI (cranial accessory nerve) and not by CN XII (hypoglossal nerve).

2. **c. Tensor veli palati**
   ❑ Most of the muscle of palate are supplied by cranial accessory nerve (via vagus accessory complex) except few.
   ❑ Tensor veli palate develops in first pharyngeal arch and supplied by mandibular branch of trigeminal nerve.

▼ Hypoglossal Nerve

Hypoglossal nerve is given by the **medulla oblongata** ventrally in the preolivary sulcus and passes through the **hypoglossal canal** to exit the cranial cavity.

❑ It loops around the occipital artery and the carotid bifurcation (**in carotid triangle**) to pass between the carotids and internal jugular vessels. Next it runs deep to the digastric posterior belly and stylohyoid muscles to enter the **submandibular triangle**.

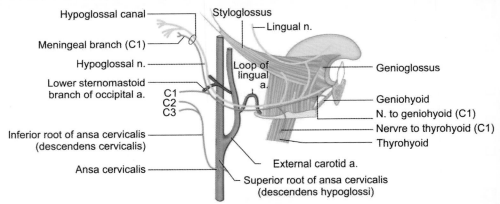

Fig. 33: Hypoglossal nerve course and distribution

❑ Between mylohyoid and hyoglossus, the hypoglossal nerve lies below the deep part of the submandibular gland, the submandibular duct and the lingual nerve, with which it communicates.

❑ It then passes on to the lateral aspect of genioglossus, continuing forwards in its substance as far as the tip of the tongue.

- Hypoglossal nerve carries sensory fibers from C1 to supply the **cranial dura mater** through the meningeal branch; to supply the **upper root of the ansa cervicalis** and the nerve to both the **thyrohyoid and geniohyoid** muscles.
- It supplies motor fibers to all of the intrinsic and extrinsic muscles of the tongue **except the palatoglossus** (which is supplied by the vagus accessory complex)
- Complete hypoglossal division causes unilateral lingual paralysis and eventual **hemiatrophy**.
- Protruded tongue **deviates to the paralyzed side**: Genioglossus muscle normally moves the tongue anterior, inferior and medial (AIM). Since muscle on the affected side is paralyzed, the normal (unaffected) muscle becomes unopposed and pushes the tongue further across the midline, and tongue deviates to the side of the lesion.
- The **larynx may deviate towards the active side** in swallowing: Hypoglossal nerve also carries the C-1 fibers to supply few muscles in the neck region, like hyoid depressors. These muscles get paralysed in nerve lesion and larynx may deviate towards the active side during swallowing.

QUESTIONS

1. **Palsy of right genioglossus causes:**
   a. Deviation of tongue to right
   b. Deviation of tongue to left
   c. Deviation of soft palate to right
   d. Deviation of soft palate to left

2. **In complete unilateral damage to Hypoglossal nerve, all are true EXCEPT:** *(AIIMS 2012)*
   a. Tongue atrophy on affected side
   b. Deviation of tongue towards the site of lesion
   c. Deviation of larynx to the contralateral side during swallowing
   d. Loss of tactile sensation on affected side

ANSWERS

1. **a. Deviation of tongue to right**
   - Genioglossus muscle moves the tongue anterior (protrusion), inferior (depression) and medial (AIM).
   - In bilateral contraction of genioglossus, the vector of medial pull is balanced (and cancelled), and there occurs protrusion and depression of tongue in midline.
   - Palsy of right genioglossus muscle deviates the tongue to the right side, due to unopposed medial pull of the left genioglossus.

2. **d. Loss of tactile sensation on affected side**
   - Tactile sensation of tongue is not carried by the hypoglossal nerve, hence there will be no such loss on the tongue.
   - Hypoglossal nerve is a pure motor nerve and supplies the tongue muscles. Lesion of the hypoglossal nerve causes unilateral lingual paralysis and eventual hemiatrophy. The protruded tongue deviates to the paralysed side, due to unopposed activity (medial pull) of the opposite (normal) side genioglossus muscle.
   - Hypoglossal nerve also carries the C-1 fibers to supply few muscles in the neck region, like hyoid depressors. These muscles get paralysed in nerve lesion and larynx may deviate towards the active side during swallowing.

▶ Cervical Sympathetic trunk

Cervical part of sympathetic trunk lies on either side of cervical vertebral column in front of the transverse processes of cervical vertebrae and neck of the 1st rib **behind the carotid sheaths**.

- The cervical sympathetic trunk ganglia receive preganglionic fibers from neurons whose cell bodies that lie in the intermediolateral column of the upper thoracic (T1-4) spinal cord; there is no preganglionic output from the cervical spinal cord.
- Postganglionic fibers reach their target tissues in the head and neck via the cervical spinal nerves and perivascular nerve plexuses distributed along the carotid and vertebral arteries.
- It has 3 cervical ganglia: Superior, middle, and inferior. They are formed by the fusion of 8 primitive ganglia, corresponding to eight cervical nerves.

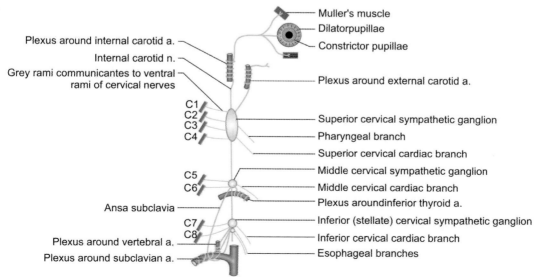

Fig. 34: Cervical sympathetic trunk, ganglia and branches

- ❏ **Superior cervical ganglion** (the largest) lies in front of the transverse processes of vertebrae C1 to C2, posterior to the internal carotid artery and anterior to the longus capitis.
  - ➤ It gives the internal carotid nerve to form the internal carotid plexus (and supply **superior tarsal muscle** and **dilator pupillae** muscles). The fibers also contribute to the formation of **deep petrosal nerve**.
  - ➤ It also gives the external carotid nerve to form the external carotid plexus; the pharyngeal branches to the **pharyngeal plexus**; and the **superior cervical cardiac nerve** to the heart.
- ❏ Middle cervical ganglion lies at the level of the cricoid cartilage (vertebra C6), just above the inferior thyroid artery.
  - ➤ It gives **middle cervical cardiac nerve**, which is the largest of the three cervical sympathetic cardiac nerves.
- ❏ Inferior cervical ganglion gets fused with the first thoracic ganglion to become the **cervicothoracic (stellate) ganglion**.
  - ➤ It lies in front of the neck of the first rib and the transverse process of vertebra C7 and behind the dome of the pleura and the vertebral artery.
  - ➤ It gives the **inferior cervical cardiac nerve**.
- ❏ Ansa subclavia connects the middle and inferior cervical sympathetic ganglia, forming a loop around the first part of the subclavian artery.
- ❏ It contains preganglionic and postganglionic sympathetic fibers, cell bodies of the post-ganglionic sympathetic fibers, and visceral afferent fibers with cell bodies in the upper thoracic dorsal root ganglia.
- ❏ Sympathetic chain gives gray rami communicantes but **receives no white rami communicantes** in the cervical region.

Cervical Sympathetic Ganglia

Characteristic features	Superior cervical ganglion	Middle cervical ganglion	Inferior cervical ganglion
Location	In front of the transverse processes of vertebrae C1,2	At the level of the cricoid cartilage (vertebra C6)	In front of the neck of the first rib and the transverse process of vertebra C7
Formed by the fusion of primitive cervical ganglia	1-4	5,6	7,8
Grey rami communicantes to ventral rami of cervical nerves	C1-4	C5,6	C7,8
Perivascular sympathetic plexus along	▪ Internal carotid artery ▪ External carotid artery	Inferior thyroid artery	Vertebral artery Subclavian artery
Branches along cranial nerves	Along cranial nerves IX,X,XI and XII		
Visceral branches	▪ Superior cervical cardiac nerve ▪ Pharyngeal plexus	▪ Middle cervical cardiac nerve ▪ Thyroid ▪ Tracheo-esophageal	Inferior cervical cardiac nerve

▼ Cervical Plexus

The upper 4 cervical **ventral rami** form the cervical plexus, whose branches collectively innervate the **infrahyoid strap muscles** and the **diaphragm**, and the skin covering the lateral and anterior parts of the neck, and the **angle of the mandible**.
Note: Some authors also mention upper part of fifth cervical ventral ramus contributing to cervical plexus.

- ❏ It gives unnamed branches to longus capitis and colli, sternocleidomastoid, trapezius, levator scapulae, and scalene muscles.
- ❏ Named branches are cutaneous and motor

Cutaneous Branches:
- ❏ **Lesser occipital nerve** (C2) ascends along the posterior border of the sternocleidomastoid to the scalp behind the auricle
- ❏ **Great auricular nerve** (C2–C3) ascends on the sternocleidomastoid to innervate the skin on auricle, behind the auricle and on the parotid gland. It also supplies the **skin on the angle of mandible**.
- ❏ **Transverse cervical nerve** (C2–C3) innervates the skin of the anterior triangle of neck.
- ❏ **Supraclavicular nerve** (C3–C4) divides into anterior, middle, and lateral branches to supply the skin over the clavicle and the shoulder.

Motor Branches:
- ❏ **Ansa cervicalis** is a nerve loop formed by the union of the superior root (C1 or C1 and C2; descendens hypoglossi) and the inferior root (C2 and C3; descendens cervicalis).
  - ➤ It is **embedded on the anterior wall** of carotid sheath in the anterior triangle of neck.
  - ➤ It innervates the strap muscles, such as the omohyoid, sternohyoid, and sternothyroid muscles (**except thyrohyoid and geniohyoid** muscles, which are supplied by C1 fibers, carried by hypoglossal nerve).
- ❏ **Phrenic nerve** takes origin from the C3-5 (chiefly C4) carries motor, sensory, and sympathetic fibers.
- ❏ Accessory phrenic nerve (C5) may occasionally be found, descends lateral to the phrenic nerve, enters the thorax by passing posterior to the subclavian vein, and joins the phrenic nerve below the first rib to supply the diaphragm.

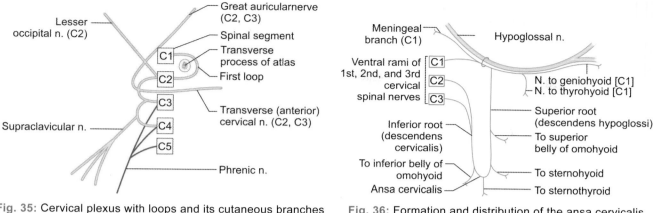

Fig. 35: Cervical plexus with loops and its cutaneous branches   Fig. 36: Formation and distribution of the ansa cervicalis

1. Ansa cervicalis supplies: *(JIPMER 2010)*
   a. Sternohyoid   b. Mylohyoid
   c. Cricothyroid   d. Stylohyoid

2. Superior cervical ganglia give gray rami communicates to:
   a. C1-C4   b. C5-C6 *(NEET Pattern 2012)*
   c. C7-C8   d. None

1. a. Sternohyoid
   ❑ Ansa cervicalis supplies numerous anterior neck muscles including sternohyoid.
   ❑ Mylohyoid develops in first pharyngeal arch and is supplied by the inferior alveolar nerve (mandibular nerve; trigeminal).
   ❑ Cricothyroid develops in fourth pharyngeal arch and is supplied by external laryngeal nerve branch of superior laryngeal nerve (vagus).
   ❑ Stylohyoid muscle develops in second pharyngeal arch and is supplied by the facial nerve.

2. a. C1-C4
   ❑ Superior cervical ganglia give gray rami communicates to C1-4 spinal nerves.
   ❑ Middle cervical ganglia give gray rami to C5,6 and inferior to C7,8 spinal nerves.

▶ Reflexes

Corneal blink reflex is closure of the eyelids in response to blowing on the cornea or touching it with a wisp of cotton.
❑ Its afferent limb is the **nasociliary nerve** (branch of the ophthalmic division trigeminal nerve) and efferent limb is the **facial nerve** (reflex arc).
❑ It leads to bilateral contraction of the **orbicularis oculi** muscles and a momentary closure of the eyelids.

Masseter reflex (jaw jerk) is elicited by hitting the mentum (mandible) down with the help of a knee hammer.
❑ It is a **proprioceptive** reflex carried by the **mandibular (trigeminal) nerve** towards the **mesencephalic sensory nucleus** of trigeminal, the fibers then reaching the **motor nucleus** of trigeminal in the pons.
❑ Motor fibers carried by the **trigeminal mandibular nerve** activates the **masseter** muscle in turn, which leads to **elevation** of the mandible.
❑ It is the only **monosynaptic reflex** are present in the brain.

Gag reflex (pharyngeal reflex) is the brisk and brief elevation of the soft palate and bilateral contraction of pharyngeal muscles evoked by touching the posterior pharyngeal wall.
❑ It helps prevent objects from entering the throat except as part of normal swallowing and helps prevent choking.
❑ Sensory limb is mediated predominantly by CN IX (glossopharyngeal nerve) and the motor limb by CN X (vagus nerve).

Stapedius reflex (acoustic reflex) is the contraction of **stapedius** muscle on exposure to **high-intensity sound** stimulus.
❑ The stapedius stiffens the ossicular chain by pulling the stapes of the middle ear away from the oval window of the cochlea, which decreases the transmission of vibrational energy to the cochlea and prevent inner ear injury.
❑ The afferent nerve is CN VIII (**cochlear nerve**) and the efferent is **facial nerve**.
❑ Neural impulses from the auditory nerves (CN VIII) ascend from both cochleae to each ipsilateral ventral cochlear nucleus (VCN). VCN send fibers to the **superior olivary complex** (SOC) before the impulses cross at the brainstem to innervate both ipsilateral and contralateral facial motor nuclei.

1. Proprioceptive impulses for masseter reflex are carried to which nucleus of trigeminal nerve   *(AIPG 2008)*
   a. Mesencephalic   b. Sensory
   c. Motor   d. Spinal

2. Which of the following reflexes test the integrity of nucleus ambiguus
   a. Jaw jerk   b. Stapedial reflex
   c. Gag reflex   d. Corneal reflex

3. Afferent component in corneal reflex is mediated by
   (NEET Pattern 2012)
   a. Optic nerve   b. Ophthalmic nerve
   c. Facial nerve   d. Oculomotor nerve

4. Centre for Stapedial reflex   *(AIIMS 2016)*
   a. Superior olivary complex   b. Lateral lemniscus
   c. Inferior colliculus   d. Medial geniculate body

ANSWERS

1. a. Mesencephalic
- ❑ **Mesencephalic nucleus** of trigeminal nerve receives the **proprioceptive** information of masseter reflex and integrates with the motor nucleus to produce contraction of jaw elevators.
- ❑ Masseter reflex is a mono-synaptic reflex where hitting on the mentum produces rapid stretching of the muscles like masseter and the jaw gets closed.
- ❑ **Main sensory** nucleus of trigeminal is chiefly concerned with the **tactile reception**, whereas, **spinal nucleus** receives the sensations of **pain and temperature**.

2. c. Gag reflex
- ❑ Gag reflex: Contraction of the constrictor muscle of the pharynx elicited by touching the back of the pharynx.

3. b. Ophthalmic nerve
- ❑ Corneal (blink) reflex is closure of the eyelids in response to touching it with a wisp of cotton.
- ❑ Its afferent limb is the **nasociliary nerve** of the ophthalmic division of the trigeminal nerve and efferent limb is the **facial nerve** (reflex arc).
- ❑ It leads to bilateral contraction of the **orbicularis oculi** muscles and a momentary closure of the eyelids.

4. a. Superior olivary complex
- ❑ Acoustic (stapedial) reflex: In response to **loud sound** contraction of the stapedius muscle stiffens the middle ear ossicles and tilts the **stapes in the oval window** of the cochlea; this effectively **decreases the vibrational energy** transmitted to the cochlea.
- ❑ The best known reflex mediated through the **superior olive** is the stapedius reflex.

▼ Cranial Nerve Injuries

QUESTIONS

1. Lacrimation is affected in injury of: (AIIMS 2010)
   a. Nasociliary nerve   b. Greater petrosal nerve
   c. Lesser petrosal nerve   d. Auriculotemporal nerve

2. Which nerve is responsible for referred pain in ear:
                                                 (NEET pattern 2012)
   a. Trochlear   b. Olfactory
   c. Glossopharyngeal   d. Abducent

3. A patient presented with vesicles in upper eye lid, forehead and nose on the right side of face consistent with herpes zoster. Which of the following nerves is likely involved:
                                                 (JIPMER 2016)
   a. Supraorbital nerve   b. Supratrochlear nerve
   c. Lacrimal nerve   d. Ophthalmic nerve

4. Which of the following clinical finding is NOT seen in lesions of structures passing through jugular foramen?
   a. Palatal paralysis   (JIPMER 2016)
   b. Difficulty in shrugging of shoulder
   c. Loss of sensation from the floor of mouth
   d. Loss of taste sensation in posterior 1/3rd of tongue

5. Injury to which of the following nerve in the diagram, may affect respiratory movements: (AIIMS 2016)
   a. A
   b. B
   c. C
   d. D

ANSWERS

1. b. Greater petrosal nerve
- ❑ Greater petrosal nerve carries the preganglionic parasympathetic fibers to the pterygopalatine ganglion, which relays them to the lacrimal, nasal and palatine glands.
- ❑ Injury of greater petrosal nerve causes dryness in the eyes, nose and palate ipsilaterally.
- ❑ Nasociliary nerve carries sensory fibers like corneal sensations.
- ❑ Lesser petrosal nerve carries the pre-ganglionic parasympathetic fibers to the otic ganglion, which relays them to the parotid gland.
- ❑ Auriculotemporal nerve carries the post-ganglionic parasympathetic fibers from otic ganglion, to the parotid gland.

2. c. Glossopharyngeal
- ❑ Glossopharyngeal nerve supplies the ear region and oral cavity region as well.
- ❑ Any pathology of the oral region may present with referred pain to the ear region.

3. d. Ophthalmic nerve
- ❑ Ophthalmic nerve (trigeminal nerve) supplies the forehead region, upper eyelid and nose and the presentation is consistent with the herpes spread along the course of the nerve.

4. c. Loss of sensation from the floor of mouth
- ❑ Sensations from the floor of mouth is carried by branches of trigeminal nerve, which is not involved in this lesion.
- ❑ Jugular foramen lets pass the cranial nerves 9, 10 and 11.
- ❑ These nerves supply the muscles of palate, pharynx and larynx, along with trapezius and sternocleidomastoid muscles.
- ❑ Difficulty in shrugging the shoulder is due to paralysis of trapezius muscles supplied by spinal accessory nerve.
- ❑ Loss of taste sensation in posterior 1/3rd of tongue is due to injury of glossopharyngeal nerve.

ANSWERS

5. a. A

- Injury to **phrenic nerve** (marker 'A') compromises **diaphragm** (and respiratory movements).
- Phrenic nerve ('A') is identified running anterior to **scalenus anterior** muscle.
- **Key**: B - Sympathetic chain; C - Vagus nerve; D - Recurrent laryngeal nerve.
- In this diagram, sternocleidomastoid muscle has been removed to expose contents of carotid sheath.
- Carotid sheath contains vagus nerve lying between (and posterior to) two vessels: internal jugular vein (lateral) and common carotid artery (medial).
- Sympathetic chain ('B') is identified lying posteromedial to carotid sheath (and the common carotid artery).
- Vagus nerve ('C') is identified between the two vessels (internal jugular vein and common carotid artery) lying posteriorly.
- Recurrent laryngeal nerve ('D') is a branch of vagus nerve, loops under the right subclavian artery and ascends superiorly, lying in tracheo-esophageal groove.

▼ Miescellaneous

QUESTIONS

1. Buccinator muscle is pierced by all EXCEPT

(AIIMS 2008, 15)

- a. Buccal branch of facial nerve/artery
- b. Mucus gland of buccopharyngeal fascia
- c. Parotid duct
- d. Buccal branch of mandibular nerve

2. Which of the following is a WRONG pair regarding features of cranial nerves:

- a. Most commonly involved in basal skull fracture: Facial nerve
- b. Most commonly involved in raised intracranial tension: Abducent nerve
- c. Most commonly affected in spinal anaesthesia: Abducent nerve
- d. Most commonly involved in intracranial aneurysm: Optic Nerve

3. Choose the INCORRECT statement about cranial nerves:

- a. Abducent has the longest intracranial course
- b. Trochlear shows internal decussation
- c. Olfactory is the shortest
- d. Vagus has largest distribution

ANSWERS

1. d. Buccal branch of facial nerve

- Buccal branch of facial nerve **supplies buccinator** but **doesn't pierce** it.
- Buccinator muscle is 'not' pierced by buccal branch of facial nerve (**or artery**).
- **Buccal branch** of mandibular nerve **does pierce** the buccinator muscle, to reach and supply the **mucous membrane** on inner cheek.
- **Molar mucous glands** of buccopharyngeal fascia **pierce** the buccinator muscle to reach the oral cavity.
- **Parotid duct** runs to the anterior border of masseter, winds round it and **pierces the buccinator** muscle, to enter the oral cavity.

2. d. Most commonly involved in intracranial aneurysm: Optic nerve

- Most commonly involved in intracranial aneurysm is **occulomotor** nerve

3. a. Abducent has the longest intracranial course

- Trochlear nerve has the **longest intracranial** course. It has **internal decussation** and supplies **contralateral** superior oblique muscle.
- **Olfactory** nerve has **shortest** length.
- Vagus nerve has the **largest distribution in the body** (supplies head, neck, thorax, abdomen).

▼ Muscles in the Head and Neck region

Table 6: Cutaneous and superficial muscles of neck

Muscle	Superior attachment	Inferior attachment	Innervation	Main action(s)
Platysma	Inferior border of mandible, skin, and subcutaneous tissues of lower face	Fascia covering superior parts of pectoralis major and deltoid muscles	Cervical branch of facial nerve (CN VII)	Draws corners of mouth inferiorly and widens it as in expressions of sadness and fright; draws skin of neck superiorly when teeth are clenched
Sternocleidomastoid (SCM)	Lateral surface of mastoid process of temporal bone and lateral half of superior nuchal line	*Sternal head:* anterior surface of manubrium of sternum *Clavicular head:* superior surface of medial third of clavicle	Spinal accessory nerve (CN X1, motor); C2 and C3 nerves (pain and proprioception)	*Unilateral contraction:* tilts head to same side (i.e., laterally flexes neck) and rotates it so face is turned superiorly toward opposite side *Bilateral contraction:* (1) extends neck at atlantooccipital joints, (2) flexes cervical vertebrae so that chin approaches manubrium, or (3) extends superior cervical vertebrae while flexing inferior vertebrae so chin is thrust forward with head kept level With cervical vertebrae fixed, may elevate manubrium and medial ends of clavicles, assisting pump-handle action of deep respiration

Sternocleidomastoid muscle takes its origin from sternum and clavicle, inserts into the mastoid process and superior nuchal line. It is supplied by the spinal accessory nerve. It turns it to the opposite side and tilts the head to the same side *(NEET Pattern 2016)*

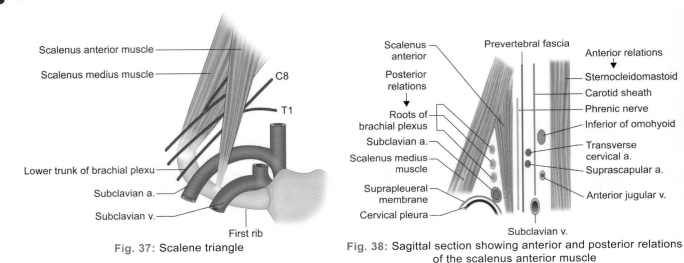

Fig. 37: Scalene triangle

Fig. 38: Sagittal section showing anterior and posterior relations of the scalenus anterior muscle

Scalene anterior muscle has **origin** from transverse processes of C3–C6 vertebrae and **insertion** into 1st rib. It is supplied by **cervical spinal nerves C4–C6** and causes **flexion of head**.

❑ **Relations** of scalenus anterior muscle:
  ➢ Anterior—Phrenic nerve, **subclavian vein,** carotid sheath, **transverse cervical artery** and suprascapular artery, prevertebral fascia, clavicle
  ➢ Posterior—**subclavian artery**, pleura, roots of brachial plexus
  ➢ Lateral—Brachial plexus.
❑ The subclavian vein and phrenic nerve pass anteriorly to the anterior scalene as the muscle crosses over the first rib. The phrenic nerve is oriented vertically as it passes in front of the anterior scalene, while the subclavian vein is oriented horizontally as it passes in front of the anterior scalene muscle.
❑ The **interscalene triangle** is present between the scalenus anterior muscle, the scalenus medius muscle and the first rib. The subclavian artery and the brachial plexus pass through this gap (subclavian vein runs anterior to scalenus anterior muscle and lies outside the triangle).
❑ A **narrow** interscalene triangle compresses the brachial plexus and subclavian artery (**scalene syndrome**) causing paresthesia, more rarely circulatory disturbances (e.g. edema, ischemia) and pain. Typically, the ulnar side and the little finger are affected.

QUESTIONS

1. **Deep injury of neck always involves:** (NEET Pattern 2015)
   a. Platysma
   b. Trapezius
   c. Sternocleidomastoid
   d. Longus colli

2. **FALSE about scalenus anterior muscle:** (NEET Pattern 2015)
   a. Covered by prevertebral fascia
   b. Related anteriorly to phrenic nerve
   c. Inserts in inner part of 1st rib
   d. Forms floor of posterior triangle

3. **TRUE statement is:**
   a. Buccinator is a muscle of mastication
   b. Digastric is an elevator of mandible
   c. Omohyoid is a suprahyoid muscle
   d. Oral diaphragm is formed by mylohyoid muscle

4. **Which suprahyoid muscle is supplied by both facial nerve and mandibular nerve:** (NEET Pattern 2012)
   a. Stylohyoid   b. Thyrohyoid
   c. Digastric   d. Stylohyoid

5. **All of the following are true about Scalenus anterior muscle EXCEPT** (AIIMS 2010)
   a. It is attached to the scalene tubercle of second rib   b. It is anterior to the transverse cervical artery
   c. It is pierced by the phrenic nerve   d. It separates the subclavian vein from the subclavian artery

ANSWERS

1. **a. Platysma**
   ❑ Platysma is a thin muscular sheet that surrounds the superficial fascia of the neck, and its integrity determines whether a PNT (penetrating neck injury) is superficial or deep. The possibility for injury to a vital organ exists when this structure is penetrated.

2. **d. Forms floor of posterior triangle**
   ❑ Phrenic nerve runs on the anterior surface of scalenus anterior muscle, covered by prevertebral fascia.
   ❑ Scalenus anterior inserts on the first rib but is not at the floor of posterior triangle of neck.
   ❑ Muscles at the floor are: Scalenus medius, levator scapulae, splenius capitis, semispinalis capitis.

3. **d. Oral diaphragm is formed by mylohyoid muscle**
   ❑ Buccinator is a muscle of facial expression (IInd pharyngeal arch; facial nerve).
   ❑ Digastric muscle pulls the mandible down on hyoid bone (depressor of mandible) to open the mouth.
   ❑ Omohyoid takes origin from scapula and insert into hyoid bone, is an infrahyoid muscle.
   ❑ Oral diaphragm is the floor of the oral cavity formed by mylohyoid muscle.

4. **c. Digastric**
   ❑ Mandibular nerve supplies anterior belly of digastric (Ist arch) and facial nerve supplies posterior belly of digastric (IInd arch).

5. a. It is attached to the scalene tubercle of second rib
- ❏ Scalenus anterior (and scalenus medius) both attach to first rib (and 'not' second).
- ❏ Phrenic descends anterior of the muscle from the lateral to the medial side (but nerve fibers may pierce the muscle **occasionally**).
- ❏ Scalenus anterior muscle is sandwiched between subclavian artery from subclavian vein and separates the two vessels. (But as a variation, the muscle may be present posterior to the artery **sometime**).
- ❏ Transverse cervical artery passes anterior to the scalenus anterior muscle (but may be found running posterior as a **variation**). Scalenus anterior muscle is considered to be an important surgical landmark in the neck region.

❏ Mandibular nerve supplies anterior belly of digastric (Ist arch) and facial nerve supplies posterior belly of digastric (IInd arch).

❏ **Styloid apparatus** is found within the parapharyngeal space, refers to the structures derived from the 2nd branchial arch along with associated ligaments and muscles: styloid process of the temporal bone, lesser horn of the hyoid bone, stylohyoid ligament, stylomandibular ligament and stylohyoid, styloglossus and stylopharyngeus muscles.

Arterial Supply in Head and Neck Region

▸ Carotid Arteries

Right common carotid artery begins at the bifurcation of the brachiocephalic artery, and the left common carotid artery, arises from the aortic arch.

❏ Common carotid artery ascends within the **carotid sheath** and divide at the level of the **upper border of the thyroid cartilage** into the external and internal carotid arteries.

❏ **Carotid pulse**: The common carotid artery pulsations may be readily felt beneath the **anterior border of sternocleidomastoid**.

❏ It is compressed against the anterior tubercle of transverse process of the 6th cervical vertebrae called carotid tubercle (**Chassaignac tubercle**) by pressing medially and posteriorly with the thumb.

❏ It is about 4 cm above the sternoclavicular joint at the level of cricoid cartilage.

❏ **Carotid body** Is a chemoreceptor lying at the bifurcation of the common carotid artery.

❏ **Carotid sinus** is a pressoreceptor (baroreceptor) presenting as a dilatation located **at the origin** of the internal carotid artery, to detect the blood pressure and can bring about a slowing of the heart rate, vasodilation and decrease in blood pressure.

Internal sarotid artery has **no branches** in the neck, ascends within the **carotid sheath** in company with the internal jugular vein and vagus nerve, enters the cranium through the **carotid canal** in the petrous part of the temporal bone. It supplies most of the ipsilateral cerebral hemisphere, eye and accessory organs, the forehead and, in part, the external nose, nasal cavity and paranasal sinuses.

External carotid artery extends from the level of the upper border of the thyroid cartilage to the neck of the mandible, where it ends in the parotid gland into two terminal branches the maxillary and superficial temporal arteries.

❏ It gives 8 branches: Anterior (3): Superior thyroid artery, lingual artery, facial artery; posterior (2): Occipital artery, posterior auricular; Medial (1): Ascending pharyngeal and Terminal (2): Maxillary, superficial temporal.

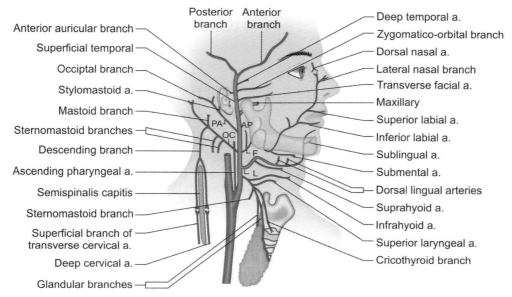

Fig. 39: Branches of External carotid artery

- **Superior thyroid artery** is the **first branch** of external carotid artery, given below the level of the greater horn of the hyoid bone, descends obliquely in the carotid triangle and passes deep to the infrahyoid muscles to reach the superior pole of the thyroid gland.
- **Lingual artery** originates at the level of the tip of the greater horn of the hyoid bone and passes deep to the hyoglossus to reach the **tongue**. It gives branches like dorsal lingual, sublingual, and deep lingual arteries.
- **Ascending pharyngeal artery** is a medial branch from the deep surface of the external carotid artery in the carotid triangle, ascends between the internal carotid artery and the wall of the pharynx. It gives branches to pharynx, palate, **tonsils** and **eustachian tube**.
- **Occipital artery** is a posterior branch given just above the level of the hyoid bone, passes deep to the digastric posterior belly, occupies the groove on the mastoid process, and appears on the skin above the occipital triangle.
- **Posterior auricular artery** is also a posterior branch, ascends superficial to the styloid process and deep to the parotid gland and ends between the mastoid process and the external acoustic meatus.
- **Superficial temporal artery** arises behind the neck of the mandible as the smaller terminal branch of the external carotid artery and ascends anterior to the external acoustic meatus into the scalp. Its pulse can be taken immediately anterior to the tragus of the pinna. It is accompanied by the auriculotemporal nerve along its anterior surface. It gives the transverse facial artery, which passes forward across the masseter between the zygomatic arch above and the parotid duct below. It divides into frontal and parietal branches approximately 2.5 cm above the zygomatic arch.

▶ Subclavian Artery

Subclavian artery is a branch of the **brachiocephalic trunk on the right** but arises **directly from the arch of the aorta** on the **left**. It is divided into **three parts** that are successively anterior, deep and lateral to **scalenus anterior** muscle, third part passes from the lateral margin of the muscle to the outer border of the first rib.

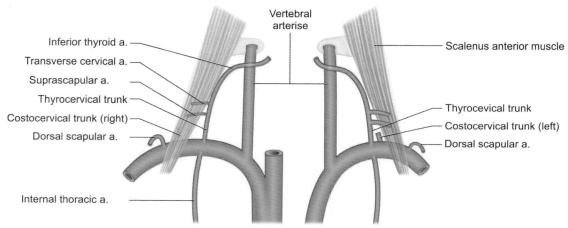

Fig. 40: Subclavian artery and branches

- First part of subclavian artery gives three branches (VIT): V - **Vertebral**, I – **Internal thoracic** artery, T - **Thyrocervical** trunk.
- Second part gives **Costocervical trunk**
- Third part gives **Dorsal scapular artery**
- Thyrocervical trunk itself gives three branches (SIT): S - **Suprascapular** artery, I - **Inferior thyroid** artery, T - **Transverse cervical** artery.

Branches

- **Suprascapular artery** passes in **front** of the scalene anterior muscle and the brachial plexus parallel to but below the transverse cervical artery. Then it passes **superior** to the superior transverse scapular ligament, whereas the suprascapular nerve passes inferior to this ligament.
- **Inferior thyroid artery** ascends in **front** of the scalene anterior muscle, turns medially behind the carotid sheath but in front of the vertebral vessels, and then arches downward to the **lower pole of the thyroid gland**. It gives ascending cervical artery, which ascends on the anterior scalene muscle medial to the phrenic nerve.
- **Transverse cervical artery** runs laterally across the anterior scalene muscle, phrenic nerve, and trunks of the brachial plexus, passing deep to the trapezius. It divides into a superficial branch and a deep branch, which **occasionally** takes the place of the dorsal (descending) scapular artery.
- **Internal Thoracic artery** arises from the first part of the subclavian artery, descends through the thorax behind the upper six costal cartilages, and ends at the sixth intercostal space by dividing into the **superior epigastric** and **musculophrenic** arteries.

- ❏ **Costocervical trunk** arises from the posterior aspect of the **second part** of the subclavian artery behind the scalene anterior muscle and divides into the following arteries:
  - ➤ **Deep cervical artery** passes between the transverse process of vertebra C7 and neck of the first rib, ascends between the semispinalis capitis and semispinalis cervicis muscles, to anastomose with the deep branch of the descending branch of the occipital artery.
  - ➤ **Superior intercostal artery** descends posterior to the cervical pleura anterior to the necks of the first two ribs and gives the **first two posterior intercostal arteries**.
- ❏ **Dorsal (descending) Scapular** artery is 'usually' given by the **third part** of the subclavian artery. Occasionally it may be replaced by the deep (descending) branch of the transverse cervical artery.

▶ Vertebral Artery

- ❏ **Vertebral artery** arises from the **first part** of subclavian artery, ascends between the scalene anterior and longus colli muscles.
- ❏ It passes through **foramina transversaria** of the upper 6 cervical vertebrae (C1 to C6), **posterior arch of atlas** and lies in suboccipital **triangle.**
- ❏ Next it passes through the posterior atlantooccipital membrane, **vertebral canal**, pierce duramater and arachnoid mater to enter the **subarachnoid space** and passes **through foramen magnum** to enter the cranial cavity.
- ❏ Two vertebral arteries join to form the **basilar artery**.

Subclavian steal syndrome: Subclavian stenosis results in **upper limb ischemia**, and it may steal blood flow from the circle of Willis, into the arm, especially during **heavy manual exercise** of the ipsilateral arm. It may increase demand on vertebral flow, producing posterior circulation TIAs. Blood flow from the carotid, circle of Willis, and basilar circulation is diverted through the vertebral artery into the subclavian artery and into the arm, causing vertebrobasilar insufficiency and thus brain stem ischemia and stroke.

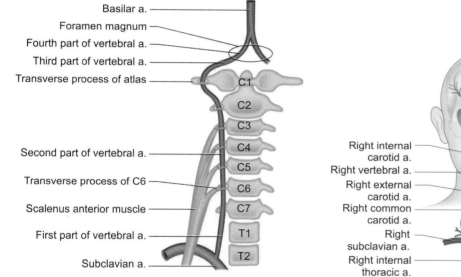

Fig. 41: Vertebral artery origin and course

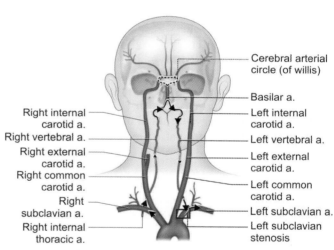

Fig. 42: Subclavian steal syndrome

Subclavian steal syndrome. Thrombosis of the proximal part of the subclavian artery (left) results in **retrograde blood flow through the ipsilateral vertebral artery** and into the left subclavian artery. Blood can be **shunted** from the **right** vertebral artery and down the **left vertebral** artery. Blood may also reach the left vertebral artery through the **carotid circulation**.

▶ Maxillary Artery

Maxillary artery is the larger **terminal** branch of external carotid artery given at the posterior border of the ramus of the mandible, runs deep to the neck of the mandible and enters the infratemporal fossa.

- ❏ It is divided into **three parts**:
  - ➤ 1st (**Mandibular**) part runs anteriorly between the neck of the mandible and the sphenomandibular ligament.
  - ➤ 2nd (**Pterygoid**) part runs anteriorly deep to the temporalis and superficial or deep to the lateral pterygoid muscle. Branches supply chiefly the muscles of mastication.
  - ➤ 3rd (**Pterygopalatine**) part runs between the two heads of the lateral pterygoid muscle and then through the pterygomaxillary fissure into the pterygopalatine fossa.

- ❑ **Middle meningeal artery** is a branch of **1st part**, passes through foramen spinosum, may be damaged in skull fracture at pterion, leading to extra (epi) dural hematoma.
- ❑ **Lower teeth** are supplied by **1st part** of maxillary artery — inferior alveolar branches.
- ❑ **Upper teeth** are supplied by **3rd part** — superior alveolar arteries.

Table 7: Branches of the maxillary artery			
	First part	**Second part**	**Third part**
Branches	Five	Four	Six
1.	Deep auricular artery	Deep temporal	Posterior superior alveolar (dental) artery
2.	Anterior tympanic artery	Pterygoid branches	Infraorbital artery
3.	Middle meningeal artery	Masseteric artery	Greater palatine artery
4.	Accessory meningeal artery	Buccal artery	Pharyngeal artery
5.	Inferior alveolar artery		Artery of pterygoid canal
6.			Sphenopalatine artery

- ❑ **Inferior alveolar artery**: Descends to enter mandibular canal of mandible via mandibular foramen; supplies mandible and upper teeth.
- ❑ **Posterior superior alveolar artery**: Descends on maxilla's infratemporal surface with branches traversing alveolar canals to supply maxillary molar and premolar teeth, adjacent gingiva, and mucous membrane of maxillary sinus.
- ❑ **Inferior orbital artery**: Traverses **inferior orbital fissure** and runs at the floor of orbit; supplies lacrimal sac, upper teeth (maxillary canines and incisors).

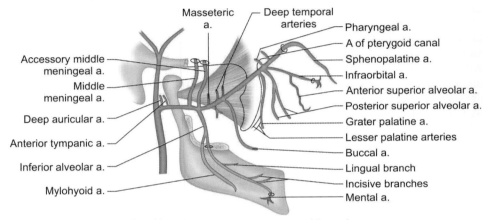
Fig. 43: Maxillary artery course and branches

- ❑ **Descending palatine artery**: Descends through palatine canal, dividing into greater and lesser palatine arteries to mucosa and glands of hard and soft palate.
- ❑ **Sphenopalatine artery**: Terminal branch of maxillary artery, traverses sphenopalatine foramen to supply walls and septum of nasal cavity; frontal, ethmoidal, sphenoid, and maxillary sinuses; and anterior most palate.

QUESTIONS

1. FALSE about subclavian artery: *(NEET Pattern 2016)*
   a. On left side arises from arch of aorta
   b. On right side arises from brachiocephalic trunk
   c. Vertebral artery arises from 2nd part
   d. Divided by scalenus anterior muscle into three parts

2. WRONG statement about branches of external carotid artery is:
   a. Anterior ethmoidal artery is a branch
   b. Maxillary artery is a terminal branch
   c. Ascending pharyngeal artery is a medial branch
   d. Superior thyroid artery is the first branch

3. Exposure of left subclavian artery by supraclavicular approach does NOT require cutting of: *(AIIMS 2007)*
   a. Sternocleidomastoid   b. Scalenus anterior
   c. Scalenus medius   d. Omohyoid

4. Which of the following is NOT a branch of first part of maxillary artery: *(NEET Pattern 2012)*
   a. Greater palatine artery   b. Middle meningeal artery
   c. Deep auricular artery   d. Inferior alveolar artery

5. Posterior superior alveolar artery is a branch of: *(NEET Pattern 2014)*
   a. Nasal branch of maxillary artery
   b. Palatal branch of maxillary artery
   c. Mandibular artery
   d. Inferior alveolar artery

6. In subclavian steal syndrome there is reversal of blood flow in:
   a. Ipsilateral vertebral artery
   b. Contralateral vertebral artery
   c. Ipsilateral subclavian artery
   d. Contralateral subclavian artery

7. First branch of external carotid artery: *(NEET Pattern 2016)*
   a. Superior thyroid artery
   b. Inferior thyroid artery
   c. Ascending pharyngeal artery
   d. Thyroid ima artery

8. Sternocleidomastoid is NOT supplied by the artery: *(AIIMS 2008)*
   a. Superior thyroid   b. Thyrocervical trunk
   c. Occipital   d. Posterior auricular artery

9. Which structure can be felt at the lower part of the medial border of sternocleidomastoid: *(NEET Pattern 2014)*
   a. Subclavian artery   b. Common carotid artery
   c. Internal mammary artery d. Maxillary artery

10. Most common site of subclavian artery stenosis is in part: *(AIPG 2009)*
   a. 1st   b. 2nd
   c. 3rd   d. Terminal

QUESTIONS

11. **Third part of vertebral artery is related to which marked area in the following diagram** *(AIIMS 2017)*
   a. A
   b. B
   c. C
   d. D

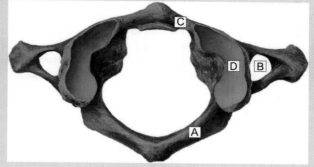

ANSWERS

1. **c. Vertebral artery arises from 2nd part**
   - ❏ Vertebral artery arises from 1st part of subclavian artery.
   - ❏ On the left side subclavian artery comes directly off the aortic arch, while on the right side it arises from the brachiocephalic trunk. It is divided by scalenus anterior muscle into three parts.

2. **a. Anterior ethmoidal artery is a branch**
   - ❏ Ophthalmic artery gives anterior ethmoidal artery which enters the anterior ethmoid foramen in the medial wall of the orbit and supplies the ethmoidal air sinuses, medial and lateral wall of nasal cavity, and dura mater.

3. **c. Scalenus medius**
   - ❏ Scalenus medius muscle lies postero-inferior to subclavian artery and is not required to be cut.

4. **a. Greater palatine artery**
   - ❏ Greater palatine artery is the continuation of descending palatine artery, which itself is the terminal branch of third part of maxillary artery.

5. **b. Palatal branch of maxillary artery**
   - ❏ Posterior superior alveolar artery arises from third part of maxillary artery just before it enters the pterygomaxillary fissure.
   - ❏ It supplies the molar and premolar teeth and mucus membrane of maxillary air sinus.
   - ❏ There is no proper option available, palatal branch appears to be most suitable for palatal (upper) teeth.

6. **a. Ipsilateral vertebral artery**
   - ❏ In subclavian steal syndrome there is retrograde flow in the vertebral artery due to an ipsilateral subclavian artery block.
   - ❏ The block results in lower pressure in the distal subclavian artery and upper limb ischemia. Consequently, blood flows from the contralateral vertebral artery to the basilar artery and then in a retrograde direction down the ipsilateral vertebral artery away from the brainstem.

7. **a. Superior thyroid artery > c. Ascending pharyngeal artery**
   - ❏ The first branch of external carotid artery is usually the superior thyroid artery, though sometimes it could be ascending pharyngeal artery (a variation).

8. **d. Posterior auricular artery**
   - ❏ It's a wrong questions, since all the four arteries mentioned supply the muscle sternocleidomastoid.
   - ❏ Posterior auricular artery has been taken as the best answer as per the latest Journals published.
   - ❏ Upper third: Occipital artery.
   - ❏ Middle third: Superior thyroid artery (53%), the external carotid artery (27%), or both (20%).
   - ❏ Lower third: Suprascapular artery (73%), Transverse cervical artery (7%), the thyrocervical trunk (13%), or the superficial cervical artery (7%).

9. **b. Common carotid artery**
   - ❏ Common carotid artery may be compressed against the prominent transverse process of the sixth cervical vertebra (Chassaignac's carotid tubercle), which sits lateral to the cricoid cartilage.
   - ❏ Above this level, the artery is superficial, and its pulsation may be readily felt beneath the anterior border of sternocleidomastoid.
   - ❏ Subclavian pulsations may be detected behind the clavicle at the lateral border of sternocleidomastoid or where it crosses the first rib.

10. **a. 1st**
   - ❏ Subclavian artery is most commonly obstructed in the proximal portion -1st part proximal to the origin of vertebral and internal thoracic artery. It is focal and is usually an extension of atherosclerotic narrowing from the aortic arch into the artery.
   - ❏ The stenosis is more common on left side - Left subclavian is involved 3 times more frequently involved than the right.
   - ❏ Subclavian artery stenosis proximal to the vertebral artery leads to subclavian steal syndrome.

11. **a. A**
   - ❏ The given diagram is atlas vertebra (superior view) and marker A shows the posterior arch of atlas, which is related to the third part of vertebral artery.
   - ❏ Key: Marker B: Foramen transversarium; C: Anterior arch; D: Superior articular facet.

▶ **Meninges and Venous drainage of Cranium**

There are three concentric membranes (meninges) that envelop the brain and spinal cord.
- ❏ The outermost layer is **dura mater** (pachymeninx) and inner are **arachnoid and pia mater** (leptomeninges).

❑ The cranial dura mater is a two-layered membrane consisting of the external **periosteal** layer (i.e., the endosteum of the neurocranium) and the internal **meningeal** layer, which is continuous with the dura of the vertebral canal and forms dural infoldings (or reflections) that divide the cranial cavity into compartments and accommodates the **dural venous sinuses**.

❑ Arachnoid mater is separated from the pia mater by the **subarachnoid space**, which contains cerebrospinal fluid (CSF) and enlarges at several locations to form **subarachnoid cisterns**.

❑ The arachnoid projects **arachnoid villi** (collections of which are called arachnoid granulations) into the cranial venous sinuses (like superior sagittal sinus), which serve as sites where **CSF reabsorption** into the venous blood.

❑ **Diploic veins** lie in the diploe of the skull and are connected with the cranial dura sinuses by the emissary veins.

❑ **Emissary veins** are the small veins connecting the venous sinuses of the dura with the diploic veins and the veins on the outside of the skull.

The cerebral arteries that run in the subarachnoid space penetrate the pia mater as they enter the brain, whereby the pia mater is reflected onto the surface of the cerebral artery continuous with the tunica adventitia.

Vasculature of the Dura

❑ The arterial supply of the dura mater is by the **middle meningeal artery** (branch of maxillary artery), which divides into an anterior branch and a posterior branch.

❑ The venous drainage of the dura mater is by middle meningeal veins, which drain into the pterygoid venous plexus.

Innervation of dura mater

❑ It is derived mainly from three sources: 1) Three divisions of **trigeminal** nerve, 2) C2 & 3 spinal nerves and 3) Cervical sympathetic trunk.

❑ **Vagus** and **hypoglossal** nerves, and possibly the facial and glossopharyngeal nerves may also supply duramater (less established).

❑ The supratentorial dura is supplied by the meningeal branches from the three divisions of the trigeminal nerve.

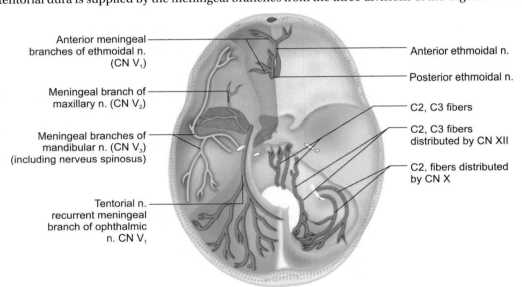

Anterior meningeal branches of ethmoidal n. (CN V₁)

Meningeal branch of maxillary n. (CN V₂)

Meningeal branches of mandibular n. (CN V₃) (including nerveus spinosus)

Tentorial n. recurrent meningeal branch of ophthalmic n. CN V₁

Anterior ethmoidal n.

Posterior ethmoidal n.

C2, C3 fibers

C2, C3 fibers distributed by CN XII

C2, fibers distributed by CN X

Fig. 44: Nerve supply of duramater

The infratentorial dura is supplied by ascending meningeal branches of C2 and 3 spinal nerves.

❑ Anterior cranial fossa: Meningeal branches of the anterior and posterior ethmoidal nerves (**ophthalmic** division of trigeminal nerve. and few additional branches of **maxillary** division of trigeminal nerve.

❑ Middle cranial fossa: Meningeal branch of the **maxillary** nerve (in the anterior part) and the **mandibular** nerve (nervus spinosus) in the posterior part.

❑ Posterior cranial fossa: Meningeal branches of the **vagus** and **hypoglossal** nerves, carrying the C1 and C2 fibers to supply the dura.

Dural Folds

❑ **Falx cerebri** is a sickle (crescent) shaped double fold of duramater that lies between the two cerebral hemispheres in the longitudinal fissure.

   ➤ Anteriorly the falx is fixed to the **crista galli**, and posteriorly it blends with the tentorium cerebelli; the **straight sinus** runs along this line of attachment to the tentorium.

   ➤ The **superior sagittal sinus** runs in upper attached margin, lower edge is free and concave, and contains the **inferior sagittal sinus**.

- Tentorium cerebelli is a tent-shaped fold of the dura mater forming the **roof** of the posterior cranial fossa.
  - It supports the **occipital lobes** of the cerebral hemispheres and **covers the cerebellum**.
  - It has two margins and two surfaces. Inner free margin is U-shaped and encloses the **tentorial notch** for the passage of the midbrain.
  - Venous sinuses enclosed in the tentorium cerebelli
- Transverse sinus, within the posterior part of the attached margin.
- Superior petrosal sinus, within the anterolateral part of the attached margin.
- **Falx cerebelli** is a small sickle-shaped dural fold in the sagittal plane projecting forward into the posterior cerebellar notch between the cerebellar hemispheres. **Occipital sinus** run along with its posterior attached part.
- **Diaphragma sellae** is a small circular horizontal fold of the inner (meningeal) layer of the dura mater forming the roof of the hypophyseal fossa **covering the pituitary gland**.

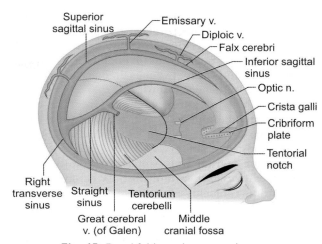

Fig. 45: Dural folds and venous sinuses

Table 8: Dural infoldings and the enclosed sinuses		
Dural fold	**Shape**	**Dural venous sinus enclosed**
Falx cerebri	Sickle shaped, separates right and left cerebral hemisphere	Superior sagittal , inferior sagittal , straight sinuses
Tentorium cerebelli	Tent shaped (semilunar), separates occipital lobes of cerebrum from cerebellum	Transverse and superior petrosal sinuses
Falx cerebelli	Sickle shaped, extends between cerebellar hemispheres	Occipital sinus
Diaphragma sellae	Horizontal fold forms the roof of the sella turcica covering the hypophysis	Anterior & posterior Intercavernous sinuses

Venous drainage of brain:

There are deep (internal) cerebral veins and superficial (external) cerebral veins in the brain.

- **Deeper circulation**:
  - Paired **internal cerebral veins** (deep cerebral veins) drain the deep parts of the hemisphere. They are formed near the interventricular foramen by the union of the thalamostriate vein and choroid veins.
  - They unite to form the **great cerebral vein of Galen**; just before their union each receives the corresponding **basal vein**.
  - Most of the blood in the deep cerebral veins collects into the great cerebral vein, which **empties into the straight sinus** located in the midline of the tentorium.
- **Superficial circulation**:
  - **Superior cerebral veins** (eight to twelve) drain the superior, lateral, and medial surfaces of the hemispheres into the **superior sagittal sinus**.
  - **Inferior cerebral veins** are veins **drain the under surface of** the cerebral hemispheres and empty into the **cavernous** and **transverse** sinuses. Those on the temporal lobe anastomose with the middle cerebral and basal veins, and join the cavernous, sphenoparietal, and superior petrosal sinuses.

Dural venous sinuses are **intradural** spaces present between the external (periosteal layer) and the internal (meningeal layer) of the dura mater, or between duplications of the meningeal layers, containing venous blood drained from the cranial cavity. They may be paired or unpaired.

- **Basilar plexus** consists of interconnecting venous channels on the basilar part of the occipital bone and connects the two inferior petrosal sinuses. It communicates with the **internal vertebral venous plexus**.
- **Sphenoparietal sinus** lies along the posterior edge of the lesser wing of the sphenoid bone and **drains into the cavernous sinus**.
- Diploic, meningeal veins and cortical veins drain into **superior sagittal sinus**.

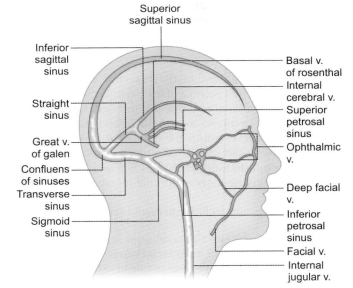

Fig. 46: Dural venous sinuses and connections

- ❏ **Two internal cerebral veins** unite behind the brainstem to form midline **great cerebral vein of Galen**.
- ❏ Vein of Galen receives **inferior sagittal sinus** and continues as **straight sinus** (in midline).
- ❏ **Straight sinus** (deeper venous drainage of brain) drains into the **confluence of sinuses**.
- ❏ **Confluence of sinuses** lies at internal occipital protuberance and receive three incoming channels (tributaries) **SOS**: Straight sinus, Occipital sinus and Superior sagittal sinus.
- ❏ **Superior sagittal sinus** enters the confluence of the sinuses (torcula), where the falx cerebri meets the tentorium cerebelli.
- ❏ **Transverse sinus** run in the attached margin of the tentorium cerebelli and drains venous blood from the confluence of sinuses to the sigmoid sinus. Usually the right, is directly continuous with the superior sagittal sinus, and the left with the straight sinus.

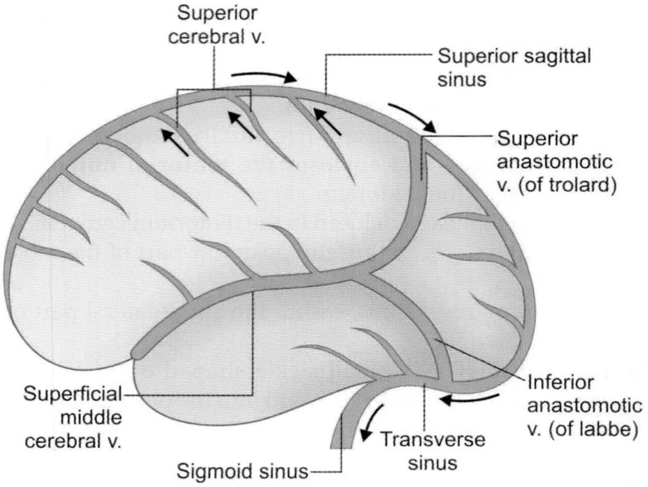

Fig. 47: Cerebral veins and connections

- ❏ **Sigmoid sinus** drains into the internal jugular vein at the jugular foramen.
- ❏ **Superior petrosal sinus** drains the cavernous sinus into the **transverse sinus** on either side.
- ❏ **Inferior petrosal sinus** is the first tributary to internal jugular vein.
- ❏ Superior petrosal sinus leaves the posterosuperior part of the cavernous sinus and runs posterolaterally in the **attached margin of the tentorium cerebelli.**
- ❏ The largest cortical vein that connects the superficial Sylvian (**middle cerebral**) vein and the **superior sagittal sinus** is the superior anastomotic vein (vein of **Trolard**).
- ❏ **Vein of Labbe** (inferior anastomotic vein) is part of the superficial cerebral veins of the brain.
- ❏ It crosses and anastomoses at its two ends with the **middle cerebral vein** and the **transverse sinus**.
- ❏ It drains its adjacent cortical regions gathering tributaries from minor veins of the temporal lobe (**not** superior cerebral veins).

◤ Cavernous Sinus

- ❏ **Cavernous sinus** is a dural venous sinus that lie on either side of the body of the sphenoid bone, in the middle cranial fossa, extending from the superior orbital fissure to the apex of the petrous temporal bone.
  - ➢ The cavity of the cavernous sinus is formed when the two layers of duramater split and enclose itself within.
  - ➢ The floor of the sinus is formed by the **endosteal** layer, while the lateral wall, roof, and medial wall by the **meningeal** layer.
  - ➢ Medially, the roof is continuous with the diaphragm sellae.

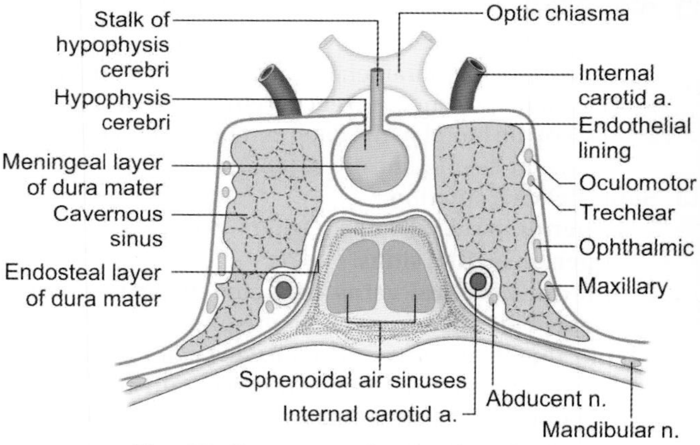

Fig. 48: Cavernous sinus and contents

Contents

- ❏ Cavernous segment of the **internal carotid artery**, associated with a perivascular **T1 sympathetic plexus**.
- ❏ Cranial nerves that run forwards through the cavernous sinus to enter the orbit via the superior orbital fissure are (above downwards) **oculomotor, trochlear** and the **ophthalmic nerve**, maxillary nerve (all lie in the lateral wall of the sinus).
- ❏ **Abducens** nerve enters the cavernous sinus by passing within a dural tunnel (Dorello's canal) and then runs on the **inferolateral** side of the horizontal portion of the cavernous carotid artery, just medial to the ophthalmic nerve.
- ❏ **Inferior ophthalmic vein** begins in a venous network at the forepart of the floor and medial (not lateral) wall of the orbit.
- ❏ It either joins the superior ophthalmic vein or passes through the superior orbital fissure to drain directly into the cavernous sinus.
- ❏ It communicates with the pterygoid venous plexus by a branch (not the parent vein) that passes through the inferior orbital fissure.
- ❏ Infections from face can send septic emboli into the cavernous sinus via **superior ophthalmic veins** (usually), **inferior ophthalmic veins** or **deep facial veins**.
- ❏ **Cavernous sinus pathology** may lead to ptosis (paralysed levator palpebrae superior), proptosis (protrusion of eyeball due to venous congestion), chemosis (swelling of the conjunctivae), periorbital edema, and extraocular dysmotility causing diplopia secondary to a combination of third, fourth and sixth cranial nerve palsies.

Table 9: Tributaries and draining channels for cavernous sinus	
Tributaries (incoming channels)	**Draining channels (outgoing channels/communications)**

▪ Brain
   – Superficial middle cerebral vein
   – Inferior cerebral vein
▪ Meninges
   – Sphenoparietal sinus
   – Anterior (frontal) trunk of middle meningeal vein
▪ Orbit
   – Superior ophthalmic vein
   – Inferior ophthalmic vein
   – Central vein of retina (occasionally)
	▪ Transverse sinus (via superior petrosal sinus)
	▪ Internal jugular vein (via inferior petrosal sinus)
	▪ Pterygoid plexus of veins (through emissary veins)
	▪ Superior ophthalmic vein
	▪ Facial vein (through pterygoid plexus & superior ophthalmic vein)
	▪ Maxillary vein (through pterygoid venous plexus)
	▪ Intercavernous sinuses
	▪ Basilar plexus of veins

Gray's Anatomy Ed 41

Unlike the ophthalmic nerve, the maxillary nerve does not run through the cavernous sinus or its lateral wall, but courses beneath the dura of the middle cranial fossa below the level of the cavernous sinus.

> Sensory disturbances in the territory of **ophthalmic** and **maxillary** divisions of the trigeminal nerve are observed and a decreased corneal reflex may also be detected, sluggish pupillary responses (due to damage of sympathetic and parasympathetic nerves).

> There may be evidence of dilated, tortuous retinal veins and papilledema.

> Any spreading infection involving the **dangerous area of face**, may lead to **septic thrombosis** of the cavernous sinuses; infected thrombus (usually *Staphylococcus*) pass from the facial vein or pterygoid venous complex into the sinus via either ophthalmic veins or emissary veins that enter the cranial cavity through the foramen ovale.

Dangerous triangle of the face includes area from the corners of the mouth to the bridge of the nose, including the nose and maxilla. It also includes upper nasal cavities, paranasal sinuses, cheek (especially near the medial canthus), upper lip, anterior nares, or even an upper incisor or canine tooth.

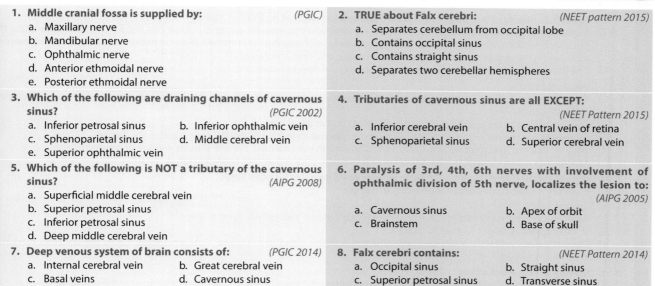

Fig. 49: Connections of cavernous sinus

❑ Venous communication between the facial vein and the cavernous sinus (via the **ophthalmic veins** and **deep facial vein**) may lead to retrograde spread of infections into the cranial cavity causing cavernous sinus thrombosis, meningitis or brain abscess.

❑ The **valveless** nature of the veins connecting the cavernous sinus causes easy spread of infection.

QUESTIONS

1. Middle cranial fossa is supplied by: *(PGIC)*
   a. Maxillary nerve
   b. Mandibular nerve
   c. Ophthalmic nerve
   d. Anterior ethmoidal nerve
   e. Posterior ethmoidal nerve

2. TRUE about Falx cerebri: *(NEET pattern 2015)*
   a. Separates cerebellum from occipital lobe
   b. Contains occipital sinus
   c. Contains straight sinus
   d. Separates two cerebellar hemispheres

3. Which of the following are draining channels of cavernous sinus?   *(PGIC 2002)*
   a. Inferior petrosal sinus   b. Inferior ophthalmic vein
   c. Sphenoparietal sinus   d. Middle cerebral vein
   e. Superior ophthalmic vein

4. Tributaries of cavernous sinus are all EXCEPT: *(NEET Pattern 2015)*
   a. Inferior cerebral vein   b. Central vein of retina
   c. Sphenoparietal sinus   d. Superior cerebral vein

5. Which of the following is NOT a tributary of the cavernous sinus?   *(AIPG 2008)*
   a. Superficial middle cerebral vein
   b. Superior petrosal sinus
   c. Inferior petrosal sinus
   d. Deep middle cerebral vein

6. Paralysis of 3rd, 4th, 6th nerves with involvement of ophthalmic division of 5th nerve, localizes the lesion to: *(AIPG 2005)*
   a. Cavernous sinus   b. Apex of orbit
   c. Brainstem   d. Base of skull

7. Deep venous system of brain consists of: *(PGIC 2014)*
   a. Internal cerebral vein   b. Great cerebral vein
   c. Basal veins   d. Cavernous sinus
   e. Straight sinus

8. Falx cerebri contains: *(NEET Pattern 2014)*
   a. Occipital sinus   b. Straight sinus
   c. Superior petrosal sinus   d. Transverse sinus

9. All are true about diploic veins EXCEPT: *(AIPG 2008)*
   a. Lined by single layer endothelium supported by elastic tissue
   b. Present in cranial bones
   c. Valveless
   d. Develop by 8th week of IUL

10. All of the following statements are true regarding cavernous sinus thrombosis EXCEPT: *(AIIMS 2014)*
   a. Loss of jaw jerk
   b. Inferior ophthalmic vein can spread infection from dangerous area of face
   c. Ethmoidal sinusitis is the most common cause
   d. Loss of sensation around the eye

11. Which is NOT true about cranial duramater? *(AIIMS 2014)*
   a. It has periosteal and meningeal layers
   b. It is supplied by 5th cranial nerve
   c. It is the outermost meningeal layer
   d. Dural venous sinuses are present inner to the meningeal layer

12. Among the following, content of cavernous sinus is:
   a. Maxillary division of trigeminal nerve   *(AIIMS 2014)*
   b. Ophthalmic division of trigeminal nerve
   c. Trochlear nerve
   d. Internal carotid artery

13. Which of the following is a direct content of cavernous sinus?
   a. Occulomotor nerve
   b. Trochlear nerve
   c. Maxillary branch of trigeminal
   d. Abducent nerve

14. TRUE about vein of Labbe: *(JIPMER 2017)*
   a. Drains into superior sagittal sinus
   b. Drains into transverse sinus
   c. Anastomotic channel for superior cerebral veins
   d. Superior anastomotic channel for superficial middle cerebral vein

15. TRUE statement(s) about inferior ophthalmic vein is/are: *(PGIC 2017)*
   a. Begins near the orbital floor and lateral wall
   b. Communicates with pterygoid venous plexus
   c. Drains into cavernous sinus
   d. Passes through superior orbital fissure
   e. Passes through inferior orbital fissure

16. Septic emboli in facial vein can cause cavernous sinus thrombosis because facial vein makes clinically important connections with the cavernous sinus. The most commonly involved communicating vein is:
   a. Superior ophthalmic
   b. Deep facial
   c. Inferior ophthalmic
   d. Pterygoid plexus of veins

1. a. Maxillary nerve; b. Mandibular nerve; c. Ophthalmic nerve
   ❑ Middle cranial fossa is supplied by meningeal branch of the maxillary nerve (in the anterior part) and the mandibular nerve in the posterior part. Medially ophthalmic nerve gives sensory branches.

2. c. Contains straight sinus
   ❑ Falx cerebri is a sickle shaped dural fold which separates right and left cerebral hemisphere and contains superior sagittal, inferior sagittal and straight sinuses in it.
   ❑ Tentorium cerebelli separates cerebellum from occipital lobes of cerebrum.
   ❑ Falx cerebelli is a sickle shaped dural fold that extends between and separate two cerebellar hemispheres and contains occipital sinus in its posterior attached part.

3. a. Inferior petrosal sinus; e. Superior ophthalmic vein
   ❑ Cavernous sinus drains by various outgoing channels including inferior petrosal sinus.
   ❑ Superior ophthalmic vein has bidirectional flow and is a tributary and a draining channel as well.

4. d. Superior cerebral vein
   ❑ Superior cerebral veins (eight to twelve) drain the superior, lateral, and medial surfaces of the hemispheres into the superior sagittal sinus.

5. d. Deep middle cerebral vein
   ❑ Deep middle cerebral vein doesn't get connected to the cavernous sinus directly.
   ❑ Superficial middle cerebral vein drains into the cavernous sinus at its anterior aspect.
   ❑ Superior and inferior petrosal sinuses are actually drainage channels for cavernous sinus but just for the sake of handling this peculiar questions, we may consider them as tributaries of cavernous sinus (when in some pathology, the intracranial pressure increases in the posterior cranial fossa and the venous drainage is reversed).
   ❑ The dural venous sinuses are valveless and the blood can flow in either direction.

6. a. Cavernous sinus
   ❑ Cranial nerves 3, 4, 6 and the ophthalmic division of trigeminal pass through the cavernous sinus together and hence any pathology in the sinus can involve all of them.
   ❑ Optic canal lies at the apex of orbit and cranial optic nerve lies there.
   ❑ Brainstem has the nerve nuclei of last 10 cranial nerves and its lesion will produce more elaborate damage.
   ❑ Base of skull has many nerves in its relation and any lesion here damage the mandibular division of trigeminal also.
   ❑ Mandibular nerve escapes the lesions of cavernous sinus, since it does not pass through it.

7. a. Internal cerebral vein; b. Great cerebral vein; c. Basal veins; e. Straight sinus
   ❑ Cavernous sinus comes under superficial circulation.

8. b. Straight sinus
   ❑ Falx cerebri is a double fold of duramater containing superior and inferior sagittal sinus.
   ❑ It also contains straight sinus at the base.
   ❑ Occipital sinus runs in the falx cerebelli, whereas superior petrosal sinus and transverse sinus run in the attached margin of tentorium cerebelli.

9. d. Develop by 8th week of IUL
   ❑ Diploic veins start developing in the cranial bones at about 2 years of age and are fully developed at the age of 35 years.
   ❑ These are lined by a single layer endothelium supported by elastic tissue and are valveless.

10. a. Loss of jaw jerk
- ❏ Cavernous sinus thrombosis does not involve the mandibular nerve of trigeminal, hence jaw jerk is intact.

11. d. Dural venous sinuses are present inner to the meningeal layer
- ❏ Dural venous sinuses are intradural spaces present between the external (periosteal layer) and the internal (meningeal layer) of the dura mater, or between duplications of the meningeal layers, containing venous blood drained from the cranial cavity.
- ❏ Dural venous sinuses are outer to meningeal layer and inner to endosteal layer.
- ❏ Inner to the meningeal layer of duramater is subdural space.

12. d. Internal carotid artery
- ❏ Cavernous sinus contains the cavernous segment of the internal carotid artery, associated with a perivascular T1 sympathetic plexus.
- ❏ The cranial nerves that run forwards through the cavernous sinus enter the orbit via the superior orbital fissure.
- ❏ In this questions all the options are ANSWERS, though the first choice preferably is internal carotid artery.

13. d. Abducent nerve
- ❏ The abducens nerve enters the cavernous sinus by passing within a dural tunnel (Dorello's canal) and then runs on the inferolateral side of the horizontal portion of the cavernous carotid artery, just medial to the ophthalmic nerve.
- ❏ Oculomotor nerve, trochlear nerve and maxillary branch of trigeminal lie in the lateral wall of cavernous sinus.

14. b. Drains into transverse sinus
- ❏ Superficial middle cerebral vein communicates with the transverse sinus via inferior anastomotic vein of Labbe).
- ❏ The vein of Labbe is inferior (not superior) anastomotic vein, which crosses and anastomoses at its two ends with the middle cerebral vein and the transverse sinus (not superior sagittal sinus). It drains its adjacent cortical regions gathering tributaries from minor veins of the temporal lobe (not superior cerebral veins).

15. b. Communicates with pterygoid venous plexus; c. Drains into cavernous sinus; d. Passes through superior orbital fissure
- ❏ Inferior ophthalmic vein begins in a venous network at the forepart of the floor and medial (not lateral) wall of the orbit. It either joins the superior ophthalmic vein or passes through the superior orbital fissure to drain directly into the cavernous sinus.
- ❏ It communicates with the pterygoid venous plexus by a branch (not the parent vein) that passes through the inferior orbital fissure.

16. a. Superior ophthalmic
- ❏ Most commonly involved vein to carry septic emboli in facial vein to cavernous sinus is **superior ophthalmic vein**.

- ▪ Superior sagittal sinus lies in the midline structure called falx cerebri and is unpaired *(NEET 2012)*
- ▪ Superior petrosal sinus is a draining channel for cavernous sinus *(NEET Pattern 2014)*
- ▪ Great cerebral vein of Galen is joined by the inferior sagittal sinus to drain into the straight sinus *(NEET Pattern 2015)*
- ▪ Superior cerebral veins (eight to twelve) drain the superior, lateral, and medial surfaces of the hemispheres into the superior sagittal sinus *(NEET pattern 2014)*
- ▪ Superficial middle cerebral vein runs along the lateral sulcus draining most of the temporal lobe into the sphenoparietal sinus or cavernous sinus *(NEET pattern 2016)*
- ▪ Abducent nerve lies infero-lateral to the internal carotid artery inside the cavernous sinus *(NEET Pattern 2016)*
- ▪ Two internal cerebral veins on each side unite to form the great cerebral vein of Galen in the midline *(NEET Pattern 2012)*

❏ **Superior ophthalmic vein** has **bidirectional** blood flow and is a **tributary** to the cavernous sinus and a **draining channel** as well. It drains venous blood of orbit into the cavernous sinus and vice versa.

Hemorrhages within the head area include: Epidural hemorrhage, subdural hemorrhage, subarachnoid hemorrhage.

❏ **Epidural** hemorrhage is caused by a **skull fracture** near the **pterion** and is associated with the middle cranial fossa.
- ➢ **Middle meningeal artery** is ruptured, and blood is collected between the skull and dura mater.
- ➢ It presents with a **medical emergency** and a **lucid interval** for a few hours is followed by death if not attended to.
- ➢ CT scan reveals a lens-shaped (**biconvex**) hyperdensity adjacent to bone.
- ➢ It is a classic medical emergency that requires a craniotomy (**burr holes**) for blood clot evacuation and coagulation of the ruptured vessel.

❏ **Subdural hemorrhage** is caused by a violent shaking of the head and commonly occurs in alcoholics and elderly.
- ➢ It is **venous bleed** from superior cerebral veins (**bridging veins**) and blood is located between the dura and arachnoid.
- ➢ CT scan shows a thin, **crescent-shaped** hyperdensity that hugs the contours of the brain; blood accumulates slowly (days to weeks after trauma).

❏ **Subarachnoid hemorrhage** is caused by a contusion or laceration injury to the brain or a **berry aneurysm**.
- ➢ CT scan shows arterial blood with the subarachnoid space; irritation of the meninges causes a sudden onset of the **'worst headache of my life'**, blood is found within the CSF in lumbar puncture.

▶ Venous drainage of Scalp, Face and Neck

❏ **Facial vein** begins as an angular vein by the confluence of the supraorbital and supratrochlear veins.

❏ The **angular vein** is continued at the lower margin of the orbital margin into the facial vein.

❏ Facial vein receives tributaries corresponding to the branches of the facial artery and also receives the infraorbital and deep facial veins.

❏ It drains either directly into the internal jugular vein or by joining the anterior branch of the retromandibular vein (RMV) to form the common facial vein, which then enters the internal jugular vein.

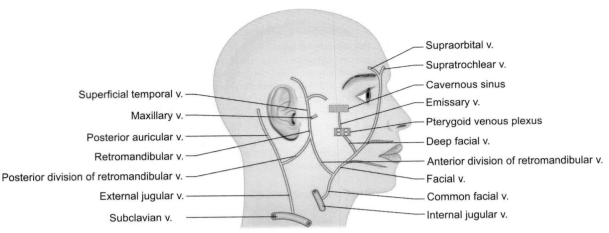

Fig. 50: Facial vein and its connections

Retromandibular vein (RMV) is formed by the union of the **superficial temporal** and **maxillary** veins behind the mandible.
- ❏ It divides into an anterior branch, which joins the facial vein to form the common facial vein, and a posterior branch, which joins the posterior auricular vein to form the external jugular vein.
- ❏ **Pterygoid venous plexus** lies on the lateral surface of the medial pterygoid muscle, receives veins corresponding to the branches of the maxillary artery and drains into the maxillary vein.
  - ➤ It communicates with the cavernous sinus by **emissary veins** (which pass through the foramen ovale), the **inferior ophthalmic vein** by a vein (which runs through the infraorbital fissure), and the facial vein by the **deep facial vein**.

External jugular vein is formed by the union of the posterior auricular vein and the posterior branch of the retromandibular vein.
- ❏ It crosses the sternomastoid obliquely under the platysma and ends in the subclavian (or occasionally in the internal jugular) vein.
- ❏ It receives the suprascapular, transverse cervical, and anterior jugular veins.

Internal jugular vein drains blood from the skull, brain, superficial face and much of the neck.
- ❏ It begins in the **jugular foramen** as a continuation of the sigmoid sinus, descends in the carotid sheath, and ends in the brachiocephalic vein.
- ❏ It has the superior bulb at its beginning and the inferior bulb just above its termination, receives multiple veins like the facial, lingual, and superior and middle thyroid veins.
- ❏ It descends in the neck **within the carotid sheath** and unites with the subclavian vein behind the sternal end of the clavicle to form the brachiocephalic vein.

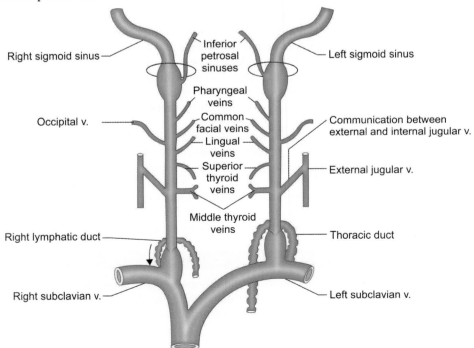

Fig. 51: Beginning and termination of the internal jugular veins along with their tributaries

❑ At its junction with the internal jugular vein, the **left venous angle** usually receives the thoracic duct, and the **right venous angle** receives the right lymphatic duct.

❑ The left brachiocephalic vein is longer, more oblique and crosses the midline to unite with right counterpart and form SVC.

1. Angular vein communicates with: *(NEET Pattern 2012)*
   a. Cavernous sinus
   b. Superior sagittal sinus
   c. Inferior sagittal sinus
   d. Straight sinus

2. NOT true about facial vein is: *(NEET Pattern 2013)*
   a. Drains into external jugular vein
   b. Largest vein of face
   c. Continuation of angular vein
   d. Has no valves

3. TRUE regarding surface anatomy of internal jugular vein: *(NEET Pattern 2012)*
   a. Line passing from ear lobule to midpoint of clavicle
   b. Line passing from ear lobule to medial end of clavicle
   c. Line joining ear lobule to lateral end of clavicle
   d. Line joining mastoid process to midpoint of clavicle

1. a. Cavernous sinus
   ❑ Angular vein is the upper most segment of the facial vein, formed by the union of the supratrochlear vein and supraorbital vein.
   ❑ It runs obliquely downward by the side of the nose, is linked with the cavernous sinus by the superior and inferior ophthalmic veins which are devoid of valves.

2. a. Drains in external jugular vein
   ❑ Facial vein is the largest vein of face with no valves.
   ❑ It begins as angular vein, joins anterior division of retromandibular vein to form common facial vein, which in turn drains into internal jugular vein.

3. b. Line passing from ear lobule to medial end of clavicle
   ❑ Surface marking for internal jugular vein is represented by a broad band from the lobule of the ear to the sternoclavicular joint, where it joins the subclavian vein.

▶ Lymphatic drainage of Head and Neck

Lymph nodes in the head and neck are arranged in **two horizontal rings** and **two vertical chains** on either side.

❑ The outer (superficial) ring consists of the occipital, preauricular (parotid), submandibular and submental nodes.

❑ The inner (deep) ring is contributed by MALT (mucosa-associated lymphoid tissue) located primarily in the nasopharynx and oropharynx (**Waldeyer's ring**).

❑ The vertical chain consists of superior and inferior groups of nodes related to the carotid sheath.

❑ All lymph vessels of the head and neck drain into the **deep cervical nodes**, either directly from the tissues or indirectly via nodes in outlying groups.

❑ Lymph reaches the systemic venous circulation via either the **right lymphatic duct** or the **thoracic duct**.

❑ Superficial lymph nodes of the head
   ➢ Lymphatics from the face, scalp, and ear drain into the occipital, retroauricular, parotid, buccal, submandibular, submental, and superficial cervical nodes, which themselves drain into the deep cervical nodes (including the jugulodigastric and juguloomohyoid nodes).

❑ Deep lymph nodes of the head
   ➢ Nasal cavity and paranasal sinuses drain into the submandibular, retropharyngeal, and upper deep cervical.
   ➢ Middle ear drains into the retropharyngeal and upper deep cervical nodes.
   ➢ **Larynx** drains into the upper and lower deep cervical; **Pharynx** drains into the retropharyngeal and upper and lower deep cervical. **Thyroid gland** drains into the lower deep cervical, prelaryngeal, pretracheal, and paratracheal nodes.

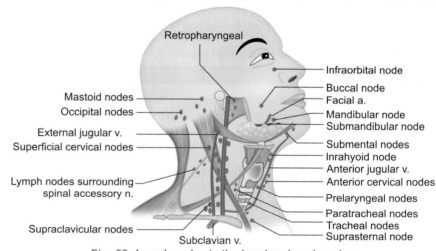

Fig. 52: Lymph nodes in the head and neck region

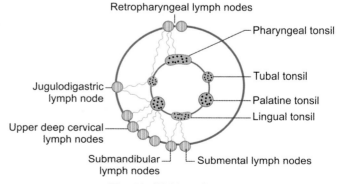

Fig. 53: Waldeyer's ring

- Superficial cervical lymph nodes lie **along the external jugular vein** in the posterior triangle and along the anterior jugular vein in the anterior triangle. They drain into the deep cervical nodes.
- Deep cervical lymph nodes are divided into two groups: Superior and inferior.
  - Superior deep cervical nodes lie along the **internal jugular vein** in the carotid triangle of the neck. They receive afferent lymphatics from the back of the head and neck, tongue, palate, nasal cavity, larynx, pharynx, trachea, thyroid gland, and esophagus.
    - The efferent vessels join those of the inferior deep cervical nodes to form the jugular trunk, which empties into the thoracic duct on the left and into the junction of the internal jugular and subclavian veins on the right.
  - Inferior deep cervical nodes lie on the **internal jugular** vein near the subclavian vein. They receive afferent lymphatics from the anterior jugular, transverse cervical, and apical axillary nodes.

Waldeyer's ring is an aggregation of MALT (mucosa-associated lymphoid tissue) located underneath the epithelial lining of pharyngeal wall, surrounding the air and food pathway.
  - It includes: Nasopharyngeal tonsil (posterosuperiorly), lingual tonsil (anteriorly), tubal and palatine tonsils (laterally).

QUESTIONS

1. Submental lymph node of drainage by all EXCEPT:
(NEET Pattern 2014; 15)
   a. Anterior palate
   b. Tip of tongue
   c. Floor of mouth
   d. Lower lip

2. Waldeyer's ring consists of all of the following EXCEPT:
(NEET Pattern 2012)
   a. Palatine tonsils
   b. Pharyngeal tonsils
   c. Tubal tonsils
   d. Postauricular nodes

ANSWERS

1. a. Anterior palate
- Submental (suprahyoid) lymph node are situated between the anterior bellies of the digastric muscle.
- They drain the central portions of the lower lip and floor of the mouth and the tip of the tongue.
- Palate drain mostly into the upper deep cervical lymph nodes and few into retropharyngeal lymph nodes.

2. d. Postauricular nodes
- Waldeyer's ring includes nasopharyngeal tonsil (posterosuperiorly), lingual tonsil (anteriorly), tubal and palatine tonsils (laterally).

- **Anterior** half of nasal cavity (including anterior part of nasal septum) drains into **submandibular nodes** *(NEET Pattern 2015)*
- **Deep** cervical nodes lie along **internal jugular vein** *(NEET Pattern 2013)*

▼ Scalp and Face

- Scalp is composed of **five layers**, which can be remembered using the mnemonic SCALP: (1) Skin, (2) Connective tissue, (3) Aponeurosis, (4) Loose areolar tissue, and (5) Pericranium. The first three layers constitute the scalp proper, which moves as a unit.
- **Skin** has abundant hair and numerous sebaceous glands.
- **Connective tissue** forms a thick, vascularized subcutaneous layer which is dense, contains numerous blood vessels and nerves, sweat glands, and hair follicles. The arteries anastomose freely and are held by the dense connective tissue around them, and thus, they tend to remain open when cut, causing **profuse bleeding**.
- Aponeurosis (**galea aponeurotica**) is a tendinous sheet that covers the vault of the skull and continues as the frontal muscle anteriorly and the occipital muscle posteriorly. Laterally, the galea aponeurotica is continuous with the temporoparietal fascia.
- Loose areolar connective tissue is known as '**dangerous layer of scalp**' because blood and pus freely tend to collect in this layer. If pus collects in this layer, the 'infection' may travel readily along emissary veins into the intracranial dural venous sinuses leading to their 'thrombosis', which may be fatal.
- Pericranium forms the periosteum of the neurocranium (skull).
- **Arterial supply**: Scalp is supplied by the supratrochlear and supraorbital branches of the ophthalmic artery (internal carotid) and by the superficial temporal, posterior auricular, and occipital branches of the external carotid arteries.

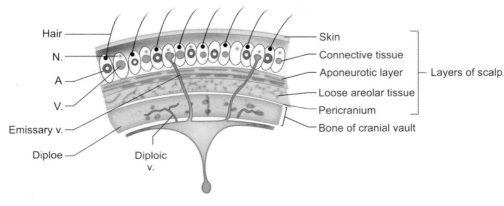

❑ **Nerve supply**: Scalp is innervated by the supratrochlear, supraorbital, zygomaticotemporal, auriculotemporal, lesser occipital, greater occipital, and third occipital nerves.

Facial artery arises from the **external carotid artery** just superior to the lingual artery (above the upper border of the hyoid bone).

❑ It ascends forward, deep to the posterior belly of the digastric and stylohyoid muscles, passes deep to the mandible, winds around the lower border of the mandible, reaches the **anterior margin of the masseter** and runs upward and forward on the face.

❑ It gives the ascending palatine, tonsillar, glandular, and submental branches in the neck and the **inferior labial, superior labial**, and **lateral nasal** branches in the face.

❑ Facial artery terminates as an **angular artery** that anastomoses with the palpebral and dorsal nasal branches of the ophthalmic artery to establish communication between the external and internal carotid arteries.

❑ **Pulse**: Facial artery can be palpated as it crosses the lower mandibular border **immediately anterior to masseter border** and on the face approximately 1 cm lateral to the angle of the mouth.

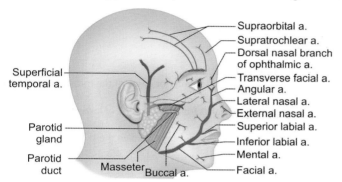 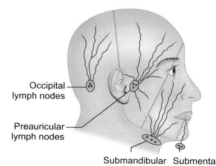

Fig. 54: Arterial supply of face (1- zygomaticotemporal, 2- zygomaticofacial, 3- infraorbital, 4- palpebral branch of lacrimal artery); Lymphatic drainage of the scalp and face

Face has **three lymphatic territories**:

❑ Upper territory includes greater part of the forehead, lateral halves of the eyelids including conjunctiva, parotid area, and adjoining part of the cheek and drain into **preauricular** (superficial parotid) lymph nodes.

❑ Middle territory includes central part of the forehead, medial halves of the eyelids, external nose, upper lip, lateral part of lower lip, medial part of cheek, and greater part of the lower jaw and drain into **submandibular** lymph nodes.

❑ Lower territory includes central part of the lower lip and chin and drain into **submental** lymph nodes.

Dermatomes of the face arise mainly from cutaneous branches of the three major divisions of the trigeminal nerve.

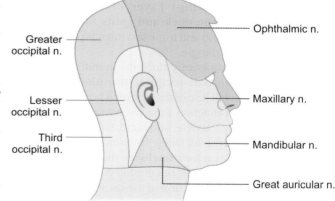

❑ The skin covering the front and sides of the neck, and over the angle of the mandible, and over the lateral scalp and posterior aspect of the pinna is supplied by branches of the cervical plexus (C2–C4), and the skin over the back of the head is supplied by the greater occipital nerve (C2, posterior primary ramus).

QUESTIONS

1. Which of the following is NOT a branch of facial artery?
   (NEET Pattern 2014)
   a. Superior labial   b. Inferior labial
   c. Lateral nasal   d. Sublingual

2. Supraorbital and Supratrochlear arteries are branches of which of the following?   *(NEET Pattern 2016)*
   a. External carotid artery   b. Internal carotid artery
   c. Ophthalmic artery   d. Maxillary artery

3. Nerve supply of tip of nose: *(NEET Pattern 2013)*
   a. External nasal branch of ophthalmic nerve
   b. Inferior orbital nerve
   c. Buccal branch of mandibular nerve
   d. Orbital branch of maxillary nerve

4. Dangerous area of scalp is: *(NEET Pattern 2016)*
   a. Superficial fascia
   b. Aponeurosis
   c. Sub-aponeurotic tissue
   d. Pericranium

5. Tissue expander in scalp is placed between:
   (NEET Pattern 2016)
   a. Skin and galea aponeurotica
   b. Subcutaneous tissue and loose areolar connective tissue
   c. Aponeurosis and periosteum
   d. Areolar tissue and bone

6. Nerve supply of scalp: *(PGIC)*
   a. Auriculotemporal nerve
   b. Zygomatic nerve
   c. Occipital nerve
   d. Supratrochlear nerve
   e. Infratrochlear nerve

1. **d. Sublingual**
   - ❑ Sublingual artery is a branch of lingual artery.
2. **c. Ophthalmic artery**
   - ❑ Supraorbital and Supratrochlear arteries are terminal branches of the ophthalmic artery.
3. **a. External nasal branch of ophthalmic nerve**
   - ❑ Tip of the nose is under the ophthalmic nerve territory, supplied by the external nasal branch.
4. **c. Sub-aponeurotic tissue**
   - ❑ The 'danger area of the scalp' is called the area of loose connective tissue. The pus and blood spread easily within it and can pass into the cranial cavity along the emissary veins. Therefore, infection can spread from the scalp to the intracranial venous sinuses.
5. **c. Aponeurosis and periosteum**
   - ❑ The plane of dissection/insertion is usually the natural relatively avascular plane beneath the subcutaneous tissue (and over the muscle fascia. in most parts of the body).
   - ❑ However, in the scalp and forehead, the tissue expander is placed in the subgaleal plane to minimize bleeding.
   - ❑ Note: The layer of loose areolar connective tissue beneath the aponeurotic layer accounts for the free mobility of the scalp proper on the underlying bone. It also provides an easy plane of cleavage.
6. **a. Auriculotemporal nerve; b. Zygomatic nerve; c. Occipital nerve; d. Supratrochlear nerve**
   - ❑ Infratrochlear nerve do not supply the region of scalp.

- Platysma develops in second pharyngeal arch and is supplied by facial nerve (cervical branch).
- The pulsations of facial artery can be felt at two sites, at the base of the mandible close to anteroinferior angle of the masseter and about 1.25 cm lateral to the angle of the mouth *(NEET Pattern 2012)*
- Lymphatics from the central part of the lower lip drain into submental lymph nodes. Lymphatics from lateral parts of lower lip and whole of upper lip drain into submandibular lymph nodes *(NEET Pattern 2016)*
- Risorius is a muscle of facial expression, to produce a smile, albeit an insincere-looking one that does not involve the skin around the eyes *(NEET Pattern 2012)*
- Palpebral part orbicularis oculi close eyelids as in blinking or winking *(NEET Pattern 2013)*

▼ Neck Fascia and Spaces

Deep cervical fascia forms a. **Investing layer**, b. **Pretracheal layer** and c. **Prevertebral layer**.

❑ Superficial (**Investing**) Layer of Deep Cervical Fascia **encircles the neck and splits** to enclose the sternocleidomastoid and trapezius muscles and is at the roof of posterior triangle.
   - ➤ It is attached superiorly along the mandible, mastoid process, external occipital protuberance, and superior nuchal line of the occipital bone.
   - ➤ Inferiorly it is attached along the acromion and spine of the scapula, clavicle, and manubrium sterni.

❑ **Pretracheal** Layer of Deep Cervical Fascia **invests the larynx and trachea, encloses the thyroid gland**, is continuous with the buccopharyngeal facia, and contributes to the formation of the carotid sheath.
   - ➤ It attaches superiorly to the thyroid and cricoid cartilages and inferiorly to the pericardium.
   - ➤ A **thyroid mass usually moves with swallowing** because the thyroid gland is enclosed by pretracheal fascia.

❑ **Prevertebral** Layer of Deep Cervical Fascia is cylindrical and **encloses the vertebral column and its associated muscles**.
   - ➤ It is attached to the external occipital protuberance and the basilar part of the occipital bone and becomes continuous with the endothoracic fascia and the anterior longitudinal ligament of the bodies of the vertebrae in the thorax.
   - ➤ It lies behind the pharynx and esophagus, envelops the phrenic nerve, scalene muscles, cervical primary rami, cervical sympathetic chain, and subclavian and vertebral arteries.

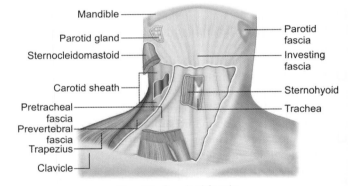

Fig. 55: Cervical fascia

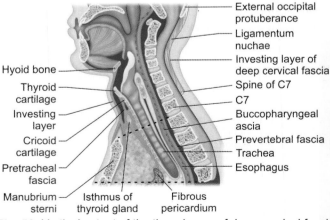

Fig. 56: Vertical extent of the three layers of deep cervical fascia and the buccopharyngeal fascia

➢ It lies at the floor of posterior triangle and extends laterally over the first rib into the axilla to form axillary sheath enveloping the divisions and cords of the brachial plexus with the axillary artery.

➢ Subclavian/axillary veins lie outside the axillary sheath and therefore can distend freely.

➢ It is said to have two layers: Alar fascia (anterior part) and Proper prevertebral fascia (posterior part). Danger space is a potential space lying between the two.

❑ **Buccopharyngeal fascia** covers the buccinator muscles and the pharynx and blends with the pretracheal fascia. It is attached to the pharyngeal tubercle and the pertygomandibular raphe.

❑ **Pharyngobasilar fascia** is the fibrous coat in the wall of the pharynx and is situated between the mucous membrane and the pharyngeal constrictor muscles.

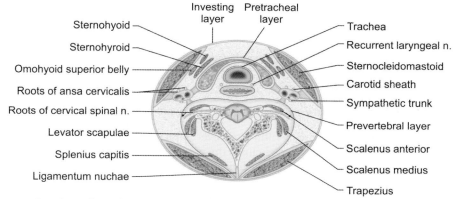

Fig. 57: Transverse section through neck at the level of the 6th cervical vertebra to show the horizontal disposition of the 3 layers of deep cervical fascia

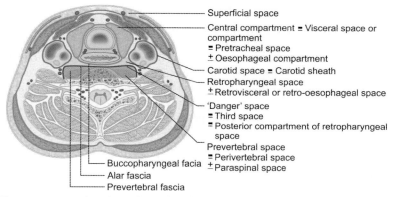

Fig. 58: Transverse section through to show layers of cervical fascia and the related spaces

❑ **Alar fascia** (anterior part of prevertebral fascia) is a coronally orientated sheet, attached to the transverse process of the cervical vertebrae.

➢ It is separated from prevertebral fascia by loose connective tissue that fills the so-called **danger space.**

➢ It lies posterior to the pharynx/esophagus and the buccopharyngeal fascia, from which it is separated by loose connective tissue that fills the **retropharyngeal space**.

➢ It passes anterolaterally to fuse with the prevertebral fascia and **extends inferiorly from the skull base** to about the level of the seventh cervical vertebra (it varies between C6 and T4), where it fuses with the visceral layer of middle cervical fascia, thereby **delimiting the lowest extent** of the retropharyngeal and danger spaces.

❑ **Posterior visceral space** lies posterior to the pharynx and cervical esophagus. It extends from the skull base down to the superior mediastinum, its caudal limit being the level of fusion between the alar and buccopharyngeal fascia.

❑ The posterior visceral space is often referred to as the **retropharyngeal space** in the upper neck.

❑ **Retropharyngeal space** is present between the buccopharyngeal fascia (anterior) and alar part of prevertebral fascia (posterior), extending from the base of the skull into the posterior mediastinum.

➢ Neck infections in front of PVF in the retropharyngeal space forms acute retropharyngeal abscess which bulges forward in the paramedian position. This is due to firm midline attachment between the buccopharyngeal fascia and the prevertebral (alar) fascia divides the space into two segments.

➢ Laterally the space is sealed by the attachments of both these fascial layers to the carotid sheath.

➢ Retropharyngeal abscess or infection may spread from the neck into the posterior mediastinum through the retropharyngeal space.

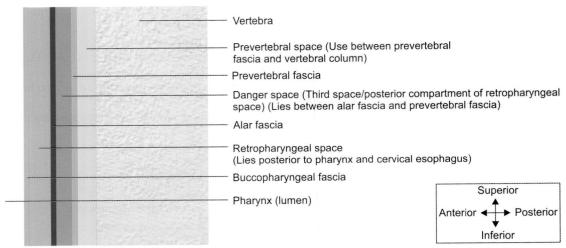

Fig. 59: Sagittal section through to show vertical disposition of layers of cervical fascia and the related spaces

- ❏ **Prevertebral space** is the potential space lying behind the prevertebral fascia and in front of the vertebral column.
  - ➢ It extends from the skull base to the coccyx and encloses the prevertebral muscles.
  - ➢ Almost all of the pathology that affects the prevertebral space arises from either the adjacent vertebrae or their intervertebral discs, or the spinal cord and associated nerve roots and spinal nerves.
  - ➢ Tuberculosis of the spine may breach the space and form a **Pott's abscess**.
- ❏ **Danger space** lies between the anterior (alar part) and posterior layers of prevertebral fascia.
  - ➢ It extends from the skull base down to the posterior mediastinum, where the alar, visceral and prevertebral layers of deep cervical fascia fuse.
  - ➢ The potential space so created is closed superiorly, inferiorly and laterally; infections can only enter by penetrating its walls.
  - ➢ The **danger space is so called because** its loose areolar tissue offers a potential route for the rapid downward spread of infection, primarily from the retropharyngeal, para-pharyngeal or prevertebral spaces, to the posterior mediastinum.
- ❏ **Carotid space** is a layer of loose connective tissue demarcated by adjacent portions of the investing layer of deep cervical fascia, the pretracheal fascia and the prevertebral fascia.
  - ➢ A potential cavity exists within the carotid sheath that permits the spread of infections from the upper neck down into the lower neck and mediastinum.
  - ➢ Infections around the carotid sheath may be restricted because, superiorly (near the hyoid bone) and inferiorly (near the root of the neck), the connective tissues adhere to the vessels.
- ❏ **Carotid sheath** has contributions from all **three layers** of deep cervical fascia: Prevertebral, pretracheal, and investing layers and is attached to the base of the skull superiorly.
- ❏ The four major structures contained in the carotid sheath are: Common carotid artery (as well as the internal carotid artery more superiorly), internal jugular vein, vagus nerve (CN X) and the deep cervical lymph nodes.
  - ➢ The **carotid artery** lies medial to the **internal jugular vein**, and the **vagus nerve** is situated posteriorly between the two vessels.
  - ➢ In the upper part, the carotid sheath also contains the glossopharyngeal nerve (IX), the accessory nerve (XI), and the hypoglossal nerve (XII), which pierce the fascia of the carotid sheath.

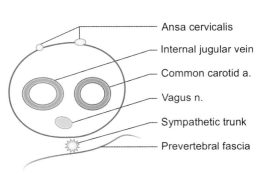

Fig. 60: Carotid sheath, contents and relations

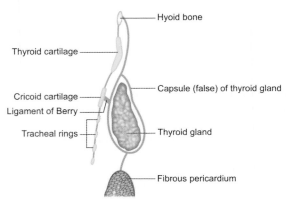

Fig. 61: Ligament of Berry

❑ The ansa cervicalis is **embedded in the anterior wall** of sheath. It is formed by "descendens hypoglossi" (C1) and "descendens cervicalis" (C2-C3). **Sympathetic trunk** lies **posterior** to it.

1. All is true about cervical fascia EXCEPT:
   a. Ligament of Berry fixes thyroid gland to cricoid cartilage
   b. Prevertebral fascia forms the roof of posterior triangle
   c. Ansa cervicalis is embedded in the anterior wall of carotid sheath
   d. Carotid sheath is formed by pretracheal and prevertebral fascia

2. Retropharyngeal abscess lies between which two layers of fascia: *(JIPMER 2017)*
   a. Between pharyngobasilar and buccopharyngeal fascia
   b. Between buccopharyngeal and alar fascia
   c. Between buccopharyngeal and prevertebral fascia
   d. Between alar and prevertebral fascia

3. In the given diagram identify the dangerous space: *(AIIMS 2016)*

   a. A
   b. B
   c. C
   d. D

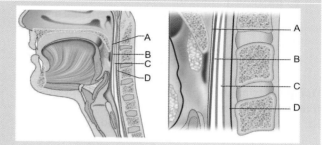

1. b. Prevertebral fascia forms the roof of posterior triangle
   ❑ Prevertebral fascia forms the floor of posterior triangle, the roof is formed by the investing layer of deep cervical fascia.

2. b. Between buccopharyngeal and alar fascia
   ❑ Retropharyngeal abscess develops in the space bounded by buccopharyngeal fascia (anteriorly) and alar fascia (posteriorly).

3. c. C
   ❑ Danger space (marker 'C') is the potential space that lies between the anterior (alar part) and posterior layers of prevertebral fascia (both shown in brown color).
   ❑ This diagram shows the sagittal section of head and neck region, layers of cervical fascia and spaces.
   ❑ Prevertebral fascia (shown in brown color) has two parts: Alar fascia (anterior part) and proper prevertebral fascia (posterior part).
   ❑ Danger space is a potential space lying between the two.
   ❑ Buccopharyngeal (visceral) fascia (shown in green color) lies behind the pharynx.
   ❑ Key: A - Un-named space; B - Retropharyngeal space; C - Danger space; D - Prevertebral space.
   ❑ Retropharyngeal Space (marker 'B') is present between the buccopharyngeal fascia (anterior) and prevertebral fascia (posterior).
   ❑ Prevertebral space (marker 'D') is the potential space lying behind the prevertebral fascia and in front of the vertebral column.

- Fascia around the brachial plexus is called as **axillary sheath** and is a derivative of **prevertebral fascia** *(AIIMS 2008; 2011)*
- **Cervical sympathetic chain** is NOT a content of carotid sheath but is closely related to posterior wall of the sheath *(JIPMER 2010)*

❑ Retropharyngeal Space of Gillette is a potential space (**filled with loose areolar tissue**) and lies between the buccopharyngeal fascia & the prevertebral fascia, extending from the base of the skull to the superior mediastinum.

▶ Neck Triangles

❑ A **quadrilateral area** is evident in the neck, limited superiorly by the inferior border of the mandible and a line continued from the angle of the mandible to the mastoid process, inferiorly by the upper border of the clavicle, anteriorly by the anterior median line, and posteriorly by the anterior border of trapezius.

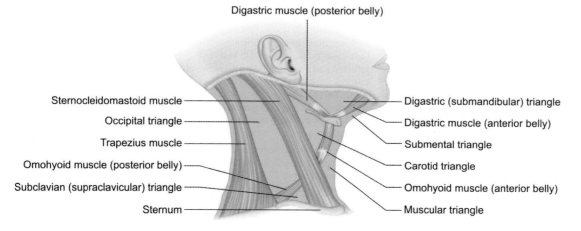

Digastric muscle (posterior belly)

Sternocleidomastoid muscle — Occipital triangle — Trapezius muscle — Omohyoid muscle (posterior belly) — Subclavian (supraclavicular) triangle — Sternum

Digastric (submandibular) triangle — Digastric muscle (anterior belly) — Submental triangle — Carotid triangle — Omohyoid muscle (anterior belly) — Muscular triangle

- ❑ It is further divided into **anterior** and **posterior** triangles by **sternocleidomastoid**, which passes obliquely from the sternum and clavicle to the mastoid process and occipital bone.
- ❑ **Anterior triangle** is further subdivided into the **carotid** triangle, **submandibular** triangle, **submental** triangle, and **muscular** triangle. The **posterior** triangle is further subdivided into the **occipital** triangle and **subclavian** triangle.
- ❑ Posterior Triangle is bounded by the posterior border of the **sternocleidomastoid** (SCM) muscle, the anterior border of the **trapezius** muscle, and the superior border of the **clavicle** (middle third).
  - ➢ Platysma and the investing layer of the deep cervical fascia lies at the **roof**.
  - ➢ The **floor** formed by prevertebral fascia overlying anterior and lateral groups of prevertebral muscles.
  - ➢ It is crossed, approximately 2.5 cm above the clavicle, by the **inferior belly of omohyoid**, which subdivides it into **occipital** and **supraclavicular** triangles.

Occipital triangle is bounded by SCM, trapezius and inferior belly of omohyoid.

- ❑ Its floor, from above down, is formed by semispinalis capitis (occasionally), splenius capitis, levator scapulae, and scaleni medius and posterior.
- ❑ The roof has skin, superficial fascia, platysma and deep fascia.

Subclavian (supraclavicular, omoclavicular) triangle is bounded by SCM, clavicle and inferior belly of omohyoid.

- ❑ It corresponds to supraclavicular fossa.
- ❑ Its floor contains the first rib, scalenus medius and the first slip of serratus anterior
- ❑ It is covered by skin, superficial and deep fasciae, and platysma, and crossed by the supraclavicular nerves.

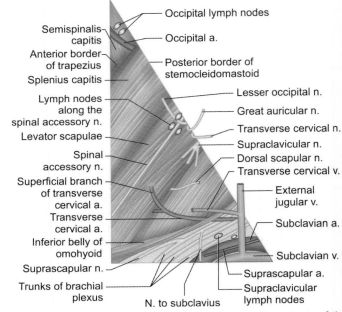

Fig. 62: Schematic diagram showing the floor and contents of the right posterior triangle

Triangle	Main contents and the underlying structures
A. Posterior triangle	
1. Occipital triangle	- Spinal accessory nerve - Dorsal scapular nerve - Cervical plexus (branches) e.g., supraclavicular nerves - Brachial plexus (uppermost part/trunks) - Superficial transverse cervical artery - Occipital artery - External jugular vein (part)
2. Supraclavicular (omoclavicular or subclavian) triangle	- Subclavian artery (3rd part)* - Subclavian vein (occasionally) - Brachial plexus (trunks)** - Nerve to subclavius - Superficial transverse cervical, suprascapular, and dorsal scapular vessels - External jugular vein (terminal part)
B. Anterior triangle	
1. Carotid triangle	- Common carotid artery bifurcation and two branches - Carotid sinus and body (at bifurcation) - Five first branches of external carotid and the corresponding veins - Last three cranial nerves (X, XI, XII) - Internal and external laryngeal nerves (vagus branches) - Carotid sheath (containing common and internal carotid artery, internal jugular vein and vagus nerve) - Ansa cervicalis (embedded on carotid sheath anteriorly) - Cervical sympathetic trunk (posterior to carotid sheath)
2. Submandibular (digastric. Triangle)	- Anterior part - Submandibular salivary gland and lymph nodes - Facial artery (superficial) and vein (deep) to submandibular gland - Hypoglossal nerve - Submental and mylohyoid vessels and nerves (lie on mylohyoid) - Posterior part - External carotid artery

Triangle	Main contents and the underlying structures
	▪ Carotid sheath and its contents ▪ Structures passing between the external and internal carotid arteries*** ▪ Parotid gland (lower part)
3. Submental triangle	▪ Submental lymph nodes ▪ Small veins that unite to form the anterior jugular vein
4. Muscular triangle	▪ Strap (ribbon) muscles: sternothyroid, sternohyoid, thyrohyoid ▪ Thyroid gland, trachea, and esophagus (deep level)

*Subclavian artery (3rd part) can be blocked on first rib in supraclavicular triangle.
**Brachial plexus can be blocked in the scalene triangle between scalenus anterior and medius.
***Internal carotid artery, internal jugular vein and vagus nerve lie deeper and are separated from the external carotid artery by styloglossus, stylopharyngeus and the glossopharyngeal nerve.

Carotid triangle is bounded posteriorly by sternocleidomastoid, anteroinferiorly by the superior belly of omohyoid and superiorly by stylohyoid and the posterior belly of digastric. At floor are seen parts of thyrohyoid, hyoglossus and inferior and middle pharyngeal constrictor muscles.

Digastric triangle is bordered superiorly by the lower border of the mandible and its projection to the mastoid process, posteroinferiorly by the posterior belly of digastric and by stylohyoid, and anteroinferiorly by the anterior belly of digastric.
It is covered by the skin, superficial fascia, platysma and deep fascia, which contain branches of the facial and transverse cutaneous cervical nerves.
Its floor is formed by mylohyoid and hyoglossus.

Submental triangle is a median triangle with **anterior belly of digastric muscles** on each side, body of hyoid bone at the base and apex is at the chin. Mylohyoid muscle is at the floor and submental lymph nodes are the content.

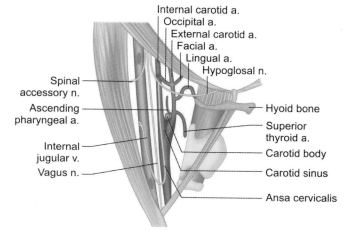

Fig. 63: Carotid triangle

Muscular triangle is limited anteriorly by the midline of neck from the hyoid bone to the sternum, posteroinferiorly by anterior margin of sternocleidomastoid and posterosuperiorly by the superior belly of omohyoid.

Suboccipital triangle is present on the back of the neck bounded by the following three muscles:
Rectus capitis posterior major (above and medially), Obliquus capitis superior (above and laterally) and Obliquus capitis inferior (below and laterally)

Note: Rectus capitis posterior minor is also in this region but does not form part of the triangle.

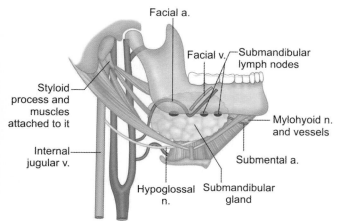

Fig. 64: Digastric triangle

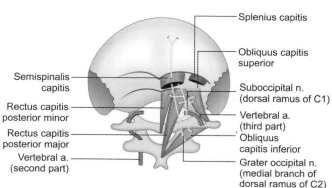

Fig. 65: Boundaries and contents of the suboccipital triangle

Suboccipital triangle is covered by a layer of dense fibro-fatty tissue, situated beneath the semispinalis capitis. The floor of the triangle is formed by the posterior atlanto-occipital membrane, and the posterior arch of the atlas.
❑ Contents of the suboccipital triangle: Third part of vertebral artery, Dorsal ramus of nerve C1- suboccipital nerve, Suboccipital venous plexus
   Vertebral artery and the suboccipital nerve lie in the deep groove on the upper surface of the **posterior arch of the atlas**.

1. **All are contents of occipital triangle EXCEPT:**
   (NEET Pattern 2013)
   a. Great auricular nerve   b. Suprascapular nerve
   c. Lesser occipital nerve   d. Occipital artery

2. **Structure superficial to mylohyoid in anterior digastric triangle are all EXCEPT:**
   a. Deep part of submandibular gland
   b. Hypoglossal nerve
   c. Part of parotid gland
   d. Mylohyoid artery and nerve

3. **All of the following are in the anterior triangle of neck EXCEPT:**
   (PGIC 2010)
   a. Digastric   b. Subclavian
   c. Muscular   d. Submental
   e. Carotid

4. **All is true about digastric triangle EXCEPT:**
   a. On either side is anterior belly of digastric muscle
   b. Floor is formed by mylohyoid muscle
   c. Floor is formed by hyoglossus muscle
   d. Contains mylohyoid nerve and vessels

5. **All the following are contents of suboccipital triangle EXCEPT:**
   a. Vertebral artery
   b. Dorsal ramus of CI nerve
   c. Sub occipital plexus of vein
   d. Occipital artery

6. **After surgery on right side of neck, a person could not raise his arm above head and also could not shrug the shoulder. What is the possible cause:**
   (PGIC 2013)
   a. Damage to spinal accessory nerve
   b. Paralysis of trapezius muscle
   c. Injury to axillary nerve
   d. Paralysis of latissimus dorsi
   e. Paralysis of deltoid muscle

7. **Chassaignac tubercle is:**   *(NEET Pattern 2014)*
   a. Erb's point
   b. Carotid tubercle on C6 vertebra
   c. Found on first rib
   d. Medial condyle of humerus

8. **Chassaignac tubercle lies at level of:**
   a. Erb's point
   b. Stellate ganglion
   c. Atlas
   d. Odontoid process

9. **Identify the vagus nerve in the transverse section of neck:**
   (AIIMS 2015)
   a. A
   b. B
   c. C
   d. D

1. **b. Suprascapular nerve**
   ❑ Cervical plexus gives branches into the posterior (occipital part) triangle, including supraclavicular nerves.
   ❑ Suprascapular nerve is a branch from the upper trunk of brachial plexus and a content of subclavian part of posterior triangle.

2. **d. Mylohyoid artery and nerve**
   ❑ Deep part of submandibular gland and hypoglossal nerve are deep to mylohyoid muscle.
   ❑ Structures passing superficial to mylohyoid in anterior part of digastric triangle are submandibular gland (superficial part), facial vein, facial artery, mylohyoid nerve and vessels, hypoglossal nerve and submandibular nodes.

3. **b. Subclavian**
   ❑ Posterior triangle of neck has two parts: Occipital & subclavian.
   ❑ Subclavian triangle is also called as supraclavicular or omoclavicular triangle.

4. **a. On either side is anterior belly of digastric muscle**
   ❑ Digastric triangle is bounded by anterior belly of digastric anteriorly and posterior belly posteriorly.
   ❑ Mylohyoid and hyoglossus muscles are at the floor.
   ❑ Digastric triangle contains mylohyoid nerve and vessels, submandibular gland, facial artery and vein, hypoglossal nerve and submandibular lymph nodes.

5. **d. Occipital artery**
   ❑ Contents of suboccipital triangle are vertebral artery (3rd part), suboccipital nerve (dorsal ramus of C1) and suboccipital venous plexus.
   ❑ Occipital artery lies in occipital triangle.

6. **a. Damage to spinal accessory nerve; b. Paralysis of trapezius muscle**
   ❑ Spinal accessory nerve is prone to iatrogenic injury in posterior triangle of neck, which leads to paralysis of trapezius muscle and difficulty in shrugging the shoulder.
   ❑ There is also weakness of overhead abduction (carried out by serratus anterior and trapezius).

7. b. Carotid tubercle on C6 vertebra
- ❑ The anterior tubercle of the sixth cervical transverse process (tubercle of Chassaignac) can be palpated medial to the sternocleidomastoid muscle, and against it the common carotid artery can be massaged to relieve the symptoms of supraventricular tachycardia.
- ❑ It separates the carotid artery from the vertebral artery and is used as a landmark for anaesthesia of the brachial plexus and cervical plexus.

8. a. Erb's point
- ❑ Chassaignac or carotid tubercle is a large anterior tubercle of the transverse process of the sixth cervical vertebra. The common carotid artery may be compressed against the tubercle, which sits lateral to the cricoid cartilage. Above this level, the artery is superficial and its pulsation may be readily felt beneath the anterior border of sternocleidomastoid.
- ❑ Erb's point is 2 to 3 cm above the clavicle and beyond the posterior border of the sternomastoid, at the level of the transverse process of the sixth cervical vertebra; stimulation here contracts various arm muscles.
- ❑ Stellate ganglion is not at the level of Chassaignac tubercle.
- ❑ Although the ganglion lies at the level of the C7 vertebra, stellate ganglion block is performed under fluoroscopy by inserting the needle at the level of the C6 vertebra to avoid piercing the pleura. The needle of the anaesthetic syringe is inserted between the trachea medially and the sternocleidomastoid muscle and the common carotid artery laterally using the cricoid cartilage (C6) and the transverse process of C6 vertebra (Chassaignac or carotid tubercle) as landmark.

9. c. C
- ❑ Vagus nerve (C) lies **inside the carotid sheath** sandwiched between common carotid artery medially and internal jugular vein laterally.
- ❑ Key: A - Sympathetic trunk lies postero-medial to the carotid sheath in the carotid triangle of neck. **Stellate ganglion block** is done here; B - Phrenic nerve, lies **anterior to scalenus anterior muscle**, covered by pre-vertebral fascia, in the posterior triangle of neck; D - Recurrent laryngeal nerve, branch of vagus running in the **tracheo-oesophageal groove**.

- ❑ The posterior belly of the digastric and stylohyoid muscles are innervated by the **facial nerve**, whereas the anterior belly of the digastric and mylohyoid muscles are innervated by the **trigeminal nerve.**
- ❑ The **geniohyoid** and **thyrohyoid** muscles are innervated by C1 through the hypoglossal nerve.

Tongue

- ❑ The dorsum (posterosuperior surface) of tongue is divided by a V-shaped **sulcus terminalis** into an anterior, **oral** (presulcal) part that faces upwards, and a posterior, **pharyngeal** (postsulcal) part that faces posteriorly.
- ❑ **Foramen cecum** is located at the apex of the V and indicates the site of origin of the **embryonic thyroglossal duct.**
- ❑ **Lingual Papillae** are of four types: **Circumvallate** papillae are arranged in the form of a V in front of the sulcus terminalis; **fungiform** papillae on the sides and the apex of the tongue; **filiform** papillae are most numerous on the dorsum and **foliate** papillae are rudimentary.

Development of Tongue and Thyroid

Tongue develops in ventral portion of pharyngeal arches (at the **floor of pharynx**) and have three components:
- ❑ **Connective tissue**: Contributed by pharyngeal arch **mesoderm**
- ❑ **Epithelium** on the anterior 2/3 of tongue is derived from surface **ectoderm** and posterior 1/3 from **endoderm**.
  - ➤ The ectoderm-endoderm junction marked by **sulcus terminalis**.
- ❑ **Muscles** of tongue develop from the **occipital myotomes** (somites). Palatoglossus muscle is an **exception**, as it develops in pharyngeal arches.

Note: Tongue has contribution from all the three germ layers.

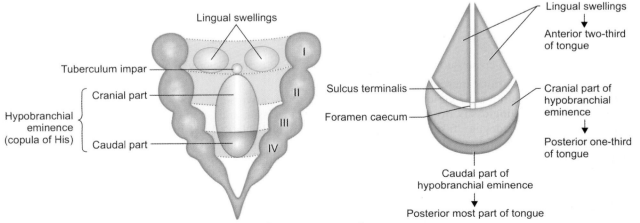

Fig. 66: Development of tongue

- ❑ Anterior two-thirds of the tongue develops in first pharyngeal arch from one median swelling (**tuberculum impar**) and two lateral **lingual swellings**.

❑ Posterior one-third of the tongue develops from the **cranial part of copula** or hypobranchial eminence that is formed by mesoderm of the pharyngeal arches 3 and 4.

❑ Posteriormost part of tongue develops from the **caudal part of hypobranchial eminence**.

❑ Intrinsic and extrinsic muscles of tongue are derived from myoblasts that migrate to the tongue region from **occipital somites** (except palatoglossus, which develops in **pharyngeal arches**).

Table 10: Development of tongue			
Embryonic precursor	**Intermediate structure**	**Adult structure**	**Innervation**
Pharyngeal arch 1	Tuberculum impar (median tongue bud) Lateral lingual swellings	Overgrown by lateral lingual swellings Mucosa (Anterior 2/3 of tongue)	General sensations[1]: Lingual branch (V$_3$) Taste sensations[2]: Chorda tympani (facial nerve)
Pharyngeal arch 2 (minimal contribution)	Copula	Overgrown by other structures	
Pharyngeal arch 3	Large, ventral part of hypopharyngeal eminence	Mucosa (posterior 1/3 of tongue)	Branch of Glossopharyngeal nerve[3]
Pharyngeal arch 4	Small, dorsal part of hypopharyngeal eminence	Mucosa of posteriormost tongue (small region on dorsal side of posterior 1/3 of tongue)	Branch of superior laryngeal nerve (Vagus)[4]
Occipital somites	Myoblasts	Muscles of tongue (except palatoglossus)	Hypoglossal nerve[5]
Pharyngeal arch mesodem	Myoblasts	Palatoglossus muscle	Cranial accessory nerve[6]

[1]**General sensations** of anterior 2/3 of tongue are carried by the lingual nerve (branch of V$_3$ Mandibular branch of trigeminal nerve)
[2]**Taste sensations** of anterior two third of tongue (except the circumvallate papillae) are carried by the chorda tympani nerve (branch of facial nerve)
[3]**General and taste sensations** from the posterior 1/3 of tongue are carried by a branch of glossopharyngeal nerve
[4]**General and taste sensations** from the posteriormost tongue are carried by a branch of superior laryngeal nerve (branch of vagus nerve)
[5]Hypoglosssal nerve supply all the tongue muscles **except palatoglossus**.
[6]alatoglossus muscle develops in pharyngeal arch mesoderm and is supplied by cranial accessory nerve (vagus accessory complex; pharyngeal plexus)
Note: tognue epithelium on the anterior 2/3 is derived from the **surface ectoderm** and the posterior epithelium is from the **endoderm**. The endoderm-ectoderm junction is marked by **sulcus terminalis**.

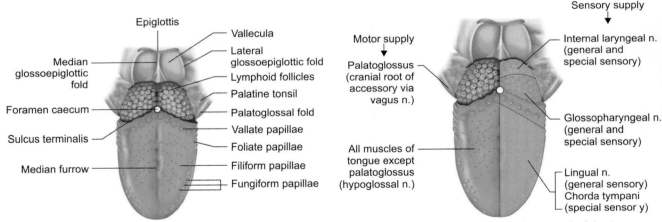

Fig. 67: Features on the dorsal surface of the tongue   Fig. 68: Neve supply (motor and sensory) of the tongue

Tongue has intrinsic and extrinsic musculature.

❑ Intrinsic muscles: Superior and inferior longitudinal, vertical, and transverse.

❑ Extrinsic muscles: **Genioglossus**, hyoglossus, styloglossus, palatoglossus, and geniohyoid.

❑ **Genioglossus**: **AIM** the tongue – Takes it **A**nterior, **I**nferior and **M**edial. Bilateral activity depresses tongue and pulls tongue anteriorly for protrusion; **unilateral** contraction deviates tongue to **contralateral** side.

❑ **Palatoglossus**: It is capable of **elevating** posterior **tongue** or depressing soft palate; most commonly acts to constrict isthmus of fauces.

❑ **Hyoglossus** is a depressor of tongue and **styloglossus** pulls the tongue back.

❑ **Clinical correlations**: Genioglossus is the chief muscle of tongue protrusion. Bilateral loss of genioglossus function, for example during deep **general anaesthesia** or as a consequence of a central neurologic lesion, results in the tongue falling against the posterior wall, with the attendant risk of upper airway obstruction and **suffocation**.

  ➤ Thus, the normally functioning genioglossi can be considered as **'safety muscles'** that aid in the patency of the upper airway.

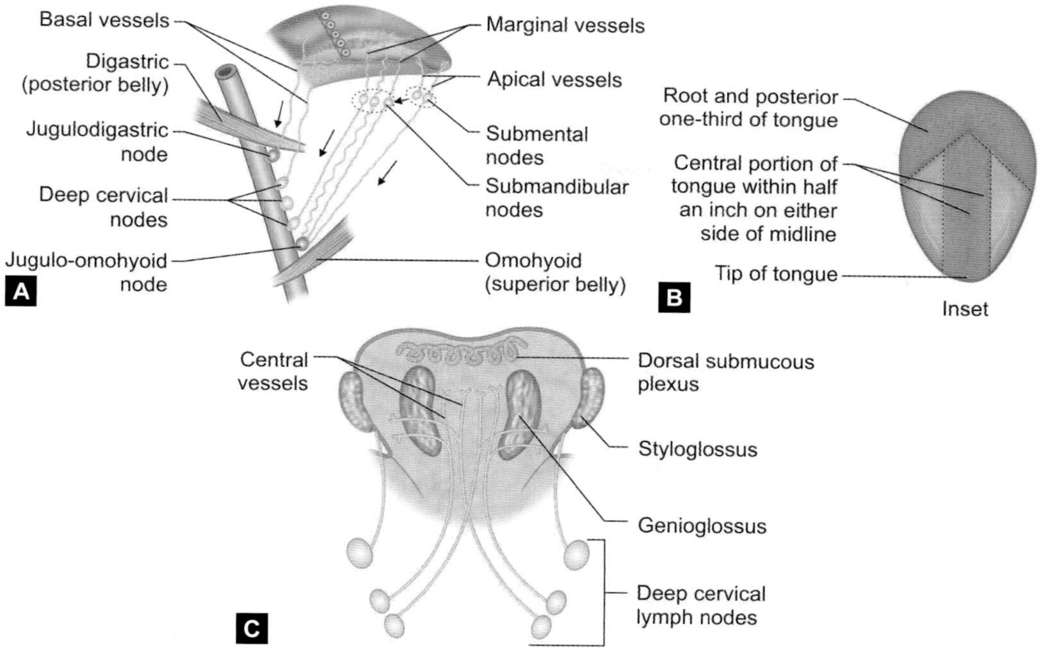

Fig. 69: Lymphatic drainage of the tongue: (A) showing course and direction of apical, marginal, and based lymph vessels; (B) showing course and direction of central lymph vessels. Figure in the inset shows areas (in red) having bilateral lymphatic drainage

➤ Genioglossus muscles are innervated with each inspiration and this important muscle activity can become defunct in certain patients with **sleep apnea syndrome** – one of the culprit muscle.

➤ In this case as the patient goes into sleep, genioglossus muscle relaxes and is unable to prevent the tongue from falling backward into the respiratory tube, leading to difficulty in breathing and the patient is forced to wake up **momentarily**, again to fall asleep.

➤ This cycle of **fall asleep → wake-up →** fall asleep continues **throughout** the sleep period.

Lymphatics are in four groups:

❑ **Apical** vessels drain the tip and inferior surface of the tongue into **submental** lymph nodes. Their efferents go to the submandibular nodes mainly, some cross the hyoid bone to reach the jugulo-omohyoid nodes.

❑ **Marginal** vessels drain the marginal portions of the anterior two-third of the tongue unilaterally into **submandibular** lymph nodes and then to the lower deep cervical lymph nodes, including **jugulo-omohyoid**.

❑ **Central** vessels drain the central portion of the anterior two-third of the tongue (i.e., area within 0.5 inch on either side of midline). They pass vertically downwards in the midline of the tongue between the genioglossus muscles and then drain bilaterally into the **deep cervical lymph nodes**.

❑ **Basal** vessels drain the root of the tongue and posterior one-third of the tongue bilaterally into upper deep cervical lymph nodes, including **jugulodigastric**.

❑ **Taste pathways**; a- geniculate ganglion of facial nerve, b- superior ganglion of glossopharyngeal nerve, c- inferior ganglion (ganglion nodosum) of vagus nerve.

❑ Cranial nerves (taste) → **nucleus tractus solitarius** → medial lemniscus → VPM thalamus → Genu of internal capsule → Parietal lobe (gustatory cortex - **area 43**).

❑ The taste area is located in the inferior part of the postcentral gyrus (**parietal lobe**).

❑ **Lemniscus:** A bundle of fibers, e.g. Lemnisci are the collections of nerve fibers passing through the brainstem. **Medial lemniscus** carries **taste** and lateral lemniscus carry auditory fibers in the brainstem.

QUESTIONS

1. Tongue develops from all EXCEPT:
   a. Tuberculum impar   b. Hypobranchial eminence
   c. Second arch   d. Lingual swellings

2. Posterior one-third of the tongue develops from:
   (NEET pattern 2012)
   a. Lingual swellings   b. Tuberculum impar
   c. Hypobranchial eminence d. Tongue bud

3. The taste pathway from circumvallate papillae of the tongue goes through:
   a. Chorda tympani branch of Facial nerve
   b. Greater petrosal nerve branch of Facial nerve
   c. Superior laryngeal branch of Vagus nerve
   d. Lingual branch of Glossopharyngeal nerve

4. Protrusion of tongue is NOT possible in damage of:
   (NEET Pattern 2015)
   a. Styloglossus
   b. Hyoglossus
   c. Palatoglossus
   d. Genioglossus

5. Taste sensation of tongue is carried by: *(PGIC 2017)*
   a. Facial nerve   b. Glossopharyngeal nerve
   c. Vagus   d. Chorda tympani
   e. Lingual nerve

6. Tip of tongue drains lymphatics into: *(JIPMER)*
   a. Occipital lymph node   b. Submental lymph node
   c. Deep cervical lymph nodes d. Tonsillar lymph nodes

1. **c. Second arch**
   - ❏ Second arch has negligible contribution in the adult tongue.

2. **c. Hypobranchial eminence**
   - ❏ Posterior one-third of the tongue develops from the cranial part of hypobranchial eminence (copula of His).

3. **d. Lingual branch of Glossopharyngeal nerve**
   - ❏ Taste sensation from anterior two-thirds of the tongue run in the chorda tympani of the facial nerve, except for the circumvallate papillae (sensation carried by the glossopharyngeal nerve).

4. **d. Genioglossus**
   - ❏ Posterior part of genioglossus pulls tongue anteriorly for protrusion.
   - ❏ It is also called safety muscle of tongue as it prevents backward fall of tongue into the oral cavity, especially if the patient is unconscious.

5. **a. Facial nerve; b. Glossopharyngeal nerve; c. Vagus; d. Chorda tympani**
   - ❏ Lingual nerve carries general (not taste) sensations.

6. **b. Submental lymph node**
   - ❏ Apical vessels drain the tip and inferior surface of the tongue into submental lymph nodes after piercing the mylohyoid muscle.
   - ❏ Their efferents go to the submandibular nodes mainly, some cross the hyoid bone to reach the jugulo-omohyoid nodes.

- ▪ Taste sensation from **anterior 2/3rd of tongue** is carried by **chorda tympani** (branch of facial nerve), towards the facial nerve and geniculate ganglion (*NEET Pattern 2012*)
- ▪ Anterior 2/3rd of the tongue is demarcated by **sulcus terminalis**, a V shape structure which divides the tongue into anterior two-thirds (oral part) and posterior one-third (pharyngeal part) (*AIIMS 2016*)

▶ Salivary Glands

Development

- ❏ Salivary glands arise bilaterally as the result of epithelial-mesenchymal interactions between the **ectodermal** epithelial lining of the oral cavity and the subjacent **neural crest-derived mesenchyme**.
- ❏ **Parotid** glands develop from **ectodermal** lining near angles of the stomodeum in the 1st/2nd pharyngeal arches. Submandibular and sublingual glands also develop from **surface ectoderm** lining the oral cavity. Some authors believe these two glands develop both from **ectoderm and endoderm**.

Parotid Salivary gland

Parotid gland is the largest of the three salivary glands and occupies the retromandibular space between the ramus of the mandible in front and the mastoid process and the sternocleidomastoid muscle behind.
  - ➤ It is invested with a dense fibrous capsule, the parotid sheath, derived from the investing layer of the deep cervical fascia.
  - ➤ It is separated from the submandibular gland by a facial extension and the stylomandibular ligament, which extends from the styloid process to the angle of the mandible. (Therefore, pus does not readily exchange between these two glands.)
- ❏ **Bed of parotid gland** is related to three bony structures:
  - ➤ **Ramus of the mandible** covered by two muscles (masseter laterally and medial pterygoid medially).
  - ➤ **Mastoid process** covered by two muscles (sternocleidomastoid laterally and posterior belly of digastric muscle medially).
  - ➤ **Styloid process** covered by three muscles (styloglossus, stylopharyngeus, and stylohyoid).
- ❏ **Relations** of parotid gland
  - ➤ **Anteromedial Surface** is deeply grooved by the posterior border of the ramus of the mandible with covering muscles and lateral aspect of the temporomandibular joint.
  - ➤ **Posteromedial surface** is moulded onto the mastoid and styloid processes and their covering muscles. The styloid process separate the gland from internal carotid artery, internal jugular vein, and last four cranial nerves.
  - ➤ **Superficial Surface** covered from superficial to deep by skin, superficial fascia containing anterior branches of greater auricular nerve, superficial parotid (preauricular) lymph nodes, platysma, parotid fascia and deeper parotid lymph nodes.
- ❏ Stensen's parotid duct crosses the masseter, pierces the buccinator muscle, and opens into the vestibule of the oral cavity opposite the upper second molar tooth.
- ❏ Parotid duct can be palpated at tense anterior margin of masseter muscle.
- ❏ Parotid gland secretes copious watery (serous) saliva by parasympathetic stimulation and produces a small amount of viscous saliva by sympathetic stimulation.
- ❏ The parasympathetic (secretomotor) innervation pathway is: Inferior salivatory nucleus → glossopharyngeal nerve → tympanic branch → tympanic plexus (middle ear cavity) → lesser petrosal nerve → foramen ovale → otic ganglion → auriculotemporal nerve (trigeminal, mandibular) → parotid gland.

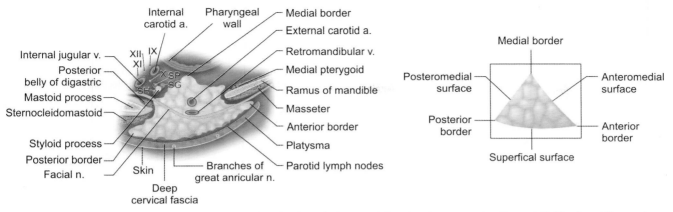

Fig. 70: Horizontal section through parotid gland showing its relations and the structures passing through it. The inset figure shows borders and surfaces of the parotid gland (SG: Styloglossus muscle, SH: Stylohyoid muscle, SP: Stylopharyngeus muscle)

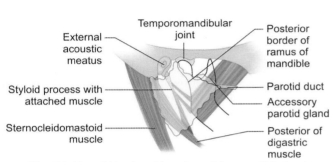

Fig. 71: Parotid bed and location of the parotid gland

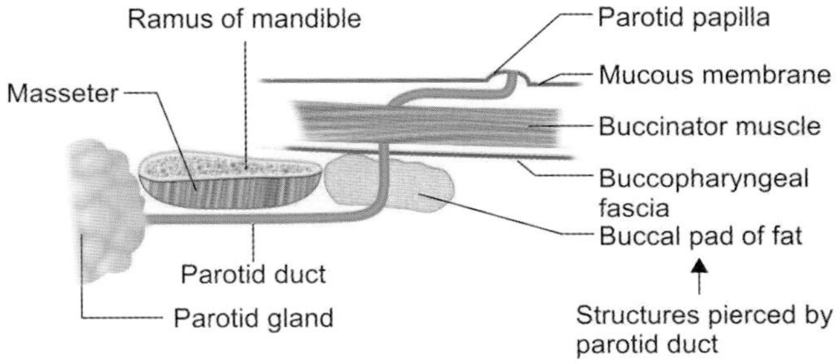

Fig. 72: Course of the parotid duct. Also note the structures pierced by it during its course from the parotid gland to the vestibule of the mouth

- ❑ Otic Ganglion lies in the infratemporal fossa, just below the foramen ovale between the mandibular nerve and the tensor veli palatini (muscle is deeper and medial).
  - ➢ Preganglionic axons originate in the inferior salivatory nucleus and travel in the glossopharyngeal nerve and its tympanic branch.

Otic ganglion is **functionally** related to the glossopharyngeal nerve, which carries the preganglionic fibers to the ganglion.

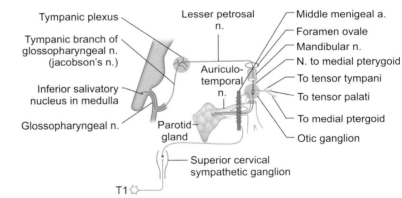

Fig. 73: Otic ganglion and its connections

It is **anatomically** (topographically) related to the mandibular nerve (branch of trigeminal), which carries post ganglionic fibers to parotid salivary gland.

- ➢ They traverse the tympanic plexus and lesser petrosal nerve, and pass through the foramen ovale to reach the otic ganglion, where they synapse.
- ➢ Postganglionic fibers pass by communicating branches to the auriculotemporal nerve, which conveys them to the parotid gland.
- ➢ Stimulation of the lesser petrosal nerve produces vasodilator and secretomotor effects.

▌▌▌ CLINICAL CORRELATIONS ▌▌▌

- ▪ Frey's syndrome (auriculotemporal nerve syndrome): Patient presents with flushing and beads of perspiration (gustatory sweating) and hyperaesthesia in and around parotid region, instead of salivation in response to taste of food after injury of the auriculotemporal nerve.
  - – Penetrating wounds of the parotid gland may damage auriculotemporal and great auricular nerves.
  - – The auriculotemporal nerve contains parasympathetic cholinergic (secretomotor), sensory, and sympathetic fibers.
  - – The great auricular nerve contains sensory and sudomotor (sympathetic cholinergic) fibers.

- When these nerves are cut, during regeneration the secretomotor fibers grow into endoneurial sheaths of fibers supplying cutaneous receptors for pain, touch and temperature, and sympathetic fibers supplying sweat glands and blood vessels.
- A stimulus intended for salivation evokes cutaneous hyperesthesia, sweating, and flushing.
- It can occur after parotid surgery and may be treated by cutting the tympanic plexus in the middle ear.
- Denervation by tympanic neurectomy or auriculotemporal nerve avulsion may be advocated, but are often not curative.
- The symptoms can be managed by the subcutaneous infiltration of purified botulinum toxin into the affected area, and use of antiperspirant.

QUESTIONS

1. INCORRECT regarding location of otic ganglion is: (AIIMS 2015)
  a. Anterior to middle meningeal artery
  b. Lateral to tensor veli palatini
  c. Lateral to mandibular nerve
  d. Inferior to foramen ovale

2. TRUE statement(s) about parotid gland is/are: (PGIC 2017)
  a. 2nd largest salivary gland
  b. Divided into two parts by facial nerve
  c. Deep lobe contains majority of lymph nodes
  d. Duct opens opposite upper 2nd molar tooth
  e. Lesser petrosal nerve innervates it

3. TRUE about parotid gland: (PGIC 2015)
  a. Enclosed by deep cervical fascia of neck
  b. Related to retromandibular vein
  c. Related to facial nerve
  d. External carotid artery enters the gland through anteromedial surface
  e. Parotid lymph node lies behind the gland

4. True regarding parotid gland is all EXCEPT: (PGIC)
  a. Accessory parotid glands is above parotid duct
  b. Mandible ramus grooves anteromedial surface
  c. Styloid and mastoid muscles are posteromedially
  d. Auriculo-temporal nerve lies superior and great auricular nerve lateral
  e. Pharynx examination is unnecessary

5. TRUE about innervation of parotid gland: (PGIC 2016)
  a. Postganglionic parasympathetic fibre- secretomotor
  b. Preganglionic parasympathetic fibre relay in otic ganglion
  c. Preganglionic parasympathetic nerve begin in inferior petrosal nucleus
  d. Sympathetic nerve are vasomotor
  e. Postganglionic parasympathetic fibers pass through the glossopharyngeal nerve

6. After removal of the parotid gland, patient is having sweating on cheeks while eating. Auriculotemporal nerve which contains parasympathetic secretomotor fibers to parotid gland have reinnervated which nerve: (AIIMS 2012)
  a. Facial
  b. Glossopharyngeal
  c. Buccal
  d. Greater auricular

ANSWERS

1. c. Lateral to mandibular nerve
  ❑ Otic ganglion is medial (not lateral) to mandibular nerve.
  ❑ Relations of otic ganglion:
   ▪ Otic ganglion lies inferior to foramen ovale.
   ▪ Mandibular nerve lies lateral to the ganglion and tensor veli palati muscles is medial (deeper).
   ▪ Anteriorly located is medial pterygoid muscle and posteriorly present is middle meningeal artery.

2. b. Divided into two parts by facial nerve; d. Duct opens opposite upper 2nd molar tooth; e. Lesser petrosal nerve innervates it
  ❑ Parotid gland is the largest of the salivary glands, divided by facial nerve into two parts: superficial and deep. Numerous intraglandular lymph nodes are present, virtually all found superficial to the facial nerve. The parotid duct opens in the oral vestibule opposite maxillary 2nd molar tooth. Lesser petrosal nerve brings secretomotor fibers to the gland.

3. a. Enclosed by deep cervical fascia of neck; b. Related to retromandibular vein; c. Related to facial nerve
  ❑ Parotid gland is enclosed in a capsule formed by investing layer of deep cervical fascia.
  ❑ Retromandibular vein and facial nerve run through the substance of parotid gland.
  ❑ External carotid artery enters the gland through posteromedial surface.
  ❑ Parotid lymph nodes lie partly in the superficial fascia and partly deep to deep fascia over the parotid gland.

4. e. Pharynx examination is unnecessary
  ❑ In pathological enlargement of parotid gland, pharynx examination is necessary since, medial border of gland is related to the lateral wall of oropharynx

5. a. Postganglionic parasympathetic fibre- secretomotor; b. Preganglionic parasympathetic fibre relay in otic ganglion; d. Sympathetic nerve are vasomotor
  ❑ Postganglionic parasympathetic fibre are secretomotor to parotid gland for secretion of saliva.
  ❑ Preganglionic parasympathetic fibers begin in the inferior salivatory (not petrosal) nucleus in the lower pons and relay in otic ganglion.
  ❑ Sympathetic nerve are vasomotor and parasympathetic fibers are secretomotor.
  ❑ Postganglionic parasympathetic fibers pass through the auriculotemporal nerve (branch of mandibular, trigeminal nerve).

6. c. Buccal
  ❑ This is a case of post-parotidectomy gustatory sweating, leading to sweating on the cheek (buccal nerve territory).
  ❑ Removal of the parotid gland damages auriculotemporal nerve which subsequently is misdirected and innervates sweat glands in the territory of buccal (cheek), greater auricular (in front of ear) and lesser occipital nerves (behind the ear).

❑ Sensory supply of parotid is derived from **auriculotemporal nerve** and **great auricular nerve** (C2 and C3). The C2 fibers are sensory to the parotid fascia.

- **Lesser petrosal nerve** derives preganglionic fibers from **tympanic nerve**, branch of glossopharyngeal nerve *(NEET Pattern 2014)*
- **Stensen's parotid duct** crosses the masseter, **pierces the buccinator muscle**, and opens into the vestibule of the oral cavity opposite the **upper second molar** tooth *(NEET Pattern 2012)*
- **Sympathetic root** of otic ganglion is from **plexus around middle meningeal artery**, which arises from the superior cervical ganglion *(NEET Pattern 2012)*
- The plane between the superficial and deep lobes in which facial nerve lie is called **Patey's facio-venous plane**. It helps the surgeons to remove the parotid tumour without damaging the **facial nerve**.
- Otic ganglion supplies Parotid gland *(NEET Pattern 2012)*

▶ Submandibular and Sublingual Glands

- **Submandibular gland** is present in the submandibular triangle covered by the investing layer of the deep cervical fascia.
  - ➤ It wraps around the posterior border of mylohyoid, has a large part superficial to the muscle and a small part which lies deep to the muscle.
  - ➤ The deep portion is located between the hyoglossus and styloglossus muscles medially and the mylohyoid muscle laterally and between the lingual nerve above and the hypoglossal nerve below.
  - ➤ **Wharton's duct** arises from the deep portion and runs forward between the mylohyoid and the hyoglossus, where it runs medial to and then superior to the lingual nerve (lingual nerve loop under submandibular duct).
    - Next it runs between the sublingual gland and the genioglossus and drains at the summit of the sublingual papilla (caruncle) at the side of the frenulum of the tongue.

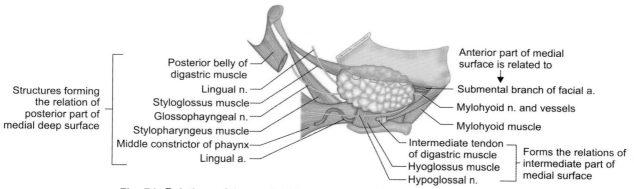

Fig. 74: Relations of the medial (deep) surface of the submandibular gland

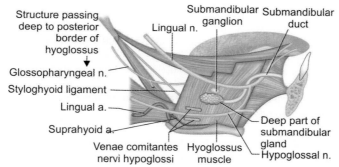

Fig. 75: Superficial relations of the hyoglossus muscle

- In between the hyoglossus muscle and the mylohyoid muscle there are several important structures (from **upper to lower**): Sublingual gland, Submandibular duct, Lingual nerve, Hypoglossal nerve and its vena comitantes.

Submandibular ganglion: The preganglionic axons originate in the superior salivatory nucleus in the pons.

- They emerge from the brainstem in the nervus intermedius and leave the main facial nerve trunk in the middle ear to join the chorda tympani, which subsequently joins the lingual nerve.
- These fibers eventually reach the submandibular ganglion, where they synapse.
- Postganglionic fibers innervate the submandibular, sublingual and lingual salivary glands; some axons re-enter the lingual nerve to access the lingual glands, while others pass directly along blood vessels to enter the submandibular and sublingual glands.
- Stimulation of the chorda tympani has a direct secretomotor effect and also dilates the arterioles in both the glands.
- **Sublingual gland** is located in the floor of the mouth between the mucous membrane above and the mylohyoid muscle below and surrounds the terminal portion of the submandibular duct.

- It empties into the floor of the mouth along the sublingual fold by 12 short ducts, few of those enter the submandibular duct.
- Like submandibular salivary gland it is served by the same neural pathway.
  - Superior salivatory nucleus sends the parasympathetic preganglionic secretomotor fibers by facial nerve → chorda tympani nerve → submandibular ganglion.
  - The post ganglionic fibers are carried by the lingual nerve (branch of mandibular, trigeminal).

QUESTIONS

1. Lobes of submandibular gland are divided by which muscle? (NEET Pattern 2015)
a. Mylohyoid
b. Genioglossus
c. Stylohyoid
d. Styloglossus

2. Structures NOT injured in submandibular gland excision: (NEET Pattern 2015)
a. Inferior alveolar nerve
b. Lingual nerve
c. Hypoglossal nerve
d. Marginal mandibular branch of facial nerve

3. Which one of the following is the CORRECT statement during operation on the submandibular gland (AIIMS 2006)
a. The submandibular gland is seen to wrap around the posterior border of mylohyoid
b. The facial artery and vein are divided as they course through the deep part of the gland
c. The hypoglossal nerve is seen to loop under the submandibular duct
d. Damage to the lingual nerve will cause loss of sensation to the posterior third of the tongue

4. TRUE about submandibular gland duct obstruction by stone (PGIC 2016)
a. Rare site of calculus formation
b. Presents as a mass below body of mandible
c. Pain starts just after starting a meal
d. Stone in Wharton duct can be palpated below mucous membrane of floor of mouth
e. Pain carried by glossopharyngeal nerve

ANSWERS

1. a. Mylohyoid
- Submandibular gland wraps around the posterior border of mylohyoid.
- It has a large part superficial to the muscle and a small part which lies deep to the muscle.

2. a. Inferior alveolar nerve
- Submandibular duct runs anteriorly **between** the lingual nerve and hypoglossal nerve, which are prone to be injured in dissection in the region.
- Marginal mandibular branch of facial nerve passes **posterior inferior to angle of jaw** and is prone to injury in the excision.

3. a. The submandibular gland is seen to wrap around the posterior border of mylohyoid
- Submandibular gland **wraps around** the posterior border of mylohyoid, a large part lies superficial to the muscle and a small part which deep to the muscle.
- It is the lingual nerve (**not hypoglossal**) which loops under the submandibular duct.
- Hypoglossal nerve **keeps running inferior** to the submandibular duct.
- Damage to the lingual nerve causes loss of sensation to the **anterior** 2/3 of the tongue.
- Posterior 1/3 of tongue is supplied by the glossopharyngeal nerve.
- Facial artery and vein are related to superficial (**not deep**) part of the gland.

4. b. Presents as a mass below body of mandible; c. Pain starts just after starting a meal; d. Stone in Wharton duct can be palpated below mucous membrane of floor of mouth
- Submandibular salivary gland is a common site of calculus formation (**not rare**). About 90% of the stones are seen in submandibular and 10% in the parotid.
- Presents as a **tense swelling** below the body of the mandible, which is greatest before or during a meal.
- The pain is sudden and intense **just after** starting a meal.
- The stone can be palpated in the duct, which **lies below** the mucous membrane of the floor of the mouth.
- Pain is carried by **lingual nerve**, branch of mandibular (trigeminal) nerve.

- Preganglionic fibers to the **submandibular ganglion** arise from **Superior salivatory** nucleus (NEET pattern 2012)
- **Lingual nerve** loops around **submandibular duct** (NEET pattern 2015)

▼ Tonsils

- Tonsils are aggregations of lymphoid tissue located in the posterior wall of the pharynx, which trap bacteria and viruses entering through the pharynx, and mount immune response to protect from infection.
- **Waldeyer Tonsillar Ring** is collection of lymphoid tissue at the oropharyngeal isthmus, formed by the **pharyngeal, palatine, tubal** and **lingual** tonsils encircling the back of the throat (refer).
  - Lower pole of the tonsil is attached to the tongue.
  - A triangular fold (**plica triangularis**) of mucous membrane extends from anterior pillar to the anteroinferior part of tonsil and encloses a space called anterior tonsillar space.
  - Upper pole of the tonsil extends into soft palate.
  - Its medial surface is covered by a semilunar mucosal fold (**Plica semilunaris**), extending between anterior and posterior pillars and enclosing a potential space called supratonsillar fossa.

➢ The **tonsillar bed** is formed (from within outwards) by: Pharyngobasilar fascia, superior constrictor muscle and buccopharyngeal fascia.

Artery supply of palatine tonsil:

❑ Tonsil is mainly supplied by the tonsillar branches of **facial artery**.

❑ **Lingual artery** is a branch of external carotid artery which gives **dorsal lingual** branches to the tonsil.

❑ **Ascending palatine artery** is a branch of facial artery, which also supplies the tonsil.

❑ The upper pole of the tonsil also receives branches from the **ascending pharyngeal artery** (branch of external carotid artery), which enter the tonsil posteriorly, and from the **descending palatine artery** (branch of maxillary artery) and its branches, the **greater and lesser palatine arteries**.

❑ **Nerve supply (palatine tonsil):** It receives branches of the glossopharyngeal nerve and the lesser palatine branch of the maxillary nerve.

➢ Since the glossopharyngeal nerve also supplies ear region, any pathology of the tonsil and tonsillar fossa may be accompanied by pain referred to the ear.

❑ **Lymphatic drainage (palatine tonsil):** Tonsillar lymphatics drain to the upper deep cervical lymph nodes directly (especially the **jugulodigastric** nodes) or indirectly through the retropharyngeal lymph nodes.

➢ The jugulodigastric nodes are enlarged in tonsillitis, and are palpable superficially 1–2 cm below the angle of the mandible.

❑ **Adenoids** (nasopharyngeal tonsil) is a subepithelial collection of lymphoid tissue at the junction of roof and posterior wall of nasopharynx.

➢ Unlike palatine tonsils adenoids have no crypts and no capsule.

➢ Adenoid are present at birth, shows physiological enlargement up to the age of six years and then tends to atrophy at puberty and almost completely disappears by the age of 20.

➢ The arterial supply is by ascending palatine branch of facial , ascending pharyngeal branch of external carotid artery, pharyngeal branch of the third part of maxillary artery, ascending cervical branch of inferior thyroid artery of thyrocervical trunk.

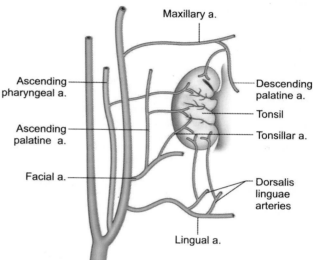

Fig. 76: Arteries supplying the tonsil

QUESTIONS

1. All are true about palatine tonsil EXCEPT: *(PGIC 2014)*
   a. Develop from 2nd pharyngeal pouch
   b. Irritation cause referred pain in ear via auricular branch of vagus
   c. Mainly supplied by facial artery
   d. Situated in the lateral wall of the oropharynx
   e. Lymphatics pass to jugulo omohyoid node

2. Palatine tonsil receives its arterial supply from all of the following EXCEPT: *(AIIMS 2005)*
   a. Facial
   b. Ascending palatine
   c. Sphenopalatine
   d. Dorsal lingual

3. All are true about adenoids EXCEPT: *(NEET Pattern 2012)*
   a. Physiological growth up to 6 years
   b. Crypta magna present
   c. Present in nasopharynx
   d. Supplied by facial artery

4. Plica triangularis is present in: *(NEET pattern 2012)*
   a. Antero inferior part of tonsil
   b. Dorsum of tongue
   c. Inlet of larynx
   d. None

5. Sensory supply to tonsil is by which nerve? *(NEET Pattern 2012)*
   a. Greater palatine nerve
   b. Lesser palatine nerve
   c. Vagus
   d. Glossopharyngeal nerve

6. TRUE about palatine tonsil: *(PGIC 2016)*
   a. Crypts are lined by squamous epithelium
   b. Supplied by IX CN
   c. Tongue depressor is used for examination
   d. Arterial supply is by tonsillar ascending branch of grater palatine artery
   e. Present in oropharynx

ANSWERS

1. b. Irritation cause referred pain in ear via auricular branch of vagus; e. Lymphatics pass to jugulo omohyoid node
   ❑ Tonsil develops in the region of pharyngeal pouch two, whose endoderm forms the tonsillar epithelium.
   ❑ It is present on each side of the oropharynx in an interval between the palatoglossal and palatopharyngeal folds and mainly supplied by facial artery branches.
   ❑ It receives branches of the glossopharyngeal nerve and the lesser palatine branch of the maxillary nerve.
   ❑ Since the glossopharyngeal nerve also supplies ear region, any pathology of the tonsil and tonsillar fossa may be accompanied by pain referred to the ear.
   ❑ Lymphatics drain to the upper deep cervical lymph nodes directly (especially the jugulodigastric nodes).

ANSWERS

2. c. Sphenopalatine
- Sphenopalatine artery is a branch of maxillary artery and does not give branches to the tonsil. It supplies the nasal septum, lateral wall of nose and the paranasal sinuses.

3. b. Crypta magna present
- Crypta magna is a remnant of the second pharyngeal pouch seen in palatine tonsil.
- Adenoids (nasopharyngeal tonsil) is a subepithelial collection of lymphoid tissue at the junction of roof and posterior wall of nasopharynx.
- Unlike palatine tonsils adenoids have no crypts and no capsule.
- Adenoid are present at birth, shows physiological enlargement up to the age of 6 years and then tends to atrophy at puberty and almost completely disappears by the age of 20.
- Ascending palatine branch of facial artery contributes to blood supply of adenoid.

4. a. Antero inferior part of tonsil
- Palatine Tonsil is present on each side of the oropharynx in an interval between the palatoglossal and palatopharyngeal folds. Plica semilunaris and plica triangularis are two developmental folds related to tonsil.

5. d. Glossopharyngeal nerve
- Tonsil is supplied by the branches of the glossopharyngeal nerve and the lesser palatine branch of the maxillary nerve.

6. a. Crypts are lined by squamous epithelium; b. Supplied by IX CN; c. Tongue depressor is used for examination; e. Present in oropharynx
- Tonsillar crypts are lined by non-keratinized stratified squamous epithelium mainly and patches of reticulated epithelium.
- Tonsil is supplied by the CN XI (glossopharyngeal nerve) and branches of maxillary (trigeminal) nerve.
- Tongue depressor is used to expose tongue, which lies in the lateral wall of oropharynx (between the palatoglossal and palatopharyngeal arches).
- Tonsil is mainly supplied by tonsillar artery (branch of facial artery). In addition, it also receive supply from, lingual, ascending palatine, ascending pharyngeal and descending palatine arteries as well.

- **Bed of tonsil** is formed by **Superior constrictor** muscle (NEET Pattern 2012)
- During **Acute tonsillitis** pain in the ear is due to involvement of **Glossopharyngeal nerve** (NEET Pattern 2018)

Palate

- Palate forms the roof of the mouth and the floor of the nasal cavity and is of two types; Hard and soft.
- **Hard palate** is the anterior four-fifths of the palate and forms a bony framework covered with a mucous membrane between the nasal and oral cavities.
  - It consists of the palatine processes of the maxillae and horizontal plates of the palatine bones.
  - It contains the incisive foramen in its median plane anteriorly and the greater and lesser palatine foramina posteriorly.
  - It receives sensory innervation through the greater palatine and nasopalatine nerves and blood from the greater palatine artery.
- **Soft palate** is a fibromuscular fold extending from the posterior border of the hard palate and makes up one fifth of the palate.
  - It moves posteriorly against the pharyngeal wall to close the oropharyngeal (faucial) isthmus while swallowing or speaking.
  - It is continuous with the palatoglossal and palatopharyngeal folds.
- **Arterial supply**: Greater and lesser palatine arteries of the descending palatine artery (branch of maxillary artery), the ascending palatine artery (branch of facial artery), and the palatine branch of the ascending pharyngeal artery.
- **Venous drainage** is into pharyngeal venous plexus and pterygoid venous plexus.
- **Lymphatic drainage** is into retropharyngeal and upper deep cervical lymph nodes.
- **Nerve supply**: Most of the palate muscles are supplied by the cranial accessory nerve, fibers carried by the vagal branches (vagus accessory complex; pharyngeal plexus), except tensor palati (which is supplied by the mandibular nerve, trigeminal).
- General sensations are carried by the lesser palatine nerves (branches of maxillary nerve; trigeminal) through pterygopalatine ganglion and glossopharyngeal nerve.
- Taste sensations are contained in lesser palatine nerves, travel through greater petrosal nerve to geniculate ganglion of facial nerve and eventually reach the nucleus tractus solitarius.

CLINICAL CORRELATIONS

- Lesion of the vagus nerve causes deviation of the uvula toward the opposite side of the lesion on phonation because of paralysis of the musculus uvulae (elevator of uvula).

QUESTIONS

1. The sensory supply of the palate is through all of the following EXCEPT *(AIPG 2002)*
   a. Facial nerve
   b. Hypoglossal nerve
   c. Glossopharyngeal nerve
   d. Vagus nerve

2. Which of the following does NOT supply the palate
   a. Tonsillar branch of facial artery
   b. Ascending palatine artery
   c. Descending palatine artery
   d. Ascending pharyngeal artery

1. **b. Hypoglossal nerve**
   - ❑ Hypoglossal nerve is a **pure motor** nerve to supply the tongue muscles.
   - ❑ General sensations of palate are carried by the **lesser palatine** nerves (branches of maxillary nerve; trigeminal) and glossopharyngeal nerve.
   - ❑ Taste sensations are contained in lesser palatine nerves, travel through greater petrosal nerve (branch of facial nerve).

2. **a. Tonsillar branch of facial artery**
   - ❑ Palate is supplied by greater and lesser palatine arteries of the descending palatine artery (branch of maxillary artery), the ascending palatine artery (branch of facial artery), and the palatine branch of the ascending pharyngeal artery.

- Sensory fibers from the **taste** buds in the hard and soft **palate** travel along **facial nerve** (AIIMS 2005)
- Soft **palate muscles** are supplied by **Cranial accessory** nerve (NEET Pattern 2012)

▶ Pharynx

- ❑ Pharynx, the upper portion of gut tube, is funnel-shaped fibromuscular tube that extends from the base of the skull to the inferior border of the cricoid cartilage.
- ❑ It conducts food to the esophagus and air to the larynx. It has three parts; **Nasopharynx, oropharynx** and **laryngopharynx**.
- ❑ **Nasopharynx** is present behind the nasal cavity above the soft palate and communicates with the nasal cavities through the nasal choanae.
- ❑ Pharyngeal tonsils are present in its postero-superior wall.
- ❑ It is connected with the tympanic cavity through the auditory (Eustachian) tube, which equalizes air pressure on both sides of the tympanic membrane.
- ❑ **Oropharynx** extends between the soft palate above and the superior border of the epiglottis below and communicates with the mouth through the oropharyngeal isthmus.
  - ➤ Palatine tonsils are located here, lodged in the tonsillar fossae and are bounded by the palatoglossal and palatopharyngeal folds.
- ❑ **Laryngopharynx** is also called hypopharynx and extends from the upper border of the epiglottis to the lower border of the cricoid cartilage.
  - ➤ It contains the piriform recesses, one on each side of the opening of the larynx, in which swallowed foreign bodies may be lodged.

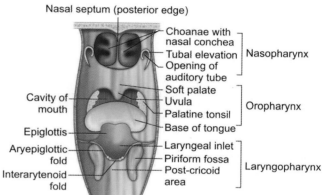

Fig. 77: Coronal view of pharynx.

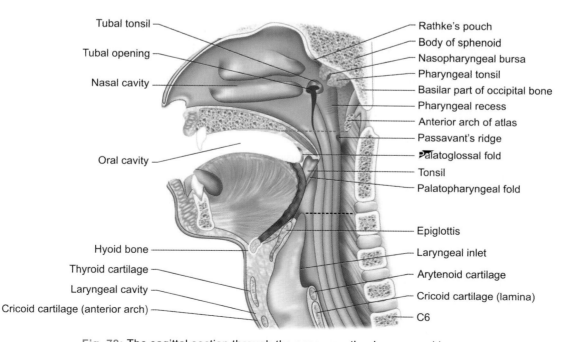

Fig. 78: The sagittal section through the nose, mouth, pharynx, and larynx

	Nasopharynx	Oropharynx	Laryngopharynx (hypopharynx)
Situation	**Behind nasal cavity**	**Behind oral cavity**	**Behind larynx**
Extent	Base of skull (body of sphenoid) to soft palate	Soft palate to upper border of epiglottis	Upper border of epiglottis to lower border of cricoid cartilage
Communications	Anteriorly with nasal cavity	▪ Anteriorly with oral cavity ▪ Superiorly with nasopharynx ▪ Inferiorly with laryngopharynx	▪ Superiorly with oropharynx ▪ Inferiorly continues as esophagus
Nerve supply	Pharyngeal branches of pterygopalatine ganglion	▪ Glossopharyngeal nerve ▪ Vagus nerve	▪ Glossopharyngeal nerve ▪ Vagus nerve
Relations Anterior	Posterior nasal aperture	Oral cavity	▪ Inlet of larynx ▪ Posterior surface of cricoid ▪ Arytenoid cartilage
Posterior	Body of sphenoid bone, pharyngeal tonsils	C2,3 vertebrae	C4,5 vertebrae
Lateral	Opening of auditory tube	Palatine tonsils (in tonsillar fossa)	Piriform fossa
Lining epithelium	Ciliated columnar	Stratified squamous (non-keratinized)	Stratified squamous (non-keratinized)
Function	Respiratory pathway	Respiratory and food pathway	Food pathway

Muscles

Table 11: Muscles of Pharynx	
Muscle	**Main action(s)**
External layer	
Superior pharyngeal constrictor	Constrict walls of pharynx during swallowing
Middle pharyngeal constrictor	
Inferior pharyngeal constrictor	
Internal layer	
Palatopharyngeus	Elevate (shorten and widen) pharynx and larynx during swallowing and speaking
Salpingopharyngeus	
Stylopharyngeus	

- ❑ **Arterial supply**: Ascending pharyngeal artery, ascending palatine branch of the facial artery, descending palatine arteries, pharyngeal branches of the maxillary artery, and branches of the superior and inferior thyroid arteries.
- ❑ **Nerve supply**: The **pharyngeal plexus** is present on the middle pharyngeal constrictor.
  - ➢ It is contributed by the pharyngeal branches of the **glossopharyngeal** and **vagus** nerves (vagus accessory complex).
  - ➢ It also receives the **sympathetic** branches from the superior cervical ganglion.
  - ➢ Its glossopharyngeal component supplies sensory fibers to the pharyngeal mucosa.
- ❑ **Vagus accessory complex**: Cranial accessory nerve fibers (from nucleus ambigus) are carried by the vagal branches to supply most of the muscles of palate, pharynx and larynx.
  - ➢ Cranial accessory nerve fibers (carried by the vagal branches) supply most of the muscles of palate, except stylopharyngeus, which is supplied by the glossopharyngeal nerve.

▋▍▎ CLINICAL CORRELATIONS ▋▍▏

- ▪ Pharyngeal lesions may irritate the glossopharyngeal and vagus nerves and the pain is referred to the ear because these nerves contribute sensory innervation to the external ear as well.
- ▪ The gaps in the pharyngeal wall has some structures passing through them.

Table 12: The gaps in the pharyngeal wall and structures passing through them	
Gap	**Structures passing through them**
Between the base of skull and the upper concave border of superior constrictor (sinus of Morgagni)	▪ Auditory tube ▪ Levator palati muscle ▪ Ascending palatine artery ▪ Palatine branch of the ascending pharyngeal artery

Gap	Structures passing through them
Between the superior and middle constrictors	▪ Stylopharyngeus muscle ▪ Glossopharyngeal nerve
Between the middle and inferior constrictors	▪ Internal laryngeal nerve ▪ Superior laryngeal vessels
Between the lower border of inferior constrictor and the esophagus (in the tracheoesophageal groove)	▪ Recurrent laryngeal nerve ▪ Inferior laryngeal vessels

❏ Nasopharyngeal Isthmus: Some fibers of the **palatopharyngeus** muscle (arising from palatine aponeurosis) sweep horizontally backwards and join the upper fibers of the **superior constrictor** muscle to form a U-shaped muscle-loop in the posterior pharyngeal wall underneath the mucosa, which is pulled forward during swallowing to form the **Passavant ridge**.

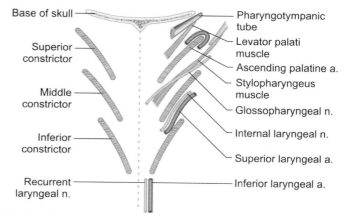
Fig. 79: Structures passing through the gaps in the pharyngeal wall

➤ During swallowing the pharyngeal isthmus (the opening between the free edges of soft palate and posterior wall) is closed by the elevation of the soft palate and pulling forward of posterior pharyngeal wall (Passavant ridge).

➤ This U-shaped muscle loop thus acts as a palatopharyngeal sphincter.

❏ **Piriform fossa** is a deep recess broad above and narrow below in the anterior part of lateral wall of the laryngopharynx, on each side of the laryngeal inlet.

➤ These recesses are produced due to bulging of larynx into laryngopharynx.

➤ Superiorly it is separated from epiglottic vallecula by lateral glossoepiglottic fold.

CLINICAL CORRELATIONS

▪ Inferior constrictor muscle has two parts: Upper thyropharyngeus made up of oblique fibers and lower cricopharyngeus made up of transverse fibers.
  – There is a potential gap posteriorly between the two parts called as pharyngeal dimple or **Killian's dehiscence**.
  – The propulsive thyropharyngeus is supplied by the pharyngeal plexus and the sphincteric cricopharyngeus is supplied by the recurrent laryngeal nerve.
  – In a case of neuromuscular incoordination the cricopharyngeus may fail to relax while the thyropharyngeus contracts, the bolus of food may get pushed backwards and tend to produce a diverticulum.
  – Through this weak area the mucosa and submucosa of the pharynx bulge to form a pharyngeal pouch or **Zenker's diverticulum**.

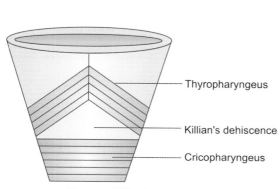
Fig. 80: Killian's dehiscence

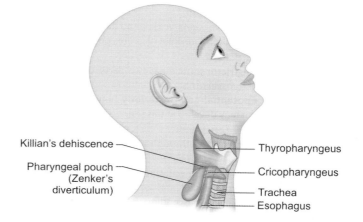
Fig. 81: Pharyngeal diverticulum

❏ Fascia and spaces related to pharynx: The two named layers of fascia in the pharynx are the Pharyngobasilar and buccopharyngeal fascia.

➤ **Pharyngobasilar Fascia** forms the submucosa of the pharynx.

- It blends with the periosteum of the base of the skull attaching to the basilar part of the occipital bone and the petrous part of the temporal bone medial to the pharyngotympanic tube, and to the posterior border of the medial pterygoid plate and the pterygomandibular raphe.
- It lies internal to the muscular coat of the pharynx.

> **Buccopharyngeal fascia** covers the muscular wall of pharynx externally, and basically is the thinner external part of the epimysium.
  - It covers the superior constrictor and passes forwards over the pterygomandibular raphe to cover buccinator.
  - Above the upper border of the superior constrictor, it blends with the pharyngobasilar fascia.

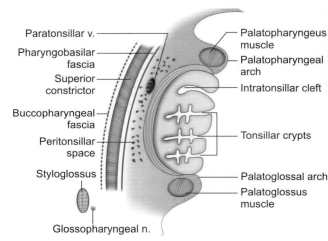

Fig. 82: Relations of tonsils (Tonsilar bed).

- ❑ **Retropharyngeal Space** is a potential space between the buccopharyngeal fascia and the prevertebral fascia, extending from the base of the skull to the superior mediastinum.
- ❑ It permits movement of the pharynx, larynx, trachea, and esophagus during swallowing.

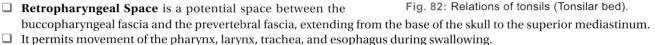

QUESTIONS

1. Which of the following structures is seen in oropharynx?
   (NEET Pattern 2014)
   - a. Pharyngotympanic tube
   - b. Fossa of Rosenmuller
   - c. Palatine tonsil
   - d. Piriform fossa

2. Which of the following part is NOT included in hypopharynx?
   - a. Pyriform sinus
   - b. Post cricoid region
   - c. Anterior pharyngeal wall
   - d. Posterior pharyngeal wall

3. Killian dehiscence is in: *(NEET Pattern 2012)*
   - a. Superior constrictor
   - b. Inferior constrictor
   - c. Middle constrictor
   - d. None

4. Eustachian tube passes between: *(NEET Pattern 2012)*
   - a. Superior and middle constrictors
   - b. Above superior constrictor
   - c. Middle and inferior constrictor
   - d. Below inferior constrictor

5. Which of the following passes between base of the skull and superior constrictor muscle *(AIIMS)*
   - a. Eustachian tube, levator palatini muscle, ascending palatine artery
   - b. Maxillary nerve and levator palatine muscle
   - c. Eustachian tube and stylopharyngeus muscle
   - d. Ascending palatine artery and glossopharyngeal nerve

ANSWERS

1. **c. Palatine tonsil**
   - ❑ Palatine tonsils are present in **tonsillar fossa** in the oropharynx.
   - ❑ Pharyngeal recess (fossa of Rosenmüller) is a deep depression behind the tubal elevation (opening of pharyngotympanic tube) in **nasopharynx**.
   - ❑ Piriform fossa is a deep recess broad above and narrow below in the anterior part of lateral wall of the **laryngopharynx**, on each side of the laryngeal inlet.

2. **c. Anterior pharyngeal wall**
   - ❑ Hypopharynx (laryngopharynx) has no description of anterior pharyngeal wall.
   - ❑ The anterior relations are: Inlet of larynx, posterior surface of cricoid and arytenoid cartilage.

3. **b. Inferior constrictor**
   - ❑ **Inferior constrictor** muscle has two parts: **Upper thyropharyngeus** made up of oblique fibers and **lower cricopharyngeus** made up of transverse fibers.
   - ❑ There is a **potential gap posteriorly** between the two parts called as pharyngeal dimple or **Killian's dehiscence**. Zenker's diverticulum may develop at this site.

4. **b. Above superior constrictor**
   - ❑ Eustachian tube passes through **sinus of Morgagni**, which is a gap between the base of skull and the upper concave border of superior constrictor muscle.

5. **a. Eustachian tube, levator palatini muscle, ascending palatine artery**
   - ❑ Between base of the skull and superior constrictor muscle lies the **Morgagni sinus**, through which passes the **auditory tube**, **levator palati** muscle, ascending palatine artery and palatine branch of the ascending pharyngeal artery.

- **Lower border** of **pharynx** is the level of **C6 vertebra** *(NEET Pattern 2015)*
- **Nasopharynx** is lined by **ciliated columnar** epithelium *(NEET Pattern 2016)*
- **Pyriformis fossa** is located in **pharyngeal part** of pharynx *(NEET Pattern 2012)*
- **Passavant ridge** is formed by **palatopharyngeus** and **superior constrictor muscle** *(NEET Pattern 2012)*
- **Sinus of Morgagni** is between **Superior constrictor** and **skull** *(NEET pattern 2014)*
- **Levator veli palati** passes through **sinus of Morgagni** *(JIPMER 2017)*

- **Rouviere's node** is the most superior of the lateral group of the **retropharyngeal** lymph nodes found at the base of the skull *(NEET Pattern 2012)*
- **Eustachian tube** opens I nasopharynx behind **posterior end** of inferior turbinate *(NEET Pattern 2012)*
- **Gerlach tonsil** is the lymphoid collection at the pharyngeal opening of **auditory tube** (tubal tonsils) *(NEET Pattern 2013)*

▶ Esophagus

Esophagus is a muscular tube (approximately 25 cm long), begins at the lower border of the pharynx at the level of the cricoid cartilage (C6), descends behind the trachea, passes through superior and posterior mediastinum and ends in the stomach at T11.

Constrictions

Site of constriction	Vertebral level	Distance from upper incisor
Beginning (pharyngo-oesophagus junction)	C6	15 cm
Aortic arch	T4	23 cm
Left principal bronchus	T6	28 cm
Esophageal hiatus in diaphragm	T10	40 cm

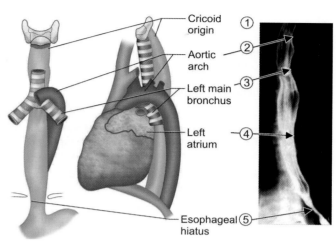

Fig. 83: The normal esophageal constrictions

- ❑ Radiology books mention an additional constriction at the level of left atrium (Not mentioned in Gray's Anatomy 41Ed)
- ❑ Esophagus is the second narrowest part of the alimentary tract, the narrowest being the vermiform appendix.
- ❑ Upper third of the esophagus, the muscularis externa is formed by skeletal muscle; in the middle third, smooth muscle fascicles intermingle with striated muscle; and this increases distally such that the lower third contains only smooth muscle (Gray's Anatomy; Ed41).
- ❑ Upper 5% of the esophagus consists of skeletal muscle only. The middle 45% of the esophagus consists of both skeletal muscle and smooth muscle interwoven together. The distal 50% has smooth muscle only (Another view)

Region	Arterial supply	Venous drainage*	Lymphatic drainage	Nerve supply
Cervical	Inferior thyroid arteries (subclavian artery → thyrocervical trunk → inferior thyroid artery)	Inferior thyroid veins → brachiocephalic veins → superior vena cava	Paratracheal (into deep cervical lymph nodes)	▪ Vagus (Recurrent laryngeal nerves) ▪ Sympathetic trunk
Thoracic	Descending thoracic aorta branches ▪ Oesophageal ▪ Bronchial arteries	▪ Azygous vein ▪ Hemiazygos veins ▪ Intercostal veins ▪ Bronchial veins	Posterior mediastinal nodes	▪ Vagus ▪ T1-4 (sympathetic)
Abdominal	▪ Left gastric artery ▪ Inferior phrenic artery (Left) ▪ Short gastric artery ▪ Posterior gastric artery	▪ Left gastric vein** ▪ Short gastric	▪ Left gastric lymph nodes ▪ Thoracic duct (directly)	▪ Vagus ▪ T5-12 (sympathetic)

*Venous drainage: Blood from the esophagus drains into a submucous plexus and thence into a peri-esophageal venous plexus, from which the esophageal veins arise.
** Left gastric vein → portal vein → hepatic sinusoids → central veins → hepatic veins → inferior vena cava.

- ❑ **Vagal parasympathetic fibers** are motor to the distal esophagus and both stimulatory and inhibitory to the lower esophageal sphincter, maintaining basal tone and coordinating distal esophageal peristalsis with relaxation of the sphincter during swallowing (the latter being mediated by intrinsic nitrergic inhibitory neurons under vagal control).
- ❑ **Sympathetic supply** of the distal esophagus originates from T5-12 spinal nerves mainly via the greater and lesser splanchnic nerves and the coeliac plexus.
- ❑ Nociceptive signals are conveyed by afferent nerves accompanying sympathetic nerves and by vagal afferents, which are also involved in mechanosensory signalling.

QUESTIONS

1. **What is the arterial supply of the thoracic esophagus:** *(NEET Pattern 2012)*
   - a. Inferior thyroid artery
   - b. Inferior phrenic artery
   - c. Bronchial artery
   - d. Left gastric artery

2. **Venous drainage of esophagus:** *(AIIMS 2014)*
   - a. Azygos vein, inferior thyroid vein, right gastric vein
   - b. Azygos vein, inferior thyroid vein, left gastric vein
   - c. Azygos vein, right gastric vein, left gastric vein
   - d. Superior thyroid vein, inferior thyroid vein, azygos vein, hemiazygos vein

QUESTIONS

3. All is true About venous drainage of esophagus EXCEPT:
(AIIMS 2016)
a. Esophageal veins drain into a submucosal plexus
b. Cervical esophagus drains directly into brachiocephalic veins
c. Thoracic esophagus drains into the azygous vein
d. Lower esophageal veins anastomose with the left gastric vein

4. Constrictions in Esophagus are present at distance of (from incisor):
(PGIC 2010)
a. 12 cm
b. 25 cm
c. 28 cm
d. 36 cm
e. 40 cm

5. Second constriction in esophagus is seen at the following site:
(NEET Pattern 2015)
a. Where it crosses left main bronchus
b. Crossing of aorta
c. At pharyngoesophageal junction
d. Where it pierces the diaphragm

6. A foreign body stuck in the oesophagus at 25 cm from upper incisors is situated at which level?
(JIPMER 2017)
a. Cricopharyngeal constriction
b. Aortic arch
c. Left principal bronchus
d. Diaphragmatic opening

1. c. Bronchial artery
❑ **Thoracic** esophagus is supplied by the branches of **descending thoracic aorta**, one of those being **bronchial** arteries.
❑ Inferior thyroid artery supplies **cervical** esophagus.
❑ Inferior phrenic artery and left gastric artery supply the **abdominal** esophagus.

2. b. Azygous vein, inferior thyroid vein, left gastric vein
❑ **Cervical** esophagus drains into inferior thyroid vein, **thoracic** into azygous venous system and **abdominal** oesophagus into the left gastric vein.

3. b. Cervical esophagus drains directly into brachiocephalic veins
❑ Cervical esophagus drains into **inferior thyroid** veins, which **eventually** drain into **brachiocephalic** veins.

4. b. 25 cm; 28 cm; 40 cm
❑ Constrictions in the oesophagus (measured from upper incisors) are: At the **beginning** of the esophagus (15 cm); crossing of **aortic arch** (23 cm); **left main bronchus** (28 cm) and **esophageal hiatus** in diaphragm (40 cm).
❑ **Shackelford's Surgery** mention a constriction at **25 cm** from the upper incisor teeth, where it is crossed by **the left main bronchus.**

5. b. Crossing of aorta
❑ Second constriction of esophagus lies at the level of crossing of arch of aorta (23 cm from upper incisors).

6. c. Left principal bronchus
❑ This is a **controversial** Questions; the answer has been taken from **Shackelford's Surgery** Pg. 101; Ed7). Other surgery textbooks mention presence of **both** arch of aorta and left principal bronchus, at **25 cm level**.

- The **cricopharyngeus** muscle, the sphincter of the upper esophageal opening, **remains closed** except during deglutition (swallowing) and emesis (vomiting).
- Physiologically, the LES is a **3-5 cm long** segment of tonically contracted **smooth muscle**, 1-2 cm of which are situated below the diaphragm. *(NEET Pattern 2016)*
- Distance of the **lower** esophageal sphincter from the upper incisors is 40 cm (some authors mention **37.5 cm**) *(NEET Pattern 2012, 16)*
- **Cricopharyngeus** muscle lies at the beginning of oesophagus at **15 cm** from upper incisors *(NEET Pattern 2016)*
- **Oesophagus** begins at the lower border of cricoid cartilage (**C6 vertebral** level) and opens into stomach at **T11 vertebral** level *(NEET Pattern 2015)*

▶ Larynx

❑ Larynx is a component of respiratory tube working as a conduit of air, protects the airway (sphincter action), is involved in phonation (speech) and help in deglutition.
❑ It is situated in front of laryngopharynx, extends from the root of the tongue to the trachea and lies in front of the C3, 4, 5 vertebrae (higher level in females and still higher in children).
❑ It has total 9 cartilages (3 paired and three unpaired). The unpaired cartilages are large and in the midline: **Thyroid, cricoid** and **epiglottis**. The paired cartilages are small and include: **Arytenoid, corniculate** and **cuneiform.**
❑ Some authors include a pair of **tritiate** cartilage under larynx skeleton.
❑ **Thyroid cartilage** is the largest cartilage of larynx and made up of hyaline variety.
❑ It has two quadrilateral laminae, which meet in front at an angle called thyroid angle forming a laryngeal prominence known as the Adam's apple (apparent in males).
❑ It is acute (90°) in males and obtuse (120°).
❑ **Cricoid cartilage** is hyaline variety and forms a complete ring (signet), lies at the level of C6 vertebra and articulates with the thyroid cartilage.
❑ Its lower border marks the end of the pharynx and larynx.
❑ **Epiglottis** is made up of elastic cartilage and is a spoon-shaped plate that lies behind the root of the tongue and forms the superior part of the anterior wall of the larynx.

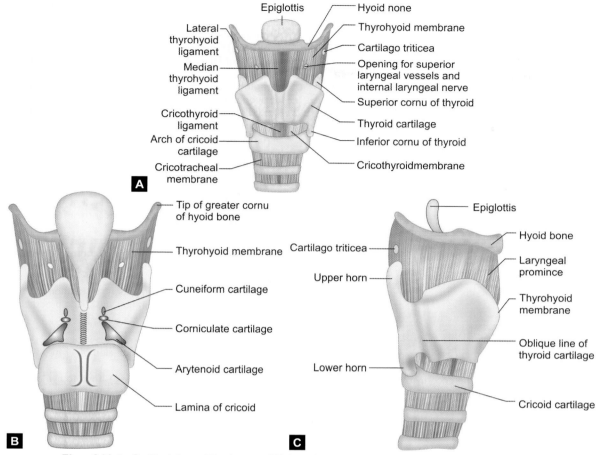

Figs. 84A to C: Skeleton of the larynx: (A) Anterior view; (B) posterior view; (C) lateral view

- ❑ The lower end attaches to the back of the thyroid cartilage.
- ❑ **Arytenoid** cartilages are paired hyaline cartilages (partly elastic).
- ❑ They are pyramid shaped, with bases that articulate with and rotate on the cricoid cartilage.
- ❑ They have vocal processes, which give attachment to the vocal ligament and vocalis muscle, and muscular processes, which give attachment to the thyroarytenoid muscle and the lateral and posterior cricoarytenoid muscles.
- ❑ It sits on the top of the cricoid cartilage and rotates to change the opening of the vocal folds (rima glottidis).
- ❑ **Corniculate** cartilages are paired elastic cartilages that lie on the apices of the arytenoid cartilages, enclosed within the aryepiglottic folds of mucous membrane.
- ❑ **Cuneiform** cartilages are also paired elastic cartilages that lie in the aryepiglottic folds anterior to the corniculate cartilages.

Table 13: Paired and unpaired cartilages of larynx	
Unpaired	Paired
Thyroid	Arytenoid
Cricoid	Corniculate
Epiglottis	Cuneiform

Table 14: Histological types of cartilages in larynx	
Hyaline cartilage	Elastic cartilage
Thyroid	Epiglottis
Cricoid	Corniculate
Basal part of arytenoid cartilage	Cuneiform
	Process of arytenoids

The ligaments of the larynx are two types: **Extrinsic** membrane or ligament attaches to the structures outside the larynx, i.e. to the hyoid bone or trachea, whereas **intrinsic** membranes join structures within the larynx but not extending to hyoid bone or trachea.

Table 15: Extrinsic and intrinsic membranes and ligaments of the larynx		
	Extrinsic	Intrinsic
Membranes	▪ Thyrohyoid	▪ Cricovocal (conus elasticus)
	▪ Cricotracheal	▪ Quadrate/Quadrangular
Ligaments	▪ Median and lateral thyroid	▪ Vocal
	▪ Cricotracheal	▪ Vestibular
		▪ Cricothyroid

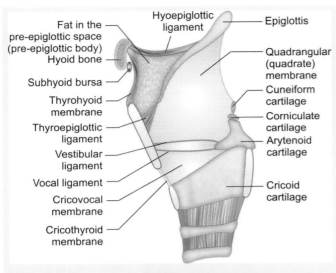

Fig. 85: Sagittal section of the larynx showing ligaments and membranes. Note the location of quadrangular and cricovocal membranes

- The cavity of larynx is divided into three parts by the vestibular and vocal folds: **Vestibule, ventricle,** and **infraglottic compartment**.
- **Vestibule** extends from the laryngeal inlet to the vestibular (ventricular) folds.
- **Ventricle** of larynx extend between the vestibular fold and the vocal fold.
- **Infraglottic compartment** extends from the rima glottidis to the lower border of the cricoid cartilage.
- **Rima Glottidis** is the space between the vocal folds and arytenoid cartilages and is the narrowest anteroposterior cleft of the laryngeal cavity. The anteroposterior diameter of glottis is 24 mm in adult males and 16 mm in adult females.
- **Vestibular Folds** (False Vocal Cords) extend from the thyroid cartilage above the vocal ligament to the arytenoid cartilage.
- **Vocal Folds** (True Vocal Cords) extend from the angle of the thyroid cartilage to the vocal processes of the arytenoid cartilages.
  - They contain the vocal ligament near their free margin and the vocalis muscle.
  - Vocal folds alter the shape and size of the rima glottidis by movement of the arytenoids and control the stream of air passing through the rima glottidis to facilitate respiration and phonation.
  - Rima glottidis becomes wide during inspiration and narrow and wedge-shaped during expiration and sound production.

CLINICAL CORRELATIONS

- Laryngotomy may be required in case of severe edema or an impacted foreign body calls for rapid admission of air into the larynx and trachea.
- It can be performed through the cricothyroid membrane (cricothyrotomy), through the thyroid cartilage (thyrotomy), or through the thyrohyoid membrane (superior laryngotomy).
- Muscles of larynx are two types: Intrinsic and extrinsic
- Intrinsic muscles: Most of the muscles in the larynx are **adductors** of vocal cord (closure of glottis), the only **abductor** muscle is **posterior cricoarytenoid**, which is called the safety muscle of larynx. It abducts the vocal cords to let pass the air through laryngeal sphincter for breathing.
- **Cricothyroid** muscle is a tensor of vocal cord and raises the pitch of voice, whereas posterior part of **thyroarytenoid** muscle is a relaxor of vocal cords while maintaining (or increasing) tension in the anterior part.
- Primary elevators of larynx are attached to the thyroid cartilage and pull it up: Stylopharyngeus, salpingopharyngeus, palatopharyngeus and thyrohyoid.
- Secondary elevators act indirectly as they are attached to the hyoid bone: Mylohyoid, digastric, stylohyoid, geniohyoid.
- Depressors of larynx are: Sternohyoid, sternothyroid and omohyoid.

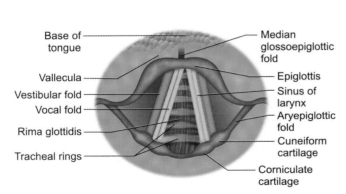

Fig. 86: The sagittal section through the nose, mouth, pharynx, and larynx

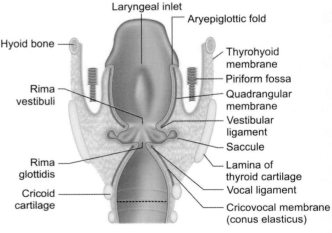

Fig. 87: Coronal section of the laryngeal cavity showing its subdivisions. A = vestibule, B = ventricle of the larynx, C = infraglottic compartment

- ❑ **Arterial** supply: Above the vocal fold by superior laryngeal artery (branch of superior thyroid artery); below the vocal fold by inferior laryngeal artery (branch of inferior thyroid artery). Rima glottidis has dual blood supply.
- ❑ **Venous** drainage: Superior laryngeal vein (drains into the superior thyroid vein) and inferior laryngeal vein (drains into the inferior thyroid vein).

Table 16: Muscles of Larynx

Muscle	Main action(s)
Cricothyroid	Stretches and tenses vocal ligament
Thyro-arytenoid[a]	Relaxes vocal ligament
Posterior crico-arytenoid	Abducts vocal folds
Lateral cricoarytenoid	Adducts vocal folds (interligamentous portion)
Transverse and oblique arytenoids[b]	Adduct arytenoid cartilages (adducting intercartilaginous portion of vocal folds, closing posterior rima glottidis)
Vocalis[c]	Relaxes posterior vocal ligament while maintaining (or increasing) tension of anterior part

[a]Superior fibers of the thyro-arytenoid muscles pass into the ary-epiglottic fold, and some of them reach the epiglottic cartilage. These fibers constitute the thyro-epiglottic muscle, which widens the laryngeal inlet.
[b]Some fibers of the oblique arytenoid muscles continue as ary-epiglottic muscles
[c]This slender muscle slip lies medial to and is composed of fibers finer than those of the thyro-arytenoid muscle.

❑ **Lymphatic drainage:** Lymphatics above the vocal cords pierce the thyrohyoid membrane, run along superior thyroid vessels and drain into upper deep cervical lymph nodes (anterosuperior group) and below the vocal cords pierce the cricothyroid membrane, reach prelaryngeal and pretracheal nodes, and drain into lower deep cervical lymph nodes (posteroinferior group).

❑ **Nerve supply:** Vagus nerve gives two branches to supply larynx: **Superior laryngeal** nerve and **recurrent laryngeal** nerve.

❑ **Superior laryngeal nerve** arises from the inferior ganglion of the vagus, runs downwards and forwards on the superior constrictor, deep to the internal carotid artery, and reaches the middle constrictor where it divides into the external and internal laryngeal nerve.

❑ **External laryngeal nerve** accompanies the superior thyroid artery, pierces the inferior constrictor and supplies the cricothyroid muscle. It also gives branches to the inferior constrictor and to the pharyngeal plexus.

❑ **Internal laryngeal nerve** passes downwards and forwards, pierces the thyrohyoid membrane and enters the larynx. It supplies the mucous membrane of the larynx up to the level of the vocal folds.

➢ **Right recurrent laryngeal nerve** is a branch of vagus given in front of the right subclavian artery, winds backwards under the artery, and they runs upwards and medially behind the subclavian and common carotid arteries to reach the tracheoesophageal groove. In the upper part of the groove it is related to the inferior thyroid artery.

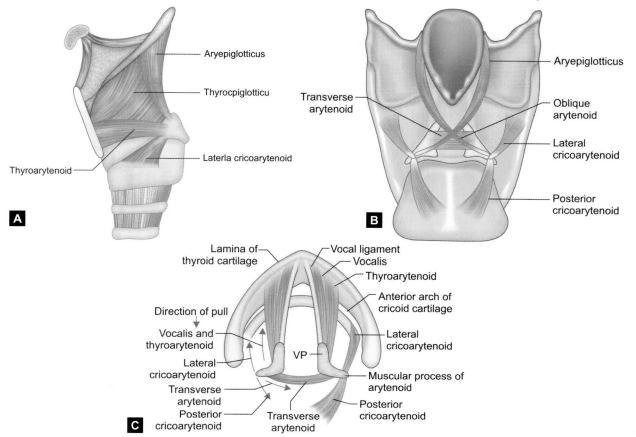

Figs. 88A to C: Intrinsic muscles of the larynx: (A) lateral view; (B) posterior view; (C) direction of pull of some intrinsic muscles (VP = vocal process of arytenoid)

❑ **Left recurrent laryngeal nerve** arises from the vagus in the mediastinum at the level of arch of aorta, loops around it and then ascends into the neck in the tracheoesophageal groove. Left nerve has a longer course than the right, passes through thoracic aperture twice and is more prone to injury statistically.

❑ All the muscles of larynx develop in sixth arch and are supplied by recurrent laryngeal nerve except the cricothyroid muscle (develops in fourth arch and supplied by external Laryngeal nerve).

Sensory supply to laryngeal mucosa above vocal cords is by internal laryngeal nerve and below the vocal cords by recurrent Laryngeal nerve.

CLINICAL CORRELATIONS

- Damage to the external laryngeal (branch of superior laryngeal) nerve can result when ligating the superior thyroid artery during thyroidectomy.
- It can be avoided by ligating the superior thyroid artery at its entrance into the thyroid gland.
- Injury to the nerve result in a weak voice with loss of projection, and the vocal cord on the affected side appears flaccid.
- Unilateral damage to the recurrent laryngeal nerve can occur while ligating inferior thyroid artery during thyroidectomy.
- It results in loss of sensation below the vocal cord and a hoarse voice, inability to speak for long periods, and movement of the vocal fold on the affected side toward the midline.
- Bilateral injury to the recurrent laryngeal nerve results in acute breathlessness (dyspnea) since both vocal folds move toward the midline and close off the air passage (and tracheostomy might be required).
- **Cricothyrotomy** is an incision through the skin and cricothyroid membrane and insertion of a tracheotomy tube into the trachea for relief of acute respiratory obstruction.
- When making a skin incision, care must be taken not to injure the anterior jugular veins, which lie near the midline of the neck.
- It is preferable for non-surgeons to perform a tracheostomy for emergency respiratory obstructions.

QUESTIONS

1. Paired laryngeal cartilage(s) is/are   *(PGIC 2014)*
   a. Thyroid   b. Arytenoid
   c. Corniculate   d. Cricoid
   e. Cuneiform

2. Which laryngeal cartilage is NOT elastic *(NEET Pattern 2012)*
   a. Epiglottis   b. Corniculate
   c. Cuneiform   d. Thyroid

3. All of the following ligaments are components of external laryngeal membrane EXCEPT   *(AIIMS 2010)*
   a. Cricothyroid
   b. Thyrohyoid
   c. Cricotracheal
   d. Hyoepiglottic

4. FALSE about larynx
   a. 9 cartilages: 3 paired and 3 unpaired cartilages
   b. Extends from C3 to C6 vertebrae
   c. External laryngeal nerve supply all larynx muscles except cricothyroid
   d. Cricothyroid is a tensor of vocal cord

5. WRONG pair of matching regarding the muscles working on vocal cords   *(NEET Pattern 2012)*
   a. Thyroarytenoid: Relaxor
   b. Lateral cricoarytenoid: Adductor
   c. Posterior cricoarytenoid: Abductor
   d. Cricothyroid: Tensor

6. Which of the following doesn't elevate the larynx
                                          (NEET 2012)
   a. Sternohyoid
   b. Thyrohyoid
   c. Mylohyoid
   d. None

7. The recurrent laryngeal nerve supplies   *(PGIC)*
   a. Vocalis muscle
   b. Posterior cricoarytenoid
   c. Cricothyroid
   d. Stylopharyngeus
   e. Omohyoid

8. During a thyroid operation, a nerve coursing along with the superior thyroid artery is injured. What can be the possible consequence(s)?   *(PGIC 2013)*
   a. Loss of sensation above vocal cord
   b. Loss of sensation below vocal cord
   c. Paralysis of lateral cricoarytenoid muscle
   d. Paralysis of cricothyroid muscle
   e. Loss of sensation in pyriform fossa

9. Which muscle is responsible for abduction of vocal cord, in the given diagram?   *(AIIMS 2016)*
   a. A
   b. B
   c. C
   d. D

1. **b. Arytenoid; c. Corniculate; e. Cuneiform**
   - ❑ **Unpaired** cartilages of larynx are in the **midline**: Epiglottis, thyroid and cricoid and paired cartilage are: Arytenoid, corniculate and cuneiform.
2. **d. Thyroid**
   - ❑ Larynx is made up of hyaline cartilage and partly elastic cartilage. **Thyroid** cartilage has **hyaline** variety.
3. **a. Cricothyroid**
   - ❑ Cricothyroid membrane **lies deep** (under laryngeal mucosa) and belongs to **internal** laryngeal membrane.
   - ❑ Cricothyroid ligament is present **between** cricoid and thyroid cartilage of the larynx.
   - ❑ The **median** cricothyroid ligament is a flat band of white tissue joining the cricoid and thyroid cartilages.
   - ❑ The **lateral** cricothyroid ligament is also known as the cricothyroid membrane (also called conus elasticus). This ligament keep the two connected cartilages together preventing them from travelling far from each other.
   - ❑ The **upper margin** of the membrane forms the **true vocal cords**.
   - ❑ The ligament is cut during **emergency cricothyrotomy**.
4. **c. External laryngeal nerve supply all larynx muscles except cricothyroid**
   - ❑ All larynx muscles are supplied by the recurrent laryngeal nerve **except** the cricothyroid muscle (supplied by the external laryngeal nerve).
5. **a. Thyroarytenoid: Relaxor**
   - ❑ The most appropriate answer is **thyroarytenoid**, though there is no perfect answer available.
   - ❑ The **posterior** part of thyroarytenoid muscle is a **relaxor of vocal cords**, while **anterior part** is a **tensor**.
   - ❑ Most of the muscles in the larynx (including lateral cricoarytenoid) are **adductors** of vocal cord.
   - ❑ Posterior cricoarytenoid is the **safety** muscle of larynx, it abducts the vocal cords to **let pass the air through** laryngeal sphincter for breathing.
   - ❑ Cricothyroid muscle is a **tensor** of vocal cord and **raises the pitch** of voice.
6. **a. Sternohyoid**
   - ❑ **Primary elevators** of larynx are attached to the thyroid cartilage and pull it up: Stylopharyngeus, salpingopharyngeus, palatopharyngeus and thyrohyoid.
   - ❑ **Secondary elevators** act indirectly as they are attached to the hyoid bone: Mylohyoid, digastric, stylohyoid, geniohyoid.
   - ❑ Depressors of larynx are: Sternohyoid, sternothyroid and omohyoid.
7. **a. Vocalis muscle, b. Posterior cricoarytenoid**
   - ❑ Recurrent laryngeal nerve supplies most of the larynx muscles (**except cricothyroid**).
8. **d. Paralysis of cricothyroid muscle**
   - ❑ The nerve coursing along with the **superior thyroid artery** is **external laryngeal nerve** (branch of superior laryngeal nerve, vagus) which supplies **cricothyroid** muscle.
   - ❑ All the muscles of larynx are supplied by recurrent laryngeal nerve **except** the cricothyroid muscle.
   - ❑ Sensory supply to laryngeal mucosa **above** vocal cords is by **internal** laryngeal nerve and **below** the vocal cords by **recurrent** laryngeal nerve.
9. **c. C**
   - ❑ This is a Questions about **posterior cricoarytenoid muscle**, which is the **only abductor** of vocal cords in larynx.
   - ❑ The diagram shows a **transverse view** of larynx, with muscles attached to various cartilages and **named accordingly**.
   - ❑ Marker 'C' is the **posteriormost muscle** called posterior cricoarytenoid, attaching to **cricoid** and **arytenoid** cartilages.
   - ❑ Marker 'A' is **lateral cricoarytenoid** muscle lying between cricoid and arytenoid cartilages. It is an **adductor** of vocal cords.
   - ❑ Marker 'B' is the **transverse** arytenoid muscle, which is also an **adductor** of vocal cords.
   - ❑ The muscle at marker 'D' is connecting thyroid cartilage with the cricoid cartilage and is called as **cricothyroid** muscle - a **tensor** of vocal cord.

- ❑ **Rima Glottidis** is the space between the vocal folds and arytenoid cartilages and is the **narrowest anteroposterior cleft** of the laryngeal cavity.
- ❑ Unilateral **vocal fold paralysis** (UVFP) occurs from a dysfunction of the **recurrent laryngeal nerve**.
- ❑ **Internal laryngeal nerve** (internal branch of superior laryngeal nerve) runs along the **superior border** of the inferior pharyngeal constrictor muscle (NEET Pattern 2013)
- ❑ Injury to **external laryngeal nerve** leads to paralysis of **cricothyroid** muscle and inability to **tense the vocal cords** resulting in weakness of voice.

- ▪ Nerve supply of larynx **above** level of vocal cord is **superior laryngeal nerve** (NEET Pattern 2015)
- ▪ Larynx has nine cartilages out of which only the **cricoid** makes a **complete ring** (signet shape) (AIIMS 2013)
- ▪ The anteroposterior diameter of glottis is **24 mm** in adult males and **16 mm** in adult females (NEET Pattern 2013)
- ▪ **Larynx** is situated in front of laryngopharynx, extends from the root of the tongue to the trachea and lies in front of the **C3, 4, 5 vertebrae** in a normal **adult male** (NEET Pattern 2015)
- ▪ **Lymphatic** drainage of the **larynx** is to the **deep cervical** nodes (NEET Pattern 2012)
- ▪ **Tensor** of vocal cord is **cricothyroid** muscle (NEET Pattern 2018)

▶ Trachea

- ❑ **Trachea** is a part of respiratory tube, beginning below the larynx (level with the **sixth cervical** vertebra), and ends at the **carina** (at the level of the **disc between T4-5 vertebra**, opposite the **sternal angle**). It may be pulled down in deep inspiration.

❑ Tracheal bifurcation in a **cadaver** placed in supine position is at **T4 vertebra**.
❑ Tracheal bifurcation is at **T3 in newborn baby**.

Note: Trachea lies in the midline but point of bifurcation is usually to the **right** side.

Dimensions:
❑ Length: 10–11 cm (within a range of 8-16 cm).
❑ External diameter: 2 cm in males and 1.5 cm in females.
❑ Internal diameter: 12 mm in adult, 1-4 mm in newborn.

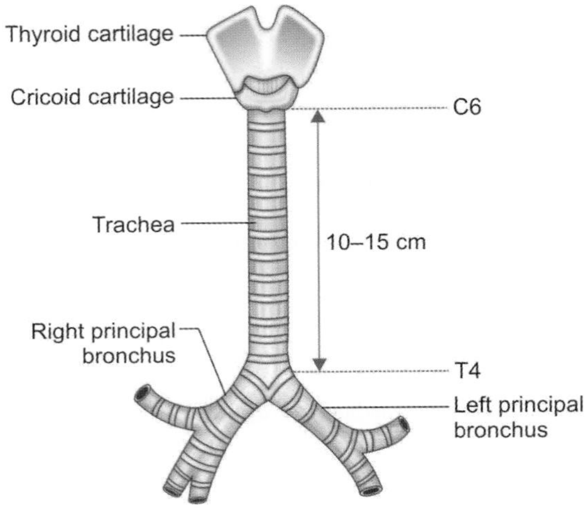

Fig. 89: Trachea-location and dimensions

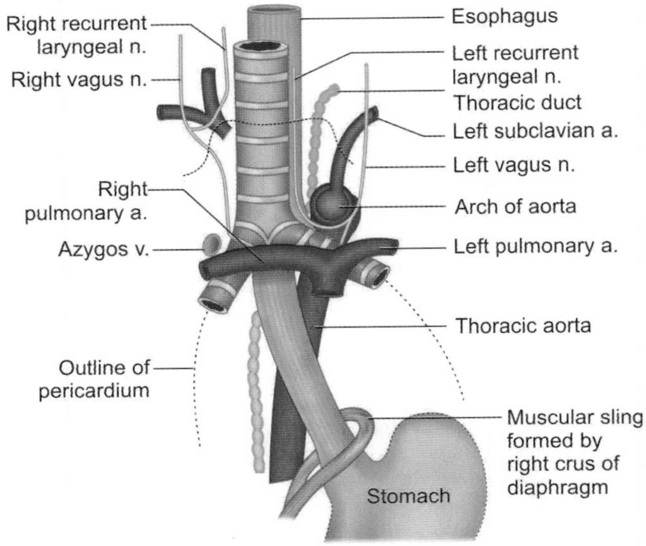

Fig. 90: Posterior and lateral relations of the trachea

❑ Structure: A long tube formed of cartilage and fibromuscular wall, and lined internally by respiratory mucosa.
❑ The anterolateral portion of the trachea consists of 16–20 U-shaped superimposed incomplete rings of hyaline cartilage and posteriorly lies the trachealis muscle.
❑ The last tracheal ring merges into the incomplete rings at the origin of each principal bronchus; the bifurcation is marked by a cartilaginous spur, the **carina**, which can be observed by bronchoscopy as a raised ridge of tissue in the sagittal plane.
   ➢ It is located about 25 cm from the incisor teeth and 30 cm from the nostrils.
❑ Arteries: Branches of the inferior thyroid arteries and their anastomosis with bronchial arteries.
❑ Veins: Inferior thyroid venous plexus.
❑ Lymphatics: Pretracheal and paratracheal lymph nodes.
❑ Nerves: Branches of the vagus, recurrent laryngeal nerves and sympathetic trunks

Tracheostomy: The **isthmus** of the thyroid gland, which normally overlies the **second and third tracheal rings**, should be divided.
❑ In emergency tracheostomy structures located in the **midline** may be damaged: Isthmus of thyroid gland, **Inferior thyroid veins**, **thyroid ima artery**, **left brachiocephalic vein**, thymus and pleura (especially infants).
❑ A high bifurcation of the **brachiocephalic trunk**, or aberrant **anterior jugular veins** (which usually lie between the midline and anterior border of sternocleidomastoid) are also prone to injury.

QUESTIONS

1. Length of trachea is *(NEET Pattern 2012)*
   a. 8-10 cm   b. 10-12 cm
   c. 12-15 cm   d. 15 cm

2. In emergency tracheostomy the following structures are damaged EXCEPT *(AIIMS 2007)*
   a. Isthmus of the thyroid   b. Inferior thyroid artery
   c. Thyroide ima artery   d. Inferior thyroid vein

ANSWERS

1. b. 10-12 cm
   ❑ Trachea has a length of about 8 to 16 cm (**10-11 cm**; Gray's Anatomy).
   ❑ It commences at the lower border of the larynx, level with the **sixth cervical** vertebra.
   ❑ Inside the trachea at the level of the **disc between T4-5 vertebra**, there is a cartilaginous ridge known as the **carina** of trachea which runs across from the front to the back of the trachea and marks the point of bifurcation into the right and left primary bronchi.
   ❑ The carina is opposite the **sternal angle** and can be positioned up to two vertebrae lower or higher, **depending on breathing**.

2. b. Inferior thyroid artery
   ❑ In emergency tracheostomy structures located in the **midline** may be damaged: Isthmus of thyroid gland, Inferior thyroid veins, thyroid ima artery, left brachiocephalic vein, thymus and pleura (especially infants).
   ❑ Inferior thyroid artery is **not damaged** in this procedure.

▶ Ear

Ear is divided into three parts—the outer ear, middle ear and the inner ear.

- ❏ Outer ear consists of the pinna and the external ear canal.
- ❏ Middle ear includes the tympanic cavity and the three ossicles. It communicates with nasopharynx via the eustachian tube.
- ❏ Inner ear sits in the bony labyrinth, has the semicircular canals (for balance and eye tracking in motion); the utricle and saccule (for balance when stationary) and the cochlea (for hearing).

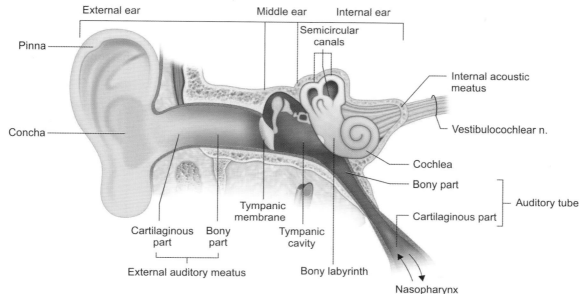

Fig. 91: The ear and its subdivisions (external, middle, and internal ear)

Ear: Development

- ❏ Internal ear develops from the **otic vesicle**, which is a derivative of the **otic placode** (surface ectoderm thickening), in the fourth week of development.
- ❏ This vesicle divides into a ventral component, which gives rise to the saccule and cochlear duct and a dorsal component, which gives rise to the utricle, semicircular canals, and endolymphatic duct.
- ❏ The epithelial structures thus formed are known collectively as the membranous labyrinth.
- ❏ Except for the cochlear duct, which forms the organ of Corti, all structures derived from the membranous labyrinth are involved with equilibrium.
- ❏ **Otic capsule** develops from the mesenchyme around the otocyst and forms the perilymphatic space, which develops into the scala tympani and scala vestibule.
- ❏ The **cartilaginous** otic capsule ossifies to form the **bony** labyrinth.
- ❏ Auricle develops from six tissue elevations (**auricular hillocks**), which form around the margins of the dorsal portion of the first pharyngeal cleft (external auditory meatus).
- ❏ First three develop on the caudal edge of the first pharyngeal (mandibular) arch and next three on the cranial edge of the second pharyngeal (hyoid) arch.

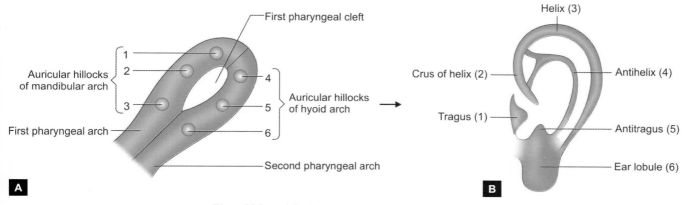

Figs. 92A and B: Development of auricle or pinna

- ❏ The tragus develops from the first arch the area of skin supplied by the mandibular nerve (trigeminal) extends little above the tragus. Helical root, and helical crus also develop in first arch.
- ❏ Second branchial arch forms major portion of the auricle which includes antihelix, antitragus, and lower helix and ear lobule.
- ❏ Faulty fusion between the first and the 2nd arch tubercles causes preauricular sinus or cyst.
- ❏ Ear ossicles: Malleus, incus and stapes develop from the neural crest cell derived secondary mesenchyme.
- ❏ Stapes bone has of dual origin, with the stapedial footplate being composed of cells of both neural crest (Reichert's cartilage) and mesodermal (otic capsule) origin.
  - ➢ If the neural crest part of the stapes fails to form the mesodermal part does not develop, indicating that the two parts are interdependent. If Reichert's cartilage fails to form, the otic capsule part does not develop.
  - ➢ The head and crus of the stapes is of neural crest origin, along with the central part of the stapedial footplate; however, the outer ring of the stapedial footplate is of mesoderm origin. This is the part of the stapes that connects to the mesodermal annular ligament. Part of the stapes is, therefore, derived from the otic capsule.
- ❏ At birth, the auditory ossicles have achieved their full adult size.

Embryonic structure	Adult derivative
Internal ear	
Otic vesicle	
Utricular portion (Ectoderm)	Utricle, semicircular ducts, vestibular ganglion of CN VIII, endolymphatic duct and sac
Saccular portion (Ectoderm)	Saccule, cochlear duct (organ of Corti), spiral ganglion of CN VIII
Middle ear	
Pharyngeal arch 1	Malleus (Mackel cartilage; neural crest cells) Incus (Meckel cartilage; neural crest cells)
	Tensor tympani muscle (mesoderm)
Pharyngeal arch 2	Stapes (Reichert cartilage; neural crest cells) Stapedius muscle (mesoderm)
Pharyngeal pouch 1	Epithelial lining of the auditory tube (endoderm) Epithelial lining of the middle ear cavity (endoderm)
Pharyngeal membrane 1	Tympanic membrane (ectoderm, mesoderm and neural crest cells, and endoderm)
External ear	
Pharyngeal groove 1	Epithelial lining of the external auditory meatus (ectoderm)
Auricular hillocks	Auricle

QUESTIONS

1. Auricular hillocks develop from pharyngeal arch:
   a. 1
   b. 2
   c. 1 and 2
   d. 2 and 3

2. Foot plate of stapes derived from:
   a. Meckel's cartilage
   b. Otic capsule
   c. Reichert's cartilage
   d. Hyoid arch

ANSWERS

1. **c. 1 and 2**
   - ❏ Auricle develops from **six** tissue elevations (auricular hillocks), **First three** develop on the caudal edge of the **first** pharyngeal (mandibular) arch and **next three** on the cranial edge of the **second** pharyngeal (hyoid) arch.

2. **c. Reichert's cartilage > b. Otic capsule**
   - ❏ Footplate of stapes has **dual origin** from the Reichert's cartilage and otic capsule.
   - ❏ If Reichert's cartilage **fails** to form, the otic capsule part does **not develop**.
   - ❏ Reichert's cartilage is the second arch cartilage (derived from the neural crest cells) and form bones like stapes, styloid process, lesser cornu and upper body of hyoid.

- ▪ **Inner ear** reaches adult form at about **10 weeks**, adult size at around **20 weeks** and adult functionality at **26th week** (NEET Pattern 2016)
- ▪ **Tympanic membrane** is derived from **all the three** germ layer (NEET Pattern 2012)

- ❏ The **tympanic cavity** and **mastoid antrum**, **auditory ossicles** and structures of the **internal ear** are all almost **fully developed at birth** and subsequently alter little; almost all of the volume changes are due to expansion of the epitympanic space.

▶ External Ear and Tympanic Membrane

- ❏ External ear consists of an **auricle** and an **external auditory meatus** and separated from the middle ear by the **tympanic membrane**.

- ❑ **Auricle** consists of cartilage connected to the skull by ligaments and muscles and is covered by skin.
  - ➢ It receives sound waves and channel them into the external auditory meatus.
  - ➢ **Helix** is the slightly curved outer rim of the auricle and **antihelix** is the broader curved eminence internal to the helix, which divides the auricle into an outer scaphoid fossa and the deeper concha.
  - ➢ **Concha** is the deep cavity in front of the antihelix and anterior to it lies a small projection called **tragus**.
  - ➢ **Lobule** is the lower portion of auricle made up of areolar tissue and fat but no cartilage.
- ❑ **Arterial supply** is from the superficial temporal and posterior auricular arteries.
- ❑ **Nerve supply:**
  - ➢ **Great auricular nerve** (C2,3), is the **major** nerve supply to auricle and supplies ear lobule and most of the cranial surface and the posterior part of the lateral surface (helix, antihelix).
  - ➢ **Lesser occipital nerve** supplies upper and cranial (posterior) part of the auricle (especially the helix).
  - ➢ **Auriculotemporal nerve** supplies the tragus, crus of the helix and the adjacent part of the helix.
  - ➢ **Auricular branch of the vagus** (Arnold's nerve) sends the axons along the **facial nerve** branches and supply small areas on both aspects of the auricle, in the depression of the concha and over its eminence.
    - ▪ These areas may show vesicles in facial nerve involvement in Ramsay Hunt syndrome (Herpes zoster).
  - ➢ **Facial nerve** itself has minimal supply in the auricle (scattered area on the depression of the concha and over its eminence).
- ❑ **External auditory meatus** is approximately 2.5 cm long, extending from the concha to the tympanic membrane.
- ❑ Its external one-third is formed by cartilage, and the internal two-thirds is formed by bone.
- ❑ The cartilaginous portion is wider than the bony portion and has numerous ceruminous glands that produce wax.
- ❑ It receives blood from the superficial temporal, posterior auricular, and maxillary arteries (deep auricular branch).
- ❑ The innervation is by the **auriculotemporal** branch of the trigeminal nerve and the **auricular branch of the vagus nerve**, which is joined by a branch of the **facial nerve** and the **glossopharyngeal nerve**.
- ❑ Anterior wall and roof is supplied by auriculotemporal nerve. Posterior wall and floor is innervated by auricular branch of vagus.

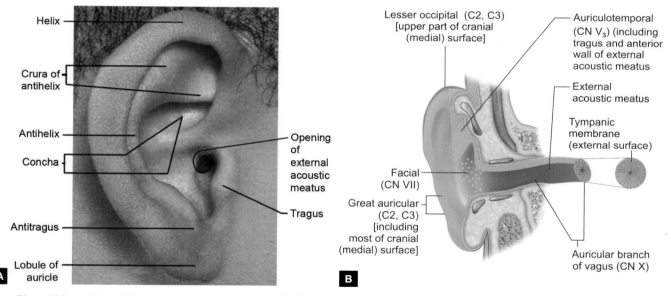

Figs. 93A and B: (A) External featurer of auricle. (B) Nerve supply to auricle, extended canal and tympanic membrane

- ❑ Posterior wall (not floor) also receives sensory fibers from facial nerve.
- ❑ **Tympanic Membrane** lies placed obliquely making an angle of about 55° with the floor of the external acoustic meatus and faces downwards, forwards, and laterally sloping medially from posterosuperiorly to anteroinferiorly; thus, the anteroinferior wall is longer than the posterosuperior wall.
- ❑ It consists of three layers: an outer (cutaneous), an intermediate (fibrous), and an inner (mucous) layer.
- ❑ It has a thickened fibrocartilaginous ring at the greater part of its circumference, which is fixed in the tympanic sulcus at the inner end of the meatus.
- ❑ The membrane has a small triangular portion between the anterior and posterior malleolar folds called the pars flaccida. The remainder of the membrane is called the pars tensa.

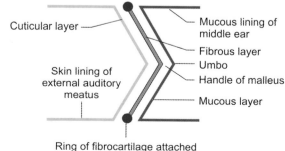

Fig. 94: Layers of the tympanic membrane.

- The cone of light is a triangular reflection of light seen in the anteroinferior quadrant. The most depressed center point of the concavity is called the umbo (knob).
- The external (lateral) concave surface is covered by skin and is innervated by the auriculotemporal branch of the trigeminal nerve and the auricular branch of the vagus nerve. The auricular branch is joined by branches of the glossopharyngeal and facial nerves.
  - ➤ This surface is supplied by the deep auricular artery of the maxillary artery.
- The internal (medial) surface is covered by mucous membrane, is innervated by the tympanic branch of the glossopharyngeal nerve, and serves as an attachment for the handle of the malleus.
  - ➤ This surface receives blood from the auricular branch of the occipital artery and the anterior tympanic artery.
- **Greater** part of auricle is supplied by **greater** auricular nerve (branch of the cervical plexus).
- **Greater auricular nerve** supplies the lobule of ear on **medial** (cranial) as well as **lateral** (outer) surface (AIIMS 2015)
- The **cartilaginous** part of external auditory canal forms the **outer one-third** (8 mm) of the meatus and the bony part forms the inner two-third (16 mm)- *(NEET Pattern 2014)*
- **Tympanic membrane** is placed obliquely making an angle of **about 55° with the floor** of the external acoustic meatus *(NEET Pattern 2013)*

▶ Middle Ear

- Middle ear is located within the petrous portion of the temporal bone and consists of the tympanic cavity with its ossicles.
- It communicates anteriorly with the nasopharynx via the auditory (Eustachian) tube and posteriorly with the mastoid air cells and the mastoid antrum through the aditus ad antrum and is traversed by the chorda tympani and lesser petrosal nerve.
- The tympanic cavity is divided into three parts:
  - ➤ **Epitympanum** (attic), a part above the pars tensa of tympanic membrane containing head of malleus, body, and short process of incus.
  - ➤ **Mesotympanum**, a part opposite to tympanic membrane containing handle of malleus, long process of incus, and stapes. It is the narrowest part of the middle ear.
  - ➤ **Hypotympanum**, a part below the tympanic membrane.

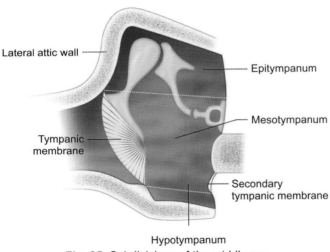

Fig. 95: Subdivisions of the middle ear

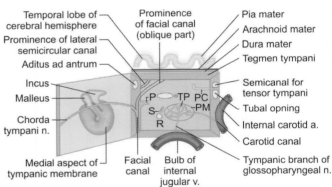

Fig. 96: Schematic diagram to show the boundaries (and their relations) of the middle ear. The middle ear is likened to a six-sided box and its lateral side is opened out (O = Oval window, P = Pyramid, PC = Processus cochleariformis, PM = Promontory, R = Round window, S = Sinus tympani, TP = Tympanic plexus)

Relations

- Middle ear cavity has a roof made up of tegmen tympani, which separates it from the middle cranial fossa.
- The floor separates it from the superior bulb of the internal jugular vein.
- The anterior wall inferior separates the middle ear from the internal carotid artery. Anterior wall shows two openings for tensor tympani and auditory tube.
- Posterior wall has an opening superiorly (aditus) through which epitympanic process communicates with the mastoid antrum.
- The lateral wall of middle ear cavity has the tympanic membrane, which separates it from the external ear canal.
- Medial wall separates it from the internal ear and present the promontory formed by the basal turn of the cochlea, the fenestra vestibuli (oval window), the fenestra cochlea (round window), and the prominence of the facial canal.
- Oval window is pushed back and forth by the footplate of the stapes and transmits the sound vibrations of the ossicles into the perilymph of the scala vestibuli in the inner ear.
- Round window is closed by the secondary tympanic (mucous) membrane of the middle ear and accommodates the pressure waves transmitted to the perilymph of the scala tympani.

Wall of middle ear	Structure/Relation
Roof (Trigeminal wall)	▪ Tegmen tympani ▪ Middle cranial fossa ▪ Temporal lobe of cerebrum
Floor (Jugular wall)	▪ Superior bulb of internal jugular vein
Anterior wall (Carotid wall)	▪ Internal carotid artery
Posterior wall (Mastoid wall)	▪ Aditus ▪ Mastoid antrum
Lateral wall (Membranous wall)	▪ Tympanic membrane ▪ External acoustic meatus
Medial wall (Labyrinthine wall)	▪ Internal ear

❑ Contents of middle ear cavity are: Chorda tympani (branch of facial nerve), ear ossicles, two muscles.
❑ Facial nerve runs in the bony canal along the medial and posterior walls of tympanic cavity and gives rise to three branches: Greater petrosal nerve, nerve to stapedius muscle and chorda tympani nerve.
❑ Ear ossicles are miniature bones namely malleus, incus, and stapes.
❑ Sound waves created vibrations in the tympanic membrane makes ossicular chain push the footplate of the stapes into the oval window, creating a traveling wave in the perilymph-filled scala vestibuli.
❑ At birth, the auditory ossicles have achieved their full adult size. They increase in density during the first years of life as marrow cavities are replaced with endosteal bone.

Table 17: Features of the three ear ossicles

	Malleus	Incus	Stapes
Resemblance	Hammer	Anvil or premolar tooth	Stirrup
Development	First pharyngeal arch cartilage	First pharyngeal arch cartilage	Second pharyngeal arch cartilage
Muscle attached	Tensor tympani	None	Stapedius
Joint/Joints	Incudomalleolar (saddle type of synovial joint)	Incudomalleolar and incudostapedial	Incudostapedial (ball and socket type of synovial joint)

❑ Muscles in the middle ear cavity are tensor tympani and stapedius.
❑ **Stapedius** muscle is the smallest of the skeletal muscles in the human body.
  ➢ It pulls the head of the stapes posteriorly, thereby tilting the base of the stapes and prevents (or reduces) excessive oscillation of the stapes and thus protects the inner ear from injury from a loud noise, and its paralysis results in hyperacusis.
❑ **Tensor tympani** draws the tympanic membrane medially and tightens it (in response to loud noises), thereby increasing the tension and reducing the vibration of the tympanic membrane.

Table 18: Muscles of the middle ear

Muscle	Origin	Insertion	Nerve supply	Action
Tensor tympani	Wall of auditory tube and wall of its own canal	Handle of malleus	Mandibular division of trigeminal nerve	Dampens down vibrations of tympanic membrane
Stapedius	Pyramid (bony projection on posterior wall of middle ear)	Neck of stapes	Facial nerve	Dampens down vibrations of stapes

❑ **Arterial supply**: Anterior tympanic (branch of maxillary artery), stylomastoid (branch of posterior auricular artery), petrosal and superior tympanic (middle meningeal artery branches), a branch from the artery of pterygoid canal and tympanic branch of the internal carotid artery.
❑ **Venous drainage** is into pterygoid venous plexus and superior petrosal sinus.
❑ **Lymphatics** drain towards retropharyngeal, parotid and upper deep cervical lymph nodes.
❑ **Nerve supply**: Tympanic Plexus is present on the promontory in the medial wall of the middle ear. It is contributed by:
❑ Tympanic branch of the glossopharyngeal nerve (Jacobson's nerve), superior and inferior caroticotympanic nerves derived from sympathetic plexus around the internal carotid artery, and a branch from geniculate ganglion.
❑ Tympanic branch of glossopharyngeal nerve enters the middle ear through a canaliculus in the floor of the tympanic cavity and contributes to the formation of tympanic plexus.
  ➢ It supplies the lining of middle ear, mastoid antrum, and auditory tube.
  ➢ It also carry the preganglionic parasympathetic secretomotor fibers to the tympanic plexus, which further sends the fibers along the lesser petrosal nerve to supply the parotid gland via otic ganglion.
❑ Mastoid antrum is an air space in the petrous portion of the temporal bone, communicating posteriorly with the mastoid cells and anteriorly with the epitympanic recess of the middle ear (via the aditus to mastoid antrum).

- Its roof is formed by tegmen tympani, which separates the antrum from middle cranial fossa.
- The floor of antrum receives the openings of mastoid air cells, posterior wall is related to sigmoid sinus and medial wall presents bulging of the lateral semicircular canal.
- The lateral wall of the antrum is formed by a plate of bone 1.5 cm thick in the adult (2 mm thick in a newborn). Its surface marking is suprameatal triangle of McEwen's.
- The mastoid air cells are innervated by a meningeal branch of the mandibular division of the trigeminal nerve.

QUESTIONS

1. Which of the following is a WRONG statement regarding middle ear cavity?
   a. Narrowest part is mesotympanum
   b. Footplate of stapes lies in epitympanum
   c. Chorda tympani is a content of epitympanum
   d. Toynbee's muscle is a content

2. Tympanic plexus is contributed by: *(NEET Pattern 2016)*
   a. Tympanic branch of glossopharyngeal nerve
   b. Vagus nerve
   c. Facial nerve
   d. Mandibular nerve

3. Stapedius pulls stapes in which direction?
   (NEET Pattern 2016)
   a. Anterior
   b. Posterior
   c. Superior
   d. Inferior

4. All of the following are true about the middle ear cavity EXCEPT: *(NEET pattern 2012)*
   a. Roof is formed by tegmen tympani
   b. Anterior wall has opening of two canals
   c. Medial wall is formed by tympanic membrane
   d. Floor has bulb of internal jugular vein

5. The distance between tympanic membrane and medial wall of middle ear at the level of center is:
   a. 3 mm
   b. 4 mm
   c. 6 mm
   d. 2 mm

6. Lateral wall of mastoid antrum is related to:
   (NEET pattern 2015)
   a. Superficial temporal artery
   b. External auditory canal
   c. Emissary vein
   d. Meningeal artery

ANSWERS

1. b. Footplate of stapes lies in epitympanum
- **Epitympanum** contains head of malleus, body, and short process of incus, along with the **chorda tympani** nerve.
- **Stapes** bone is present in **mesotympanum**, which is the **narrowest** part of middle ear cavity.
- There are two muscles in the middle ear cavity: Stapedius and tensor tympani (**Toynbee's** muscle).

2. a. Tympanic branch of glossopharyngeal nerve
- Tympanic plexus is contributed by **tympanic branch** of the glossopharyngeal nerve
- Jacobson's nerve); superior & inferior caroticotympanic nerves (sympathetic plexus around the internal carotid artery), and a branch from geniculate ganglion.

3. b. Posterior
- Stapedius reduces the oscillatory range of stapes by **pulling it posteriorly**. Tensor tympani **reduces the amplitude** of the tympanic membrane's oscillations by pulling the handle of the malleus medially to tense the membrane.

4. c. Medial wall is formed by tympanic membrane
- Tympanic membrane is present on the **lateral wall** of middle ear cavity.

5. d. 2 mm
- Middle ear cavity is shaped like a cube, compressed from side to side. In coronal section it resembles a biconcave disc.
- The vertical and anteroposterior diameters are 15 mm each, and transverse diameters are: 6 mm (at roof), 4 mm (at floor) and **2 mm (in the centre).**

The shape and dimensions of the middle ear cavity.

6. b. External auditory canal
- The lateral wall of mastoid antrum corresponds to the suprameatal triangle of MacEwen's on the outer surface of the skull, which is related to posterosuperior margin of the external auditory meatus.

- Type of **joints between ear ossicles** are **synovial** joints *(AIPG 2008)*
- **Mastoid antrum** is present in **petrous** portion of the temporal bone *(NEET Pattern 2015)*
- **Tympanic branch** of the middle ear contributes to **tympanic plexus** and is derived from **glossopharyngeal** nerve *(NEET pattern 2012)*
- Distance between tympanic membrane (lateral wall) and promontory (medial wall) of middle ear cavity is **2 mm**
- The **footplate of stapes** closes the **oval window** and is attached to its margin by annular ligament *(AIIMS 2003)*
- The medial wall of middle ear cavity shows **promontory**, a rounded prominence in the centre produced by **first (basal) turn** of the cochlea.
- The **floor** of middle ear cavity is formed by a thin plate of bone, which separates the tympanic cavity from the jugular bulb/**internal jugular vein** *(NEET Pattern 2012)*
- The **tympanic end** of Eustachian tube is situated in the **anterior wall** of the middle ear *(NEET Pattern 2013)*
- **Superior wall** (roof) of middle ear is formed by a thin plate of bone called **tegmen tympani,** which separates the tympanic cavity from the middle cranial fossa *(NEET Pattern 2015)*
- Muscle entering middle ear from pyramid apex is **Stapedius** *(NEET pattern 2012)*

Eustachian Tube

- ❏ **Eustachian (pharyngo-tympanic) tube** connects the middle ear to the nasopharynx and maintains the equilibrium of air pressure on either side of the tympanic membrane for its proper vibration and sound conduction.
- ❏ It has a length of **36 mm** and communicates the middle ear cavity with the nasopharynx.
- ❏ Lateral 1/3 (12 mm) is bony and begins at the *anterior* wall of middle ear cavity.
- ❏ Medial 2/3 (24 mm) is made up of **elastic** cartilage and opens in the nasopharynx, behind the **inferior turbinate** of nasal cavity.
- ❏ From its tympanic end it runs anterior, inferior and medial at an angle of 45° with the sagittal plane and 30° with the horizontal.
- ❏ The cartilaginous part lies in the groove between the petrous part of the temporal bone and the posterior border of the greater wing of the sphenoid bone.
- ❏ The pharyngeal end is relatively large and slit-like (vertically).
- ❏ It is situated in the lateral wall of the pharynx, about 1.25 cm behind the posterior end of inferior nasal concha.
- ❏ Eustachian tube is opened during movements like swallowing by dilator tubae (tensor veli palatini) and aided by salpingopharyngeus.
- ❏ The fibers of origin of tensor palati muscles are attached to lateral wall of the tube and its contraction during swallowing, yawning and sneezing opens the tube and helps in maintaining equality of air pressure on both sides of tympanic membrane.
- ❏ Contraction of levator palati muscles which runs below the floor of cartilaginous part also helps in opening the tube.
- ❏ The diameter of the tube is greatest at the pharyngeal orifice, least at the junction of the two parts (the isthmus), and widens again towards the tympanic cavity.
- ❏ **Arterial supply**: The osseous part of the auditory tube is supplied by the tubal artery (branch of the accessory meningeal artery) and the caroticotympanic (branches of the internal carotid artery).
- ❏ The cartilaginous part of the tube is supplied by the deep auricular and pharyngeal branches of the maxillary artery, the ascending palatine artery (usually a branch of the facial artery, occasionally given directly by the external carotid artery) and the ascending pharyngeal branch of the external carotid artery.
- ❏ Some authors also mention the artery of the pterygoid canal and the middle meningeal artery as the source of arterial supply.
- ❏ **Venous drainage**: The veins of the pharyngotympanic tube usually drain to the **pterygoid venous plexus**.
- ❏ **Nerve supply** is by tympanic plexus and from the pharyngeal branch of the pterygopalatine ganglion.

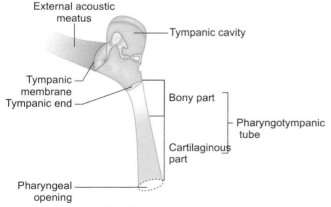

Fig. 97: Pharyngotympanic tube

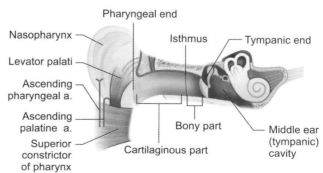

Fig. 98: Bony and cartilaginous parts, isthmus, tympanic, and pharyngeal ends of the pharyngotympanic tube

Table 19: Differences between the Eustachian tube of an infant and an adult

	Infant	Adult
Length	18 mm	36 mm
Direction	More or less horizontal (makes an angle of 10° with the horizontal plane)	Oblique, directed downwards, forwards and medially (makes an angle of 45° with the horizontal plane)
Angulation of isthmus	No angulation	Angulation present

QUESTIONS

1. TRUE about pharyngotympanic tube is/are *(PGIC 2015)*
   a. 36 mm in length
   b. 1/3 cartilaginous and 2/3 bony
   c. Runs anteromedially making an angle of 30° with the sagittal plane
   d. Tensor veli palati opens it
   e. Narrowest diameter is at the isthmus

2. Blood supply of the Eustachian tube is by all EXCEPT *(NEET 2012)*
   a. Ascending pharyngeal artery
   b. Middle meningeal artery
   c. Artery of pterygoid canal
   d. Facial artery

3. Eustachian tube is supplied by *(PGIC 2005)*
   a. Tympanic plexus
   b. Caroticotympanic nerve
   c. Glossopharyngeal nerve
   d. Pterygopalatine ganglion
   e. All

4. TRUE about anatomy of Eustachian tube *(PGIC 2014)*
   a. Aerate middle ear
   b. Open during swallowing
   c. Larger and wider in adult than children
   d. More horizontal in infant and children
   e. Open in oropharynx

ANSWERS

1. a. 36 mm in length; d. Tensor veli palati opens it; e. Narrowest lumen is at the isthmus
   ❑ Eustachian (pharyngo-tympanic) tube has a **length of 36 mm**.
   ❑ It **communicates** the middle ear cavity with the nasopharynx.
   ❑ Lateral 1/3 (12 mm) is **bony** and begins at the anterior wall of middle ear cavity.
   ❑ Medial 2/3 (24 mm) is made up of **elastic cartilage** and opens in the nasopharynx, **behind the inferior turbinate** of nasal cavity.
   ❑ It runs anterior, inferior and medial **(AIM) at an angle of 45°with the sagittal** plane and 30°with the horizontal.
   ❑ It is opened by dilator tubae (**tensor veli palatini**) and aided by salpingopharyngeus.
   ❑ Levator veli palatini **might allow** passive opening.
   ❑ The diameter of the tube is greatest at the pharyngeal orifice, **least at the junction** of the two parts (the isthmus) and widens again towards the tympanic cavity.

2. d. Facial artery
   ❑ Arteries to the pharyngotympanic tube arise from the **ascending palatine artery**, the pharyngeal branch of the maxillary artery, **ascending pharyngeal artery**, middle meningeal artery and the artery of the pterygoid canal.
   ❑ Ascending palatine artery is usually a branch of the facial artery but occasionally given directly by the external carotid artery.

3. e. All
   ❑ Eustachian tube is supplied by **tympanic plexus** and from the pharyngeal branch of the pterygopalatine ganglion.
   ❑ Tympanic plexus itself is contributed by tympanic branch of the glossopharyngeal nerve, superior and inferior **caroticotympanic** nerves derived from sympathetic plexus around the internal carotid artery, and a branch from geniculate ganglion.

4. a. Aerate middle ear; b. Open during swallowing; d. More horizontal in infant and children
   ❑ Eustachian tube communicates the nasopharynx with the middle ear cavity and **aerates** it.
   ❑ In infants the tube is shorter, relatively wider and **more horizontal** than adult.
   ❑ It opens during movements like **swallowing**, yawning and sneezing.

▶ Inner Ear

❑ Inner ear consists of the **cochlea** housing the cochlear duct for auditory sensation, and the **vestibule** housing the utricle and saccule, and the **semicircular canals** housing the semicircular ducts for the sense of balance and position.
❑ The membranous labyrinth is a closed system of fluid filled intercommunicating membranous sacs and ducts filled with endolymph.
❑ It lies within the complex intercommunicating bony cavities and canals (**bony labyrinth**) in the petrous part of the temporal bone.
❑ The space between the membranous and bony labyrinth is filled with perilymph.

Table 20: Structure and function of internal ear components.

Bony labyrinth component (Containing perilymph and the membranous labyrinth)	Membranous labyrinth component (Within bony labyrinth and containing endolymph)	Structures and sensory receptors	Major function
Vestibule	Utricle, saccule	Maculae	Detect linear movements and static position of the head
Semicircular canals	Semicircular ducts	Cristae ampullares	Detect rotational movements of the head
Cochlea	Cochlear duct	Spiral organ	Detect sounds

- ❑ The **bony labyrinth** has three parts: Cochlea, vestibule and **semicircular canals** (three).
- ❑ **Cochlea** consists of a central pillar called modiolus, and a bony cochlear canal.
  - ➢ The apex (cupula) is directed towards the medial wall of the tympanic cavity and the base is towards the bottom of the internal acoustic meatus.
- ❑ **Vestibule** is a central ovoid cavity of bony labyrinth between cochlea in front and three semicircular canals behind.
  - ➢ It lies medial to the middle ear cavity.
- ❑ **Semicircular canals** (kinetic labyrinth) are three bony semicircular canals: anterior (superior), posterior, and lateral (horizontal).
- ❑ They lie in three planes at right angles to each other and open in the vestibule by five openings.
- ❑ Each canal is about two-third of a circle and is dilated at one end to form the ampulla.
  - ➢ **Anterior** semicircular canal lies in a vertical plane at right angle to the long axis of the petrous temporal bone, is convex upwards and its position is indicated on the anterior surface of the petrous temporal bone as arcuate eminence.
  - ➢ **Posterior** semicircular canal also lies in a vertical plane parallel to the long axis of petrous temporal bone.
  - ➢ **Lateral** semicircular canal lies in the horizontal plane. The lateral semicircular canals of two sides lie in the same plane.
- ❑ The anterior semicircular canal of one side lies parallel to the posterior semicircular canal of the other side.
- ❑ The anterior and posterior semicircular canals, lying across and along the long axis of the petrous temporal bone, are each at 45° with the sagittal plane.
- ❑ **Membranous labyrinth:** The **cochlear duct** lies within the bony cochlea, the saccule, and utricle lie within the bony vestibule, and three semicircular ducts lie within the three bony semicircular canals.
- ❑ The cochlear duct (basal turn) is connected to saccule by **ductus reuniens**.
- ❑ The saccule and utricle are connected to each other by Y-shaped **utriculo-saccular duct**, which expands to form ductus and saccus endolymphaticus.
- ❑ The utricle is connected to three semicircular ducts through five openings.

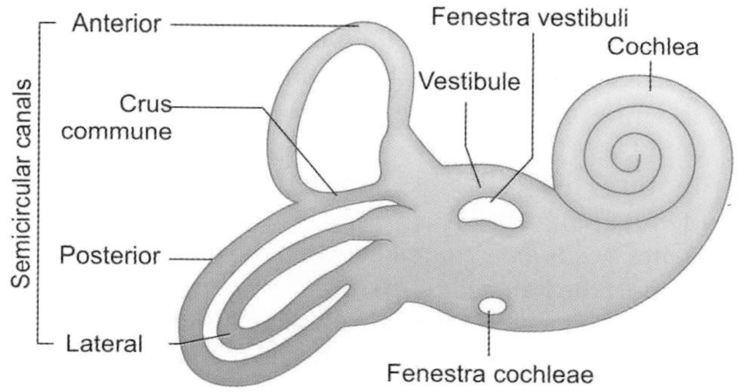

Fig. 99: Parts of the bony labyrinth.

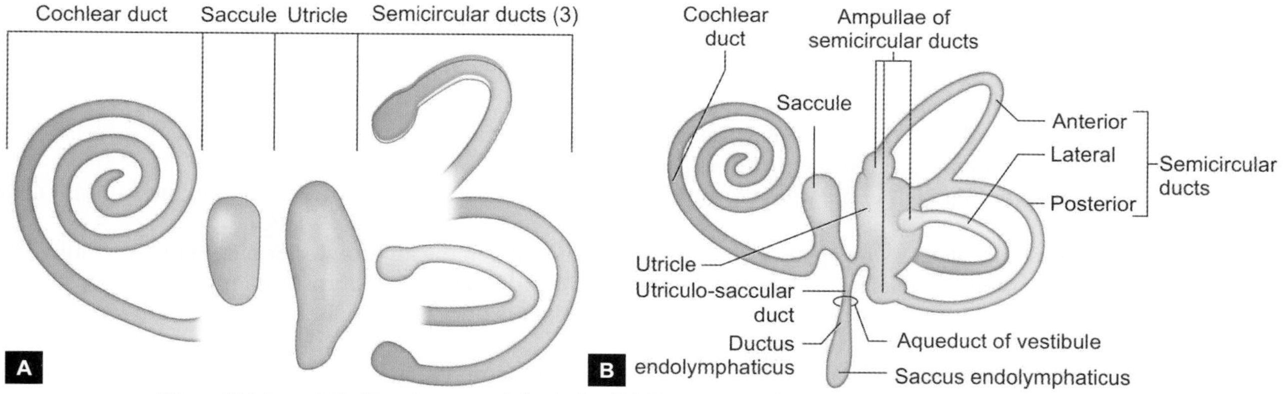

Figs. 100A and B: Membranous labyrinth: (A) Four parts of labyrinth. (B) Complete labyrinth

- ❑ **Cochlear system:** The sensory receptor within **cochlear duct** is spiral organ of Corti which sends the auditory information by the cochlear nerve (CN VIII).
- ❑ Cochlear Duct (Scala Media) is a spiral anterior part of the membranous labyrinth having two and three-fourth turns.
- ❑ It lies in the middle part of the cochlear canal between scala vestibuli and scala tympani.
- ❑ The cochlear duct contains spiral organ of Corti and appears triangular in shape in cross section.
- ❑ Base is formed by the osseous spiral lamina (medially) and basilar membrane (laterally).

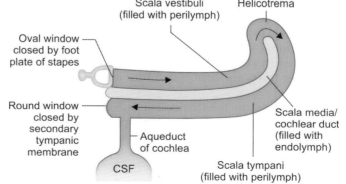

Fig. 101: Diagrammatic representation of the cochlear duct within cochlear canal. Note that cochlear duct is filled with endolymph and scala vestibuli and scala tympani are filled with perilymph (CSF = Cerebrospinal fluid).

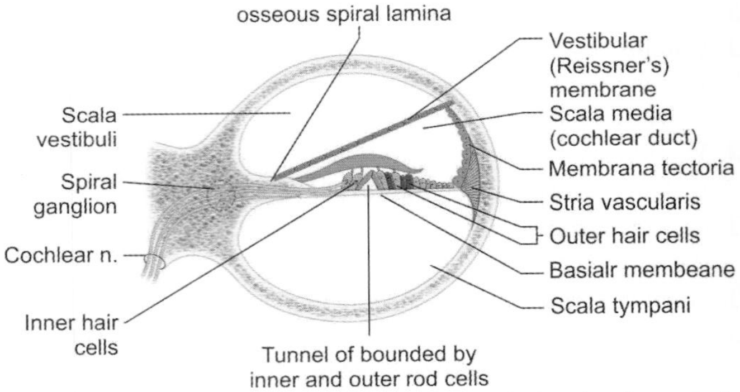

- Vestibular membrane (Reissner's membrane) is at the roof, which passes from upper surface of spiral lamina to the wall of cochlea.
- Laterally it is bounded by the outer wall of cochlear canal.
- The scala vestibuli and scala tympani containing perilymph lie above and below basilar membrane respectively.
- Cochlear duct (containing endolymph) is bathed above and below by the perilymph within the two scalae.
- The two scalae are continuous with each other through a narrow opening at the apex of cochlear duct called **helicotrema**.
- **Spiral Organ of Corti** has a tunnel of Corti formed by the inner and outer rod cells. It contains a fluid called corticolymph.

Fig. 102: Cross-section of the cochlear canal showing boundaries of the cochlear duct and organ of Corti within it.

- The hair cells are the receptor cells of hearing located on basilar membrane and their apices possess stereocilia (hair), which are overlaid by tectorial membrane.
- The inner cells are flask shaped and arranged in a single row while outer cells are cylindrical and arranged in 3 or 4 rows.
- Sound vibrations create fluid waves in perilymph of scala vestibuli, which pass to the perilymph of scala tympani, in the process the basilar membrane bulge and the overlying hair cells are stimulated.
- The inner hair cells are richly supplied by the cochlear nerve fibers and are responsible for transmission of auditory impulses.
- The outer hair cells are innervated by efferent fibers from the olivary complex and are concerned with modulation function of inner hair cells.
- Deiter's cells are situated between the outer hair cells and provide support. The Hansen's cells lie outside the hair cells also support the hair cells.
- Membrana tectoria is made up of gelatinous substance and overlies the hair cells. Medially it is attached to osseous spiral lamina. The shearing force between the hair cells and tectorial membrane stimulate the hair cells.
- **Basilar membrane** separates the cochlear duct from the scala tympani.
- The pitch localization along its length is 20 Hz at the apex and 20,000 Hz at the base of the cochlea.
- Its vibration results in deformation of the hair cell microvilli against the tectorial membrane and the stimulus is further carried to CNS.
- Ninety percent of afferent fibers (peripheral processes of bipolar neurons of spiral ganglion) supply the inner hair cells while only 10% supply the outer hair cells.
- The spiral ganglion is located in the spiral canal within the modiolus near the base of the spiral lamina.
- The central processes of bipolar ganglion cells form the cochlear nerve (CN VIII).
- Efferent fibers to the outer hair cells come from olivocochlear bundle. Their cell bodies are located in the superior olivary complex.
- **Vestibular system**: The saccule is a small globular membranous sac lying in the anteroinferior part of the vestibule.
- The utricle is an oblong membranous sac, is larger than the saccule and lies in the posterosuperior part of the vestibule.
- The saccule is connected in front to the basal turn of cochlear duct by the ductus reuniens and behind with the utricle by a Y-shaped utriculo-saccular duct.
- The vertical limb of Y continues as endolymphatic duct (ductus endolymphaticus) and its dilated blind terminal end is called saccus endolymphaticus.
- The **endolymphatic duct** passes through a bony canal (aqueduct of vestibule) in the posterior part of petrous temporal bone and its dilated terminal end projects on the posterior surface of petrous temporal bone beneath the dura mater of the posterior cranial fossa.
- The endolymph is absorbed by the epithelial cells lining the saccus and drains into extradural vascular plexus.
- The utricle receives the three semicircular ducts posteriorly through five openings.
- **Semicircular Ducts** are three in number : anterior, posterior, and lateral and lie within the corresponding semicircular canals.
- They open into the utricle by five openings. Each duct has one dilated end called ampulla.
- It corresponds to the ampulla of the corresponding semicircular canal.
- The ampullary end of each duct bears a raised crest (crista ampullaris), which projects into its lumen.
- Peripheral receptors in vestibular system are: **Maculae** are located in the medial walls of saccule and utricle.
- They sense position of head in response to gravity and linear acceleration, i.e. static balance.
- **Cristae** are located in the ampullated ends of the three semicircular ducts.
- They detect angular acceleration, i.e., kinetic balance.
- The information of balance is carried by the vestibular nerve (CN VIII).

QUESTIONS

1. **NOT a part of bony labyrinth** *(NEET Pattern 2015)*
   a. Cochlea
   b. Vestibule
   c. Utricle
   d. Semi-circular canal

2. **TRUE about internal ear anatomy**
   a. Three semi-circular canals here 6 opening into the vestibule
   b. The angle between anterior and posterior SCC is 180°
   c. Vestibule is the central chamber
   d. Spiral canal makes 2 turns

3. **Infection of CNS spreads in inner ear through** *(AIIMS 2010)*
   a. Cochlear aqueduct
   b. Endolymphatic sac
   c. Vestibular aqueduct
   d. Hyrtl's fissure

4. **A child with CSOM develops recurrent meningitis. The spread of infection to CNS is most probably through**
   a. Fissure of Santorini *(JIPMER 2017)*
   b. Hyrtl's fissure
   c. Foramen of Luschka
   d. Persistent petro-squamous septum

5. **Which area is innervated by the peripheral processes of the spiral ganglion** *(AIIMS 2016)*
   a. A
   b. B
   c. C
   d. D

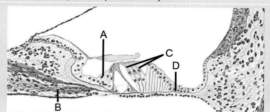

1. **c. Utricle**
   ❑ **Utricle** belongs to **membranous** labyrinth.
   ❑ Bony labyrinth components (containing perilymph and the membranous labyrinth) are **vestibule**, **semi-circular canals** and **cochlea**.

2. **c. Vestibule is the central chamber**
   ❑ Vestibule is the **central** part of bony labyrinth. Semi-circular canal forms **2/3rd of a circle** and are at **right angle** to each other.
   ❑ The utricle receives the three semi-circular ducts posteriorly through **five openings**.

3. **a. Cochlear aqueduct**
   ❑ Perilymph filled cochlear aqueduct is in direct continuation with CSF and may serve as a channel of **spread of infection** between inner ear and CNS.
   ❑ **Vestibular aqueduct** contains endolymphatic duct filled with endolymph, which does not communicate freely with CSF.
   ❑ The endolymphatic duct passes through the bony canal (**aqueduct of vestibule**) in the posterior part of petrous temporal bone and its dilated terminal end projects on the posterior surface of petrous temporal bone **beneath the dura mater** of the posterior cranial fossa.
   ❑ The endolymph is absorbed by the epithelial cells lining the saccus and drains into extradural vascular plexus.
   ❑ **Hyrtl's fissure** connects middle ear to **subarachnoid space.**

4. **b. Hyrtl's fissure**
   ❑ Hyrtl's fissure is an anatomic landmark allowing a **transient embryonic communication** between the subarachnoid space and the middle ear. It is also known as tympano-meningeal fissure, maybe a very rare cause of **spontaneous CSF otorrhea** and meningitis.

5. **a. A**
   ❑ The **inner hair cells** (marker 'A') are innervated by the peripheral processes of the spiral ganglion.
   ❑ This is a diagram of **organ of Corti** in the inner ear, showing inner and outer cells, basilar membrane and spiral ganglion cells.
   ❑ The hair cells of the organ of Corti are innervated by the peripheral processes of bipolar cells of the **spiral ganglion** (marker 'B'). They are stimulated by vibrations of the **basilar membrane** (marker 'D').
   ❑ **Inner hair cells** (marker 'A') are the chief sensory elements; they synapse with dendrites of myelinated neurons whose axons make up **90% of the cochlear nerve.**
   ❑ **Outer hair cells** (marker 'C') synapse with dendrites of unmyelinated neurons whose axons make up **10% of the cochlear nerve.** They reduce the threshold of the Inner hair cells.

▪ Inner ear is present in **petrous** part of temporal bone *(NEET pattern 2014)*

❑ **Horizontal** semi-circular canal is also called **lateral** semi-circular canal.

▶ Internal Auditory Meatus

❑ Internal auditory meatus is a canal within the petrous part of the temporal bone of the skull between the posterior cranial fossa and the inner ear.

❑ The falciform (or transverse) crest separates the superior part from the inferior part.

❑ A vertical projection from the roof divides the superior part into two sections: Anterosuperior and posterosuperior section.

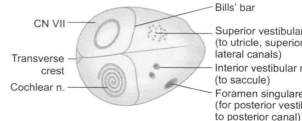

Fig. 103: Inner aspect of lateral end of internal auditory canal with structures passing through different areas.

- The anterosuperior part transmits the facial nerve (along with nervus intermedius) and is separated from the posterosuperior section, which transmits the superior vestibular nerve, by Bill's bar.
- The cochlear nerve runs anteroinferiorly and the inferior vestibular nerve runs posteroinferiorly.
- Labyrinthine vessels also pass through the meatus.
- **Bill's bar**: A **vertical crest** that separates the superior fundus in the **internal auditory canal** into anterior and posterior portions containing the facial nerve (& nervus intermedius) and the superior vestibular nerve, respectively. (AIIMS 2011)

Vestibulocochlear Nerve

- Vestibulocochlear nerve leaves the pontocerebellar angle laterally and enters the internal acoustic meatus (with the facial nerve) and remains within the temporal bone to supply sensory fibers to the sensory cells of the inner ear.
- The cochlear portion (for hearing) derives from bipolar neurons in the spiral (cochlear) ganglion that innervate the hair cells of the cochlea (organ of Corti).
- The vestibular portion (for equilibrium) arises from bipolar neurons in the vestibular ganglion that innervate sensory cells of the ampullae of the semicircular ducts as well as the utricle and saccule.

Auditory Pathway

- Auditory information is an exteroceptive sensation, which belongs to SSA (special somatic afferent), detecting sound frequencies from 20 Hz to 20,000 Hz.
- The primary afferents of the auditory pathway arise from cell bodies in the spiral ganglion of the cochlea.
- The bipolar cells of the spiral (cochlear) ganglion project peripherally to the hair cells of the organ of Corti.
- They project centrally as the cochlear nerve to the cochlear nuclei. The cochlear nerve [cranial nerve (CN) VIII] extends from the spiral ganglion to the cerebellopontine angle, where it enters the brainstem.
- The cochlear nuclei project contralaterally to the superior olivary nucleus and lateral lemniscus.
- The superior olivary nucleus, which plays a role in sound localization, receives bilateral input from the cochlear nuclei and projects to the lateral lemniscus.
- The trapezoid body (ventral pons) contains decussating fibers from the ventral cochlear nuclei.
- The ventral cochlear nucleus projects via the trapezoid body or the intermediate acoustic stria to relay centres in either the superior olivary complex, the nuclei of the lateral lemniscus, or the inferior colliculus.
- The lateral lemniscus receives input from the contralateral cochlear nuclei and superior olivary nuclei and project to the nucleus of inferior colliculus.
- The medial geniculate body receives input from the nucleus of the inferior colliculus.
- It projects through the internal capsule (sublentiform fibers) as the auditory radiation to the primary auditory Cortex.
- The medial geniculate body is connected reciprocally to the primary auditory cortex, which lies in the posterior half of the superior temporal gyrus and also dives into the lateral sulcus as the transverse temporal gyri (Heschl's gyri).
- Connections also run from the nucleus of the lateral lemniscus to the deep part of the superior colliculus, to coordinate auditory and visual responses.

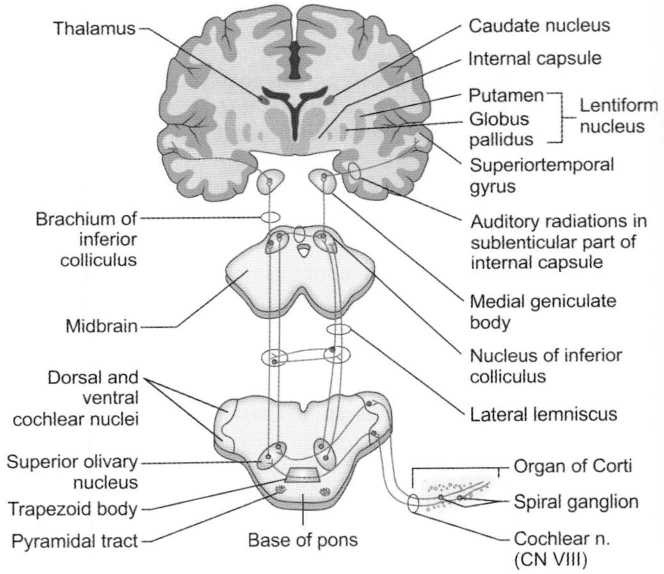

Auditory pathway (Mnemonic: SLIM – 41,42.)
Figs. 104: Superior olivary nucleus, L: Lateral lemniscus, I: Inferior colliculus, M: Medial geniculate body, 41,42: Temporal auditory cortex. Organ of Corti (inner ear) → cochlear (spiral) ganglion and nerve → cochlear nuclei → trapezoid body → superior olivary nucleus → lateral lemniscus → inferior colliculus → medial geniculate body → sublentiform fibers of internal capsule → auditory cortex (41, 42 Brodmann area)

CLINICAL CORRELATIONS

- Presbycusis results from degenerative disease of the organ of Corti in the first few millimeters of the basal coil of the cochlea (high-frequency loss of 4,000 to 8,000 Hz).

Vestibular Pathway

- Vestibular nuclei project fibers to:

- Flocculonodular lobe of the cerebellum
- CN III, IV, and VI through the medial longitudinal fasciculus (MLF)
- Spinal cord through the lateral vestibulospinal tract
- Ventral posteroinferior and posterolateral nuclei of the thalamus, both of which project to the postcentral gyrus.

QUESTIONS

1. Auditory pathway consists of all of the following EXCEPT
   a. Lateral geniculate body
   b. Superior olivary nucleus
   c. Trapezoid body
   d. Inferior colliculus

2. All are true about vestibular nerve EXCEPT *(PGIC 2016)*
   a. It has two divisions- superior and inferior vestibular
   b. Vestibular nuclei are situated at junction of pons and medulla
   c. Nerve fibers relay at Scarpa's ganglion
   d. Nucleus lies in midbrain near aqueduct

ANSWERS

1. a. Lateral geniculate body
   ❑ Medial (**not lateral**) geniculate body is related to auditory pathway. Lateral geniculate body comes in visual pathway.
   ❑ Trapezoid body is present in the **ventral pons** and contains the crossing fibers from the cochlear nuclei towards the superior olivary nucleus.

2. d. Nucleus lies in midbrain near aqueduct
   ❑ Vestibular nerve nuclei lie at the **pontomedullary junction**.
   ❑ It arises from **bipolar cells** in the vestibular ganglion, **ganglion of Scarpa**, which is situated in the upper part of the outer end of the internal auditory meatus.
   ❑ The vestibular nerve enters the brain stem at the **pontomedullary junction** and contains two divisions, the **superior and inferior** vestibular nerves. The superior vestibular nerve innervates the utricle, as well as the superior and lateral canals. The inferior vestibular nerve innervates the posterior canal and the saccule.
   ❑ Most of the afferent fibers then terminate in one of the four **ventricular nuclei**, which contain the cell bodies of the second-order neurons of the vestibular nerve. These nuclei are located on lateral floor and wall of the **fourth ventricle** in the pons and medulla.

Histology of Ear Region

Histology

❑ The auricle (pinna) is made up of elastic cartilage and is covered by skin (stratified squamous epithelium).
❑ External auditory canal is covered by skin with sebaceous glands and ceruminous glands (modified apocrine sweat glands that produce wax).
❑ Tympanic membrane is lined by skin (stratified squamous epithelium) on its external surface and simple cuboidal epithelium on its inner surface.

Nose

Surface Anatomy of Nose

❑ **Glabella** is a small horizontal ridge, which is easily palpable between the superciliary arches.
❑ It is the most forward projecting point of the forehead in the midline at the level of the supraorbital ridge
❑ **Nasion** is the intersection of the frontal bone and two nasal bones. It is present between the eyes, just superior to the bridge of the nose and just inferior to the glabella.
❑ **Radix**: The junction between the frontal bone and the nasal bone (dorsum of the nose).
❑ **Rhinion**: It is the soft-tissue correlate of the osseocartilaginous junction of the nasal dorsum. It is the anterior tip at the end of the suture of the nasal bones.
❑ **Columella**: Column between the nostrils at the base of nose.
❑ Nasal cavity has the function to warm, clean, humidify, filter the inhaled air for respiration, and appreciate the special senses of smell and taste.
❑ It opens to the exterior on the face through the anterior nasal apertures (nostrils) and communicates posteriorly with the nasopharynx through the choanae.
❑ Vestibule is a slight dilatation inside the aperture of each nostril, lined with skin containing hair, sebaceous glands, and sweat glands.
❑ **Roof** is formed by the bones : Nasal, frontal, cribriform plate of ethmoid, and body of sphenoid.
   - The axons of olfactory nerves pass through the cribriform plate of ethmoid to reach the olfactory bulb in brain.
❑ **Floor** is contributed by the palatine process of the maxilla and the horizontal plate of the palatine bone.

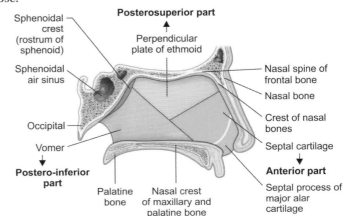

Fig. 105: Formation of the nasal septum.

➢ It has the incisive foramen, which transmits the nasopalatine nerve and terminal branches of the sphenopalatine artery.
❑ **Medial wall** is the **nasal septum** formed by the perpendicular plate of the ethmoid bone, vomer, and septal cartilage.
➢ It also get contributions by processes of the palatine, maxillary, frontal, sphenoid, and nasal bones.
❑ **Lateral wall of nose** is subdivided into three parts:
➢ **Vestibule** is a small depressed area in the anterior part, lined by modified skin containing hair called vibrissae
➢ **Atrium** of the middle meatus is the middle part.
➢ The posterior part contains the **conchae** and the spaces under each called the respective **meatus**.
➢ The skeleton of the lateral wall is partly bony, partly cartilaginous, and partly made up only of soft tissues.
➢ The bony part is formed from before backwards by the following bones (1) Nasal, (2) frontal process of maxilla (3) Lacrimal, (4) Labyrinth of ethmoid bone with superior and middle conchae; (5) Inferior nasal concha; (6) Perpendicular plate of the palatine bone together with its orbital and sphenoidal processes, and (7) Medial pterygoid plate.
➢ The cartilaginous part is formed by: (a) The superior nasal cartilage; (b) the inferior nasal cartilage; and 3 or 4 small cartilages of the ala.

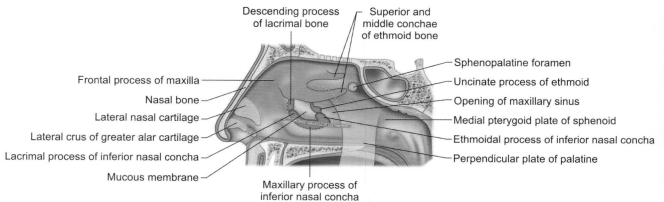

Fig. 106: Formation of the lateral wall of the nasal cavity. Red circle indicates the position of maxillary air sinus

❑ **Inferior turbinate** is an independent facial bone (not a part of ethmoid), which extends horizontally along the lateral wall of the nasal cavity and articulates with bones like maxilla, palatine, lacrimal and **ethmoid**.
❑ It is the largest of the three turbinates.
❑ The inferior meatus lies underneath the inferior concha, and is the **largest** of the three meatuses.
❑ The **nasolacrimal duct** opens into it at the junction of its anterior one-third and posterior two-thirds.
❑ This opening is guarded by the lacrimal fold, or Hasner's valve.
❑ The middle meatus lies underneath the middle concha.
❑ It presents the following features: (1) The ethmoidal bulla, is a rounded elevation produced by the underlying middle ethmoidal sinuses, (2) The hiatus semilunaris, is a deep semicircular sulcus below the bulla, (3) The infundibulum is a short passage at the anterior end of the hiatus, (4) The opening of the frontal air sinus is seen in the anterior part of the hiatus semilunaris, (5) The opening of the maxillary air sinus is located in the posterior part of the hiatus semilunaris. It is often represented by two openings, (6) The opening of the middle ethmoidal air sinus is present at the upper margin of the bulla.
❑ The superior meatus lies below the superior concha.
❑ This is the shortest and shallowest of the three meatuses.
❑ It receives the openings of the posterior ethmoidal air sinuses.
Openings in the lateral wall of nasal cavity:

Table 21: The openings in the lateral wall of the nose	
Sites	**Openings**
Sphenoethmoidal recess	Opening of the sphenoidal air sinus
Superior meatus	Opening of the posterior ethmoidal air sinuses
Middle meatus ▪ On bulla ▪ In hiatus semilunaris	Opening of the middle ethmoidal air sinuses
– Anterior part	Opening of the frontal air sinus
– Middle part	Opening of the anterior ethmoidal air sinuses
– Posterior part	Opening of the maxillary air sinus
Inferior meatus	Opening of the nasolacrimal duct (in the anterior part of meatus)

❑ Some authors mention the opening of the frontal sinus into the infundibulum.
❑ Sphenopalatine Foramen is the opening into the pterygopalatine fossa; transmits the sphenopalatine artery and nasopalatine nerve.

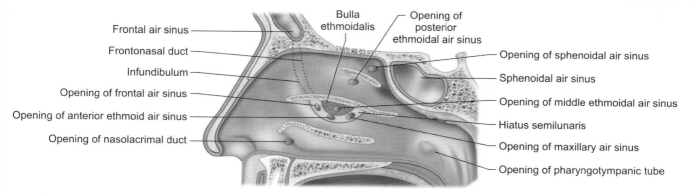

Fig. 107: Lateral wall of the nose with conchae removed showing openings of various sinuses and nasolacrimal duct

- ❏ Mucous membrane of nose has three regions: **Vestibule**, **respiratory** region and **olfactory** region.
  - ➢ **Vestibule** is present at the entrance of nostrils, bound by the alar cartilages and lined by skin with hair.
  - ➢ **Respiratory** area occupies the lower two-thirds of the nasal cavity.
  - ➢ **Olfactory** Region is located at the roof of nasal cavity, includes the superior nasal concha and the upper one-third of the nasal septum.
    - ▪ It has neuroepithelium, whose axons constitutes olfactory nerves, which enter the cranial cavity passing through the cribriform plate of the ethmoid bone to synapse in the olfactory bulb.
- ❏ Arterial supply:
  - ➢ The **sphenopalatine** artery (branch of maxillary artery) is the most important supply to the nasal cavity, giving posterior lateral nasal and posterior septal branches.
  - ➢ ly there are other contributions: Lateral nasal branches of the anterior and posterior **ethmoidal** arteries of the ophthalmic artery; the **greater palatine** branch (its terminal branch reaches the lower part of the nasal septum through the incisive canal) of the descending palatine artery of the maxillary artery; the septal branch of the **superior labial artery** of the facial artery and the **lateral nasal** branch of the facial artery.
- ❏ **Little's area** is a highly vascular area located in the anteroinferior part of the nasal septum just above the vestibule.
- ❏ Four (or five) arteries anastomose here to form a vascular plexus called **Kiesselbach's plexus**.
- ❏ It is exposed to the drying effect of inspiratory current and to finger nail trauma and is the usual site for epistaxis.
- ❏ Participating arteries are: Septal branch of the anterior ethmoidal artery (a branch of ophthalmic artery), Septal branch of the sphenopalatine artery (a branch of maxillary artery), septal branch of the greater palatine artery (a branch of maxillary artery) and septal branch of the superior labial artery (a branch of facial artery). Occasionally septal branch of the posterior ethmoidal artery (a branch of ophthalmic artery) may also contribute to the plexus.
- ❏ **Woodruff's plexus** is a **venous** plexus just inferior to the posterior end of the inferior turbinate, is considered as a frequent source of **posterior epistaxis**.

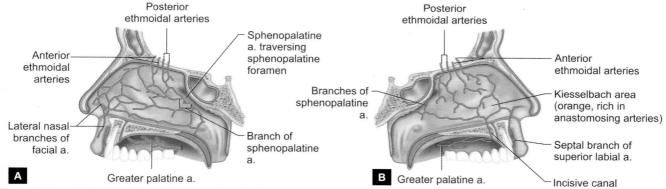

Figs. 108A and B: Arterial supply of nasal cavity. An open-book view of the lateral and medial walls of the right side of the nasal cavity is shown. The left "page" shows the lateral wall of the nasal cavity. The sphenopalatine artery (a branch of the maxillary) and the anterior ethmoidal artery (a branch of the ophthalmic) are the most important arteries to the nasal cavity. The right "page" shows the nasal septum. An anastomosis of four to five named arteries supplying the septum occurs in the antero-inferior portion of the nasal septum (Kiesselback area, orange) an area commonly involved in chronic epistaxis (nosebleeds)

▌▌▌ CLINICAL CORRELATIONS ▌▌▌

- ▪ **Epistaxis** is a nosebleed resulting usually from rupture of the sphenopalatine artery.
- ▪ It may occur from nose picking, which tears the veins in the vestibule of the nose.
- ▪ It also occurs from the anterior inferior part of nasal septum (Kiesselbach's area or plexus), where branches of the sphenopalatine (from maxillary), greater palatine (from maxillary), anterior ethmoidal (from ophthalmic), and superior labial (from facial) arteries converge.

- The sphenopalatine artery may be ligated under endoscopic visualization as it enters the nose through the sphenopalatine foramen.
- The ethmoidal arteries are exposed within the orbit and ligated.
- The maxillary artery is exposed surgically behind the posterior wall of the maxillary sinus and ligated.
- Nerve supply:
  - Smell sensation is carried by olfactory nerve under special somatic afferent (**SSA**) neural column.
  - General sensation under general somatic afferent (**GSA**) column is carried by the **anterior ethmoidal** branch of the ophthalmic nerve; the **nasopalatine**, posterior–superior, and posterior–inferior lateral nasal branches of the maxillary nerve via the pterygopalatine ganglion; and the anterior-superior alveolar branch of the infraorbital nerve.

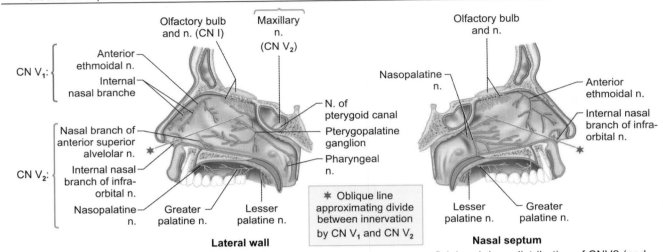

Fig. 109: Lateral wall and septum of the right nasal cavity demonstrates superficial and deep distribution of CNV2 (and, incidentally, CN I) to the nasal and upper over the midline of the head

Elevators	Procerus, levator labii superioris alaeque nasi
Depressors	Alar nasalis, depressor septi nasi
Compressors	Transverse nasalis (compressor naris)
Dilators	Alar nasalis (dilator naris)

Table: Nasal Muscles

Olfactory Nerve

Olfactory nerve (CN I) is derived from the embryonic **nasal placode** and is unusual among cranial nerves because it is **capable of some regeneration** if damaged. It is the **shortest** (length) cranial nerve.

It consists of approximately 20 bundles of **unmyelinated** afferent fibers (**special visceral afferent**) that arise from neurons in the olfactory area, the upper **one-third of the nasal mucosa**, and carry the sense of smell (olfaction).

- ❑ The axons pass through the **foramina in the cribriform plate** of the ethmoid bone and synapse in the **olfactory bulb**.
- ❑ The olfactory nerve fibers synapse with **mitral cells** in the olfactory bulb. The axons of these secondary neurons form the **olfactory tract**. The olfactory bulbs and tracts are **anterior extensions of the forebrain**.
- ❑ Each olfactory tract divides into **lateral** and **medial** olfactory striae. The **lateral** olfactory stria terminates in the **piriform cortex** of the anterior part of the **temporal lobe**, and the **medial** olfactory stria projects through the **anterior commissure** to **contralateral** olfactory structures.
- ❑ This mainly direct pathway to the neocortex, for the **most part bypasses the thalamus**.
- ❑ A **newer** olfactory pathway **that passes through the thalamus**, passing to the dorsomedial thalamic nucleus and then to the latero-posterior quadrant of the orbito-frontal cortex, has been found. This newer system probably helps in **the conscious analysis of odor.**
- ❑ **Olfactory nerve** is **pure sensory** for the sensation of smell *(NEET Pattern 2016)*
- ❑ The **shortest** (length) cranial nerve is **olfactory** nerve (CN I).

Paranasal Sinuses

- ❑ Skull bones around nasal cavity develop pneumatization and spaces called paranasal sinuses, which help in reduction of weight and resonance for voice.
- ❑ At birth, both small **ethmoidal** and **maxillary** sinuses are present, but the **frontal** sinus is nothing more than an out-pouching from the nasal cavity, and there is no pneumatization of the **sphenoid** bone.
- ❑ **Ethmoidal air sinus** shows numerous ethmoidal air cells, within the ethmoidal labyrinth between the orbit and the nasal cavity.

- Sinus pathology may erode through the thin orbital plate of the ethmoid bone (lamina papyracea) and enter into the orbit.
- Three groups are identified: **Posterior** ethmoidal air cells, drain into the superior nasal meatus, **middle** ethmoidal air cells, drain into the summit of the ethmoidal bulla (middle meatus) and **anterior** ethmoidal sinus drain into the anterior aspect of the hiatus semilunaris (middle meatus).
- **Frontal air sinus** is located in the frontal bone and opens into the hiatus semilunaris of the middle nasal meatus by way of the frontonasal duct (or infundibulum). It is innervated by the supraorbital branch of the ophthalmic nerve.
- **Maxillary air sinus** is the largest of the paranasal air sinuses and is the only paranasal sinus that may be present at birth.
- It lies in the maxilla bone lateral to the lateral wall of the nasal cavity and inferior to the floor of the orbit, and drains into the posterior aspect of the hiatus semilunaris in the middle meatus.
- **Sphenoidal air sinus** is located within the body of the sphenoid bone and drains into the spheno-ethmoidal recess of the nasal cavity.
- It is innervated by branches from the maxillary nerve and by the posterior ethmoidal branch of the nasociliary nerve.
- Pituitary gland lies in the sella turcica in the body of sphenoid above this sinus and can be reached by the trans-sphenoidal approach, which follows the nasal septum through the body of the sphenoid.

Sinus	Drainage
Frontal sinus	Middle meatus (through frontonasal duct) Into hiatus semilunaris (anterior part)
Maxillary sinus	Middle meatus Into hiatus semilunaris (posterior part)
Sphenoidal sinus	Spheno-ethmoidal recess
Anterior ethmoidal sinus	Middle meatus Into hiatus semilunaris
Middle ethmoidal sinus	Middle meatus Surface of bulla ethmoidalis
Posterior ethmoidal sinus	Superior meatus (posterior part)

QUESTIONS

1. **TRUE about anatomy of lateral wall of nose:** *(PGIC 2013)*
   a. Superior turbinate is a separate bone
   b. Ethmoid bone forms an important part of the lateral wall
   c. Middle turbinate is formed by medial process of the ethmoidal labyrinth
   d. Opening of inferior meatus is present
   e. Inferior turbinate is a separate bone

2. **Bony nasal septum is formed by all EXCEPT:** *(NEET Pattern 2012)*
   a. Vomer
   b. Sphenoid
   c. Ethmoid
   d. Nasal spine of nasal bone

3. **Uncinate process arises from:** *(NEET Pattern 2014)*
   a. Ethmoid bone
   b. Palatine bone
   c. Nasal bone
   d. Maxilla bone

4. **One of the following opens in the middle meatus of the nose:** *(NEET Pattern 2015)*
   a. Naso-lacrimal duct
   b. Eustachian tube
   c. Sphenoidal air sinus
   d. Maxillary air sinus

5. **Ethmoidal sinus opens into which of the following:** *(NEET Pattern 2012)*
   a. Hiatus semilunaris
   b. Middle meatus
   c. Superior meatus
   d. All of the above

6. **Which of the following sinuses open into middle meatus?** *(PGIC 2014)*
   a. Frontal sinus
   b. Anterior ethmoidal sinus
   c. Posterior ethmoidal sinus
   d. Maxillary sinus
   e. Sphenoid sinus

7. **Arterial supply of little's area are:** *(PGIC 2015)*
   a. Greater palatine artery
   b. Septal branch of superior artery
   c. Anterior ethmoidal artery
   d. Septal branch of sphenopalatine artery
   e. Nasal branch of sphenopalatine artery

8. **Onodi cells and Haller cells of ethmoid labyrinth seen in relation to following respectively:** *(AIIMS 2009)*
   a. Optic nerve and floor of orbit
   b. Optic nerve and Internal carotid artery
   c. Optic nerve and nasolacrimal duct
   d. Orbital floor and nasolacrimal duct

9. **Which of the following artery is NOT ligated in a case of epistaxis?** *(AIIMS 2017)*
   a. Anterior ethmoidal artery
   b. Maxillary artery
   c. Internal carotid artery
   d. External carotid artery

10. **Which of the following are NOT a branch of external carotid artery in Kiesselbach's plexus?** *(AIIMS 2017)*
   a. Sphenopalatine artery
   b. Anterior ethmoidal artery
   c. Greater palatine artery
   d. Septal branch of superior labial artery

ANSWERS

1. **b. Ethmoid bone forms an important part of the lateral wall; c. Middle turbinate is formed by medial process of the ethmoidal labyrinth; d. Opening of inferior meatus is present; e. Inferior turbinate is a separate bone**
   - Ethmoid bone has **major contribution** in the nose formation, including **lateral wall** of nose.
   - Superior and middle concha are formed by medial process of the **ethmoidal** labyrinth, whereas inferior concha is an **independent** bone.

2. **d. Nasal spine of nasal bone**
   - Bony nasal septum is contributed by the **nasal spine of frontal bone**.
   - It is the **crest** of nasal bone which contributes to nasal septum.

3. a. Ethmoid bone
- ❑ In the ethmoid bone, a **curved lamina**, the uncinate process, projects downward and backward from the labyrinth; it forms a small part of the medial wall of the maxillary sinus and articulates with the ethmoidal process of the inferior nasal concha.
- ❑ It can be seen in the middle meatus (**lateral wall** of nose).

4. d. Maxillary air sinus
- ❑ Maxillary sinus opens **posterior to the hiatus semilunaris** of middle meatus near the roof of the sinus.
- ❑ Nasolacrimal duct opens into the **anterior part of inferior meatus** closed by a mucosal flap called **Hasner's valve**.
- ❑ Eustachian tube opens into the lateral wall of nasopharynx, about **1.25 cm behind** the posterior end of inferior nasal concha.
- ❑ Sphenoid air sinus opens into **spheno-ethmoidal recess** of nasal cavity.

5. d. All of the above
- ❑ **Anterior** ethmoidal sinus opens into **hiatus semilunaris** (middle meatus).
- ❑ **Middle** ethmoidal sinus opens into surface of **bulla ethmoidalis** (middle meatus).
- ❑ **Posterior** ethmoidal sinus opens into **superior** meatus (posterior part).

6. a. Frontal sinus; b. Anterior ethmoidal sinus; d. Maxillary sinus
- ❑ Middle meatus has hiatus semilunaris with openings of some sinuses: **Frontal** sinus opens at the **front** of hiatus semilunaris, **anterior** ethmoidal sinus in the **middle** and maxillary sinus in the posterior part.
- ❑ Middle ethmoidal sinus opens in the middle meatus at the bulla.

7. a. Greater palatine artery, b. Septal branch of superior artery, c. Anterior ethmoidal artery, d. Septal branch of sphenopalatine artery
- ❑ In Little's area septal branches of the **anterior ethmoidal**, **sphenopalatine**, **greater palatine**, and **superior labial** arteries anastomose to form a vascular plexus called **Kiesselbach's plexus**.

8. b. Optic nerve and Internal carotid artery
- ❑ Ethmoid bone is a pneumatic bone and has numerous air cells around the nose.
- ❑ **Onodi cell** is the most **posterior ethmoidal cell** that is present superior and lateral to the sphenoid sinus and is intimately related to the optic nerve and internal carotid artery.
- ❑ Optic nerve may be seriously damaged in ESS (Endoscopic sinus surgery).
- ❑ Haller cell represents an extension of anterior ethmoidal air cells extending into the infra-orbital margin (roof of maxillary sinus).

9. c. Internal carotid artery
- ❑ Arteries which can be ligated in a case of epistaxis are: Anterior and posterior **ethmoids** artery, sphenopalatine artery (SPA). **More rarely** the internal maxillary artery or the external carotid artery can be ligated.

10. b. Anterior ethmoidal artery
- ❑ Anterior ethmoidal artery is a branch of **ophthalmic artery** (which itself is a branch of **internal carotid** artery).

- ▪ **Kiesselbach's plexus** is the commonest site of bleeding (90% of cases). It is situated in the **anterior inferior** part of nasal septum, just above the vestibule.
- ▪ **Little's area** is present on **anteroinferior** nasal septum *(NEET Pattern 2015)*
- ▪ **Woodruff's plexus** is situated in relation to **posterior end of inferior turbinate**. It is a site of **posterior epistaxis** in adults. The plexus is **venous in origin** and have no muscle walls leading to poor haemostasis.
- ▪ **Inferior turbinate** is a facial bone which extends horizontally along the lateral wall of the nasal cavity and **articulates** with bones like **ethmoid, maxilla**, palatine and lacrimal bones *(NEET pattern 2012)*
- ▪ Parts of ethmoid bone are Agger nasi, Bulla ethmoidalis, Uncinate process but **not Inferior turbinate** *(NEET Pattern 2014)*
- ▪ **Olfactory** region in nose is **above** superior turbinate *(NEET Pattern 2013)*
- ▪ The **roof** of nasal cavity, formed by the cribriform plate of ethmoid bone, has olfactory epithelium *(NEET Pattern 2014)*
- ▪ **Rhinion** is the soft-tissue correlate of the **osseocartilaginous junction** of the nasal dorsum *(NEET Pattern 2012)*
- ▪ **Muscles of nose** are Procerus, Compressor naris, Depressor septi but **not Angularis oris** *(NEET Pattern 2016)*
- ▪ **Anguli oris** is a facial muscle associated with **frowning**.
- ▪ **Posterior** ethmoidal sinus opens in the **superior** meatus.
- ▪ **Nasolacrimal duct** opens in the **inferior meatus**, on **anterior** aspect, covered by Hasner's valve.
- ▪ **Lacrimal bone** does **not** contribute to the formation of **Nasal septum** *(AIPG 2008)*
- ▪ Lymphatic drainage of nose is towards Submandibular nodes, Retropharyngeal nodes and Upper (not lower) deep cervical nodes *(NEET Pattern 2016)*
- ▪ Nose lymphatic **do not** drain into **lower** deep cervical nodes.
- ▪ **Haller cell** represents an extension of anterior ethmoidal air cells extending into the infra-orbital margin (roof of maxillary sinus) *(AIIMS 2009)*.

▶ Orbit and Eyeball

❑ Orbit is the socket in the skull where the eye and its appendages are present.

▶ Bony Orbit

☐ Walls of orbit:
- ➤ **Medial wall** (4 bones) is formed by maxilla, lacrimal bone, ethmoid and the sphenoid (body).
- ➤ **Lateral wall** (2 bones) is contributed by the zygomatic bone, and sphenoid (greater wing).
- ➤ **Roof** (2 bones) has frontal bone and sphenoid (lesser wing)
- ➤ Floor (3 bones) is formed by maxilla, zygomatic and palatine bones.

☐ The thickest wall is lateral and the thinnest is medial.

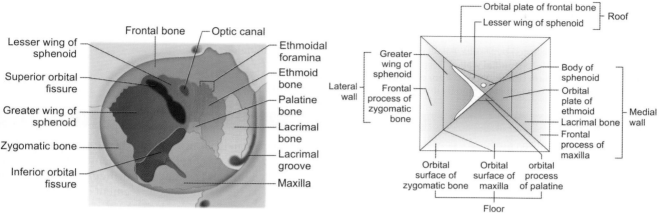

Figs. 110: Bones of the orbit

Fissures, Canals, and Foramina Related with Orbit

☐ **Superior orbital fissure** is present between the lateral wall and the roof of orbit.
- ➤ It communicates with the middle cranial fossa and is bounded by the greater and lesser wings of the sphenoid.
- ➤ It transmits the oculomotor, trochlear, abducens, three branches of ophthalmic nerve and the ophthalmic (superior and inferior) veins.

☐ **Inferior orbital fissure** is formed between the medial wall and the floor of orbit.
- ➤ It is bounded by the greater wing of the sphenoid (above) and the maxillary and palatine bones (below) and bridged by the orbitalis (smooth) muscle.
- ➤ It communicates with the infratemporal and pterygopalatine fossae and transmits the maxillary nerve and its zygomatic branch and the infraorbital vessels.
- ➤ Maxillary nerve passes through it to run at the floor of the orbit as inferior orbital nerve.

☐ **Optic Canal** is formed by the two roots of the lesser wing of the sphenoid, lies in the posterior part of the roof of the orbit and connects the orbit with the middle cranial fossa.
- ➤ It transmits the optic nerve and ophthalmic artery.

☐ **Infraorbital groove** and foramen transmit the infraorbital nerve and vessels.

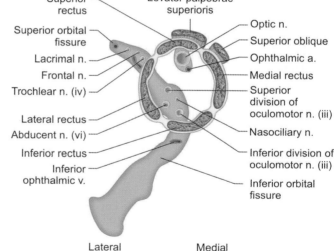

Fig. 111: Structures passing through the orbital fissures.

☐ **Supraorbital notch**/foramen transmits the supraorbital nerve and vessels.

☐ Anterior and posterior **ethmoidal Foramina** are present at the junction of roof and medial wall of orbit and transmit the anterior and posterior ethmoidal nerves and vessels, respectively.

☐ Nasolacrimal canal is formed by the maxilla, lacrimal bone, and inferior nasal concha. It transmits the nasolacrimal duct from the lacrimal sac to the inferior nasal meatus.

QUESTIONS

1. **Choose the WRONG statement concerning the wall of the orbit**
   a. Roof: Frontal bone
   b. Roof: Greater wing sphenoid
   c. Medial wall: Ethmoid bone
   d. Medial wall: Sphenoid bone

2. **TRUE statement about orbital articulation is** *(AIPG)*
   a. Medial wall of orbit is formed by maxilla, sphenoid, ethmoid and the lacrimal bone
   b. Floor is formed by maxilla, zygomatic and ethmoid
   c. Lateral wall of orbit is formed by the frontal bone, zygomatic bone, and greater wing of sphenoid
   d. Inferior orbital fissure is formed between the medial wall and the floor of orbit

ANSWERS

1. **b. Roof: Greater wing sphenoid**
   - Greater wing of sphenoid is present in the lateral wall (**not roof**) of orbit.
2. **a. Medial wall of orbit is formed by maxilla, sphenoid, ethmoid and the lacrimal bone**
   - Medial wall of orbit is formed by (in **anterior to posterior** order): Maxilla, lacrimal, ethmoid and sphenoid body.
   - **Floor** is formed by maxilla and zygomatic bones, with small contribution from palatine bone.
   - **Lateral** wall is contributed by the greater wing of sphenoid and zygomatic bone.
   - Inferior orbital fissure is present between the **lateral wall** and floor of orbit.

- **Lamina papyracea** separates nose from orbit *(NEET pattern 2013, 15)*
  - It is a **bone plate** which forms the lateral surface of the labyrinth of the ethmoid bone, covers in the middle and posterior ethmoidal cells and forms a large part of the **medial wall of the orbit**.
- **Floor of orbit** is contributed by Maxilla, Palatine and Zygomatic (bone **but not Ethmoid**)- *(AIIMS 2013)*
  - Ethmoid bone forms the **medial wall** of the orbit.
- **Maxilla** gives **maximum** contribution to **floor of orbit** *(NEET Pattern 2012)*
- **Blow out fracture** of orbit most commonly involves **floor** > medial wall. *(NEET Pattern 2018)*

Eyeball Development

- Development of the eye involves a series of inductive interactions between neighbouring tissues in the embryonic head.
- These are the **neurectoderm** of the forebrain (which forms the sensory retina and accessory pigmented structures), the **surface ectoderm** (which forms the lens and the anterior corneal epithelium) and the intervening **neural crest and their mesenchyme** (which contributes to the fibrous coats of the eye and to tissues of the anterior segment of the eye) and the **primary mesenchyme**.
- Note: Previously it was believed that neuroectoderm give rise to **neural crest cells**, but recently it has been mentioned that they are the **fourth germ layer** (derivative of epiblast ?).
- The first morphological sign of eye development is a thickening of the diencephalic neural folds at 29 days post ovulation, when the embryo has seven to eight somites, by 32 days, the optic vesicles are formed. The development continues through the tenth week.
- PAX6 is the master gene for eye development, is expressed in the single eye field at the neural plate stage. The eye field is separated into two optic primordia by SHH (Sonic HedgeHog), which upregulates PAX2.
- **Neuroectoderm** of the diencephalon (forebrain) evaginates to form the **optic vesicle**, which in turn invaginates to form the **optic cup** and **optic stalk**.
- The inner layer of the optic cup is made of neuroepithelium (**neural retina**), while the outer layer is composed of **retinal pigment epithelium** (RPE). The middle portion of the optic cup develops into the ciliary body and iris.
- Optic cup forms: Retina, epithelium of iris and ciliary body and iris muscles (sphincter and dilator pupillae).
- Optic stalk forms the optic nerve, optic chiasma and optic tract.
- The optic vesicles contact the surface ectoderm and induce the formation of **lens placode**, which eventually separates from the ectoderm to form the **lens vesicle** (and eye lens) at the open end of the optic cup. Surface ectoderm also forms the **anterior epithelium of cornea**.
- Through a groove at the bottom of the optic vesicle known as choroid fissure the **hyaloid blood vessels** enter the eye. Hyaloid artery and vein form the **central artery and vein of the retina**.
- The extracellular mesenchyme (mostly neural crest derived secondary mesenchyme and a small portion of primary mesenchyme) forms the **sclera**, the **corneal endothelium** and **stroma**, **blood vessels**, muscles, and **vitreous**.
- Three **preotic myotomes**, each supplied by its own nerve (cranial nerve Ill, IV and VI), form the extrinsic muscles of the eye.
- Conjunctiva (bulbar and palpebral) is derived from **surface ectoderm** and so are the skin of eye and glands like lacrimal gland.
- Connective tissue and bony structure of the orbit are derived from **neural crest cells**.

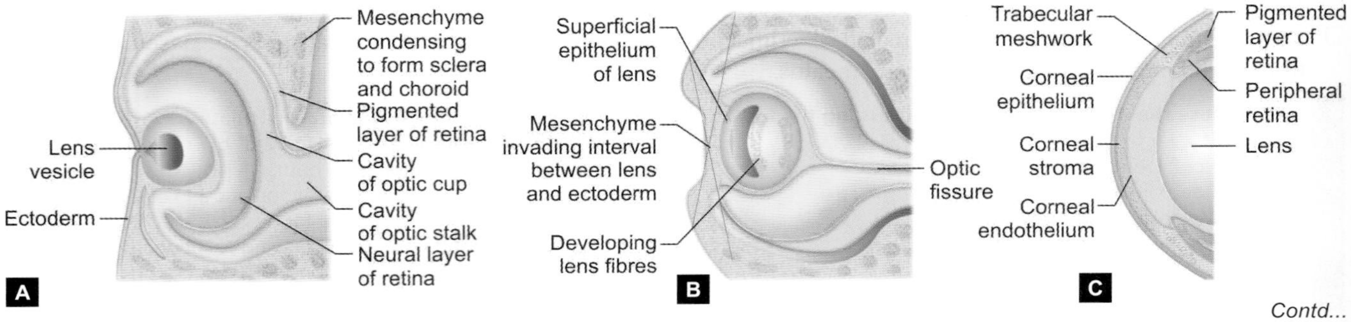

Contd...

Contd...

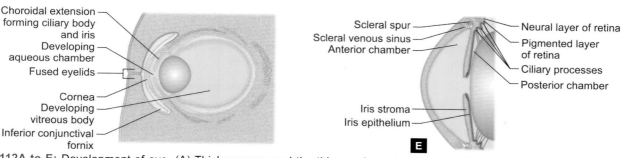

Fig. 112A to E: Development of eye. (A) Thick nervous and the thinner pigmented layers of the developing retina and the lens are evident. The two layers of the embryonic optic cup are separated by the intraretinal space. (B) The surface ectoderm anterior to the lens forms the corneal epithelium, whereas the corneal stroma and endothelium will differentiate from the invading mesenchyme (of neural crest and mesodermal origin). (C) The development of the anterior aqueous chamber is apparent with choroidal extensions and iris visible. The eyelids have developed and are fused; the extent of the conjunctival formices can be seen. (D) Anterior growth of the peripheral retina, pigmented layer of the retina and mesenchymal proliferation at the anterior part of the retina will give rise to the ciliary body and iris. The surface ectoderm anterior to the lens forms the corneal epithelium, whereas the corneal stroma and endothelium will differentiate from invading mesenchyme (of neural crest and mesodermal origin). (E) Details of the developing uveal tract. Note the development of the anterior and posterior aqueous chambers, separated by the iris, and the attachment of the lens to the ciliary body

❏ **Ocular Muscles:** Extrinsic eye muscles are derived from mesenchymal cells near the prechordal plate.

Precursor	Derivatives
Neural (plate) ectoderm	Retina (Including neural and pigment epithelium) Optic nerve Smooth muscle of the iris (sphincter pupillae and dilator pupillae) Epithelium of ciliary body and iris Vitreous (partly)
Surface ectoderm	First layer of cornea (surface epithelium) Eye lens Bulbar and palpebral conjunctiva Lacrimal glands Tarsal glands
Neural crest cells	Cornea: Descemet's membrane and endothelium Sclera Uveal and conjunctival melanocytes Meningeal sheaths of the optic nerve Smooth muscular layer of the ocular and orbital blood vessels Ciliary ganglion Orbital bones
Secondary mesenchyme (derived from neural crest cells)	Cornea: Bowman's membrane and stroma Choroid Iris (includes stroma, excludes epithelium) Ciliary body (includes stroma, ciliaris muscle, excludes epithelium) Vitreous (partly)
Primary mesenchyme	Endothelial lining of blood vessels of the eye Blood vessels in sclera and choroid Trabecular meshwork endothelium Vitreous (partly) Extraocular muscles (somitomeres)

Iris	
Derivatives	**Precursor**
Epithelium	Neural plate ectoderm
Stroma (connective tissue)	Neural crest cell derived mesenchyme
Muscles (sphincter pupillae and dilator pupillae	Neural plate ectoderm

Ciliary body	
Derivatives	**Precursor**
Epithelium	Neural plate ectoderm
Stroma (connective tissue)	Neural crest cell derived mesenchyme
Muscles (ciliaris)	Neural crest cell derived mesenchyme

Cornea

Derivatives	Precursor
Surface epithelium (first layer of cornea)	Surface ectoderm
Bowman's membrane and stroma	Mesenchyme (mostly neural crest cell derived)
Descemet's membrane and endothelium	Neural crest cells

QUESTIONS

1. **Ciliaris muscle is derived from:**
   a. Neural crest cells
   b. Neural plate ectoderm
   c. Surface ectoderm
   d. Mesoderm

2. **Stroma of cornea develops from:** *(NEET Pattern 2013, 14, 15)*
   a. Neural ectoderm
   b. Surface ectoderm
   c. Mesoderm
   d. Neural crest

3. **Corneal stroma is derived from:** *(NEET Pattern 2013)*
   a. Paraxial mesoderm
   b. Intermediate mesoderm
   c. Lateral plate mesoderm
   d. Ectoderm

4. **All are derived from neuroectoderm EXCEPT:** *(NEET Pattern 2012)*
   a. Dilator pupillae
   b. Lens vesicle
   c. Optic nerve
   d. Posterior layers of retina

5. **All of the following are mesodermal in origin EXCEPT:** *(AIPG)*
   a. Dilators of iris
   b. Iris stroma
   c. Ciliary body
   d. Choroid

6. **Which of the following is NOT a derivative of neural ectoderm?** *(AIIMS 2013)*
   a. Sphincter pupillae
   b. Dilator pupillae
   c. Ciliary muscle
   d. Retina

7. **All are derived from neural crest EXCEPT:** *(NEET Pattern 2015)*
   a. Adrenal medulla
   b. Pigment cell in skin
   c. Corneal stroma
   d. Retinal pigmented epithelium

8. **Optic cup is surrounded by:** *(NEET Pattern 2016)*
   a. Ectoderm
   b. Mesoderm
   c. Endoderm
   d. Neuroectoderm

ANSWERS

1. **a. Neural crest cells > d. Mesoderm**
   - Neural crest cells form **secondary** mesenchyme (mesoderm) to give **ciliaris** muscle.

2. **d. Neural crest > c. Mesoderm**
   - Stroma of cornea develops from **neural crest cells** derived (secondary) mesenchyme/**mesoderm**.
   - The role of primary mesenchyme/mesoderm is **minimal**.

3. **d. Ectoderm**
   - Stroma of cornea develops from neural crest cells derived (secondary) mesenchyme.
   - Note: Neural crest cells are the fourth germ layer, derived from epiblast. **Some authors** consider neural crest cells are derived from neuro**ectoderm**.

4. **b. Lens vesicle**
   - Lens vesicle develops from the **surface ectoderm**.
   - Neuroectoderm evaginates to form the optic vesicle, which in turn invaginates to form the optic cup and optic stalk.
   - **Optic cup** forms: Retina, iris muscles (sphincter and dilator pupillae) and epithelium of iris and ciliary body.
   - **Optic stalk** forms the optic nerve.

5. **a. Dilators of iris**
   - Muscles of iris: sphincter and dilator pupillae are derived from the **neural plate ectoderm**.
   - Iris stroma, ciliary body and choroid develop from **mesoderm** (neural crest cells derived).

6. **c. Ciliary muscle**
   - Ciliary muscle is derived from secondary mesenchyme formed by **neural crest cells**.
   - Neural ectoderm forms the retina and iris muscles (sphincter and dilator pupillae).

7. **d. Retinal pigmented epithelium**
   - Compared with neural crest-derived melanocytes, retinal pigment epithelium (RPE) cells in the back of the eye are pigment cells of a **different kind**. They are a part of the brain itself.
   - The neural retina and retinal pigment epithelium (RPE) originate from different portions of the optic vesicle, the more distal part developing as the **neural retina** and the proximal part as **retinal pigment epithelium**.

8. **b. Mesoderm**
   - Optic vesicle which develops from the diencephalon (neuroectoderm), changes to optic cup, and is **surrounded by mesenchyme** (mesoderm).
   - Optic cup contributes to retinal layers, whereas the mesenchyme forms the **connective tissue component** of eyeball.

☐ **Vascular tissue** of the developing eye forms by local angiogenesis of **angiogenic mesenchyme.**

- **Optic vesicle** is derived from an evagination developing on either side of the forebrain **neuroectoderm** (NEET Pattern 2016)
- Optic vesicle forms the **optic cup** and optic stalk (NEET Pattern 2015)
- **Optic cup** forms inner **neural retinal epithelium** and outer **pigmented layer** of the retina (NEET Pattern 2015)
- **Corneal endothelium** develops from **neural crest cells**.
- **Crystalline lens** develops from **surface ectoderm** (NEET Pattern 2012)
- **PAX6** is the **key regulatory gene** for eye and brain development (NEET Pattern 2016)
- **Surface ectoderm** forms the eye lens, first layer of cornea and glands exterior to eyeball like lacrimal gland (**but** sclera is a derivative of **neural crest cells**)- AIIMS 2006

▼ Eyeball

- ❏ **Cornea** has five layers:
  - ➢ Corneal epithelium is non-keratinized stratified squamous epithelium.
    - ▪ It is continuous with the conjunctival epithelium.
  - ➢ Bowman's layer (anterior limiting membrane) is an acellular layer, composed of mainly type I collagen.
  - ➢ Corneal stroma (substantia propria) makes 90% of the corneal thickness and has regularly arranged collagen (type I) fibers along with sparsely distributed interconnected keratocytes (for repair and maintenance).
  - ➢ Descemet's membrane (posterior limiting membrane) is the thin acellular layer that serves as the modified basement membrane of the corneal endothelium, composed mainly of collagen type IV fibrils, (less rigid than collagen type I).
  - ➢ Corneal endothelium is a simple squamous or low cuboidal epithelium, responsible for regulating fluid and solute transport between the aqueous and corneal stromal compartments.
    - ▪ The cells of the endothelium do not regenerate, instead, they stretch to compensate for dead cells which reduces the overall cell density of the endothelium, which may affect fluid regulation.
- ❏ Cornea is supplied by the ophthalmic division of the trigeminal nerve by long & short ciliary nerves.
- ❏ **Aqueous humor** is formed by the ciliary processes and provides nutrients for the avascular cornea and lens.
  - ➢ It passes through the pupil from the posterior chamber (between the iris and the lens) into the anterior chamber (between the cornea and the iris) and is drained into the scleral venous plexus through the canal of Schlemm at the iridocorneal angle.
  - ➢ Impaired drainage causes an increased intraocular pressure, leading to atrophy of the retina and blindness.
- ❏ Fascia bulbi (Tenon's capsule. is a thin membrane which envelops the eyeball from the optic nerve to the limbus, separating it from the orbital fat and forming a socket in which it moves.
  - ➢ It is perforated by the tendons of the ocular muscles, and is reflected backward on each as a tubular sheath.
  - ➢ The expansions from the sheaths of the lateral rectus and medial rectus are strong, especially that from the latter muscle, and are attached to the zygomatic bone and lacrimal bone respectively.
    - ▪ They check the actions of these two Recti, hence called medial and lateral check ligaments.
  - ➢ **Suspensory ligament of Lockwood** is the thickening of the lower part of the fascia bulbi .
    - ▪ It is slung like a hammock below the eyeball, being expanded in the centre, and narrow at its extremities which are attached to the zygomatic and lacrimal bones respectively.

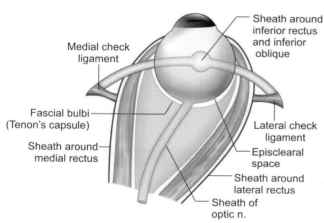

Fig. 113: Fascia bulbi (Tenon's capsule)

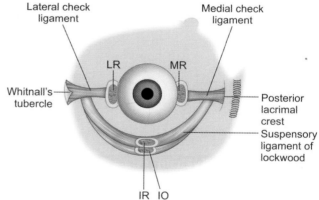

Fig. 114: Suspensory and check ligaments of the eye (IO = inferior oblique, IR = inferior rectus, LR = lateral rectus, MR = medial rectus)

- ❏ The tarsal plates are made up of condensed fibrous tissue, and form the skeleton of the eyelids.
  - ➢ **Meibomian** tarsal glands are modified sebaceous glands, partly embedded on the deeper aspects of the tarsal plates.
- ❏ Levator palpebrae superioris is a skeletal muscle inserting on the skin of the upper eyelid, as well as the superior tarsal plate.
- ❏ Superior tarsal muscle is a smooth muscle, attached to the levator palpebrae superioris, also insert on the superior tarsal plate itself.
- ❏ There are two types of ciliary glands opening into the follicles of eyelashes:
  - ➢ Glands of Zeis, the modified sebaceous glands.
  - ➢ Glands of Moll, the modified sweat glands.

QUESTIONS

1. **Thinnest area of sclera** *(AIIMS 2009)*
   a. Limbus
   b. Behind rectus insertion
   c. Equator
   d. In front of rectus insertion

2. **Continuation of inner layer of choroid is** *(NEET Pattern 2012)*
   a. Nonpigmented layer of retina
   b. Sclera
   c. Pigmented layer of retina
   d. None

1. b. Behind rectus insertion
- ❏ Sclera is the **thinnest** (weakest) **behind** the attachment of **4 recti muscle** into the sclera.
- ❏ Sclera is the **thickest posteriorly**. The thickness gradually decrease towards the attachment of recti and the again increases anteriorly towards the **limbus**.

2. c. Pigmented layer of retina
- ❏ Inner surface of choroid is smooth, brown and lies **in contact with pigmented epithelium** of the retina.
- ❏ The outer surface is rough and lies in **contact with sclera**.

- ▪ Sclera is thinnest **posterior** to attachment of superior rectus *(NEET Pattern 2012)*
- ▪ **Ligament of Lockwood's** is the suspensory ligament of eyeball, **between** the medial and lateral check ligaments and **enclosing** the inferior rectus and inferior oblique muscles of the eye *(NEET Pattern 2015)*
- ▪ Cornea has an outer epithelium at surface lined by non-keratinized stratified squamous epithelium *(NEET Pattern 2012)*
- ▪ **Intra-orbital length** of optic nerve is **30 mm** *(NEET Pattern 2016)*
- ▪ The total length of the optic nerve averages 50 mm: 1 mm for the intraocular segment, **25 mm for the intra-orbital segment**, 10 mm for the intra-canalicular segment, and 14 mm for the intracranial segment

---

▼ Lacrimatory Apparatus

- ❏ **Lacrimal gland** lies in the upper lateral region of the orbit on the lateral rectus and the levator palpebrae superioris muscles.
- ❏ Tears enter the lacrimal canaliculi through their lacrimal puncta (which is on the summit of the lacrimal papilla) before draining into the lacrimal sac, nasolacrimal duct, and finally, the inferior nasal meatus.
- ❏ The nasolacrimal duct opens into the inferior meatus is partially covered by a mucosal fold (valve of Hasner).
  - ➤ Excess tears flow through nasolacrimal duct which drains into the inferior nasal meatus.
  - ➤ It is directed downward, backward and laterally.
- ❏ **Valve of Rosenmuller** is a fold of mucous membrane at the **junction between** canaliculus and lacrimal sac (NEET Pattern 2015)

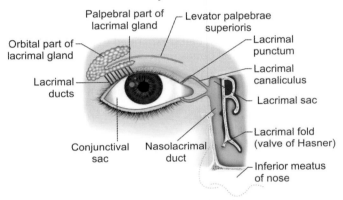

Fig. 115: Lacrimal apparatus

▼ Arterial Supply (Eyeball)

- ❏ Ophthalmic artery is a branch of the internal carotid artery (cerebral part), enters the orbit through the optic canal beneath the optic nerve.
  - ➤ It gives numerous ocular and orbital vessels
- ❏ **Central artery of the retina** travels in the optic nerve, divides into superior and inferior branches to the optic disk, and each of those further divides into temporal and nasal branches.
  - ➤ It is an **end artery** that does not anastomose with other arteries, and thus, its occlusion results in blindness.
- ❏ Long posterior ciliary arteries (branches of ophthalmic artery) pierce the posterior part of the sclera at some distance from the optic nerve, and run forward, between the sclera and choroid, to the ciliary muscle, where they divide into two branches.
  - ➤ They form an arterial circle, the **circulus arteriosus major** (around the circumference of the iris), from which numerous converging branches run, in the substance of the iris, to its pupillary margin, where they form a second (incomplete) arterial circle, the **circulus arteriosus minor**.
- ❏ **Haller's circle** (zinn/zonula): An (often incomplete) vascular circle within the sclera, formed by branches of the short *posterior ciliary arteries*, whose centripetal branches supply the laminar region of the optic nerve head.
  - ➤ It is associated with the fibrous extension of the ocular tendons (annulus of Zinn).
- ❏ Ophthalmic artery gives **anterior** and **posterior ethmoidal** arteries which pass through ethmoidal foramina to supply ethmoidal air cells, frontal sinus, nasal cavity, and skin on dorsum of nose.
- ❏ Other branches of ophthalmic artery: Short posterior ciliary, anterior ciliary, Supraorbital, Supratrochlear, Lacrimal, Dorsal nasal.

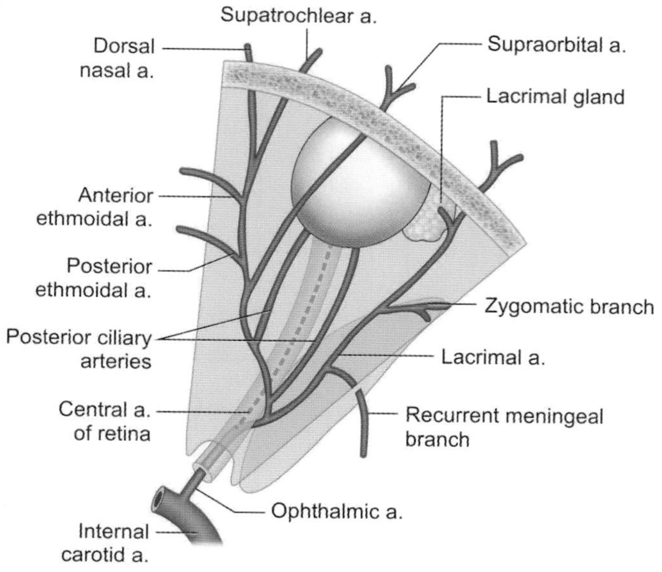

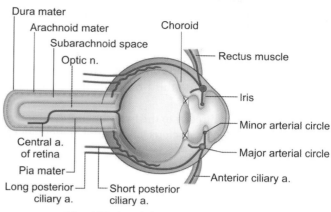

Fig. 116: Ophthalmic artery

Fig. 117: Arterial supply of the eyeball

Labels (Fig. 116): Supratrochlear a., Dorsal nasal a., Supraorbital a., Lacrimal gland, Anterior ethmoidal a., Posterior ethmoidal a., Zygomatic branch, Posterior ciliary arteries, Lacrimal a., Central a. of retina, Recurrent meningeal branch, Ophthalmic a., Internal carotid a.

Labels (Fig. 117): Dura mater, Arachnoid mater, Subarachnoid space, Optic n., Choroid, Rectus muscle, Iris, Minor arterial circle, Major arterial circle, Central a. of retina, Pia mater, Anterior ciliary a., Long posterior ciliary a., Short posterior ciliary a.

QUESTIONS

1. **NOT a branch of ophthalmic artery** *(JIPMER 2010)*
   a. Dorsal nasal artery
   b. Superficial temporal artery
   c. Central artery of retina
   d. Supratrochlear artery

2. **Which of the following is WRONG regarding ophthalmic artery** *(NEET Pattern 2015)*
   a. Present in dura along with optic nerve
   b. Supplies anterior ethmoidal sinus
   c. Artery to retina is end artery
   d. Leaves orbit through inferior orbital fissure

ANSWERS

1. **b. Superficial temporal artery**
   - Superficial temporal artery is a terminal branch of **external carotid artery**.
   - Ophthalmic artery gives central artery of retina, supraorbital & supratrochlear arteries, along with dorsal nasal artery.

2. **d. Leaves orbit through inferior orbital fissure**
   - Ophthalmic artery arises from internal carotid artery as it emerges from the roof of the cavernous sinus, enters the orbit through optic canal inferolateral to the optic nerve, both **lying in a common dural sheath.**
   - Gives central artery to retina (an **end artery**), and also supplies **ethmoidal sinuses** by giving ethmoidal arteries.

Venous Drainage (Eyeball)

Ophthalmic Veins:
- **Superior ophthalmic vein** is formed by the union of the supraorbital, supratrochlear, and angular veins.
  - It receives branches corresponding to most of those of the ophthalmic artery and, in addition, receives the inferior ophthalmic vein before draining into the cavernous sinus.
- **Inferior ophthalmic vein** begins by the union of small veins in the floor of the orbit.
  - It communicates with the pterygoid venous plexus and often with the infraorbital vein and terminates directly or indirectly into the cavernous sinus.

Optic Nerve and Visual Pathway

- Optic nerve is formed by the axons of ganglion cells of the retina, which converge at the optic disk.
  - Optic nerve is not a true nerve and is actually a CNS tract, myelinated by oligodendroglia.
  - Optic nerve axons are covered by a membrane continuous with the dura and leave the orbit by passing through the optic canal.
  - It carries SSA (special somatic afferent) fibers for vision from the retina to the brain and mediates the afferent limb of the pupillary light reflex, whereas parasympathetic fibers in the oculomotor nerve mediate the efferent limb.
  - It joins the optic nerve from the corresponding eye to form the optic chiasma, which contains fibers from the nasal retina that cross over to the opposite side of the brain.
  - The fibers from the temporal retina pass ipsilaterally through the chiasma.
- Retina constitute a chain of three neurons that project visual impulses via the optic nerve and the lateral geniculate body (LGB) to the visual cortex.

➤ Rods and cones are the first-order receptor cells that respond directly to light stimulation.
  ▪ Rods contain rhodopsin (visual purple) are sensitive to low-intensity light and work for night vision.
  ▪ Cones contain the iodopsin, operate at high illumination levels, are concentrated in the fovea centralis and responsible for high visual acuity, day vision and color vision.
➤ Bipolar neurons are the second-order neurons that relay stimuli from the rods and cones to the ganglion cells.
➤ Ganglion cells are the third-order neurons that form the optic nerve.
  ▪ They project directly to the hypothalamus, superior colliculus, pretectal nucleus, and lateral geniculate body.
➤ Three other type of cells are present in retina: Horizontal, Amacrine and Muller cells.
  ▪ Horizontal cells are the laterally interconnecting neurons in the inner nuclear layer of the retina. They interconnect photoreceptors and bipolar cells, inhibit neighboring photoreceptors (lateral inhibition) and play a role in the differentiation of colors.
  ▪ Amacrine cells operate at the inner plexiform layer (IPL), receive input from bipolar cells and project inhibitory signals to ganglion cells.
  ▪ Muller cells are the retinal glial cells, that serve as support cells for the neurons of the retina, they extend from the inner limiting layer to the outer limiting layer.

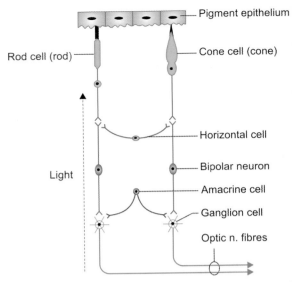

Fig. 118: Three basic layers of retina and their constituent cells. The arrow (on the left side) indicates the direction of light falling on the retina. It is important to note that several rods and cones converge on a single bipolar neuron and several bipolar neurons activate one ganglion cells. The one-to-one relationship between rods and cones, bipolar neurons and ganglion cells shown in this figure is only for the sake of simplicity.

Optic pathway

❑ **Optic nerve**, constituted by the axons of ganglion cells in retina, project from the nasal hemiretina to the contralateral lateral geniculate body and from the temporal hemiretina to the ipsilateral lateral geniculate body.
❑ **Optic chiasma** contains decussating fibers from the two nasal hemiretinas and non-crossing fibers from the two temporal hemiretinas and projects fibers to the suprachiasmatic nucleus of the hypothalamus.
❑ **Optic tract** contains fibers from the ipsilateral temporal hemiretina and the contralateral nasal hemiretina. It projects to the ipsilateral lateral geniculate body, pretectal nuclei, and superior colliculus.
❑ **Lateral geniculate body** is a six-layered nucleus. Layers 1, 4, and 6 receive crossed fibers; layers 2, 3, and 5 receive uncrossed fibers.
  ➤ It receives fibers from the ipsilateral temporal hemiretina and the contralateral nasal hemiretina
  ➤ It also receives input from layer VI of the striate cortex (Brodmann's area 17).
  ➤ It projects through the optic radiation (geniculo-calcarine tract) to layer IV of the primary visual cortex (Brodmann's area 17), through two divisions.

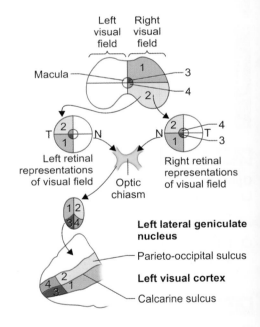

  ▪ Upper division projects to the upper bank of the calcarine sulcus (cuneus). It contains input from the superior retinal quadrants, which represent the inferior visual-field quadrants.
  ▪ Lower division loops from the lateral geniculate body anteriorly (Meyer's loop), then posteriorly, to terminate in the lower bank of the calcarine sulcus (lingual gyrus). It contains input from the inferior retinal quadrants, which represent the superior visual field quadrants.
❑ **Visual cortex** (Brodmann's area 17) is located on the banks of the calcarine fissure.
  ➤ Cuneus is the upper bank and lingual gyrus is the lower bank.
  ➤ It has a retinotopic organization: The posterior area receives macular input (central vision); intermediate area receives paramacular input (peripheral input) and the anterior area receives monocular input.

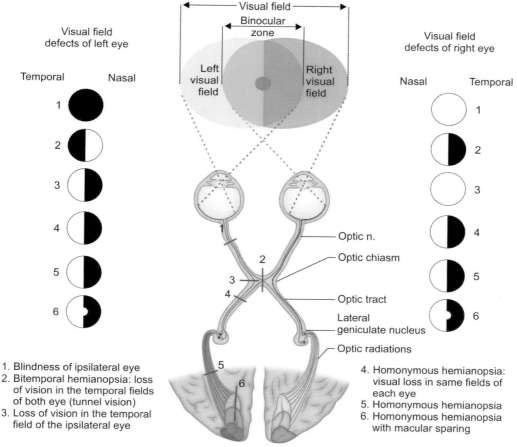

Fig. 119: Visual pathway and lesions

Visual field defects of left eye

Temporal   Nasal

1. Blindness of ipsilateral eye
2. Bitemporal hemianopia: loss of vision in the temporal fields of both eye (tunnel vision)
3. Loss of vision in the temporal field of the ipsilateral eye

Visual field defects of right eye

Nasal   Temporal

4. Homonymous hemianopsia: visual loss in same fields of each eye
5. Homonymous hemianopsia
6. Homonymous hemianopsia with macular sparing

❑ Optic pathway lesions:
1. Optic nerve injury—leads to ipsilateral blindness, with no direct pupillary light reflex.
2. Midline lesions (like pituitary tumor) results in bitemporal hemianopia (tunnel vision)
3. Bilateral lateral compression causes binasal hemianopia (nasal visual field is lost). One of the etiology is calcified internal carotid artery.
4. A lesion in the optic tract results in contralateral homonymous hemianopia. A lesion on the left side, compromises the visual field on right side i.e., right half of each eye is blind (nasal vision of left eye and temporal vision of right eye is lost).
5. A lesion in the optic radiation (geniculo-calcarine tract) again results in contralateral homonymous hemianopia. But
   a. Transection of upper division of geniculo-calcarine tract causes a contralateral lower quadrantanopia.
   b. Transection of lower division of geniculo-calcarine tract causes a contralateral upper quadrantanopia (pie in the sky).
6. Lesions of visual cortex leads to contralateral hemianopia with macular sparing. One case is cortical blindness due to a block in posterior cerebral artery resulting in contralateral homonymous hemianopia with macular sparing (macular area on brain has additional supply from middle cerebral artery).

QUESTIONS

1. **Which order neuron is bipolar cell in the retina?**
   (NEET Pattern 2012)
   a. First order   b. Second order
   c. Third order   d. Fourth order

2. **Optic nerve is which order neuron?**
   a. First   b. Second
   c. Third   d. Fourth

ANSWERS

1. **b. Second order**
   ❑ Rods and cones are the **first-order** receptor cells that respond directly to light stimulation.
   ❑ Bipolar neurons are the **second-order neurons** that relay stimuli from the rods and cones to the ganglion cells.
   ❑ Ganglion cells **third-order** neurons that form the optic nerve (CN II).

2. **c. Third**
   ❑ **Rods and cones** are the first order neurones, synapsing with the **bipolar cell** (second order neurone), which in turn synapse on the **ganglion cell neurone** (third order neurone).
   ❑ Optic nerve is collection of the axons of ganglion cell neurone, which is third order neurone in the visual pathway.

◤ Eyeball Muscles

Eyeball has two types of muscles—smooth and skeletal muscles:

❑ Smooth muscles: Iris (dilator & sphincter pupillae), Muller muscle
 ➢ Dilator pupillae is a smooth muscle with radial arrangements of fibers in the iris.
  ▪ It is innervated by the sympathetic system, which acts by releasing noradrenaline, which acts on α1-receptors.
  ▪ In threatening stimuli that activates the fight-or-flight response, this innervation contracts the muscle and dilates the iris (mydriasis), thus temporarily letting more light/information reach the retina.

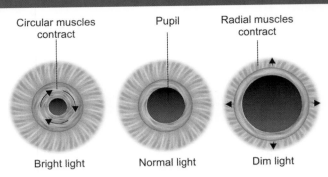

Fig. 120: Smooth muscles of iris and their functions.

 ➢ Sphincter pupillae is present in circular arrangement on the iris, is supplied by the cholinergic fibers of parasympathetic nervous system, via oculomotor nerve.
  ▪ Its contraction leads to miosis of pupil.
 ➢ Muller muscle in the eyeball is supplied by the T1 sympathetic pathway. One of its component is superior tarsal muscle, which elevates the upper eyelid.
❑ Skeletal muscles

Table 22: Extra-ocular muscles of orbit

Muscle	Origin	Insertion	Innervation	Main action[a]
Levator palpebrae superioris	Lesser wing of sphenoid bone, superior and anterior to optic canal	Superior tarsus and skin of superior eyelid	Oculomotor nerve (CN III); deep layer (superior tarsal muscle) is supplied by sympathetic fibers	Elevates superior eyelid
Superior oblique (SO)	Body of sphenoid bone	Its tendon passes through a fibrous ring a trochlea, changes its direction, and inserts into sclera deep to superior rectus muscle	Trochlear nerve (CN IV)	Abducts, depresses, and medially rotates eyeball
Inferior oblique (IO)	Anterior part of floor of orbit	Sclera deep to lateral rectus muscle		Abduts, elevates, and laterally rotates eyeball
Superior rectus (SR)			Oculomotor nerve (CN III)	Elevates, adducts, and rotates eyeball medially
Inferior rectus (IR)	Common tendinous ring	Sclera just posterior to corneoscleral junction		Depresses, adducts, and rotates eyeball laterally
Medial rectus (MR)				Adducts eyeball
Lateral rectus (LR)			Abducent nerve (CN VI)	Abducts eyeball

[a] The actions described are for muscles acting alone, starting from the primary position (gaze directed anteriorly). In fact, muscles rarely act independently and almost always work together in synergistic and antagonistic groups. Clinical testing requires maneuvers to isolate muscle actions. Only the actions of the medial and lateral rectus are tested, starting from the primary position.

Muscle	Primary action	Secondary action
Superior rectus	Elevation	Adduction and intorsion
Inferior rectus	Depression	Adduction and extorsion
Medial rectus	Adduction	
Lateral rectus	Abduction	
Superior oblique*	Intorsion	Abduction and depression
Inferior oblique	Extorsion	Abduction and elevation

* The primary (main) action of the superior oblique muscle is intorsion (internal rotation), the secondary action is depression (primarily in the adducted position) and the tertiary action is abduction (lateral rotation).

❑ Superior oblique is inserted into the posterior part of the eyeball; when it contracts, the back of the eyeball is elevated, and the front of the eyeball is depressed (particularly in the adducted position).
❑ **Intorsion** is the medial (inward) rotation of the upper pole (12 o'clock position) of the cornea, carried out by the superior oblique and superior rectus muscles (Mnemonic; SIN - Superiors are intortors).

- **Extorsion** is the lateral (outward) rotation of the upper pole of the cornea, caused by the inferior oblique and inferior rectus muscles.

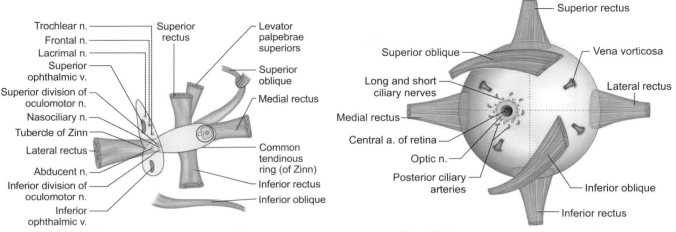

Fig. 121: Extraocular muscles: Origin

Fig. 122: Extraocular muscles: Insertion

- Common tendinous Ring of Zinn is a fibrous ring that surrounds the optic canal and the medial part of the superior orbital fissure.
- Muscles of the eye movement are innervated by the oculomotor, trochlear, and abducens nerves. Formula to remember innervation of extraocular eye muscles is (LR6, SO4)3 (Superior Oblique – CN4; Lateral Rectus – CN6; All Other eye movement muscles – CN3).
- It is the common tendinous origin of the four rectus muscles of the eye and transmits the following structures through it : Oculomotor nerve (superior & inferior division), abducent nerves and nasociliary nerve (branch of ophthalmic division of trigeminal nerve) as they pass through the superior orbital fissure.
- It also encloses the optic nerve, ophthalmic artery, and central artery and vein of the retina, which enter the orbit through the optic canal within the tendinous ring.
- LFT nerves are left outside the tendinous ring: Lacrimal & frontal nerves (branches of ophthalmic division of trigeminal nerve) and trochlear nerve as they pass through the superior orbital fissure.
- The ophthalmic (superior & inferior) veins usually lies outside the ring while they pass the fissure.

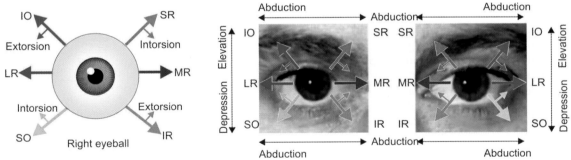

Fig. 123: Eyeball muscles and their respective movements

QUESTIONS

1. **Which of the following muscles produce intorsion of eye ball**   (NEET Pattern 2015)
   a. Superior rectus and superior oblique
   b. Inferior rectus and inferior oblique
   c. Inferior rectus and superior oblique
   d. Superior rectus and inferior oblique

2. **TRUE about inferior oblique muscle**   (PGIC 2016)
   a. Supplied by inferior division of 3rd CN
   b. Primary eye action—Extorsion, abduction & depression
   c. The muscle pass below inferior rectus
   d. Origin from lacrimal bone
   e. Nerve enters the muscle from ocular surface

ANSWERS

1. **a. Superior rectus and superior oblique**
   - **Both the Superiors** are INtortors (**Mnemonic**: SIN).
   - Superior rectus and superior oblique muscles cause **inward rotation** (intortion) of the eyeball.

2. **a. Supplied by inferior division of 3rd CN; c. The muscle pass below inferior rectus**
   - The **lower division** of occulomotor nerve supplies the **inferior oblique** by entering its posterior border (**not the ocular** surface).
   - The muscle carries out **extortion**, abduction and elevation (**not depression**).
   - The muscle takes its origin from the orbital surface of maxilla (**not the lacrimal bone**), passes laterally **below** the inferior rectus and inserts into the sclera on the lateral surface (**deep to lateral rectus** muscle).

- **Superior oblique** is the **longest** and **thinnest** extraocular muscle *(NEET Pattern 2012)*
- **Primary** action of **superior oblique** is inward rotation (**intortion**) of the eyeball *(NEET Pattern 2012)*
  - Secondary actions are depression and abduction.
- **Primary** action of **inferior oblique** is outward rotation (**extortion**) of the eyeball *(NEET Pattern 2015)*
  - Secondary actions are elevation and abduction.
- **Primary** action of superior rectus is **elevation** of eyeball *(NEET Pattern 2012)*
  - Secondary actions are adduction and intorsion.
- **Inferior oblique** is supplied by the **third** cranial nerve *(NEET Pattern 2012)*
- Constrictor pupillae is supplied by the **parasympathetic** fibers from Edinger Westphal nucleus, carried by occulomotor nerve *(NEET Pattern 2016)*

□ **Oculomotor nerve** arises from the midbrain, runs in the lateral wall of cavernous sinus, enters the orbit through the superior orbital fissure and divides into a superior division, which innervates the superior rectus and levator palpebrae superioris muscles, and an inferior division, which innervates the medial rectus, inferior rectus, and inferior oblique muscles.
  ➢ Its inferior division also carries preganglionic parasympathetic fibers (with cell bodies located in the Edinger–Westphal nucleus) to the ciliary ganglion.
□ Oculomotor nuclear complex is present in the upper midbrain (at the level of superior colliculi).
□ Motor nucleus (GSE, general somatic efferent) sends axons to supply all the muscles of eyeball (except superior oblique and lateral rectus).
□ Edinger Westphal nucleus (GVE, general visceral efferent) is a parasympathetic nucleus, sends fibers to the smooth muscles—sphincter pupillae and ciliaris.
□ **Course**: Oculomotor nerve emerges at the midbrain on the medial side of the crus of the cerebral peduncle and passes between the superior cerebellar and posterior cerebral arteries and runs forward in the interpeduncular cistern on the lateral side of the posterior communicating artery to reach cavernous sinus.
  ➢ It enters the cavernous sinus by piercing the posterior part of the roof on the lateral side of the posterior clinoid process, descends along the lateral dural wall of the cavernous sinus, dividing into superior and inferior divisions which run beneath the trochlear and ophthalmic nerves.
□ **Superior rectus** muscle is supplied contralaterally by the occulomotor nerve. Left occulomotor nucleus gives fibers, which cross the midline and join the right oculomotor nerve to supply the right superior rectus. Similarly right occulomotor nucleus supplies the left superior rectus muscle.
□ **Levator palpebrae superioris** has a single central sub-nucleus, which sends fibers through each oculomotor nerve to supply respective sided muscle.

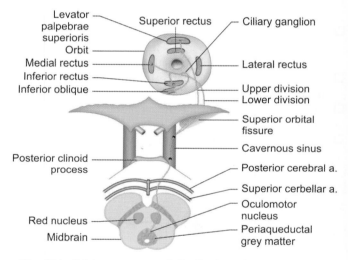

Fig. 124: Origin, course, and distribution of the oculomotor.

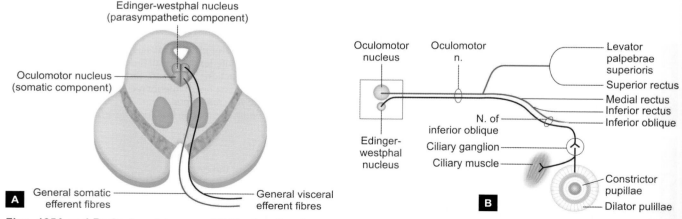

Figs. 125A and B: Oculomotor nerve: (A) The functional components and nuclei of the oculomotor nerve (B) The distribution of the constitutional fibers of the oculomotor nerve

- Occulomotor nerve lesions leads to paralysis of the levator palpebrae superioris (ptosis) and a wrinkled brow due to the inability to raise the eyelid; fixed dilated pupil (with loss of light and accommodation reflex) due to paralysed constrictor pupillae muscle & ciliary muscles; and downward and outward position of the eye (strabismus) due to the unopposed action of the superior oblique and lateral rectus muscles.

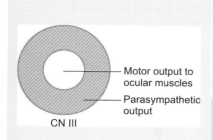

CN III has both motor (central) and parasympathetic (peripheral) components.

Motor output to ocular muscles—affected primarily by vascular disease (e.g., diabetes mellitus: glucose → sorbitol) due to ↓ diffusion of oxygen and nutrients to the interior fibers from compromised vasculature that resides on outside of nerve. Signs: ptosis, 'down and out' gaze (A)

Parasympathetic output—fibers on the periphery are 1st affected by compression (e.g., posterior communicating artery aneurysm, uncal herniation). Signs: diminished or absent pupillary light reflex, 'blown pupil' often with 'down-and-out' gaze.

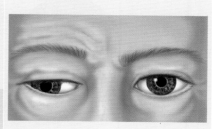

- ❑ **Medial rectus** is supplied by **inferior division** of oculomotor nerve (NEET Pattern 2016)
- ❑ Occulomotor nerve palsy causes lateral (**not medial**) deviation of the eyeball.
- ❑ Occulomotor nerve **passes between** posterior cerebral artery **and** superior cerebellar artery (JIPMER 2017)
  - ➤ It might be involved in an **aneurysm** of the two related arteries.

QUESTIONS

1. **All are characteristics of 3rd nerve EXCEPT:** *(AIIMS 2006)*
   a. Carries parasympathetic nerve
   b. Supplies inferior oblique
   c. Enters orbit through the inferior orbital fissure
   d. Causes miosis

2. **Which of the following statement is /are TRUE about oculomotor nerve?** *(PGIC 2014)*
   a. Arise from pons
   b. Edinger- Westphal nucleus gives rise to parasympathetic supply
   c. Arise from medulla
   d. Passes through interpeduncular fossa
   e. Related to medial wall of cavernous sinus

ANSWERS

1. **c. Enters orbit through the inferior orbital fissure**
   - ❑ Oculomotor nerve passes through superior (**not inferior**) orbital fissure to enter the orbit.
   - ❑ It carries preganglionic **parasympathetic** fibers to supply muscles like sphincter pupillae which causes **miosis**.
   - ❑ It also carries motor fibers to supply eyeball muscles like **inferior oblique**.

2. **b. Edinger- Westphal nucleus gives rise to parasympathetic supply; d. Passes through interpeduncular fossa**
   - ❑ Oculomotor nerve nuclei are present in the **midbrain**, send axons which exit ventrally from midbrain and pass through the **interpeduncular fossa** before they pass through **lateral wall** of cavernous sinus and enter orbit eventually.
   - ❑ **Edinger Westphal nucleus** sends parasympathetic fibers to the two smooth muscles in the eyeball: sphincter pupillae and ciliaris.

▼ Trochlear Nerve

- ❑ **Trochlear nerve** is a motor nerve carrying general somatic efferent (GSE) fibers to supply the **superior oblique muscle**.
  - ➤ Its axons arise from the midbrain, decussates in the **superior medullary velum**, runs in the lateral wall of cavernous sinus, enters the orbit through the superior orbital fissure (outside the tendinous ring of Zinn) and innervates the superior oblique muscle.
  - ➤ Trochlear nerve innervates the **contralateral** superior oblique.
    - ▪ Left trochlear nucleus gives the axons which decussate within the brainstem (internal decussation) and become the right trochlear nerve (hypothetically it is left trochlear nerve, but for all practical purposes, it is called as left trochlear nerve).
    - ▪ Similarly left trochlear nerve arises from the neuron bodies on the right (right oculomotor nucleus). Lesion of right trochlear nucleus (left trochlear nerve) paralyses the left superior oblique muscle.

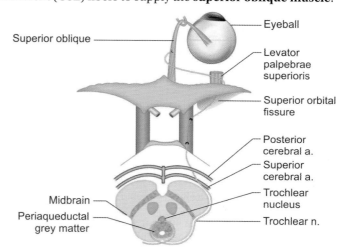

Fig. 126: Origin, course, and distribution of the trochlear nerve.

❑ Trochlear nerve is the only cranial nerve which **exits dorsally** from the brainstem.
  ➤ This nerve exits dorsally/posteriorly, loops around the brainstem and turns anteriorly to move along with other cranial nerves — which all exit the brainstem anteriorly.
  ➤ Trochlear nerve gains additional length as it goes dorsal and then comes ventral, whereas other nerves were simply exiting ventrally. Thus the nerve has the **longest intracranial course**. It is also having the longest intracranial (**subarachnoid**) course.

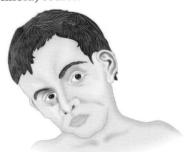

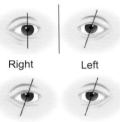

Lesion of the left superior oblique: left eye elevated and extorted, vertical and torsional diplopia

Right   Left

Head tilted to the right (away from the paralyzed left S O)
Head also flexed

Eye position when head is tilted to the right and flexed
No diplopia

Fig. 127: Paralysis of left superior oblique muscle leads to contralateral head tilt (to right side)

❑ Trochlear nerve is rarely paralyzed alone. Severe head injury may lead to torn trochlear nerve (due to its long intracranial course) and the patient presents with paralysed superior oblique.
  ➤ It results in **vertical diplopia** (double vision) on looking down, and difficulty in reading/going downstairs.
  ➤ This happens because the superior oblique normally assists the inferior rectus in pulling the eye downward, especially when the eye is in a medial (adducted) position.
  ➤ 'Head tilt test' is a cardinal diagnostic feature - Diplopia is reduced on turning the head away from the site of lesion.
❑ The patient develops **contralateral** (not ipsilateral) head tilt to compensate for *extorted eye* on the side of lesion.
❑ Trochlear nerve has very few axons and is the **smallest**, **slimmest** and **most slender** of all cranial nerves. It is the only cranial nerve, which has **dorsal exit** from the brain. Most of its fibers undergo **internal decussation** to supply contralateral superior oblique muscle. It has **longest** intracranial (subarachnoid course).

CN IV damage	Eye moves upward, particularly with contralateral gaze (B) and head tilt toward the side of the lesion (problems going down stairs, may present with compensatory head tilt in the opposite direction).	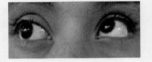

1. All is true about Trochlear nerve EXCEPT
  a. Slender most cranial nerve
  b. Has longest intradural course
  c. Innervates contralateral superior oblique
  d. Shows internal decussation

2. Which of the following is NOT true about the trochlear nerve? *(AIPG 2009; AIIMS 2011)*
  a. Has the longest intracranial course
  b. Supplies the ipsilateral superior oblique muscle
  c. Only cranial nerve that arises from the dorsal aspect of the brainstem
  d. Enters orbit through the superior orbital fissure outside the annulus of Zinn

3. TRUE about Trochlear Nerve *(PGIC 2016)*
  a. Nucleus of the trochlear nerve is located in the caudal mesencephalon beneath the cerebral aqueduct
  b. Arise from ventral aspect of brainstem
  c. Enters orbit through annulus of Zinn
  d. Lesion causes diplopia
  e. Damage causes ipsilateral palsy of superior oblique muscle

4. All is true about trochlear nerve EXCEPT
  a. Innervates contralateral superior oblique
  b. Causes depression of eyeball in adducted position
  c. Lies outside the ring of Zinn
  d. Patient attains ipsilateral head tilt, in lesion

1. b. Has longest intradural course
  ❑ Trochlear nerve has longest intracranial (**not intradural**) course.
  ❑ **Abducent** nerve has got the **longest intradural** course, since it **pierces dura mater** relatively **early** in its intracranial course.

2. c. Supplies the ipsilateral superior oblique
  ❑ It is mentioned in **Harrison Medicine**, that trochlear nerve innervates contralateral superior oblique. Hence the answer.
  ❑ **But more precisely** they should have mentioned trochlear nucleus (**not nerve**) innervated the contralateral superior oblique muscle.
  ❑ Trochlear nerve has **internal decussation** and supplies **contralateral superior oblique muscle**.
  ❑ It is the only cranial nerve with **dorsal exit** from the brain, has the **longest intracranial course**, enters orbit through the superior orbital fissure **lying outside** the annulus of Zinn.

3. **a. Nucleus of the trochlear nerve is located in the caudal mesencephalon beneath the cerebral aqueduct; d. Lesion causes diplopia**
   - ❑ Trochlear nucleus is located in the **caudal mesencephalon**, at the level of the **inferior colliculus**, anterior to the cerebral aqueduct.
   - ❑ Trochlear **nucleus**, send fibers to innervate the **contralateral superior oblique muscle**. The nerve fibers exit the brainstem on the **dorsal aspect** and pass through the superior orbital fissure staying **outside** the ring of Zinn.
   - ❑ Injury to **trochlear nucleus** paralyses the **contralateral** superior oblique muscle. Whereas, injury to trochlear **nerve** causes paralysis of **ipsilateral** superior oblique muscle.
   - ❑ It results in **vertical diplopia** (double vision) on **looking down**, e.g. while going down stairs.

4. **d. Patient attains Ipsilateral head tilt, in lesion**
   - ❑ The patient develops contralateral (**not ipsilateral**) head tilt to **compensate for extorted eye** on the affected side.
   - ❑ Trochlear **nucleus** in the midbrain, send fibers to innervate the **contralateral** superior oblique muscle.
   - ❑ Superior oblique muscle causes inward rotation (**intortion**) of the eyeball. Additionally, it also causes **depression** and **abduction** of eyeball.
   - ❑ It is the **chief muscle** to cause depression of the **adducted eye** and is **assisted by inferior rectus** for the movement.
   - ❑ Trochlear nerve passes through the superior orbital fissure staying **outside** the ring of Zinn.
   - ❑ Trochlear nerve is rarely paralyzed alone. It results in vertical diplopia (double vision) on looking down, e.g. when going down stairs. This happens because the superior oblique normally assists the inferior rectus in pulling the eye downward, especially when the eye is in a medial (adducted) position. The patient develops **contralateral** (not ipsilateral) head tilt to compensate for extorted eye on the affected side.

❑ **Right** trochlear **nucleus** gives the axons which decussate within the brainstem (**internal decussation**) and **become the left trochlear nerve** and supply **left superior oblique muscle**. Similarly, **left** trochlear **nucleus** give fibers, which become **right** trochlear **nerve** and supply **right superior oblique muscle**.
   - ➤ **Lesion of right** trochlear **nucleus** will paralyse the **left superior oblique**.
   - ➤ **Lesion** of **right** trochlear nerve paralyzes **right superior oblique.**

❑ **Injury to the trochlear nerve** cause weakness of downward eye movement with consequent **vertical diplopia** (double vision).
   - ➤ The affected eye **drifts upward** relative to the normal eye, due to the unopposed actions of the remaining extraocular muscles.
   - ➤ The patient sees **two visual fields** (one from each eye), **separated vertically**.
   - ➤ To compensate for this, patients learn to tilt the head forward (**tuck the chin in**) in order to bring the fields back together – **to fuse** the two images into a single visual field. This accounts for the '**dejected**' appearance of patients with '**pathetic nerve**' palsies.

▼ Abducent Nerve

❑ **Abducent nerve** nucleus is in the pons, axons leave the brain at the pontomedullary junction anteriorly and then pierces the dura on the dorsum sellae of the sphenoid bone.

❑ It passes through the cavernous sinus lying inferolateral to internal carotid artery and enters the orbit through the supraorbital fissure to supply motor fibers (GSE) to the lateral rectus.

❑ Abducent nerve pierces dura mater relatively early in its intracranial course and has got the longest intradural course, among the cranial nerves.

❑ It is the earliest nerve to get involved in raised intracranial tension.

❑ Abducent nerve has the longest intracranial (intradural) course. Because of the long course, it is often stretched when intracranial pressure rises and causes weakness/paralysis of the lateral rectus muscle of the eye and loss of the lateral gaze. The patient will present with a medial deviation of the affected eye (internal strabismus) or diplopia on lateral eye movement.

❑ Lesion of the abducens nerve may result from a sepsis or thrombosis in the cavernous sinus. If the opposite side of the body is affected, there is a brainstem tumor or midline pontine stroke.

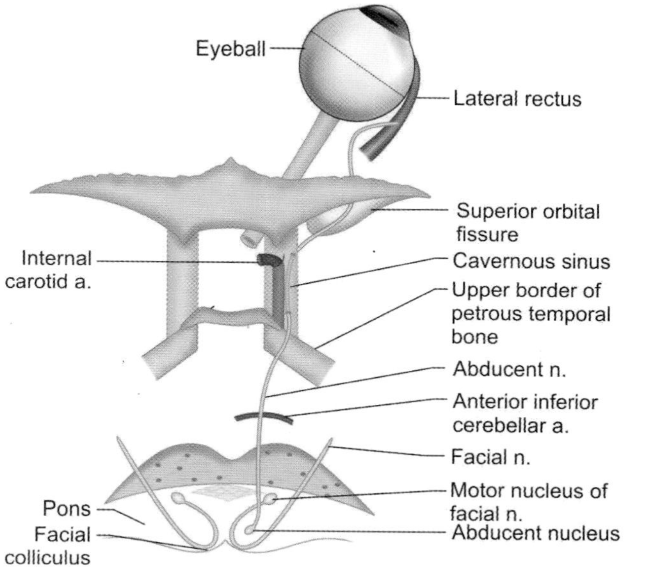

Labels (figure): Eyeball — Lateral rectus — Superior orbital fissure — Cavernous sinus — Upper border of petrous temporal bone — Abducent n. — Anterior inferior cerebellar a. — Facial n. — Motor nucleus of facial n. — Abducent nucleus — Internal carotid a. — Pons — Facial colliculus

Fig. 128: Origin, course, and distribution of the abducent nerve.

CN VI damage	Medially directed eye that cannot abduct

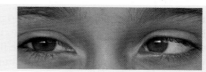

Lesions of cranial nerve supplying eyeball

QUESTIONS

1. Which extraocular muscle is supplied by opposite side nucleus? *(AIIMS 2014)*
   a. Lateral rectus
   b. Medial rectus
   c. Superior rectus
   d. Inferior rectus

2. Ptosis is due to lesion of
   a. Facial nerve
   b. Somatic fibers of occulomotor nerve
   c. Superior cervical ganglion
   d. Edinger Westphal nucleus

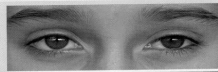

3. Which cranial nerve is involved in the clinical presentation shown below? *(AIIMS 2017)*
   a. Occulomotor
   b. Trochlear
   c. Abducent
   d. Facial

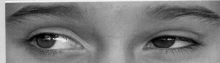

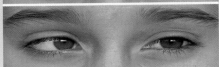

4. The cranial nerve nucleus, supplying the marked muscle with arrow, lies at the level of *(AIIMS 2017)*
   a. Superior colliculus
   b. Inferior colliculus
   c. Facial colliculus
   d. Olive

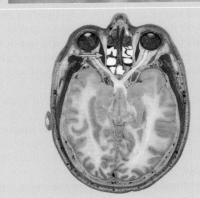

ANSWERS

1. **c. Superior rectus**
   ❑ **Both the superiors** are supplied by the **contralateral nucleus**.
   ❑ **Occulomotor** nucleus supplies **contralateral superior rectus** muscle and **trochlear** nucleus supplies **contralateral** superior oblique muscle.
   ❑ A lesion in the brainstem at the level of **left superior colliculi** will damage the **left sided occulomotor nuclei** and causes **paralysis of the right superior rectus** muscle.
   ❑ A lesion at the level of left **inferior colliculi** compromises the trochlear nucleus and leads to paralysis of the right **superior oblique muscle**.

2. **b. Somatic fibers of Occulomotor nerve > c. Superior cervical ganglion**
   ❑ Ptosis occurs due to paralysis of **levator palpebrae superioris**, the **skeletal** part of whose is supplied by **occulomotor** nerve.
   ❑ **Partial ptosis** may result due to paralysis of **superior tarsal muscle** (part of **Muller muscle**), due to interruption of T1 sympathetic pathway (a feature of Horner syndrome). For e.g., superior cervical ganglion lesion.

3. **c. Abducent**
   ❑ This is a case of **left abducent** nerve palsy, which paralyses the left **lateral rectus** muscle and patient is **unable to move** eye outward **beyond midline.**

4. **a. Superior colliculus**
   ❑ The marked muscle is **medial rectus**, which is supplied by **occulomotor nucleus** in the midbrain, at the level of **superior colliculus**.

▪ A lesion of **abducent nerve** paralyses the **lateral rectus** muscle and patient is **unable to move eye outward beyond midline** *(NEET Pattern 2012)*

◤ Nerves of Orbit and Ciliary Ganglion

❑ **Ophthalmic nerve** is the first division of trigeminal nerve, provides sensory innervation to the eyeball, tip of the nose, and skin of the face above the eye and mediates the afferent limb of the corneal reflex.
❑ It is given by the trigeminal ganglion at the floor of the middle cranial fossa.
❑ It is a pure sensory nerve, passes in the lateral wall of cavernous sinus and gives three branches, which pass through the superior orbital fissure: **Lacrimal**, **frontal** and **nasociliary** nerves.

➤ **Lacrimal nerve e**nters the orbit through the superior orbital fissure and reach the lacrimal gland, giving branches to the lacrimal gland, conjunctiva, and the skin of the upper eyelid.
  ▪ Its terminal part is joined by the zygomaticotemporal nerve that carries postganglionic parasympathetic and sympathetic GVE fibers.
➤ **Frontal nerve** enters the orbit through the superior orbital fissure, runs superior to the levator palpebrae superioris.
  ▪ It divides into the **supraorbital nerve**, which passes through the supraorbital foramen (supplies the scalp, forehead, frontal sinus, and upper eyelid) and the **supratrochlear nerve**, which passes through the trochlea (supplies the scalp, forehead, and upper eyelid).
➤ **Nasociliary nerve** enters the orbit through the superior orbital fissure, within the common tendinous ring. Branches:

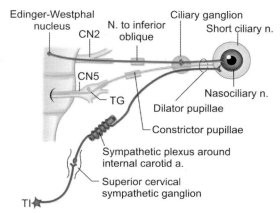

Fig. 129: Roots and distribution of the ciliary ganglion.

  ▪ **Anterior and posterior ethmoidal nerves, infratrochlear nerve, long and short ciliary nerves, meningeal** branch to supply dura in the anterior cranial fossa and a **communicating** branch is given to the ciliary ganglion.
  ▪ **Anterior ethmoidal nerve** is given in the orbit, passes out of orbit into the anterior cranial fossa (through anterior ethmoidal foramen) and supplies the duramater there. It runs in proximity to the cribriform plate of ethmoid bone and supplies the ethmoidal air cells. The nerve then enters the nasal cavity (passing a foramen close to crista galli), gives external and internal nasal branches to supply internal nasal cavity, nasal septum as well as the skin on the exterior of nose.
  ▪ **Posterior ethmoidal nerve** passes through the posterior ethmoidal foramen to the sphenoidal and posterior ethmoidal sinuses.
  ▪ **Infratrochlear nerve** innervates the eyelids, conjunctiva, skin of the nose, and lacrimal sac.
❑ **Short ciliary nerves** carry both parasympathetic and sympathetic nerve fibers.
  ➤ The parasympathetic fibers arise from the Edinger-Westphal nucleus and synapse in the ciliary ganglion via the oculomotor nerve, the postganglionic fibers leave the ciliary ganglion in the short ciliary nerve and supply the **ciliary muscle** and **sphincter pupillae**.
  ➤ Sympathetic fibers are provided by the superior cervical ganglion and they reach the ganglion either as branches of the nasociliary nerve or directly from the extension of the plexus on the ophthalmic artery (sympathetic branch to ciliary ganglion).
❑ **Long ciliary nerves** provide sensory innervation to the eyeball, including the cornea (reflex).
  ➤ In addition, they carry sympathetic fibers from the superior cervical ganglion to the **dilator pupillae** muscle.
  Note: The sympathetic fibers to the dilator pupillae muscle mainly travel in the nasociliary nerve but there are also sympathetic fibers in the short ciliary nerves that pass through the ciliary ganglion without forming synapses.
❑ **Ciliary ganglion** is a parasympathetic ganglion situated behind the eyeball, between the optic nerve and the lateral rectus muscle.
  ➤ Preganglionic axons originate in the Edinger–Westphal preganglionic nucleus of the midbrain.
  ➤ They travel via a branch of the oculomotor nerve (nerve to the inferior oblique) to the ciliary ganglion, where they synapse.
  ➤ Postganglionic fibers travel in the short ciliary nerves, which pierce the scleral coat of the eyeball and run forwards in the perichoroidal space to enter the ciliary muscle and sphincter pupillae.
  ➤ Their activation mediates accommodation of the eye to near objects and pupillary constriction.
❑ **Lacrimatory pathway:** Superior **salivatory nucleus** → facial nerve → pterygopalatine ganglion → maxillary & ophthalmic nerve (trigeminal) → **lacrimal gland.**

1. **A muscle with radially arranged fibers in iris is supplied by**
   (AIIMS 2011)
   a. Oculomotor nerve
   b. Short ciliary nerve
   c. Sympathetic supply from cervical plexus nerve from cervical sympathetic chain
   d. Parasympathetic supply

2. **Anterior ethmoidal nerve supplies all EXCEPT**   *(AIIMS 2010)*
   a. Dura mater in anterior cranial fossa
   b. Ethmoidal air cells
   c. Internal nasal cavity
   d. Maxillary sinus lining

1. **c. Sympathetic supply from cervical plexus nerve from cervical sympathetic chain**
   ❑ **Dilator pupillae** is a smooth muscle with **radial arrangements** of fibers in the iris and is supplied by the **T-1 sympathetic** fibers, which arise from the lateral horn cells of the spinal cord.
   ❑ These fibers ascend up in the sympathetic chain and synapse in **superior cervical ganglion**.
   ❑ The post-ganglionic fibers pass through around the branches of **carotid arteries** to reach the eyeball muscles like dilator pupillae.

2. d. Maxillary sinus lining
- ❑ Anterior ethmoidal nerve **does not supply** the maxillary sinus lining.
- ❑ Anterior ethmoidal nerve is a branch of **nasociliary nerve** (Trigeminal – **ophthalmic**) given in the orbit, passes out of orbit into the **anterior cranial fossa** (through anterior ethmoidal foramen) and supplies the **dura mater** there.
- ❑ It runs in proximity to the cribriform plate of ethmoid bone and supplies the **ethmoidal air cells**.
- ❑ The nerve then enters the **nasal cavity** (passing a foramen close to crista galli), gives **external and internal** nasal branches to supply internal nasal cavity, nasal septum as well as the **skin on the exterior** of nose.

- ▪ **Parasympathetic** fibers to eye come via **Ciliary** ganglion *(NEET Pattern 2015)*
  - Parasympathetic supply to eye is meant to control the smooth muscles sphincter pupillae and ciliaris.
- ▪ **Cornea** is supplied by **Nasociliary** branch of ophthalmic nerve *(AIIMS 2015)*
  - It is supplied by long and short **ciliary nerves** branches of **nasociliary** nerve, which itself is a branch of **ophthalmic** division of the trigeminal nerve.
- ▪ Lesion of the **ophthalmic division** cannot mediate the **afferent** limb of the **corneal reflex** by way of the nasociliary branch (the facial nerve mediates the efferent limb).

◤ Pterygopalatine Ganglion

- ❑ Pterygopalatine Ganglion lies in the pterygopalatine fossa just below the maxillary nerve, lateral to the sphenopalatine foramen, anterior to the pterygoid canal and behind the perpendicular plate of palatine bone.
  - ➤ It has neuron bodies of parasympathetic postganglionic GVE fibers and receives preganglionic parasympathetic fibers from the facial nerve by way of the greater petrosal nerve and the nerve of the pterygoid canal.
  - ➤ It sends postganglionic parasympathetic fibers to the nasal and palatine glands and to the lacrimal gland through the maxillary, zygomatic, and lacrimal nerves.
  - ➤ It also receives postganglionic sympathetic fibers (by the deep petrosal nerve and the nerve of the pterygoid canal), which are distributed along with the postganglionic parasympathetic fibers.
- ❑ Maxillary nerve branches which pass through the pterygopalatine ganglion without synapse carrying its own GSA fibers and also the general visceral afferent and efferent (GVA and GVE) fibers from the facial nerve to the nasal mucosa and the palate. The branches are:

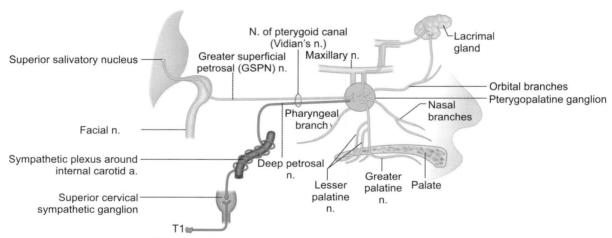

Fig. 130: Pterygopalatine ganglion, its roots and branches

- ➤ **Orbital** (innervate orbit and posterior ethmoidal and sphenoidal sinuses); **pharyngeal** branch run in palatovaginal canal (supply the roof of the pharynx and sphenoidal sinus); posterior superior **lateral nasal** branches (supply the nasal septum, posterior ethmoidal air cells, and superior and middle conchae).
- ➤ **Greater palatine nerve** descends through the palatine canal and emerges through the greater palatine foramen to innervate the hard palate and the inner surface of the maxillary gingiva; **lesser palatine nerve** descends through the palatine canal and emerges through the lesser palatine foramen (innervate the soft palate and the palatine tonsil), carries visceral sensory (GVA) and taste fibers (for the soft palate) that belong to the facial nerve and have their cell bodies in the geniculate ganglion.
- ➤ It also contains postganglionic parasympathetic and sympathetic GVE fibers that come from the facial nerve via the greater petrosal and vidian nerves and supply mucus glands in the nasal cavity and the palate; **nasopalatine nerve** runs obliquely downward and forward on the septum (innervates the nasal septum, hard palate, incisors, the skin of the philtrum and the gums).

Clinical Correlates

❑ Vidianectomy (carried out for vasomotor rhinitis cases) lesions the nerve of the pterygoid canal and results in vasodilation; a lack of secretion of the lacrimal, nasal, and palatine glands; and a loss of general and taste sensation of the palate.

❑ **Pterygopalatine** ganglion supplies **lacrimal** gland (NEET Pattern 2012)

▶ Pituitary

❑ Anterior pituitary (or adenohypophysis) is a lobe of the gland that regulates several physiological processes (including stress, growth, reproduction, and lactation).
  ➢ It develops from the Rathke's pouch, an ectodermal diverticulum of the primitive oral cavity (stomodeum).
  ➢ It includes the pars tuberalis, pars intermedia, and pars distalis.
  ➢ Intermediate lobe synthesizes and secretes melanocyte-stimulating hormone.

❑ The posterior pituitary (or neurohypophysis) is a lobe of the gland that is functionally connected to the hypothalamus by the median eminence via a small tube called the pituitary stalk (also called the infundibular stalk or the infundibulum).
  ➢ It develops from a ventral evagination of the hypothalamus.
  ➢ It includes the median eminence, infundibular stem, and pars nervosa.

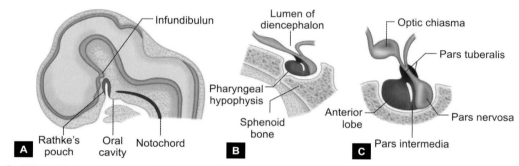

Figs. 131A to C: (A) Sagittal section through the cephalic part of a 6 week embryo showing Rathke's pouch as a dorsal outpocketing of the oral cavity and the infundibulum as a thickening in the floor of the diencephalon. (B and C) Sagittal sections through the developing hypophysis in the 11th and 16th weeks of development, respectively, Note formation of the pars tuberalis encircling the stalk of the pars nervosa

❑ Pituitary gland rests upon the hypophysial fossa of the sphenoid bone in the floor of the middle cranial fossa and is surrounded by a small bony cavity (sella turcica) covered by a dural fold (diaphragma sellae).

❑ Arterial supply: Superior and inferior hypophyseal arteries supply the pituitary gland.

❑ Venous Drainage: There are three routes for venous drainage of neurohypophysis: To adenohypophysis via long and short portal vessels; into dural venous sinuses via inferior hypophyseal veins and to hypothalamus via capillaries passing to median eminence. Venous blood carries the hormones to the target sites.

Table 23: Pituitary gland derivation and terminology.

Derivation	Tissue eye	Part	Lobe
Oral ectoderm			
Hypophyseal diverticulum from the roof of the stomodeum	Adenohypophysis (glandular tissue)	Pars anterior Pars tuberalis Pars intermedia	Anterior lobe
Neuroectoderm			
Neurohypophyseal diverticulum from the floor of the diencephalon	Neurohypophysis (nervous tissue)	Pars nervosa Infundibular stem Median eminence	Posterior lobe

QUESTIONS

1. All are derivatives of Rathke's pouch EXCEPT
   (NEET Pattern 2015)
   a. Pars intermedia
   b. Pars tuberalis
   c. Neurohypophysis
   d. Pars distalis

2. Venous drainage from neurohypophysis is routed through all of the following EXCEPT   *(AIIMS 2004)*
   a. Portal vessels to adenohypophysis
   b. Superior hypophyseal veins to ventricular tanycytes
   c. Inferior hypophyseal veins to dural venous sinuses
   d. Capillaries to median eminence and hypothalamus

ANSWERS

1. **c. Neurohypophysis**
   ❑ Neurohypophysis (posterior lobe) develops from a ventral evagination of the hypothalamus (diencephalon).
   ❑ It includes the median eminence, infundibular stem, and pars nervosa.
   ❑ Rathke's pouch gives rise to the various components of the anterior pituitary including pars anterior, pars tuberalis, pars intermedia.

2. b. Superior hypophyseal veins to ventricular tanycytes
- ❑ There are no vessels by the name superior hypophyseal veins.
- ❑ There are three routes for venous drainage of neurohypophysis: To adenohypophysis via long and short portal vessels; into dural venous sinuses via inferior hypophyseal veins and to hypothalamus via capillaries passing to median eminence.

- ▪ **Anterior lobe** (adenohypophysis) of pituitary develops from **Rathke's pouch** (ectodermal diverticulum of the primitive oral cavity) *(NEET Pattern 2013)*
- ▪ **Herring bodies** are neurosecretory structures present in the **neurohypophysis** (posterior pituitary) *(NEET Pattern 2012)*

▼ Thyroid and Parathyroid

- ❑ Thyroid gland is an endocrine gland that produces thyroxine and thyrocalcitonin, which are essential for metabolism and growth.
  - ➤ It takes iodine from food to produce thyroid hormones and is controlled by thyroid-stimulating hormone produced by the pituitary gland.
- ❑ Thyroid gland consists of right and left lobes connected by the isthmus, which crosses the second, third (and fourth) tracheal rings (most precisely third).
- ❑ A remnant of the thyroglossal duct (pyramidal lobe) may extend upward from the isthmus, usually to the left of the midline and may be anchored to the hyoid bone as a fibrous or muscular band called levator glandulae thyroideae.
- ❑ The Ligament of Berry is the superior suspensory ligament of the thyroid gland located adjacent to the cricoid cartilage on the posterior surface of the thyroid gland.

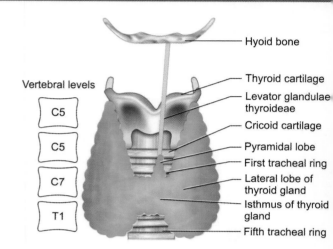

Fig. 132: Parts and extent of the thyroid gland.

Relations

- ❑ Anteriorly: Pretracheal fascia, sternohyoid muscle and the superior belly of omohyoid muscle. Inferiorly it is overlapped by the anterior border of the sternocleidomastoid muscle.
- ❑ Posteriorly: Prevertebral fascia, carotid sheath, parathyroid glands and trachea.
- ❑ Laterally: Thyroid gland is covered by the sternothyroid muscle, which is attached to the oblique line of the thyroid cartilage preventing the upper pole of the gland from extending onto the thyrohyoid muscle.
- ❑ Medially: Recurrent laryngeal nerve, trachea, larynx and oesophagus. The superior pole of the gland contacts the inferior pharyngeal constrictor and superior part of cricothyroid. The external laryngeal nerve runs medial to the superior pole to supply the cricothyroid muscle.
- ❑ The isthmus is covered by sternothyroid and is separated from it by pretracheal fascia. The superior thyroid arteries anastomose along its upper border and the inferior thyroid veins leave the thyroid gland at its lower border.
- ❑ Arterial supply: Superior and inferior thyroid arteries and the thyroid ima artery (in 10% of population).
  - ➤ External carotid artery via the superior thyroid artery.
  - ➤ Subclavian artery/thyrocervical trunk via the inferior thyroid artery.
  - ➤ Arch of the aorta via the thyroid ima artery.
- ❑ Note: Thyroid ima artery has variable origin and may arise from brachiocephalic trunk, common carotid artery, Subclavian artery, etc.
- ❑ Venous drainage: Superior and middle thyroid veins drain into the internal jugular vein and the inferior thyroid vein drain into the brachiocephalic vein.
- ❑ Lymphatic drainage
  - ➤ The upper group of lymphatics follow superior thyroid artery and lower lymphatics follow the inferior thyroid arteries.
    - ▪ The upper lymphatics drain into the prelaryngeal and upper deep cervical (jugulodigastric) lymph nodes.

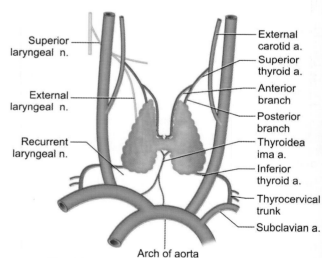

Fig. 133: Arterial supply of the thyroid gland.

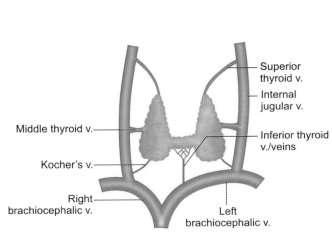

Fig. 134: Venous drainage of the thyroid gland

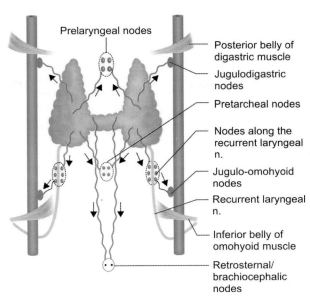

Fig. 135: Lymphatic drainage of the thyroid gland

➤ The lower group drains into pretracheal and lower deep cervical lymph nodes and group of lymph nodes along the recurrent laryngeal nerves. Those from lower part of isthmus drain into retrosternal or brachiocephalic nodes lying in the superior mediastinum.

❏ **Parathyroid Glands** are endocrine glands that play a vital role in the regulation of calcium and phosphorus metabolism and are controlled by the pituitary and hypothalamus.

❏ Parathyroid glands are 4 small ovoid bodies that lie against the dorsum of the thyroid under its sheath but with their own capsule.

➤ The superior parathyroid glands are consistently located on the posterior surface of the upper thyroid lobes near the inferior thyroid artery.

➤ The inferior parathyroid glands are located on the lateral surface of the lower thyroid lobes (not constant).

❏ Arterial supply: Each parathyroid gland receives blood supply from inferior thyroid artery, and also from the anastomosis between superior and inferior thyroid arteries.

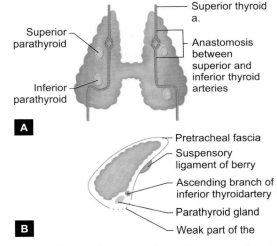

Figs. 136A and B: Location of the parathyroid glands: (A) Posterior aspect of the thyroid gland. (B) Section through thyroid lobe along with its capsule.

CLINICAL CORRELATIONS

■ Thyroid surgery is a potential risk for vital nerves which include superior laryngeal nerve and recurrent laryngeal nerve.
  – Superior thyroid artery and the external laryngeal nerve diverge from each other near the apex.
    ■ Therefore, during operative procedure, the superior thyroid artery should be ligated as close to the apex of thyroid lobe as possible to avoid injury to the external laryngeal nerve.
  – The recurrent laryngeal nerve lies very close to the inferior thyroid artery near the base of the thyroid lobe.
    ■ Therefore, during thyroidectomy, in olden times it was advocated that the inferior thyroid artery should be ligated as away from the base of the thyroid lobe as possible to avoid injury to the recurrent laryngeal nerve.
  – But recently it has been realized inferior thyroid artery supplies recurrent laryngeal nerve and parathyroid glands as it nears the thyroid gland and the advocated method compromises blood supply to recurrent laryngeal nerve and also the parathyroid glands.
    ■ So, the latest approach is that ligation is being done at capsular level by identifying every small branch entering the gland (capsular ligation of inferior thyroid artery, closest to the gland), to retain the blood supply of parathyroids and the nerve as well.

QUESTIONS

1. **NOT true is**   (AIIMS 2009)
   a. Superior thyroid artery is branch of external carotid
   b. Parathyroid artery is branch of posterior division of superior thyroid artery
   c. Inferior thyroid artery is branch of thyrocervical trunk
   d. Thyroid ima artery is invariably a branch of arch of aorta

2. **TRUE statement(s) about thyroid gland is/are**   (PGIC 2017)
   a. Ensheathed by pretracheal layer of deep cervical fascia
   b. Attached to cricoid cartilage by Berry ligament
   c. Isthmus lies at level of second and third tracheal cartilage
   d. Superior thyroid artery is related to recurrent laryngeal nerve
   e. Thyroidea ima artery mostly arises from subclavian artery

1. **d. Thyroid ima artery is invariably a branch of arch of aorta**
   - ❑ Thyroid ima artery is present in a small group of population and has a **variable origin** (may be a branch of **arch of aorta**, **subclavian artery**, **common carotid artery**).
   - ❑ **Superior thyroid artery** is a branch of **external carotid** artery and contributes partly towards the parathyroid blood supply.
   - ❑ Parathyroid arteries are **usually** branches of inferior thyroid artery. In **some population**, parathyroid artery may be a branch of **posterior division of superior thyroid artery**.
   - ❑ Inferior thyroid artery is a branch of **thyrocervical trunk** and is the main source of blood supply to the parathyroids.

2. **a. Ensheathed by pretracheal layer of deep cervical fascia; b. Attached to cricoid cartilage by Berry ligament; c. Isthmus lies at level of second and third tracheal cartilage**
   - ❑ Superior thyroid artery is related to external (**not recurrent**) laryngeal nerve. Thyroidea ima artery has a **variable origin**. It mostly arises from the brachiocephalic trunk but may also originate from the aortic arch or even subclavian artery.
   - ❑ Thyroid gland is **ensheathed** by the pretracheal layer of the deep cervical fascia anterior to the trachea. This fascia condenses and attaches the thyroid gland to the cricoid cartilage and is known as the **Berry's ligament**. Isthmus of thyroid gland lies at level of **second and third** tracheal cartilage.

- **Isthmus** of thyroid gland usually anterior to the **second, third and fourth** tracheal cartilages ring (*NEET Pattern 2015*)
  - Some authors mention it as **second and third ring**, most precisely **3rd ring**.
- **Isthmus** of thyroid gland lies at **C7 vertebral** level (*NEET Pattern 2015*)
- **Superior thyroid artery** runs alongwith **external laryngeal** nerve towards the thyroid gland (*NEET Pattern 2016*)
- **Inferior** thyroid artery supplies the **recurrent** laryngeal nerve and lies very close to the near the base of the thyroid lobe.
- **Inferior** thyroid artery is a branch of **thyrocervical** trunk (*NEET Pattern 2015*)
- **Inferior** thyroid vein drain into the **brachiocephalic** vein (*NEET Pattern 2012*)
  - **Superior** and **middle** thyroid veins drain into the **internal jugular vein.**
- Ligament of **Berry** in thyroid fixes to **Cricoid** cartilage (*NEET Pattern 2014*)
- Lymphatic drainage of **thyroid gland** is mainly into **deep cervical** nodes (*NEET Pattern 2015*)

TM Joint

- ❑ **Temporomandibular joint** is a bicondylar synovial joint. Some authors consider it as a combined gliding and hinge type of the synovial joint (ginglymoid–diarthrodial compound synovial joint).
- ❑ The articular surfaces of the bones are covered by fibrocartilage (not hyaline), hence it is considered as atypical synovial joint.
- ❑ It has two (superior and inferior) synovial cavities divided by an articular disk.
  - ➤ There is an upper gliding joint between the articular tubercle and mandibular fossa above and the articular disk below where forward gliding (protrusion) and backward gliding (retraction/translation) take place.

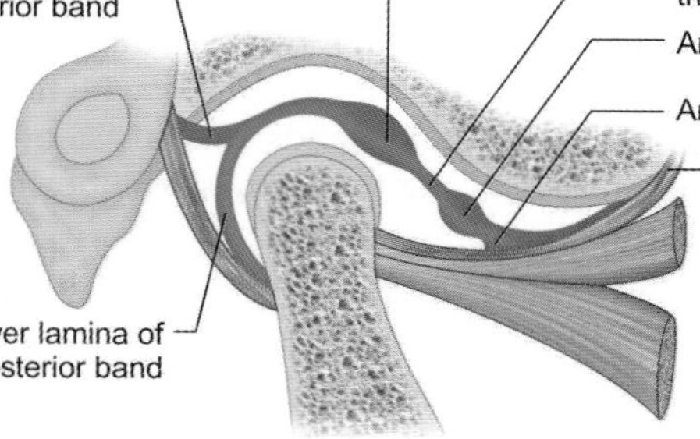

Fig. 137: Parts of the intra-articular disc.

  - ➤ The lower hinge joint is between the disk and the mandibular head (condyle) where elevation (closing) and depression (opening) of the jaw take place. During yawning, the disc and the head of the mandible glide across the articular tubercle.
- ❑ TM joint has an **articular capsule** that extends from the articular tubercle and the margins of the mandibular fossa to the neck of the mandible.
- ❑ It is reinforced by the **lateral (temporomandibular) ligament**, which extends from the tubercle on the zygoma to the neck of the mandible, and the **sphenomandibular ligament**, which extends from the spine of the sphenoid bone to the lingula of the mandible.
- ❑ **Stylomandibular ligament** extends from the styloid process to the posterior border of the ramus of the mandible, near the angle of the mandible, separating the parotid from the submandibular gland.
- ❑ Pterygomandibular raphe is a ligamentous band between the buccinator muscle and the superior pharyngeal constrictor, extends between the pterygoid hamulus superiorly and the posterior end of the mylohyoid line of the mandible inferiorly.
- ❑ TM joint is innervated by the auriculotemporal and masseteric branches of the mandibular nerve.
- ❑ The arterial supply is by the superficial temporal, maxillary (middle meningeal and anterior tympanic branches), and ascending pharyngeal arteries.

Table 24: Movements of temporomandibular joint.

Movements of mandible	Muscle(s)
Elevation (close mouth)	Temporalis, masseter, and medial pterygoid
Depression (open mouth)	Lateral pterygoid, suprahyoid, and infrahydoid muscles[a]
Protrusion (protrude chin)	Lateral pterygoid, masseter, and medial pterygoid[b]
Retrusion (retrude chin)	Temporalis (posterior oblique and near horizontal fibers) and masseter
Lateral movements (grinding and chewing)	Temporalis of same side, pterygoids of opposite side, and masseter

[a] The prime mover is normally gravity; these muscles are mainly active against resistance.
[b] The lateral pterygoid is the prime mover here, with minor secondary roles played by the masseter and medial pterygoid.

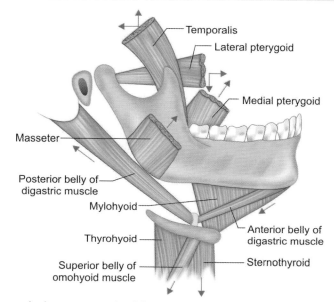

Fig. 138: Muscles of mastication producing movements of the temporomandibular joint. The arrows indicate the direction of their actions. Chief muscles of mastication are labelled in bold

CLINICAL CORRELATIONS

- Dislocation of the temporomandibular joint occurs anteriorly as the mandible head glides across the articular tubercle during yawning and laughing.
- Upper fibers of lateral pterygoid muscles insert onto anterior aspect of articular disc as well as on to the head of mandible; spasms of this muscle in activities like yawning can result in dislocation of mandible by pulling the disc anterior to the articular tubercle.

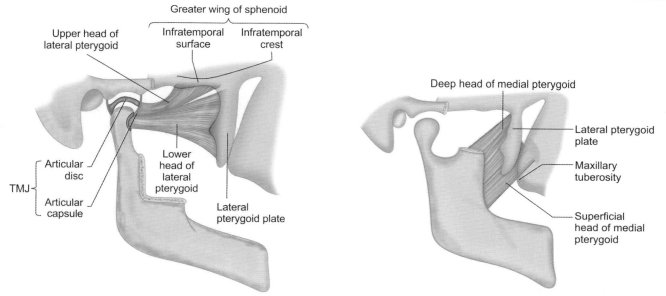

Fig. 139: Origin and insertion of the lateral pterygoid muscle   **Fig. 140:** Origin and insertion of the medial pterygoid muscle

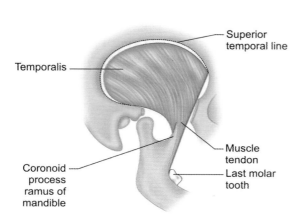

Fig. 141: Origin and insertion of the temporalis muscle

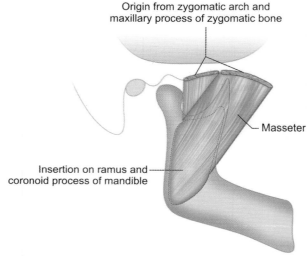

Fig. 142: Origin and insertion of the masseter muscle

1. **A person having difficulty in opening in mouth but not in closing the mouth. Which of the following statement is CORRECT about concerned muscle?** *(PGIC 2013)*
   a. Origin from lateral pterygoid plate
   b. Origin from medial pterygoid plate
   c. Insertion to anterior margin of articular disc
   d. Supplied by mandibular nerve
   e. Depress mandible while opening it

2. **Following are the TM Joint ligaments EXCEPT:**
   (NEET Pattern 2014)
   a. Stylomandibular
   b. Temporomandibular
   c. Tympanomandibular
   d. Sphenomandibular

3. **Identify muscle causing opening of jaw in the diagram:**
   (AIIMS 2015)
   a. A
   b. B
   c. C
   d. D

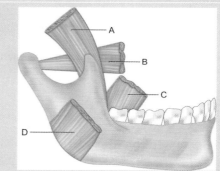

4. **What is the function of the marked muscle in the following diagram?** *(AIIMS 2017)*
   a. Protraction
   b. Retraction
   c. Elevation
   d. Depression

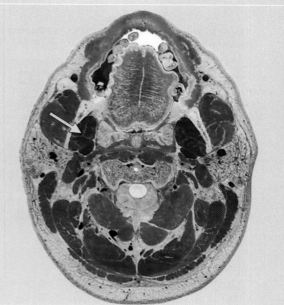

QUESTIONS

QUESTIONS

5. Which of the following marked muscles is involved in opening of jaw? *(AIIMS 2017)*
   a. A
   b. B
   c. C
   d. D

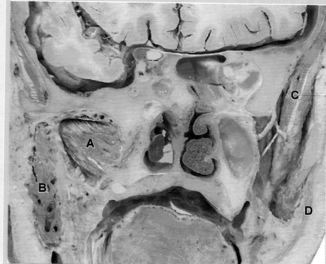

ANSWERS

1. a. Origin from lateral pterygoid plate; c. Insertion to anterior margin of articular disc; d. Supplied by mandibular nerve; e. Depress mandible while opening it
   - ❑ Lateral pterygoid muscle takes its origin from lateral pterygoid plate and **inserts into the pterygoid fovea** on the neck of mandible along with the **anterior margin of articular disc.**
   - ❑ Lateral pterygoid is supplied by the **mandibular nerve** and causes **protrusion** and **depression** of mandible, helping to **open** the mouth.

2. c. Tympanomandibular
   - ❑ TM joint has a **capsular ligament strengthened** by temporomandibular, sphenomandibular, and stylomandibular ligaments.

3. b. B
   - ❑ Lateral pterygoid muscle causes **protrusion** and **depression** of mandible bone and **open the jaw.**
   - ❑ Lateral pterygoid muscle inserts into the pterygoid fovea on the neck of mandible and **pulls mandible forward** and down (protrusion and depression) to help **open the mouth.**
   - ❑ **MTM** (Masseter, temporalis and medial pterygoid) muscles are **elevators** of mandible (close the jaw), whereas, lateral pterygoid is a depressor.

4. c. Elevation
   - ❑ The given diagram is a **transverse section** of the head region at the tongue level, showing the **medial pterygoid** muscle at the area marked by the arrow. The major function of this muscle is **elevation of the mandible.**

5. a. A
   - ❑ This a **coronal section** of head showing some marked **muscles** involved in **mastication.**
   - ❑ Muscle involved in **opening of jaw** is **lateral pterygoid** (maker A).
   - ❑ Key- A: Lateral pterygoid; B: Masseter; C: Temporalis; D: Buccinator
   - ❑ Masseter and temporalis muscles are the elevators of mandible.
   - ❑ **Buccinator** compresses the cheeks **against the teeth** (assistant muscle of mastication).

- ▪ **Elevation** of mandible is brought about by the contraction of **MTM** (Masseter, Temporalis and Medial pterygoid) muscles.
- ▪ Depression is carried out by digastric, geniohyoid and the mylohyoid muscles **along with the lateral pterygoids.**
- ▪ **Lateral pterygoid** is attached to **intra articular disc** of temporomandibular joint *(NEET Pattern 2016)*
  - – **Spasm** or excessive contraction of **lateral pterygoid** can result in **dislocation of mandible** *(AIIMS 2003)*
- ▪ **Lateral pterygoid** is depressor of mandible to **open the mouth** *(NEET Pattern 2012, 14)*
- ▪ TM joint has a capsular ligament strengthened by **temporomandibular, sphenomandibular,** and **stylomandibular** ligaments (but not by Tympanomandibular ligament) *(NEET Pattern 2014)*
- ▪ The **central** part of the **articular disc** in TM joint is **avascular** and **not innervated** *(AIIMS 2002)*

Surface Marking

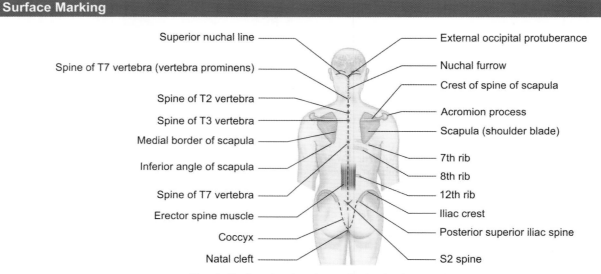

Superior nuchal line

Spine of T7 vertebra (vertebra prominens)

Spine of T2 vertebra

Spine of T3 vertebra

Medial border of scapula

Inferior angle of scapula

Spine of T7 vertebra

Erector spine muscle

Coccyx

Natal cleft

External occipital protuberance

Nuchal furrow

Crest of spine of scapula

Acromion process

Scapula (shoulder blade)

7th rib

8th rib

12th rib

Iliac crest

Posterior superior iliac spine

S2 spine

Fig. 1: Surface landmarks on the back of the body

Table 1: Approximate levels of some spines on the back of the body	
Vertebral spine	**Level**
T2	Superior angle of the scapula
T3	Where crest of spine of the scapula meets its medial border
T7	Inferior angle of the scapula
L4	Highest point of iliac crest
S2	Posterior-superior iliac spine

❑ **Inion** is the point situated on the external occipital protuberance in the median plane.

❑ The spinous process of C2 is the first palpable midline feature, located several centimeters inferior to the inion.

❑ The **ligamentum nuchae** terminates inferiorly at the spine of the seventh cervical vertebra (C7, vertebra prominens), which is the most superior visible projection in this region.

❑ The spine of the first thoracic vertebra (T1) is palpable immediately inferior to C7 and is usually more prominent than the spine of C7.

❑ In the thoracic regions, tips of the thoracic **spines lie opposite the body of the next lower vertebra**. For example, tip of the T4 thoracic spine lies at the level of T5 vertebral body.

❑ The inferior margin of the posterior superior iliac spines (PSIS) lies at level of the second sacral spine (ranges from the L5–S1 vertebral junction to the S2 spinous process). It serves as a useful landmark for the inferior limit of the adult dural sac.

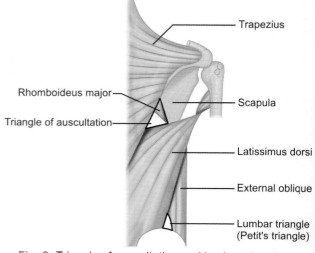

Trapezius

Rhomboideus major

Triangle of auscultation

Scapula

Latissimus dorsi

External oblique

Lumbar triangle (Petit's triangle)

Fig. 2: Triangle of auscultation and lumbar triangle.

❑ The triangle of auscultation lies between the upper border of latissimus dorsi, the lower inferolateral border of trapezius and the inferomedial border of rhomboid major; although for simplicity, the medial border of the scapula is often substituted for the latter muscle.

❑ The lumbar (Petit's) triangle, one of the sites of the rare primary lumbar hernia, lies inferiorly just lateral ot the highest point of the iliac crest, between the inferolateral border of latissimus dorsi, the posterior-free border of external oblique and the iliac crest.

1. Not a boundary of Triangle of Auscultation: *(AIIMS 2008)*
  a. Scapula
  b. Trapezius
  c. Latissimus dorsi
  d. Serratus anterior

2. TRUE about boundary of triangle of auscultation is:
  a. Lateral boundary by latissimus dorsi   *(NEET Pattern 2015)*
  b. Medial boundary by scapula
  c. Lateral boundary by latissimus dorsi
  d. Medial boundary by trapezius

3. Boundaries of petit triangle are formed by all EXCEPT:
  a. Inguinal ligament   *(NEET Pattern 2016)*
  b. External oblique muscle
  c. Iliac crest
  d. Latissimus dorsi

4. Floor of Petit's triangle is formed by: *(NEET Pattern 2016)*
  a. Sacrospinalis
  b. Internal oblique
  c. Rectus abdominis
  d. Fascia transversalis

1. d. Serratus anterior
  ❑ Serratus anterior is inserted on the medial border of scapula **but lies anterior** to scapula. Hence, it is **not** in the triangle of auscultation.
  ❑ Triangle of Auscultation is bounded by **2 muscles and scapula**. Superiorly – Trapezius, Inferiorly – Latissimus dorsi and Laterally – medial wall of Scapula.
  ❑ Rib 7 and Rhomboideus major lie in the **floor** of the triangle. Since **minimal muscle** fibers lie over the triangle, **auscultation** by stethoscope is **better** over this triangle, especially, the sounds of swallowed fluids. **Cardiac end of the stomach** lies deep to this triangle.

2. c. Lateral boundary by latissimus dorsi
  ❑ Triangle of auscultation has trapezius (**superior**), latissimus dorsi (**inferior**) and medial wall of scapula (as **lateral** boundary).

3. a. Inguinal ligament
  ❑ Petit's (lumbar) triangle lies just lateral to the highest point of the iliac crest, between the inferolateral border of **latissimus dorsi**, the posterior-free border of **external oblique** and the **iliac crest**.

4. b. Internal oblique
  ❑ **Internal abdominal oblique** muscle is present at the floor of Petit's triangle.

◤ Vertebrae

Cervical vertebra: Presence of foramen transversarium (FT); Body is oval shaped; Vertebral canal is triangular (Δ); Superior articular facet is directed backward & upward (BU); Bifid spine.

Thoracic vertebra: Presence of rib facet on body and transverse process; Body is triangular (Δ); Vertebral canal is oval; Superior articular facet is directed backward, upward & lateral (BUL).

Lumbar vertebra: Body is oval; Vertebral canal is triangular (Δ); Superior articular facet is directed backward & medial.

Note: (1) Cervical and lumbar vertebra **both** have oval Body is **oval** and **triangular** (Δ) Vertebral canal.

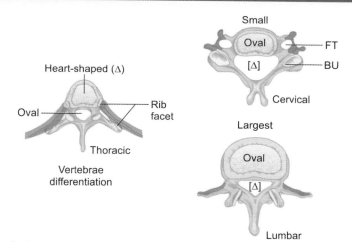

Fig. 3: Differentiating features among cervical, thoracic and lumbar vertebra

Table 2: Cervical vertebrae*	
Part	**Characteristics**
Vertebral body	Small and wider from side to side than anteroposteriorly: superior surface concave with uncus of body (uncinate process); inferior surface convex
Vertebral foramen	Large and triangular
Transverse processes	Foramina transversaria and anterior and posterior tubercles; vertebral arteries and accompanying venous and sympathetic plexuses pass through foramina transversaria of all cervical vertebrae except C7, which transmits only small accessory vertebral veins

Part	Characteristics
Articular processes	Superior facets directed superoposteriorly; inferior facets directed inferoanteriorly; obliquely placed facets are most nearly horizontal in this region
Spinous processes	Short (C3–C5) and bifid (C3–C6); process of C6 long, that of C7 is longer (thus, C7 is called 'vertebra prominens')

*The C1, C2 and C7 vertebrae are atypical.

Table 3: Thoracic vertebrae

Part	Characteristics
Vertebral body	Heart-shaped; one or two costal facets for articulation with head of rib
Vertebral foramen	Circular and smaller than those of cervical and lumbar vertebrae (admits the distal part of a medium-sized index finger)
Transverse processes	Long and strong and extend posterolaterally; length diminishes from T1 to T12 (T1–T10 have facets for articulation with tubercle of rib)
Articular processes	Nearly vertical articular facets: superior facets directed posteriorly and slightly laterally; inferior facets directed anteriorly and slightly medially; planes of facets lie on an arc centered in the vertebral body
Spinous processes	Long; slope posteroinferiorly; tips extend to level of vertebral body below

Table 4: Lumbar vertebrae

Part	Characteristics
Vertebral body	Massive; kidney-shaped when viewed superiorly
Vertebral foramen	Triangular; larger than in thoracic vertebrae and smaller than in cervical vertebrae
Transverse processes	Long and slender; accessory process on posterior surface of base of each process
Articular processes	Nearly vertical facets; superior facets directed posteromedially (or medially); inferior facets directed anterolaterally (or laterally); mammillary process on posterior surface of each superior articular process
Spinous processes	Short and sturdy; thick, broad, and hatchet-shaped

◤ Cervical vertebra

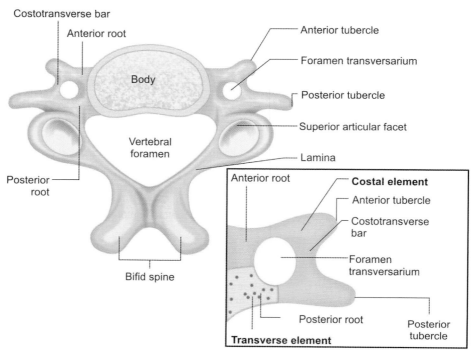

Fig. 4: Typical cervical vertebra (superior aspect); inset on the right side shows the costal and transverse elements of the transverse process

Table 5: Osteologic features of the vertebral column

	Body	Superior articular facets	Inferior articular facets	Spinous processes	Vertebral canal	Transverse processes	Comments
Atlas (C1)	None	Concave, face generally superior	Flat to slightly concave, face generally inferior	None, replaced by a small posterior tubercle	Triangular, largest of cervical region	Largest of cervical region	Two large lateral masses, joined by anterior and posterior arches
Axis (C2)	Tall with a vertical projecting dens	Flat to slightly convex, face generally superior	Flat, face anterior and inferior	Largest of cervical region, bifid	Large and triangular	Form anterior and posterior tubercles	Large superior articular processes that support the atlas and cranium
C3–C6	Wider than deep; have uncinate processes	Flat, face posterior and superior	As above	Bifid	Large and triangular	End as anterior and posterior tubercles	Considered typical cervical vertebrae
C7	Wider than deep	As above	Transition to typical thoracic vertebrae	Large and prominent, easily palpable	Triangular	Thick and prominent, may have a large anterior tubercle forming an 'extra rib'	Often called 'vertebral prominens' because of large spinous process

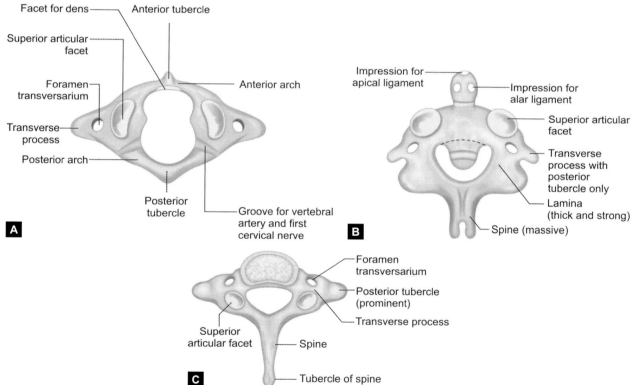

Figs. 5A to C: Atypical cervical vertebrae: (A) Atlas vertebra (superior aspect); (B) Axis vertebra (Posterosuperior aspect); (C) Seventh cervical vertebra (superior aspect)

1. **Difference between typical cervical & thoracic vertebra:**
   a. Has a triangular body   *(AIPG 2007)*
   b. Has a foramen transversarium
   c. Superior articular facet directed backwards & upwards
   d. Has a large vertebral body

2. **Which cervical vertebra has lateral mass:**
   (NEET Pattern 2016)
   a. Atlas   b. Axis
   c. C5   d. C7

QUESTIONS

3. All of the following characteristics differentiate a typical cervical vertebra from a thoracic vertebra EXCEPT:
(AIIMS 2007)
a. Has a triangular vertebral canal
b. Has foramen transversarium
c. Superior articular facet is directed backwards & upwards
d. Has a large vertebral body

4. Typical cervical vertebrae can be differentiated from thoracic vertebra by all EXCEPT: *(AIIMS 2012)*
a. Triangular vertebral canal
b. Foramen transversarium
c. Superior articular facet directed backwards and upwards
d. Small vertebral body

ANSWERS

1. b. Has a foramen transversarium
- Cervical vertebra is characterized by foramina in its transverse process—**foramen transversarium**
- **Cervical & lumbar** vertebrae have **oval bodies** and are triangular in thoracic region.
- Superior articular facets are directed **backwards & upwards in both** the cervical as well as thoracic vertebrae.
- **Cervical** vertebra has a **small body;** the lumbar vertebra bodies are the largest.

2. a. Atlas
- **Lateral masses** are the most bulky and solid parts of the **atlas**, in order to support the weight of the head. Each carry two articular facets, a superior and an inferior.

3. d. Has a large vertebral body
- Vertebral body is the **smallest** in the **cervical** region. Large vertebral body is present at the level of lumbar vertebra.
- Vertebral foramen is **triangular** and **large** in the cervical vertebra.
- The foramen is small and circular in thoracic vertebra.
- Cervical vertebrae are identified by the **foramen transversarium** in their transverse process.
- Superior articular facets are directed **backwards & upwards** in the cervical and thoracic regions.

4. c. Superior articular facet directed backwards and upwards
- Superior articular facet is directed **backwards & upwards in both** the cervical as well as thoracic vertebrae, and **hence cannot help us to differentiate** the two from each other. Thoracic vertebra is in **addition directed laterally** (BUL – backward/upward/lateral).
- The vertebral canal in **cervical** vertebrae is **triangular**, which is oval in thoracic vertebrae.
- Vertebral vessels (artery & vein) pass through the **upper six foramina** transversaria present in the cervical vertebrae.
- Cervical vertebrae have the **smallest bodies**, whereas, lumbar are the largest.

▶ Curvatures

The **cervical** curve is convex anteriorly **(lordosis)** and extends from the first cervical to the second thoracic vertebra; the **thoracic** curvature is convex posteriorly **(kyphosis)** and extends from the second to the twelfth thoracic vertebra.

The **lumbar curvature** is convex anteriorly **(lordosis)** and extends from the twelfth thoracic vertebra to the lumbosacral prominence and the **sacral curve** is convex posteriorly **(kyphosis)**.

The **primary curves** form during fetal development. The **secondary curves** develop after birth.

- Primary curvatures are present at birth and are due to shape of the vertebral bodies. These are **thoracic** and **sacral** and are concave forward (or convex dorsally).
- Secondary curvatures are acquired after birth consequent to changes in the posture with age and are mainly due to the shape of the intervertebral disc. These are **cervical** and **lumbar** and are convex forwards.
- The cervical curvature appears during the months of **neck-holding** and acquired at 4 to 5 months after birth.
- The lumbar curvature appears while the **upright posture** is being attained during the age of 12 to 18 months.

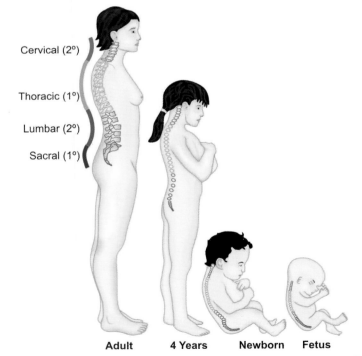

Cervical (2°)
Thoracic (1°)
Lumbar (2°)
Sacral (1°)

Adult   4 Years   Newborn   Fetus

Fig. 6: Curvatures of vertebral column. The four curvatures of the adult vertebral column: cervical, thoracic, lumbar, and sacral are contrasted with the C-shaped curvature of the column during fetal life, when only the primary (1°) curvatures exist. The secondary (2°) curvatures develop during infancy and childhood.

1. Number of vertebrae in vertebral column:

(NEET Pattern 2013)

a. 25
b. 27
c. 29
d. 33

2. Which vertebral segment is numerically most constant?

(AIIMS 2012)

a. Cervical
b. Thoracic
c. Lumbar
d. Sacral

3. Which of these parts of vertebral canal will show secondary curves with concavity backwards: *(AIPG 2007)*

a. Cervical
b. Thoracic
c. Sacral
d. Coccyx

4. Which of the following is TRUE regarding vertebral column curvature?

(PGIC 2015)

a. Primary curves are concave forward
b. Lumbar curve is primary
c. Thoracic curve develops when infant starts walking
d. Cervical appears when the infant starts supporting its head
e. Lumbar curve appears when the child assumes the upright posture

1. d. 33

❏ There are total **thirty-three** vertebrae, upper twenty-four are articulating and separated from each other by intervertebral discs, seven cervical vertebrae, twelve thoracic vertebrae and five lumbar vertebrae.
❏ The lower nine are fused, five in the sacrum and four in the coccyx.
❏ The number of vertebrae in a region can vary but overall the number remains the same. The number of those in the **cervical region** however is **only rarely changed**.

2. a. Cervical

❏ The number of vertebrae in a region can vary but overall the number remains the same. The number of those in the **cervical region however is only rarely changed**.

3. a. Cervical

❏ **Cervical** curvature is a **secondary curvature**, with a posterior concavity.
❏ Secondary curvatures develop **after birth**-like cervical & lumbar curvatures.
❏ These curvatures are **convex anteriorly** and concave backwards.
❏ Primary curvatures like thoracic and sacral & coccygeal curvatures are present **since birth** and are concave anteriorly.

4. a. Primary curves are concave forward; d. Cervical appears when the infant starts supporting its head; e. Lumbar curve appears when the child assumes the upright posture

❏ Vertebral column has **four curvatures** that occur in the cervical, thoracic, lumbar, and sacral regions.
❏ The **fetal** thoracic and sacral **kyphoses** are concave anteriorly, whereas the **acquired** cervical and lumbar **lordoses** are concave posteriorly.
❏ The cervical lordosis becomes evident when an infant begins to **raise (extend) the head** while prone and to hold the head erect while sitting.
❏ The lumbar lordosis becomes apparent when the child **learns to assume the upright posture** for standing and walking.
❏ **Thoracic** curve is a **Primary** curve *(NEET Pattern 2016)*

Table 6: Cranio–Vertebral Joints: Articulation between occipital condyles (cranium) and atlas & axis (vertebrae)

Joints included	Atlanto–Occipital joint	Atlanto–Axial joint
Type of joint	Ellipsoid (Condylar) syovial joint	▪ One median atlanto-axial joint- Pivot synovial joint ▪ Two lateral atlanto-axial joints-Plane synovial joints

Articular surfaces	▪ Occipital condyles
	▪ Atlas (superior articular surface)
		▪ Median atlanto-axial joint
		  – Odontoid process of axis
		  – Anterior arch and transverse ligament of atlas
		▪ Lateral atlanto-axial joint
		  – Inferior facet on lateral mass of atlas
		  – Superior articular facet on axis

Permitted movements	▪ Flexion & extension (Yes/nodding movement of head)[1] ▪ Lateral flexion[2] ▪ Rotation	▪ Rotation ('No' movement)

Ligaments	▪ Fibrous capsule
	▪ Accessory ligaments (conncet the cranium and the atlas)
	  – Anterior atlanto-occipital membrane
	  – Posterior atlanto-occipital membrane
		▪ Median atlanto-axial joint
		  – Fibrous capsule
		  – Cruciform ligament (2 parts)
		    - Transverse Ligament[3]
		    - Longitudinal Ligament[4]
		  – Ligaments between axis and occipital bone
		    - Apical ligament of dens[5]
		    - Alar ligaments[6]
		    - Membrana tectoria[7]

1. **Flexion** is carried out by: Longus capitis & rectus capitis anterior and **extension** by: Rectus capitis posterior major & minor; semispinalls and splenius capitits; trapezius (upper fibers)
2. **Lateral flexion** is carried out by rectus capitis lateralis

3. **Transverse Ligament** is present between lateral massess of the atlas, arching over the posterior aspect of dens of the axis
4. Longitudinal Ligament extends from the dens of axis to anterior aspect of the foramen magnum (superior band) and to body of the axis (inferior band).
5. Apical ligament of dens extends from the apex of the dens to the anterior aspect of the foramen magnum (of the occipital bone).
6. **Alar ligament** extend from the apex of the dens to the tubercle on the medial side of the occipital condyle.
7. Membrana tectoria is a **continuation of the posterior longitudinal ligament**[Q]. It covers the posterior surface of the dens and the apical, alar, and cruciform ligaments.

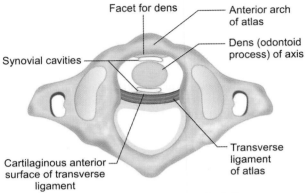

Fig. 7: Median atlantoxial articulation.

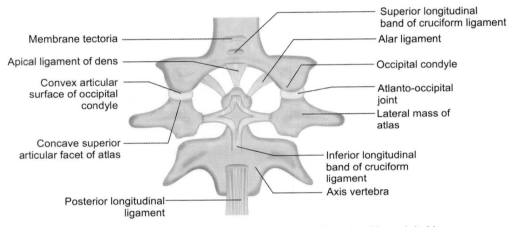

Fig. 8: Posterior view of the ligaments connecting the axis with occipital bone.

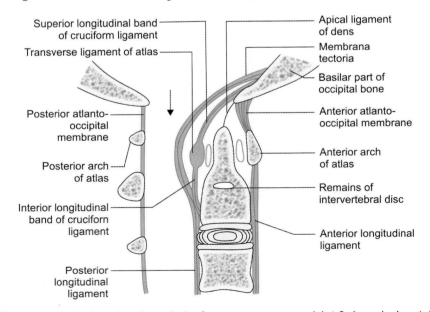

Fig. 9: Median sagittal section through the foramen magnum and 1st-3rd cervical vertebraes

Questions

1. The movement at the following joint permits a person to look towards the right or left: *(AIPG 2004)*
   a. Atlanto-occipital joint
   b. Atlantoaxial joint
   c. C2-C3 joint
   d. C3-C4 joint

2. Membrana tectoria is continuation of: *(AIIMS 2014)*
   a. Anterior atlanto-occipital membrane
   b. Posterior atlanto-occipital membrane
   c. Anterior longitudinal ligament
   d. Posterior longitudinal ligament

3. Transverse ligament of atlas is part of: *(AIIMS)*
   a. Cruciform ligament
   b. Ligamenta flava
   c. Anterior longitudinal ligament
   d. Posterior longitudinal ligament

4. Cranio-vertebral joint does NOT include: *(AIIMS 2015)*
   a. Atlas
   b. Axis
   c. Wings of sphenoid
   d. Basi-occiput

5. Dislocation of the vertebra is uncommon in thoracic region because in this region: *(AIIMS 2004)*
   a. The articular processes are interlocked
   b. The vertebral body is long
   c. Anterior longitudinal ligament is strong
   d. Spinous process is long and pointed

6. TRUE about atlanto-axial joint: *(PGIC 2016)*
   a. Vertebral artery passes through groove on arch of atlas vertebrae to foramen magnum
   b. Permits flexion & extension
   c. Permits side to side movement of head
   d. Permits flexion only
   e. Permits rotation

Answers

1. **b. Atlantoaxial joint**
   - Looking towards right or left ('**NO' movement** of head) occurs at the **atlantoaxial joint**.
   - '**YES' movement** occurs at the **atlanto-occipital** joint and involves flexion & extension of head over vertebra.
   - C2-C3 and C3-C4 joints allow mainly flexion & extension of the neck and a small degree of rotation is also possible.

2. **d. Posterior longitudinal ligament**
   - Membrana tectoria is continuation of **posterior longitudinal ligament** into the cranial cavity through the foramen magnum.
   - It is attached inferiorly to the posterior surface of the body of **axis** and has superior attachment to the **basiocciput** in the cranial cavity.

3. **a. Cruciform ligament**
   - Transverse ligament forms the **horizontal part of cruciform ligament**.

4. **c. Wings of sphenoid**
   - Sphenoid bone has **no articulation** in cranio-vertebral joints.

5. **a. The articular processes are interlocked**
   - The superior articular process is directed **backward, upward and laterally** (BUL) in the thoracic region.
   - It **interlocks** with the corresponding inferior articular facet making a **strong articulation** rendering dislocation in the thoracic region **uncommon**.

6. **a. Vertebral artery pass through grove on arch of atlas vertebrae to foramen magnum; c. Permits side to side movement of head; e. Permits rotation.**
   - The atlantic parts of the vertebral arteries pass through **groove on arch** of atlas vertebra, perforate the dura and arachnoid and pass through the **foramen magnum**.
   - Atlanto-axial joint is a **pivot synovial** joint, which permits **rotation** and **side to side** ('NO') movement.
   - Flexion and extension ('YES') movement occurs at **atlanto-occipital** joint. It also allows lateral bending.

▶ Movements

- Flexion, extension, lateral flexion and rotation are the movements that occur in cervical, thoracic and lumbar spine. **'Yes'** (nodding) movement happens at atlanto-occipital joint and **'No'** movement at atlantoaxial joint. Sacral and coccygeal spine has **no movements**.

Movement	Spine region
Maximum flexion	Cervical
Maximum extension	Lumbar
Maximum lateral flexion	Cervical & lumbar
Maximum rotation	Thoracic
Least rotation	Lumbar
No movements	Sacrum & coccyx

- **Flexion** of the vertebral column is maximum in the **cervical** region. **Extension** of the vertebral column is most marked in the **lumbar** region (more extensive than flexion). However, the **interlocking** articular processes here **prevent rotation**. The lumbar and cervical region intervertebral discs that are large relative to the size of the vertebral bodies, whereas thoracic region has thin intervertebral discs. **Rotation is maximum** in **thoracic** region but flexion is limited, including lateral flexion.

QUESTIONS

1. The lumbar region of the vertebral column permits all the following movements EXCEPT: *(AIPG 2003)*
a. Flexion
b. Extension
c. Lateral flexion
d. Rotation

2. Maximum Flexion in thoracic vertebrae occurs at: *(NEET Pattern 2016)*
a. Upper thoracic
b. Middle thoracic
c. Lower thoracic
d. Same at all level

ANSWERS

1. d. Rotation
❏ Lumbar region shows **restricted rotation** movement.
❏ The **interlocking** articular processes **prevent** rotation.

2. c. Lower thoracic
❏ Maximum thoracic flexion occurs in the **lower thoracic** spine because the vertebrae **start to orient their facets** similar to the lumbar spine where the most flexion and extension occurs.
❏ Also, the lower thoracic spine is **not as cemented in place** by the floating ribs

▼ Muscles

Muscle	Proximal attachment	Distal attachment	Nerve supply	Main action(s)
Superficial posterior axio-appendicular (extrinsic shoulder) muscles				
Trapezius	Medial third of superior nuchal line; external occipital protuberance; nuchal ligament; spinous processes of C7–T12 vertebrae	Lateral third of clavicle; acromion and spine of scapula	Spinal accessory nerve (CN XI) (motor fibers) and C3, C4 spinal nerves (pain and proprioceptive fibers)	Descending part elevates; ascending part depresses; and middle part (or all parts together) retracts scapula; descending and ascending parts act together to rotate glenoid cavity superiorly
Erector Spinae Iliocostalis Longissimus Spinalis	Arises by a broad tendon from posterior part of iliac crest, posterior surface of sacrum, sacroiliac ligaments, sacral and inferior lumbar spinous processes, and supraspinous ligament	*Iliocostalis:* Lumborum, thoracis, cervicis; fibers run superiorly to angles of low ribs and cervical transverse processes *Longissimus:* Thoracis, cervicis, capitis; fibers run superiorly to ribs between tubercles and angles to transverse processes in thoracic and cervical regions, and to mastoid process of temporal bone *Spinalis:* Thoracis, cervicis, capitis; fibers run superiorly to spinous processes in the upper thoracic region and to cranium	Posterior rami of spinal nerves	*Acting bilaterally:* Extend vertebral column and head, as back is flexed, control movement via eccentric contraction *Acting unilaterally:* Laterally flex vertebral column

QUESTIONS

1. Shape of trapezius muscle is: *(AIIMS 2017)*
a. Triangular
b. Quadrilateral
c. Trapezium
d. Quadrangular

2. Trapezius is attached to all structures EXCEPT: *(AIPG)*
a. First rib
b. Clavicle
c. Scapula
d. Occiput

3. All are true about erector spinae EXCEPT: *(NEET Pattern 2016)*
a. Causes flexion of trunk
b. Causes lateral flexion and rotation of trunk
c. Includes ilio-costalis, longissimus and spinalis
d. All are correct

ANSWERS

1. a. Triangular
❏ Trapezius is a flat, **triangular** muscle that extends over the back of the neck and upper thorax. The paired trapezius muscles form a **diamond shape**, from which the **name is derived**.

2. a. First rib
❏ **Origin: Occipital** bone, ligamentum nuchae, spinous processes of seventh cervical and all thoracic vertebrae
❏ **Insertion: Clavicle**, acromion, spine of **scapula**

3. a. Causes flexion of trunk
❏ Erector spinae **extends** the vertebral column (**antagonist** muscle to rectus abdominis). Acting unilaterally, it causes **lateral flexion** and **rotation** of trunk.
❏ It has **three parts:** lateral (Ilio-costalis), an intermediate (Longissimus), and a medial (Spinalis).

▼ Lumbar Puncture

❏ A line is then taken between the **highest points** of the iliac crests: this line almost always intersects the vertebral column at the **L4 vertebral** body or L4/L5 intervertebral disc level.

❑ With the spines now identified, the skin is anesthetized and a needle is inserted between the spines of L3 and L4 (or L4 and L5).

❑ In order: subcutaneous tissue, **supraspinous** ligament, **interspinous** ligament, **ligamentum flavum**, epidural space containing the internal vertebral venous plexus, dura, arachnoid, and finally, the subarachnoid space.

Newborn

❑ The **supracristal plane** intersects the vertebral column slightly higher (L3–L4).

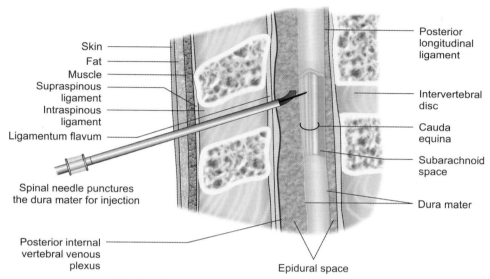

Fig. 10: Structures pierced during lumbar puncture

Structures pierced during lumbar puncture are: Skin → subcutaneous tissue → supraspinous and interspinous ligament → Ligament flavum → Dura mater → Arachnoid mater.

1. In lumbar puncture, which ligament is NOT pierced:
  a. Anterior longitudinal
  b. Ligamentum flava
  c. Posterior longitudinal
  d. Supraspinous

2. Popping sensation felt on doing Lumbar puncture is while piercing: *(AIIMS 2015)*
  a. Ligamentum flavum
  b. Supraspinous ligament
  c. Interspinous ligament
  d. Dura mater

1. c. Posterior longitudinal
  ❑ In lumbar puncture **posterior longitudinal** ligament is **not pierced**. Though it may be reached accidently if the needle has been **advanced too far anteriorly**.

2. a. Ligamentum flavum > d. Dura mater
  ❑ The classical "popping" sensation occurs when the needle has passed through the **ligamentum flavum**.
  ❑ The needle then be advanced in 2 mm intervals until a second pop is felt (**dura mater** is pierced) and CSF is obtained.

► Surface Marking and Landmarks

The horizontal **sternal plane** is 'traditionally' reported to pass through the **intervertebral disc between** the fourth and fifth thoracic vertebrae posteriorly.

❑ Here lies the **sternal angle (of Louis)**, which is at the junction between manubrium and body of the **sternum**.
   ➢ It indicates the level where (1) the **second rib** (costal cartilage) articulate with the sternum, (2) the **aortic arch** begins and ends, (3) the **trachea bifurcates** into the right and left primary bronchi, (4) **Pulmonary trunk** divides into right and left pulmonary arteries, (5) Upper border of heart, (6) the site where the **superior vena cava penetrates** the pericardium to enter the right atrium, (7) it marks the plane of separation between the **superior** and **inferior mediastinum**, (8) **Azygos vein arches** over the root of right lung to end in the superior vena cava.

<table>
<tr><td>QUESTIONS</td><td>

1. TRUE about tracheal bifurcation: *(NEET Pattern 2016)*
   a. At lower border of T4
   b. A ridge of cartilage is present
   c. Lies carina
   d. All of the above

</td><td>

2. At Saint Louis angle what crosses: *(NEET Pattern 2012)*
   a. Arch of aorta
   b. Azygos vein
   c. Common carotid artery
   d. Innominate vein

</td></tr>
</table>

<table>
<tr><td>ANSWERS</td><td>

1. **d. All of the above**
   ❑ At lower border of T4, a ridge of cartilage is present called **carina**, which marks the bifurcation of trachea into two bronchi.

2. **a. Arch of aorta > b. Azygos vein**
   ❑ At **sternal angle of Louis** arch of aorta begins (anteriorly) and ends (posteriorly), crosses from right to left.
   ❑ **Azygos vein** arches over the root of right lung to end in the superior vena cava at this level.

</td></tr>
</table>

❑ Arch of aorta beginning, and ending is at the **same level** - T4 vertebra.

► Development of Cardiovascular System

The heart is formed from tissues derived from the midline **splanchnopleuric coelomic epithelium** with later contributions from **neural crest mesenchyme.**

❑ The splanchnopleuric **coelomic epithelium** gives rise to the myocardium, including the **conduction system** of the heart.
❑ The **endocardium**, including its derived cardiac mesenchymal population, which produces the valvular tissues of the heart.
❑ Splanchnopleuric coelomic epithelium is also the source of the **epicardium**, coronary arteries and interstitial fibroblasts.

On approximately **day 16**, heart progenitor cells migrate through the **primitive streak** to a position cranial to the neural folds where they establish a horseshoe-shaped region in the **splanchnic layer of lateral plate mesoderm** called the primary heart forming regions.

❑ This cardiogenic area is at the **cephalic end** of embryo between the septum transversum and prochordal plate.
❑ The intraembryonic celom lying in this area forms **pericardial cavity** and the splanchnopleuric mesoderm underneath the pericardial cavity forms the **heart tube**.
❑ During formation of **head fold** the heart tube comes to lie on the roof of the pericardial cavity.

Mesoderm around the endocardium forms the myocardium. The myocardial cells secrete some extracellular matrix rich in hyaluronic acid called **cardiac jelly**.

❑ Cardiac jelly a gelatinous substance **secreted by cardiac myocytes**, is present between the endothelium and myocardium of the embryonic heart, which transforms into the **connective tissue of the endocardium**.
❑ It has been called a gelatinoreticulum, a myoepicardial reticulum and, more recently, the myocardial basement membrane.
❑ Cardiac jelly accumulates within the endocardial cushions, which are **precursors of cardiac valves**. (*Gray's Anatomy - Ed41*)
❑ Mesoderm that migrates from the coelomic wall near the liver into the cardiac region forms the **epicardium**.

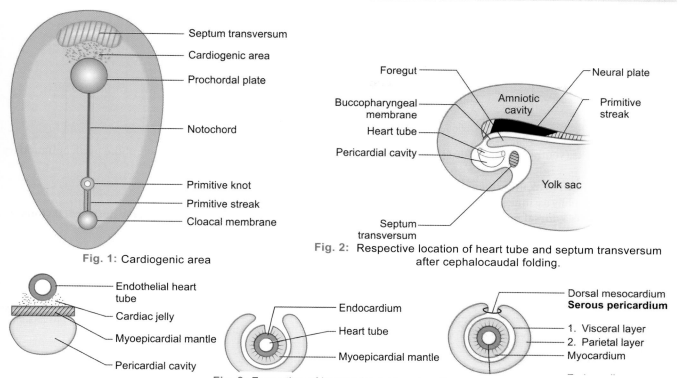

Fig. 1: Cardiogenic area

Fig. 2: Respective location of heart tube and septum transversum after cephalocaudal folding.

Fig. 3: Formation of heart tube and pericardium

The **heart beat begins** at the end of the third week and beginning of fourth week of intrauterine life (day 22).

❑ The blood flow during the fourth week can be visualized by Doppler ultrasonography. The heart tube develops **five dilatations**: sinus venosus, primitive atrium, primitive ventricle, bulbus cordis and the truncus arteriosus.

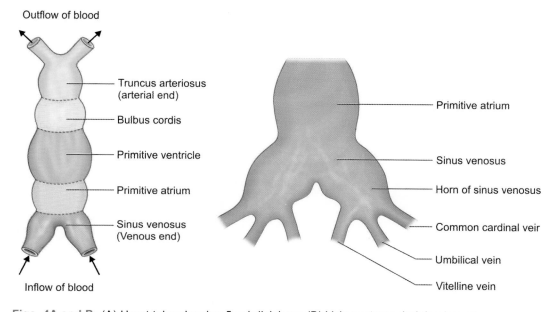

Figs. 4A and B: (A) Heart tube showing 5 subdivisions; (B) Vein systems draining into sinus venosus.

Table 1: Embryonic dilatation and their derivatives	
Embryonic dilatation	**Adult derivatives**
1. Truncus arteriosus	Ascending aorta Pulmonary trunk
2. Bulbus cordis	Smooth upper part of the right ventricle (Conus arteriosus) Smooth upper part of the left ventricle (aortic vestibule)

Embryonic dilatation	Adult derivatives
3. Primitive ventricle	Trabeculated part of the right ventricle Trabeculated part of the left ventricle
4. Primitive atrium	Trabeculated part of the right atrium Trabeculated part of the left atrium
5. Sinus venosus	Smooth part of the right atrium (sinus venarum) Coronary sinus Oblique vein of the left atrium

Truncus arteriosus (ventral aorta) divides into ascending aorta and pulmonary trunk by formation of the aorticopulmonary (AP) septum.

- ❏ During the fourth week these dilations undergo **dextral looping** which is complete by day 28.
- ❏ The **atria** gradually assume **posterior** location and the ventricles move into a more anterior position.
- ❏ Initially there is a **dorsal mesocardium** suspending the heart tube, which later develops **transverse pericardial sinus.**

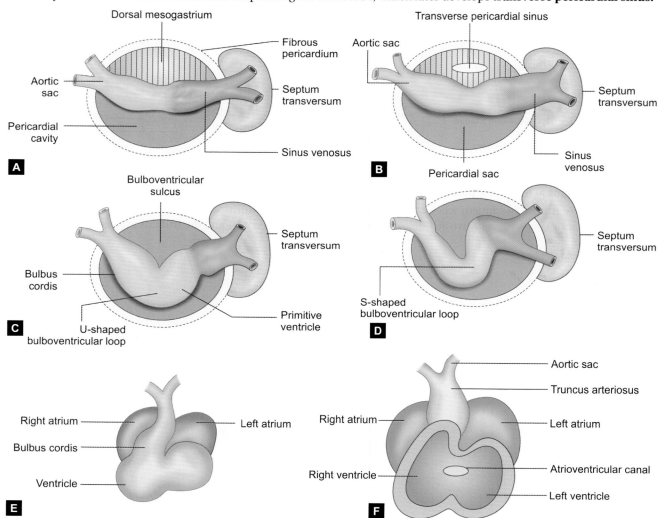

Figs. 5A to F: Development of the heart tube into adult components

The **right horn of sinus venosus** gets absorbed into the **posterior aspect of primitive atrium** to form the **sinus venarum** (posterior smooth wall of right atrium), whereas the **rough anterior wall** of right atrium develops from the **primitive atrium anteriorly.**

- ❏ The **sulcus terminalis** is the junction of the smooth and rough (trabeculated) part of the right atrium, indicated internally by the **crista terminalis**.
- ❏ **Crista terminalis** is a vertical muscular ridge running anteriorly along the **right atrial wall** from the opening of the SVC to the opening of the IVC, providing the origin of the pectinate muscles.
- ❏ The **left horn** of sinus venosus forms the **coronary sinus** which opens into the **posterior wall** of right atrium.

- Superior vena cava and inferior vena cava develop from the **cardinal veins** and open into the right atrium.
- **Pulmonary veins** develop in the dorsal mesocardium and open into the **posterior wall of left atrium**.
- Coronary arteries and veins are considered as the **vasa-vasorum of heart**.

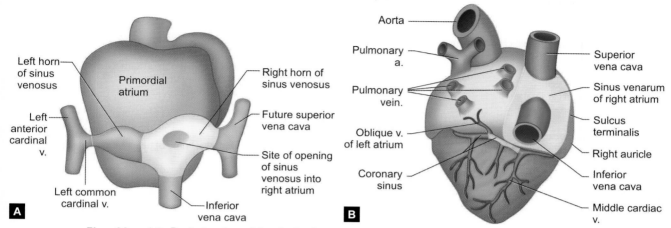

Figs. 6A and B: Posterior view of developing heart showing incorporation of sinus venosus into heart

The opening of **sinus venosus** into the primitive atrium is guarded by **Left and Right Venous Valves**.

- **Left** venous valve along with septum spurium gets **fused with the interatrial septum**.
- The **right** venous valve is greatly **stretched** out and becomes subdivided into **three parts** by formation of two muscular bands: the superior and inferior limbic bands.
- Three parts of right venous valves (from above to downward) form: (a) **crista terminals,** (b) valve of IVC (**Eustachian**), and (c) valve of coronary sinus **Thebesian**.

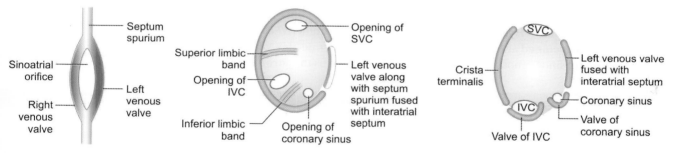

Fig. 7: Right and left venous valves and their derivatives

- Inferior vena cava opening is guarded by a rudimentary semilunar valve called **Eustachian** valve, which develops partly from right venous valve and partly from sinus septum.
- Opening of coronary sinus has an incomplete semi-circular valve called the **Thebesian** valve, which develops from the lower part of the right venous valve.

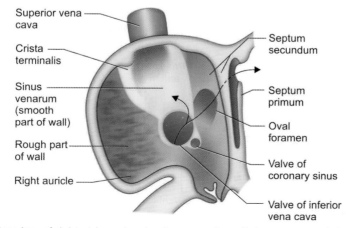

Fig. 8: Interior view of right atrium showing incorporation of sinus venosus into posterior wall

1. UNTRUE about cardiac jelly: *(AIIMS 2006)*
   a. Secreted by cardiac myocytes surrounding primitive heart tube
   b. Found exterior to endothelium
   c. Forms myocardium
   d. Transforms into the connective tissue of the endocardium

2. Heart begins to beat in the week:
   a. 4
   b. 5
   c. 6
   d. 7

3. Sinus venosus receives blood from all EXCEPT: *(NEET Pattern 2015)*
   a. Vitelline vein
   b. Umbilical vein
   c. Common cardinal vein
   d. Subcardinal vein

4. What is TRUE about sinus venosus: *(NEET Pattern 2012)*
   a. Forms rough wall of right atrium
   b. Forms smooth wall of right atrium
   c. Forms right coronary sinus
   d. Forms left leaflet of coronary sinus

1. c. Forms myocardium
   ❑ **Cardiac jelly** is secreted by the cardiac myocytes (**myocardium**) around the endothelial lining of heart tube and transforms into the **connective tissue of endocardium**.

2. a. 4
   ❑ Heart beat begins by **day 22 post-ovulation** and can be detected by Doppler ultrasound.
   ❑ It is week 4 post-ovulation (or fertilization) and week 6 from LMP (Last Menstrual Period).

3. d. Subcardinal vein
   ❑ Sinus venosus is the venous end of the heart tube having right and left horns.
   ❑ Each horn receives blood from following three pair of veins. **Vitelline** veins (from yolk sac), **Umbilical** veins (from placenta) and common **cardinal** veins (from body wall).

4. b. Forms smooth wall of right atrium
   ❑ **Sinus venosus** is a paired structure but shifts towards right associating only with the right atrium as the embryonic heart develops.
   ❑ The left portion shrinks in size and eventually forms the **coronary sinus** and oblique vein of the left atrium, whereas the right part becomes incorporated into the right atrium to form the **sinus venarum** (smooth part of right atrium).

❑ Heart tube is formed at day 22 (**week 4**) of development *(NEET Pattern 2016)*
❑ Heart tube is formed in **Hyaluronic acid** secreted by myocardium *(NEET Pattern 2016)*
❑ Heart is **fully developed** at 10th week (3rd month) of intrauterine life *(NEET Pattern 2013)*
❑ The **left horn** of sinus venosus undergoes regression and forms the **coronary sinus** *(NEET Pattern 2013)*

▼ Septa Formation

Heart divides into its four chambers by formation of its septum and valves.

❑ Four **main septa** involved in dividing the heart include the AV septum, the atrial septum, the IV septum and the AP septum.
❑ Septum formation in the heart in part arises from development of **endocardial cushion** tissue in that atrioventricular canal (**atrioventricular cushions**) and in the cono-truncal region (**cono-truncal swellings**).

AV Septum

❑ Four endocardial cushions surround the atrioventricular canal.
❑ The dorsal and ventral AV endocardial cushions fuse to form the AV septum, which divides the orifice into right and left atrioventricular canals.
❑ Cushion tissue then becomes fibrous and forms the **mitral** (bicuspid) valve on the left and the **tricuspid** valve on the right.

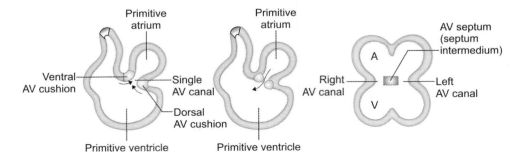

Fig. 9: Development of atrioventricular (AV) septum

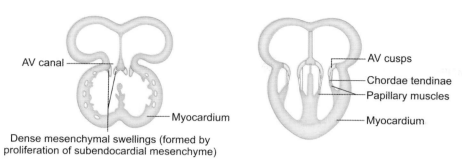

Fig. 10: Formation of atrioventricular valves

◤ Development of Atria and Interatrial Septum

Atrial development is dependent upon expansion of the original atrial region and incorporation of additional structures.

❑ On the right, the sinus venosus is incorporated and forms the **smooth-walled** portion of the right atrium, which is separated from the **trabeculated portion** by the **crista terminalis**.

❑ On the left, the **pulmonary vein,** which forms in the **dorsal mesocardium**, is positioned into the posterior wall of the left atrium when cells in the dorsal mesenchyme proliferate and accompany the septum primum as this structure grows toward the floor of the atrium.

❑ Later, the root of the **pulmonary vein** is incorporated into the left atrium by atrial expansion until the vein's **four branches** enter the atrium on its posterior wall. This portion constitutes the **smooth-walled** region of the left atrium.

Table 2: Adult components of right and left atria and their embryonic source of development	
Adult component	**Embryonic sources of development**
Right atrium	
▪ Rough trabeculated part (atrium proper) in front of crista terminalis	Primitive atrium (right half)
▪ Right auricle	
▪ Smooth part behind crista terminalis (sinus venarum)	Sinus venosus
▪ Crista terminalis valve of IVC and valve of coronary sinus	From right venous valve
▪ Most ventral smooth part	Right half of AV canal
Left atrium	
▪ Posterior smooth part between the openings of pulmonary veins	Absorption of pulmonary veins near the atria
▪ Anterior rough part and left auricle	Left half of primitive atrium
▪ Most ventral smooth part	Left half of the AV canal

Development of Interatrial Septum

In fetal circulation, the oxygenated blood from placenta (mother) enters the right atrium and flows **directly into the left atrium** bypassing the lungs. (**Lungs are non-functional** in fetal stage).

❑ The primitive atrium is divided first by a **septum primum**, which grows down from the superior wall to the **atrio-ventricular cushions**.

❑ The septum primum is a sickle-shaped crest descending from the roof of the atrium, begins to divide the atrium in two but leaves a lumen, the **ostium primum**, for communication between the two sides.

❑ Later, when the ostium primum is **obliterated** by fusion of the septum primum with the endocardial cushions, the **ostium secundum** is formed by cell death that creates an **opening in the septum primum**.

❑ **Rightward** of the septum primum, a second **septum secundum** membrane grows down from the ventral-cranial wall toward—but not reaching—the cushions, and covering most, but not all, of the ostium secundum, resulting in a **flap of the foramen ovale. Blood keep flowing from the right atrium to left continually.**

❑ **At birth**, when pressure in the left atrium increases, the two septa **press against each other** and close the communication between the two atria, completed at around 3 months after birth.

❑ As the septum primum and septum secundum get fused with each other, **foramen ovale** in septum secundum is apposed and **closed by septum primum**.

Formation of the atrial septum

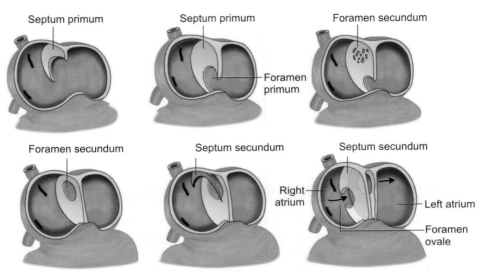

Fig. 11: Formation of the atrial septum. The arrows in 6 indicate the direction of blood flow from the right atrium to the left atrium across the fully developed atrial septum. Septum primum blue, septum secundum green

Fossa ovalis is an oval depression on the interatrial portion consisting of the valve of the fossa ovalis (a central sheet of thin fibrous tissue) on the floor, which is a **remnant of septum primum**.

❑ **Limbus fossa ovalis** is the prominent horseshoe-shaped **margin** of the fossa ovalis; it represents the edge of the **fetal septum secundum**.

Atrial Septal Defect (ASD): Shunts blood from the left atrium to the right atrium and causes hypertrophy of the right atrium, right ventricle, and pulmonary trunk, and thus mixing of oxygenated and deoxygenated blood, producing cyanosis. It is basically of two types:

❑ In **ostium primum** type ASD, blood keep flowing from left atrium into right atrium, through **foramen (ostium) primum**.
  ➤ If septum primum fails to fuse with endocardial cushions, the defect lies immediately above the atrioventricular (AV) boundary (may also be associated with a ventricular septal defect).
  ➤ It is **less common** than secundum ASD and is due to a **failure** of the septum primum to **fuse** with the endocardial cushions.

❑ **Ostium secundum** type ASD is the most common ASD.
  ➤ If septum secundum is too short to cover foramen secundum, it allows shunting of blood from left to right atrium, through **foramen (ostium) secundum**.
  ➤ It is caused by either an excessive resorption of the Septum primum (**large foramen secundum**) or an underdevelopment and reduced size of the Septum secundum (**large foramen ovale**).

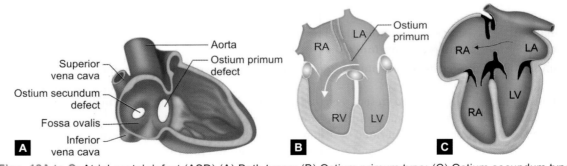

Figs. 12A to C: Atrial septal defect (ASD) (A) Both types; (B) Ostium primum type; (C) Ostium secundum type

Development of Pulmonary veins

Pulmonary vein forms in the **dorsal mesocardium** and is incorporated into the left atrium by atrial expansion until the vein's four branches enter the atrium on its posterior wall.

❑ This portion constitutes the **smooth-walled region of the left atrium**.

- Some authorities believe that the **pulmonary vein develops as an outgrowth of the dorsal atrial wall**, just to the left of the septum primum.

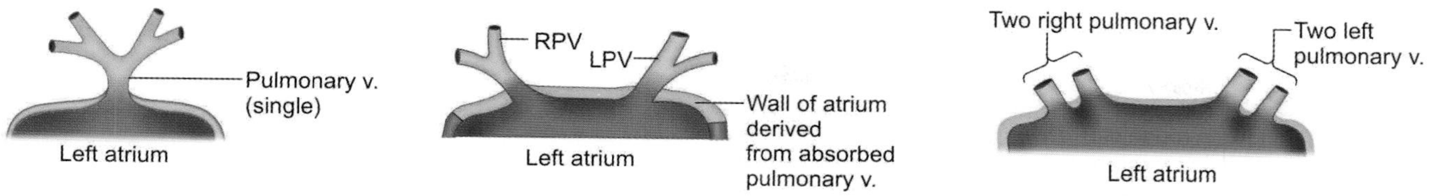

Fig. 13: Absorption of pulmonary veins into the left atrium. RPV = right pulmonary vein; LPV = left pulmonary vein.

QUESTIONS

1. **NOT true about right atrium:** *(NEET Pattern 2015)*
   a. Posterior part is smooth
   b. Anterior part is derived from absorption of right horn of sinus venosus
   c. Fossa ovalis represent remnant of foramen ovale
   d. Anterior and posterior parts are divided by crista terminalis

2. **Septum secundum arises from:** *(NEET Pattern 2016)*
   a. Bulbus cordis
   b. Primitive ventricle
   c. Primitive atrium
   d. Sinus venosus

3. **Fossa ovalis is a remnant of:** *(NEET Pattern 2012)*
   a. Septum primum
   b. Septum secundum
   c. Ductus arteriosus
   d. Ductus venosus

4. **FALSE about limbus fossa ovalis:** *(NEET Pattern 2016)*
   a. Derived from septum primum
   b. Seen in right atrium
   c. Situated above fossa ovalis
   d. Also called Annulus ovalis

5. **Limbus fossa ovalis and floor of fossa ovalis represents:**
   a. Septum Primum
   b. Septum secundum
   c. Septum primum and septum secundum
   d. Septum secundum and septum primum

6. **Pulmonary veins develop from:**
   a. Sixth aortic arch
   b. Primitive left atrium
   c. Left common cardinal vein
   d. Left vitelline vein

ANSWERS

1. **b. Anterior part is derived from absorption of right horn of sinus venosus**
   - **Right horn** of sinus venosus contributes to **sinus venarum** (posterior smooth part of right atrium).
   - Anterior part of right atrium is **rough** (derived from the **primitive atrium**).

2. **c. Primitive atrium**
   - Septum secundum grows down from the **roof of the common atrium** toward the atrioventricular endocardial cushions.

3. **a. Septum primum**
   - Fossa ovalis is an oval depression on the interatrial portion consisting of the **valve of the fossa ovalis** (a central sheet of thin fibrous tissue) which is a remnant of septum primum, and the **limbus of the fossa ovalis** (a horseshoe-shaped muscular rim), which is a remnant of the septum secundum.

4. **a. Derived from septum primum**
   - Limbus (annulus) fossa ovalis is a horseshoe-shaped muscular **rim**, situated above fossa ovalis. It is a **remnant of the septum secundum**.

5. **d. Septum secundum and septum primum**
   - **Limbus** fossa ovalis is the margin of foramen ovale (present in **septum secundum**).
   - As viewed from right atrium, the **floor** of fossa ovalis is formed by **septum primum**.

6. **b. Primitive left atrium**
   - According to some authorities, pulmonary veins develop from the **left atrial wall**.
   - There is **no consensus** about whether the pulmonary vein as a branch from the left atrium obtains a connection to the lung plexus or the pulmonary vein forms as a solitary vessel in the dorsal mesocardium and is only secondarily incorporated into the atrium.

- **Foramen ovale closes** because of fusion of Septum primum + Septum secundum *(NEET Pattern 2012)*

Development of Ventricles and Interventricular Septum

The interventricular (IV) septum consists of **three parts** (superior to inferior): (a) Bulbar, (b) Membranous, (c) Muscular part

- **Bulbar part** develops from right and left **bulbar ridges.** (Some authors use the term **conus swelling** for bulbar ridges.)
- **Membranous IV septum** forms by (1) inferior endocardial atrioventricular cushion, (2) right bulbar ridge, and (3) left bulbar ridge.
- **Muscular IV septum** develops as outgrowth of **muscular wall in the floor** of the primitive ventricle and **grows toward the AV septum** but stops to create the IV foramen, leaving the septum incomplete.
- The membranous IV septum closes the IV foramen, **completing** partition of the ventricles.

Table 3: Adult components of right and left ventricles and their embryonic source of development	
Adult component	Embryonic source of development
Right ventricle	
▪ Inflowing rough part	Primitive ventricle
▪ Out flowing smooth part (infundibulum)	Bulbus cordis
Left ventricle	
▪ Inflowing rough part	Primitive ventricle
▪ Outflowing smooth part (aortic vestibule)	Bulbus cordis

❏ If the three components fail to fuse, it may result in an **open interventricular foramen** (VSD).
❏ It occurs commonly in the membranous part of the IV septum, resulting in **left-to-right shunting** of blood through the IV foramen, which increases blood flow to the lungs and causes **pulmonary hypertension** and **congestive heart failure**.

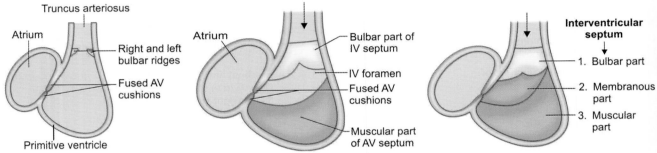

Fig. 14: Formation of interventricular septum.

▶ AP Septum and Anomalies

Partition of the Truncus Arteriosus and Bulbus Cordis

❏ The truncal ridges and the bulbar ridges (derived from **neural crest mesenchyme**) grow in a **spiral fashion** and fuse to form the AP septum.
❏ The **truncus arteriosus** region is divided by the **spiral aorticopulmonary septum** into the proximal segments of the **aorta** and **pulmonary artery**. The resultant vessels also spiral each other.
❏ The bulbus is divided into the smooth-walled portion of the right ventricle and the conus and truncus arteriosus.

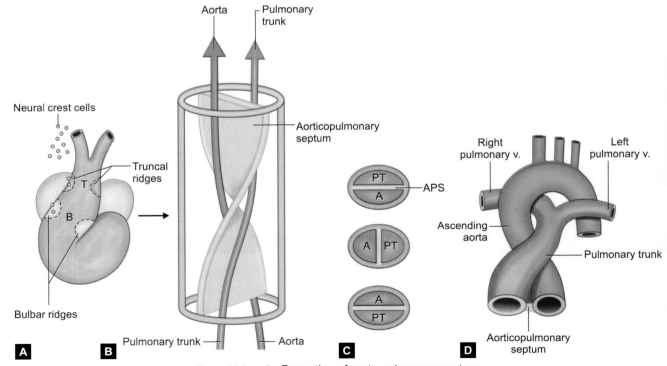

Figs. 15A to D: Formation of aorta-pulmonary septum.

AP septum anomalies may result from abnormal division of the cono-truncal region.

❑ AP septum anomalies like PTA, TGV and TOF present with **right to left shunt**, blood reaches systemic circulation without proper oxygenation, hence leading to **cyanosis**.

Persistent truncus arteriosus (PTA)

❑ **Failure** of cono-truncal ridge to **fuse and descend** towards the ventricles result in absence of AP septum – Persistent truncus arteriosus.

❑ There is **absence** of **ascending aorta** and **pulmonary trunk**, and the primitive truncus arteriosus is present with **mixing** of blood, resulting in **cyanosis**.

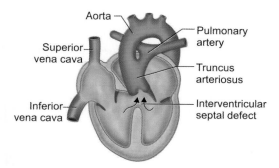

Fig. 16: Persistent truncus arteriosus (PTA)

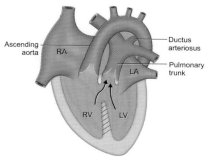

Fig. 17: Transposition of great vessels (TGV)

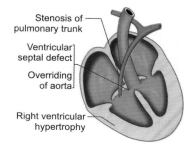

Fig. 18: Tetralogy of Fallot (TOF)

Transposition of great vessels (TGV)

❑ If the **AP septum is not spiral**, the great **vessels are not spiral,** and they **open in the opposite** ventricles (transposition of great vessels).

❑ The aorta arises from the right ventricle, and the pulmonary artery emerges leftward and posteriorly from the LV (two separate parallel circulations).

❑ This results in **right-to-left shunting** of blood and **cyanosis** and some communication between them must exist after birth to sustain life.

❑ Most patients have an interatrial communication, two-thirds have a **patent ductus arteriosus**, and about one-third have an associated VSD.

Tetralogy of fallot (TOF)

❑ It occurs when the AP septum fails to align properly (migrates anteriorly) with the AV septum, resulting in (1) **pulmonary stenosis** (obstruction to right ventricular outflow), (2) **VSD**, (3) **overriding aorta** (dextraposition of aorta), and (4) **right ventricular hypertrophy**.

❑ It is characterized by **right-to-left shunting** of blood and **cyanosis**.

❑ **Overriding aorta** (dextraposition of aorta) is that the aorta (its outlet) lies over both ventricles (instead of over the left ventricle), directly above the VSD, causing the **aorta to arise from both ventricles**.

1. **Transposition of great vessels occurs due to:**
   a. Failure of cono-truncal ridge to fuse and descend towards the ventricles
   b. Anterior displacement of aortico-pulmonary septum
   c. Aortico-pulmonary septum not following its spiral course
   d. Migration of neural crest cells towards truncal and bulbar ridges

2. **All are essential components of tetralogy of Fallot EXCEPT:**
   (AIIMS 2007)
   a. Valvular pulmonic stenosis
   b. Right ventricular hypertrophy
   c. Infundibular stenosis
   d. Aorta overriding

3. **Cardiac defects causing right to left shunt, leading to early cyanosis are all EXCEPT:**
   a. Transposition of great vessels
   b. Tetralogy of Fallot
   c. Patent ductus arteriosus
   d. Persistent truncus arteriosus

4. **Pentalogy of Fallot is characterized by:**
   (AIIMS)
   a. Ventricular septal defect
   b. Patent ductus arteriosus
   c. Atrial septal defect
   d. Pulmonary stenosis

1. **c. Aortico-pulmonary septum not following its spiral course**
   - ❑ If the AP septum is **not spiral**, the great vessels are not spiral, and they open in the opposite ventricles (transposition of great vessels).
   - ❑ The **aorta arises from the right ventricle**, and the pulmonary artery emerges leftward and posteriorly from the LV (two separate parallel circulations).

2. **a. Valvular pulmonic stenosis**
   - ❑ In tetralogy of Fallot **infundibular stenosis** occurs due to anterior deviation of the infundibular septum causing hypoplasia of the sub-pulmonary infundibulum, leading to narrowing of RVOT (Right Ventricular Outflow Tract).

3. **c. Patent ductus arteriosus**
   - ❑ Patent ductus arteriosus carries the blood towards the lungs and promotes oxygenation thus, **reduces cyanosis**.
   - ❑ AP septum anomalies like PTA, TGV and TOF present with **right to left shunt**, blood reaches systemic circulation without proper oxygenation, hence leading to **cyanosis**.

4. **c. Atrial septal defect > b. Patent ductus arteriosus**
   - ❑ The pentalogy of Fallot is a variant of the more common tetralogy of Fallot, comprising the **classical four features with** the addition of an atrial septal defect/patent foramen ovale or patent ductus arteriosus.

- ▪ **Absence** of Aorta Pulmonary (AP) septum (also called cono-truncal septum) leads to **persistent (patent) truncus arteriosus**.
- ▪ **Unequal division of the conus cordis** resulting from **anterior displacement** of the cono-truncal septum gives rise to a narrow pulmonary trunk-**pulmonic stenosis** and a wide aorta. This leads to the complex of **tetralogy of Fallot**. *(AIIMS 2003)*

◢ Foetal Circulation

❑ Oxygenated and nutrient-enriched blood returns to the fetus from the placenta via the **left umbilical vein**.

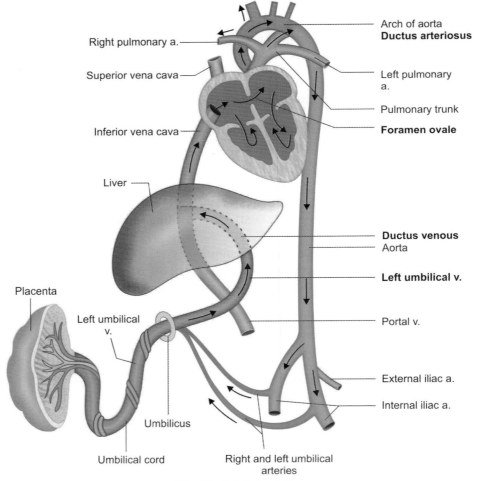

Fig. 19: Fetal circulation

❑ Most of the blood **bypasses** the liver sinusoids by passing through the **ductus venosus** and enters the inferior vena cava (IVC).

❑ From the IVC, blood enters the right atrium, where most of the blood **bypasses** the right ventricle (and hence **lung**) through the **foramen ovale** to enter the left atrium. From the left atrium, blood enters the **left ventricle** and is delivered to fetal tissues via the **aorta**.

❑ Deoxygenated fetal blood is sent back to the placenta via **right and left umbilical arteries** (branches of internal iliac arteries).

❑ Some blood in the right atrium enters the right ventricle; blood in the right ventricle enters the pulmonary trunk, but most of the blood **bypasses the lungs** through the **ductus arteriosus**.

❑ **At birth**, when the baby breathes, the left atrial pressure rises, pushing the septum primum against the septum secundum and **closing the foramen ovale**. Blood flow through the pulmonary artery increases and becomes poorly oxygenated as it now receives systemic venous blood. Pulmonary vascular resistance is abruptly lowered as **lungs inflate** and the **ductus arteriosus is obliterated** over the next few hours to days.

❑ Changes include **closure** of the **right and left umbilical arteries**, left umbilical vein, ductus venosus, ductus arteriosus, and **foramen ovale**.

❑ At removal of placenta, ligation of the umbilical cord causes thrombosis of the umbilical arteries (becomes **medial umbilical ligaments**), vein (becomes **ligamentum teres**) and ductus venosus (becomes **ligamentum venosum**). These embryological remnants raise corresponding peritoneal folds on the **anterior abdominal wall**.

Peritoneal folds on the anterior abdominal wall:

❑ **Falcform ligament** contains **ligamentum teres** (adult remnant of left umbilical vein) towards liver.

❑ **Medial umbilical fold is raised by Medial umbilical ligament** (adult remnant of distal umbilical arteries).

❑ **Median umbilical fold** is raised by urachus (adult remnant of allantois).

❑ **Lateral umbilical fold** is raised by inferior epigastric vessels.

❑ **Note: Proximal portion** of **umbilical artery** persists in adults as superior vesical arteries.

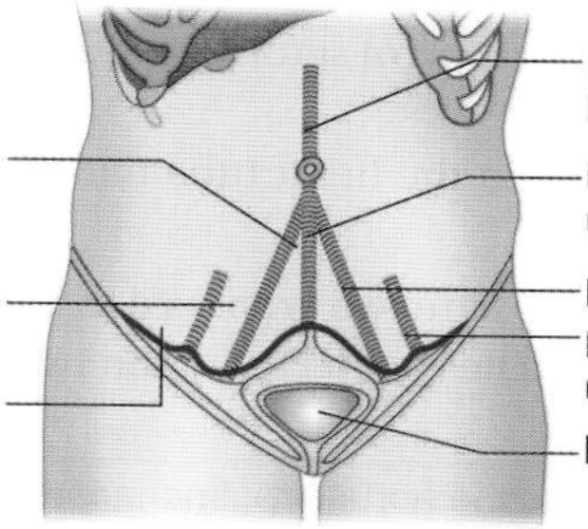

Fig. 20: Peritoneal folds on the anterior abdominal wall

❑ **Physiological closure** of ductus arteriosus occurs within 1–4 days of birth. Often a small shunt of blood stays for 24–48 hours in a normal full-term infant. At the end of 24 hours (one day), 20% ducts are functionally close, 82% by 48 hours and 100% at 96 hours (4 days).

❑ **Anatomical closure** of ductus arteriosus occurs within 2–12 postnatal weeks (1 month to 3 months). DA is closed by 8 weeks in 88% of children with a normal cardiovascular system. Anatomical closure involves **tunica intima** proliferation and fibrosis.

Note: Authorities consider the patent ductus to be abnormal **only after 3 months** (12 weeks) of age.

QUESTIONS

1. **Anatomical closure of ductus arteriosus occurs at:**
   a. Birth   b. 3–4 days
   c. 10 days   d. 30 days

2. **Anatomical closure of ductus arteriosus occurs at:**
   a. 2 weeks   b. 4 weeks
   c. 12 weeks   d. 16 weeks

3. **Ductus venosus connects:**   (NEET Pattern 2012)
   a. Pulmonary trunk and descending aorta
   b. Right atrium and left atrium
   c. Portal vein and IVC
   d. Pulmonary trunk and ascending aorta

ANSWERS

1. **d. 30 days**
   ❑ **Anatomical closure** of ductus arteriosus occurs within **2–12 postnatal weeks** (1 month to 3 months).
   ❑ DA is closed by 8 weeks in 88% of children with a normal cardiovascular system.
   ❑ Authorities consider the patent ductus to be **abnormal only after 3 months** (12 weeks) of age.

2. **c. 12 weeks**
   ❑ Anatomical closure of ductus arteriosus occurs within 2–12 postnatal weeks (1 month to 3 months). Maximum: 12 weeks, beyond that its pathology.

3. **c. Portal vein and IVC**
   ❑ In fetal circulation, ductus venosus shunts a portion of the left umbilical vein blood flow directly to the inferior vena cava.
   ❑ It allows oxygenated blood from the placenta to bypass the liver.
   ❑ The only related option appears to be choice c.

- Remnant of umbilical artery is **medial umbilical ligament** *(NEET Pattern 2016)*
- **Ligamentum teres** is the adult remnant of left umbilical vein *(NEET Pattern 2016)*
- Lateral umbilical fold of peritoneum is produced by **Inferior epigastric vessels** *(NEET Pattern 2016)*
- **Median** umbilical ligament is derived from **urachus** *(NEET Pattern 2013)*

▶ Development of Pericardium and Sinuses

- ❑ The pericardial cavity is derived from the part of **intraembryonic coelom**. The heart tube invaginates the pericardial cavity from the dorsal aspect and is suspended within the pericardial cavity by a double-layered fold of the layer of the pericardial cavity called **dorsal mesocardium.**

- ❑ **Visceral layer** of serous pericardium is derived from **splanchnopleuric mesoderm**, whereas **parietal** layer of serous pericardium (and fibrous pericardium) is derived from **somatopleuric** mesoderm.

- ❑ With the folding (looping) of the heart tube, the **arterial and venous ends come close**. The **dorsal mesogastrium disappears** to form **transverse sinus** of pericardium.

- ❑ Later the parietal and visceral layers of serous pericardium become continuous with each other at the arterial and venous ends of the heart tube, i.e. serous pericardium gets arranged into **two tubes: arterial** - the one enclosing the aorta and pulmonary trunk, and **venous**: the other enclosing the superior vena cava, inferior vena cava, and four pulmonary veins.

- ❑ The two tubes are separated by the **transverse sinus** of pericardium.

- ❑ The definitive reflections of the pericardium in accordance with the rearrangement of SVC, IVC, and pulmonary veins at the venous end lead to the formation of an isolated pouch of pericardium called **oblique sinus** of the pericardium.

- ❑ Oblique sinus is a recess of serous pericardium that passes **upward behind the left atrium** and between the left and right pulmonary veins.

  As mentioned, when the heart tube folds, a space develops between arterial and venous end—**transverse pericardial sinus**.

- ❑ Anterior to the sinus are two arteries derived from truncus arteriosus: **ascending aorta** and **pulmonary trunk**.

- ❑ Superior vena cava lies **posterior** to the sinus and bifurcation of pulmonary trunk is superior to it.

Note: During surgery on the aorta or pulmonary artery, a **surgeon can pass a finger** and make a ligature through the transverse sinus between the arteries and veins, thus stopping the blood circulation with the ligature.

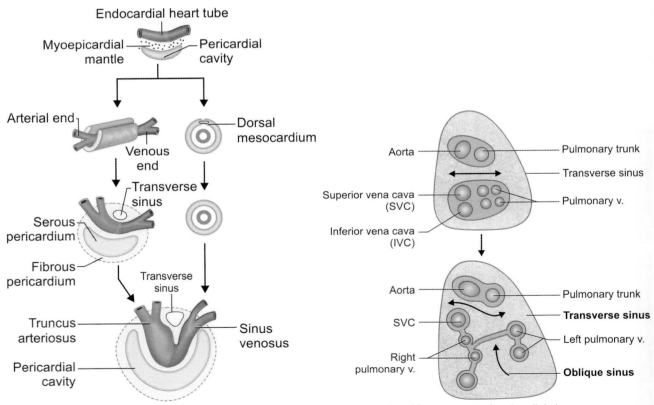

Fig. 21: Formation of pericardial cavity and sinuses.   Fig. 22: Formation of pericardial sinuses

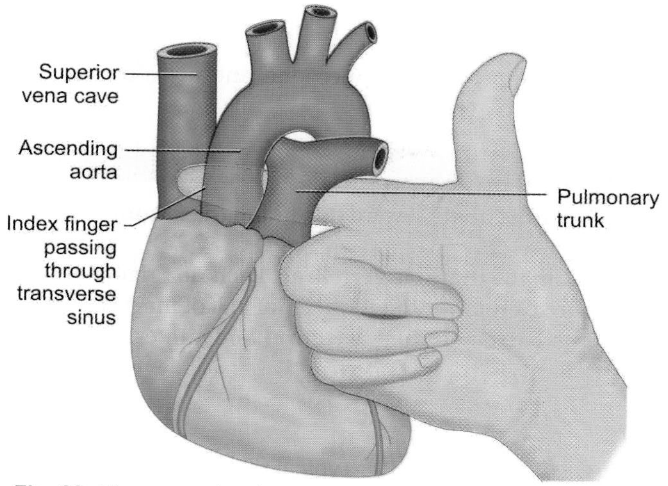

Superior vena cave

Ascending aorta

Index finger passing through transverse sinus

Pulmonary trunk

Fig. 23: Finger passing through the transverse pericardial sinus.

1. The structure present anterior to transverse pericardial sinus is: *(NEET Pattern 2012)*
   a. Inferior vena cava   b. Superior vena cava
   c. Aorta   d. Pulmonary artery

2. Posterior to transverse pericardial sinus is: *(NEET Pattern 2015)*
   a. Aorta   b. Pulmonary trunk
   c. SVC   d. Left atrium

1. c. Aorta
   ❑ As the heart tube folds, a space develops between **arterial** and **venous** end – transverse pericardial sinus.
   ❑ **Anterior** to the sinus are two arteries derived from truncus arteriosus: **ascending aorta** and **pulmonary trunk** (and not pulmonary artery).
   ❑ A finger can be put into the sinus to pull the two major arteries and a ligature put around, during cardiothoracic surgeries.
   ❑ Superior vena cava lies **posterior** to the sinus and bifurcation of pulmonary trunk is superior to it.

2. c. SVC
   ❑ Transverse pericardial sinus lies between the aorta and pulmonary trunk **anteriorly** and the superior vena cava **posteriorly**.

▪ Transverse pericardial sinus lies between arterial and venous tubes *(NEET Pattern 2016)*

◤ Development of Respiratory System

❑ A laryngotracheal groove appears in the floor of the pharynx (**ventral wall of foregut**), which evaginates to form the laryngotracheal (**respiratory**) **diverticulum**.

❑ A tracheoesophageal **septum** divides the foregut into a **ventral** portion, the laryngotracheal tube and a dorsal portion (primordium of the oropharynx and esophagus).

❑ The ventral portion forms the **larynx, trachea**, and **lung** buds.

❑ The **lung buds** are invested by **splanchnopleuric mesenchyme** derived from the medial walls of the pericardioperitoneal canals, whereas the lateral walls produce **somatopleuric mesenchyme**, which contributes to the body wall.

❑ **Epithelium and glands** in the respiratory tube are derived from the **endoderm of foregut**.

❑ Smooth muscles, connective tissue and visceral pleura are derived from **visceral** (splanchnic) **lateral plate mesoderm**.

❑ **Parietal** pleura is derived from **somatic** lateral plate mesoderm.

Tracheoesophageal fistula: Faulty partitioning of the foregut by the tracheoesophageal septum causes esophageal atresias and tracheoesophageal fistulas.

❑ **Development of lungs:** After a **pseudoglandular** (5 to 17 weeks) and **canalicular** (13 to 25 weeks) phase, cells of the cuboidal-lined respiratory bronchioles change into thin, flat **cells, type I alveolar** epithelial cells, intimately associated with blood and lymph capillaries.

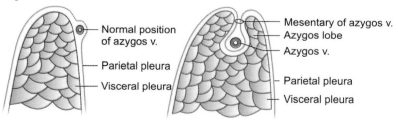

Normal position of azygos v.

Parietal pleura

Visceral pleura

Mesentery of azygos v.

Azygos lobe

Azygos v.

Parietal pleura

Visceral pleura

Fig. 24: Azygos lobe of the lung.

❑ **Azygos lobe of lung:** The **azygos vein** may sometimes course in a more lateral position, within a four-layered pleural septum within the superior lobe, creating an 'azygos lobe'.
❑ Azygos lobe is an anatomically separated part of the upper lobe, and **not a true or accessory lobe** of lung, as it has no bronchi, veins and arteries of its own.

▶ Ribs

❑ Development: Ossification begins **near the angle** toward the **end of the second month** of fetal life and is seen **first in the sixth and seventh** ribs.
❑ Ribs usually develop in association with the **thoracic vertebrae**. Each rib originates from lateral **sclerotome** populations, and forms from the **caudal** half of one sclerotome and the **cranial** half of the next subjacent sclerotome.
❑ The **head** of a rib articulates with the **corresponding vertebral body**, intervertebral disc and **higher** (upper) vertebral body.

Types of ribs

❑ **Typical ribs**: 3–9 and **Atypical ribs**: 1, 2, 10, (11 and 12). Typical ribs have same general features, whereas the atypical ribs have special features.
❑ **True ribs**: 1–7 (i.e. upper 7 ribs) and **False ribs**: 8–12 (i.e. lower 5 ribs)
    Note: True ribs articulate with the sternum anteriorly, whereas **false ribs do not articulate with the sternum** anteriorly. False ribs articulate with more superior costal cartilage and form the anterior **costal margin**.
❑ **Vertebro-sternal** ribs: 1–7. These ribs articulate posteriorly with **vertebrae** and anteriorly with the **sternum**.
❑ **Vertebro-chondral** ribs: 8–10. These ribs articulate posteriorly with vertebrae and anteriorly their cartilages join the cartilage of the higher (upper) rib.
❑ **Vertebral** (floating) ribs: 11 and 12 (articulate with vertebral bodies but **do not articulate with the sternum**)
    Note: The first 7 'true' ribs attach to the sternum by costal cartilages, whereas, the remaining lower 5 'false' ribs either join the respective costal cartilage (8–10) or 'float' free at their anterior ends (11–12).

Joints

❑ Sternochondral (called as Sternocostal) joints are the articulation of the sternum with the **first seven** cartilages.
❑ Costal cartilage of **first rib** attaches to manubrium sternii by a plate of fibrocartilage and hence it is **not a typical** primary cartilagenous (**synchondrosis**) joint. It does not permit any movement.
❑ Second to seventh costal cartilages form **plane synovial** joints with the sternum and are **freely mobile**.

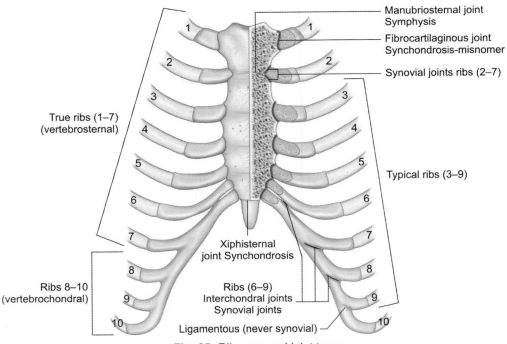

Fig. 25: Rib cage and joint types

- First rib attachment to sternum (first sterno-costal joint) is an unusual variety of **synarthrosis** and is often **inaccurately** called a primary cartilaginous (**synchondrosis**) joint.
- Ribs 2–7 attach with the **sternum** by **synovial** joints
- Ribs 6–9 attach with **each other** by **synovial** joints (Interchondral joints). At some points, there are **fibrous** attachments as well.
- 8, 9 and 10th ribs are attached to 7th rib by **synovial** joint.
- **Manubriosternal** joint is **symphysis** (secondary cartilaginous) joint.

   Xiphisternal joint is a primary cartilaginous (**synchondrosis**) joint. Some authors mention it as symphysis.

Note: The joints between anterior end of rib and costal cartilage (**costo-chondral** joint) are primary cartilagenous (**synchondrosis**) joints. They do **not permit** any movement.

- First rib is the **broadest and shortest** of the true ribs. It has two **grooves** for the subclavian artery and vein.

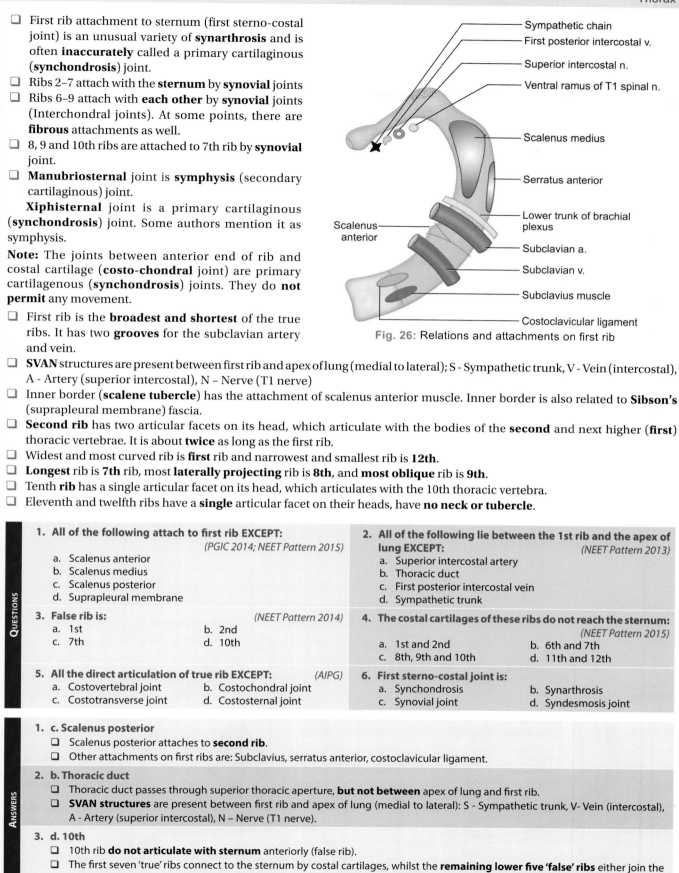

Fig. 26: Relations and attachments on first rib

- **SVAN** structures are present between first rib and apex of lung (medial to lateral); S - Sympathetic trunk, V - Vein (intercostal), A - Artery (superior intercostal), N – Nerve (T1 nerve)
- Inner border (**scalene tubercle**) has the attachment of scalenus anterior muscle. Inner border is also related to **Sibson's** (suprapleural membrane) fascia.
- **Second rib** has two articular facets on its head, which articulate with the bodies of the **second** and next higher (**first**) thoracic vertebrae. It is about **twice** as long as the first rib.
- Widest and most curved rib is **first** rib and narrowest and smallest rib is **12th**.
- **Longest** rib is **7th** rib, most **laterally projecting** rib is **8th**, and **most oblique** rib is **9th**.
- Tenth **rib** has a single articular facet on its head, which articulates with the 10th thoracic vertebra.
- Eleventh and twelfth ribs have a **single** articular facet on their heads, have **no neck or tubercle**.

QUESTIONS

1. All of the following attach to first rib EXCEPT:
   (PGIC 2014; NEET Pattern 2015)
   a. Scalenus anterior
   b. Scalenus medius
   c. Scalenus posterior
   d. Suprapleural membrane

2. All of the following lie between the 1st rib and the apex of lung EXCEPT: *(NEET Pattern 2013)*
   a. Superior intercostal artery
   b. Thoracic duct
   c. First posterior intercostal vein
   d. Sympathetic trunk

3. False rib is: *(NEET Pattern 2014)*
   a. 1st   b. 2nd
   c. 7th   d. 10th

4. The costal cartilages of these ribs do not reach the sternum: *(NEET Pattern 2015)*
   a. 1st and 2nd   b. 6th and 7th
   c. 8th, 9th and 10th   d. 11th and 12th

5. All the direct articulation of true rib EXCEPT: *(AIPG)*
   a. Costovertebral joint   b. Costochondral joint
   c. Costotransverse joint   d. Costosternal joint

6. First sterno-costal joint is:
   a. Synchondrosis   b. Synarthrosis
   c. Synovial joint   d. Syndesmosis joint

ANSWERS

1. **c. Scalenus posterior**
   - Scalenus posterior attaches to **second rib**.
   - Other attachments on first ribs are: Subclavius, serratus anterior, costoclavicular ligament.

2. **b. Thoracic duct**
   - Thoracic duct passes through superior thoracic aperture, **but not between** apex of lung and first rib.
   - **SVAN structures** are present between first rib and apex of lung (medial to lateral): S - Sympathetic trunk, V- Vein (intercostal), A - Artery (superior intercostal), N – Nerve (T1 nerve).

3. **d. 10th**
   - 10th rib **do not articulate with sternum** anteriorly (false rib).
   - The first seven 'true' ribs connect to the sternum by costal cartilages, whilst the **remaining lower five 'false' ribs** either join the suprajacent (upper) costal cartilage (8–10) or 'float' free at their anterior ends as relatively small and delicate structures tipped with cartilage.

4. c. 8th, 9th and 10th > d. 11th and 12th
- ❑ Ribs 8 - 10 are **vertebro-chondral** with no direct articulation to sternum.
- ❑ Their costal cartilages articulate with each other and with 7th costal cartilage.
- ❑ Ribs 11 and 12 have free anterior ends (**floating ribs**) and definitely they are never going to reach the sternum., but this statement is never mentioned in textbooks.

5. d. Costosternal joint
- ❑ Ribs directly articulate with vertebral body by costovertebral joint, with transverse process by costotransverse joint and with costal cartilage by costochondral joint.
- ❑ It is the **costal cartilage** which attaches the ribs to the sternum, hence the costosternal joint is a **misnomer**, and correctly should be mentioned as chondrosternal joint.

6. b. Synarthrosis > a. Synchondrosis
- ❑ The first sterno-costal joint is an unusual variety of **synarthrosis** (fibrous) and is often **inaccurately** called a 1° cartilaginous (**synchondrosis**).

- ▪ **Ossification of ribs begins** toward the end of the second month of fetal life (**8–10 weeks**) (*NEET Pattern 2016*)
- ▪ **Scalene tubercle** is a feature of 1st rib (*NEET Pattern 2015*)
- ▪ 8, 9 and 10th ribs are attached to 7th rib by **synovial** joint (*NEET Pattern 2014*)
- ▪ 8th rib do not articulate with sternum and is a vertebrocondral rib, as it attaches to the costal cartilage of the next higher rib anteriorly (*NEET Pattern 2014*)
- ▪ All **costochondral** joints are 1° cartilaginous (**synchondrosis**) joints (*AIPG 2004*)
- ▪ 10th rib is **false rib**, since it does not attach to the sternum (*NEET Pattern 2013*)

▶ Nervous Supply of Thorax

Thoracic spinal nerves

- ❑ There are **twelve pairs** of thoracic spinal nerves, contributing to **intercostal nerves**. They supply muscles in and skin over **intercostal space.**; lower nerves supply muscles and skin of **anterolateral abdominal wall**.
- ❑ **Intercostal nerves** are the anterior (**ventral**) primary rami of the first 11 thoracic spinal nerves. 12th is the **subcostal nerve**, which arises from ventral ramus of T12.
- ❑ These nerves run **between** the internal and innermost layers of muscles, with the intercostal veins and arteries.
- ❑ They are lodged in the **costal grooves** on the inferior surface of the ribs and give **muscular** branches and lateral and anterior **cutaneous** branches.
- ❑ **Typical** intercostal nerves are 3rd, 4th, 5th, and 6th. They remain **confined** to their own intercostal spaces.
- ❑ **Atypical** intercostal nerves are 1st, 2nd, 7th, 8th, 9th, 10th and 11th. They **extend beyond** the thoracic wall and partly or entirely supply the other regions.

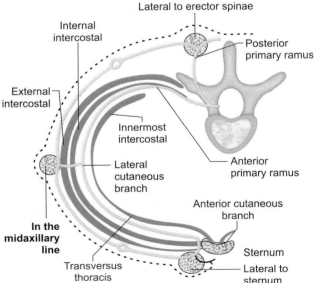

Fig. 27: Transverse view of thoracic region showing spinal nerve and intercostal nerve

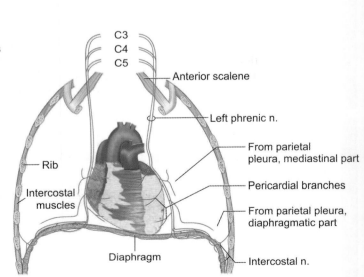

Fig. 28: Phrenic nerve: origin, course and supply.

❏ T1-T2: Also supply **upper limb** via brachial plexus (T1) and intercostabrachial nerve (T2).

❏ T7-T11: Also supply **abdominal wall.**

❏ T12: Also supplies abdominal wall and skin of **buttock.**

Intercostobrachial nerve is the lateral cutaneous branch of the **2nd intercostal nerve**. It supplies the skin of the floor of axilla and upper part of the medial aspect of arm.

❏ It is often the source of **referred cardiac pain.**

❏ It may sometime get damaged in **axillary node clearance** (ANC), such as that done for breast cancer surgery.

Subcostal nerve (T-12) arises from **ventral ramus of T12.** It follows **inferior border** of 12th rib and passes into abdominal wall. It is distributed to the **abdominal wall** and the **gluteal skin.**

Phrenic nerve takes origin from the anterior primary rami of C3-C5 (chiefly C4) carries motor, sensory, and sympathetic fibers.

❏ It descends on the **anterior surface** of the scalene anterior muscle under cover of the sterno-cleido-mastoid muscle, at the root of the neck and enters the thorax, where it is **joined b**y the pericardio-phrenic artery.

❏ It then passes **anterior to the root** of the lung (hilum) **lying between** the mediastinal pleura and fibrous pericardium and supplying them.

❏ Right phrenic nerve is **shorter** and **more vertical**, left is longer and has a more oblique course.

❏ **Right dome** of diaphragm is at **higher** level (pushed up by liver) and the **left dome** of diaphragm is **lower** (pushed down by heart).

❏ It is the **sole motor supply** to diaphragm.

❏ It carries sensation from the central portion of **diaphragm, peritoneum, pleura** and **pericardium** along the course

❏ The pain of **pericarditis** originates in the parietal layer only and is transmitted by the **phrenic nerve.**

❏ The fibrous and parietal layer of serous pericardium are supplied by the phrenic nerve, **visceral** layer is **insensitive to stretch.**

QUESTIONS

1. **TRUE about left phrenic nerve is:** *(AIIMS)*
   a. Arise from dorsal rami of C3, 4, 5
   b. Descends in the left pleural space
   c. Supplies mediastinal and diaphragmatic pleura on left side and diaphragmatic peritoneum
   d. Passes through the vena caval opening in the diaphragm

2. **All are true about intercostal nerves EXCEPT:**
   a. The relationship from above downward is nerve, vein, artery
   b. T4, T5, T6 are called typical intercostal nerve
   c. Lie between the innermost intercostal and internal intercostal muscle
   d. T7 to T11 supply the abdominal wall

3. **Subcostal nerve is:** *(NEET Pattern 2016)*
   a. Dorsal ramus of T6
   b. Ventral ramus of T6
   c. Dorsal ramus of T12
   d. Ventral ramus of T12

4. **All of the following are true about phrenic nerve EXCEPT**
   a. It is a purely motor nerve
   b. It arises mainly from C4 spinal nerve
   c. It is formed at the lateral order of scalenus anterior
   d. Accessory phrenic nerve is commonly a branch from the nerve to subclavius

ANSWERS

1. **c. Supplies mediastinal and diaphragmatic pleura on left side and diaphragmatic peritoneum**
   ❏ Phrenic nerve arises from the anterior (**ventral**) primary rami of C-2, 3, 4, descends lying between the mediastinal pleura and fibrous pericardium.
   ❏ It provides motor supply to diaphragm and carries sensations from central portion of the diaphragm.
   ❏ Additionally, it also carries sensations from mediastinal pleura, pericardium and peritoneum.

2. **a. The relationship from above downward is nerve, vein, artery**
   ❏ The relationship from above downward is vein, artery, nerve.

3. **d. Ventral ramus of T12**
   ❏ Subcostal nerve is **ventral ramus** of T12

4. **a. It is a purely motor nerve**
   ❏ Phrenic nerve is a **mixed** (sensory motor nerve).

▪ **Intercostal nerve** is a branch of **ventral rami** of thoracic spinal nerves *(NEET Pattern 2015)*

▪ **Intercostobrachial nerve** is a branch of 2nd intercostal nerve *(JIPMER 2002)*

▪ Intercostal nerve 2 is **atypical** nerve, since it innervates **upper limb** (by contributing to intercosto-brachial nerve) *(NEET Pattern 2013)*

▪ Left phrenic nerve runs **anterior to scalenus anterior** *(AIIMS 2009)*

▪ Pain of **pericarditis** is carried by **phrenic** nerve *(AIIMS 2007)*

▪ Phrenic nerve supplies **peritoneum under diaphragm** *(NEET Pattern 2016)*

▼ **Arterial Supply in Thorax**

☐ **Internal Thoracic Artery** arises from the **first part** of the subclavian artery and descends directly behind the **first six** costal cartilages, just **lateral to the sternum**.

➤ It gives **two anterior intercostal** arteries in each of the **upper six** intercostal spaces and **terminates at the sixth** intercostal space by dividing into the **musculophrenic** and **superior epigastric** arteries.

➤ **Pericardiophrenic artery** is a branch of internal thoracic artery, which accompanies the **phrenic nerve** between the pleura and the pericardium to the diaphragm and supplies the pleura, pericardium, and diaphragm (upper surface).

☐ **Anterior intercostal arteries** that supply intercostal **spaces 1 to 6** are branches of the internal thoracic artery, **7 to 9** are given by the musculophrenic artery.

➤ There are **two anterior intercostal** arteries in each of the intercostal spaces that run laterally, one each at the upper and lower borders of each space.

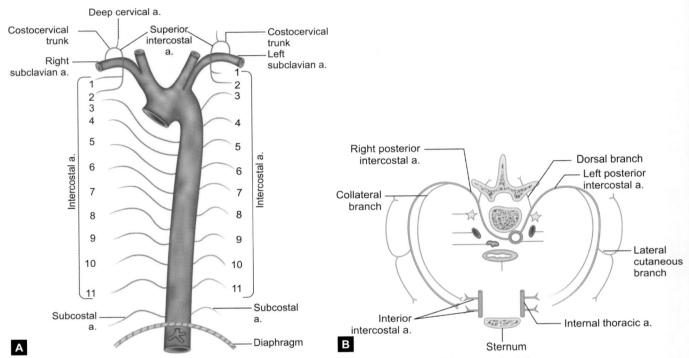

Figs. 29A and B: Posterior intercostal arteries: (A) Origin; (B) Course and relations.

➤ The **upper** artery in each intercostal space **anastomoses** with the **posterior intercostal artery**, and the lower one joins the collateral branch of the posterior intercostal artery.

➤ They give muscular branches to the intercostal, serratus anterior, and pectoral muscles.

➤ Their anterior Perforating Branches (second, third, and fourth) give medial **mammary branches to breast**.

☐ **Musculophrenic Artery** follows the costal arch on the inner surface of the costal cartilages, gives rise to **two anterior intercostal** arteries in the 7–9th spaces; perforates the diaphragm; and ends in the 10th intercostal space, where it anastomoses with the deep circumflex iliac artery.

➤ It supplies the pericardium, diaphragm, and muscles of the abdominal wall.

☐ **Superior Epigastric Artery** descends on the deep surface of the rectus abdominis muscle within the rectus sheath; supplies this muscle and **anastomoses** with the **inferior epigastric artery** (in rectus sheath).

➤ It supplies the diaphragm, peritoneum, and anterior abdominal wall.

☐ **Posterior intercostal arteries** that supply intercostal spaces 1 and 2 are branches of the **superior intercostal artery** (that arises from the **costocervical trunk** of the subclavian artery), **spaces 3 to 11** are branches of the **descending thoracic aorta**.

➤ In the intercostal space, they pass **between** internal and innermost intercostal muscles, **lie between** the intercostal vein above and the intercostal nerve below. They supply the of the intercostal muscles, overlying skin and parietal pleura.

➤ **Right** posterior intercostal arteries are **longer** than the left.

➤ Mammary branches arise from posterior intercostals arteries of the **2nd, 3rd, and 4th** intercostal spaces and supply the **mammary gland.**

➤ **Right** bronchial artery arises from **right 3rd** posterior intercostal artery.

Superior (highest) intercostal artery is a branch of costocervical trunk and descends in front of the neck of the first two ribs and gives rise to posterior intercostal arteries to the first two intercostal spaces.

▼ Aorta

- ❏ **Ascending Aorta** arises from the **left ventricle** within the pericardial sac and ascends behind the sternum to end at the level of the **sternal angle** (approximately).
  - ➤ It lies in the **middle mediastinum**, has **three aortic sinuses** located immediately above the cusps of the aortic valve, and gives off the right and left **coronary arteries**.
- ❏ **Arch of aorta** continues from the ascending aorta. Its origin, slightly to the right, is level with the superior border of the right **second sternocostal joint**.
  - ➤ It runs upwards, backwards, and to the left, **in front** of the bifurcation of the trachea then turns downwards behind the left bronchus finally descending to the left of the **fourth thoracic vertebral** body, continuing as the descending thoracic aorta.
  - ➤ It terminates level with the sternal end of the **left second costal cartilage** and so lies wholly within the **superior mediastinum** (behind the **lower half** of manubrium sterni).
  - ➤ It gives **three branches**: Brachiocephalic, left common carotid, and left subclavian arteries.
  - ➤ **Origin** and termination of arch of aorta is at the same level: **2nd costal cartilage** and **T4 vertebra**.
- ❏ **Descending thoracic aorta** begins at the level of the fourth thoracic vertebra.
  - ➤ It descends on the **left side** of the vertebral column and then approaches the median plane to end in front of the vertebral column by passing through the **aortic hiatus** of the diaphragm (T12 vertebral level).
  - ➤ It gives origin to **nine pairs** of posterior intercostal arteries and **one pair of subcostal** arteries.
  - ➤ It also gives rise to pericardial, **bronchial** (one right and two left), esophageal, mediastinal, and **superior phrenic** branches.

Coarctation (narrowing) of aorta is due to defect in the tunica media, which forms a shelf-like projection into the lumen, most commonly in the region of the ductus arteriosus.

- ❏ It is of three types:
  - ➤ **Pre-ductal** coarctation: The narrowing is **proximal** to the ductus arteriosus. If severe, blood flow to the aorta distal (to lower body) to the narrowing is dependent on a patent ductus arteriosus, and hence **its closure can be life-threatening**.
  - ➤ **Ductal** coarctation: The narrowing occurs **at the insertion** of the ductus arteriosus. This kind usually appears when the ductus arteriosus closes.
  - ➤ **Post-ductal** coarctation: The narrowing is **distal** to the insertion of the ductus arteriosus. Even with an open ductus arteriosus blood flow to the lower body can be impaired.

The postductal type of coarctation may permit years of normal life, allowing the development of an extensive **collateral circulation** to the aorta distal to the stenosis.

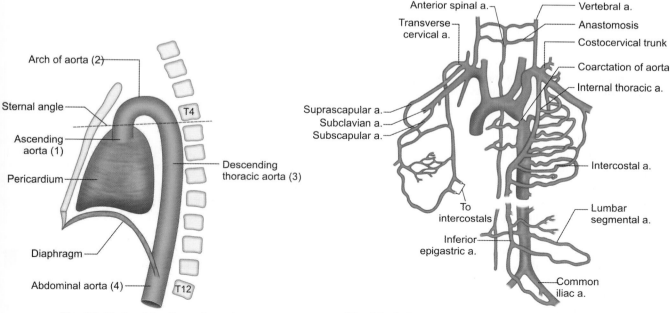

Fig. 30: Parts of the thoracic aorta   Fig. 31: Collaterals in coarctation of aorta (a = artery)

❑ Arch of aorta → subclavian artery → internal thoracic artery → **anterior intercostal artery** → **posterior intercostal artery** → descending thoracic aorta → thorax, abdomen, pelvis and lower limb.

❑ Arch of aorta → subclavian artery → **costocervical trunk** → superior intercostal artery → third posterior intercostal artery → descending thoracic aorta → thorax, abdomen, pelvis and lower limb.

❑ **Scapular anastomosis** → dorsal scapular artery → posterior intercostal artery → descending thoracic aorta → thorax, abdomen, pelvis and lower limb.

❑ Arch of aorta → subclavian artery → internal thoracic artery → **superior epigastric** artery → **inferior epigastric** artery iliac artery → Pelvis and **lower limb**.

❑ Arch of aorta → subclavian artery → **vertebral artery** → anterior spinal artery → segmental artery → thoracic and abdominal aorta → thorax, abdomen, pelvis and lower limb.

QUESTIONS

1. TRUE about anterior intercostal artery: *(NEET Pattern 2015)*
   a. Present in 1st to 12th intercostal space
   b. Each intercostal space has two anterior intercostal arteries
   c. Branch of internal thoracic artery
   d. Branch of aorta

2. TRUE about internal thoracic artery: *(NEET Pattern 2016)*
   a. Arises from 1st part of subclavian artery
   b. Pericardiophrenic is a terminal branch
   c. Divides in the 4th intercostal space
   d. Descends at posterior end of intercostal space

3. In post-ductal coarctation of aorta, collaterals are formed by all EXCEPT: *(AIIMS 2008, AIPG 2010)*
   a. Vertebral artery
   b. Subscapular/suprascapular artery
   c. Posterior intercostal artery
   d. Internal thoracic artery

4. In post-ductal Coarctation of the aorta, blood flow to the lower limbs in maintained by increased blood flow through: *(AIIMS 2007)*
   a. Inferior phrenic and pericardiophrenic artery
   b. Intercostal and Superior epigastric artery
   c. Subcostal and umbilical artery
   d. Vertebral and anterior spinal artery

ANSWERS

1. b. Each intercostal space has two anterior intercostal arteries
   ❑ Each of upper nine intercostal spaces (1 to 9) have **one posterior** and **two anterior** intercostal arteries.
   ❑ The 10th and 11th spaces have one posterior intercostal artery, but **no anterior intercostal artery**.
   ❑ Anterior intercostal arteries for upper six spaces arise from **internal thoracic artery**.
   ❑ For 7th to 9th spaces, these are branches of **musculophrenic artery**.

2. a. Arises from 1st part of subclavian artery
   ❑ Internal thoracic artery is a branch from **1st part** of subclavian artery, has a vertical course inferiorly running at the anterior (**not posterior**) end of intercostal space. At the **sixth-to-seventh** costal cartilages it bifurcates into two terminal branches - musculophrenic artery and superior epigastric artery.

3. a. Vertebral artery
   ❑ This Questions has no answer, as all of the given arteries participate in the anastomosis.
   ❑ Since Gray's anatomy has **no mention of vertebral artery** in the topic, that becomes the answer of choice.

4. b. Intercostal and superior epigastric artery > d. Vertebral and anterior spinal artery
   ❑ **Lower limb** may be supplied by the channel:
   ❑ Arch of aorta → subclavian artery → internal thoracic artery → **superior epigastric** artery → inferior epigastric artery iliac artery → Pelvis and lower limb.
   ❑ Arch of aorta → subclavian artery → internal thoracic artery → anterior **intercostal artery** → posterior **intercostal artery** → descending thoracic aorta → thorax, abdomen, pelvis and lower limb.
   ❑ Arch of aorta → subclavian artery → **vertebral artery** → **anterior spinal artery** → segmental artery → thoracic and abdominal aorta → thorax, abdomen, pelvis and lower limb.

- **Superior intercostal artery** is a branch of **costocervical trunk.**
- **Upper two** posterior intercostal arteries arise from Superior intercostal artery *(NEET Pattern 2015)*
- **Vasa Vasorum** of ascending aorta arises from **left coronary artery** *(NEET Pattern 2015)*
- **Arch of aorta** arises from ascending aorta *(NEET Pattern 2016)*
- **Posterior intercostal arteries** are branches of **descending thoracic aorta** *(NEET Pattern 2015)*
- **Largest** branch of the arch of aorta is **brachiocephalic** trunk.
- Commonest **variation** in the origin of great arteries from the arch of aorta is the **origin of left common carotid** artery from the brachiocephalic trunk.
- **Aortic knuckle** is the projection at the upper end of the left margin of the cardiac shadow in PA view of X-ray chest.
- **Sinuses of Valsalva** are three dilatations in the ascending aorta above the semilunar valves.

▶ Venous Drainage in Thorax

❑ The left and right **brachiocephalic veins** are formed posterior to the **sternoclavicular joints.**
❑ Right brachiocephalic vein descends almost vertically, whereas the left brachiocephalic vein passes **obliquely posterior to the manubrium sterni.**

- **Superior vena cava** is formed at the lower border of the right **1st** costal cartilage by the union of right and left brachiocephalic (innominate) veins.
- SVC pierces the pericardium at the level of the right **2nd** costal cartilage and terminates into the right atrium at the lower border of the right **3rd** costal cartilage (**Mnemonic: 1, 2, 3**).

  Superior Vena Cava is formed by the union of the **right and left** brachiocephalic veins and drains blood from all structures **superior to the diaphragm** (EXCEPT the lungs and heart).

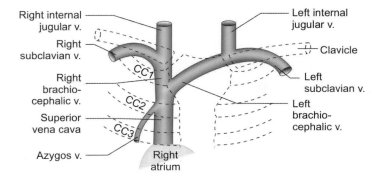

Fig. 32: Surface marking for the veins (v = vein)

- It descends on the right side of the ascending aorta, receives the azygos vein, and enters the right atrium.
- Its upper (extra-pericardial) part lies in the **superior** mediastinum and lower (intra-pericardial) part in the **middle** mediastinum.

  The **intercostal veins** accompany the similarly named arteries in the intercostal spaces.
- The small **anterior intercostal veins** are tributaries of the **internal thoracic** and **musculophrenic veins**; the internal thoracic veins drain into the respective **brachiocephalic vein**.
- **Posterior Intercostal Veins** run in the **costal groove** of the rib and **majorly** drain the thoracic wall.
  - They drain backwards, and most drain directly or indirectly into the **azygos vein** on the right and the **hemiazygos or hemiazygos** veins on the left.
- **Internal Thoracic Vein** is formed by the confluence of the **superior epigastric** and **musculophrenic veins**, ascends on the medial side of the artery, receives the **upper six** anterior intercostal and **pericardiophrenic** veins, and **ends in the brachiocephalic** vein.
- **Thoracoepigastric Vein** is a venous communication between the **lateral thoracic vein** and the **superficial epigastric vein** (or femoral vein) that runs superficially on the anterolateral aspect of the trunk.
  - This vein connects the **inferior** and **superior** caval areas of drainage and may be **dilated** and visible in cases of **vena caval obstruction**.

Azygos Venous System

- **Azygos** (unpaired) vein is formed by the union of the **right subcostal** and **right ascending lumbar** veins.
  - Its lower end communicates **with IVC**.
  - It enters the thorax by passing through the **right crus** of diaphragm (through the aortic opening **sometimes**).
  - It arches over the root of the right lung and empties into the SVC (**T4 vertebra; costal cartilage 2**).
  - It is the **first tributary of SVC**.
  - Tributaries of the azygos vein are: **Lower 7** right posterior intercostal veins, **right superior** intercostal vein (formed by union of 2nd, 3rd, and 4th right posterior intercostal veins), **hemiazygos vein** (at the level of T7/T8 vertebra), **accessory** hemiazygos vein (at the level of T8/T9 vertebra), **right bronchial vein**, esophageal veins, mediastinal veins, pericardial veins.
- **Hemiazygos Vein** represents the left-sided equivalent of the more inferior part of the azygos vein.
  - It is formed by the union of the **left subcostal** and **left ascending lumbar** veins.
  - Its lower end may be connected to the **left renal vein**.
  - It ascends on the left side of the vertebral bodies, pass through the **left crus** of diaphragm, receives the **lower** posterior intercostal veins (9th, 10th, and 11th).
  - It crosses the midline to drain into azygos vein (at the level of **T8 vertebra**).
  - **Accessory Hemiazygos Vein** is the left-sided mirror image of the superior portion of the azygos vein.
  - It begins at the fourth or fifth intercostal space; descends, receiving the **5th to 8th intercostal veins**.
  - It drains into **Azygos vein** (at the level of T7/T8 vertebra).
- **Superior Intercostal Vein** is formed by the union of the **2nd to 4th** posterior intercostal veins and drains into the azygos vein on the right and the brachiocephalic vein on the left.
- **Right** bronchial veins drain into **azygos vein** and **left** bronchial veins drain into the **left superior intercostal** vein or the **accessory hemiazygos vein**.

Table 4: Mode of termination of right and left posterior intercostal veins	
Right posterior intercostal veins	**Left posterior intercostal veins**
1st (highest) drains into the right brachiocephalic vein	1st (highest) drains into left brachiocephalic vein
2nd, 3rd, and 4th join to form right superior intercostal vein, which in turn drains into the azygos vein	2nd, 3rd, and 4th join to form left superior intercostal vein, which in turn drains into left brachiocephalic vein
5th–11th drain into the azygos vein	5th–8th drain into accessory azygos vein 9th–11th drain into hemiazygos vein
Subcostal vein drains into the azygos vein	Subcostal vein drains into the hemiazygos vein

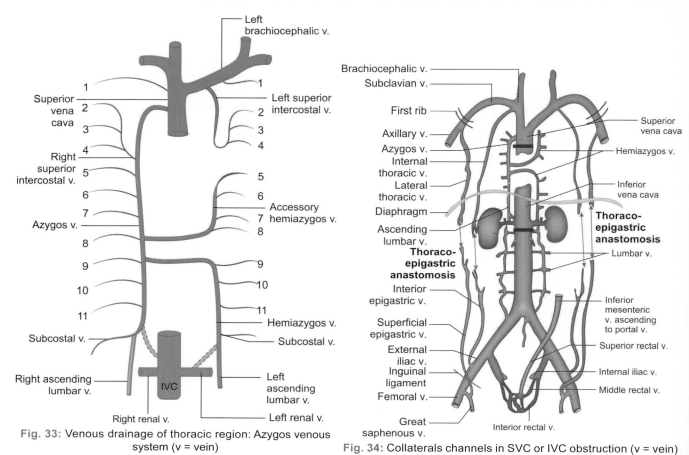

Fig. 33: Venous drainage of thoracic region: Azygos venous system (v = vein)

Fig. 34: Collaterals channels in SVC or IVC obstruction (v = vein)

Collateral pathways in **vena cava obstruction**

❑ The SVC may be obstructed at two sites: **Above** the opening of azygos vein (superior mediastinum) or **below** the opening of azygos vein (middle mediastinum).

❑ In case of SVC obstruction **above** the opening of azygos vein, the venous blood from the upper half of the body is shunted to right atrium through **azygos vein**.

  ➢ The **collateral channel** is: Subclavian vein → Internal thoracic vein → anterior intercostal vein → posterior intercostal vein → azygos vein → SVC.

❑ In case SVC obstruction is **below** the opening of the azygos vein, the venous blood from the upper half of the body is returned to the right atrium through inferior vena cava through various collateral pathways, formed between the tributaries of superior and inferior vena cavae (**caval-caval shunt**).

  ➢ The patient develops prominent subcutaneous **anastomotic venous communications** due to dilatation of various anastomotic venous channels between upper and lower body. Few of them are shown below:

   ▪ SVC → Azygos vein → lumbar azygos vein/ascending lumbar vein → IVC.

   ▪ SVC → subclavian vein → internal thoracic vein → superior epigastric vein → inferior epigastric vein → iliac vein → IVC.

   ▪ SVC → subclavian vein → axillary vein → lateral thoracic vein → thoracoepigastric vein → superficial epigastric vein → femoral vein → IVC.

❑ In a corresponding manner, in **IVC Obstruction** as well, the **same anastomosing channels** are dilated between IVC and SVC (**caval–caval shunt**) so that the blood could be returned to the **right atrium**.

Table 5: Veins draining into SVC and IVC

Veins draining into SVC	Veins draining into IVC
<ul><li>Superior epigastric - internal thoracic vein - subclavian vein</li><li>Lateral thoracic vein - axillary vein</li><li>Posterior intercostal vein- azygos and hemiazygos veins</li></ul>	<ul><li>Inferior epigastric vein - external iliac vein</li><li>Superficial epigastric - great saphenous - femoral vein</li><li>Superficial circumflex iliac - femoral vein</li><li>Deep circumflex iliac - external iliac vein</li><li>Iliolumbar vein - common iliac vein</li></ul>

QUESTIONS

1. NOT true about superior vena cava: *(NEET Pattern 2015)*
   a. Opens into right atrium
   b. Pierces pericardium at 3rd costal cartilage
   c. Enters the heart of level of 3rd costal cartilage
   d. Receives azygos vein behind sternal angle

2. In IVC obstruction, all of the following collaterals help EXCEPT: *(AIIMS 2006)*
   a. Superior epigastric and inferior epigastric vein
   b. Superficial epigastric and iliolumbar vein
   c. Azygos and ascending lumbar vein
   d. Lateral thoracic and prevertebral vein

3. IVC obstruction presents with:
   a. Esophageal varices
   b. Hemorrhoids
   c. Para-umbilical dilatation
   d. Thoraco-epigastric dilatation

4. Which of the following veins drains into the brachiocephalic vein:
   a. Internal thoracic vein
   b. Hemiazygos vein
   c. Right superior intercostal vein
   d. Left superior intercostal vein

5. The last tributary of the azygos vein is: *(NEET Pattern 2014)*
   a. Right superior intercostal vein
   b. Hemi-azygos vein
   c. Right bronchial vein
   d. Accessory azygos vein

6. True about hemiazygos vein are all EXCEPT: *(NEET Pattern 2016)*
   a. Formed by right lumbar azygos and right ascending lumbar veins
   b. Pierces left crus of diaphragm
   c. Drains esophageal vein
   d. At T8 level drains into azygos vein

ANSWERS

1. **b. Pierces pericardium at 3rd costal cartilage**
   - ❑ Superior vena cava pierces the pericardium at the level of the **right 2nd costal cartilage**
   - ❑ **Mnemonic: 1, 2, 3:**
     - Superior vena cava is formed at the lower border of the right **1st** costal cartilage by the union of right and left brachiocephalic veins. It pierces the pericardium at the level of the right **2nd** costal cartilage and terminates into the right atrium at the lower border of the right **3rd** costal cartilage.
   - ❑ **Azygos vein** terminates in the superior vena cava at the level of the 2nd costal cartilage (behind **sternal angle**).

2. **b. Superficial epigastric and iliolumbar vein**
   - ❑ In IVC obstruction, collaterals open up to drain blood into SVC and thence to the heart (right atrium).
   - ❑ Since, superficial epigastric and iliolumbar vein **both drain into IVC**, they are **not helping** the cause.

3. **d. Thoraco-epigastric dilatation**
   - ❑ In IVC obstruction the blood needs to be drained into SVC through various **collaterals**.
   - ❑ One of the collateral channel is: IVC → femoral vein → superficial **epigastric** vein → thoracoepigastric vein → lateral **thoracic** vein → axillary vein → subclavian vein → SVC.

4. **d. Left superior intercostal vein**
   - ❑ First posterior intercostal vein on **each side** drains into brachiocephalic vein.
   - ❑ Posterior intercostal veins of left intercostal space 2, 3 and 4 drains into the **left superior intercostal vein**, which itself drains into the **left brachiocephalic vein**.
   - ❑ Internal thoracic vein drains into subclavian vein and hemi-Azygos vein drains into Azygos vein.

5. **c. Right bronchial vein**
   - ❑ Right bronchial vein opens into the Azygos vein **near its termination** into SVC.

6. **a. Formed by right lumbar azygos and right ascending lumbar veins**
   - ❑ Hemiazygos vein is formed by the confluence of the **left ascending lumbar** and **left subcostal veins**.

- **Left superior intercostal vein** drains into left brachiocephalic vein *(NEET Pattern 2015)*
- Right bronchial vein drains into azygos vein *(NEET Pattern 2016)*
- Hemiazygos vein crosses left to right at the level of T8 vertebra *(NEET Pattern 2012)*
- **Direct tributary** of superior vena cava is **Azygos vein** *(NEET Pattern 2016)*
- Azygos vein and hemiazygos veins lie in **posterior mediastinum** *(NEET Pattern 2016)*
- **Superior vena cava** opens into right atrium at the level of **T5 vertebra** *(NEET Pattern 2012)*

▶ Lymphatic Drainage

Right upper half of the body above diaphragm (**right upper quadrant**) of the body drains the lymphatics into the **right lymphatic duct** and **rest** of the body drains **into thoracic duct**.

- ❑ The **confluence** of lymph trunks receives lymph from **four main lymphatic trunks**: The right and left **lumbar** lymph trunks and the right and left **intestinal** lymph trunks.

❑ In a small percentage of population this abdominal confluence of lymph trunks is represented as a dilated sac called **the cisterna chyli**. It is present in the **abdomen at L-1, 2** vertebral levels.

    Thoracic (Pecquet) Duct is the largest lymphatic vessel and begins in the abdomen at **T-12 vertebral level** as the continuation of cisterna chyli.

❑ It is usually **beaded** because of its numerous **valves** and often forms double or triple ducts.

❑ It drains the **body below diaphragm** (lower limbs, pelvis, abdomen) and **left half of the body above** diaphragm (thorax, upper limb and the head and neck).

❑ Thoracic duct passes through the **aortic hiatus** in the diaphragm and ascends through the **posterior mediastinum** between the aorta and the azygos vein.

❑ At **T-5 vertebral level** it deviates to **left side of midline** and keep ascending up to pass the **thoracic inlet**. It arches laterally over the apex of the left pleura and empties into the **left venous angle** — junction of the left internal jugular and subclavian veins (Beginning right brachiocephalic vein).

❑ Tributaries of thoracic duct:
 ➢ Bilateral (right and left) **descending thoracic** lymph trunks, which convey lymph from the **lower intercostal spaces** (6 to 11).

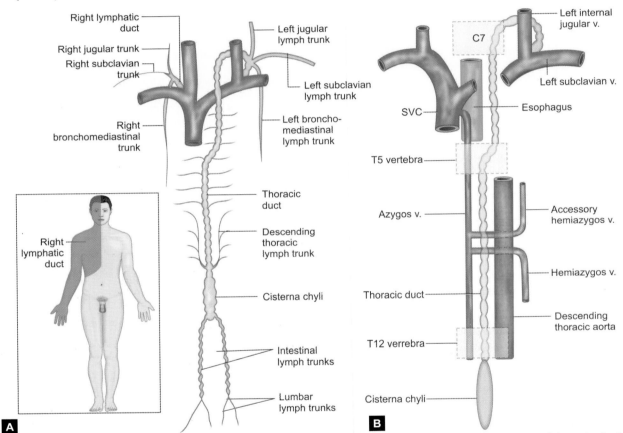

Figs. 35A and B: (A) Thoracic duct and right lymphatic duct; (B) Formation, course and termination of thoracic duct

 ➢ **Right and Left upper intercostal** lymph trunks, which convey lymph from the upper intercostal spaces (1 to 5).
 ➢ Mediastinal lymph trunks
 ➢ Left subclavian lymph trunk
 ➢ Left jugular lymph trunk
 ➢ Left bronchomediastinal lymph trunk

    Right lymphatic duct is a short vessel that drains the **right upper half of the body above** diaphragm.

❑ It receives the lymphatic drainage majorly from **three sources**: Right half of the head and neck (**Jugular** lymphatic trunk); Right upper limb (right **subclavian** lymphatic trunk) and the right thoracic cavity (right **broncho-mediastinal** lymphatic trunk).

❑ It drains into the **right venous angle** - junction of the right internal jugular and subclavian veins (Beginning of left brachiocephalic vein).

❑ Right lymphatic duct drains **right side** of the **head and neck**, **upper limb**, **thorax** (including breast and lung.

QUESTIONS

1. Thoracic duct opens into: *(NEET Pattern 2015)*
   a. Subclavian vein
   b. Internal jugular vein
   c. Right brachiocephalic vein
   d. Left brachiocephalic vein

2. The thoracic duct receives tributaries from all of the following EXCEPT: *(AIIMS 2008)*
   a. Bilateral ascending lumbar trunk
   b. Bilateral descending thoracic trunk
   c. Left upper intercostal duct
   d. Right bronchomediastinal lymphatic trunk

ANSWERS

1. d. Left brachiocephalic vein
   ❑ Thoracic duct opens into the left venous (jugulo-subclavian) angle, at the **beginning of** left brachio-cephalic vein.

2. d. Right bronchomediastinal lymphatic trunk
   ❑ **Right bronchomediastinal** lymphatic trunk drains into **right lymphatic duct** (not thoracic duct).
   ❑ **Theme:** Right half of the body above diaphragm (right upper quadrant) drains the lymphatics into the **right lymphatic duct** and rest of the body drains into thoracic duct (with few exceptions).
   ❑ **Right lymphatic duct** receives the lymphatic drainage majorly from **three sources**: Right half of the head and neck (**Jugular** lymphatic trunk); Right upper limb (right **subclavian** lymphatic trunk) and the Right thoracic cavity (right **bronchomediastinal** lymphatic trunk).
   ❑ **Thoracic duct** receives three major lymphatic vessels at its commencement: Bilateral **ascending lumbar** ducts; Bilateral **descending thoracic** ducts and Intestinal lymphatic trunks.
   ❑ Bilateral descending thoracic ducts drain the lower 6 intercostal spaces and empty into the thoracic duct.
   ❑ Upper 6 intercostal spaces (upper **intercostal duct**) on the **both sides** drain into thoracic duct.

- Thoracic duct commences **at T 12** vertebral level *(NEET Pattern 2016)*
- Thoracic duct does NOT drain **right upper part of body** *(NEET Pattern 2013)*
- Thoracic duct passes through **posterior** and **superior** mediastinum.

▶ Intercostal Space

There are eleven intercostal spaces that lie between the two adjacent ribs (and their costal cartilages). The 3rd–6th spaces are called **typical intercostal spaces** because the blood and nerve supply of 3rd–6th intercostal spaces is confined only to thorax.

Contents

Three intercostal muscles: **External** intercostal, **internal** intercostal and **innermost** intercostal (intercostalis intimi).

The neurovascular bundle (Intercostal nerves, arteries, veins and lymphatics) lies between the internal intercostal and innermost intercostal muscles. The arrangement of the structures is Intercostal Vein → Artery → Nerve (Mnemonic VAN goes down, superior to inferior).

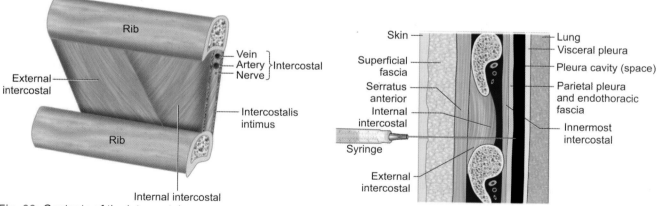

Fig. 36: Contents of the intercostal space

Fig. 37: Intercostal drainage for pleural aspiration

Intercostal Drainage

Thoracentesis (pleuracentesis or pleural tap) is a surgical procedure to collect pleural effusion for analysis. A needle or tube is inserted through thoracic wall into the pleural cavity posterior to the midaxillary line one or two intercostal spaces below the fluid level but not below the 9th space.

The ideal site is seventh, eighth, or ninth intercostal space, as this site avoids possible accidental puncture of the lung, liver, spleen, and diaphragm. To avoid damage to the intercostal nerve and vessels, the needle is inserted superior to the rib, high enough to avoid the collateral branches.

The needle penetrates the following structures: Skin → superficial fascia → serratus anterior muscle → external intercostal muscle → internal intercostal muscle → innermost intercostal muscle → endothoracic fascia → parietal pleura.

❑ Few authors mention posterior mid-scapular line as a common site for aspiration.

Intercostal Nerve Block is performed to relieve pain associated with a rib fracture or herpes zoster (shingles). A needle is inserted at the posterior angle of the rib **along the lower border** of the rib in order to inject the anesthetic near the intercostal nerve. In addition, the collateral branches of the intercostal nerve are also anesthetized.

QUESTIONS	
1. **Relationship of neurovascular bundle from above downward in intercostal space:** *(NEET Pattern 2015)* a. Nerve → Artery → Vein b. Artery → Nerve → Vein c. Vein → Nerve → Artery d. Vein → Artery → Nerve	2. **Intercostal injection is given at:** *(NEET Pattern 2016)* a. In the center of the intercostal space b. In anterior part of intercostal space c. Upper border of the rib d. Lower border of the rib

ANSWERS

1. **d. Vein → Artery → Nerve**
   ❑ The arrangement of neurovascular bundle in the costal groove **superior to inferior** is posterior intercostal Vein, posterior intercostal Artery and intercostal Nerve (VAN goes down, superior to inferior).

2. **d. Lower border of the rib**
   ❑ While giving intercostal block, the needle is passed along the **lower border** of rib (unlike pleural aspiration), so that the anesthetic drug reaches the intercostal nerve well, which **lies close** to the lower border.

- While doing **thoracentesis**, it is advisable to introduce needle along **upper border** of the rib.
- The order of neurovascular bundle in intercostal space from above to below is: **vein-artery-nerve**. This order is NOT observed in **first** intercostal space *(AIIMS 2013)*
- **Pleural tapping** in the mid-axillary line, muscle NOT pierced is **transversus thoracis** *(AIIMS 2007)*
- **Intercostal block** is given at **lower border** of the rib *(NEET Pattern 2016)*

▶ Diaphragm

Diaphragm is a curved musculotendinous sheet attached to the circumference of the thoracic outlet and to the upper lumbar vertebrae, which forms the floor of the thoracic cavity, separating it from the abdominal cavity.

It is relatively flat centrally and domed peripherally, rising higher on the right side than on the left, an asymmetry that reflects the relative densities of the underlying liver and gastric fundus, respectively.

Some authors mention the presence of heart leads to lower positioning of left dome of diaphragm.

The diaphragm is higher in the supine (compared to the erect) position, and the dependent half of the diaphragm is considerably higher than the uppermost one in the decubitus position.

It is at the lowest position while sitting posture, allows maximum excursion of lungs and explains patients of asthma being most comfortable in sitting posture.

Diaphragm takes origin from three parts: Sternal, costal and vertebral.

Sternal part consists of two fleshy slips, which arise from the posterior surface of the xiphoid process.

Costal part on each side consists of six fleshy slips, which arise from the inner surface of lower six ribs near their costal cartilages. Lumbar part arises by means of right and left crura of diaphragm and five arcuate ligaments.

Insertion is into the central tendon of diaphragm.

Diaphragm is the chief muscle of inspiration, descends when it contracts, causing an increase in thoracic volume by increasing the vertical diameter of the thoracic cavity.

Crura

Right crus attaches to anterior aspects of the upper three lumbar vertebrae and intervening intervertebral discs.

Left crus (shorter in length) attaches to anterior aspects of the upper two lumbar vertebrae and intervening intervertebral discs.

Medial fibers of the right crus embrace the esophagus where it passes through the diaphragm, the more superficial fibers ascend on the left, and deeper fibers cover the right margin.

In 30% population a superficial muscular bundle from the left crus contributes to the formation of the right margin of the hiatus.

Arcuate ligaments

❑ **Median arcuate ligament** is an arched fibrous band connecting the upper ends of two crura.
❑ **Medial arcuate ligament** (Medial Lumbocostal Arch) is the thickened upper margin of the psoas sheath. It extends from the side of the body of L2 vertebra to the tip of the transverse process of L1 vertebra.
❑ **Lateral arcuate ligament** (Lateral Lumbocostal Arch) is the thickened upper margin of fascia covering the anterior surface of the quadratus lumborum. It extends from the tip of transverse process of L1 vertebra to the 12th rib.

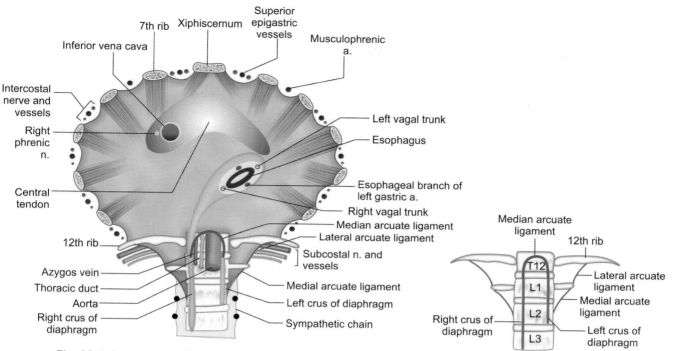

Fig. 38: Inferior view of diaphragm showing its multiple attachments, openings and the passing structures

Table 6: Diaphragmatic openings

Opening	Location	Shape/type	Vertebral level	Structures passing through
Vena caval (tendinous)	▪ Central tendon of diaphragm ▪ Right side of midline ▪ Between central and right posterior leaflet	Quadrangular/Square	T8 (lower border)	▪ **IVC** ▪ Branches of right phrenic nerve
Esophageal (muscular)	▪ Left side of midline ▪ Through the right crus of diaphragm	Oval/Elliptical	T10 (body)	▪ **E**sophagus ▪ Right and left vagal trunk ▪ Esophageal branches of left gastric artery
Aortic hiatus (osseo-aponeurotic)	▪ Midline ▪ Behind the diaphragm ▪ Posterior to median arcuate ligament	Circular/round	T12 (lower border)	▪ **A**orta ▪ Azygos vein (sometimes) ▪ Thoracic duct

Mnemonic: VOA (Voice of Anatomy) at T8,10,12; V (IVC), O (Oesophagus or esophagus), A (Aorta).

Minor Openings:

Costo-xiphoid gap (space of Larry) is present between the muscular slips arising from xiphoid process and 7th costal cartilage. Superior epigastric vessels pass through it.

Musculophrenic artery passes through the gap between the slips of origin from 7th to 8th ribs.

Sympathetic chain passes deep to the medial arcuate ligament, subcostal nerves and vessels pass deep to the lateral arcuate ligament.

Greater, lesser, and least splanchnic nerves pass by piercing the crus of diaphragm to enter the abdomen.

Azygos vein pierces right crus of diaphragm to enter thorax, hemiazygos vein pierces the left crus.

◤ Neurovascular Bundle

Table 7: Neurovascular structures of diaphragm

Vessels and nerves	Superior surface of diaphragm	Inferior surface of diaphragm
Arterial supply	Superior phrenic arteries from thoracic aorta Musculophrenic and pericardiophrenic arteries from internal thoracic arteries	Inferior phrenic arteries from abdominal aorta

Innervation	Motor supply: phrenic nerves (C3–C5) Sensory supply: centrally by phrenic nerves (C3–C5), peripherally by intercostal nerves (T5–T11) and subcostal nerves (T12)

IVC, inferior vena cava.

QUESTIONS

1. Which of the following statements is/are TRUE about diaphragm: *(PGIC)*
- a. Left side pushed down by heart
- b. Left side lower than the right
- c. Right side lower than the left
- d. Right side pushed up by liver

2. Diaphragmatic hernia can occur through all the following EXCEPT: *(AIPG)*
- a. Esophageal opening
- b. Costovertebral triangle
- c. Costal and sternal attachment of diaphragm
- d. Inferior vena cava opening

3. The structures passing posterior to diaphragm are all EXCEPT: *(AIIMS 2006)*
- a. Aorta
- b. Azygos vein
- c. Thoracic duct
- d. Greater splanchnic nerve

4. Blood supply of diaphragm is through all EXCEPT: *(NEET Pattern 2016)*
- a. Middle phrenic artery
- b. Inferior phrenic artery
- c. Musculophrenic artery
- d. Pericardiophrenic artery

ANSWERS

1. a. Left side pushed down by heart; b. Left side lower than the right; d. Right side pushed up by liver
- ❑ Left side of diaphragm is lower, since it is **pushed down** by heart, whereas right side of diaphragm is higher, since **pushed up by liver** (Subject experts in different fields have contradictory views, and the topic **remains controversial**).

2. d. Inferior vena cava opening
- ❑ There is no description of hernia through tendinous opening for IVC in literature.

3. d. Greater splanchnic nerve > b. Azygos vein
- ❑ Aorta and thoracic duct pass through the aortic hiatus, which lies **posterior** to the diaphragm.
- ❑ Azygos vein **may pass** through this opening **sometimes**, usually it **pierces through the crus** of diaphragm to enter the thorax.
- ❑ Greater splanchnic nerve usually **pierces through the crus** of diaphragm to enter the thorax.

4. a. Middle phrenic artery
- ❑ Diaphragm is supplied by **superior** phrenic arteries (from thoracic aorta), **musculophrenic** and **pericardiophrenic** arteries (from internal thoracic arteries) and **inferior** phrenic arteries (from abdominal aorta).

- ▪ Structures NOT passing through aortic opening is **vagus nerve** *(NEET Pattern 2018)*
- ▪ The opening in **central tendon** of diaphragm transmits **inferior vena cava** *(AIIMS 2017)*
- ▪ The opening in **central tendon** of diaphragm transmits **right phrenic** nerve branch *(NEET Pattern 2013)*
- ▪ Content(s) of **aortic hiatus** are azygos vein, thoracic duct and aorta (PGIC 2016)
- ▪ **Oesophagus** enters through **muscular** part of diaphragm *(NEET Pattern 2014)*
- ▪ Structure NOT passing through esophageal hiatus is **left phrenic nerve** *(AIIMS 2011)*
- ▪ **Sensory supply** to diaphragm is through **both** intercostal nerve and phrenic nerve *(NEET Pattern 2016)*
- ▪ Aorta and thoracic duct (and Azygos vein **sometimes**) pass **posterior** to the diaphragm. Whereas, **greater splanchnic nerve** does **not pass posterior** to diaphragm, it actually pierces through the crus of the diaphragm to enter the abdomen. *(AIIMS 2006)*
- ▪ Most common site of **Morgagni hernia** is right anteromedial (RAM). *(AIIMS 2009)*

▸ Tracheobronchial Tree

- ❑ **Conducting Portion** of airway includes the nasal cavity, nasopharynx, larynx, trachea, bronchi, bronchioles (possess no cartilage), and **terminal bronchioles**.
- ❑ **Respiratory portion** includes the **respiratory bronchioles**, alveolar ducts, atria, and alveolar sacs.

Details of trachea have been discussed in **head and neck region**. In this section the details of **thoracic trachea** are mentioned.

- ❑ **Trachea** bifurcates into bronchi at the level of the **disc between T4-T5 vertebra**, opposite the **sternal angle** (Most authors).
- ❑ Trachea bifurcation is seen at **T4 vertebral** level in **cadavers**.
- ❑ **Carina** is a ridge of cartilage in the trachea bifurcation, which lies between the division of the two main bronchi.
  - ➢ Carina lies at tracheal bifurcation, which is usually at the level of the **disc between T4-T5 vertebra**, in line with the sternal angle, but may raise or descend up to two vertebrae higher or lower with breathing.
  - ➢ Tracheobronchial injury, an injury to the airways, occurs **within 2.5 cm** of the carina 60% of the time.

The long axis of right principal bronchus deviates about **25° from the long axis of the trachea**, whereas long axis of the left principal deviates about 45° from the long axis of the trachea.

- ❑ **Right principal bronchus** is **short** (length), **wide** (lumen) and **more vertical** (in line with trachea), as compared with the left principal bronchus.
  - ➢ It branches into 3 lobar bronchi (upper, middle, and lower) and finally into **10 segmental bronchi**.
  - ➢ The first branch, the **superior lobar** bronchus, then enters the right lung opposite the fifth thoracic vertebra.

- The **azygos vein** arches over it, and the right pulmonary artery lies at first inferior, then anterior to it (hence the name **eparterial bronchus**).
- Next right principal enters the pulmonary hilum and divides into **middle** and **inferior** lobar bronchi.

❑ **Left principal bronchus** is narrower, longer, and more horizontal than the right.

- It is about 2 inches (5 cm) long and does not lie in line with the trachea.
- It runs inferolaterally inferior to the arch of the aorta, crosses anterior to the esophagus and thoracic aorta and posterior to the left pulmonary artery.

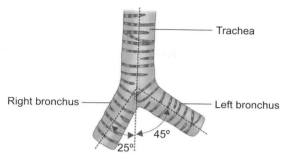

Fig. 39: Trachea and principal bronchi

- It divides into 2 lobar or secondary bronchi, the **upper** and **lower**, and finally into **8 to 10 segmental bronchi.**

Note: The branching of **segmental bronchi** corresponds to the **bronchopulmonary segments** of the lung.

QUESTIONS

1. Tracheal bifurcation is at:
   a. Upper border of T4
   b. Lower border of T4
   c. Upper border of T5
   d. Lower border of T5

2. At what level does the trachea bifurcates:
   (NEET Pattern 2012)
   a. Upper border of T4
   b. Lower border of T4
   c. 27.5 cm from the incisors
   d. Lower border of T5

3. Trachea bifurcates at the vertebra level:
   a. T2
   b. T3
   c. T4
   d. T5

4. Carina is situated at which level: *(NEET Pattern 2015)*
   a. T3
   b. T4
   c. T6
   d. T9

ANSWERS

1. **c. Upper border of T5 > b. Lower border of T4**
   ❑ Trachea bifurcates at the disc between T4/T5 vertebra (Most of the authors).
   ❑ Trachea bifurcates at T4 in cadavers.

2. **b. Lower border of T4**
   ❑ The most appropriate option has been taken as the answer.
   ❑ Trachea bifurcates into bronchi at the level of the disc between T4-T5 vertebra, opposite the sternal angle (Most authors).
   ❑ Carina (at tracheal bifurcation) is located about 25 cm from the incisor teeth and 30 cm from the nostrils.

3. **d. T5 > c. T4**
   ❑ Trachea bifurcates at the disc between T4/T5 vertebra (Most of the authors).
   ❑ Trachea bifurcates at T4 in cadavers.

4. **b. T4**
   ❑ **Carina** lies at tracheal bifurcation, which is usually at the level of the **disc between T4-T5 vertebra**, in line with the sternal angle, but may raise or descend up to two vertebrae higher or lower with breathing.

- **Angle** of right principal bronchus from midline is 25° *(NEET Pattern 2016)*

▶ Pleura

Pleura is a thin serous membrane around the lungs that consists of a parietal and a visceral layers.

Parietal Pleura lines the inner surface of the thoracic wall and the mediastinum and has costal, diaphragmatic, mediastinal, and cervical parts.

❑ Parietal pleura is separated from the thoracic wall by the endothoracic fascia, which is an extrapleural fascial sheet lining the thoracic wall.
❑ It forms the pulmonary ligament, a two-layered vertical fold of mediastinal pleura, which extends along the mediastinal surface of each lung from the hilus to the base (diaphragmatic surface) and ends in a free falciform border.
❑ It supports the lungs in the pleural sac by retaining the lower parts of the lungs in position.

Visceral Pleura (Pulmonary Pleura) adheres intimately to the lung surfaces and dips into all of the fissures.

❑ It is reflected at the root of the lung and continues as parietal pleura.
❑ Pleural cavity is a potential space between the parietal and visceral pleurae.
❑ It contains a film of fluid that lubricates the surface of the pleurae and facilitates the movement of the lungs.

Pleural Recesses

❑ **Costodiaphragmatic recess** is slit-like space formed by the reflection of the costal and diaphragmatic parietal pleurae, allows expansion of the lungs inferiorly during inspiration.

➤ Excess fluid within the pleural cavity accumulates in the costodiaphragmatic recess and costodiaphragmatic angle is blunted (PA radiograph) in erect posture.

❑ **Costomediastinal recess** is slit-like spaces between the costal and mediastinal parietal pleura.

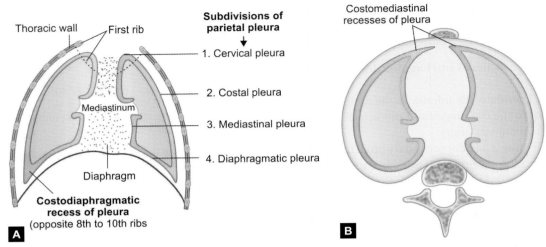

Figs. 40A and B: Reflection of the pleura in thoracic cavity. (A) Vertical section; (B) Transverse section

❑ During inspiration, the anterior borders of both lungs expand and enter the right and left costomediastinal recesses.

❑ In addition, the lingula of the left lung expands and enters a portion of the left costomediastinal recess, causing that portion of the recess to appear radiolucent (dark) on radiographs.

According to the surface it lines parietal pleura is divided into the following four parts : Costal, diaphragmatic, mediastinal and cervical.

❑ The cervical pleura (cupula) is the dome of the pleura, projecting into the neck above the neck of the first rib.

❑ It is reinforced by Sibson fascia (suprapleural membrane), which is a thickened portion of the endothoracic fascia, and is attached to the first rib and the transverse process of the seventh cervical vertebra.

Table 8: Details of pleura of pleura		
Type	**Visceral**	**Parietal**
Location	Lines the surface of the lung	Lines the thoracic wall and mediastinum
Development	Lateral plate mesoderm (Splanchnopleuric layer)	Lateral plate mesoderm (Somatopleuric layer)

Nerve supply	▪ Autonomic (pain insensitive)*:
	  – Sympathetic (T1-T5)
	  – Parasympathetic (vagus)
		▪ Somatic (pain sensitive):
		  – **Intercostal nerves (T2-T5)** supply peripheral costal pleura and peripheral portion of diaphragmatic pleura
		  – **Phrenic nerve** supplies mediastinal central pleura and central portion of the diaphragmatic pleura

Arterial supply	▪ Internal thoracic ▪ Superior phrenic ▪ Posterior intercostal ▪ Superior intercostal arteries	▪ Bronchial arteries
Venous drainage	Systemic veins	Pulmonary veins

*Visceral pleura is sensitive to stretch (may be involved in respiratory reflexes).

 CLINICAL CORRELATIONS

▪ Pleuritis (inflammation) involving visceral pleura present with no pain, whereas parietal pleuritis is associated with sharp local pain and referred pain, felt in the thoracic wall (intercostal nerves) and root of the neck (phrenic nerve (C3,4,5).
▪ Surgical posterior approach to the kidney may damage the pleura in case 12th rib is very short and 11th rib is mistaken for 12th rib.

QUESTION

1. **UNTRUE about visceral pleura:**   *(NEET Pattern 2013)*
   a. Develops from splanchnopleuric mesoderm
   b. Has three borders
   c. Supplied by phrenic nerve
   d. Pain insensitive

ANSWER

1. **c. Supplied by phrenic nerve**
   ❑ **Visceral pleura** develops from **splanchnopleuric** layer of the lateral plate of mesoderm, supplied by the **autonomic** (sympathetic) nerves (T1–T5) and is **insensitive to pain by stretch.**

Lungs

Lungs are attached to the heart and trachea by their roots and the pulmonary ligaments.

❑ The lung bases rest on the convex surface of the diaphragm, descend during inspiration, and ascend during expiration.

Right Lung has an apex that projects into the neck and a concave base that sits on the diaphragm.

❑ It is larger and heavier than the left lung, but is **shorter and wider** because of the higher right dome of the diaphragm and the inclination of the heart to the left.

❑ It is divided into upper, middle, and lower lobes by the **oblique** and **horizontal** fissures.

❑ It has 3 lobar (secondary) bronchi and 10 segmental (tertiary) bronchi.

❑ The diaphragmatic surface consists of the middle lobe and lower lobe.

❑ There are specific impressions evident, created by various related structures (e.g. SVC, arch of azygos vein, esophagus).

Left Lung is divided into upper and lower lobes by an **oblique fissure**, is usually more vertical in the left lung than in the right lung.

❑ **Lingula** is a tongue-shaped portion present in the upper lobe that corresponds to embryologic counterpart to the right middle lobe.

❑ Left lung has 2 lobar (secondary) bronchi and **8 to 10 segmental bronchi**.

❑ It shows a cardiac impression, a **cardiac notch** (a deep indentation of the anterior border of the superior lobe), and grooves for various structures (e.g. aortic arch, descending aorta, left subclavian artery).

Hilum and Mediastinal Surface

The arrangement of structures in the hilum of left lung is remembered by the mnemonic **ABV (Atal Bihari Vajpayi)** in superior to inferior direction. Artery (pulmonary) → Bronchus (principal) → Vein (pulmonary).

❑ It is the same sequence in right lung as well but with the addition of a bronchus above the artery **(epiarterial bronchus)**.

❑ In all these structures bronchus is the most posterior structure at the lung hilum.

❑ There are 2 veins which are named anterior and inferior according to their location at the hilum. (Similar arrangement on both sides).

❑ Bronchus and bronchial arteries are always **posterior** most structures at the hila of both lungs.

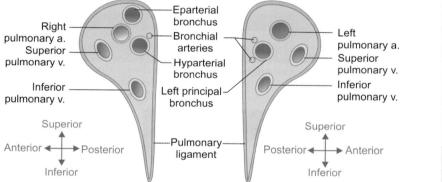

Table 9: Arrangement of structures at the lung hilum	
Right side	**Left side**
▪ Eparterial	Pulmonary artery
▪ Pulmonary artery	Left principal bronchus
▪ Hyparterial bronchus	Inferior pulmonary vein
▪ Inferior pulmonary vein	

Fig. 41: Arrangement of structures in the roots of right and left lungs (a = artery; v = vein)

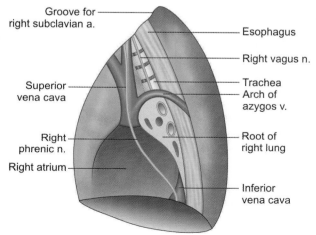

Fig. 42: Relations of the mediastinal surface of the right lung
(a = artery; n = nerve; v = vein)

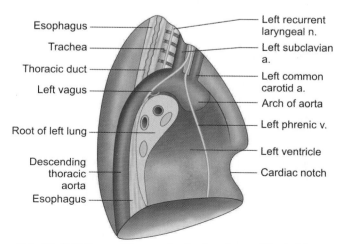

Fig. 43: Relations of the mediastinal surface of the left lung
(a = artery; n = nerve; v = vein)

Table 10: Relations of the mediastinal surfaces of the right and left lungs

Mediastinal surface of the right lung	Mediastinal surface of the left lung
Right atrium	Left ventricle
Superior and inferior vena cavae	Ascending aorta
Azygos vein	Arch of aorta and descending thoracic aorta
Right brachiocephalic vein	Left subclavian and left common carotid arteries
Esophagus and trachea	Esophagus and thoracic duct
Three neural structures	Four neural structures
▪ Right phrenic nerve	▪ Left phrenic vein
▪ Right vagus nerve	▪ Left vagus nerve
▪ Right sympathetic chain	▪ Left recurrent pharyngeal nerve
	▪ Left sympathetic chain

QUESTIONS

1. **Which is the most superior structure at hilum of left lung:**
   (AIIMS 2007)
   a. Pulmonary vein
   b. Pulmonary artery
   c. Bronchus
   d. Bronchial artery

2. **Superior most structure in hilum of right lung:**
   (NEET Pattern 2016)
   a. Eparterial bronchus
   b. Hyparterial bronchus
   c. Pulmonary artery
   d. Pulmonary vein

3. **Which of the following are related to the mediastinal part of right lung?** *(NEET Pattern 2013)*
   a. Arch of aorta
   b. SVC
   c. Pulmonary trunk
   d. Left ventricle

4. **Inferior most structure of right hilum is:**
   (NEET Pattern 2014)
   a. Bronchus
   b. Inferior pulmonary vein
   c. Pulmonary artery
   d. Inferior bronchial vein

5. **The root of the right lung does NOT lie behind which one of the following:**
   a. Right atrium
   b. Right vagus
   c. Superior vena cava
   d. Phrenic nerve

6. **Which is NOT a lobe of lung:** *(NEET Pattern 2015)*
   a. Azygos
   b. Superior
   c. Inferior
   d. Lingula

ANSWERS

1. **b. Pulmonary artery**
   ❑ The arrangement of structures in the hilum of left lung is remembered by the mnemonic ABV (Atal Bihari Vajpayi) in **superior to inferior** direction. **Artery** (pulmonary) → Bronchus (principal) → Vein (pulmonary).
   ❑ Pulmonary artery is uppermost whereas, pulmonary vein is inferior most.

2. **a. Eparterial bronchus**
   ❑ In right lung, **one bronchus** is located above the pulmonary artery (called as **eparterial bronchus**) and is the uppermost structure in the hilum.

3. **b. SVC**
   ❑ Arch of aorta and left ventricle are related to the mediastinal surface of **left lung.**
   ❑ **Pulmonary trunk** is not related to any of the two lungs (mediastinal surfaces).

4. **b. Inferior pulmonary vein**
   ❑ Inferior pulmonary vein is the **lowermost** structure in the hila of each lung.

5. **b. Right vagus**
   ❑ Root of lung is related to phrenic nerve anterior and **vagus nerve posterior**.

6. **d. Lingula**
   ❑ Right lung has three lobes (superior, middle and inferior) and left lung has two (**superior** and **inferior**).
   ❑ Lingula is **a portion** of the left upper lobe.
   ❑ **Azygos lobe** is an anatomically separated part of the upper lobe, and **not a true or accessory** lobe of lung, as it has no bronchi, veins and arteries of its own.

▪ Hilum of the right lung is arched by **azygos vein** *(AIPG)*

▶ Bronchopulmonary Segments

❑ The **bronchopulmonary segment** is the anatomical, functional, and surgical **unit** of the lungs.
❑ It is the **wedge shaped** largest subdivision of a lobe, named according to the **segmental bronchus** supplying it, and is surgically resectable.
❑ It contains a segmental (tertiary or lobular) **bronchus**, a branch of the **pulmonary artery**, and a branch of the **bronchial artery**, which run together through the central part of the segment, surrounded by a delicate connective tissue (intersegmental) septum.
❑ The tributaries of pulmonary veins are **intersegmental** and lie at the margins of

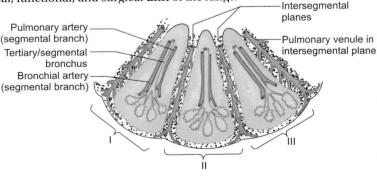

Fig. 44: Branchopulmonary segments

bronchopulmonary segments. They create **surgical planes**, which a surgeon can follow for **segmental resection**, with minimal tissue damage.

- ❑ There are **10 bronchopulmonary segments** in each lung.
  - ➤ Often **medial basal segment is absent in left lung** as anterior and medial basal of left lower lobe combine into anteromedial basal segment (**9 BPS in left lung**).
  - ➤ Occasionally apical and posterior BPS of left upper lobe typically combine into apicoposterior segment (**8 BPS in left lung**).

Table 11: Bronchopulmonary segment in lungs		
	Right lung	**Left lung**
Upper lobe	Apical (I), Posterior (II); Anterior (III)	Apical (I), Posterior (II), Anterior (III), Superior lingular (IV); Inferior lingular (V)
Middle lobe	Lateral (IV); Medial (V)	Absent
Lower lobe	Superior/Apical (VI), Medial basal* (VII), Anterior basal (VIII), Lateral basal (IX); Posterior basal (X)	Superior/Apical (VI), Medial basal*** (VII), Anterior basal*** (VIII), Lateral basal (IX); Posterior basal (X)

Note: Medial basal (VII) is also called as the cardiac BPS of right lung.
Apical and posterior of left upper lobe typically combine into apicoposterior segment.
Anterior and medial basal of left lower lobe often combine into anteromedial basal segment.

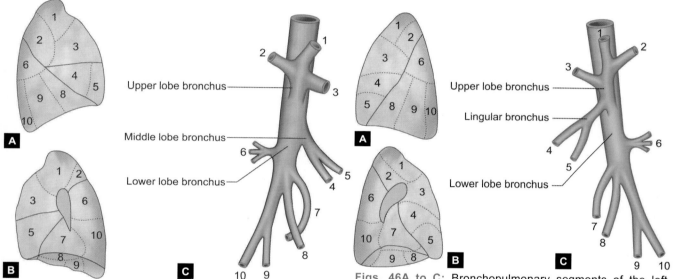

Figs. 45A to C: Bronchopulmonary segments of the right lung. (A) Lateral view; (B) Medial view; (C) Lobar and segmental bronchi.

Figs. 46A to C: Bronchopulmonary segments of the left lung. (A) Lateral view; (B) Medial view; (C) Lobar and segmental bronchi.

Foreign Body Aspiration

Location of the foreign body aspirate depends upon the **posture** of the patient and decided by the gravity factor as well (most dependent location).

- ❑ Most of the aspirations occur in **supine posture** (coma, post anesthesia) and the aspirate moves into right lower lobar bronchus to be found in the **apical (VI) BPS of right lower lobe**. Some books additionally mention the collection in **posterior (II) BPS of right upper lobe** as well.
- ❑ If aspiration occur in **erect** (sitting or standing) posture, aspirated material most commonly enters the **posterior basal (X) BPS of right lower lobe**.
- ❑ If a person is lying in **right lateral position**, the aspirate most commonly enters the right upper lobar bronchus and lodges within the **posterior (II) BPS of right upper lobe**.
- ❑ In **left lateral position** aspirated material most commonly enters the left upper lobar bronchus and lodges within the **inferior lingular (V) bronchopulmonary segment of the left upper lobe**.

QUESTIONS

1. Bronchopulmonary segments in right and left lungs respectively: *(NEET Pattern 2015)*
   - a. 9, 11
   - b. 11, 9
   - c. 10, 10
   - d. 8, 10

2. Bronchopulmonary segments in right and left lungs respectively: *(NEET Pattern 2015)*
   - a. 9, 11
   - b. 11, 9
   - c. 10, 8
   - d. 8, 10

3. All of the following are characteristic of a bronchopulmonary segment EXCEPT: *(AIIMS 2014)*
   a. It is surgically resectable
   b. It is named according to the segmental bronchus supplying it
   c. It is drained by independent intrasegmental branch of pulmonary vein
   d. It is the largest subdivision of a lobe

4. An inhaled foreign body is likely to lodge in the right lung due to all of the following features EXCEPT: *(AIPG)*
   a. Right lung is shorter and wider left lung
   b. Right principal bronchus is more vertical than the left bronchus
   c. Tracheal bifurcation directs the foreign body to the right lung
   d. Right inferior lobar bronchus is in continuation with the principal bronchus

5. A patient presents with chest pain due to aspiration pneumonitis. On examination there is dullness on percussion in area medial to the medial border of scapula on elevation of arm. Which part of the lung is most likely to be affected? *(AIIMS 2000)*
   a. Right superior BPS
   b. Right posterior BPS
   c. Left superior BPS
   d. Right apical BPS

6. A bed-ridden patient on liquid diet develops aspiration pneumonia. Which of the following is bronchopulmonary segment is most likely affected?
   a. Posterior of right upper lobe
   b. Inferior lingular of left upper lobe
   c. Apical of right lower lobe
   d. Posterior of right lower lobe

1. **c. 10,10**
   - Right principal bronchus branches into 3 lobar bronchi (upper, middle, and lower) and finally into **10 segmental bronchi** (and bronchopulmonary segments).
   - Left principal bronchus branches into 2 lobar or secondary bronchi, the upper and lower, and finally into **8 to 10 segmental bronchi** (and bronchopulmonary segments).

2. **c. 10, 8**
   - Right principal bronchus branches into 3 lobar bronchi (upper, middle, and lower) and finally into **10 segmental bronchi** (and bronchopulmonary segments).
   - Left principal bronchus branches into 2 lobar or secondary bronchi, the upper and lower, and finally into **8 to 10 segmental bronchi** (and bronchopulmonary segments).

3. **c. It is drained by independent intrasegmental branch of pulmonary vein**
   - The branches of pulmonary veins are **intersegmental** (not intra) and lie at the margins of bronchopulmonary segments and drain adjacent segments.
   - Each segment drains into **more than one** vein and each vein drain **more than one** segment.

4. **a. Right lung is shorter and wider left lung**
   - Foreign bodies are more likely to lodge in right lung because, right principal bronchus (**not lung**) is **shorter** and **wider** and **more vertical** in disposition.

5. **a. Right superior BPS**
   - Upon elevation of arm, medial border of scapula **corresponds to the oblique fissure** of lung on the posterior thorax. Medial to that lies the **apex of lower lobe** of the lung.
   - This is the location of the **apical (superior) BPS of right lower lobe**, which is a common site of **aspiration pneumonitis**.
   - Right posterior BPS is the **posterior BPS of right upper lobe**.
   - Left superior BPS is the **superior (apical) BPS of left lower lobe**.
   - Right apical BPS is **apical BPS of right upper lobe**, though it may also be the **superior (apical) BPS of right lower lobe**.

6. **c. Apical of right lower lobe > a. Posterior of right upper lobe**
   - Aspiration in supine (bed-ridden) posture most commonly involves the right lower lobar bronchus and aspirate lodges within the **superior (apical) bronchopulmonary segment of the right lower lobe**. It is found at the posterior BPS of the right upper lobe as well (**Harrison's Medicine Ed19**).
   - In erect/upright posture (sitting or standing) aspirated material most commonly enters the right lower lobar bronchus and lodges within the **posterior basal bronchopulmonary** segment (no. 10) of the right lower lobe.

- The right lower lobar bronchus is most vertical, most nearly continues the direction of the trachea, and is larger in diameter than the left, and therefore, small **aspirated objects** commonly lodge and the fluid aspirations reach the **right lower lobes** more often.
- A BPS is aerated by **tertiary bronchus** *(NEET Pattern 2015)*
- **Medial** bronchopulmonary segment is a part of **middle lobe of right** lung *(NEET Pattern 2016)*
- **Cardiac BPS** of right lung is **medial basal** BPS.
- Medial basal (cardiac) BPS is **often absent** in the left lung.
- Segments of **upper lobe** in the **right** lung are **apical**, **anterior** and **posterior** *(NEET Pattern 2013)*

▶ Pulmonary Vasculature

Lung is supplied by **two arterial systems**: Bronchial and Pulmonary arteries.

- **Bronchial arteries** carry oxygen to tracheobronchial tree and lungs and supplies **till the level of respiratory bronchiole**.

> They perfuse the proximal air conducting pathways including tertiary and terminal bronchioles and reach till the beginning of respiratory unit.
- **Pulmonary arteries** alone vascularize the further distal pathways, including alveolar ducts and the alveoli.
  > There are pre-capillary anastomoses between bronchial and pulmonary arteries, **at the level of respiratory bronchioles**, thus strengthening the **dual vasculature** of lungs.

Bronchial System of Arteries

- Bronchial arteries carry **oxygenated blood** to the lung and the **visceral pleura**.
  > **Right** bronchial artery is a branch of a **posterior intercostal artery**.
  > There are **two left bronchial arteries** given by the **descending thoracic aorta**.

Lung is supplied by **two venous systems**: Pulmonary and Bronchial veins

Bronchial System of Veins

- Bronchial veins carry **deoxygenated** blood from the bronchial arteries that supply large bronchi.
  > **Right** bronchial veins drain into the **azygos** vein, **left** into the **accessory** hemiazygos vein (or the left superior intercostal vein).

Pulmonary System of Veins

- **Pulmonary** veins carry **oxygenated** blood from the pulmonary capillary plexus and deoxygenated bronchial blood to the **left atrium.**
  > **Four** pulmonary veins open into the **posterior aspect of the left atrium.**
  > **Within** the lung pulmonary veins are **intersegmental** (found at the periphery of the bronchopulmonary segments), not accompanied by branches of bronchi, pulmonary arteries, or bronchial arteries.

Lymphatic vessels drain the bronchial tree, pulmonary vessels, and connective tissue septa.

They run along the bronchiole and bronchi **toward the hilum** to drain into the pulmonary and then bronchopulmonary nodes, which in turn drain to the inferior (carinal) and superior **tracheobronchial** nodes, the tracheal (paratracheal) nodes, **bronchomediastinal** nodes and trunks, and eventually to the **thoracic duct** (on the left) and **right lymphatic duct** (on the right).

Note: Lymphatics are **absent** in the walls of the pulmonary alveoli.

QUESTIONS

1. Bronchial artery supplies lungs up to:
   (AIPG 2008; NEET Pattern 2016)
   a. Tertiary bronchioles
   b. Respiratory bronchiole
   c. Alveolar ducts
   d. Terminal bronchiole

2. Rasmussen's aneurysm involves: *(AIIMS 2008)*
   a. Bronchial artery
   b. Pulmonary artery
   c. Intercostal artery
   d. Aorta

ANSWERS

1. **b. Respiratory bronchioles**
   - Bronchial arteries carry oxygen to tracheobronchial tree and lungs and supplies **till the level of respiratory bronchiole.**
   - **Pulmonary arteries** alone vascularize the **further distal pathways**, including alveolar ducts and the alveoli.

2. **b. Pulmonary artery**
   - Rasmussen's aneurysm refers to an aneurysm of the small to medium **pulmonary artery branches** that develop in the vicinity of a tuberculous cavity.
   - It is an inflammatory **pseudo-aneurysmal dilatation** of a branch of pulmonary artery adjacent to a tuberculous cavity may lead to **life-threatening** massive hemoptysis occasionally.

Nerve Supply of Lungs

Pulmonary plexuses are anterior and posterior to the other structures at the hila of the lungs.
- They are formed by cardiac branches from the second to fifth (or sixth) thoracic sympathetic ganglia and from the vagus and cervical sympathetic cardiac nerves.
- The left plexus also receives branches from the left recurrent laryngeal nerve.
- Vagus nerve carrying parasympathetic fibers that innervate the smooth muscle and glands of the bronchial tree are excitatory (bronchoconstrictor and secretomotor).
- Vagus also carry sensation of stretching of the lung during inspiration and is concerned in the reflex control of respiration.
- **Sympathetic** fibers innervate blood vessels, smooth muscle, and glands of the bronchial tree are inhibitory (bronchodilator and vasoconstrictor).

Respiratory Movements

Breathing involves changing the **thoracic volume** by altering the **vertical**, **transverse** and **anteroposterior** diameters of the thorax.

- ❑ **Inspiration** involves muscles that **elevate** the thoracic cage (ribs and sternum) and **increase the diameters** of thoracic cavity for **lung expansion.**
  - ➢ **Diaphragm** is the chief muscle of **inspiration**, pulls the dome inferiorly into the abdomen, thereby **increasing the vertical diameter** of the thorax and **expansion** of lung (**air moves in**).
- ❑ **Expiration** is a passive process caused by the **elastic recoil** of the lungs. **Forced expiration** requires contraction of the anterior abdominal muscles and few others.
  - ➢ Muscles of expiration are depressors of rib and decrease the diameters of thoracic cavity and lung compression.

Pump Handle Movement

- ❑ Elevation of **upper** 6 (vertebrosternal) ribs causes sternum to be pushed forward and upward, which increases the **anteroposterior diameter** of the thorax and lungs expand (**inspiration**).

Bucket Handle Movement

- ❑ The **lower** (vertebrochondral) ribs elevate by swinging upward and laterally leading to an increase in the **transverse** (lateral) **diameter** of the thorax for lung expansion (**inspiration**).

Table 12: Respiratory muscles

Type of respiration	Inspiration (rib elevators)	Expiration (rib depressors)
Quiet respiration	▪ Diaphragm (chief muscle) ▪ External intercostal muscles	Passive
Deep inspiration	▪ **External intercostal muscles** ▪ **Scalene muscles** ▪ Sternocleidomastoid ▪ Levator costarum ▪ **Serratus posterior superior** ▪ Innermost intercostal	Passive
Forced expiration	▪ Levator scapulae ▪ Trapezius ▪ Rhomboids ▪ Pectoral muscles ▪ **Serratus anterior**	▪ Anterior abdominals* ▪ Quadratus lumborum ▪ **Internal intercostal (costal part) muscles**** ▪ Transverse thoracis ▪ Serratus posterior inferior

*Anterior abdominals are : External and internal oblique muscles along with transversus abdominis.

**Internal intercostal (interchondral part) participates in inspiration.

- ❑ **Mnemonic:** Remember (SIT - Q depressors) for expiration: S – Serratus posterior inferior, I – Internal intercostals, T – Transversus thoracis and Q – quadratus lumborum. They work along with anterior abdominals for expiration.

Table 13: Factors responsible for the increase in various diameters of the thoracic cavity during inspiration

Diameter	Factors responsible for increase
Vertical	Descent (contraction) of the diaphragm
Anteroposterior	**Pump-handle movement** of the sternum (brought about by the elevation of vertebrosternal ribs)
Transverse	**Bucket-handle movement** of the vertebrochondral ribs

QUESTIONS

1. **All are accessory muscles of inspiration EXCEPT:**
   - a. Serratus anterior
   - b. Serratus posterior
   - c. Latissimus dorsi
   - d. Scalene

2. **Muscle of expiration:** *(NEET Pattern 2015)*
   - a. External intercostal
   - b. Diaphragm
   - c. Internal intercostal
   - d. Serratus anterior

3. **Which of the following do NOT elevate the ribs:** *(NEET Pattern 2014)*
   - a. Serratus posterior superior
   - b. Serratus posterior inferior
   - c. External intercostals
   - d. Levator costarum

4. **Function of external intercostal muscles:** *(NEET Pattern 2016)*
   - a. Elevation of ribs
   - b. Depression of ribs
   - c. Expiration
   - d. All of the above

ANSWERS

1. **c. Latissimus dorsi**
   - ❑ Accessory muscles of inspiration are **elevators of rib** and **increase the diameters** of thoracic cavity for **lung expansion**.

2. **c. Internal intercostal**
   - ❑ Muscles of expiration are **depressors of rib** and **decrease the diameters** of thoracic cavity and **lung compression**.
   - ❑ Internal intercostal (**costal part**) helps in **expiration**, whereas the interchondral part participates in inspiration.
   - ❑ **Diaphragm** is the chief muscle of **inspiration**, assisted by external intercostal and serratus anterior.

3. **b. Serratus posterior inferior**
   - ❑ Muscles that elevate the ribs work for inspiration, whereas serratus posterior inferior **depress** the ribs (for **expiration**).
   - ❑ Remember (SIT - Q depressors) for expiration: S – Serratus posterior inferior, I – Internal intercostals, T – Transversus thoracis and Q – quadratus lumborum. They work along with **anterior abdominals** for expiration.

4. **a. Elevation of ribs**
   - ❑ External intercostal muscles **elevate** ribs during **forced inspiration**.

- External intercostals, **interchondral portions** of the internal intercostals and the **levator costae** may elevate the ribs during inspiration.
- The internal intercostals except **for the interchondral portion** and the **transversus thoracic** may depress the ribs or cartilages during **expiration**.

▶ Pleura and Lung (Surface Marking)

Surface Marking for Pleura

- **Apical pleura:**
  - ➤ Starting in the midline at the sternal angle, the anterior reflections of the parietal pleura may be traced superiorly along a curved line that diverges from the midline and extends up and outwards to the apex of the lung and pleural cavity.
  - ➤ The line lies 3–4 cm above the anterior end of the first rib; the surface marking is posterior to the medial third of the clavicle in level with the seventh cervical vertebra.
- **Anterior border of pleura:**
  - ➤ The right and left pleurae are in contact retrosternally in the midline from the second to the fourth costal cartilages, at which point they diverge.
  - ➤ The pleura on the right descends vertically to the xiphisternum, whereas the pleura on the left deviates laterally by 3–5 cm and then passes inferiorly to cross the anterior end of the sixth rib.
  - ➤ This deviation produces an area between the heart and the sternum that is free of pleura; a needle puncture (pericardiocentesis) of the heart can be performed at this site without risk of damaging the pleura.
- **Inferior border of pleura:**
  - ➤ The **costodiaphragmatic reflections** of the right pleurae follows around the chest wall from the midpoint of xiphisternal angle anteriorly to the eighth rib in the mid-clavicular line, tenth rib in the mid-axillary line and twelfth rib at paravertebral line.
  - ➤ It is almost the same for left lung but with **one exception**: It begins from the sixth rib/costal cartilage anteriorly to the eighth rib in the mid-clavicular line, tenth rib in the mid-axillary line and twelfth rib at paravertebral line.
- **Posterior border of pleura:**
  - ➤ In posterior view, the medial edges of the pleurae lies along a line joining the transverse processes of the second to the twelfth thoracic vertebrae on either side.

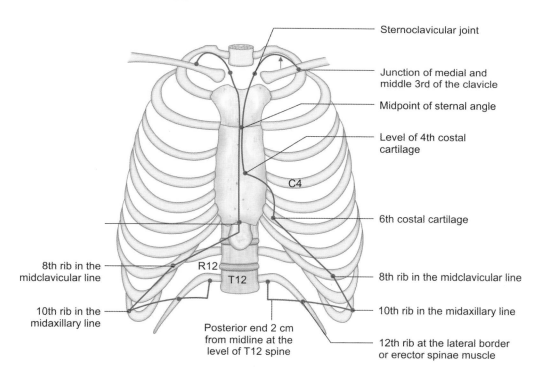

Fig. 47: Surface marking of pleura on bony cage

Surface marking for lung

- The surface markings of both the apex and costovertebral border of the **lung** correspond to those of the **parietal pleura**.
  - ➤ However there are few differences between the two which need the detailed description.
  - ➤ Pleura lies two rib lower than lung to allow lung expansion during inspiration.

Table 14: Surface marking for lungs and pleural		
Level	Costodiaphragmatic line (inferior border of pleura)	Lower border of lung (2 ribs higher)
Mid-clavicular line	8th rib	6th rib
Mid-axillary line	10th rib	8th rib
Paravertebral line	12th rib	10th rib

- ❏ Conventionally, the surface projection of the lower border of the lung is represented by a curved line that crosses the mid-clavicular line at the sixth rib, the mid-axillary line at the eighth rib and the tenth rib just lateral to the vertebral column.
- ❏ CT data reveal considerable variation, redefining the lower lung border.
- ❏ Lower anterior border of the right lung is at seventh rib in the mid-clavicular line and left lung at fifth rib in the mid-clavicular line.
- ❏ **Oblique fissure:**
  - ➤ On each side, the upper and lower lobes of the lung are separated by the oblique fissure.
  - ➤ It is marked by a line that runs anteroinferiorly from the posterior end of the fourth rib (spinous process of the third thoracic vertebra), crosses the fifth rib in the mid-axillary line and continues inferiorly, crossing sixth rib on both sides at the mid-clavicular line (i.e. 7–8 cm lateral to the midline).
  - ➤ The oblique fissure follows the medial border of the scapula when the upper limb is in full abduction. The left oblique fissure may be slightly more vertical than the right.
- ❏ **Horizontal fissure:** It lies between the upper and middle lobes of the right lung.
  - ➤ It extends from the fourth costal cartilage at the right sternal border to intersect the oblique fissure at mid-axillary line.
- ❏ The **right middle lobe** may be projected on to the thoracic wall using three points namely: The fourth costal cartilage at the right parasternal edge, the fifth rib at the mid-axillary line and the sixth rib at the mid-clavicular line.

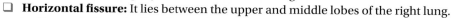

Fig. 48: Surface markings of the lung and pleura on the front

Labels in Fig. 48: Site of sternal angle; Sternoclavicular joint; Level of 4th costal cartilage; Area of superficial cardiac dullness; 6th costal cartilage; 6th rib; 8th rib; Just above the xiphisternal joint

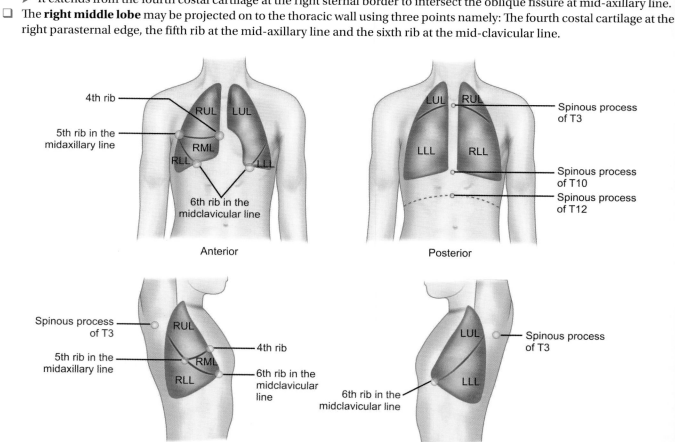

Fig. 49: Surface projection of different lobes of lungs (RUL = right upper lobe, LUL = left upper lobe, RML = right middle lobe, RLL = right lower lobe, LLL = left lower lobe)

❑ The upper and middle lobes lie anterior to the oblique fissure and are clinically examined from in front and to the side.
❑ The lower lobes lie **posteriorly** and should be examined from behind.

1. Surface marking of the oblique fissure of lung include all EXCEPT: *(NEET Pattern 2013)*
   a. T3 vertebra   b. 5th rib
   c. 7th rib   d. 6th costal cartilage

2. The right costophrenic line extends up to the level of which rib in the mid-axillary line: *(NEET Pattern 2014)*
   a. 6th   b. 8th
   c. 10th   d. 12th

1. c. 7th rib
   ❑ 7th rib does not come in the surface marking of oblique fissure.
   ❑ Oblique fissure passes anteroinferiorly from the **spinous process of the T3** vertebra to cross the **fifth rib** in the midaxillary line and further continues inferiorly, crossing the sixth rib (**and costal cartilage**) at the mid-clavicular line.

2. c. 10th
   ❑ Right costophrenic line measures approximately 5 **cm vertically** and extends from the **eighth to the tenth rib** along the midaxillary line.

❑ Area of **superficial cardiac dullness** is between **4th and 6th** costal cartilages.

Pericardium and Cavity

❑ Pericardium is a fibroserous sac that enloses the heart and the roots of the great vessels and occupies the middle mediastinum pericardium.
   ➤ Fibrous pericardium is the outer dense, fibrous layer that blends with the adventitia of the roots of the great vessels and the central tendon of the diaphragm.
   ➤ Parietal layer of serous pericardium lines the inner surface of the fibrous pericardium, and reflects as the visceral layer on the outer surface of heart forming epicardium.
❑ Arterial supply: Pericardiophrenic, bronchial, and esophageal arteries.
❑ Nerve supply: Phrenic nerve, vagus nerves and the sympathetic trunks.
❑ Clinical correlation: Pain sensation carried by the phrenic nerves is often referred to the skin (C3 to C5 dermatomes) of the ipsilateral supraclavicular region.

Table 15: Differences between the parietal and serous pericardium

Parietal pericardium	Visceral pericardium (epicardium)
It is adherent to the fibrous pericardium	It is adherent to the myocardium of the heart
It develops from somatopleuric mesoderm	It develops from splanchnopleuric mesoderm
It is innervated by the somatic nerve fibers	It is innervated by the autonomic nerve fibers
It is sensitive to pain	It is insensitive to pain

Pericardial cavity is a potential space between the visceral and parietal layers of the serous pericardium, lined by mesothelium.
❑ It normally contains a small amount of pericardial fluid (20 mL), which allows friction-free movement of the heart during diastole and systole.
❑ The reflections of the serosal layer are arranged as two complex 'tubes'; the aorta and pulmonary trunk are enclosed in one, and the venae cavae and four pulmonary veins lie in the other.
❑ The perivenous tube is an inverted J; the cul-de-sac within its curve posterior to the left atrium is termed the oblique sinus.
❑ The transverse sinus is a passage between the two pericardial tubes; the aorta and pulmonary trunk are anterior, and the atria and their great veins are posterior.

Table 16: Pericardial sinuses

Pericardial sinus	Location	Relations
Transverse	Lies between arterial and venous sleeves of pericardial reflection	▪ Anterior: Ascending aorta and pulmonary trunk ▪ Posterior: Superior vena cava and atria ▪ Superior: Bifurcation of pulmonary trunk ▪ Inferior: Upper surface of left atrium
Oblique	It is a recess of serous pericardium behind the base of the heart, lies within the venous sleeve of pericardial reflection	▪ Anterior: Left atrium ▪ Posterior: Parietal layer of pericardium* ▪ Superior: Upper margin on left atrium ▪ Left: Left pair of pulmonary veins ▪ Right: Right pair of pulmonary veins and IVC

*Pericardium separates the oblique sinus from esophagus.

▼ Heart: Surface, Borders, Grooves and Chambers

The heart has the following three surfaces: Sternocostal (anterior), diaphragmatic (inferior) and left surface.

- ❑ **Anterior (sternocostal)** surface is formed mostly by right ventricle and right auricle and partly by left ventricle and left auricle.
  - ➢ Anterior interventricular groove is evident on this surface which separates right and left ventricle.
  - ➢ The left atrium is hidden on the front by the ascending aorta and pulmonary trunk.
- **The base** (posterior surface) is formed primarily by the **left atrium** (2/3) and partly by the posterior part of **right atrium** (1/3).
  - ➢ It is directed backwards and to the right (i.e. opposite to the apex).
  - ➢ It lies in front of the middle four thoracic vertebrae (T5–T8) in the lying-down position and descends one vertebra in the erect posture (T6–T9).
  - ➢ The base is separated from vertebral column by the oblique pericardial sinus, esophagus, and aorta.
  - ➢ Some authors consider the base of the heart as the upper border of the heart where great blood vessels (superior vena cava, ascending aorta and pulmonary trunk) are attached.
- ❑ **Cardiac apex** is the blunt rounded extremity of the heart formed by the left ventricle, which is directed anteroinferiorly and to the left.
  - ➢ It is overlapped by the left lung and pleura.
  - ➢ The apex is located most commonly behind the fifth left intercostal space, near or a little medial to the midclavicular line.
- ❑ **Diaphragmatic surface** is flat and rests on the central tendon of the diaphragm.
  - ➢ It is formed mainly by the left ventricle (2/3) and partly right ventricle (1/3) which are separated from each other by the posterior interventricular groove.
- ❑ Left surface is formed mainly by the left ventricle and partly by the left atrium and auricle.
  - ➢ It is directed upwards, backwards, and to the left.

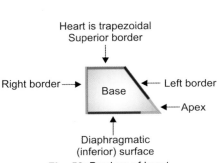

Fig. 50: Borders of heart.

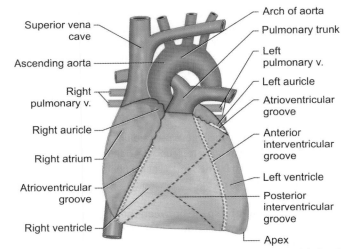

Fig. 51: Anterior (sternocostal) surface of the heart is formed mainly by the right ventricle and partly by the right atrium, left ventricle and left auricle

Grooves/Sulci

- ❑ **Coronary (atrioventricular) sulcus** is present on the external surface of the heart, in a circumferential manner around the heart, marks the division between the atria and the ventricles.
- ❑ The **crux** is the point at which the interventricular and interatrial sulci cross the coronary sulcus.
- ❑ Coronary sulcus is divided into anterior and posterior parts.
- ❑ The right half of anterior part is large and lodges right coronary artery.
- ❑ Left half of anterior part is small and lodges circumflex branch of left coronary artery.

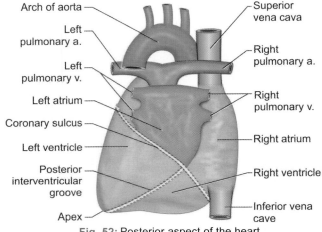

Fig. 52: Posterior aspect of the heart

Table 17: Heart sulci and their contents

Sulcus/Groove	Location	Contents
Coronary (atrioventricular) sulcus*	Between atria and ventricles, circumferentially around the heart	**Right side** ▪ Right coronary artery ▪ Small cardiac vein **Left side** ▪ Left coronary artery ▪ Circumflex artery ▪ Great cardiac vein ▪ Coronary sinus
Anterior interventricular sulcus	Between right and left ventricles; marks the interventricular septum, anteriorly	▪ Left anterior descending (anterior interventricular) artery ▪ Great cardiac vein
Posterior interventricular sulcus	Delineates the interventricular septum posteriorly	▪ Posterior interior interventricular artery ▪ Middle cardiac vein

*Coronary sulcus marks the annulosus fibrosus that supports the valves.

QUESTIONS

1. Base of the heart is formed by: *(NEET Pattern 2013)*
   a. Left atrium
   b. Right atrium
   c. Left ventricle
   d. Right ventricle

2. True about atrioventricular groove are all EXCEPT: *(NEET Pattern 2015)*
   a. Contains left anterior descending coronary artery
   b. Also called coronary sulcus
   c. Contains right coronary artery
   d. Contains circumflex branch of left coronary artery

ANSWERS

1. **a. Left atrium > b. Right atrium**
   ❑ **Base** of the heart is the posterior surface of heart and is mainly contributed by **left atrium** and partly **right atrium**.

2. **a. Contains left anterior descending coronary artery**
   ❑ **Left anterior descending coronary artery** runs in the anterior **interventricular** (not atrioventricular) groove.
   ❑ Atrioventricular groove (coronary sulcus) **separates** atria from ventricles.
   ❑ Right coronary artery lodges in right part of coronary sulcus and left coronary artery gives circumflex branch in left part of coronary sulcus.

- ▪ Posterior to sternum is **right ventricle** *(NEET Pattern 2013)*
- ▪ **Apex** of the heart is formed by **left ventricle** *(NEET Pattern 2016)*
- ▪ **Lower half** of arch of aorta lies **behind manubrium sternum**.
- ▪ **Right border** of heart is formed by SVC, **right atrium** and IVC *(NEET Pattern 2016)*
- ▪ **Most fixed** part of the heart is **base of the heart**.

◢ Heart Chambers

Right atrium has an anterior rough-walled portion (atrium proper and the auricle) lined with pectinate muscles and a posteriorly situated smooth-walled (sinus venarum) into which the two vena cavae open.

❑ Sulcus terminalis is a groove on the external surface of the right atrium (embryologic junction of the sinus venosus and primitive atrium) corresponding to crista terminalis on internal surface.

❑ Crista terminalis is a vertical muscular ridge running anteriorly along the right atrial wall from the SVC to IVC opening and provide the origin of the pectinate muscles.

❑ Pectinate muscles are the prominent ridges of atrial myocardium located in the interior of both auricles and the right atrium.

Table 18: Differences between the smooth and rough parts of the right atrium

Smooth part (sinus venarum)	Rough part (atrium proper)
Developmetally it is derived from right horn of the sinus venosus	Development it is derived from primitive atrium
All the venous channels *EXCEPT* anterior cardiac veins open into this part (e.g., SVC, IVC, coronary sinus., and venae cordae minimi)	Presents series of transverse ridges, the musculi pectinati which arise from the *crista terminalis* and run forwards towards the auricle. The interior of auricle presents reticular sponge-like network of the muscular ridges

Right atrium is larger but thinner than the left atrium.

❑ Right auricle is the conical muscular pouch of the upper anterior portion of the right atrium, it covers the proximal part of the right coronary artery.

❑ Posterior smooth-wall (sinus venarum) receives the opening of SVC, IVC and coronary sinus.

❑ **Eustachian valve** of the IVC and the **Thebesian valve** of the coronary sinus are evident on the interior.

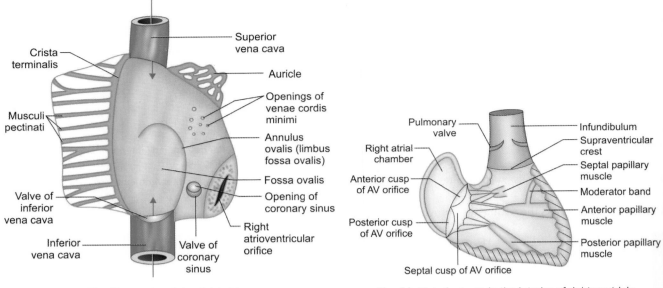

Fig. 53: Interior of the right atrium   Fig. 54: Main features in the interior of right ventricle

- ❑ **Fossa ovalis** is an oval-shaped depression in the interatrial septum and represents the site of the foramen ovale, through which blood runs from the right atrium to the left atrium in fetal circulation. It has an upper rounded (horseshoe-shaped) margin known as **limbus fossa ovalis**.

Left atrium has smooth wall, except for a few pectinate muscles in the auricle.
- ❑ It is the most posterior of the four chambers lying posterior to the right atrium but anterior to the esophagus and shows no structural borders on a posteroanterior (PA) radiograph.
- ❑ Four valveless pulmonary veins from lungs (oxygenated blood) open into the left atrium.

Right ventricle is largely evident anteriorly and contributes to the major portion of the sternocostal surface of the heart.
- ❑ The trabeculated inflow tract of the RV receives venous blood from the right atrium posteriorly through the tricuspid valve while the smooth outflow tract conus arteriosus (infundibulum) expels blood superiorly and to the left into the pulmonary trunk.
- ❑ **Trabeculae carneae** are irregular anastomosing muscular ridges, which form the trabeculated part of the ventricles (inflow tract) and develop embryologically from the primitive ventricle.
- ❑ **Supraventricular crest** (a C-shaped internal muscular ridge), marks the junction between the trabeculated part and smooth part of the right ventricle.
- ❑ **Papillary muscles** are cone-shaped muscles enveloped by endocardium, extend from the anterior and posterior ventricular walls and the septum, and their apices are attached to the chordae tendineae.
- ❑ These contract to tighten the chordae tendineae, preventing the cusps of the tricuspid valve from being everted into the atrium, preventing regurgitation of ventricular blood into the right atrium.
- ❑ Chordae tendineae extend from one papillary muscle to more than one cusp of the tricuspid valve.
- ❑ **Septomarginal trabecula** is an isolated band of trabeculae carneae that forms a bridge between the intraventricular (IV) septum and the base of the anterior papillary muscle of the anterior wall of the right ventricle.
- ❑ It is called the **moderator band** for its ability to prevent overdistention of the ventricle and carries the right limb (Purkinje fibers) of the atrioventricular bundle from the septum to the sternocostal wall of the ventricle.
- ❑ Interventricular septum gives origin of the septal papillary muscle. It has a small membranous upper part and lower muscular part.

Table 19: Differences of inflowing and outflowing parts of the right ventricle	
Inflowing lower part	**Outflowing upper part**
It develops from primitive ventricle	It develops from bulbus cordis
It is large in size and lies below the supraventricular crest	It is small in size and lies above the supraventricular crest
It is rough due to presence of the muscular ridges—the *trabeculae carneae*. It forms most of the right ventricular chamber	It is smooth and forms upper 1 inch conical part of the right ventricular chamber—the infundibulum, which gives rise to pulmonary trunk

Left ventricle is mainly evident at the posterior view of the heart, its apex is directed downward, forward, and **towards the left.**
- ❑ The trabeculated inflow tract of the LV receives oxygenated blood from the left atrium through the mitral valve while the smooth outflow tract of the LV expels blood superoanteriorly into the ascending aorta.

- It is divided into the left ventricle proper and the aortic vestibule, which is the upper anterior part of the left ventricle, leading into the aorta.
- It has two papillary muscles (anterior and posterior) with their chordae tendineae and a meshwork of muscular ridges, the trabeculae carneae cordis.
- Left ventricle has a **thicker (three times)** wall, and is longer, narrower, and more conical-shaped than the right ventricle.

Table 20: Differences between the inflowing and outflowing parts of the left ventricle

Inflowing part	Outflowing part
It develops from primitive ventricle	It develops from bulbus cordis
It lies below the aortic vestibule	It lies between the membranous part of the interventricular part of the interventricular septum and anterior cusp of the mitral valve
It is rough due to presence of trabeculae carneae and forms most of the left ventricular chamber	It is smooth and forms smooth small upper part—the aortic vestibule, which gives rise to the ascending aorta

Table 21: Differences between the right and left ventricles

Right ventricle	Left ventricle
Receives deoxygenated blood from right atrium and pumps it to the lungs through pulmonary trunk	Receives oxygenated blood from left atrium and pumps it to the whole body through aorta
Wall of right ventricle is thinner than that of left ventricle (ratio 1: 3)	Wall of left ventricle is thicker than that of right ventricle (ratio 3:1)
Possesses three papillary muscles (anerior, posterior, and septal)	Possesses two papillary muscles (anterior and posterior)
Moderator band present	Moderator band absent
Cavity of righ ventricle is crescentic in shape in cross section	Cavity of left ventricle is circular in shape in cross section

QUESTIONS

1. **WRONG statement about right atrium is:** *(PGIC)*
   a. Related to central tendon of diaphragm at T10 level
   b. AV node is present in muscular atrioventricular septum
   c. Auricle is present superolaterally
   d. Crista terminalis divides right atrium in two parts
   e. Coronary sinus lies between fossa ovalis and IVC

2. **Torus aorticus is seen due to:** *(NEET Pattern 2015)*
   a. Atrium bulging into the aorta
   b. Aortic sinus bulging into left atrium
   c. Aortic sinus bulging into right atrium
   d. Aortic wall tear

3. **Trabeculae carneae are present in:** *(NEET Pattern 2016)*
   a. Left atrium
   b. Right atrium
   c. Left ventricle
   d. Right ventricle

4. **NOT true about right atrium:** *(NEET Pattern)*
   a. Fossa ovalis represent remnant of foramen ovale
   b. Anterior and posterior parts are divided by Crista terminalis
   c. Anterior part is derived from absorption of right horn of sinus venosus
   d. Posterior part is smooth

ANSWERS

1. **a. Related to central tendon of diaphragm at T10 level; c. Auricle is present superolaterally; e. Coronary sinus lies between fossa ovalis and IVC**
   - Right atrium is related to central tendon of diaphragm at **T8 vertebra** level, at the IVC opening.
   - AV node is present in atrial component of the **muscular** atrioventricular septum in Koch's triangle.
   - Auricle in the right atrium lies **superomedially**. Crista terminalis **divides** right atrium into smooth posterior part and rough anterior part.
   - Coronary sinus opening lies between fossa ovalis **and tricuspid orifice**.

2. **c. Aortic sinus bulging into right atrium**
   - Torus aorticus (aortic mound) is the prominent region of the **right atrial septum**, which marks the projection of the **noncoronary aortic sinus** into the right atrial wall.
   - The bulge is superior to the coronary sinus and anterior to the fossa ovalis.
   - The right coronary artery arises from the anterior ('right coronary') aortic sinus; The left coronary artery arises from the left posterior (left coronary) aortic sinus.

3. **c. Left ventricle > d. Right ventricle**
   - **Trabeculae carneae** are rounded or irregular muscular columns which project from the inner surface of the **left and right ventricles** of the heart.
   - These are different from the **pectinate muscles**, which are present in the **atria** of the heart.

4. **c. Anterior part is derived from absorption of right horn of sinus venosus**
   - **Anterior** part of right atrium is derived from **primitive atrium**. Posterior **smooth** part (sinus venarum) is derived from absorption of right horn of sinus venosus. **Crista terminalis** is the boundary line between the two parts.

- **Supraventricular crest** lies between right ventricular **inlet** and **outlet** *(JIPMER 2017)*
- **Right ventricle** rests on **central tendon** of diaphragm, forms anterior **surface** of heart has a wall thickness is **3–5 mm** and is **crescent shape** in cross section *(NEET Pattern 2016)*
- In **TEE** (transesophageal echocardiography) most commonly evaluated is **left atrium** *(JIPMER 2016)*
- Openings in the right atrium: Inferior vena cava opening is guarded by **Eustachian valve** (rudimentary), coronary sinus by **Thebesian valve** and atrioventricular opening by **tricuspid valve.**
- **SA node** is situated in the **upper part** of crista terminalis *(NEET Pattern 2015)*

▼ Heart Valves

Heart valves are situated around the **fibrous rings** of the cardiac skeleton and are **lined with endocardium**.

- ❑ There are two pairs of valves in the heart: (a) a pair of **atrioventricular** valves, and (b) a pair of **semilunar** valves.
- ❑ **Pulmonary valve** is the semilunar valve that lies between the right ventricle and the pulmonary artery and has **three cusps** (anterior, right, and left).
- ❑ **Aortic valve** is the semilunar valve located between the left ventricle and the aorta and is composed of **three cusps** (posterior, right, and left).
- ❑ **Tricuspid valve** lies between the right atrium and ventricle, has anterior, posterior, and septal cusps, which are attached by the **chordae tendineae** to three **papillary muscles** that keep the valve closed.
- ❑ Mitral valve lies between the left atrium and ventricle, has **two cusps**: a larger anterior and a smaller posterior both of which are tethered to papillary muscles (anterolateral and posteromedial) by chordae tendineae.
- ❑ First (lubb) heart sounds is caused by the **closure** of the mitral and tricuspid valves (M1T1) at the onset of ventricular systole.
- ❑ Second (dup) heart sound is caused by the **closure** of the aortic and pulmonary valves (A2P2) at the onset of ventricular diastole.

▼ Conduction System of Heart

Conduction system of the heart is constituted by the specialized cardiac muscle cells that lie immediately beneath the endocardium and carry impulses throughout the cardiac muscle, signaling the heart chambers to contract in the proper sequence.

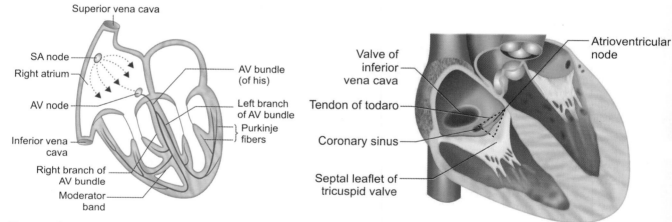

Fig. 55: Conducting system of the heart (SA = sinuatrial, AV = atrioventricular)

Fig. 56: Triangle of Koch, at the apex of which lies the atrioventricular node

Sinuatrial node is located at the **junction** of the SVC and right atrium. It is present in the **sub-epicardial region.** Some authors mention its presence in **myocardium**.

- ❑ Embryologically it develops at the **upper end of crista terminalis** (junction between the sinus venosus and the atrium proper).
- ❑ It is the **dominant pacemaker** of the heart. It initiates the cardiac impulse, **simply because** it generates impulses slightly faster than the other areas with pacemaker potential.

    Atrioventricular node is located within the right side (atrial component) of the muscular **atrioventricular septum** near the ostium of the coronary sinus.

- ❑ It is present in the **subendocardial** region, more precisely at the **apex of Koch's triangle**.

    Triangle of Koch: A roughly triangular area on the septal wall of the right atrium, bounded by the **septal leaflet of the tricuspid valve** inferiorly, the anteromedial margin of the **orifice of the coronary sinus** as a base, and the **tendon of Todaro** superiorly.

❑ It **contains the AV node** and the proximal penetrated portion of the bundle of His.
   ➤ In a case of AV nodal **re-entry tachycardia**, radiofrequency ablation of this triangular area improves the symptoms.
   From the SA node, the impulse spreads throughout the right atrium and to the AV node via the anterior, middle, and posterior **internodal tracts** and to the left atrium via the **Bachmann bundle**.

❑ **AV bundle of His** begins at the AV node (at the apex of Koch's triangle) and runs along the right side of the **membranous** part of the interventricular septum.

❑ It splits into **right** and **left bundle branches**, which descend into the muscular part of the interventricular septum.

❑ **Left** bundle branch (LBB) is **thicker** than the RBB.

❑ A portion of the RBB enters the **moderator band (septomarginal trabecula)** to reach the anterior papillary muscle.

❑ Both bundle branches terminate in a complex network of intramural **Purkinje myocytes** to spread out into the ventricular walls.

Table 22: Showing the components of conducting system and their location in heart	
Component of conduction system	**Location**
SA node	▪ Subepicardial (? myocardium) ▪ Right atrium – Upper end of crista terminalis – Near opening of SVC
AV node	▪ Triangle of Koch's – In the atrioventricular septum – Near lower part interatrial septum – Sub-endocardial
AV bundle of His	Membranous part of interventricular septum
RBB	Right surface of interventricular septum
LBB	Left surface of interventricular septum
Purkinje fibers	Sub-endocardial plexus of ventricular conduction cells

QUESTIONS

1. **Boundary of Koch's triangle is NOT formed by:**
   (AIIMS; PGIC; NEET Pattern 2013)
   a. Tricuspid valve
   b. Tendon of Todaro
   c. Limbus fossa ovalis
   d. Coronary sinus

2. **Koch's triangle is bounded by all EXCEPT:**   *(JIPMER 2017)*
   a. Coronary sinus ostium
   b. IVC opening
   c. Tendon of Todaro
   d. Septal cusp of tricuspid valve

ANSWERS

1. **c. Limbus fossa ovalis**
   ❑ Limbus fossa ovalis is **not in the boundary** of Koch's triangle.
   ❑ The boundaries are: Septal cusp of tricuspid valve; tendon of Todaro (fibrous skeleton of heart) and coronary sinus opening.

2. **b. IVC opening**
   ❑ Koch's triangle is bounded in front by the base of septal leaflet of tricuspid valve, behind by anterior margin of the opening of coronary sinus and above by the tendon of Todaro.

▪ **SA node** is present in the **sub-epicardial region**. Some authors mention its presence in **myocardium**.
▪ **Purkinje fibers** are modified **cardiac muscle** *(NEET pattern 2014)*

▶ Fibrous Skeleton of heart

Running at the **ventricular base** is a complex framework of **dense collagen** with membranous, tendinous and **fibroareolar extensions**, intimately related to **atrioventricular valves** and the **aortic orifice** (pulmonary valve is **not** contained in it).

❑ The skeleton **does not provide support** for the cardiac valves, as such.

❑ It serves as the **origin and insertion sites** of cardiac myocytes and forms an **electrical barrier** between the atria and ventricles so that they contract independently.

❑ The right and left fibrous rings of heart (**annulus fibrosus cordis**) surround the atrioventricular and arterial orifices.

❑ The right fibrous ring is known as the annulus fibrosus **dexter** cordis, and the left is known as the annulus fibrosus **sinister** cordis.

❑ The fibrous skeleton is **strongest** at the junction of the aortic, mitral and tricuspid valves, the so-called **central fibrous body**.

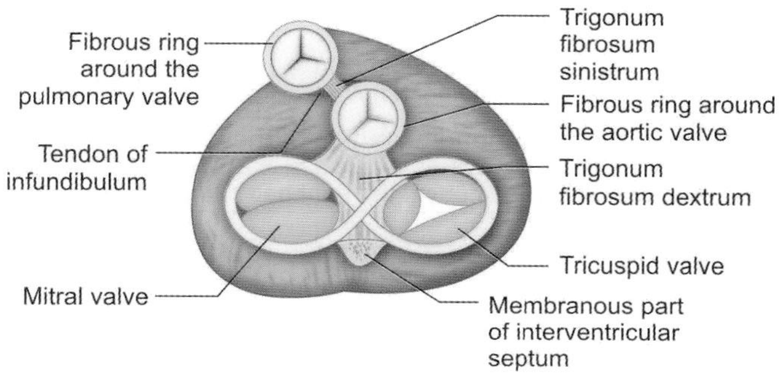

Fig. 57: Fibrous skeleton of heart

QUESTIONS

1. TRUE statement(s) regarding fibrous skeleton of heart is/are: *(PGIC 2017)*
  a. Framework of collagen fibers and fibroareolar extensions
  b. Related to atrioventricular valves and the aortic and pulmonary valves
  c. Provide support for cardiac valves
  d. Tendon of Todaro is a part of it
  e. Maintains electrophysiological discontinuity between the atria and ventricles

ANSWERS

1. a. Framework of collagen fibers and fibroareolar extensions; e. Maintains electrophysiological discontinuity between the atria and ventricles
  ❏ Fibrous skeleton of heart is intimately related to atrioventricular valves and the aortic orifice (**but pulmonary valve is not** contained in it). It **does not provide support** for cardiac valves. **Tendon of Todaro** is a persistent continuation of the embryonic venous valves (**not a part of fibrous skeleton** of heart).

❏ **Strongest** fibrous ring of the **skeleton** of heart is around the **aortic orifice.**

▶ Surface Marking of Heart

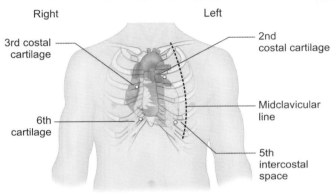
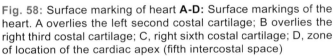

Fig. 58: Surface marking of heart **A-D:** Surface markings of the heart. A overlies the left second costal cartilage; B overlies the right third costal cartilage; C, right sixth costal cartilage; D, zone of location of the cardiac apex (fifth intercostal space)

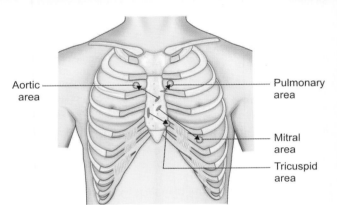

Fig. 59: Surface marking of heart valves

Upper border; It slopes from the 2nd left costal cartilage to the 3rd right costal cartilage
  ❏ **Right border:** Is a curved line, convex to the right, running from the 3rd to the 6th right costal cartilages, usually 1–2 cm lateral to the sternal edge.
  ❏ **Inferior (acute) border:** Runs leftwards from the sixth right costal cartilage to the cardiac apex, located approximately 9 (8.7±1) cm lateral to the midline (in the left fifth intercostal space).
  ❏ **Left (obtuse) border:** Is convex laterally and extends from the cardiac apex to meet the 2nd left costal cartilage approximately 1 cm from the left sternal edge.

Table 23: Cardiac valves and auscultatory areas		
Cardiac valves	**Surface marking (orifice)**	**Auscultatory area**
Pulmonary	Horizontal line (2.5 cm) over the superior border of the left third costal cartilage*	Sternal end of the left second intercostal space
Aortic	Oblique line (2.5 cm) running inferolaterally and to the right from the medial end of the left third intercostal space*	Sternal end of the right second intercostal space
Tricuspid	Vertical line (4 cm) that starts near the midline just below the level of the right (CC-4) fourth costal cartilage and passes down and slightly to the right*	Over the left lower sternal border at the level of the fifth intercostal space
Mitral	Oblique line (3 cm) opposite the left fourth costal cartilage and descending to the right*	Near the cardiac apex ⊠ 9 (8.7±1) cm lateral to the midline (in the left fifth intercostal space)

*and behind the corresponding region of the sternum

Note: Tricuspid valve lies behind the right half of the sternum opposite to the 4th and 5th intercostal spaces.

The cardiovascular silhouette (shadow), is the contour of the heart and great vessels seen on posterior–anterior **chest radiographs.**
  ❏ Its right border is formed by the SVC, the right atrium, and the IVC.
  ❏ The **left border** is formed by the aortic arch (which produces the aortic knuckle), the pulmonary trunk, the left auricle, and the left ventricle.
  ❏ Its **inferior border** is formed by the right ventricle, and the left atrium shows no border.

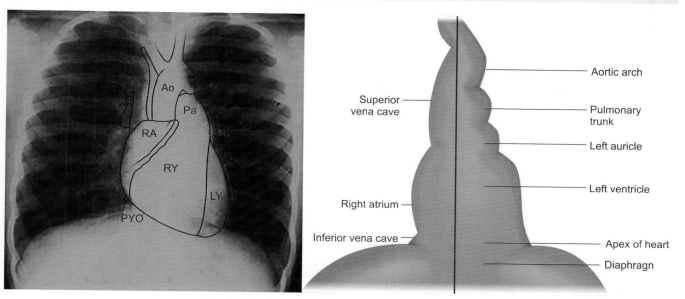

Fig. 60: Borders of cardiac silhouette on chest X-ray

QUESTIONS

1. **Which of the following represents the surface marking of the aortic valve:** *(NEET Pattern 2012)*
   a. Sternal end of the left 3rd costal cartilage
   b. Sternal end of the right 3rd costal cartilage
   c. Behind the sternum in left 3rd intercostal space
   d. Behind the sternum in right 3rd intercostal space

2. **Surface marking of the mitral valve is:** *(NEET Pattern 2012)*
   a. Behind sternal end of the left 4th costal cartilage
   b. Behind sternal end of the right 4th costal cartilage
   c. Left 4th intercostal space in midclavicular line
   d. Left 3rd intercostal space in midclavicular line

ANSWERS

1. **c. Behind the sternum in left 3rd intercostal space**
   ❑ Aortic valve is represented by an oblique line (2.5 cm) running inferolaterally and to the right from the medial end of the **left third intercostal space** (and behind the corresponding region of the sternum).

2. **a. Behind sternal end of the left 4th costal cartilage**
   ❑ The orifice of the mitral valve is level with the left half of the sternum opposite the **left fourth costal cartilage** and is represented by an oblique line approximately 3 cm long and descending to the right.

❑ **Right border** of heart is formed by the **SVC**, **IVC** and the **right atrium**. Some authors mention **ascending aorta** in the right border of heart, as well.

▼ Arterial Supply of Heart

Coronary arteries arise from the sinus (of Valsalva) in the ascending aorta and are filled with blood during the **ventricular diastole**.

❑ They have maximal blood flow during diastole and minimal blood flow during systole because of compression of the arterial branches in the myocardium during systole.
❑ **Right coronary artery** takes origin from the anterior (right) aortic sinus of the ascending aorta, runs between the root of the pulmonary trunk and the right auricle, and then descends in the right coronary sulcus, and majorly supplies the right atrium and ventricle. Branches (table)
❑ **Left coronary artery** takes origin from the left aortic sinus of the ascending aorta, just above the aortic semilunar valve.
   ➢ It is shorter than the right coronary artery and usually is distributed to more of the myocardium.
❑ **Circumflex artery** is a branch of left coronary artery, runs in the coronary sulcus, gives off the left marginal artery, supplies the left atrium and left ventricle, and anastomoses with the terminal branch of the right coronary artery.

Table 24: Arteries of heart and their area of distribution

Artery/branches	Distribution
Right coronary artery	▪ Right ventricle
▪ Acute marginal	▪ Right atrium
▪ Posterior interventricular (posterior descending)	▪ Interventricular septum (posterior 1/3)
▪ Right conus (infundibular)	▪ Left ventricle (partly)*
▪ SA nodal artery (65% population)	▪ SA Node (65% population)
▪ AV nodal artery (80% population)	▪ AV node (20% population)
▪ Atrial, anterior and posterior ventricular	▪ Bundle of His (partly)
	▪ Left bundle branch (partly)

Artery/branches	Distribution
Left coronary artery ▪ Anterior interventricular (left anterior descending) ▪ Circumflex ▪ Left diagonal ▪ Obtuse marginal (left marginal) ▪ Left conus ▪ SA nodal artery (35% population) ▪ AV nodal artery (20% population) ▪ Atrial, anterior and posterior ventricular	▪ Left ventricle ▪ Left atrium ▪ Interventricular septum (anterior 2/3) ▪ Right ventricle (partly)** ▪ SA Node (35% population) ▪ AV node (80% population) ▪ Bundle of His (major portion) ▪ Left bundle branch ▪ Right bundle branch

*Small part of left ventricle adjoining posterior interventricular groove
**Small part of right ventricle adjoining anterior interventricular groove

SA node receives blood supply from the SA node artery, a branch of the right coronary artery in the majority (about 60–70%) of hearts, and a branch of the left coronary artery (usually the left circumflex artery) in about 20–30% of hearts, fewer than 10% of nodes receive a bilateral supply.

Table 25: Arterial supply to conduction system

Part of conduction system	Arterial supply
SA node	Right coronary artery (65%) Left coronary artery (35%)
AV node	Right coronary artery (80%) Left coronary artery (20%)
AV bundle of His	Left coronary artery Right coronary artery (partly)
Left bundle branch	Left coronary artery Right coronary artery (partly)

Table 26: Arterial supply to heart

Artery/branch	Origin	Course	Distribution	Anastomoses
Right coronary artery (RCA)	Right aortic sinus	Follows coronary (AV) sulcus between atria and ventricles	Right atrium, SA and AV nodes, and posterior part of IVS	Circumflex and anterior IV branches of LCA
SA nodal`	RCA near its origin (60%)	Ascends of SA node	Pulmonary trunk and SA node	
Right marginal	RCA	Passes to inferior margin of heart and apex	Right ventricle and apex of heart	IV branches
Posterior interventicular	RCA (in 67%)	Runs in posterior IV groove to apex of heart	Right and left ventricles and posterior third of IVS	Anterior IV branch of LCA (at apex)
AV nodal	RCA near origin of posterior IV artery	Passes to AV node	AV node	
Left coronary artery (LCA)	Left aortic sinus	Runs in AV groove and gives off anterior IV and circumflex branches	Most of left atrium and ventricle, IVS, and AV bundles; may supply AV node	RCA
SA nodal	Circumflex branch of LCA (in 40%)	Ascends on posterior surface of left atrium to SA node	Lelf atrium and SA node	
Anterior interventricuar	LCA	Passes along anterior IV groove to apex of heart	Right and left ventricles and anterior two thirds of IVS	Posterior IV branch of RCA (at apex)
Circumflex	LCA	Passes to left in AV sulcus and runs to posterior surface of heart	Left atrium and left ventricle	RCA
Left marginal	Circumflex branch of LCA	Follow left border of heart	Left ventricle	IV branches
Posterior interventricular	LCA (in 33%)	Runs in posterior IV groove to apex of heart	Right and left ventricles and posterior third of IVS	Anterior IV branch of LCA (at apex)

SA nodal artery passes between the right atrium and the root of the ascending aorta, encircles the base of the SVC, and supplies the SA node and the right atrium.

❑ The first branch of right coronary artery is called as conus artery.
  ➤ This is sometimes termed a 'third coronary' artery (may arise separately from the anterior aortic sinus in 36% of individuals or may be a branch of left coronary artery occasionally).

Applied anatomy:

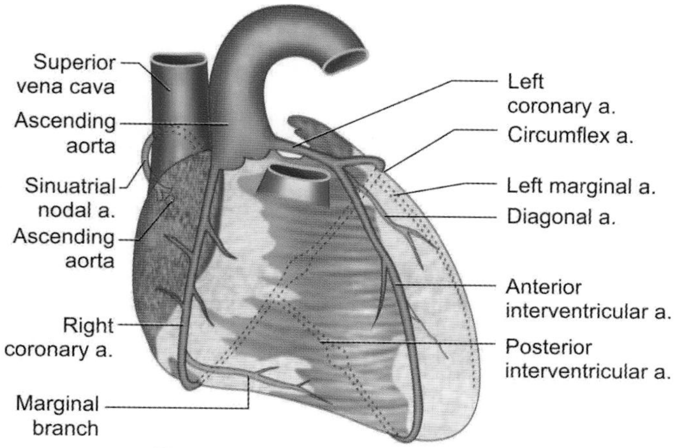

Fig. 61: Arterial supply of the heart

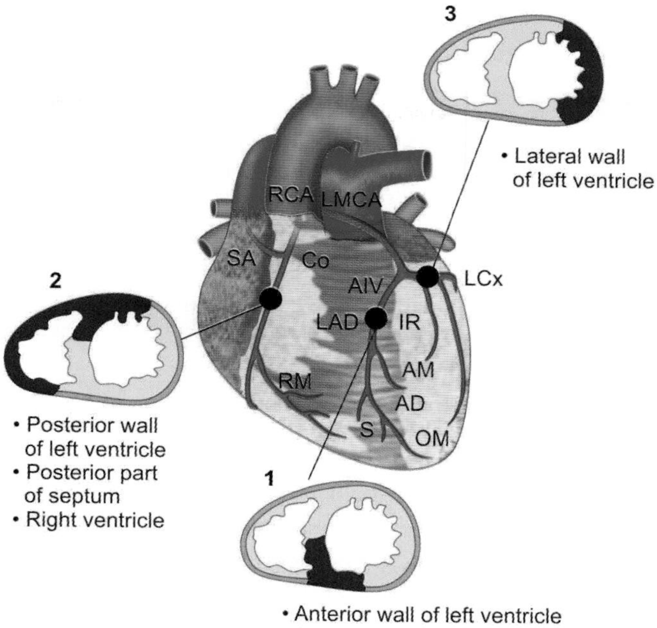

Fig. 62: Sites of infarct in coronary artery blocks

Myocardial infarction due to thrombotic occlusion of a coronary artery involves a localized area, as depicted in the diagram. **Most commonly** involved is LAD-left anterior descending artery (50%), followed by the RCA—right coronary artery (30%), and then the LCx—left circumflex artery (15%). This is indicated by the numbers 1, 2, and 3.

QUESTIONS

1. **Occlusion of the LAD will lead to infarction of which area:** *(NEET pattern 2012)*
   a. Posterior part of the interventricular septum
   b. Anterior wall of the left ventricle
   c. Lateral part of the heart
   d. Inferior surface of right ventricle

2. **Right coronary artery supplies all of the following parts of conducting system in the heart EXCEPT:** *(NEET Pattern 2013)*
   a. SA node
   b. AV node
   c. AV bundle
   d. Right bundle branch

3. **All of the following arteries are common sites of occlusion by a thrombus EXCEPT:** *(AIIMS 2005)*
   a. Anterior interventricular
   b. Posterior interventricular
   c. Circumflex
   d. Marginal

4. **TRUE statement about right coronary artery is/are:**
   a. Diameter less than LCA *(PGIC 2010)*
   b. RCA arises from anterior aortic sinus
   c. RCA supplies major part of right atrium and right ventricle
   d. RCA gives rise to circumflex coronary branch
   e. RCA supplies RBB

5. **Branch of right coronary artery is/are:** *(PGIC 2003)*
   a. Obtuse marginal
   b. Acute marginal
   c. Posterior interventricular
   d. Diagonal
   e. Conus artery

6. **Artery supply to Koch's triangle is from:** *(NEET Pattern 2012)*
   a. Right coronary artery
   b. Left coronary artery
   c. Left anterior descending artery
   d. Artery from anterior aortic sinus

ANSWERS

1. **b. Anterior wall of left ventricle**
   ❑ LAD (Left anterior descending) artery is also known as anterior interventricular artery and runs in the same named groove, supplying anterior 2/3 of interventricular septum lying deep to it and also the **adjacent anterior wall of the left ventricle**.
   ❑ Posterior part of the interventricular septum and inferior surface of right ventricle is supplied by PIVA (posterior interventricular artery).
   ❑ Left lateral surface of the heart is supplied by circumflex artery.

2. **d. Right bundle branch**
   ❑ **Right bundle branch** is present in that region of the interventricular septum, which is **exclusively supplied by left coronary** artery. (Note: Right coronary artery does not supply right bundle branch).
   ❑ SA node and AV node are supplied by **right coronary artery** in most of the population.
   ❑ **Major portion** of bundle of His is supplied by **left coronary artery**, and partly supplied by right coronary artery.

3. **d. Marginal**
   - ❑ Marginal arteries are **rarely** the sites of coronary vaso-occlusive disease.
   - ❑ There are two main marginal arteries: 1. Acute marginal (branch of right coronary) and 2. Obtuse marginal (branch of circumflex, left coronary artery).

4. **a. Diameter less than LCA; b. RCA arises from anterior aortic sinus; c. RCA supplies major part of right atrium and right ventricle**
   - ❑ Right coronary artery has **smaller lumen** as compared with left coronary artery (left ventricle is thicker than right).
   - ❑ Right coronary artery arises from the **anterior aortic sinus**, supplies major portion of right atrium and ventricle.
   - ❑ Circumflex artery is a branch of left coronary artery and is the exclusive supply to the **right bundle branch**.

5. **b. Acute marginal; c. Posterior interventricular; e. Conus artery**
   - ❑ Left coronary artery gives **obtuse marginal** artery, **diagonal** artery and **left conus** artery, in addition to few more.

6. **a. Right coronary artery > b. Left coronary artery**
   - ❑ **Koch's triangle** (and AV node) is supplied by **right coronary** artery in majority of population.

- ▪ **Coronary arteries** anastomoses cannot rapidly provide collateral routes sufficient to circumvent sudden coronary obstruction, so they are called as **'functional' end arteries**.
- ▪ **Endocardium** is most vulnerable to ischemia when flow through a major epicardial coronary artery is compromised, though the **endocardium** chiefly receives oxygen and nutrients by diffusion or microvasculature **directly from the chambers** of the heart.
- ▪ **Right coronary artery** (RCA) arises from the **right (anterior) aortic sinus** of the ascending aorta.
- ▪ **Left** coronary artery (LCA) arises from the **left (posterior)** aortic sinus of the ascending aorta.
- ▪ **Coronary arteries** are filled with blood **during the ventricular diastole**. They have maximal blood flow during diastole and minimal blood flow during systole because of compression of the arterial branches in the myocardium during systole.
- ▪ **Third coronary artery** is **conus artery** (NEET Pattern 2016)
- ▪ Arterial supply of **ventral 2/3rd** of interventricular septum of heart is by **left coronary artery** (NEET pattern 2015)
- ▪ **Coronary dominance** is determined by **posterior interventricular artery** (NEET pattern 2013)
- ▪ If the **circumflex artery gives** off the **posterior interventricular artery**, then the arterial supply is called **left dominance** (AIIMS 2007)
- ▪ **Posterior interventricular artery** is a branch of right coronary artery in most of the people (right dominance). In **10% population** it arises from **circumflex artery.**
- ▪ **Kugel's artery** is an arterial channel formed by the anastomosis of **atrial branch** of circumflex artery and similar **atrial branch** of right coronary artery.
- ▪ **Annulus of Vieussens** is the circular anastomotic channel around the infundibulum between right and left **conus arteries**.

▼ Venous Drainage of Heart

Cardiac veins and coronary sinus
- ❑ **Coronary sinus** is the largest vein draining the heart lying in the coronary sulcus, that separates the atria from the ventricles.
- ❑ It opens into the right atrium **between** the opening of the IVC and the tricuspid valve opening.
- ❑ It has **Thebesian valve**, which is one-cusp valve at the right margin of its aperture.
- ❑ Coronary sinus receives the great, middle, and small cardiac veins; the oblique vein of the left atrium; and the posterior vein of the left ventricle.
- ❑ **Great cardiac vein** begins at the apex of the heart and ascends in the anterior interventricular groove (along with the anterior interventricular branch of the left coronary artery), turns to the left to lie in the coronary sulcus and continues as the coronary sinus.
- ❑ **Middle cardiac vein** begins at the cardiac apex and ascends in the posterior interventricular groove (accompanying the posterior interventricular branch of the right coronary artery), drains into the right end of the coronary sinus.
- ❑ **Small cardiac vein** runs along the right margin of the heart in company with the acute marginal artery and then posteriorly in the coronary sulcus (along with right coronary artery) to end in the right end of the coronary sinus.
- ❑ **Oblique vein** of the left atrium descends to enter the coronary sinus, near its left end.
- ❑ **Anterior cardiac veins** drain the anterior right ventricle, crosses the coronary groove, and enter into the anterior wall of right atrium.
- ❑ **Smallest cardiac veins** (venae cordis minimae) are multiple veins, begin in the substance (endocardium and innermost layer of the myocardium) of all four chambers and empty directly into the same chambers.

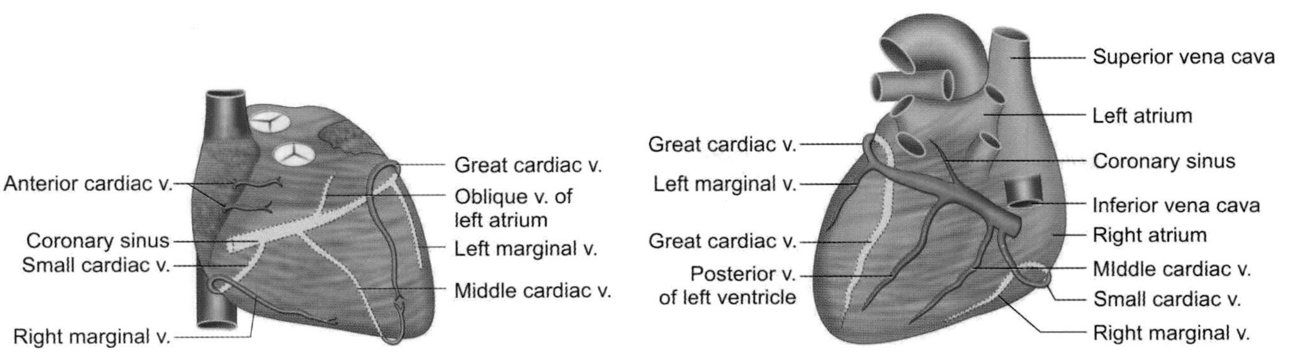

Fig. 63: Venous drainage of heart (v = vein)

QUESTIONS

1. All opens into coronary sinus EXCEPT: *(NEET Pattern 2014)*
   a. Middle cardiac vein
   b. Small cardiac vein
   c. Anterior cardiac vein
   d. Great cardiac vein

2. All veins open in sinus venarum EXCEPT:
   (NEET Pattern 2016)
   a. Coronary sinus
   b. Anterior cardiac vein
   c. Great cardiac vein
   d. SVC

3. Thebesian veins drain into: *(NEET Pattern 2016)*
   a. Right atrium
   b. Coronary sinus
   c. Great cardiac vein
   d. Anterior cardiac vein

4. All are true about coronary sinus EXCEPT:
   (NEET Pattern 2016)
   a. Develops from left horn of sinus venosus
   b. Opening is guarded by semilunar valve
   c. Situated in anterior part of coronary sulcus
   d. Directly opens into right atrium

5. The coronary sinus: *(JIPMER 2005)*
   a. Lies in anterior part of the coronary sulcus
   b. Ends in right atrium
   c. Has venae cordis minimae as its tributaries
   d. Develops from right anterior cardinal vein

6. WRONG about venous drainage of heart:
   a. Coronary sinus is guarded by Thebesian valve
   b. Middle cardiac vein lies in posterior atrioventricular groove
   c. Great cardiac vein accompanies left anterior descending artery
   d. Venae cordis minimi open into all four chambers

ANSWERS

1. c. Anterior cardiac vein
   ❑ Anterior cardiac veins open into the **anterior wall of right atrium**. They are not affected in case of coronary sinus thrombosis, where other cardiac veins are dilated.

2. c. Great cardiac vein
   ❑ Great cardiac vein drains into **coronary sinus** and not sinus venarum (posterior smooth wall of right atrium).

3. a. Right atrium
   ❑ Thebesian veins drain into **all the four** chambers of heart, are **most abundant in the right atrium** and least in the left ventricle.

4. c. Situated in anterior part of coronary sulcus
   ❑ Coronary sinus is located in **posterior** part of coronary sulcus.

5. b. Ends in right atrium
   ❑ Coronary sinus drains the venous blood of the heart into the **right atrium**.
   ❑ Coronary sinus develops from the **left horn** of the sinus venosus, lies in the **posterior part** of coronary sulcus.
   ❑ Venae cordis minimi drain **directly** into the nearest heart chamber (drain into all the 4 chambers).

6. b. Middle cardiac vein lies in posterior atrioventricular groove
   ❑ Middle cardiac vein lies in posterior interventricular (**not atrioventricular**) groove.

- **Coronary sinus** is guarded by **Thebesian** valve. *(NEET Pattern 2013)*
- **Great cardiac vein** accompanies anterior interventricular artery (Left anterior descending artery) in the **anterior interventricular groove**. *(NEET Pattern 2013, 16)*
- **Middle** cardiac vein accompanies posterior interventricular artery in the **posterior interventricular groove** *(AIPG 2003)*

◤ Innervation of Heart

Initiation of the cardiac cycle is myogenic, originating in the SA node. It is modulated in rate, force and output **by autonomic nerves**.

❑ Preganglionic sympathetic axons arise from T1-T5 spinal segment. Few fibers synapse in the corresponding thoracic sympathetic ganglia, others ascend to synapse in the **cervical ganglia; postgang**lionic fibers from these ganglia form the sympathetic cardiac nerves. Sympathetic fibers cause **cardio-stimulation** and dilate **the coronary arteries.**

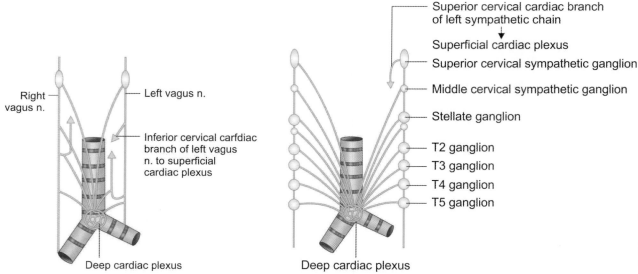

Figs. 64A and B: Deep cardiac plexus: (A) Parasympathetic contribution; (B) Sympathetic contribution (n = nerve)

❑ Preganglionic parasympathetic fibers from **dorsal nucleus of vagus** (and nucleus ambigus) run in vagal cardiac branches to synapse in the cardiac plexuses and atrial walls. Postganglionic axons are distributed to the SA node, AV node, atrial myocytes (not ventricular myocytes), and smooth muscle of coronary arteries, causing **cardio inhibition:** Deceleration in the SA node (decrease in heart rate), decrease in speed of conduction through the AV node, decreased force of contraction of atrial myocytes and coronary vasoconstriction.

❑ Cardiac plexus receives the superior, middle, and inferior cervical and thor**acic cardiac nerves from t**he sympathetic trunks and vagus nerves.

❑ Superficial cardiac plexus is located inferior to the aortic arch and anterior to the right pulmonary artery.

❑ It is contributed by: (a) superior cervical cardiac branch of left cervical sympathetic trunk, and (b) inferior cervical cardiac branch of left vagus nerve. The cardiac ganglion (of Wrisberg) is present in this plexus immediately **below the aortic ar**ch, to the right of the ligamentum arteriosum.

❑ Deep cardiac plexus is located **posterior to the aortic arch and anterior to the tracheal bifurcation**. It is contributed by: (a) all the cardiac branches derived from three cervical and upper 5 thoracic ganglia of the sympathetic chains and (b) all the cardiac branches of vagus and recurrent laryngeal nerves. The only cardiac nerves that do not join it are those that join the superficial part of the plexus.

❑ **Right** sympathetic and parasympathetic branches terminate chiefly in the region of the **SA node**, and the left branches end chiefly in the region of the AV node. The cardiac muscle fibers are devoid of motor endings and are activated by the conducting system.

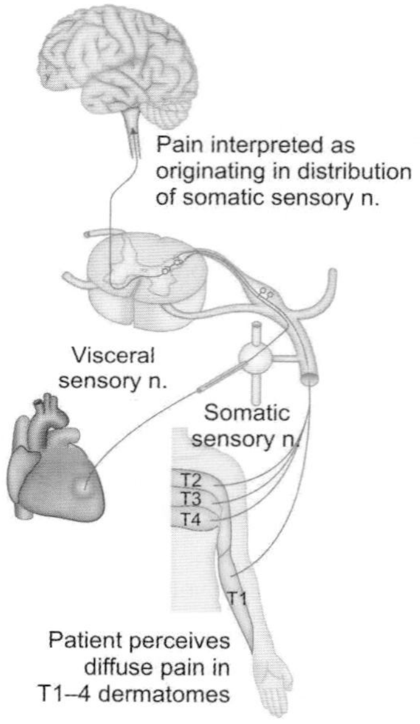

Fig. 65: Pain pathway for heart and referred pain to the precordium and upper inner arm

Sensory Fibers

Chemoreception: The neuronal cell bodies are located in the inferior (nodose) ganglia of CN X. These neurons send a peripheral process to chemoreceptors (specifically the aortic bodies) via CN X and a central process to the **nucleus tractus solitarius** in the brain. These neurons transmit changes in the partial pressure of arterial oxygen (PaO_2).

    Pressoreception: The neuronal cell bodies are located in the inferior (nodose) ganglia of CN X. These neurons send a peripheral process to baroreceptors in the great veins, atria, and aortic arch via CN X and a central process to the **nucleus tractus solitarius** in the brain. These neurons transmit changes in blood pressure.

    Nociception: The neuronal cell bodies are located in the dorsal root ganglia at T1 to T5 spinal cord levels. These neurons send a peripheral process to the heart via the sympathetic fibers and a central process to the spinal cord.

    Cardiac nociceptive impulses enter the spinal cord in the first to fifth thoracic spinal nerves, mainly via the **middle and inferior cardiac nerves**, but some fibers pass through **thoracic splanchnic** (cardiac) nerves. The pain associated with angina pectoris may be referred over the T1 to T5 dermatomes (precordium and referred pain down the left arm). Cardiac pain may be referred to the neck and mandible, because of the connection of sympathetic fibers with the cervical nerves. Sometime it is felt retrosternal and in the epigastrium due to communicating fibers with greater splanchnic nerves (T5-T9).

QUESTIONS

1. **Angina pectoris is carried by:**
   a. Superior cervical cardiac nerve
   b. Middle and inferior cervical cardiac nerve
   c. Thoracic splanchnic nerve
   d. Vagus

2. **In angina pectoris, the pain radiating down the left arm is mediated by increased activity in afferent fibers contained in the:** *(AIIMS 2003)*
   a. Carotid branch of the glossopharyngeal nerve
   b. Phrenic nerve
   c. Vagus nerve and recurrent laryngeal nerve
   d. Thoracic splanchnic nerve

3. **A 59-year-old man complains of recurrent attacks in the region of left shoulder radiating to sternum and the pit of stomach. The attacks of pain came at lengthy intervals until the last two days when it became continuous. The physician diagnosed it as an angina pectoris. In this case the pain pathway from the heart is carried by:** *(AIIMS)*
   a. Superior cervical cardiac nerve
   b. Middle and inferior cervical cardiac nerve
   c. Thoracic splanchnic nerve
   d. Vagus

4. **Cardiac ganglion is situated:** *(NEET Pattern 2015)*
   a. Below arch of aorta
   b. Above arch of aorta
   c. Left side of ligamentum arteriosum
   d. Posterior to ligamentum arteriosum

5. **True about SA node are all EXCEPT:** *(NEET Pattern 2015)*
   a. Supplied by nodal artery
   b. Primary pacemaker
   c. Supplied by left vagus nerve
   d. Made up of nodal cells and connective tissue

6. **The following statements are true regarding the SA node EXCEPT:** *(AIIMS 2005)*
   a. Is located at the right border of the ascending aorta
   b. In contains specialized nodal cardiac muscle
   c. It is supplied by the atrial branches of the right coronary artery
   d. It initiates cardiac conduction

ANSWERS

1. **b. Middle and inferior cervical cardiac nerve > c. Thoracic splanchnic nerve**
   ❑ Angina pectoris sensory impulses enter the spinal cord in the **first to fifth thoracic spinal nerves**, mainly via the middle and inferior **cervical cardiac nerves** and through **thoracic cardiac nerves** (some authors mention them as thoracic splanchnic nerves).

2. **d. Thoracic splanchnic nerve**
   ❑ In this case of angina pain, radiating to left arm (T2), the cardiac nociceptive impulses enter the spinal cord through **thoracic cardiac nerves** (some authors mention them as **thoracic splanchnic nerves**).

3. **c. Thoracic splanchnic nerve**
   ❑ This is a case of inferior wall MI and the pain fibers are carried along the **thoracic splanchnic nerve** (greater splanchnic with **root value T5-T9**), hence referred pain is felt in retrosternal and **epigastric** (T7) region.

4. **a. Below arch of aorta**
   ❑ The cardiac ganglion (of Wrisberg) is present in the **superficial cardiac plexus** immediately **below** the aortic arch to the right of the ligamentum arteriosum.

5. **c. Supplied by left vagus nerve**
   ❑ Of all the cells in the heart, those of the sinu-atrial node generate the most rapid rhythm, and therefore function as the **cardiac pacemaker**.
   ❑ It is supplied by **SA nodal artery** (generally a branch of right coronary artery).
   ❑ The heart receives parasympathetic input to the SA node via the **right vagus nerve**, and to the AV node via the left vagus nerve.
   ❑ **Nodal cells** are packed within a dense matrix of **connective tissue** as interlacing strands of **myocytes**.
   ❑ They are smaller, paler and more empty-looking than working atrial myocardial fibers.

6. **a. Is located at the right border of the ascending aorta**
   ❑ SA node is located at the right border of the superior vena cava (**not ascending aorta**).
   ❑ It contains specialized cardiac muscle having **fastest rate** of impulse generation and initiates the cardiac conduction (hence called **pacemaker** of the heart).
   ❑ SA node is supplied by the **nodal branch** of right coronary artery in about 65% of population, whereas, 35 % of the population receives the nodal branch from the circumflex branch of left coronary artery.

▪ Sympathetic nerve supply to heart arises from **T1- T5** and is excitatory to SA node. *(NEET Pattern 2013, 14)*

◢ Mediastinum

❑ **Mediastinum** is the space between the pleural cavities in the thorax, bounded laterally by the pleural cavities, anteriorly by the sternum, and posteriorly by the twelve thoracic vertebra.
   ➢ It is divided into a superior division and an inferior division by a line from the **sternal angle of Louis** to the T4 to T5 intervertebral disc.
   ➢ The inferior division is then further divided into the anterior, middle, and posterior divisions.

- ❑ **Superior mediastinum** lies between the manubrium sterni anteriorly and the upper thoracic vertebrae posteriorly.
  - ➤ Its inferior boundary is a slightly oblique plane that passes backwards from the manubriosternal joint to the lower part of the body of the fourth thoracic vertebra.
- ❑ **Inferior mediastinum** is divided into three parts—anterior, in front of the pericardium; middle, containing the pericardium and its contents; and posterior, behind the pericardium.
  - ➤ **Anterior mediastinum** is bounded anteriorly by the sternum (and transversus thoracis muscle and the fifth to seventh left costal cartilages) and posteriorly by the pericardium.
    - ▪ **Contents: Thymus, small mediastinal branches of the internal thoracic artery, lymphatic vessels and nodes, etc.**
  - ➤ **Middle mediastinum**
  - ➤ **Posterior mediastinum** is bounded anteriorly by the pericardium above and the posterior surface of the diaphragm below, posteriorly from the fifth to the twelfth thoracic vertebrae.

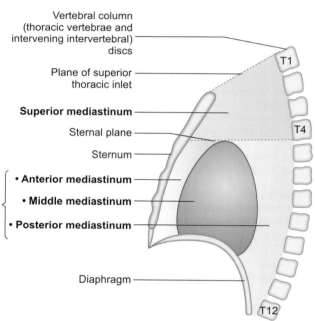

Fig. 66: Divisions of the mediastinum

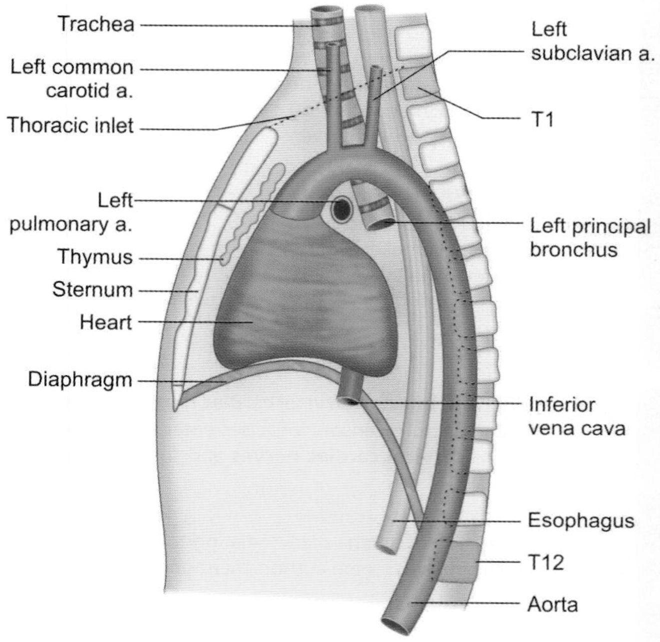

Fig. 67: Boundaries and contents of the mediastinum

Table 27: Major structures of the thoracic cavity

Mediastinum	Superior mediastinum		Thymus, great vessels, trachea, esophagus, and thoracic duct
	Inferior mediastinum	Anterior	Thymus
		Middle	Heart, pericardium, and roots of great vessels
		Posterior	Thoracic aorta, thoracic duct, esophagus, and azygos venous system

Table 28: Contents of the mediastinum

		Inferior mediastinum		
	Superior mediastrinum	**Anterior**	**Middle**	**Posterior**
Organs	▪ Thymus ▪ Esophagus ▪ Trachea	▪ Thymus	▪ Heart ▪ Pericardium	▪ Esophagus
Arteries	▪ Aortic arch ▪ Brachiocephalic trunk ▪ Left common carotid artery ▪ Left subclavian artery	▪ Smaller vessels	▪ Ascending aorta ▪ Pulmonary trunk and branches ▪ Pericardiacophrenic arteries	▪ Thoracic aorta and branches
Veins and lymph vessels	▪ Superior vena cava ▪ Brachiocephalic veins ▪ Thoracic duct	▪ Smaller vessels, lymphatics, and lymph nodes	▪ Superior vena cava ▪ Azygus vein ▪ Pulmonary veins ▪ Pericardiacophrenic veins	▪ Azygos vein ▪ Hemiazygos vein ▪ Thoracic duct
Nerves	▪ Vagus nerves ▪ Left recurrent laryngeal nerve ▪ Cardiac nerves ▪ Phernic nerves	▪ None	▪ Phrenic nerve	▪ Vagus nerves

QUESTIONS

1. **All are true about mediastinum EXCEPT:** *(PGIC 2015)*
   a. Heart passes through superior mediastinum
   b. Heart passes through middle mediastinum
   c. Thymus remnant may present in middle mediastinum
   d. Posterior boundary of posterior mediastinum corresponds to T1-T4 vertebrae
   e. Lower border of anterior mediastinum is extended more than posterior mediastinum

2. **Esophagus is present in all EXCEPT:** *(NEET Pattern 2013)*
   a. Superior mediastinum
   b. Middle mediastinum
   c. Anterior mediastinum
   d. Posterior mediastinum

ANSWERS

1. **a. Heart passes through superior mediastinum; c. Thymus remnant may present in middle mediastinum; d. Posterior boundary of posterior mediastinum corresponds to T1-T4 vertebrae; e. Lower border of anterior mediastinum is extended more than posterior mediastinum**
   - Heart is present in the **middle** mediastinum.
   - Thymus remnants may be found in **superior** and **anterior** mediastinum.
   - Posterior boundary of posterior mediastinum is from **T5-T12 vertebra**.
   - Lower border of **posterior** mediastinum extends **quite lower (inferior)** as compared with anterior mediastinum.
2. **c. Anterior mediastinum > b. Middle mediastinum**
   - Esophagus enters the **superior** mediastinum and lies between trachea (anterior) and vertebra (posterior).
   - Inferiorly it continues into the **posterior** mediastinum, pass through the diaphragm and open into stomach.

- **Trachea** lies in **superior** mediastinum.
- **Lower limit** of superior mediastinum lies at **T4 vertebral** level *(NEET Pattern 2016)*

Thoracic Outlet Syndrome

Superior thoracic aperture is also called as thoracic inlet (some authors call it thoracic outlet).

- It is bounded by **manubrium** anteriorly, **first rib** laterally, and the **first thoracic vertebrae** posteriorly.
- Structures passing through superior thoracic aperture are:
  - Muscles: Sternohyoid, sternothyroid, longus cervicis/longus colli.
  - Arteries: Right and left internal thoracic arteries, brachiocephalic trunk/artery, left common carotid artery, left subclavian artery, right and left superior intercostal arteries.
  - Nerves: Right and left vagus nerves, **left recurrent laryngeal nerve**, right and left phrenic nerves, right and left first thoracic nerves, right and left sympathetic chains.
  - Veins: Right and left brachiocephalic veins, right and left 1st posterior intercostal veins, inferior thyroid veins.
  - Lymphatics: **Thoracic duct**.
  - Viscera: Apices of lungs (with cervical pleura), trachea, esophagus.
  - Others: Anterior longitudinal ligament.

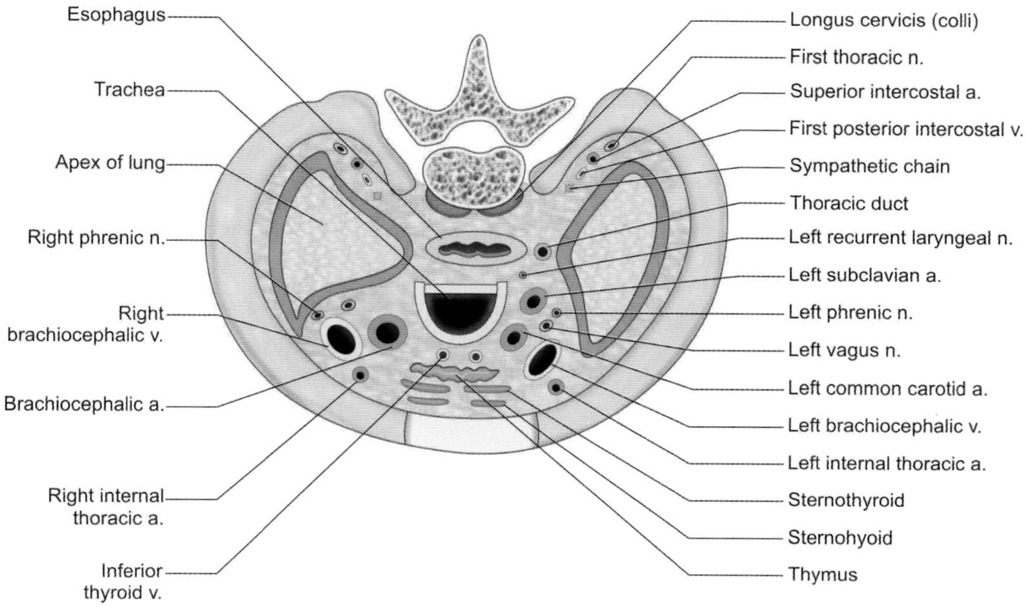

Fig. 68: Transverse section of thorax, structures passing through the thoracic inlet (a = artery; n = nerve; v= vein)

Thoracic outlet syndrome is the compression of neurovascular structures such as the subclavian artery, the brachial plexus (lower trunk or C8 and T1 nerve roots), or less often the axillary vein or subclavian vein, by thoracic outlet abnormalities such as a drooping shoulder girdle, a cervical rib or fibrous band, an abnormal first rib, or occasionally compression of the edge of the scalenus anterior muscle.

❏ Continual hyperabduction of the arm may cause another variety **(hyperabduction syndrome)**.

❏ Arterial compression leads to ischemia, paresthesia, numbness, and weakness of the affected arm, sometimes with **Raynaud phenomenon** of the arm.

❏ Nerve compression causes atrophy and weakness of the **muscles of the hand** and, in advanced cases, of the forearm, with pain and sensory disturbances in the arm.

❏ **Cervical rib** is a small additional rib which may develop in the root of the neck in association with the seventh cervical vertebra.

  ➢ It is often fibrous (may be ossified). It may cause compression of the neurovascular bundle, leading to pain, paresthesia and even pallor of the affected upper limb in thoracic outlet syndrome.

❏ **Sibson's fascia** (suprapleural membrane) is a thickening of connective tissue that **covers the apex** of each human lung.

  ➢ It is an extension of the **endothoracic fascia** that exists between the parietal pleura and the thoracic cage.

  ➢ It attaches to the internal border of the **1st rib**, its costal cartilage and the **transverse processes** of vertebra C7.

  ➢ It extends approximately an inch more superiorly than the superior thoracic aperture, along with the lungs to extend higher than the top of the rib cage.

  ➢ Morphologically, it is regarded as the flattened tendon of the **scalenus minimus**.

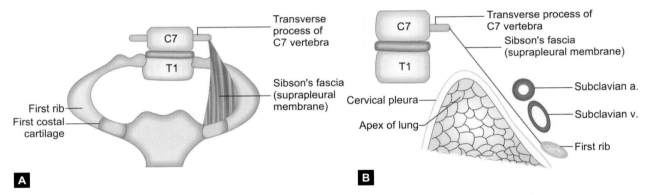

Figs. 69A and B: Suprapleural membrane (Sibson's fascia): (A) Attachments; (B) Relations

1. Structures passing through superior thoracic aperture are all EXCEPT: *(AIIMS 2005)*
   a. Right recurrent laryngeal nerve
   b. Left common carotid artery
   c. Left sympathetic trunk
   d. Thoracic duct

2. Which structure does NOT pass through superior thoracic aperture: *(NEET Pattern 2016)*
   a. Right vagus
   b. Brachiocephalic artery
   c. Thoracic duct
   d. Right recurrent laryngeal nerve

3. TRUE about attachment of suprapleural membrane: *(PGIC 2014)*
   a. Attached to clavicle
   b. Attached to 1st rib and its costal cartilage
   c. Attached to 2nd rib and its costal cartilage
   d. Attached to junction of manubrium and body of sternum
   e. Attached to tip of the transverse process of the 7th cervical vertebrae

4. Compression of cervical rib can cause: *(PGIC 2014)*
   a. Thenar hypertrophy
   b. Neurovascular symptom
   c. Raynaud's phenomenon
   d. C8; T1 paresthesia
   e. Weakness of forearm muscles

5. 5. All are true about Sibson's fascia EXCEPT: *(NEET Pattern 2018)*
   a. Attached to inner of first rib
   b. Covers supraclavicular part of lung
   c. Modified inner part of scalenus anterior
   d. Attached to transverse process of C7

1. a. Right recurrent laryngeal nerve
   ❏ Left (**not right**) recurrent laryngeal nerve passes through the superior thoracic aperture.
   ❏ Right recurrent laryngeal nerve **hooks around the right subclavian artery** in the neck region and ascends up in the tracheoesophageal groove to supply larynx.
   ❏ **Left common carotid artery** is given by the arch of aorta in the superior mediastinum (thorax) and pass through
   ❏ Thoracic aperture to enter the neck region.
   ❏ Sympathetic trunk begins at the **foramen magnum, it** passes through the **thoracic aperture** to reach the thorax, then go through **opening in the diaphragm** to reach the abdomen and terminates in **front of the coccyx**.
   ❏ Thoracic duct passes through the thoracic aperture and **enters the neck region** to terminates in the neck veins.

2. **d. Right recurrent laryngeal nerve**
   - Left (**not right**) recurrent laryngeal nerve passes through the superior thoracic aperture.
   - **Both** Vagii pass through the thoracic aperture.
   - **Brachiocephalic artery** is given by the arch of aorta in the superior mediastinum (thorax) and pass through thoracic aperture to enter the neck region.
   - **Thoracic duct** passes through the thoracic aperture and enters the neck region to terminates in the neck veins.

3. **b. Attached to 1st rib and its costal cartilage; e. Attached to tip of the transverse process of the 7th cervical vertebrae**
   - Suprapleural membrane (Sibson's fascia) attaches to the **internal border** of the 1st rib, its costal cartilage and the transverse processes of vertebra C7.

4. **b. Neurovascular symptom; c. Raynaud's phenomenon; d. C8; T1 paresthesia; e. Weakness of forearm muscles**
   - **Cervical rib** may result in thoracic outlet syndrome leading to compression of neurovascular structures such as the **subclavian artery**, the brachial plexus (**lower trunk** or C8 and T1 nerve roots).
   - Arterial compression leads to ischemia, paresthesia, numbness, and weakness of the affected arm, sometimes with **Raynaud phenomenon** of the arm. Nerve compression causes atrophy and weakness of the **muscles of the hand** and, in advanced cases, of the forearm, with pain and **sensory disturbances** in the arm.

5. **c. Modified inner part of scalenus anterior**
   - The suprapleural membrane (Sibson's fascia) is an extension of the endothoracic fascia.
   - Morphologically it represents the spread out degenerated tendon of scalenus minimus muscle.
   - It is attached anteriorly to the inner border of the first rib, and posteriorly to the anterior border of the transverse process of the 7th cervical vertebra.
   - It covers the apical pleura and intervenes between it and the subclavian vessels.

■ Attachment of **Sibson's** fascia is at **C7 vertebra** (*NEET Pattern 2015*).

Upper Limb

▶ **Embryology of Upper Limb**

❑ Upper limb buds appear by the **end of week 4** (regulated by **Hox genes**). Lower limb buds appear **2 days later** (beginning of week 5).
❑ Upper limbs rotate **laterally by 90 degrees**, so that the thumb becomes lateral and little finger medial.

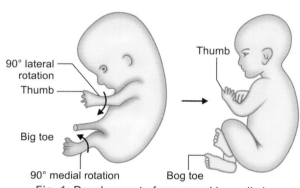

Fig. 1: Development of upper and lower limb

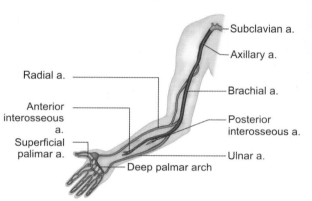

Fig. 2: Development of arteries of upper limb

❑ The **flexor** compartment comes **anterior** and the extensor compartment becomes posterior.
❑ Developmentally, **radius** bone is a **preaxial** bone and radial artery is **preaxial artery**. Ulna bone is postaxial bone with ulnar artery as postaxial artery.
❑ Subclavian artery represents the lateral branch of the **seventh intersegmental artery**. Its main continuation, the axial artery of the upper limb, becomes the axillary and brachial arteries. The original axial vessel ultimately persists as the **anterior interosseous artery** and the deep palmar arch.

▶ **Clavicle**

❑ The only long bone, **positioned in a horizontal plane** and is **subcutaneous throughout** its extent.
❑ Has **no medullary cavity**. (**Gray's Anatomy** mentions: There is a medullary cavity in its medial two-thirds).
❑ A **nutrient foramen** is found in the lateral end of the subclavian groove, running in a lateral direction; the nutrient artery is derived from the **suprascapular artery**.
❑ **Ossification**. Clavicle is the first bone to begin ossification (between the 5th and 6th week of intrauterine life) and is the **last bone to complete** it (at 25 years).
❑ It is the only long bone which ossifies by **two primary centers**. It **ossifies mostly in membrane** except sternal and acromial zones (true cartilage). **Note**: Long bones generally ossify in cartilage.

QUESTIONS

1. **FALSE about clavicle**   *(NEET Pattern 2012)*
   a. Ossifies in membrane
   b. Horizontal bone
   c. No medullary cavity
   d. Most common site of fracture is the junction of medial 1/3rd with lateral 2/3rd

ANSWER

1. **d. Most common site of fracture is the junction of medial 1/3rd with lateral 2/3rd**
   ❑ The fracture clavicle is most often in the **middle third** (at the junction of lateral 1/3rd and medial 2/3rd) and results in upward displacement of the proximal fragment pulled by the sternocleidomastoid muscle and downward displacement of the distal fragment by the deltoid muscle and gravity.

Scapula

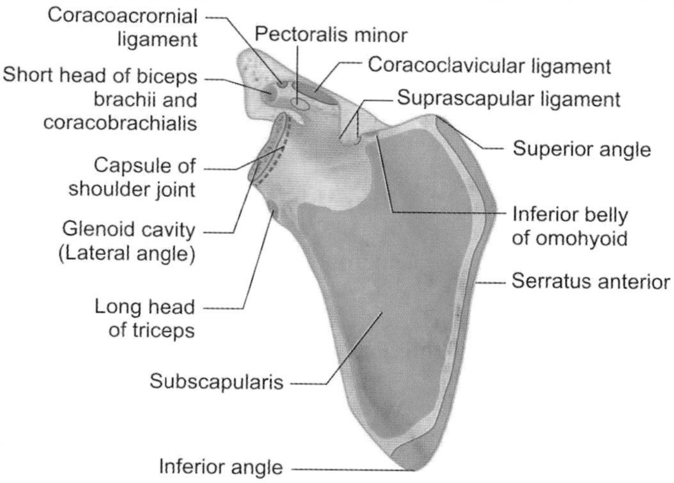

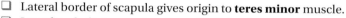

Fig. 3: Scapula (Anterior view)

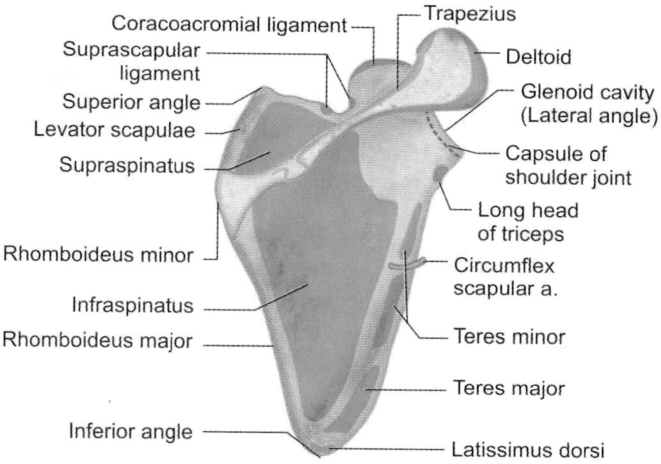

Anterior view labels:
- Coracoacrornial ligament
- Pectoralis minor
- Short head of biceps brachii and coracobrachialis
- Coracoclavicular ligament
- Suprascapular ligament
- Capsule of shoulder joint
- Superior angle
- Glenoid cavity (Lateral angle)
- Inferior belly of omohyoid
- Long head of triceps
- Serratus anterior
- Subscapularis
- Inferior angle

Fig. 4: Scapula (Posterior view)

Posterior view labels:
- Coracoacromial ligament
- Suprascapular ligament
- Superior angle
- Levator scapulae
- Supraspinatus
- Rhomboideus minor
- Infraspinatus
- Rhomboideus major
- Inferior angle
- Trapezius
- Deltoid
- Glenoid cavity (Lateral angle)
- Capsule of shoulder joint
- Long head of triceps
- Circumflex scapular a.
- Teres minor
- Teres major
- Latissimus dorsi

- ❑ Lateral border of scapula gives origin to **teres minor** muscle.
- ❑ Long head of triceps arises from the **infraglenoid tubercle** on the lateral border of scapula.
- ❑ Infraspinatus attaches to the dorsal surface and subscapularis to the ventral surface of scapula.
- ❑ Coracoid process
  - ➢ The tip gives origin to coracobrachialis (medially) and short head of the biceps (laterally).
  - ➢ The upper surface receives insertion of **pectoralis minor**.

1. Which of the marked structures is palpable in the infraclavicular fossa *(AIIMS 2017)*
- a. A
- b. B
- c. C
- d. D

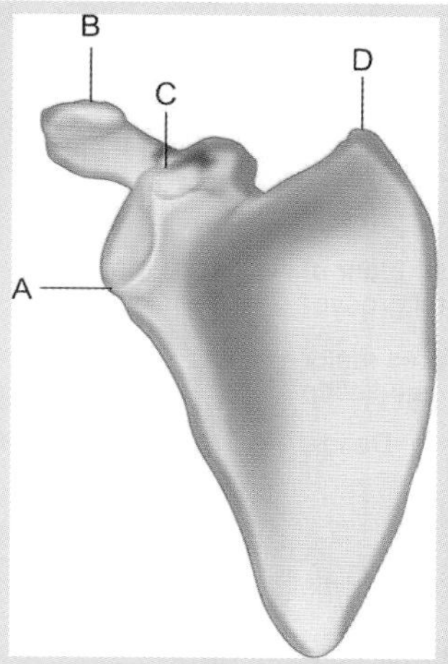

2. Muscle inserting on medial border of scapula *(NEET Pattern 2016)*
- a. Subscapularis
- b. Serratus anterior
- c. Teres minor
- d. Latissimus dorsi

3. The following muscles are attached to the coracoid process of the scapula EXCEPT:
- a. Coracobrachialis
- b. Short head of biceps
- c. Pectoralis minor
- d. Long head of triceps

4. Which border of scapula is NOT palpable *(NEET Pattern 2015)*
- a. Medial
- b. Lateral
- c. Inferior
- d. Superior

5. Superior angle of scapula lies at which level *(NEET Pattern 2015)*
- a. C5
- b. T2
- c. T7
- d. T12

1. c. C
- ❑ The **tip of coracoid process** can be palpated 2.5 cm below the junction of lateral 1/4 and medial 3/4 of the clavicle (in the infraclavicular fossa).
- ❑ Key: A- Infraglenoid tubercle; B- Acromion process; C-Coracoid process; D-Superior angle of scapula.

2. b. Serratus anterior
- ❑ Serratus anterior is inserted on the medial border of scapula (**costal aspect**).

3. d. Long head of triceps
- ❑ Long head of triceps attaches to the **infraglenoid tubercle** (NEET Pattern 2015)

4. b. Lateral > d. Superior
- ❏ The lateral border separates the attachments of subscapularis and teres minor and major. These muscles project beyond the bone and, with latissimus dorsi below, **cover it so completely** that it cannot be felt through the skin.
- ❏ Even the superior border and angle of the scapula are deep to soft tissue and is **not readily palpable**.

5. b. T2
- ❏ Superior angle lies at the junction of superior and medial borders, and lies over the **2nd rib and 2nd thoracic** vertebra.
- ❏ The inferior angle is opposite the spine of the 7th thoracic vertebra and overlies the inferior border of 7th rib.

- ❏ **Retraction** of scapula (bring scapula back to the midline) is carried out by muscles: **Trapezius, rhomboideus** major and minor.
- ❏ **Protraction** of scapula (take scapula away from midline as happens in pushing a wall in front) is brought about by muscles: **Serratus anterior**, pectoralis minor.
- ❏ **Serratus anterior** takes origin from the lateral surface of upper 8 ribs and is inserted to the anterior surface of **medial border** of scapula. It pulls the scapula forward (protraction). It also pulls on the inferior angle of scapula to help in lateral **scapular rotation**.

▶ Humerus

- ❏ SIT (Supra-spinatus, Infraspinatus, Teres minor) muscles 'sit' on greater tubercle. Subscapularis attaches to the lesser tubercle of humerus.
- ❏ Three muscles are attached in the region of bicipital (intertubercular) groove: **Pectoralis Major** on the lateral lip of the groove, **teres major** on the medial lip of the groove and **latissimus dorsi** in the floor of the groove. (**Mnemonic**: Lady between two Majors).
- ❏ The capsular ligament of the elbow joint is attached to the lower end along a line that reaches the upper limits of the radial and coronoid fossae anteriorly and of the olecranon fossa posteriorly (these fossae are **intracapsular**).

■ The nerves related closely to the humerus are: Axillary, radial, ulnar *(NEET Pattern 2015)*

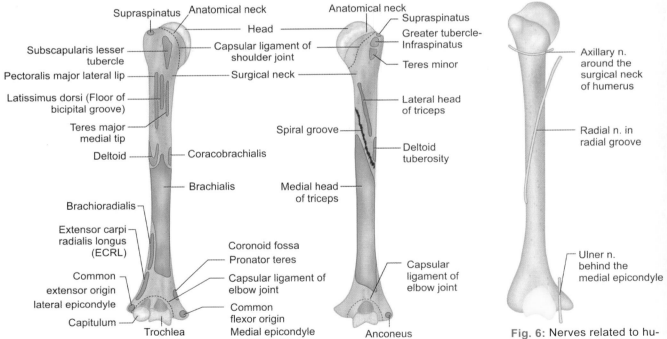

Fig. 5: Attachments on humerus (anterior and posterior aspect)

Fig. 6: Nerves related to humerus

Nutrient artery is a branch of profunda brachii artery, arises near the **mid-level** of the upper arm and enters the nutrient canal near the attachment of coracobrachialis, posterior to the deltoid tuberosity; it is **directed distally**.

1. Which of the following is NOT intracapsular
(NEET Pattern 2015)?
- a. Coronoid fossa
- b. Radial fossa
- c. Olecranon fossa
- d. Lateral epicondyle

2. Contents of bicipital groove are *(PGIC 2009,15)*
- a. Synovial membrane of shoulder joint
- b. Ascending branch of anterior circumflex artery
- c. Ascending branch of posterior circumflex artery
- d. Radial artery
- e. Coracobrachialis muscle

Answers

1. **d. Lateral epicondyle**
   - ❑ Lateral (and medial) epicondyles are **outside** the capsular ligament. They are **traction epiphysis**.
2. **a. Synovial membrane of shoulder joint; b. Ascending branch of anterior circumflex artery**
   - ❑ Synovial membrane of shoulder joint forms a tubular sheath around the tendon of biceps brachii where it lies in the bicipital groove of the humerus.
   - ❑ Anterior circumflex artery sends an ascending branch upwards in the groove.
   - ❑ Note: Tendon of long head of biceps is intracapsular, and extrasynovial, but enclosed in the synovial sheath.

▼ Forearm Bones

Questions

1. **About radius bone TRUE is**   (NEET Pattern 2013)
   a. Radial groove is present
   b. Major contributor to wrist joint
   c. Radial artery lies medial to styloid process of radius
   d. Medial bone of forearm

2. **The structure that lies lateral to distal radial tubercle**
   a. Extensor pollicis longus   (NEET Pattern 2014)
   b. Extensor carpi radialis longus
   c. Brachioradialis
   d. Extensor carpi ulnaris

Answers

1. **b. Major contributor to wrist joint > c. Radial artery lies medial to styloid process of radius**
   - ❑ Radius articulates with carpal bones to form radiocarpal (wrist) joint. It is the **major contributor** in the joint.
   - ❑ The **medial bone ulna** is excluded from this articulation by an articular disc.
   - ❑ Radial artery lies **medial to styloid** process of radius, then winds laterally around the styloid process to **enter** the anatomical snuff box.
   - ❑ Radial (spiral) groove is present on **humerus** bone.
2. **b. Extensor carpi radialis longus**
   - ❑ Distal end of radius has **Lister's tubercle** on the dorsal side.
   - ❑ The tendon of extensor carpi radialis longus (and Brevis) pass **lateral** to the tubercle.
   - ❑ The tendon of extensor pollicis longus passes **medial** to the Lister's tubercle.

- ■ At the base of the radial styloid process, there is insertion of **brachioradialis** tendon. (NEET Pattern 2012)

Questions

1. **FALSE statement/s regarding upper limb bones is/are** (PGIC)
   a. Most common site of fracture clavicle is the junction of intermediate 1/3rd with lateral 1/3rd
   b. Teres minor attaches to lateral border of scapula
   c. Lateral epicondyle of humerus is intracapsular
   d. Tendon of extensor carpi radialis longus pass medial to the Lister's tubercle
   e. Radius is the main contributor to wrist joint

2. **All the pairs about bony attachments around shoulder joint are correctly matched EXCEPT**   (PGIC)
   a. Latissimus dorsi: Floor of intertubercular sulcus
   b. Short head of biceps: Tip of coracoid process
   c. Subscapularis: Lesser tubercle
   d. Teres major: Greater tubercle
   e. Radial styloid process: Brachioradialis

Answers

1. **c. Lateral epicondyle of humerus is intracapsular; d. Tendon of extensor carpi radialis longus pass medial to the Lister's tubercle**
   - ❑ Lateral (and medial) epicondyles are **outside** the capsular ligament.
   - ❑ Tendon of extensor carpi radialis longus pass **lateral** to the Lister's tubercle.
   - ❑ Most common site of fracture clavicle is the junction of medial 2/3rd with lateral 1/3rd. It **may also be considered** as junction of intermediate 1/3rd with lateral 1/3rd.
   - ❑ Lateral border of scapula gives origin to **teres major & minor** muscles.
   - ❑ Wrist joint is called radio-carpal joint and formed by articulation of the distal end of the radius with the proximal row of carpal bones.
2. **d. Teres major: Greater tubercle**
   - ❑ Attachment on greater tubercle is teres minor **(not major)**. Teres major attached to the medial lip of bicipital groove on humerus.

- ■ Nutrient arteries to both ulna & radius are branches of **anterior interosseus artery** branch of ulnar artery.
- ■ Most commonly fractured bone in the body is **Clavicle**. It occurs at the junction of its lateral one-third and medial two-third

▼ Joints of Upper Limb

Table 1: Joints of upper limb

Joint	Type	Joint	Type
Sternoclavicular	Saddle	Wrist	Ellipsoid > Condylar
Acromioclavicular	Plane	1st carpometacarpal	Saddle (sellar)
Shoulder	Ball and socket	Metacarpophalangeal	Ellipsoid > Condylar
Elbow	Hinge	Intercarpal and midcarpal	Plane
Superior and inferior radioulnar	Pivot (trochoid)	Interphalangeal	Hinge
Middle radioulnar	Syndesmosis		

Weight Transmission

❑ Weight of the upper limb is transmitted to the axial skeleton by various bones, joints and ligaments.

❑ Weight of the hand is transmitted to the radius via the wrist joint. From radius the line of transmission of weight passes to the ulna via interosseous ligament (**middle radioulnar joint**). From ulna the weight is transmitted to the humerus via elbow joint.

❑ Humerus transmits the weight to the scapula via the shoulder joint. Scapula transmits the **weight of upper limb** to the clavicle via the **coracoclavicular ligament** and acromioclavicular joint.

❑ Clavicle transmits the weight of the upper limb to the **axial skeleton** (rib and sternum) via the sternoclavicular joint and ligaments like **costoclavicular ligament**.

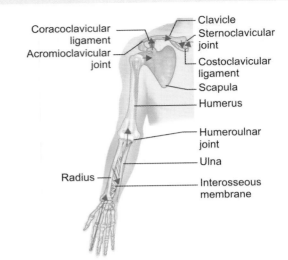

Fig. 7: Line of weight transmission: Hand → Radius→ Ulna→ Humerus→ Scapula→ Clavicle → Sternum and ribs→ Vertebral column

Table 2: Movements at shoulder joint			
Movement	Prime mover(s)	Synergists	Additional points
Flexion	Pectoralis major (clavicular head); deltoid (clavicular and anterior acromial parts)	Coracobrachialis (assisted by biceps brachii)	From fully extended position to its own (coronal) plane, sternocostal head of pectoralis major is major force
Extension	Deltoid (spinal part)	Teres major; latissimus dorsi; long head of triceps brachii	Latissimus dorsi, (sternocostal head of pectoralis major, and long head of triceps brachii) act from fully flexed position to their own (coronal) planes
Abduction	Deltoid (as a whole, but especially acromial part)	Supraspinatus	Supraspinatus is particularly important in initiating movement; also, upward rotation of scapula occurs throughout movement, making a significant contribution
Adduction	Pectoralis major; latissimus dorsi	Teres major; long head of triceps brachii	In upright position and in absence of resistance, gravity is prime mover
Medial rotation	Subscapularis	Pectoralis major; deltoid (clavicular part); latissimus dorsi; teres major	With arm elevated. "synergists" become more important than prime movers
Lateral rotation	Infraspinatus	Teres minor; deltoid (spinal part)	
Tensors of articular capsule (to hold head of humerus against the glenoid cavity)	Subscapularis; infraspinatus (simultaneously)	Supraspinatus; teres minor	Rotator cuff (SITS) muscles acting together; when "resting", their tonus adequately maintains integrity of joint
Resisting down-ward dislocation (shunt muscles)	Deltoid (as a whole)	Long head of triceps brachii; coracobrachialis; short head of biceps brachii	Used especially when carrying heavy objects (suitcases, buckets)

❑ The total range of shoulder abduction is 180°. Abduction up to 90° occurs at the **shoulder joint**, further 90° to 120° occurs as **humerus is rotated laterally**, 120° to 180° range is added by **lateral rotation of scapula**.

❑ **Supraspinatus** initiates abduction and causes initial 15° of abduction; **deltoid** is the main abductor from 15° to 90° of abduction, sequentially humerus is laterally rotated by the **infraspinatus and teres minor** muscles and next overhead abduction (90°–180°) is carried out by the 2 muscles mainly – **trapezius** and **serratus anterior**.

❑ During abduction, trapezius and serratus anterior cause lateral rotation of scapula and glenoid cavity eventually faces **upwards**.

❑ Humerus and scapula move in the **ratio of 2:1** during abduction, i.e., for every 15° elevation, the humerus moves 10° and scapula moves 5°.

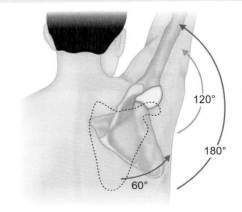

Fig. 8: Shoulder abduction (range of movement)

- Abduction at shoulder involves **rotation of clavicle** at its longitudinal axis, which occurs at both the **sternoclavicular** and the **acromioclavicular** joints. This contributes about 60° rotation to the clavicle in total.
- Both supraspinatus and deltoid are involved **throughout** the range of abduction, including the initiation of the movement.

> - Pectoralis minor is an accessory muscle of inspiration, which stabilizes scapula by pulling it anteriorly and inferiorly. It doesn't participate in shoulder joint movements as such *(NEET Pattern 2014)*

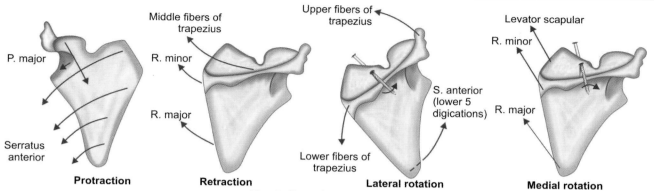

Fig. 9: Scapular movements

Movement	Muscles producing the movements
Protraction	▪ Serratus anterior ▪ Pectoralis minor (assists)
Retraction	▪ Trapezius (middle fibres) ▪ Rhomboideus minor ▪ Rhomboideus major
Elevation	▪ Trapezius (upper fibres)
Depression	▪ Pectoralis minor ▪ Trapezius (lower fibres) ▪ Latissimus dorsi ▪ Weight of the upper limb
Medial rotation	▪ Levator scapulae ▪ Rhomboideus minor ▪ Rhomboideus major
Lateral rotation	▪ Trapezius (upper and lower fibres) ▪ Serratus anterior (lower 5 digitations)

Table 3: Movements at elbow joint	
Movements	**Muscles involved**
Flexion	Primary muscles: Brachialis, biceps (in supination), brachioradialis (in mid prone). Supportive muscles: Pronator teres, flexor carpi radialis.
Extension	Triceps, Anconeus

- The transverse axis of elbow joint is not transverse but oblique being directed downwards and medially. This is because medial flange of trochlea lies **about 6 mm below** its lateral flange.
- Consequently, when the elbow is extended the arm and forearm do not lie in straight line, rather forearm is deviated slightly laterally.
- This angle of deviation of long axis of forearm from long axis of arm is termed **carrying angle**.
- The carrying angle disappears during pronation and full flexion of forearm.
- The carrying angle varies from 5° to 15° and is more pronounced in females

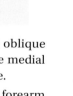

Lateral (outward) deviation of extended and supinated forearm

Fig. 10: Carrying elbow at elbow

Table 4: Movements at radio-ulnar joints	
Movements	**Muscles involved**
Pronation	Pronator quadratus (strong pronator), pronator teres (Rapid pronator), brachioradialis*
Supination	Supinator (in extended elbow), Biceps (in flexed elbow), brachioradialis*

Note: Flexor carpi radialis, palmaris longus and gravity help in pronation.

Table 5: Movements at wrist joint		
Movements	**Joint involved**	**Muscles involved**
Flexion	Midcarpal and wrist (in order of involvement)	Flexor carpi radialis, flexor carpi ulnaris, palmaris longus assisted by flexor digitorum superficialis and profundus, and flexor pollicis longus
Extension (dorsiflexion)	Wrist and midcarpal joint (in order of involvement)	Extensor carpi radialis longus and brevis, extensor carpi ulnaris, assisted by extensor digitorum, extensor pollicis longus, extensor indicis and extensor digiti minimi
Adduction (Ulnar deviation)	Wrist	Flexor carpi ulnaris and extensor carpi ulnaris
Abduction (Radial deviation)	Mainly occurs at midcarpal joint	Flexor carpi radialis, extensor carpi radialis longus and brevis, abductor pollicis longus and extensor pollicis brevis

*Wrist adduction has greater range than abduction.

❑ Wrist joint is a synovial, biaxial and **ellipsoid** joint. Some authors consider it as **condylar** variety.

❑ It is formed by articulation of the **distal end of the radius** and the **articular disc** of the triangular fibrocartilage with the **proximal row of carpal bones**- scaphoid, lunate, and rarely triquetrum.

❑ Ulna bone **do not participate** in wrist joint and is excluded from this articulation by an articular disc.

QUESTIONS

1. **UNTRUE statement/s about upper limb joints**   *(PGIC)*
   a. Pectoralis minor has no action at shoulder joint
   b. Pectoralis major is an abductor at shoulder joint
   c. Serratus anterior muscle causes retraction of scapula
   d. Flexor pollicis longus is a flexor at elbow joint
   e. Flexor carpi ulnaris causes ulnar deviation at wrist joint

2. **TRUE about abduction at shoulder joint**   *(PGIC 2016, 17)*
   a. Supraspinatus initiates abduction
   b. Serratus anterior and trapezius are involved
   c. Multipennate deltoid clavicular fibre is main abductor
   d. Axillary nerve injury has no effect on abduction
   e. Musculotendinous cuff stabilizes shoulder joint

3. **Which are NOT the flexors of forearm**   *(PGIC 2010)*
   a. Pronator teres   b. Brachialis
   c. Brachioradialis   d. Anconeus
   e. Flexor pollicis longus

4. **Wrist is which type of synovial joint**
   a. Condylar   b. Ellipsoid
   c. Hinge   d. Trochoid

5. **Abduction of Hand is caused by**   *(NEET Pattern 2015)*
   a. Flexor carpi radialis
   b. Flexor carpi ulnaris
   c. Flexor digitorum profundus
   d. Flexor digitorum superficialis

6. **Weight transmission from upper limb to axial skeleton is done by all EXCEPT**   *(AIIMS)*
   a. Costoclavicular ligament   b. Coracoacromial ligament
   c. Coracoclavicular ligament   d. Interclavicular ligament

ANSWERS

1. **b. Pectoralis major is an abductor at shoulder joint; c. Serratus anterior muscle causes retraction of scapula; d. Flexor pollicis longus is a flexor at elbow joint**
   ❑ Pectoralis major muscle is an adductor (and not abductor) at shoulder joint.
   ❑ Serratus anterior muscle causes protraction of scapula. Retractors are: Rhomboideus major and minor muscles.
   ❑ Flexor pollicis longus do not cross (and act) at elbow joint. It flexes the phalanges and carpometacarpal joint of the thumb.
   ❑ Pectoralis minor stabilizes scapula by pulling it anteriorly and inferiorly. It doesn't participate in shoulder joint movements.
   ❑ Flexor carpi ulnaris causes flexion at the wrist joint and ulnar deviation (adduction) as well.

2. **a. Supraspinatus initiates abduction; b. Serratus anterior and trapezius also help in abduction; e. Musculotendinous cuff stabilizes shoulder joint**
   ❑ Both supraspinatus and deltoid are involved throughout the range of abduction, including the initiation of the movement.
   ❑ Serratus anterior and trapezius help in overhead abduction.
   ❑ The multipennate acromial (not clavicular) fibres of deltoid are the powerful abductors of arm at the shoulder joint.
   ❑ Axillary nerve injury paralyses the deltoid; hence abduction is seriously compromised. Musculotendinous rotator cuff stabilizes the shoulder joints posterosuperiorly and partly anteriorly as well (but inferiorly it is deficient).

3. **d. Anconeus; e. Flexor pollicis longus**
   ❑ Anconeus muscle is an extensor at elbow joint (with triceps) and flexor pollicis longus muscle do not cross (and act) at elbow joint.
   ❑ Biceps brachii is a powerful supinator and causes elbow flexion as well.
   ❑ Brachioradialis is a flexor at elbow joint especially in mid-prone position. Humeral head of pronator teres crosses elbow joint, hence participate in elbow flexion.
   ❑ Chief action of brachialis is elbow flexion

4. **b. Ellipsoid > a. Condylar**
   ❑ The wrist (radiocarpal) joint is an ellipsoid type of synovial joint, though some authors consider it as condylar variety.
   ❑ Internal pudendal vessels pass through greater and lesser sciatic foramina (not through obturator foramen).

5. **a. Flexor carpi radialis**
   ❑ Abduction of the hand occurs at the wrist joint, carried out by the muscles like Flexor carpi radialis.
   ❑ Flexor carpi ulnaris works for adduction of hand at wrist joint.

6. b. Coracoacromial ligament

- ☐ Coracoacromial ligaments attaches to bone scapula at different points and is not attached to the previous or next bone in line of weight transmission.
- ☐ Ligaments involved in weight transmission connect one bone with the next bone, in line of weight transmission.
- ☐ There are numerous ligaments which help in weight transmission of upper limb to the axial skeleton, frequently mentioned is coracoclavicular, attached the conoid tubercle and trapezoid line, transmit the weight of the upper limb to the clavicle.

- ☐ Only point of bony contact between the upper limb and chest **Sternoclavicular joint**
- ☐ **Strongest** ligament of the upper limb is Coracoclavicular ligament

▶ Nerve Supply of Upper Limb

Table 6: Segmental innervation of the muscles of the upper limb

Nerves	Muscles
C3, 4	Trapezius, levator scapulae
C5	Rhomboids, deltoids, supraspinatus, infraspinatus, teres minor, biceps
C6	Serratus anterior, latissimus dorsi, subscapularis, teres major, pectoralis major (clavicular head), biceps, coracobrachialis, brachialis, brachioradialis, supinator, extensor carpi radialis longus
C7	Serratus anterior, latissimus dorsi, pectoralis major (sternal head), pectoralis minor, triceps, pronator teres, flexor carpi radialis, flexor digitorum superficialis, extensor digit minimi
C8	Pectoralis major (sternal head), pectoralis minor, triceps, flexor digitorum superficialis, flexor digitorum profundus, flexor pollicis longus, pronator quadratus, flexor carpi ulnaris, extensor carpi ulnaris, abductor pollicis longus, extensor pollicis longus, extensor pollicis brevis, extensor Indicis, abductor pollicis brevis, flexor pollicis brevis, opponens pollicis
T1	Flexor digitorum profundus, intrinsic muscles of the hand (except abductor pollicis brevis, flexor pollicis brevis, opponens pollicis)

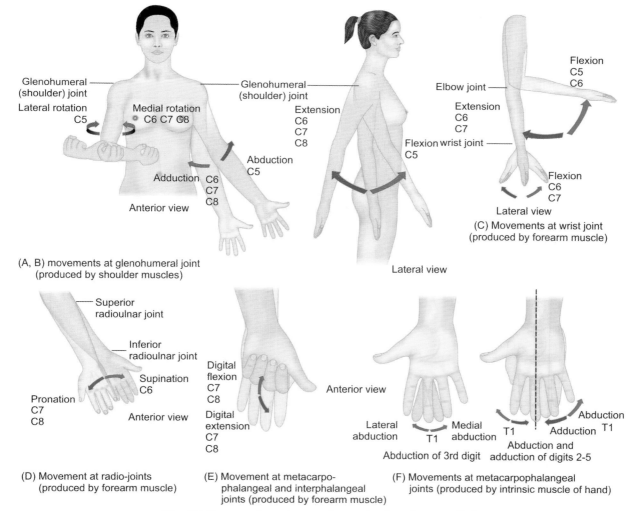

Fig. 11: Movements and respective root values in upper limb

Table 7: Muscle groups and their root values in upper limb joints

Territory	Muscles	Nerves
Shoulder	Abductors and lateral rotators	C5
	Adductors and medial rotators	C6–8
Elbow	Flexors	C5, 6
	Extensors	C7, 8
Forearm	Supinators	C6
	Pronators	C7, 8
Wrist	Flexors and extensors	C6, 7
Digits	Long flexors and extensors	C7, 8
Hand	Intrinsic muscles	C8, T1

▶ Brachial Plexus

Brachial Plexus

- ❑ **Brachial plexus** is contributed by the ***ventral* primary rami** of the lower four cervical nerves and the first thoracic nerves (C5–8; T1).
- ❑ It has roots and trunks (in the **neck**), divisions (passing behind clavicle), cords and branches (in the **axilla**).
- ❑ It is covered by a prolongation of **prevertebral fascia** (axillary sheath) around the nerves in the axilla.
- ❑ The rami enter the **posterior triangle of the neck** between scalenus anterior and medius.
- ❑ **Upper trunk** is formed by C5 and C6, where these nerves emerge from deep to scalenus anterior. The **middle trunk** is the continuation of C7. The **lower trunk** is contributed by C8 and T1, where these nerves cross anterior to the first rib.
- ❑ The trunks divide into anterior and posterior **divisions**, which pass behind the clavicle to enter the axilla.
- ❑ The **cords** are formed by the confluence of divisions: the **lateral cord** from the anterior divisions of the upper and middle trunks; the **posterior cord** by all three posterior divisions; and the **medial cord** by the anterior division of the lower trunk.
- ❑ The **posterior** divisions and posterior cord innervate **postaxial** (extensor) musculature; the anterior divisions and the lateral and medial cords innervate preaxial (flexor) musculature.

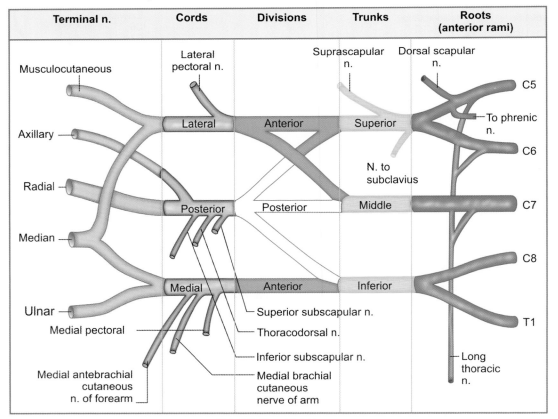

Fig. 12: Brachial plexus

- Branches from the **cords** are mentioned in the table.
- **Radial nerve** is a branch of posterior cord (STARS) and supplies posterior (**extensor**) compartment of upper limb.
- **Ulnar** nerve is a branch of medial cord (UM4) and runs on the ulnar (medial) side of the limb.
- **Median nerve** runs in the midline of the limb and has contributions from **both** medial and lateral cords.

Branches

- **Two** branches are given directly from the **roots** in the neck: **Dorsal scapular nerve** (C5), which supplies **rhomboid major and minor** and **levator scapulae** muscles descends along with the dorsal scapular artery on the deep surface of the rhomboid muscles along the medial border of the scapula (JIPMER 2007; NEET Pattern 2014)
- **Long thoracic nerve of Bell** (C5–C7), which is given in the neck, enters axilla and descends on the external surface of the *serratus anterior* muscle and supplies it.
- **Upper Trunk** gives rise to two branches:
  1. **Suprascapular** Nerve (C5–C6) passes deep to the trapezius and joins the suprascapular artery in a course towards the shoulder. Passes through the scapular notch under the superior transverse scapular ligament and supplies the supraspinatus and infraspinatus muscles.
  2. **Nerve to the Subclavius** (C5) descends in front of the plexus and behind the clavicle to innervate the subclavius.

Table 8: Branches of the cords of brachial plexus		
Lateral cord (LML)	Lateral pectoral	C5, 6, 7
	Musculocutaneous	C, 6, 7
	Lateral root of median	C(5), 6, 7
Medial cord (UM4)	Medial pectoral	8, T1
	Medial cutaneous of forearm	C8, T1
	Medial cutaneous of arm	C8, T1
	Ulnar	C(7), 8, T1
	Medial root of median	C8, T1
Posterior cord (STARS)	Upper subscapular	C5, 6
	Thoracodorsal	C6, 7, 8
	Lower subscapular	C5, 6
	Axillary	C5, 6
	Radial	C5, 6, 7, 8, (T1)

Brachial Plexus Lesions

- **Erb-Duchenne paralysis** It is injury to **upper trunk** of brachial plexus caused due to **undue separation** of head and neck as may happen during a breech delivery or a violent displacement of the head from the shoulder (e.g., a fall from a motorcycle).
- It results in a **loss** of abduction, flexion, and lateral rotation of the arm, producing a **policeman/waiter's tip hand deformity**, in which the arm tends to lie in medial rotation, forearm in extension and pronation.

Table 9: Erb's palsy		
Nerves involved	**Cause of injury**	**Clinical features**
Erb-Duchenne palsy (upper turnk; C-5L, 6 injury) ■ Supra-scapular nerve ■ Axillary nerve ■ Musculocutaneous nerve ■ Radial	Undue separation of head and neck ■ Fall on shoulder ■ Birth injury	Policeman tip hand deformity

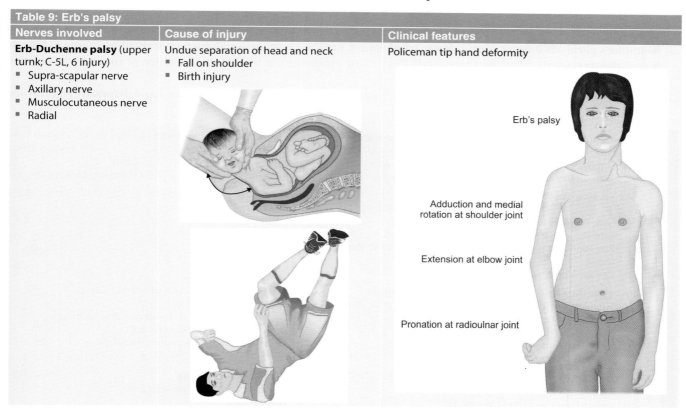

Erb's palsy

Adduction and medial rotation at shoulder joint

Extension at elbow joint

Pronation at radioulnar joint

Erb's point is a meeting point of **six nerves**: ventral rami of C-5 root, ventral rami of C-6 root, suprascapular nerve, nerve to subclavius, anterior division of upper trunk and posterior division of upper trunk.

Table 10: Klumpke's palsy

Nerves involved	Cause of injury	Clinical features
(**Lower trunk**; C-8; T-1 injury) ▪ Median nerve ▪ Ulnar nerve ▪ T-1 Sympathetic fibres	**Hyper-abduction** of arm ▪ Holding a branch while fall from a tree ▪ Birth injury	**Claw hand deformity**

Horner syndrome

Affected eyelid droops ("ptosis")
Smaller pupil

Horner syndrome

❏ **Klumpke's paralysis** It occurs due to **lower trunk** injury, may be caused **hyperabduction** at shoulder during a difficult breech delivery, sports injury, by a cervical rib (cervical rib syndrome), or by abnormal insertion or spasm of the anterior and middle scalene muscles (scalene syndrome).

❏ The patient presents with paralysed hand muscles (lumbrical and interossei) leading to **claw hand deformity** and **Horner syndrome** (due to lesioned T1 sympathetic fibres).

1. Which among the following is a branch from the trunk of brachial plexus   *(NEET Pattern 2013,16)*
   a. Suprascapular nerve   b. Long thoracic nerve
   c. Anterior thoracic nerve   d. Nerve to subclavius

2. Which of the following nerves carries fibres from all the roots of brachial plexus   *(NEET Pattern 2013)*
   a. Axillary   b. Ulnar
   c. Median   d. Musculocutaneous

3. All are true about brachial plexus EXCEPT   *(NEET pattern 2014)*
   a. Lower trunk is formed by root C8 and T1
   b. Lateral cord is formed by upper and middle trunk
   c. Posterior cord is formed by posterior divisions of all three trunks
   d. C4 root is post fixed to plexus

4. Posterior cord supplies   *(NEET Pattern 2015)*
   a. Teres minor
   b. Pectoralis minor
   c. Coracobrachialis
   d. Long head of biceps

5. Injury to the upper trunk of brachial plexus results in
   a. Supination of forearm   *(PGIC 2012)*
   b. External rotation of arm
   c. Inability to initiate abduction
   d. Decreased sensation on medial side of hand
   e. Paralysis of deltoid muscle

6. TRUE about the upper trunk of brachial plexus
   a. Carries root value C-5, 6, 7
   b. Can be blocked medial to scalenus anterior muscle
   c. Long thoracic nerve arises from it
   d. Lesion leads to partial injury of radial nerve

7. FALSE regarding Klumpke's paralysis is   *(JIPMER 2008)*
   a. Claw hand deformity
   b. Intrinsic muscles of hand involved
   c. Horner's syndrome
   d. Upper trunk of brachial plexus involved

8. WRONG about Erb's palsy   *(AIIMS 2002)*
   a. Loss of abduction at shoulder joint
   b. Loss of lateral rotation
   c. Loss of pronation at radioulnar joint
   d. Loss of flexion at elbow joint

9. Fall on shoulder resulted in arm held in medially rotated position and forearm pronated. The following facts concerning this patient are correct, EXCEPT   (AIIMS 2004)
   a. The injury was at Erb's point
   b. A lesion of C5 and C6 was present
   c. The median and ulnar nerves were affected
   d. Supraspinatus, infraspinatus, subclavius and biceps brachii were paralysed

10. Concerning brachial plexus, which of the following facts are TRUE   (PGIC 2008;15)
   a. Formed by spinal nerve C4-C7
   b. Most common site of injury is upper trunk
   c. Injury may occur during breech delivery
   d. Radial nerve is branch of medial cord
   e. Lower trunk injury results in hand deformity

1. d. Nerve to subclavius > a. Suprascapular nerve
   ❏ Most of the authors mention two branches of from the upper trunk of brachial plexus: Suprascapular nerve and nerve to subclavius.
   ❏ Gray's anatomy mentions that the slender nerve to subclavius (C5, 6) springs from the upper trunk.
   ❏ Suprascapular nerve (C5, 6) usually arises as the first branch of the upper trunk but it frequently springs directly from the ventral primary ramus of C5. It innervates supra and infraspinatus muscles.

2. c. Median
   ❏ Median nerve is contributed by two roots given by lateral cord: C6, 7 and medial cord: C8; T1. It appears to be the best answer.
   ❏ Axillary nerve- C5,6; Ulnar nerve - C (7) 8, T1; Musculocutaneous nerve- C5,6,7.
   ❏ Radial nerve (C5, 6, 7, 8, T1) carries fibres from all the roots of brachial plexus.

3. d. C4 root is post fixed to plexus
   ❏ Contribution by C4 to brachial plexus is pre-fixed brachial plexus. Post-fixed brachial plexus has contribution by T2
   ❏ Upper trunk has C5,6; Middle trunk: C7 and Lower trunk: C8 and T1 root values.
   ❏ Lateral cord is formed by anterior divisions of upper and middle trunk.
   ❏ Medial cord by anterior division of lower trunk and Posterior cord by posterior divisions of upper, middle and lower trunks.

4. a. Teres minor
   ❏ Posterior cord gives five branches, including axillary nerve which supplies teres minor muscle.

5. c. Inability to initiate abduction; e. Paralysis of deltoid muscle
   ❏ Injury to upper trunk of brachial plexus results in Erb's palsy resulting in policeman tip hand deformity: Adduction and medial (internal) rotation at shoulder joint; extension at elbow joint and pronation at radioulnar joint.
   ❏ Initiation of shoulder abduction (supraspinatus paralysed) and raising the arm to 90° (deltoid paralysed) is not possible.
   ❏ Outer (lateral) surface of the upper limb (C-5, 6 dermatome) has sensory disturbance.
   ❏ Decreased sensation on medial side of hand (C-8 dermatome) occurs in Klumpke's palsy.

6. d. Lesion leads to partial injury of radial nerve
   ❏ Upper trunk of brachial plexus carries C-5, 6 root values.
   ❏ Trunks of brachial plexus pass in the scalene triangle bounded by scalenus anterior and medius muscle, it lies lateral (and not medial) to the scalenus anterior muscle, where a block can be carried out.
   ❏ Long thoracic nerve arises directly from the roots of brachial plexus (C-5, 6, 7).
   ❏ Lesion of upper trunk of brachial plexus (e.g., Erb's palsy) leads to partial (C5,6) injury of radial nerve (C-5, 6, 7, 8; T1).

7. d. Upper trunk of brachial plexus involved
   ❏ In Klumpke's palsy there is a lesion in the lower trunk of brachial plexus, leading to claw hand deformity due to paralysis of hand muscles, including intrinsic muscles like lumbrical and interossei. Features of Horner syndrome are evident due to injury of T1 sympathetic fibres.

8. c. Loss of pronation at radioulnar joint
   ❏ Pronation at the radioulnar joint is carried by the pronator teres and pronator quadratus muscle, supplied by the median nerve with root value C-7 mainly. Hence, there will be no loss of pronation in Erb's paralysis.
   ❏ In Erb's palsy there is a weakness of supination due to the paralysed biceps brachii secondary to the lesioned musculocutaneous nerve (C-5 and 6).

9. c. The median and ulnar nerves were affected
   ❏ This is a case of Erb's paralysis, where C-5 and 6 roots are damaged.
   ❏ Median nerve carries the root value C5-8; T-1 and ulnar nerve has the root value C-7, 8; T-1. Hence it is evident that ulnar nerve escapes in such a lesion, whereas, median nerve is partially injured (left with some residual functionality).
   ❏ Supraspinatus, infraspinatus, subclavius and biceps brachii are all supplied by the nerves carrying root value C-5,6 are paralysed.

10. b. Most common site of injury is upper trunk, c. Injury may occur during breech delivery, e. Lower trunk injury result in hand deformity
   ❏ Brachial plexus is contributed by the spinal nerve C5-8; T1.
   ❏ Radial nerve is a branch of the posterior cord of brachial plexus.
   ❏ Most common site of injury is upper trunk. Obstetric brachial palsy following breech delivery is a typical group: upper lesions predominating with a great number of upper root avulsions and phrenic nerve lesions. Lower trunk (C-8; T1) injury results in claw hand deformity.

- Three trunks (upper, middle and lower), dorsal divisions join to form the **posterior cord** of brachial plexus *(NEET Pattern 2015)*
- The roots of C-5, 6, 7 contribute to the long thoracic nerve (of Bell) in the neck region (supraclavicular portion of brachial plexus) *(NEET Pattern 2013)*
- Radial nerve is the **largest** branch of brachial plexus and is the continuation of **posterior cord** (C5-8; T1) *(NEET pattern 2014)*
- Root value of ulnar nerve - C (7),8; T1 *(NEET Pattern 2015)*
- Roots of brachial plexus are present in neck region (and **not axilla**) *(NEET Pattern 2013)*
- Arterial supply to brachial plexus is from the branches of **subclavian** and **vertebral** arteries.
- Erb's point is at the junction of C5 and C6 roots *(NEET Pattern 2013)*

▼ Axillary Nerve

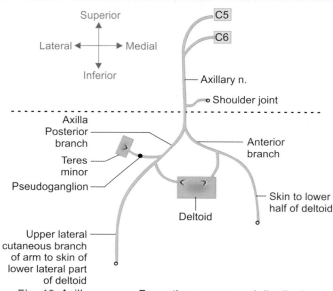

Fig. 13: Axillary nerve: Formation, course and distribution

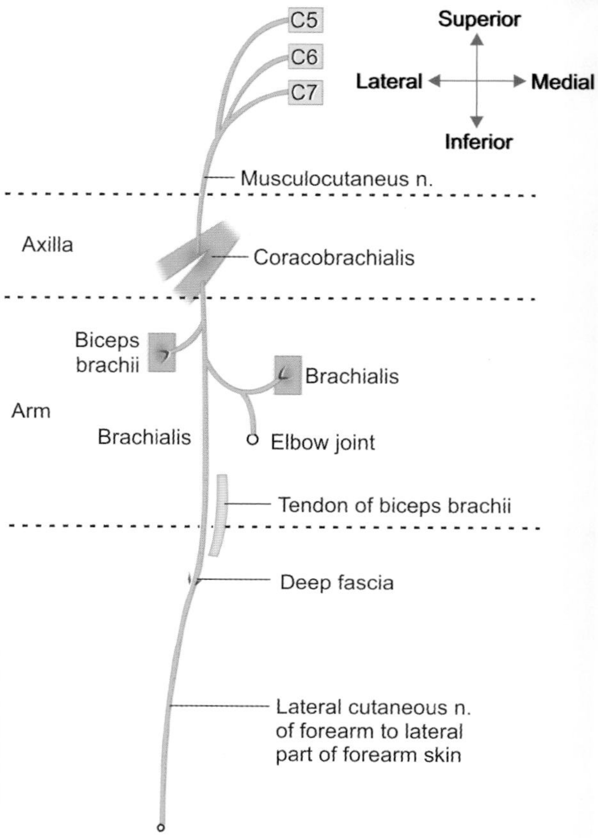

Fig. 14: Musculocutaneous nerve: Formation, course and distribution

- ❑ **Axillary** (circumflex) **nerve** is a branch of **posterior cord** of brachial plexus given in the axilla, pass almost horizontally through the **quadrangular space**, accompanied by the posterior circumflex humeral vessels *(NEET Pattern 2015)*
- ❑ It innervates **teres minor** and **deltoid**, and the skin on the lateral aspect of the shoulder overlying lower half of deltoid.
- ❑ **Injury** to the axillary nerve may be caused by a **fracture of the surgical neck** of the humerus or **inferior dislocation** of the humerus results in the weakness of abduction especially (15-90°) and lateral rotation of the arm. Regimental batch anaesthesia (loss of sensation on skin over the lower half of deltoid – C5) is also observed.

▼ Musculocutaneous Nerve

- ❑ It arises from **lateral cord** of the brachial plexus (C5, C6, and C7). It provides motor innervation to the muscles on the front of the arm and sensory innervation to the skin of the lateral part of the forearm.
- ❑ It supplies: Biceps brachii, Brachialis and Coracobrachialis muscles *(NEET Pattern 2012)*
- ❑ Coracobrachialis is **pierced** and supplied by musculocutaneous nerve *(NEET Pattern 2013)* Radial nerve

▼ Radial Nerve

Radial nerve is a continuation of the **posterior cord** of brachial plexus in the axilla, carries fibres from **all the roots** (C5-8; T1) of brachial plexus.

- ❑ It is **the largest nerve** in the upper limb and the **most commonly damaged**.
- ❑ In the axilla it lies **posterior** to the third part of the axillary artery. It gives three branches in the axilla: **Posterior cutaneous nerve of arm** (cutaneous innervation on the back of the arm up to the elbow); **nerve to the long head of triceps** and **nerve to the medial head of triceps.**

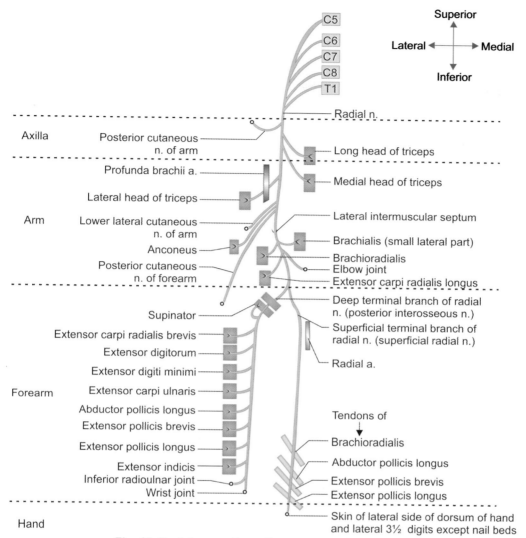

Fig. 15: Radial nerve: Formation, course and distribution

❑ It enters the arm at the lower border of the teres major and passes between the long and medial heads of triceps to enter the **lower triangular space**, through which it reaches the **radial (spiral) groove** along with profunda brachii vessels and lies in direct contact with the humerus.

❑ In the radial groove, it gives **five branches**: Lower lateral cutaneous nerve of the arm (innervation on the lateral surface of the arm up to the elbow); posterior cutaneous nerve of the forearm (innervation down the middle of the back of the forearm up to the wrist); nerve to lateral head of triceps; nerve to medial head of triceps and nerve to anconeus (passes through medial head of triceps to reach the anconeus).

❑ At the lower end of the spiral groove, radial nerve **pierces the lateral muscular septum** of the arm, enters the anterior compartment of the arm and give nerve to **brachialis** (small lateral part).

❑ Nerve to **brachioradialis** is given about three fingers' breadths above the lateral epicondyle, and the nerve to **extensor carpi radialis longus** 1 cm more distally. One nerve to **extensor carpi radialis brevis** leaves the main nerve about 1 cm proximal to the lateral epicondyle, and another leaves at the site of division into **two terminal branches**.

❑ Radial nerve is a **content of cubital fossa** and in front of the lateral epicondyle terminates into two branches: Superficial (**cutaneous**) and Deep (**motor**) *(NEET Pattern 2015)*

❑ The **deep branch** supplies two muscles, extensor carpi radialis brevis and supinator, passes through supinator to enter and supply the posterior compartment of the forearm, named as **posterior interosseous nerve**. It also gives articular branches to the distal radioulnar, wrist, and carpal joints.

❑ The **superficial branch** descends inferiorly deep to brachioradialis, passes posteriorly at about 7 cm above wrist, emerge from under the tendon of brachioradialis, proximal to the radial styloid process and then passes over the tendons and roof of **anatomical snuff-box** (subcutaneously) and supply skin over the lateral part of the dorsum of hand and dorsal surfaces of lateral 3½ digits (**excluding** the nail beds).

Table 11: Radial nerve injuries

Site of injury	Lesion	Motor loss	Sensory loss
Axilla (Very high lesion)	• Crutch palsy • Saturday night palsy (arm draped over chair)	• Loss of elbow extension (triceps paralysis) • Wrist drop (loss of wrist extension) • Finger drop (loss of finger extension) • Difficulty in supination*	• Over the posterior surface of the lower part of the arm and forearm • Over the lateral part of the dorsum of hand and dorsal surfaces of lateral 3½ digits (excluding the nail beds), especially a small patch on the dorsum around the anatomical snuffbox.
Spiral groove (High lesion)	• Fracture midshaft of humerus • IM injection • Saturday night palsy	• Elbow extension possible (triceps spared) • Wrist drop (loss of wrist extension) • Finger drop (loss of finger extension) • Difficulty in supination*	• Over the lateral part of the dorsum of hand and dorsal surfaces of lateral 3½ digits (excluding the nail beds), especially a small patch on the dorsum around the anatomical snuffbox.
At the elbow (Low lesion)	• Fracture/dislocations • Entrapment injury (radial tunnel syndrome)	• No wrist drop (ECRL spared)** • Finger drop (loss of finger extension) • Difficulty in supination	• No cutaneous loss

* Difficulty in supination in extended elbow (supinator and brachioradialis paralysis); supination is possible in flexed elbow (functional biceps brachii).

Wrist extension is preserved because the branch to the extensor carpi radialis longus **arises proximal to the elbow.

In radial nerve injuries there is weakness of abduction and adduction of the hand (paralysed extensor carpi and ulnaris muscles).

❑ In radial nerve injuries, extension at PIP and DIP may be possible carried out by **lumbrical and interossei** (supplied by median and ulnar nerve).

❑ In wrist drop, the patient is given cock-up splint to prevent the resulting deformities.

- Radial nerve gives branch to anconeus muscle in the groove *(JIPMER 2009)*
- Two cutaneous nerves, the **lower lateral cutaneous nerve of the arm** and the posterior cutaneous nerve of the forearm are given by radial nerve in the radial groove *(NEET Pattern 2014)*
- A long, slender branch of radial nerve (to medial head of triceps), lies close to the ulnar nerve as far as the lower third of the arm, is frequently called as ulnar collateral nerve *(NEET Pattern 2013)*
- Injury to radial nerve at wrist leads to Sensory loss on dorsum of 1st web space.

1. **Which of the following is NOT seen with lower radial nerve injury** *(AIPG 2008)*
   a. Weakness of brachioradialis
   b. Inability to extend fingers
   c. Paralysis of extensor carpi radialis brevis
   d. Loss of sensations over dorsum of hand

2. **Finger drop with no wrist drop is caused by lesion of** *(NEET Pattern 2015)*
   a. Radial nerve in the radial groove
   b. Posterior interosseous nerve
   c. Anterior interosseous nerve
   d. Ulnar nerve behind medial epicondyle

3. **All are affected in low radial nerve palsy EXCEPT** *(AIPG 2011)*
   a. Extensor carpi radialis longus
   b. Extensor carpi radialis brevis
   c. Finger extensors
   d. Sensation on dorsum of hand

4. **Injury to radial nerve in lower part of spiral groove may result in all EXCEPT** *(AIIMS 2003)*
   a. Spare nerve supply to extensor carpi radialis longus
   b. Results in paralysis of anconeus muscle
   c. Leaves extension at elbow joint intact
   d. Weakens supination movement

5. **Damage to the radial nerve in the spiral groove spares which muscle**
   a. Lateral head of biceps   b. Long head of triceps
   c. Medial head of triceps   d. Anconeus

6. **Which of the following movements of thumb are NOT affected in radial nerve injury** *(PGIC 2009)*
   a. Opposition   b. Abduction
   c. Adduction   d. Extension
   e. Flexion

1. **a. Weakness of brachioradialis**
   ❑ Lower radial nerve injury (as in fracture lower end of humerus) means damage to the nerve just before its terminal divisions at the front of humeral lateral epicondyle.
   ❑ It spares the brachioradialis as it is supplied by the nerve after it exits the radial groove and the branch lies quite higher than the lateral epicondyle.
   ❑ Radial nerve at its lower end supplies extensor carpi radialis brevis and then divides into two terminal branches: Posterior interosseous nerve (muscular) and superficial cutaneous branch of radial nerve.
   ❑ Posterior interosseous nerve supplies the finger extensors, which have got paralysed in this case.
   ❑ The superficial cutaneous branch of radial nerve supplies the lateral dorsum of hand, showing sensory loss in this injury.
   ❑ Lower radial nerve injury also leads to paralysis of extensor carpi radialis brevis as its radial branch is quite low.

2. **b. Posterior interosseous nerve**
   - ❑ Injury to posterior interosseous nerve results in paralysis of extensor muscles in the posterior forearm.
   - ❑ Finger drop (loss of finger extension at metacarpophalangeal joint) occurs, along with weakening of wrist extension.
   - ❑ Wrist extension is still possible (no wrist drop) because of the functional ECRL (Extensor Carpi Radialis Longus) muscle, a powerful wrist extensor, already supplied by a branch of radial nerve proximal to the site of injury.

3. **a. Extensor carpi radialis longus**
   - ❑ Low radial nerve injuries occur around the elbow joint (e.g., fracture humerus at lower end) and may spare the ECRL (Extensor Carpi Radialis Longus) muscle.
   - ❑ All the muscles supplied by radial nerve distal to the lesion get paralysed and there is sensory loss over the dorsum of hand.

4. **a. Spare nerve supply to extensor carpi radialis longus**
   - ❑ Injury to radial nerve in lower part of radial groove results in paralysis (not sparing) of ECRL (Extensor Carpi Radialis Longus).
   - ❑ Triceps receive branches of radial nerve in axilla and radial groove, hence it will be spared, and elbow extension is intact.
   - ❑ Anconeus may (or may not) be paralysed, depending upon the involvement of the branch in the fracture.
   - ❑ Supinator muscle is paralysed, hence there will be difficulty in supination.

5. **b. Long head of triceps > c. Medial head of triceps**
   - ❑ Radial nerve in radial groove gives branches to long head of triceps and medial head of triceps as well.

6. **a. Opposition; c. Adduction; e. Flexion**
   - ❑ Radial nerve supplies the extensors of thumb and abductor pollicis longus (lateral abduction).
   - ❑ Opposition and flexion of thumb is carried out by muscles supplied by median and ulnar nerve.
   - ❑ Adductor pollicis is supplied by ulnar nerve.

▸ Median Nerve

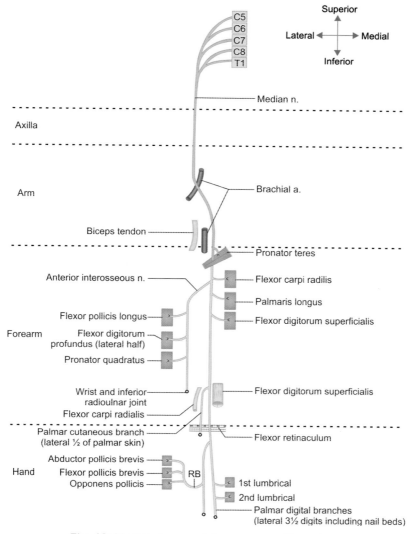

Fig. 16: Median nerve: origin, course and branches.

❏ About 5 cm proximal to the flexor retinaculum, it emerges from the lateral side of the FDS and becomes superficial, **lying lateral to the tendons of FDS** and palmaris longus.

❏ The most commonly damaged nerve in wrist slash injury is median nerve, less commonly ulnar nerve may also be damaged.

❏ **Wrist slash injury** (suicidal attempts) A deep laceration on the radial side of the wrist may cut the following structures: Radial artery, **median nerve**, flexor carpi radialis tendon, and palmaris longus tendon.

❏ A deep laceration on the ulnar side of the wrist may cut the following structures: Ulnar artery, **ulnar nerve**, and flexor carpi ulnaris tendon.

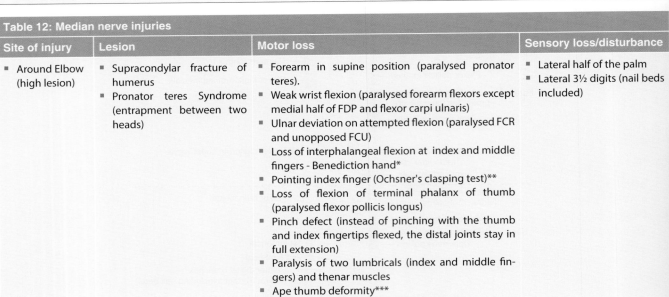

Fig. 17: Median nerve at the wrist

Median nerve is formed by the union of the lateral root (C5, 6, 7) from the **lateral cord**, and the medial root (C8, T1) from the **medial cord**, which meet **anterior** to the third part of the axillary artery.

❏ It enters the arm at the lower border of teres major, **initially** lies lateral to brachial artery and **then crosses in front** of the artery from lateral to medial side **at the level of midhumerus** (i.e., level of insertion of coracobrachialis).

❏ After crossing, it runs downwards to **enter cubital fossa**, lies medial to the brachial artery and tendon of biceps brachii and gives muscular branches to supply all the superficial flexors of the forearm (flexor carpi radialis, palmaris longus, and flexor digitorum superficialis) **except** flexor carpi ulnaris. It leaves the fossa by passing between the two heads of **pronator teres** and gives off anterior interosseous nerve.

❏ **Anterior interosseous nerve** is a pure motor nerve, accompanied by the anterior interosseous vessels, dives deeply to pass down **along the interosseous membrane** and supplies 2½ muscles: Flexor pollicis longus, pronator quadratus and **lateral half** of the flexor digitorum profundus (FDP).

❏ In the forearm, the **median nerve** runs deep to the flexor digitorum superficialis (FDS).

❏ The **palmar cutaneous nerve** arises about 3-7 cm proximal to the flexor retinaculum (and proximal wrist crease), passes lateral to the main nerve and **superficial to the flexor retinaculum** to supply the skin over the thenar eminence and lateral aspect of the palm.

❏ Median nerve enters the palm by passing through carpal tunnel where it lies **deep to flexor retinaculum** and superficial to the tendons of FDS, FDP, and FPL and their associated ulnar and radial bursae.

❏ In the palm, the median nerve divides into lateral and medial divisions. The lateral division gives a **recurrent branch**, which curls upwards to supply thenar muscles except the deep head of flexor pollicis brevis.

❏ It gives five **palmar digital nerves** which supply first and second lumbricals and skin of the palmar aspect of the lateral 3½ digits and skin on the dorsal aspect of distal phalanges (**nail beds**).

▪ Median nerve is also called as **Labourer's nerve** as it supplies the anterior forearm muscles and anterior thumb muscles. These muscles help to **push, pull, lift heavy loads** by the labourers and if the nerve is damaged they are helpless to carry out all such movements (*NEET Pattern 2012*)

Table 12: Median nerve injuries			
Site of injury	**Lesion**	**Motor loss**	**Sensory loss/disturbance**
▪ Around Elbow (high lesion)	▪ Supracondylar fracture of humerus ▪ Pronator teres Syndrome (entrapment between two heads)	▪ Forearm in supine position (paralysed pronator teres). ▪ Weak wrist flexion (paralysed forearm flexors except medial half of FDP and flexor carpi ulnaris) ▪ Ulnar deviation on attempted flexion (paralysed FCR and unopposed FCU) ▪ Loss of interphalangeal flexion at index and middle fingers - Benediction hand* ▪ Pointing index finger (Ochsner's clasping test)** ▪ Loss of flexion of terminal phalanx of thumb (paralysed flexor pollicis longus) ▪ Pinch defect (instead of pinching with the thumb and index fingertips flexed, the distal joints stay in full extension) ▪ Paralysis of two lumbricals (index and middle fingers) and thenar muscles ▪ Ape thumb deformity***	▪ Lateral half of the palm ▪ Lateral 3½ digits (nail beds included)

Site of injury	Lesion	Motor loss	Sensory loss/disturbance
▪ Distal forearm/ Wrist	▪ Wrist slash injury/suicidal attempts	▪ Paralysis of two lumbricals (index and middle fingers) and thenar muscles ▪ Ape thumb deformity	▪ Lateral half of the palm ▪ Lateral 3½ digits (nail beds included)
▪ Carpal tunnel (syndrome)	▪ Tenosynovitis of flexor tendons due to repeat stress injury (e.g., data entry) ▪ Myxedema (deficiency of thyroxine) ▪ Oedema in pregnancy ▪ Anterior dislocation of lunate bone ▪ Osteoarthritis at wrist ▪ Rheumatoid arthritis	▪ Paralysis of two lumbricals (index and middle fingers) and thenar muscles ▪ Ape thumb deformity (later stages)	▪ Lateral 3½ digits (nail beds included) ▪ No sensory loss over the lateral half of the palm (palmar cutaneous branch is spared)

*__Benediction hand__: When patient attempts to make a fist, the index and middle fingers remain straight (loss of flexion at PIP and DIP joints due to paralysed superficial and deep flexors).

**__Pointed index finger__: When the patient is asked to clasp both his hands. The index finger on the affected side will stand pointing out instead of being flexed.

***__Ape thumb deformity__ presents with thenar atrophy and thumb remains laterally rotated and adducted (paralyzed thenar muscles and intact adductor pollicis).

Note: Division of the median nerve **distal** to the origin of its palmar cutaneous branch, arises 3 and 7 cm proximal to the flexor retinaculum, leave intact the sensation over the thenar eminence and radial side of the proximal part of the hand.

❑ **Benediction hand deformity** It may result due to median nerve injury. **While trying to make a fist**, patient can only partially flex index and middle finger.

❑ The ability to flex the digits 2–3 at the metacarpophalangeal joints is **lost** as is the ability to flex the proximal and distal interphalangeal joints. This is due to the loss of innervation of the **lateral 2 lumbricals** of the hand and the **lateral half of the flexor digitorum profundus** which are supplied by the median nerve.

❑ **Flexion** at the proximal interphalangeal joints of digits 4–5 is **weakened**, but flexion at the metacarpophalangeal joints and distal interphalangeal joints remains **intact**.

❑ The extensor digitorum is left **unopposed** and the metacarpophalangeal joints of **digits 2–3 remain extended** while attempting to make a fist.

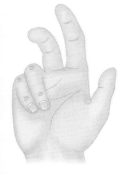

Fig. 18: Benediction hand deformity

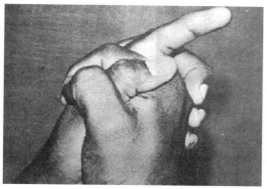

Fig. 19: Ochsner's clasping test

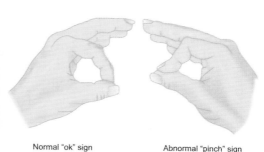

Normal "ok" sign   Abnormal "pinch" sign

Fig. 20: Clinical testing for median nerve injury

❑ **Ochsner's clasping test** assesses the function of the median nerve for lesions in the cubital fossa or above, by testing for the function of long flexors to index finger (flexor digitorum superficialis and profundus). When the **patient is asked to clasp both his hands**, the index finger on the affected side will stand **pointing out** instead of being flexed.

❑ **Pinch defect:** Instead of pinching with the thumb and index fingertips flexed, the distal joints **stay in full extension**. It is observed in median nerve injury, due to **paralysis of long flexors** to thumb and digits.

❑ **Carpal tunnel syndrome** It is caused by compression of the median nerve due to the reduced size of the osseofibrous carpal tunnel, resulting from **inflammation or thickening** of the synovial sheaths of the flexor tendons (tenosynovitis) due to repeat stress injury (e.g., data entry), inflammation of the flexor retinaculum, or arthritic changes in the carpal bones (particularly rheumatoid arthritis).

➤ It is usually **idiopathic** though it is associated with soft tissue thickening, as may occur in **myxoedema** and **acromegaly**; it may also be associated with oedema, obesity or **pregnancy**. Anterior dislocation of lunate may compress the median nerve leading to features of carpal tunnel syndrome.

➤ It leads to pain and paresthesia (tingling, burning, and numbness) in the hand in the area supplied by the median nerve, **worse at night** and on gripping objects. It may also lead to **atrophy** of the thenar muscles in cases of severe compression. However, **no paresthesia occurs over the thenar eminence** of skin because this area is supplied by the palmar cutaneous branch of the median nerve, **already given** before the nerve enters tunnel.

➤ The structures that pass **through the carpal tunnel** include the flexor digitorum superficialis tendons, flexor digitorum profundus tendons, flexor pollicis longus tendon, and median nerve. No arteries pass through the carpal tunnel.

❑ Clinical signs include **sensory loss** on the palmar aspects of the index, middle, and half of the ring fingers and palmar aspect of the thumb. Patient presents with **ape thumb deformity**, **Tinel** & **Phalen** test are positive (see following sections for detail). Treatment is usually surgical decompression of the nerve by **dividing the flexor retinaculum**, if conservative management (like **splinting** at night) fails.

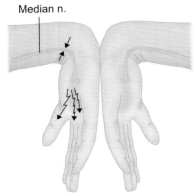

Fig. 21: Phalen test

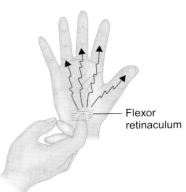

Fig. 22: Tinel's sign

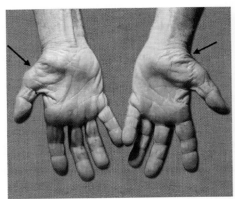

Fig. 23: Ape thumb deformity

QUESTIONS

1. A patient is trying to make a fist, but can only partially flex index and middle finger. Which nerve is damaged most probably *(AIIMS; JIPMER pattern 2016)*
a. Median
b. Ulnar
c. Radial
d. Anterior interosseous nerve

2. Median nerve injury at wrist, is commonly tested by
a. Contraction of abductor pollicis brevis
b. Contraction flexor pollicis brevis
c. Contraction opponens pollicis
d. Loss of sensation on palm

3. Which of the following muscle is supplied by median nerve *(PGIC 2016)*
a. Opponens pollicis
b. Adductor pollicis
c. Lateral half of the flexor digitorum profundus
d. Superficial head of flexor pollicis brevis
e. Deep part of flexor pollicis brevis

4. Anterior interosseous nerve supplies *(PGIC 2017)*
a. Brachioradialis
b. Flexor pollicis longus
c. Flexor carpi ulnaris
d. Flexor digitorum superficialis
e. Pronator teres

ANSWERS

1. a. Median
❑ Median nerve injury leads to 'benediction hand' deformity, as observed in this patient.

2. a. Contraction of abductor pollicis brevis
❑ Median nerve injury at wrist is commonly subjected to pen test—the patient lies his hand flat on a table with his palm facing upwards.
❑ The patient is asked to abduct his thumb to touch the examiner's pen which is held above it. This test is for the function of abductor pollicis brevis, supplied by median nerve.
❑ Flexor pollicis brevis and opponens pollicis have dual nerve supply: supplied by median and ulnar nerve.

3. a. Opponens pollicis; c. Lateral half of the flexor digitorum profundus; d. Superficial head of flexor pollicis brevis
❑ Opponens pollicis is usually mentioned to innervated by the lateral terminal branch of the median nerve (but Gray's anatomy mentions that it also receives a branch of the deep terminal branch of the ulnar nerve).
❑ Adductor pollicis is supplied by ulnar nerve.
❑ Lateral half of the Flexor digitorum profundus is supplied by the median nerve, whereas ulnar nerve supplies the medal half.
❑ The superficial head of flexor pollicis brevis is innervated by the lateral terminal branch of the median nerve and the deep part by the deep branch of the ulnar nerve.

ANSWERS

4. b. Flexor pollicis longus
- ❑ Anterior interosseous nerve supplies the deep muscles of the anterior forearm: Flexor pollicis longus, pronator quadratus and radial half of flexor digitorum profundus.
- ❑ Brachioradialis: Radial nerve; Flexor carpi ulnaris: Ulnar nerve; Flexor digitorum superficialis and Pronator teres: Median nerve.

▼ Ulnar Nerve

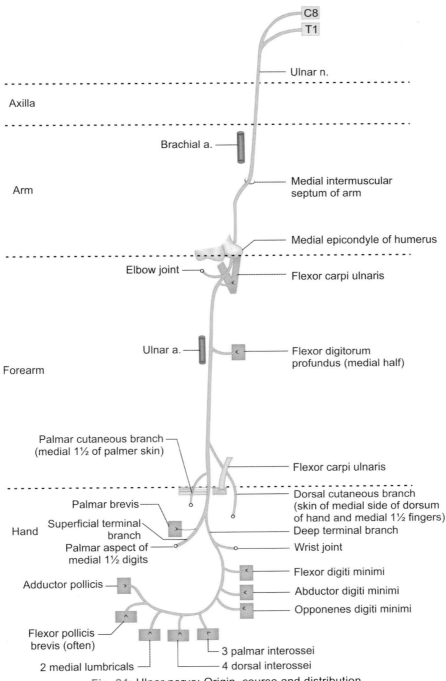

Fig. 24: Ulnar nerve: Origin, course and distribution

❑ Ulnar nerve enters the forearm by passing **between** the two heads of flexor carpi ulnaris, descend down in the forearm with ulnar artery on the lateral side.
  - ➢ **Branches** In **upper** forearm: Flexor carpi ulnaris, and medial half of flexor digitorum profundus.
  - ➢ In **distal** forearm: Dorsal cutaneous branch (given 6 cm proximal to the wrist), supply dorsum of medial third of the hand and medial 1½ fingers.

- ➤ Near the wrist: Palmar cutaneous branch, passes superficial to flexor retinaculum & supply hypothenar eminence.
- ➤ Ulnar nerve passes **superficial** to the flexor retinaculum lying just lateral to the pisiform, covered by a fascial band (volar carpal ligament) through the **Guyon's ulnar tunnel.** Just distal to pisiform, the ulnar nerve divides into its terminal superficial and deep branches. The **superficial** terminal branch supplies palmaris brevis and provide sensory innervation to the skin on the palmar surface of medial 1½ fingers.
- ➤ The **deep** branch of ulnar nerve runs laterally within concavity of deep palmar arterial arch, is purely motor and supplies all the intrinsic muscles of the hand (except first two lumbricals & abductor pollicis brevis).

Ulnar nerve is the continuation of the **medial cord** of brachial plexus (**C8 and T1**) and receives a contribution from the ventral ramus of **C7** (which supply flexor carpi ulnaris).

- ❑ It does not give any branch in the axilla and in the arm. In the axilla it lies **medial** to third part of axillary artery (between axillary artery and vein).
- ❑ In the arm, it runs distally along the medial side of the brachial artery up to the **midarm** (level of insertion of coracobrachialis), inclines posteromedially to **perforate** the medial intermuscular septum (10 cm proximal to the medial epicondyle) and passes through a fibrous canal, the 'arcade of Struthers' (length-5 cm).
- ❑ The walls of the canal include the medial intermuscular septum and the fascial sheath investing the medial head of triceps brachii. It is accompanied by the **superior collateral ulnar vessels** in the lower third of the arm and distally by the **posteroinferior ulnar collateral vessels**.
- ❑ Behind the **medial epicondyle**, it is lodged in a groove where it can be easily palpated. The groove is converted into 'cubital **tunnel**' by a fibrous band extending between medial epicondyle and olecranon process. The **ulnar nerve** crosses the ulnar collateral ligament in the **floor** of the tunnel.

Note: Ulnar nerve gives no muscular branches in the arm.

- ❑ The medial part of the elbow where ulnar nerve passes behind medial epicondyle of humerus is termed 'funny bone' because as it hits a hard surface, tingling funny sensations is felt along the ulnar side of the forearm and hand.
- ❑ Ulnar nerve division at the wrist paralyses all the intrinsic muscles of the hand (apart from the radial two lumbricals, abductor pollicis brevis, and part of flexor pollicis brevis & opponens pollicis).
- ❑ Ulnar nerve is called as '**musician's nerve**' as it innervates most of the intrinsic muscles involved in the **fine intricate** finger movements for playing musical instruments.

Table 13: Ulnar nerve injuries			
Site of injury	**Lesion**	**Motor loss**	**Sensory loss/disturbance**

Elbow (high lesion)	▪ Fracture/dislocation of the medial epicondyle (humerus)
	 ▪ Cubital tunnel syndrome
	 ▪ Compression between the two heads of flexor carpi ulnaris
	 ▪ Tardy ulnar nerve palsy (valgus deformity)
		▪ Claw-hand deformity*
		
		 ▪ Hypothenar and interosseous wasting
		 ▪ Loss of
		   – Abduction and adduction of the fingers (card test positive)
		   – Flexion of the metacarpophalangeal joints
		   – Adduction of the thumb (Froment sign positive)
		 ▪ Weakness of wrist flexion (hand deviates to radial side upon flexion)
			▪ Over the palmar and dorsal surfaces of medial third of the hand and medial 1½ fingers (little finger and the ulnar half of the ring finger)

Wrist (low lesion)	▪ Wrist laceration/ slashing
	 ▪ Guyon's canal syndrome
		▪ Claw hand deformity (more pronounced)**
		 ▪ Hypothenar and interosseous wasting
		 ▪ Loss of
		   – Abduction & adduction of the fingers (card test positive)
		   – Adduction of the thumb (Froment sign positive)
			▪ Over the palmar and dorsal surfaces of medial 1½ fingers (little finger and the ulnar half of the ring finger)
			 ▪ No sensory loss over the ulnar aspect of the dorsum of the hand (dorsal cutaneous branch is spared)

*****Claw-hand deformity** (main en griffe) affecting ring and little fingers. Extension at metacarpophalangeal joint & flexion at the interphalangeal joints.

Claw hand deformity is **more pronounced in low injury, since FDP (flexor digitorum profundus) is not paralysed; therefore there is a marked flexion of DIP joints. The sensation over the ulnar aspect of the dorsum of the hand is **spared** because the dorsal branch of the ulnar nerve is given off approximately 5 cm proximal to the wrist joint.

- ❑ **Cubital tunnel syndrome**
    - ➤ It may result from **compression on the ulnar nerve** in the cubital tunnel behind the medial epicondyle, causing **numbness and tingling** in the ring and little fingers.

➤ The cubital tunnel is formed by the **medial epicondyle**, ulnar collateral ligament, and two heads of the flexor carpi ulnaris, and transmits the ulnar nerve and **superior ulnar collateral artery**.

❑ **Guyon's canal** (pisohamate tunnel)
➤ It is a fibro-osseous canal, 4 cm long, on the anteromedial side of the wrist for passage of **ulnar artery and nerve** into the hand.

Ulnar boundary: **Pisiform bone**, flexor carpi ulnaris and abductor digiti minimi

Medial boundary: **Hook of hamate**, extrinsic flexor tendons, the transverse carpal ligament.

Roof: Palmar carpal ligament and palmaris brevis.

Floor: Flexor retinaculum and pisohamate ligaments (more distally, pisometacarpal ligaments and flexor digiti minimi)

Contents: Ulnar nerve and artery

➤ Ulnar nerve **divides within it** at the level of the hook of the hamate into a **deep, lateral motor** branch and a **superficial, medial sensory** branch. If the nerve is compressed in the tunnel, both modalities will be affected.

❑ **Guyon's canal syndrome**
➤ Entrapment of the **ulnar nerve** in the Guyon's canal, causing pain, numbness, and tingling in the ring and little fingers, and motor weakness in later stages.
➤ It is seen in cases of prolonged pressure upon the outer part of the palm like long distance **cyclists** and road workers using **vibrating drills**. It can be treated by **surgical decompression** of the nerve.

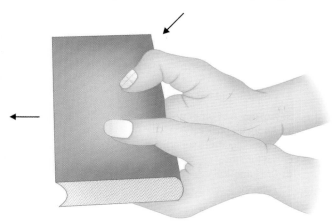

Fig. 25: Froment's sign (book test)

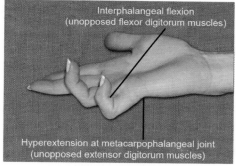

Interphalangeal flexion
(unopposed flexor digitorum muscles)

Hyperextension at metacarpophalangeal joint
(unopposed extensor digitorum muscles)

Fig. 26: Ulnar claw hand

❑ **Froment's sign**
➤ The patient is instructed to grasp a book/paper **between the thumb and index finger**. Normally he grasps the book firmly with thumb extended, taking full advantage of the **adductor pollicis** and the first dorsal interosseous muscles.
➤ In ulnar nerve **injury**, powerful flexion of the thumb interphalangeal joint signals **weakness of adductor pollicis** and first dorsal interosseous with overcompensation by the flexor pollicis longus (supplied by median nerve).

Ulnar Claw Hand

❑ Injury to ulnar nerve presents with ulnar claw hand: **hyperextension** of metacarpophalangeal and **flexion** of interphalangeal joints of ring and little finger.

❑ Ulnar nerve supplies medial 2 lumbricals (ring and little finger) in the hand. Lumbricals have a combined action of MCP (Metacarpophalangeal) flexion and IP (Interphalangeal) extension (glass holding posture).

❑ In **ulnar nerve injury**, since the lumbricals are not functional, the **forearm muscles are unopposed**.

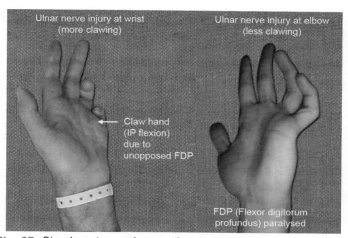

Ulnar nerve injury at wrist
(more clawing)

Ulnar nerve injury at elbow
(less clawing)

Claw hand
(IP flexion)
due to
unopposed FDP

FDP (Flexor digitorum
profundus) paralysed

Fig. 27: Simply put, as reinnervation occurs along the ulnar nerve after a high lesion, the deformity will get worse (FDP reinnervated) as the patient recovers—hence the use of the term 'paradox'

❑ MCP joint goes into **hyperextension** (unopposed activity of extensor digitorum muscles, posterior forearm) and IP joints go into **flexion** (unopposed activity of flexor digitorum muscles, anterior forearm) and they bring the deformity called **ulnar claw hand**.

Ulnar Paradox

❑ The **higher** the lesion of the ulnar nerve injury, the **less prominent** is the deformity and vice versa, because in higher lesions the long finger flexors are also paralysed (which were causing interphalangeal flexion/clawing). The loss of finger flexion makes the deformity look less obvious/less clawing.

❑ Ulnar nerve injury at wrist causes '**more**' clawing (severe interphalangeal flexion deformity, due to unopposed flexor digitorum profundus).

❑ Ulnar nerve injury at elbow paralyses flexor digitorum profundus and leads to '**less**' clawing (less interphalangeal flexion deformity).

This is known as the '**ulnar paradox**'– normally we would **expect** a more pronounced deformity, due to ulnar nerve injury at elbow (as compared with wrist level) but in fact the **opposite** is observed.

QUESTIONS

1. All are true about ulnar nerve EXCEPT *(PGIC 2014)*
   a. Root value C8; T1
   b. Pass through flexor digitorum superficialis
   c. Supply flexor digitorum superficialis
   d. Supply flexor carpi ulnaris
   e. Passes behind medial epicondyle

2. FALSE regarding ulnar nerve is *(PGIC 2014)*
   a. C7 fibers arise from lateral cord
   b. Root value: C7,8; T1
   c. No branch in arm
   d. Passes between supinator heads
   e. Lies superficial to FDP and flexor retinaculum

3. Ulnar paradox means *(NEET Pattern 2016)*
   a. High level injury- less severe claw hand
   b. Low level injury-less severe claw hand
   c. High level injury-more severe claw hand
   d. Low level- more severe claw hand

4. Ulnar injury in the arm leads to all EXCEPT *(AIIMS 2007)*
   a. Sensory loss of the medial 1/3rd of the hand
   b. Weakness of the hypothenar muscles
   c. Claw hand
   d. Adduction of thumb

5. Superficial branch of ulnar nerve supplies *(JIPMER 2013)*
   a. Palmaris brevis
   b. Abductor pollicis
   c. Abductor digiti minimi
   d. Opponens pollicis

6. Deep branch of ulnar nerve supplies *(PGIC 2009)*
   a. Adductor pollicis
   b. Flexor digitorum superficialis
   c. 1st lumbrical
   d. 3rd lumbrical
   e. Palmaris brevis

ANSWERS

1. b. Pass through flexor digitorum superficialis; c. Supply flexor digitorum superficialis
   ❑ Ulnar nerve carries the root value C (7),8; T1. It Passes through the cubital tunnel behind the medial epicondyle and enters the forearm by passing between the two heads of flexor carpi ulnaris and innervates it. It doesn't pass through or supply flexor digitorum superficialis.

2. d. Passes between supinator heads
   ❑ Ulnar nerve is the continuation of medial cord (C8; T1), may receive C7 fibres from lateral cord.
   ❑ It gives no branch in arm, enters the forearm by passing between the two (humeral and ulnar) heads of origin of flexor carpi ulnaris, descends on the medial side of forearm lying superficial to flexor digitorum profundus and deep to flexor carpi ulnaris, runs with ulnar artery to pass superficial to flexor retinaculum to enter the palm.

3. a. High level injury- less severe claw hand
   ❑ Ulnar paradox- The higher the lesion of the median and ulnar nerve injury, the less prominent is the deformity and vice versa, because in higher lesions the long finger flexors are also paralysed (which were causing interphalangeal flexion/clawing). The loss of finger flexion makes the deformity look less obvious/ less clawing.
   ❑ Note: Option d) 'Low level- more severe claw hand' is equally good answer, as mentioned by few authors.

4. d. Adduction of thumb
   ❑ Ulnar nerve supplies the adductor pollicis muscle and hence it will be paralysed in its lesion.
   ❑ Hence, adduction of thumb is not a clinical finding in ulnar nerve palsy.

5. a. Palmaris brevis
   ❑ The superficial branch of ulnar nerve in hand supplies palmaris brevis muscle and skin on the palmar aspect of medial
   ❑ 1 1/2 fingers.

6. a. Adductor pollicis; d. 3rd lumbrical
   ❑ Flexor digitorum superficialis is supplied by median nerve in the forearm. 1st lumbrical is also supplied by the median nerve.
   ❑ The deep branch of ulnar nerve is purely motor and supplies all the intrinsic muscles of the hand (including adductor pollicis) except the muscles of thenar eminence and first two lumbricals. Palmaris brevis is supplied by superficial terminal branch of ulnar nerve.

▶ **Cutaneous Innervation**

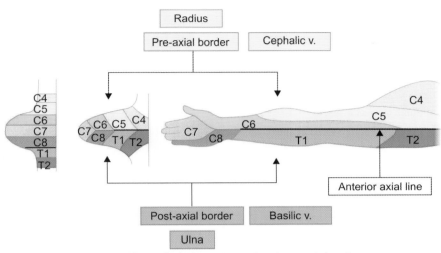

Fig. 28: Upper limb dermatome developmental pattern

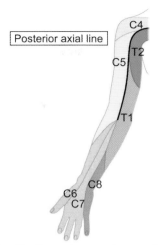

Fig. 29: Dermatomes of upper limb
(Posterior view)

❑ Developmentally, **radius bone** is a **preaxial bone** and ulna is postaxial. Similarly, **radial artery** is preaxial along with **cephalic vein**, whereas ulnar artery is postaxial along with the basilic vein.

❑ The preaxial vein becomes the **cephalic vein** and drains into the axillary vein in the axilla. The **postaxial vein** becomes the basilic vein, which passes deep in the arm to continue as the axillary vein.

❑ The **anterior axial line** reaches till the **wrist joint**, whereas posterior axial lines stops at the elbow joint (NEET Pattern 2014).

❑ Five root values of brachial plexus (C5-8; T1) are pulled into the upper limb bud and distributed in a definite **segmental pattern**.

❑ Lateral aspect of upper limb (**superior aspect** of the abducted arm) has **upper dermatomes** (C-5,6) and medial (inferior aspect of abducted arm) has lower dermatomes (C-8; T1).

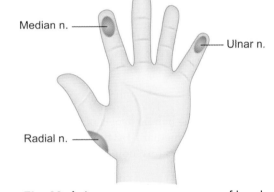

Fig. 30: Autonomous sensory areas of hand

Note: Angina pain is felt radiating down the medial side of the left arm (T1,2).

- Nerve root supplying cutaneous distribution of index finger is C7 *(NEET Pattern 2016)*
- Dermatome of thumb and index finger is C6; C7 *(AIIMS 2013)*
- Base of little finger is supplied by C8 dermatome *(AIPG 2012)*
- The nerve supply of nail bed of index finer is median nerve *(NEET Pattern 2013)*
- Injury at C7 root, leads to sensory loss at Posterior forearm *(NEET Pattern 2013)*

Table 14: Upper Limb dermatomal pattern	
Spinal segment	**Dermatomal area**
C3, 4	Region at the base of neck, extending laterally over tip of shoulder
C5	Lateral aspect of arm (superior aspect of the abducted arm)
C6	Lateral foream and thumb
C7	Middle three figers and centre of posterior aspect of forearm
C8	Little finger, medial side of the hand & forearm (inferior aspect of abducted arm)
T1	Medial aspect of the forearm & arm
T2	Medial aspect of arm & axilla

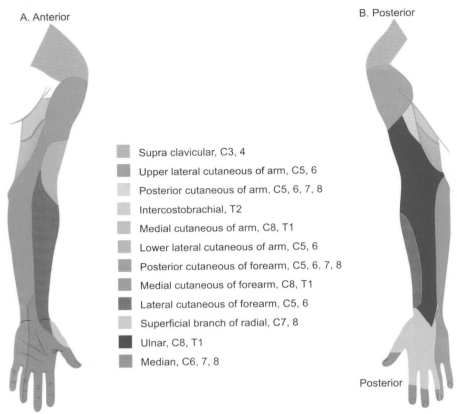

Fig. 31: Upper limb cutaneous innervation

- Sensations on the palmar aspect of lateral 3 1/2 fingers (including nail beds) are carried by **median nerve**.
- Palmar aspect of medial 1 1/2 fingers (including nail beds) is supplied by **ulnar nerve**.
- Lateral 3 1/2 fingers (excluding nail beds) on the dorsum of hand is supplied by radial nerve and medial 1 1/2 fingers by ulnar nerve.

Note: As a **variation**, some individuals have lateral 2 1/2 fingers on the dorsum of hand supplied by radial nerve and medial 2 1/2 fingers by ulnar nerve.

▸ Reflexes

- **Biceps jerk (C5, 6):** The elbow is flexed to a right angle and slightly pronated. A finger is placed on the biceps tendon and struck with a knee hammer; this should elicit **flexion and slight supination** of the forearm.
- **Triceps jerk (C6–8):** The arm is supported at the wrist and flexed to a right angle. Triceps tendon is struck with a knee hammer just proximal to the olecranon; this should elicit **extension of the elbow**.
- **Supinator (brachioradialis):** Reflex is elicited by striking the brachioradialis tendon at its **insertion at the base** of the wrist into the radial styloid process with knee hammer, while the forearm is supported in midprone position. This reflex is carried by the radial nerve (C5,6) and results in **supination** along with slight **wrist extension** and **radial deviation**, and slight **elbow flexion** as well.
- **Inverted supinator reflex** indicates spinal cord disease **at the C5 to C6 level**. In a positive response, tapping on the brachioradialis muscle fails to flex the elbow but instead flexes the fingers. The lesion at C5 to C6 **eliminates** the brachioradialis reflex (lower motor neuron) but **exaggerates** all reflexes below that level (upper motor neuron), including the finger flexion reflexes (C8), which are stimulated by mechanical conduction of the blow on the brachioradialis.

QUESTIONS

1. **There is loss of sensation of lateral 3 and 1/2 finger. The likely nerve injured is/are** *(PGIC 2013)*
   a. Only median nerve
   b. Median nerve plus ulnar nerve only
   c. Median nerve plus radial nerve only
   d. Ulnar and radial nerve only
   e. Median, radial and ulnar nerve

2. **Claw hand is caused by lesion of** *(AIPG 2007)*
   a. Ulnar nerve
   b. Median nerve
   c. Axillary nerve
   d. Radial nerve

3. A person is unable to adduct his thumb. The nerve involved is characterized by *(PGIC 2013)*
   a. Having C7,8 T1 root value
   b. Arise from medial cord of brachial plexus
   c. Arise from lateral cord of brachial plexus
   d. Musician's nerve
   e. Supplies 1st two lumbricals

4. Following an incised wound in the front of wrist, the subject is unable to oppose the tips of the little finger and the thumb. The nerve(s. involved is/are *(NBEP Pattern 2014)*
   a. Ulnar nerve alone
   b. Median nerve alone
   c. Median and ulnar nerves
   d. Radial and ulnar nerves

5. A boy presents with injury to medial epicondyle of the humerus. Which of the following would NOT be seen *(AIIMS 2002)*
   a. Weakness of the ulnar deviation and flexion
   b. Complete paralysis of the IIIrd and IVth digits
   c. Atrophy of the hypothenar eminence
   d. Decreased sensation of the hypothenar eminence

6. In an accident, the musculocutaneous nerve was completely severed, but still the person was able to weakly flex the elbow joint. All of the following muscles are responsible for this flexion EXCEPT *(AIIMS 2004)*
   a. Brachioradialis
   b. Flexor carpi radialis
   c. Ulnar head of pronator teres
   d. Flexor carpi ulnaris

7. A patient arrives in the emergency room after having attempted suicide by lacerating his wrist. No major artery was damaged, but the nerve that is immediately lateral to the flexor digitorum superficialis tendon is cut. Which of the following actions will no longer be possible
   a. Abduction of the second digit
   b. Adduction of the second digit
   c. Flexion at the interphalangeal joint of the thumb
   d. Opposition of the thumb

8. A 16 years old girl failed in her final examination disgusted with life, she cut across the front of wrist at the flexor retinaculum. She was rushed to hospital. The surgeon noticed that cut was superficial. All the following structures would have been damaged EXCEPT *(AIIMS 2002)*
   a. Ulnar nerve
   b. Median nerve
   c. Palmar cutaneous branch of median nerve
   d. Superficial branch of radial artery

9. Most common nerve damaged in supracondylar fracture is
   a. Median
   b. Anterior interosseous
   c. Radial
   d. Ulnar

10. After radical mastectomy there was injury to the long thoracic nerve. The integrity of the nerve can be tested at the bedside by asking the patient to *(AIIMS 2002; NEET Pattern 2012)*
    a. Shrug the shoulders
    b. Raise the arm above the head on the affected side
    c. Touch the opposite shoulder
    d. Lift a heavy object from the ground

11. During knife fight a person gets injured in the neck region and presents to emergency department with weakness in raising right arm above head. On further examination winging of right scapula is noted. The injury has damaged
    a. Spinal accessory nerve
    b. Long thoracic nerve of Bell
    c. Suprascapular nerve
    d. Dorsal scapular nerve

12. Pronator teres syndrome is due to involvement of which of the following nerve *(NEET Pattern 2013; AIIMS 2015)*
    a. Radial nerve
    b. Anterior interosseous nerve
    c. Ulnar nerve
    d. Median nerve

13. Nerve injury causing hyperextension of metacarpophalangeal and flexion of interphalangeal joints of ring and little finger *(AIIMS 2015)*
    a. Radial nerve
    b. Ulnar nerve
    c. Anterior interosseus nerve
    d. Posterior interosseus nerve

14. Damage to C7 nerve root causes weakness of *(NEET Pattern 2016)*
    a. Elbow flexion
    b. Supination
    c. Wrist flexion
    d. Finger abduction

15. An Injection was given in the deltoid muscle and has injured a nerve. Which of the following statements are TRUE *(PGIC 2012)*
    a. Loss of rounded contour of shoulder
    b. Loss of sensation on skin over the upper half of deltoid
    c. Loss of overhead abduction
    d. Atrophy of deltoid muscle
    e. Axillary nerve injury

16. A patient is brought to the emergency with history of trauma to his right upper limb. Extension of metacarpophalangeal is lost. There is no wrist drop and extension of IP joint is normal. The most likely nerve involved is
    a. Ulnar nerve
    b. Median nerve
    c. Radial nerve
    d. Posterior interosseous nerve

17. Patient exhibits weakness of Pinch grip; other thumb movements are normal. There is no sensory loss in the hand. The probable cause is damage to
    a. Posterior interosseous nerve
    b. Anterior interosseous nerve
    c. Deep branch of ulnar nerve
    d. Median nerve proximal to flexor retinaculum

18. A lesion involving C8 nerve root will affect *(JIPMER 2007)*
    a. Extensors of wrist and fingers
    b. Flexors of wrist and fingers
    c. Small muscles of hand
    d. None of the above

19. Medial epicondyle fracture leads to *(PGIC 2011)*
 a. Loss of sensation of thenar eminence
 b. Atrophy of hypothenar eminence
 c. Wrist drop
 d. Radial deviation of hand on attempted flexion
 e. Ulnar deviation of hand on attempted flexion

20. A patient presents with numbness in little and ring fingers along with atrophy of hypothenar eminence. Which of the following is injured *(AIIMS)*
 a. Posterior cord of the brachial plexus
 b. Palmar cutaneous branch of the ulnar nerve
 c. Deep branch of the ulnar nerve
 d. Ulnar nerve before division into superficial and deep branches

21. A bookshelf falls on a person's arm laterally. He presents with inability to extend his wrist. On examination he is unable to make a strong hand grip and there is loss of sensation on dorsum of the hand and fingers. Which of the following nerve is injured *(AIIMS 2012)*
 a. Brachial plexus
 b. Radial nerve
 c. Posterior cord
 d. Ulnar nerve

22. A patient woke up from sleep with difficulty in extending fingers. He can make a grip and hold a pen. Wrist extension was possible. No sensory disturbance was found, injury could be at *(AIIMS 2013)*
 a. C8, T1
 b. Posterior interosseous nerve
 c. Lower part of brachial plexus
 d. Hand area in motor cortex

23. A 30-year-old male underwent excision of the right radial head. Following surgery, the patient developed in ability to extend the fingers and thumb of the right hand. He did not have any sensory deficit. Which one of the following is the most likely cause
 a. Injury to posterior interosseus nerve
 b. Iatrogenic injury to common extensor origin
 c. Injury to anterior interosseus nerve
 d. High radial nerve palsy

24. All of the following muscles undergo paralysis after injury to C5 and C6 spinal nerves EXCEPT *(AIIMS 2004)*
 a. Biceps
 b. Coracobrachialis
 c. Brachialis
 d. Brachioradialis

25. A person while skiing catches a tree to stop and suffered a hyperabduction injury. The neural involvement is/are
 a. C8; T1 nerve root *(PGIC 2012)*
 b. Upper trunk of brachial plexus
 c. Lower trunk of brachial plexus
 d. Ulnar nerve
 e. Median nerve

26. All of the following muscles strictly receive nerve supply from anterior interosseous nerve EXCEPT
 a. Pronator quadrates
 b. Flexor pollicis longus
 c. Flexor digitorum profundus of index finger
 d. Flexor digitorum profundus of middle finger

27. A patient presented with inability to flex distal interphalangeal joint of fourth and fifth finger, and is unable to hold a card between his fingers. Fracture at which of the following site might have damaged the nerve, leading to this set of clinical features *(AIIMS 2017)*
 a. A
 b. B
 c. C
 d. D

28. Following pairs describe the muscles producing flexion at elbow joint and their respective nerve. Choose the WRONG pair *(AIPG)*
 a. Biceps brachii: Musculocutaneous nerve
 b. Brachioradialis: Median nerve
 c. Flexor carpi ulnaris: Ulnar nerve
 d. Flexor carpi radialis: Median nerve

29. Finger by which all three major nerves of the upper limb can be tested *(PGIC)*
 a. Index
 b. Ring
 c. Thumb
 d. Middle
 e. Little

1. c. Median nerve plus radial nerve only
 ❑ Sensations on the palmar aspect of lateral 3 1/2 fingers (including nail beds) are carried by median nerve.
 ❑ Palmar aspect of medial 1 1/2 fingers (including nail beds) is supplied by ulnar nerve.
 ❑ Lateral 31/2 fingers (excluding nail beds) on the dorsum of hand are supplied by radial nerve and medial 1 1/2 fingers by ulnar nerve.

2. a. Ulnar nerve > b. Median nerve
- ❏ Claw hand (Main en griffe) occurs due to the paralysis of the lumbricals, which flex the metacarpophalangeal joints and extend the inter-phalangeal joints.
- ❏ The patient has hyperextension at the metacarpophalangeal joints (due to unopposed long extensors of posterior forearm) and flexion at the inter-phalangeal joints (due to unopposed long flexors of anterior forearm).
- ❏ In ulnar nerve palsy, only the medial two fingers develop clawing, while in median and ulnar nerve palsies all the four fingers develop clawing (total claw hand).

3. a. Having C7,8 T1 root value; b. Arise from medial cord of brachial plexus
- ❏ d) Musician's nerve
- ❏ Loss of thumb adduction occurs due to paralysis of adductor pollicis (ulnar nerve lesion).
- ❏ Ulnar nerve has C (7), 8; T1 root value, is the continuation of medial cord of brachial plexus, supplies intrinsic muscles of the hand like all interossei and medial two lumbricals, hence controls finer movement of fingers for playing musical instruments (appropriately called musician's nerve).

4. c. Median and ulnar nerves
- ❏ Incised wounds in front of the wrist damages median nerve often, but ulnar nerve may also get involved.
- ❏ Opposition of the tips of little finger and thumb requires opponens pollicis (median nerve) and opponens digiti minimi (ulnar nerve) as well.

5. b. Complete paralysis of the IIIrd and IVth digits
- ❏ Injury to medial epicondyle damages ulnar nerve, leading to paralysis of flexor carpi ulnaris (loss of ulnar deviation) and medial half of flexor digitorum profundus (loss of DIP flexion).
- ❏ It also leads to hypothenar muscle paralysis (and atrophy) and sensory loss on the hypothenar eminence.
- ❏ But flexor digitorum superficialis (supplied by median nerve for finger flexion) and extensor digitorum (supplied by radial nerve for finger extension) are still functional.

6. c. Ulnar head of pronator teres
- ❏ Ulnar head of pronator teres do not cross (or act) at elbow joint.
- ❏ Elbow flexion is carried out by brachialis and biceps brachii muscles (supplied by musculocutaneous nerve) are paralysed in this patient.
- ❏ Brachioradialis (radial nerve), flexor carpi radialis (median nerve), flexor carpi ulnaris (ulnar nerve) are accessory muscles for elbow flexion.

7. d. Opposition of the thumb
- ❏ Median nerve gets damaged more often in suicidal wrist slashing, which lies lateral to the tendon of flexor digitorum superficialis.
- ❏ Opponens pollicis has been paralysed due to the injured median nerve at wrist leading to loss of opposition of the thumb.
- ❏ Abduction and adduction of digits is carried out by the interossei, which are supplied by the ulnar nerve.
- ❏ Flexion at the interphalangeal joint of thumb is carried out by the flexor pollicis longus, supplied by the anterior interosseous nerve (given by median nerve in the forearm).

8. a. Ulnar nerve
- ❏ Statistically it has been observed that the median nerve is cut more often than the ulnar in suicidal wrist slashing.
- ❏ In wrist slashing the attempted cuts are made proximal to the flexor retinaculum and mostly in radial to ulnar direction. The median nerve lies quite superficial in this region, before it enters the carpal tunnel and is frequently cut here.
- ❏ Wrist slashing injures the superficial branch of radial artery and the palmar cutaneous branch of median nerve very often.

9. b. Anterior interosseous
- ❏ Anterior interosseous nerve is the most common nerve to be injured in supracondylar fracture.
- ❏ The fracture damages few axons of the median nerve which enter the anterior interosseous branch.
- ❏ Radial nerve may also get damaged, but less often.
- ❏ Ulnar nerve is damaged rarely, in this fracture, and most of the time it is iatrogenic injury, while inserting the nail, to treat the fracture (percutaneous pinning through the medial epicondyle).

10. b. Raise the arm above the head on the affected side
- ❏ Injury to long thoracic nerve paralyses serratus anterior and the patient finds difficulty in overhead abduction.
- ❏ Shrugging of shoulder is mainly carried out by trapezius, which is supplied by the spinal accessory nerve (it also works alongwith serratus anterior for overhead-abduction).
- ❏ Pectoralis major causes flexion at the shoulder joint and is involved in touching the opposite shoulder.

11. a. Spinal accessory nerve > b. Long thoracic nerve of Bell
- ❏ Spinal accessory nerve is quite superficial in the neck region and is damaged more often as compared to long thoracic nerve of Bell (which gets damaged in the axilla region more commonly).
- ❏ Both the muscles are involved in overhead abduction (90-180°)
- ❏ Both the muscles (Serratus anterior and Trapezius) if paralysed can produce winging of scapula.

12. d. Median nerve
- Pronator teres syndrome is a nerve entrapment syndrome, caused by compression of the median nerve near the elbow.
- The nerve may be compressed between the heads of the pronator teres as a result of trauma, muscular hypertrophy, or fibrous bands.
- Patient presents with pain and tenderness in the proximal aspect of the anterior forearm, and hypoesthesia (decreased sensation) of palmar aspects of the lateral three and half fingers and adjacent palm.
- Symptoms often follow activities that involve repeated pronation.
- The patient may also present with weakness in the distal anterior forearm muscles (flexor and pronator) and thumb (thenar) muscles supplied by median nerve.

13. b. Ulnar nerve
- Injury to ulnar nerve presents with ulnar claw hand: hyperextension of metacarpophalangeal and flexion of interphalangeal joints of ring and little finger
- Ulnar nerve supplies medial 2 lumbricals (ring and little finger) in the hand. Lumbricals have a combined action of MCP (Metacarpophalangeal) flexion and IP (Interphalangeal) extension (glass holding posture).
- In ulnar nerve injury, since the lumbricals are not working, the forearm muscles are unopposed. MCP joint goes into hyperextension (unopposed activity of extensor digitorum muscles, posterior forearm) and IP joints go into flexion (unopposed activity of flexor digitorum muscles, anterior forearm) and they bring the deformity called ulnar claw hand.

14. c. Ans. Wrist flexion
- Elbow flexion and supination is under C5,6 root value, which gets compromised in Erb's palsy.
- Finger abduction is under hand muscles interossei, supplied by C8; T1 root value, compromised in Klumpke's palsy.

15. a. Loss of rounded contour of shoulder, d. Atrophy of deltoid muscle, e. Axillary nerve injury
- This patient has damage of axillary nerve leading to paralysis of deltoid muscle. Since deltoid undergoes atrophy, rounded contour of shoulder is lost. Loss of sensation is on skin over the lower half of deltoid (C5).

16. d. Posterior interosseous nerve
- Extension of metacarpophalangeal (knuckle joint is carried out by the posterior interosseous nerve-PIN).
- PIN supplies the posterior forearm muscles including the extensor digitorum, which help in extension at 4 joints – Wrist, MCP, PIP and DIP.
- In this patient the injury must be below the lateral epicondyle of humerus, where main trunk of radial nerve terminates as 2 branches, one of them being a muscular branch-PIN and other a cutaneous.
- ECRL is functional in the patient because it is supplied it the main trunk of radial nerve before the nerve divides. ECRL is a strong extensor at wrist joint so, no wrist drop is evident here.
- Extension at MCP is the job of posterior forearm muscles supplied by PIN, hence, it is lost.
- Extension at interphalangeal joint(s) is carried by the dorsal digital expansion present on the dorsal aspect of digits. This expansion is a modification of extensor digitorum, and receives the contributions from 12 muscles of the palm (8 interossei and 4 lumbricals).
- Here extension of IP joint is normal because the 12 muscles of the palm (supplied by the median & ulnar nerves) are still functional, despite the paralysed extensor digitorum (PIN).

17. b. Anterior interosseous nerve
- Weakness of pinch grip is due to involvement of Flexor Pollicis Longus (FPL) and Flexor digitorum profundus (FDP) of index finger.
- Anterior interosseous nerve supplies FDP to index and middle finger and FPL.
- Median nerve injury proximal to retinaculum results in loss of sensation to palmar radial 3 1/2 digits. Thumb opposition (OP), abduction of thumb (APB) and flexion of MCP joint thumb (FPB) also get affected.
- QUESTIONS clearly says that other movements of thumb are not affected (i.e., abduction and opposition are normal) and no sensory loss, so median nerve injury above wrist is ruled out.

18. b. Flexors of wrist and fingers
- Small muscles of hand are supplied by C8; T1, more precisely T1.
- Wrist (and Finger) extensors—C6(7)
- Wrist (and Finger) flexors—C7(8)
- Intrinsic muscles of hand—C8; T1

19. b. Atrophy of hypothenar eminence, d. Radial deviation of hand on attempted flexion
- Fracture at medial epicondyle may damage the ulnar nerve, leading to atrophy of hypothenar muscles.
- Since flexor carpi ulnaris supplied by ulnar nerve is paralysed, on attempted flexion at wrist, radial deviation occurs (unopposed flexor carpi radialis muscle).

20. d. Ulnar nerve before division into superficial and deep branches
- Medial cord of brachial plexus gives ulnar nerve which has been injured before it divides into two terminal branches in the hand (inside Guyon's canal).
- The deep branch supplies hypothenar muscles and superficial branch innervates skin of palmar surface of little finger and medial half of ring finger.

21. b. Radial nerve
- Loss of wrist extension occurs in radial nerve injury, in this case, it has been injured in radial groove.
- For making a strong hand grip by long flexors, slight dorsiflexion of wrist is required (carried out by ECRL and ECRB). In this case ECRL and ECRB are paralysed, hence the hand grip is not strong.

22. b. Posterior interosseous nerve
- ❑ Injury to posterior interosseous nerve leads to loss of finger extension at metacarpophalangeal joint.
- ❑ Lower part of brachial plexus carries C-8; T1 root value and supplies long flexors of finger and intrinsic muscles of hand for making a grip and holding a pen (intact in the patient).

23. a. Injury to posterior interosseus nerve
- ❑ The patient has a motor nerve injury in the proximity to radial head - posterior interosseous nerve, hence leading to paralysis of posterior forearm muscles (extensors of thumb and fingers).

24. b. Coracobrachialis
- ❑ Coracobrachialis (a flexor and adductor of the abducted arm) is innervated through the anterior division of C5, 6 and (predominantly) 7 segmental levels (Gray's Anatomy Ed 41). Hence, a lesion at C5 and 6 may not paralyse coracobrachialis completely.
- ❑ Brachioradialis is supplied by root value C-5 and 6, and hence is paralysed and so are biceps brachii (C-5,6) and brachialis: C-5,6,7 (But the dominant vale is C-6).

25. a. C8; T1 nerve root; c. Lower trunk of branchial plexus; d. Ulnar nerve; e. Median nerve
- ❑ This is a case of Klumpke's paralysis, which may be caused by hyperabduction of the arm, as occurs in catching a tree to stop, while in fast motion.
- ❑ The lower trunk of brachial plexus is pulled, and compromises first thoracic nerve is usually torn, though often C8 is also injured.
- ❑ The nerve fibres from this segment run in ulnar and median nerves to supply the small muscles of the hand.

26. d. Flexor digitorum profundus of middle finger
- ❑ Radial half of flexor digitorum profundus (index & middle fingers) is supplied by anterior interosseous nerve (median nerve) and medial half (ring & little fingers) by ulnar nerve.
- ❑ Flexor digitorum profundus of middle finger is supplied by ulnar nerve in 20% of the population (variation), hence the answer.

27. d. D
- ❑ This is a case of ulnar nerve injury, which might be consequent in a fracture at medial epicondyle (marker D) of humerus. The patient has inability to flex distal interphalangeal joint of fourth and fifth finger, due to paralysis of medial half of flexor digitorum profundus. He is unable to hold a card between his fingers because of the paralysed palmar interossei muscles, which help in finger adduction.
- ❑ **Key**: Marker A: Surgical neck (Relation- Axillary nerve); B: Mid-shaft (Relation- Radial nerve); C: Lateral epicondyle (Relation- Radial nerve).

28. b. Brachioradialis: Median nerve
- ❑ Brachioradialis muscle belongs to posterior compartment of forearm, supplied by radial nerve branch.
- ❑ Muscles crossing the elbow joint anteriorly, cause flexion e.g., biceps brachii, brachialis, flexor carpi radialis, flexor carpi ulnaris, pronator teres etc.
- ❑ Brachioradialis, flexor of the forearm, is unusual in that it is located in the posterior compartment, but crosses the elbow joint anteriorly.

29. c. Thumb
- ❑ Three major nerves work for the varied movements of thumb.

Movements	Muscles involved (nerve supply)
Flexion (accompanied by medial rotation)	Flexor pollicis brevis (median and ulnar nerves), flexor pollicis longus (median nerve). Opponens pollicis (median and ulnar nerves)
Extension (accompanied by lateral rotation)	Extensor pollicis longus (radial nerve). Extensor pollicis brevis (radial nerve). Abductor pollicis longus (radial nerve).
Abduction	Abductor pollicis brevis (median nerve). Abductor pollicis longus (radial nerve).
Adduction	Adductor pollicis (ulnar nerve).
Opposition	Abductor pollicis brevis (median nerve)→ Opponens pollicis (median and ulnar nerve)→ Flexor pollicis brevis (median and ulnar nerves)

- ▪ **Abduction** and **lateral rotation** of shoulder is carried out by **C5,6** root value, which gets compromised in Erb's palsy.
- ▪ Injury to the suprascapular nerve is characterized by atrophy of the supraspinatus and infraspinatus muscles. Deficits will include difficulty in initiation of arm **abduction** and weakness in **external rotation** of the arm.
- ▪ Injury to the **long thoracic nerve** results in paralysis of the **serratus anterior** muscle, causing a **winged scapula** (the medial border of the scapula moves or protrudes posteriorly away from the thoracic wall) when pushing against resistance. It may also cause **difficulty in raising the arm above the head**.
- ▪ Posterior interosseous nerve has **pseudoganglion** at the termination.
- ▪ Root value of supinator jerk is C5, 6 (NEET Pattern 2015)
- ▪ During sentinel lymph node biopsy, the nerves at risk are: intercostobrachial nerve (most common), long thoracic nerve, thoracodorsal nerve.

▶ Muscles of Upper Limb

Table 15: Posterior axioappendicular muscles

Muscle	Proximal attachment	Distal attachment	Innervation	Muscle action
Superficial posterior axioappendicular (extrinsic shoulder) muscles				
Trapezius	Medial third of superior nuchal line; external occipital protuberance; nuchal ligament; spinous processes of C7–T12 vertebrae	Lateral third of clavicle; acromion and spine of scapula	Spinal accessory nerve (CN XI) (motor fibers) and C3, C4 spinal nerves (pain and proprioceptive fibers)	Descending part elevates; ascending part depresses; and middle part (or all parts together) retracts scapula; descending and ascending parts act together to rotate glenoid cavity superiorly
Latissimus dorsi	Spinous processes of inferior 6 thoracic vetebrae, thoracolumbar fascia, iliac crest, and inferior 3 or 4 ribs	Floor of intertubercular sulcus of humerus	Thoracodorsal nerve (**C6, C7**, C8)	Extends, adducts, and medially rotates humerus; raises body towards arms during climbing

Trapezius is triangular shape muscle, appears trapezium shaped as looked upon both halves together (AIIMS 2016).

❑ It causes Retraction of scapula, shrugging of shoulder, overhead abduction (along with serratus anterior).

❑ Paralysis of trapezius results in: **Drooped shoulder** (NEET Pattern 2014) and **slight winging of scapula** (the superior angle of scapula becomes more prominent).

Latissimus dorsi is an upper limb muscle, which has migrated to lower back muscle for improved functionality (AIIMS 2013)

❑ It is inserted on the floor of intertubercular sulcus

❑ Helps in shoulder extension, medial rotation and adduction (scratching the back).

❑ Is also called climber's muscle, as it becomes more evident due to contraction while climbing (like trees). (NEET Pattern 2015)

❑ The axis of pull of latissimus dorsi doesn't cross the shoulder joint and cannot have a shunt action on the joint.

❑ It is supplied by Thoracodorsal nerve (C6, 7, 8), which is a branch of the posterior cord of brachial plexus (NEET Pattern 2013)

❑ Mastectomy may damage thoracodorsal nerve leading to paralysis of latissimus dorsi.

❑ **Rotator (Musculotendinous) cuff**

➤ It fuses with the joint capsule, formed by blending of tendons of four muscles (**SITS**): **S**upraspinatus (superiorly); **I**nfraspinatus and **T**eres minor (posteriorly) and **S**ubscapularis (anteriorly).

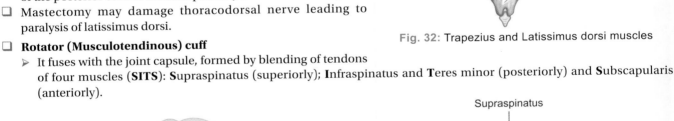

Fig. 32: Trapezius and Latissimus dorsi muscles

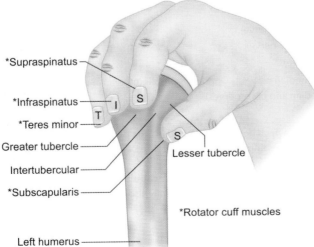

Fig. 33: Rotator cuff: A dynamic stabilizer of shoulder joint

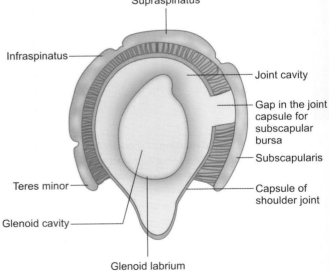

Fig. 34: Rotator cuff muscles (Lateral view of glenoid cavity)

- It reinforces the capsule posterosuperiorly, but weak anteroinferiorly—Shoulder dislocations are more commonly **anteroinferior**.
- The most common tendon injured in rotator cuff injury is **supraspinatus**. Complete tear of supraspinatus is characterized by **difficulty to initiate abduction**, but further abduction is possible if limb is abducted passively to 15°.
- Rotator cuff injury (also called subacromial bursitis or **painful arc syndrome)**, most commonly it involves the tendon of the supraspinatus muscle and the subacromial bursa.
- **Subscapularis** is often it is neglected in the clinical literature, hence called as **'forgotten** tendon'.

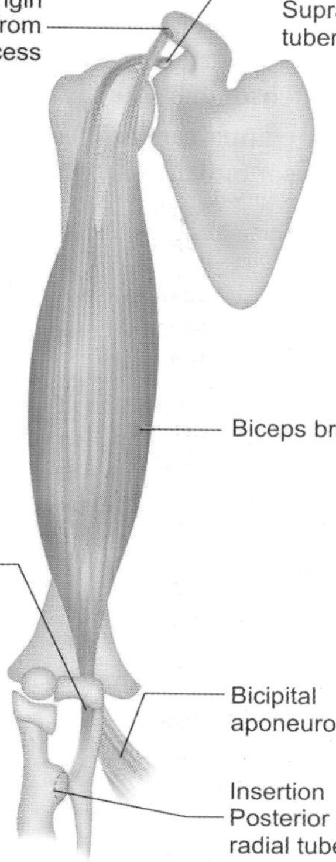

Muscles of Arm

- Anterior: Biceps brachii, Coracobrachialis, Brachialis
- Posterior: Triceps brachii
- ❏ Biceps brachii short head takes origin from the **tip of coracoid process** and the long head from the supraglenoid tubercle.
- ❏ Insertion: **Radial tuberosity** (NEET Pattern 2015)
- ❏ Origin of long head of biceps brachii is **intracapsular and extrasynovial**, but enclosed by a prolongation of synovial membrane of shoulder joint (NEET Pattern 2015)
- ❏ Innervation: Musculocutaneous nerve
- ❏ Action: Biceps brachii is a flexor at elbow joint, but it is also a **powerful supinator** (NEET Pattern 2015)
- ❏ It crosses both shoulder and elbow joint, and cause flexion at both.
- ❏ Biceps brachii is a powerful supinator at the superior radioulnar joint and helps in screw-driving movements.
- ❏ While carrying a heavy suitcase the downward dislocation of glenohumeral joint is resisted by the **shunt muscles** like biceps.
- ❏ When a heavy object in hand is lowered, the extension at the elbow is brought about by active relaxation **(lengthening)** of the flexors - biceps (antagonist).

Fig. 35: Origin and insertion of biceps brachii

Muscles of Forearm

- Anterior compartment **(Superficial)** (5): Flexor carpi radialis, Flexor digitorum superficialis, Flexor carpi ulnaris, Pronator teres and palmaris longus.

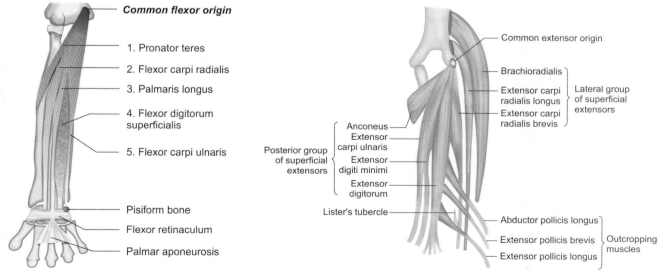

Fig. 36: Anterior forearm muscles (superficial)

Fig. 37: Posterior forearm muscles

➤ Anterior compartment **(Deep)** (3): Flexor digitorum profundus, Flexor pollicis longus, pronator quadratus (NEET Pattern 2013)

➤ Posterior compartment **(Superficial)**: Anconeus, brachioradialis, extensor carpi radialis longus, extensor carpi radialis brevis, extensor digitorum, extensor digiti minimi and extensor carpi ulnaris.

➤ Posterior compartment **(Deep)**: Supinator, abductor pollicis longus, extensor pollicis brevis, extensor pollicis longus and extensor indicis.

QUESTIONS

1. Deltoid muscle causes all EXCEPT   *(NEET Pattern 2015)*
   a. Flexion of shoulder
   b. Extension of shoulder
   c. Internal rotation of shoulder
   d. Adduction of shoulder

2. All of the following muscles causes retraction of scapula EXCEPT   *(AIIMS 2010; NEET Pattern 2014)*
   a. Trapezius
   b. Levator scapulae
   c. Rhomboideus major
   d. Rhomboideus minor

3. After surgery on right side of neck, a person could not raise his arm above head and also could not shrug the shoulder. What are the possible causes   *(PGIC 2013)*
   a. Damage to spinal accessory nerve
   b. Paralysis of trapezius muscle
   c. Injury to axillary nerve
   d. Paralysis of latissimus dorsi
   e. Paralysis of deltoid muscle

4. INCORRECT about serratus anterior   *(NEET Pattern 2015)*
   a. Forms medial wall of axilla
   b. Causes protraction of scapula
   c. Causes rotation of scapula
   d. Supplied by thoracodorsal nerve

5. TRUE about anconeus muscle is   *(NEET Pattern 2014)*
   a. Posterior forearm muscle
   b. Helps in screwing movement
   c. Helps in forearm supination
   d. Supplied by ulnar nerve

6. Muscle in extension compartment of forearm which causes flexion of elbow   *(NEET Pattern 2014)*
   a. Brachioradialis
   b. Abductor pollicis longus
   c. Extensor pollicis longus
   d. Extensor carpi radialis longus

7. The nerve supply to pronator muscle of distal radioulnar joint is   *(JIPMER 2003)*
   a. Median nerve
   b. Ulnar nerve
   c. Anterior interosseous nerve
   d. Posterior interosseous nerve

8. Muscles causing supination of forearm   *(NEET Pattern 2015)*
   a. Biceps brachii
   b. Brachioradialis
   c. FDS
   d. Anconeus

9. All of the following muscles have dual nerve supply EXCEPT   *(NEET Pattern 2015)*
   a. Subscapularis
   b. Pectoralis major
   c. Pronator teres
   d. Flexor digitorum profundus

10. When a heavy object in hand is lowered, the extension at the elbow is brought about by   *(AIIMS 2003)*
    a. Active shortening of the extensors.
    b. Passive shortening of the extensors
    c. Active lengthening of the flexors
    d. Active shortening of the flexors

11. While carrying a heavy suitcase the downward dislocation of glenohumeral joint is resisted by the following muscles EXCEPT   *(AIIMS 2002)*
    a. Deltoid
    b. Coracobrachialis
    c. Short head of biceps
    d. Latissimus dorsi

12. C8, T1 supplies following muscles EXCEPT
    a. Extensor indicis
    b. 3rd and 4th lumbrical(s)
    c. Abductor pollicis brevis
    d. Palmar interossei

13. After mastectomy, patient is NOT able to extend, adduct and internally rotate the arm. Nerve supply to which of the following muscles is damaged   *(AIIMS 2012)*
    a. Pectoralis major
    b. Teres minor
    c. Latissimus dorsi
    d. Long head of Triceps

14. Oblique cord is related to   *(NEET Pattern 2014)*
    a. Supinator
    b. Long flexors
    c. Short flexors
    d. Lumbricals

15. A man cannot do abduction and internal rotation of arm. Which of the following muscle is responsible for the both movements   *(PGIC 2013)*
    a. Pectoralis major
    b. Subscapularis
    c. Deltoid
    d. Supraspinatus
    e. Teres major

16. Insertion of extensor carpi ulnaris   *(NEET Pattern 2016)*
    a. Base of proximal phalanx of thumb
    b. Base of distal phalanx of thumb
    c. Scaphoid base
    d. Base of 5th Metacarpal

17. Posterior interosseous nerve supplies all EXCEPT   *(PGIC 2016)*
   a. Extensor carpi radialis longus
   b. Extensor carpi ulnaris
   c. Extensor digitorum
   d. Extensor indices
   e. Flexor carpi ulnaris

1. d. Adduction of shoulder
   ❑ Deltoid muscle is a powerful abductor at shoulder joint, using middle (lateral) fibres.
   ❑ It causes flexion and medial rotation (by anterior fibres) and extension & lateral rotation (by posterior fibres).

2. b. Levator scapulae
   ❑ Levator scapulae muscle is mainly an elevator (not retractor) of scapula.
   ❑ Retraction of scapula (bring scapula back to the midline) is carried out by muscles: Trapezius, rhomboideus major and minor.
   ❑ Protraction of scapula (take scapula away from midline as happens in pushing a wall in front) is brought about by muscles: Serratus anterior, pectoralis minor.

3. a. Damage to spinal accessory nerve, b. Paralysis of trapezius muscle
   ❑ Spinal accessory nerve runs very superficial in the posterior triangle of neck and is prone to iatrogenic injury, leading to paralysis of trapezius muscle and difficulty shrugging the shoulder, as well as overhead abduction.

4. d. Supplied by thoracodorsal nerve
   ❑ Long thoracic nerve (of Bell) supplies serratus anterior muscle.
   ❑ Serratus anterior pulls the scapula forward (protraction). It also pulls on the inferior angle of scapula to help in lateral scapular rotation, the glenoid cavity is turned to face more directly upwards as the arm is raised from the side and carried above the head against gravity.

5. a. Posterior forearm muscle > b. Screwing movements
   ❑ Anconeus is a muscle of posterior compartment of the forearm, though some sources consider it to be part of the posterior compartment of the arm.
   ❑ Anconeus assists triceps in extending forearm (major action); stabilizes elbow joint; may abduct ulna during pronation. Some authors mention it helping in screwing movements as well.
   ❑ Anconeus muscle: Assists triceps in extending forearm; stabilizes elbow joint; may abduct ulna during pronation

6. a. Brachioradialis
   ❑ Muscle of extensor compartment but causing elbow flexion in midprone position is brachioradialis muscle.

7. c. Anterior interosseous nerve
   ❑ Pronator teres muscle (median nerve) causes pronation at proximal radioulnar joint.
   ❑ Pronation at distal radioulnar joint is carried out by pronator quadratus, supplied by the anterior interosseous nerve.

8. a. Biceps brachii > b. Brachioradialis
   ❑ Biceps brachii is a powerful supinator, especially when the elbow is in flexion.
   ❑ Supination in extended elbow is carried out by supinator muscle.
   ❑ Brachioradialis causes elbow flexion, especially in mid-prone position. It can bring the forearm in midprone position by carrying out slight pronation and supination. It is the muscle tested for supinator reflex.

9. c. Pronator teres
   ❑ Pronator teres is supplied by median nerve.
   ❑ Subscapularis is supplied by upper subscapular nerve & lower subscapular nerve
   ❑ Pectoralis major is supplied by medial pectoral nerve & lateral pectoral nerve.
   ❑ Medial half of flexor digitorum profundus is supplied by ulnar nerve & lateral half by anterior interosseus nerve.

10. c. Active lengthening of the flexors
   ❑ When a heavy object in hand is lowered, the extension at the elbow is brought about by active relaxation (lengthening) of the flexors - biceps (antagonist).
   ❑ The antagonist muscle opposes (antagonizes) the concerned movement to makes it more controlled and precise. Though it is opposing the movement but does it with partial resistance, so that the resultant movement becomes smooth. For example, biceps opposing extension at elbow partially, so that extension becomes slow and smooth, as occurs in lowering down a heavy object in hand.
   ❑ Normal extension at the elbow is by active contraction (shortening) of the extensor - triceps (agonist).

11. d. Latissimus dorsi
   ❑ The axis of pull of latissimus dorsi doesn't cross the shoulder joint and cannot have a shunt action on the joint.
   ❑ Shunt muscles are those which stabilise the corresponding joint, when they are not producing a movement at the joint.
   ❑ For example, while carrying a heavy suitcase the downward dislocation of glenohumeral joint is resisted by the muscles like deltoid, coracobrachialis and short head of biceps.

12. **a. Extensor indicis**
   - ❑ The muscle of the back of forearm, extensor indicis is supplied by the radial nerve branch-PIN (posterior interosseous nerve - C7, 8 fibres).
   - ❑ All the hand muscles like 3 and 4 lumbricals, abductor pollicis brevis, palmar interossei are supplied by C-8 and T-1 root values.

13. **c. Latissimus dorsi**
   - ❑ Mastectomy may damage thoracodorsal nerve leading to paralysis of latissimus dorsi. The patient finds difficulty in shoulder extension, medial rotation and adduction.

14. **a. Supinator**
   - ❑ Oblique cord is a small fibrous band on the deep head of supinator which extends lateral side of ulnar tuberosity to the lower part of radial tuberosity. Its fibres run inferolaterally (opposite to the interosseous membrane).
   - ❑ It is considered as the degenerate tendon of flexor pollicis longus. Its function is unclear.

15. **c. Deltoid**
   - ❑ Deltoid is a power abductor at the shoulder joint, which is carried out by the lateral fibres.
   - ❑ Anterior fibres of deltoid act for flexion and medial rotation at shoulder joint and posterior fibres for extension and lateral rotation.
   - ❑ Pectoralis major work for adduction (not abduction).
   - ❑ Subscapularis and teres major muscles are not involved in abduction, though both of them carry out medial rotation.

16. **d. Base of 5th Metacarpal**
   - ❑ Extensor carpi ulnaris is present on the ulnar (little finger) side and is inserted on the base of 5th metacarpal. The other options are present o the radial (thumb side) side.
      - ■ Origin: Lateral epicondyle of humerus and posterior border ulna.
      - ■ Insertion: Base of 5th metacarpal (NEET Pattern 2016)
      - ■ Nerve supply: Posterior interosseous nerve.
      - ■ Action: Extension (dorsiflexion) and adduction (ulnar deviation) at wrist joint.

17. **a. Extensor carpi radialis longus; e. Flexor carpi ulnaris**
   - ❑ Posterior interosseous nerve (branch of radial nerve) supplies muscles of posterior forearm, which are chiefly extensors.
   - ❑ Extensor carpi radialis longus is already supplied by radial nerve (main trunk) and flexor carpi ulnaris is supplied by ulnar nerve.

- ▪ **Rhomboid** muscles and levator scapulae are supplied by the **dorsal scapular nerve** (NEET Pattern 2015,16)
- ▪ The four tendons of flexor digitorum profundus give origin to four **lumbricals** (NEET Pattern 2015)
- ▪ Teres major is supplied by the **lower subscapular nerve**, which also supplies subscapularis muscle. (NEET Pattern 2014)
- ▪ **Anconeus** is a small muscle on in posterior compartment of forearm. It originates from the humerus (posterior surface of lateral condyle and inserts into ulna (on posterior surface and olecranon). It is innervated by a branch of the radial nerve (C7,8) in the radial groove of the humerus.
- ▪ **Winging of scapula** is undue prominence of medial border of scapula, especially when an attempt is made for scapular protraction, occurs due to paralysis of serratus anterior muscle. Winging of scapula is also caused by trapezius and rhomboid palsy involving the accessory nerve and the dorsal scapular nerve, respectively. (NEET Pattern 2012)
- ▪ **Flexor digitorum superficialis** tendon splits into medial and lateral bands, which pass around the **flexor digitorum profundus** tendon and insert on the base of the middle phalanx, while the flexor digitorum profundus tendon inserts on the base of the distal phalanx as a single tendon.

▼ Arterial Supply of Upper Limb

The axial vessel for the upper limb is the **subclavian artery,** which arises from the brachiocephalic trunk on the right and directly from the arch of the aorta on the left.

- ❑ It is divided into **three parts** that are successively anterior, deep and lateral to **scalenus anterior**. The second and third parts are in close relation to the primary ventral rami of C7, C8 and T1, and to the middle and lower trunks of the brachial plexus.
- ❑ The subclavian artery becomes the axillary artery at the **lateral border of the first rib**. The axillary artery passes along with the divisions of the brachial plexus deep to the clavicle, and is intimately related to the cords below it. It passes deep to **pectoralis minor** (which divides it into three parts) and becomes the brachial artery at the lower border of teres major.
- ❑ The **brachial artery** is closely related to the median nerve in the arm, both **reach cubital fossa**, on the anterior aspect of the elbow, lying medial to the tendon of biceps brachii and deep to the bicipital aponeurosis. The artery divides into the **radial** and **ulnar** arteries in the cubital fossa, just distal to the elbow.
- ❑ The larger branch **ulnar artery** gives common interosseous artery arises close to its origin and subsequently divides into the anterior and posterior interosseous arteries. **Anterior interosseous artery** (and nerve) descend inferiorly on the anterior aspect of interosseous membrane. The posterior interosseous artery is separated from the membrane by the deep extensor muscles.

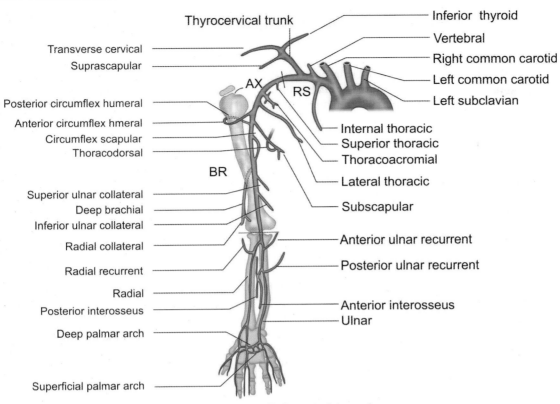

Fig. 38: Upper limb – arterial supply

❑ Ulnar artery is the **major artery** to hand and continues as **superficial palmar arch**, whereas radial artery contributes to deep palmar arch.

▼ Collateral Circulation

➢ Collateral circulation formed by branches of the thyrocervical trunk with the circumflex humeral and subscapular arteries allow survival of **upper limb** in cases of blockage in subclavian or axillary arteries.

➢ rofunda brachii accompanies the radial nerve and contributes to the collateral circulation **about the elbow** with the ulnar collateral and recurrent vessels and the radial collateral and recurrent vessels.

➢ Anastomosis between superficial and deep palmar arches **in hand.**

➢ **Thyrocervical trunk** is a branch from the *first part* of subclavian artery. It gives three branches **SIT**: S – Supra-scapular artery; I – Inferior thyroid artery and T – Transverse cervical artery.

❑ **Suprascapular Artery** is a branch of the thyrocervical trunk, passes over the superior transverse scapular ligament. It supplies the supraspinatus and infraspinatus muscles and the shoulder and acromioclavicular joints. It also participates in **scapular anastomosis**.

❑ **Dorsal Scapular Artery:** In the majority of population, the dorsal scapular artery arises from the **third** (or less often the second) part of the subclavian artery. Occasionally it is given by **first** part of subclavian artery. It may be given by first part of subclavian via thyrocervical trunk → transverse cervical artery (deep branch) → dorsal scapular artery. It is **accompanied by** the dorsal scapular nerve and supplies the levator scapulae, rhomboids, and serratus anterior muscles.

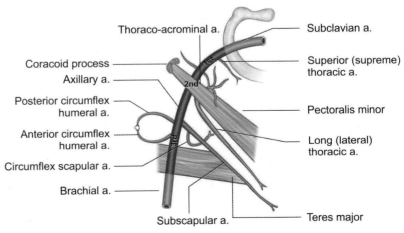

Fig. 39: Axillary artery

▶ Axillary Artery

❑ **Axillary artery** extends from the **lateral border** of the first rib to the **lower border** of the teres major muscle, where it becomes the **brachial artery**.

❑ It is followed by the **axillary vein on medial side**, is divided into three parts by the **pectoralis minor** muscle.

❑ It has three parts and **six branches**. First part (1 branch – superior thyroid artery); second part (2 branches – thoracoacromial and lateral thoracic artery) and third part (3 branches – anterior and posterior circumflex humeral arteries and subscapular artery).

Branches of axillary artery

❑ **Superior Thoracic Artery** supplies the intercostal muscles in the first and second anterior intercostal spaces.

❑ **Thoracoacromial Artery** is a short branch from the second part of the axillary artery and has pectoral, clavicular, acromial, and deltoid branches. It **pierces the clavipectoral fascia**.

❑ **Lateral Thoracic Artery** runs along the lateral border of the pectoralis minor muscle, supplies the pectoralis major, pectoralis minor, serratus anterior muscles and send branches to **mammary gland**.

❑ **Subscapular Artery** is the largest branch of the axillary artery, divides into the thoracodorsal and circumflex scapular arteries. **Thoracodorsal Artery** accompanies the thoracodorsal nerve and supplies the latissimus dorsi muscle and the lateral thoracic wall.

❑ **Circumflex Scapular Artery** passes posteriorly into the **upper triangular space**, ramifies in the infraspinous fossa and **anastomoses** with branches of the dorsal scapular and suprascapular arteries.

❑ **Anterior Humeral Circumflex Artery** passes anteriorly around the surgical neck of the humerus, anastomoses with the posterior humeral circumflex artery.

❑ **Posterior Humeral Circumflex Artery** runs posteriorly with the axillary nerve through the **quadrangular space**, anastomoses with the anterior humeral circumflex artery and an ascending branch of the profunda brachii artery.

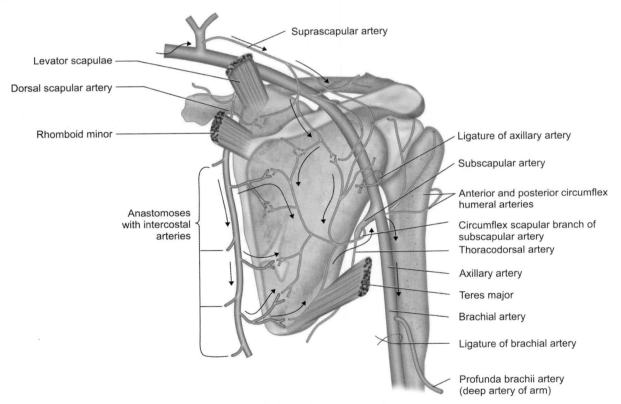

Fig. 40: Scapular anastomosis

▶ Scapular Anastomosis

Scapular anastomosis is an arterial system connecting each **subclavian artery** and the corresponding **axillary artery**, forming a collateral circulation around the scapula.

❑ It allows blood to flow past the shoulder joint regardless of the position of the arm and also provides a **collateral** pathway towards the limb in case of **blockage** at the subclavian or axillary artery.

- ❏ The participating arteries are:
  - ➤ Branches from the **subclavian artery**
    - ▪ Suprascapular artery
    - ▪ Dorsal scapular artery
  - ➤ Branches from the **axillary artery**
    - ▪ Subscapular artery (and its branch circumflex scapular artery)
    - ▪ Anterior circumflex humeral artery
    - ▪ Posterior circumflex humeral artery
- ❏ There are numerous anastomosing arteries, but **two major channels** are prominent.
  - ➤ Subclavian artery (Ist part) → thyrocervical trunk → suprascapular artery → circumflex scapular artery → subscapular artery → axillary artery (IIIrd part)
  - ➤ Subclavian artery (IIIrd part) → dorsal scapular artery → subscapular artery → axillary artery (IIIrd part)
- ❏ In the majority of population, the **dorsal scapular artery** arises from the third (or less often the second. part of the subclavian artery. **Occasionally** it is given by first part of subclavian via thyrocervical trunk → transverse cervical artery (deep branch) → dorsal scapular artery → subscapular artery → axillary artery (scapular anastomosis).
- ❏ A minor anastomosis is present on the acromion process between acromial branches of
  - ➤ Suprascapular artery (branch of 1st part of subclavian artery)
  - ➤ Thoracoacromial artery (branch of 2nd part of axillary artery)
  - ➤ Posterior circumflex humeral artery (branch of 3rd part of axillary artery)

▶ Brachial Artery

Brachial artery extends from the **inferior border** of the teres major muscle to its bifurcation in the cubital fossa.

- ❏ It is accompanied by the basilic vein in the middle of the arm, descends down to the center of the cubital fossa, **medial to the biceps tendon**, lateral to the median nerve, deep to the bicipital aponeurosis.
- ❏ The **stethoscope** is placed on this artery while taking **blood pressure** and listening to the arterial pulse. It divides into the **radial** and **ulnar arteries** at the level of the radial neck (1 cm below elbow bend) in the cubital fossa.
- ❏ It gives three branches in the arm:
  - ➤ **Profunda** (deep) **Brachial artery** descends posteriorly in the **radial groove** (with radial nerve. and gives off an ascending branch, which anastomoses with the descending branch of the posterior humeral circumflex artery. It divides into two branches:
    - ▪ Middle collateral artery (posterior descending branch of the profunda brachii artery)
    - ▪ Radial collateral artery (anterior descending branch of the profunda brachii artery)
  - ➤ **Superior Ulnar Collateral Artery** pierces the medial intermuscular septum and accompanies the ulnar nerve behind the septum and medial epicondyle.
  - ➤ **Inferior Ulnar Collateral Artery** (supratrochlear artery) arises just above the elbow and descends in front of the medial epicondyle.

▶ Radial Artery

Radial artery is the smaller lateral branch of the brachial artery in the **cubital fossa** and descends laterally under cover of the brachioradialis muscle, with the superficial radial nerve on its lateral side.

- ❏ It curves over the radial side of the carpal bones **deep to the tendons of** the abductor pollicis longus muscle, the extensor pollicis longus and brevis muscles, and over the surface of the scaphoid and trapezium bones.
- ❏ It becomes **a content of anatomical snuffbox** and enters the palm by passing between the two heads of the first dorsal interosseous muscle and then between the heads of the adductor pollicis muscle, and divides into the **princeps pollicis artery** and the **deep palmar arch.**
- ❏ **Radial artery pulse** is felt proximal to wrist, in front of the distal end of the radius between the tendons of the brachioradialis and flexor carpi radialis. It may also be palpated in the anatomical snuffbox between the tendons of the extensor pollicis longus and brevis muscles.
- ❏ **Branches**:
  - ➤ **Radial Recurrent Artery** arises from the radial artery just below its origin and anastomoses with the radial collateral branch of the profunda brachii artery.
  - ➤ **Palmar Carpal Branch** joins the palmar carpal branch of the ulnar artery and forms the palmar carpal arch.
  - ➤ **Superficial Palmar Branch** passes through the thenar muscles and anastomoses with the superficial branch of the ulnar artery to complete the **superficial palmar arterial arch**.
  - ➤ **Dorsal Carpal Branch** joins the dorsal carpal branch of the ulnar artery and the dorsal terminal branch of the anterior interosseous artery to form the dorsal carpal rete.

- ➢ **Princeps Pollicis** descends along the ulnar border of the first metacarpal bone and divides into two proper digital arteries for each side of the thumb.
- ➢ **Radialis Indicis** may arise from the deep palmar arch or the princeps pollicis artery.

▼ Ulnar Artery

Ulnar artery is the **larger** medial branch of the brachial artery **in the cubital fossa**. It descends in the forearm and enters the hand **anterior to the flexor retinaculum**, lateral to the pisiform bone, and medial to the hook of the hamate bone.

- ❏ It divides into the **superficial palmar arch** (refer) and the deep palmar branch (which join the radial artery to complete the deep palmar arch.
- ❏ Branches:
  - ➢ **Anterior Ulnar Recurrent Artery** anastomoses with the inferior ulnar collateral artery.
  - ➢ **Posterior Ulnar Recurrent Artery** anastomoses with the superior ulnar collateral artery.
  - ➢ **Common Interosseous Artery** arises from the lateral side of the ulnar artery and divides into the anterior and posterior interosseous arteries.
    - ▪ **Anterior Interosseous Artery** descends with the anterior interosseous nerve in front of the interosseous membrane, perforates the interosseous membrane **to anastomose with** the posterior interosseous artery and join the dorsal carpal network.
    - ▪ **Posterior Interosseous Artery** gives rise to the interosseous recurrent artery, which anastomoses with a middle collateral branch of the profunda brachii artery. It descends behind the interosseous membrane in company with the posterior interosseous nerve and **anastomoses with** the dorsal carpal branch of the anterior interosseous artery.
  - ➢ **Palmar Carpal Branch** joins the palmar carpal branch of the radial artery to form the palmar carpal arch.
  - ➢ **Dorsal Carpal Branch** passes around the ulnar side of the wrist and joins the dorsal carpal rete.

▼ Elbow Anastomosis

Elbow anastomosis: Collateral circulation around the elbow involves the following pathways.

- ❏ Superior ulnar collateral artery → posterior ulnar recurrent artery
- ❏ Inferior ulnar collateral artery → anterior ulnar recurrent artery
- ❏ Radial collateral artery → recurrent radial artery
- ❏ Middle collateral artery → recurrent interosseus artery

1. Which of the following statement(s. is TRUE regarding axillary artery   *(PGIC 2015)*
   a. Start from upper border of clavicle
   b. Ulnar nerve lies medially to distal 1/3 of artery
   c. Radial nerve lies posteriorly distal 1/3 of artery
   d. Axillary vein lies laterally to proximal 1/3 of the artery
   e. End at lower border of pectoralis minor

2. In a subclavian artery block at the outer border of first rib all of the following arteries help in maintaining the circulation to upper limb EXCEPT   *(AIIMS 2008; 2011)*
   a. Thyrocervical trunk
   b. Suprascapular
   c. Subscapular
   d. Superior thoracic

3. Anastomosis around the shoulder is between branches of   *(NEET Pattern 2014)*
   a. 1st part of subclavian and 1st part of axillary artery
   b. 1st part of subclavian and 3rd part of axillary artery
   c. 3rd part of subclavian and 2nd part of axillary artery
   d. 3rd part of subclavian and 3rd part of axillary artery

4. Occlusion occurs at the 2nd part of axillary artery, blood flow is maintained by anastomosis between   *(AIIMS 2007)*
   a. Anterior and posterior circumflex humeral artery
   b. Circumflex scapular and posterior circumflex humeral artery
   c. Deep branch of transverse cervical artery and subscapular artery
   d. Anterior circumflex humeral and subscapular artery

5. Which branch of subclavian contributes to scapular anastomosis
   a. Vertebral
   b. Internal thoracic
   c. Thyrocervical truck
   d. Dorsal scapular

6. Interosseous membrane of forearm is pierced by   *(NEET Pattern 2013)*
   a. Brachial artery
   b. Anterior interosseous artery
   c. Posterior interosseous artery
   d. Ulnar recurrent artery

7. Branches of brachial artery are all EXCEPT   *(NEET Pattern 2014)*
   a. Profunda brachii
   b. Superior ulnar collateral
   c. Inferior ulnar collateral
   d. Radial collateral

8. Artery forming anastomosis around the surgical neck of humerus is a branch of   *(NEET Pattern 2014)*
   a. 1st part of axillary artery
   b. 2nd part of axillary artery
   c. 3rd part of axillary artery
   d. Subclavian artery

9. Interosseous recurrent artery is a branch of
(NEET Pattern 2014)
   a. Anterior interosseous artery
   b. Posterior interosseous artery
   c. Common interosseous artery
   d. Radial artery

11. Patient presented with fall on outstretched hand. X-ray taken is shown below. Which of the following vessel is most likely involved
(AIIMS 2017)
   a. Ulnar artery
   b. Radial artery
   c. Brachial artery
   d. Cubital vein

10. Which of the following arteries supply pectoralis major muscle
(PGIC 2009)
   a. Pectoral branches of thoracoacromial artery
   b. Intercostal artery
   c. Lateral thoracic artery
   d. Subclavian artery
   e. Internal mammary artery

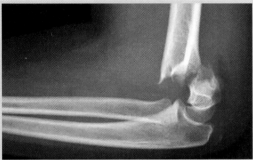

1. **b. Ulnar nerve lies medially to distal 1/3 of artery; c. Radial nerve lies posteriorly distal 1/3 of artery**
   ❑ Subclavian artery crosses the outer border of first rib to continue as axillary artery, which itself continue as brachial artery at the lower border of teres major.
   ❑ It is crossed and covered by pectoralis minor, which divides the artery into three parts.
   ❑ Axillary vein lies medial (not lateral) to the distal part of the artery in the axilla.

2. **d. Superior thoracic**
   ❑ In this case scapular anastomosis helps in maintaining the circulation to upper limb.
   ❑ Superior thoracic artery does not participate in scapular anastomosis.

3. **b. 1st part of subclavian and 3rd part of axillary artery > d. 3rd part of subclavian and 3rd part of axillary artery**
   ❑ Anastomosis around the shoulder (scapular anastomosis) is generally mentioned between first part of subclavian artery and third part of axillary artery.
   ❑ But since dorsal scapular artery (which participate in scapular anastomosis) is often a branch of third part of subclavian artery, it is also an anastomosis between third part of subclavian artery and third part of axillary artery.

4. **c. Deep branch of transverse cervical artery and subscapular artery**
   ❑ Scapular anastomosis is present between branches of subclavian artery (deep branch of transverse cervical) and axillary artery (subscapular), which continue supplying the ischemic region.
   ❑ Anterior and posterior circumflex arteries are branches of third part of axillary artery.
   ❑ Circumflex scapular and posterior circumflex humeral artery are branches of third part of axillary artery.
   ❑ Anterior circumflex humeral and subscapular are branches of third part of axillary artery.

5. **d. Dorsal scapular > c. Thyrocervical truck**
   ❑ Conventionally described the deep transverse cervical artery (a branch of the thyrocervical trunk of the first part of the subclavian artery) takes part in the scapular anastomosis.
   ❑ Recently it has been established that the dorsal scapular artery (a branch of third part of subclavian artery) being more constant than the deep cervical artery, takes part in scapular anastomosis.
   ❑ Thyrocervical trunk also participate in scapular anastomosis by giving suprascapular artery and transverse cervical artery.

6. **b. Anterior interosseous artery**
   ❑ Anterior interosseous artery (a branch of common interosseous artery) runs on the anterior surface of interosseous membrane.
   ❑ At the proximal border of pronator quadratus, it pierces the interosseous membrane to reach posterior forearm and anastomose with posterior interosseous artery.

7. **d. Radial collateral**
   ❑ Radial collateral artery is anterior descending branch of the profunda brachii artery, not a direct branch of brachial artery.

8. **c. 3rd part of axillary artery**
   ❑ Arteries forming anastomosis around the surgical neck of humerus are anterior and posterior circumflex humeral arteries (branches from 3rd part of axillary artery).

9. **b. Posterior interosseous artery**
   ❑ Ulnar artery gives common interosseous artery, which divides into anterior and posterior interosseous arteries.
   ❑ Posterior interosseous artery gives the interosseous recurrent artery.

10. **a. Pectoral branches of thoracoacromial artery; b. Intercostal artery; c. Lateral thoracic artery; e. Internal mammary artery**
   ❑ Subclavian artery does not supply pectoralis major muscle.
   ❑ The thoraco-acromial artery provides its major blood supply, while the intercostal perforators arising from the internal mammary artery provide a segmental blood supply. It is also supplied by lateral thoracic artery.
   ❑ Despite the extensive use of pectoralis major flaps in reconstructive surgery, certain pectoralis major musculocutaneous flaps may suffer from partial distal necrosis.
   ❑ The blood supply that provides circulation to these muscles perforates through to the breast parenchyma, thus also supplying blood to the breast.

11. c. Brachial artery
- ❑ This is a case of supracondylar fracture, with distal condylar fragment displaced in anterior direction.
- ❑ It can lead to tear or entrapment of the brachial artery. If left untreated could lead to Volkmann's contracture (permanent flexion contracture of the hand at the wrist, resulting in a claw-like deformity of the hand and fingers).

▶ Venous Drainage of Upper Limb

❑ Upper limb is drained by **superficial** and **deep** groups of vessels.

❑ Superficial veins are subcutaneous and deeper veins accompany the arteries, usually as venae comitantes.

❑ The deep group of veins drains the tissues beneath the deep fascia of the upper limb and is connected to the superficial system by **perforating veins.**

❑ **Superficial Veins**
  ➢ The **dorsal venous network** located on the dorsum of the hand gives rise to the **cephalic vein** and **basilic vein**. The palmar venous network located on the palm of the hand gives rise to the median antebrachial vein.

❑ **Cephalic Vein** begins as a radial continuation of the dorsal venous arch, runs on **roof of anatomical snuff box**, courses along the anterolateral surface of the forearm and arm and then between the deltoid and pectoralis major muscles along the **deltopectoral groove** (along with deltoid branch of the thoracoacromial artery). It pierces the costocoracoid membrane (of **clavipectoral fascia**) and ends in the axillary vein. It is often connected with the basilic vein by the **median cubital vein** in front of the elbow.

❑ **Basilic vein** drains the ulnar end of the arch, passes along the medial aspect of the forearm, pierces the deep fascia at the elbow, and joins the **venae comitantes** of the brachial artery to form the **axillary vein**, at the lower border of the teres major muscle.

❑ **Median Cubital Vein** connects the cephalic vein to the basilic vein at the **roof of cubital fossa**. It lies superficial to the bicipital aponeurosis and is **used for intravenous injections**, blood transfusions, and withdrawal.

  ➢ **Median Antebrachial Vein** arises in the palmar venous network, ascends on the front of the forearm, empties into the basilic vein or median cubital vein.

  ➢ **Dorsal Venous arch** is a network of veins formed by the dorsal metacarpal veins that receive dorsal digital veins and continues proximally as the cephalic vein and the basilic vein.

❑ **Deep veins**
  ➢ The **radial veins** receive the dorsal metacarpal veins. The **ulnar veins** receive tributaries from the deep palmar venous arches. The **brachial veins** are the vena comitantes of the brachial artery and are joined by the **basilic vein** to form the **axillary vein** and subsequently the **subclavian vein**.

  ➢ Axillary Vein is formed at the lower border of the teres major muscle by the union of the brachial veins (venae comitantes of the brachial artery) and the basilic vein and ascends along the medial side of the axillary artery. It continues as the subclavian vein at the lateral border of the first rib.

  ➢ **Subclavian vein** is the continuation of the **axillary vein**. It starts at the inferior margin of the first rib, crosses superiorly, joins the internal jugular vein to form the **brachiocephalic** behind the sternoclavicular joint.

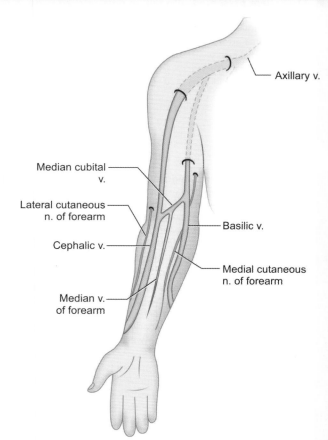

Median cubital v.

Lateral cutaneous n. of forearm

Cephalic v.

Median v. of forearm

Axillary v.

Basilic v.

Medial cutaneous n. of forearm

Fig. 41: Venous drainage of upper limb

1. **Cephalic vein drains into**   *(NEET Pattern 2013)*
   - a. Brachial vein
   - b. Subclavian vein
   - c. Axillary vein
   - d. Basilic vein

2. **All of the following are postaxial veins EXCEPT**
   - a. Cephalic vein
   - b. Basilic vein
   - c. Axillary vein
   - d. Subclavian vein

1. **c. Axillary vein > d. Basilic vein**
   - ❑ Cephalic vein drains into axillary vein by two routes:
   - ❑ Cephalic vein drains into axillary vein after piercing clavipectoral fascia.
   - ❑ Some amount of venous blood is drained into basilic vein through median cubital vein.
   - ❑ Basilic vein joins brachial veins to drain into axillary vein eventually.

2. **a. Cephalic vein**
   - ❑ Cephalic vein is a preaxial vein, embryologically, runs along the preaxial bone radius.

❑ **Median cubital vein** is the most preferred vein for routinely giving intravenous injections and for withdrawing blood from the donors.

❑ Basilic vein is preferred for **cardiac catheterization**.

Axilla and Spaces Around Shoulder Joint

❑ Axilla (armpit) is a **pyramid-shaped** space between the upper thoracic wall and the arm.

Table 16: Axilla: Boundaries and contents

Anterior wall	Pectoralis major and minor and subclavius muscle; clavipectoral fascia
Posterior wall	Subscapularis, teres major and latissimus dorsi
Medial wall	Serratus anterior and ribcage*
Lateral wall	Inter-tubercular sulcus and coracobrachialis and short head of biceps muscle
Apex	Interval between the clavicle, first rib, and upper border of the scapula
Base	Axillary fascia and skin
Contents	▪ Axillary artery, vein and lymphatics ▪ Brachial plexus (cords and branches) ▪ Long thoracic nerve, intercostobrachial nerve ▪ Axillary tail (of Spence)**

*Medial wall includes upper 4 ribs and intercostal muscles.
**Axillary tail (of Spence) is a superolateral extension of the mammary gland.

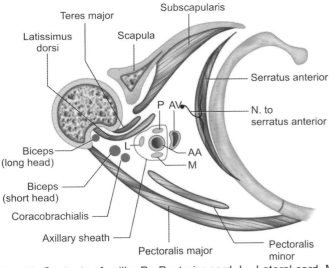

Fig. 42: Contents of axilla. P - Posterior cord, L - Lateral cord, M - Medial cord of brachial plexus; AA - Axillary artery; AV - Axillary vein

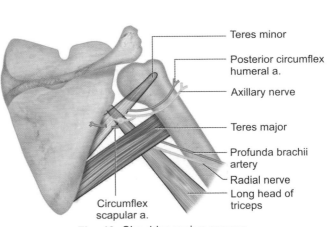

Fig. 43: Shoulder region spaces

Table 17: Spaces around shoulder region

Space	Boundary	Contents
Quadrangular (foramen of Velpeau)	Superior: **Teres minor** (and capsule of shoulder joint) Inferior: Teres major Medial: Long head of triceps Lateral: Surgical neck of humerus	**Axillary nerve** and **posterior circumflex humeral** vessels

Space	Boundary	Contents
Upper triangular	Superior: Teres minor Inferior: Teres major Lateral: Long head of triceps	**Circumflex scapular** vessels
Lower triangular	Superior: Teres major Medial: Long head of triceps Lateral: Shaft of humerus (and medial head of triceps)	**Radial nerve** and the **profunda brachii** (deep brachial) vessels

*Subscapularis muscle is anterior relation to all the three spaces and teres minor posterior. The posterior relation of lower triangular space is teres major.

▶ Fascia

- ❑ **Axillary Sheath** is a tubular fascial prolongation of the **prevertebral layer of the deep cervical fascia** into the axilla, enclosing cords and branches of brachial plexus and axillary artery. Axillary vein is outside the axillary sheath.
- ❑ **Axillary Fascia** forms the floor of axilla and is continuous anteriorly with the **pectoral** and **clavipectoral fasciae** (suspensory ligament of the axilla), laterally with the **brachial fascia**, and posteromedially with the fascia over the latissimus dorsi.
- ❑ Roots of brachial plexus are in the neck region (not in axilla).
- ❑ Muscle forming the medial wall of axilla is serratus anterior.
- ❑ **Clavipectoral fascia** (costocoracoid membrane; coracoclavicular fascia)
  - ➤ It is situated under cover of the clavicular portion of the pectoralis major and **occupies the interval between** the pectoralis minor and subclavius, and **protects** the axillary vein and artery, and axillary nerve.
  - ➤ It is the cranial continuation of the deep lamina of the **pectoral fascia** and the medial continuation of the parietal layer of the **subscapular bursal fascia.**
  - ➤ ts lower part splits to enclose the pectoralis minor muscle. Below this muscle it extends downwards as the **suspensory ligament of axilla**, which is attached to the dome of the axillary fascia. The suspensory ligament keeps the dome of axillary fascia pulled up, thus maintaining the concavity of the axilla.

Superiorly	Fuses with cervical fascia
Inferiorly	Fuses with axillary fascia
Laterally	Continuous with coracoacromial ligament (above and lateral to coracoid) Envelops coracoid process, short head of biceps and coracobrachialis
Medially	Attached to first rib and costoclavicular ligament Blends with external intercostal membrane of upper two intercostal spaces

- ❑ Clavipectoral fascia is traversed by: Cephalic vein, Lateral pectoral nerve, Thoracoacromial vessels and Lymphatics: passing between infraclavicular and apical nodes of the axilla

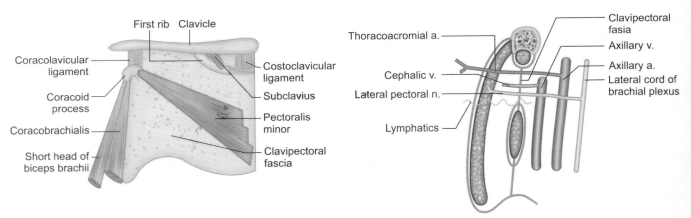

Fig. 44: Clavipectoral fascia: Front view   Fig. 45: Structures piercing clavipectoral fascia (Sagittal section)

- ❑ The portion of clavipectoral fascia extending from the first rib to the coracoid process is called **costo-coracoid ligament**.

Cubital Fossa

- Boundaries: **B**rachioradialis laterally, **pronator teres** medially; superiorly by **an imaginary horizontal line** connecting the two epicondyles of the humerus.
- Floor: **B**rachialis and **supinator** muscles
- **Contents** (in medial to lateral order): **Median nerve, brachial artery, biceps tendon** and **radial nerve.**
- **Ulnar nerve** passes behind the medial epicondyle and is **not a content** of cubital fossa (*NEET Pattern 2012*)
- At its lower end, the **brachial artery** divides into the **radial** and **ulnar arteries**.
- From medial to lateral, the **basilic, median cubital** and **cephalic veins** lie in the superficial fascia (at the roof).
- Fascial roof is strengthened by the bicipital aponeurosis on which runs the **antecubital vein** draining cephalic vein into the basilic vein.

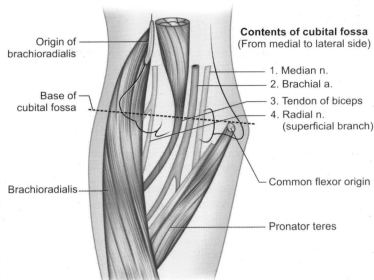

Contents of cubital fossa (From medial to lateral side)

Origin of brachioradialis

Base of cubital fossa

1. Median n.
2. Brachial a.
3. Tendon of biceps
4. Radial n. (superficial branch)

Common flexor origin

Brachioradialis

Pronator teres

Fig. 46: Cubital fossa: Boundaries and contents

1. **Boundaries of quadrilateral space include all EXCEPT**
   (NEET Pattern 2014)
   a. Teres major
   b. Long head of triceps
   c. Neck of humerus
   d. Deltoid

2. **Boundaries of upper triangular space include all EXCEPT**
   (NEET Pattern 2012)
   a. Teres minor
   b. Teres major
   c. Subscapularis
   d. Triceps

3. **The accompanying artery with axillary nerve in the quadrangular space is**
   a. Anterior circumflex humeral artery
   b. Posterior circumflex humeral artery
   c. Profunda brachii artery
   d. Circumflex scapular artery

4. **Structure related to deltopectoral groove**
   (NEET Pattern 2015)
   a. Axillary artery
   b. Cephalic vein
   c. Basilic vein
   d. Radial nerve

5. **Clavipectoral fascia is derived from which ligament**
   (NEET Pattern 2013)
   a. Coracoacromial
   b. Coracoclavicular
   c. Costoclavicular
   d. Costocoracoid

6. **Clavipectoral fascia splits to enclose subclavius and pectoralis minor, and continues as** *(NEET Pattern 2015)*
   a. Axillary sheath
   b. Costocoracoid ligament
   c. Costoclavicular ligament
   d. Suspensory ligament

7. **WRONG about clavipectoral fascia** *(PGIC)*
   a. Situated under clavicular portion of the pectoralis minor
   b. Fuses with the deep cervical fascia superiorly
   c. Costocoracoid membrane is a modification
   d. Continue downward to join the axillary fascia
   e. Laterally joins fascia over the short head of the biceps brachii

8. **Bicipital aponeurosis lies over which structure in cubital fossa** *(NEET Pattern 2015)*
   a. Median cubital vein
   b. Radial nerve
   c. Brachial artery
   d. Anterior interosseous artery

9. **TRUE about cubital fossa is/are**
   a. Medial boundary is flexor carpi ulnaris
   b. Base is imaginary line connecting humeral epicondyles
   c. Floor is brachialis muscle
   d. Brachial artery is medial to biceps tendon ·
   e. Antecubital vein is a content

(PGIC)

1. **d. Deltoid**
   - The quadrangular space is bounded by the teres minor (superiorly), teres major (inferior), triceps (medial), and the humerus (laterally).

2. **c. Subscapularis**
   - Subscapularis muscle is anterior relation (not boundary) of upper triangular space

3. b. Posterior circumflex humeral artery
- ❏ Axillary nerve and posterior circumflex humeral artery pass through quadrangular space and then wind around the surgical neck of humerus.

4. b. Cephalic vein
- ❏ Deltopectoral groove is an indentation between the deltoid muscle and pectoralis major, through which the cephalic vein passes and where the coracoid process is most easily palpable (below clavicle).

5. d. Costocoracoid
- ❏ Occasionally, the clavipectoral fascia thickens to form a band between the first rib and coracoid process, the costocoracoid ligament, under which the lateral cord of the brachial plexus is closely applied.

6. d. Suspensory ligament
- ❏ Below pectoralis minor muscle, clavipectoral fascia extends downwards as the suspensory ligament of axilla, which attach and pulls up the dome of the axillary fascia (and maintain the concavity of the axilla).

7. a. Situated under clavicular portion of the pectoralis minor
- ❏ Clavipectoral fascia is situated under clavicular portion of the pectoralis major and it splits to enclose pectoralis minor.

8. c. Brachial artery
- ❏ Bicipital aponeurosis passes superficial to the brachial artery and median nerve. It lies deep to superficial veins.
- ❏ It provides some protection for the deeper structures during venepuncture at cubital fossa.

9. b. Base is imaginary line connecting humeral epicondyles, c. Floor is brachialis muscle; d. Brachial artery is medial to biceps tendon
- ❏ Medial boundary of cubital fossa is pronator teres muscle; Antecubital vein is at the roof (it is not a content).

▶ Mammary Gland

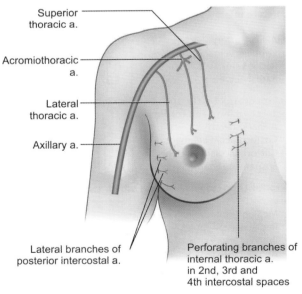

Fig. 47: Arterial supply to mammary gland

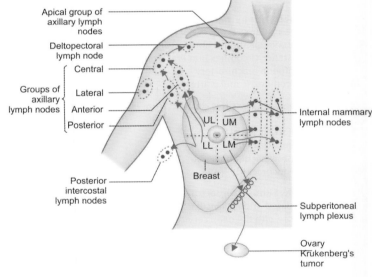

Fig. 48: Lymphatic drainage of the breast (UL, Upper lateral quadrant; LL, Lower lateral quadrant; UM, Upper medial quadrant; LM, Lower medial quadrant)

- ❏ Mammary gland is a modified apocrine sweat gland. It extends over the **second to sixth ribs** and from the sternum to the midaxillary line, **nipple** lies at the level of the **fourth intercostal space**.
- ❏ It lies in the superficial fascia, supported by the **suspensory ligaments (of Cooper)**, strong fibrous attachments, that run from the dermis of the skin to the deep layer of the superficial fascia **(pectoral fascia)** running through the breast.
- ❏ There are 15 to 20 lobes of glandular tissue, each lobe opens by a lactiferous duct onto the tip of the nipple, which enlarges to form a lactiferous sinus (stores milk).
- ❏ During surgery radial incisions should be put to avoid damaging the lactiferous ducts.

- **Arterial supply:**
  - Internal thoracic artery (branch of first part of subclavian artery)
  - Branches of **axillary artery** (all the three parts): Superior thoracic artery, Thoraco-acromial trunk; Lateral thoracic artery; Subscapular artery
  - Posterior intercostal arteries (branches of **descending thoracic aorta**)
- **Venous drainage**: Drained by the identically named veins accompanying the arteries, mainly into the **axillary vein** via **lateral thoracic vein**. Additional venous drainage from the breast is to the **internal thoracic vein** via medial mammary veins, **anterior intercostal veins**, and **posterior intercostal veins** (drain into the azygos system).
- **Nerve supply**: Anterior and lateral cutaneous branches of the **second to the sixth intercostal nerves**.
- **Lymphatic drainage**: Lymph Drainage from the **Lateral Quadrant** Majority of the lymph (>75%) drains as follows: Axillary nodes (humeral, subscapular, pectoral, central, and apical) → infraclavicular and supraclavicular nodes → right subclavian lymph trunk (for the right breast) or left subclavian lymph trunk (for the left breast).
- Lymph Drainage from the **Medial Quadrant** Parasternal nodes → right bronchomediastinal lymph trunk (for the right breast) or left bronchomediastinal lymph trunk (for the left breast). May also drain into the opposite breast.
- Lymph Drainage from the **Inferior Quadrant** Into the nodes of the upper abdomen (e.g., inferior phrenic lymph nodes).
- Breast cancer in advanced stages: Infiltrates Cooper's ligaments, produces shortening of the ligaments, causing depression or dimpling of the overlying skin. Advanced sign of inflammatory breast cancer, **peau d'orange** (texture of orange peel) is the edematous swollen and pitted breast skin due to obstruction of the subcutaneous lymphatics.

QUESTIONS

1. **All is true about mammary gland EXCEPT**
   (NBEP Pattern 2013)
   a. Is a modified sweat gland
   b. Extends from the 2-6 ribs vertically
   c. Supplied by internal mammary artery
   d. Nipple is supplied by sixth intercostal nerve

2. **How many lactiferous ducts open in nipple**
   (NEET Pattern 2015, 16)
   a. 0–10
   b. 15–20
   c. 25–50
   d. 50–75

3. **Lymphatic drainage of upper outer quadrant of breast**
   (NEET Pattern 2013)
   a. Anterior axillary
   b. Posterior axillary
   c. Lateral axillary
   d. Para sterna

4. **All are true regarding axillary lymph nodes EXCEPT**
   (AIPG Pattern 2013)
   a. Posterior group lies along subscapular vessels
   b. Lateral group lies along lateral thoracic vessels
   c. Apical group lies along axillary vessels
   d. Apical group is terminal lymph nodes

5. **The terminal axillary lymph nodes are**
   (AIIMS 2005, NEET Pattern 2016)
   a. Apical   b. Central
   c. Lateral   d. Pectoral

6. **Mammary gland is supplied by**   *(PGIC 2012)*
   a. Subscapular artery   b. Musculophrenic artery
   c. Internal mammary artery   d. Superior thoracic artery
   e. Superior epigastric artery

ANSWERS

1. **d. Nipple is supplied by sixth intercostal nerve**
   - Nipple lies in the fourth intercostal space and is supplied by fourth intercostal nerve.

2. **b. 15–20**
   - The parenchyma of the breast consists of about 15–20 lobes arranged in a radial fashion and converge towards the nipple as lactiferous ducts.

3. **a. Anterior axillary**
   - Lymphatics from upper outer quadrant of breast drain into anterior (pectoral) axillary lymph nodes.

4. **b. Lateral group lies along lateral thoracic vessels**
   - Lateral group of axillary lymph nodes lie along the axillary vein.

5. **a. Apical**
   - Anterior (pectoral), posterior (subscapular) and lateral (humeral) groups drain the lymph into the central group of lymph nodes, which eventually drain into the terminal apical lymph nodes (near the apex of axilla).

6. **a. Subscapular artery; c. Internal mammary artery; d. Superior thoracic artery**
   - Mammary gland receives blood from the axillary artery branches (subscapular and superior thoracic); internal mammary artery branches and the posterior intercostal arteries.
   - The terminal branches of internal thoracic artery: superior epigastric artery and musculophrenic artery do not supply the mammary gland.

Most of the lymph from breast is drained into **Anterior axillary** lymph nodes

Subareolar **plexus of Sappey** is the Plexus of lymph vessels deep to the areola which drain into anterior axillary lymph nodes

▼ Anatomical Snuff Box

- ❑ **Anatomical snuff box** is an elongated triangular depression seen on lateral aspect of the wrist immediately distal to the radial styloid process, gets **more prominent when** the thumb is fully extended.
- ❑ The superficial radial nerve, can be rolled from side to side on the tendon of extensor pollicis brevis
- ❑ The tenderness in the anatomical box indicates **fracture of scaphoid** bone.
- ❑ **De Quervain's tenosynovitis**: Inflammation of the two tendons forming anterolateral boundary of anatomical snuff box. The tendons involved are **abductor pollicis longus** and **extensor pollicis brevis** and Finkelstein test becomes positive.

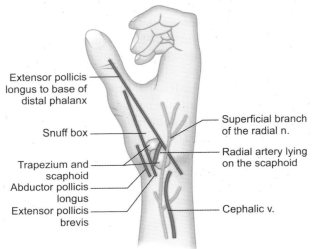

Fig. 49: Anatomical snuff box

Boundaries	▪ Anterolaterally (Radial)
	  – Tendons of abductor pollicis longus
	  – Extensor pollicis brevis
	▪ Posteromedially (ulnar)
	  – Tendon of extensor pollicis longus

Borders	▪ Proximal border
	  – Styloid process of the radius
	▪ Distal border
	  – Apex of the schematic snuffbox isosceles triangle

Floor	Scaphoid, trapezium and base of first metacarpal bone*
Roof	▪ Skin and superficial fascia ▪ Cephalic vein (subcutaneous) ▪ Radial nerve branches (subcutaneous)
Contents	Radial artery (pulse)

* At the floor, two joints are partly evident - the wrist joint and the first carpometacarpal joint.

▼ Flexor and Extensor Retinacula

- ❑ **Flexor Retinaculum** It forms the carpal (osteofascial) tunnel on the anterior aspect of the wrist, is attached **medially** to the triquetrum, the pisiform, and the hook of the hamate and **laterally** to the tubercles of the scaphoid and trapezium. It serves as an origin for muscles of the thenar eminence.
- ❑ Structures passing **superficial** to flexor retinaculum are: Ulnar artery and nerve; Palmar cutaneous branch of median nerve; Tendon of Palmaris longus muscle
- ❑ Structures passing **deep** to flexor retinaculum are: **Median nerve;** Tendons of **Flexor digitorum superficialis and profundus muscles;** Tendon of flexor pollicis brevis; Ulnar and radial bursae

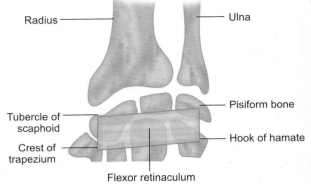

Fig. 50: Carpal tunnel and flexor retinaculum

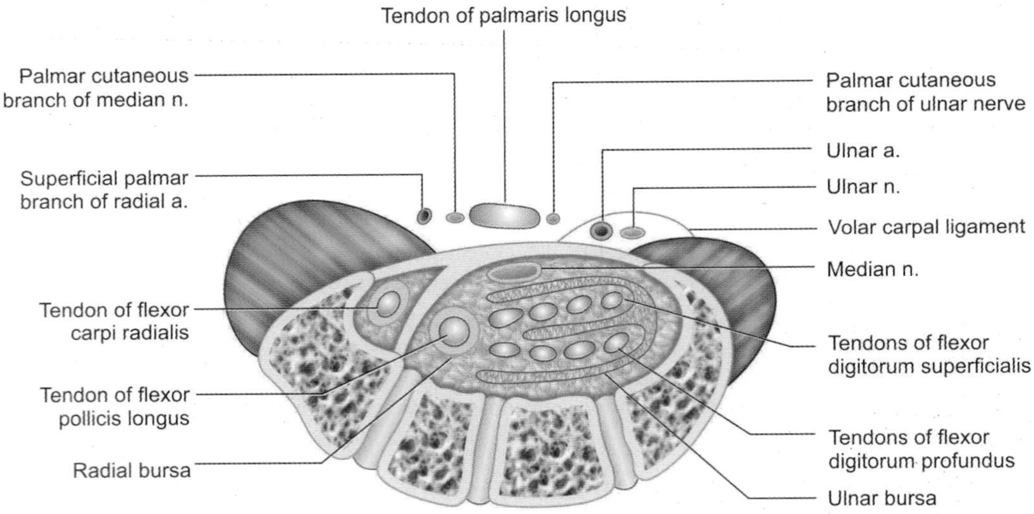

Fig. 51: Structures related to carpal tunnel and flexor retinaculum

- ❑ **Extensor Retinaculum** It is a thickening of the antebrachial fascia on the **back of the wrist**, subdivided into compartments, and places the **extensor tendons beneath** it.
- ❑ It extends from the lateral margin of the radius to the styloid process of the ulna, the pisiform, and the triquetrum and is crossed superficially by the **superficial branch of the radial nerve**.

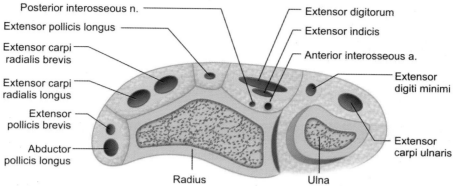

Fig. 52: Extensor retinaculum compartments and contents

Compartment	Structure/structures, passing through
I	▪ Abductor pollicis longus (APL) ▪ Extensor pollicis brevis (APB)
II	▪ Extensor carpi radialis longus (ECRL) ▪ Extensor carpi radialis brevis (ECRB)
III	▪ Extensor pollicis longus (EPL)
IV	▪ Extensor digitorum (ED) ▪ Extensor indicis (EI) ▪ Posterior interosseous nerve ▪ Anterior interosseous artery
V	▪ Extensor digiti minimi (EDM)
VI	▪ Extensor carpi ulnaris (EUC)

- ❑ 4th compartment has the extensor digitorum and extensor indicis tendons pass through the 4th compartment along with the posterior interosseous nerve and anterior interosseous artery.

1. Boundaries of anatomical snuff box are all EXCEPT
(JIPMER 2010; NEET Pattern 2015)
a. Abductor pollicis longus
b. Extensor pollicis longus
c. Extensor pollicis Brevis
d. Extensor carpi ulnaris

2. The carpal tunnel contains all of the following important structures EXCEPT
(AIPG 2005)
a. Median Nerve
b. Flexor pollicis longus
c. Flexor carpi radialis
d. Flexor digitorum superficialis

3. Carpal tunnel contains all EXCEPT *(NEET Pattern 2015)*
a. Median nerve
b. FDS tendon
c. FPL tendon
d. FCU tendon

4. First extensor compartment of wrist has which of the following structures
(PGIC 2008)
a. Extensor pollicis brevis
b. Extensor carpi radialis longus
c. Extensor carpi radialis brevis
d. Extensor digiti minimi
e. Abductor pollicis longus

5. 3rd extensor compartment of wrist contains tendon of
(NEET Pattern 2015)
a. ECRL
b. ECRB
c. EPL
d. EPB

6. Nerve damaged due to anterior dislocation of lunate
(NEET Pattern 2016)
a. Median and ulnar
b. Median
c. Ulnar
d. Radial

1. d. Extensor carpi ulnaris

2. c. Flexor carpi radialis
- ❑ The tendon of flexor carpi radialis passes through a tunnel created by a fascial slip on the roof of flexor retinaculum.
- ❑ It passes neither superficial nor deep to the flexor retinaculum, it is actually embedded within the retinaculum.
- ❑ Median nerve, flexor pollicis longus and flexor digitorum superficialis all pass deep to the flexor retinaculum and are contents of carpal tunnel.

3. d. FCU tendon
- ❑ Nine flexor tendons pass under the flexor retinaculum along with the median nerve.
- ❑ FCU insertion is into the pisiform bone and then via ligaments into the hamate bone (pisohamate ligament) and 5th metacarpal bone-forming pisometacarpal ligament.

4. a. Extensor pollicis brevis; e. Abductor pollicis longus
- ❑ First extensor compartment of wrist has two tendons: Abductor pollicis longus and extensor pollicis brevis.
- ❑ These two tendons form the anterolateral boundary of anatomical snuff box and are involved in de Quervain's tenosynovitis.

5. c. EPL
- ❑ Third compartment of extensor retinaculum let pass the tendon of extensor pollicis longus.

6. b. Median
- ❑ Anterior dislocation of lunate may lead to carpal tunnel syndrome and compression of medial nerve.

▶ Hand Bones

- ❑ **Carpal Bones:** There are 8 carpal bones in the upper limb. **Mnemonic:** She Looks Too Pretty; Try To Catch Her.
  - ➤ **Proximal row** (lateral to medial): Scaphoid, Lunate, Triquetral, Pisiform
  - ➤ **Distal row:** Trapezium, Trapezoid, Capitate, Hamate
- ❑ **Capitate** begins to ossify in the **second month**; hamate at the end of the third month; triquetrum in the third year; and the lunate, scaphoid, trapezium and trapezoid in the fourth year in females (fifth year in males).
- ❑ **Pisiform** begins to ossify in the ninth or tenth year in females, and the **twelfth in males**.
- ❑ Some authors mention: **Lunate-4th year**, Scaphoid and trapezoid—5th year and trapezium-6th year

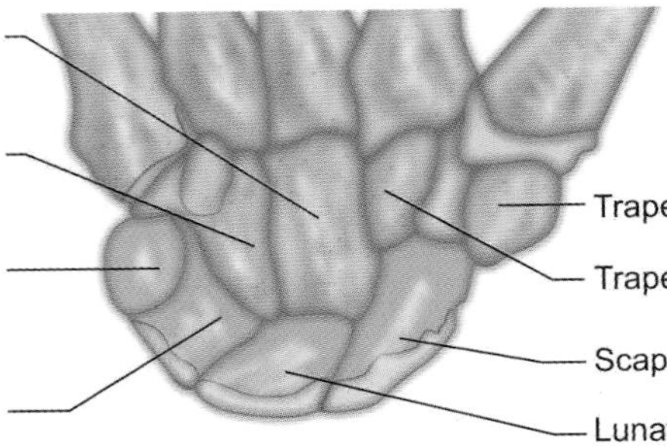

Capitate is the largest carpal bone, first carpal bone to ossify and articulates with maximum number of bones. It **occupies the center** of the wrist (NEET Pattern 2016)

Capitate: second month
Hamate: third month
Pisiform: 9-12 years
Triquetrum: third year
Trapezium
Trapezoid
Scaphoid
Lunate
4 to 5 years

Fig. 53: Carpal bones: Age of appearance of ossification centres

- ❑ Pisiform bone ossifies at 9-12 years. The dorsal surface of pisiform has an oval articular surface for **triquetral** bone (NEET Pattern 2015)
- ❑ Scaphoid is the **most commonly fractured** carpal bone. A fracture leads to **osteonecrosis** of the scaphoid bone (proximal fragment) because the blood supply to the scaphoid bone flows from distal to proximal. There is **tenderness** at the floor of the anatomical snuff box.
- ❑ Most commonly dislocated carpal bone is **Lunate**
- ❑ All metacarpals have epiphysis at their distal end (i.e., head) **except First metacarpal**, which has epiphysis at its proximal end (i.e., base)
- ❑ Shortest and stoutest metacarpal is **First metacarpal**.

1. Which of the following has epiphysis at head
(NEET Pattern 2013)
- a. Distal phalanx
- b. Middle phalanx
- c. Thumb metacarpal
- d. Third metacarpal

2. Capitate bone articulates with all EXCEPT
(NEET Pattern 2016)
- a. Second metacarpal
- b. Lunate
- c. Trapezium
- d. Scaphoid

3. WRONG about the first metacarpal is *(NEET Pattern 2013)*
- a. Epiphysis is at the head
- b. Base is convexo-concave for sellar synovial joint
- c. Doesn't articulate with other metacarpals
- d. More anterior and medially rotated

4. TRUE about blood supply of scaphoid *(NEET Pattern 2015)*
- a. Mainly through ulnar artery
- b. Major supply from ventral surface
- c. Major supply from dorsal surface
- d. Proximal supply in antegrade fashion

1. d. Third metacarpal
- ❑ Epiphysis is present on the heads of all metacarpals, except first metacarpal (epiphysis is at the base).
- ❑ Epiphysis at the head of the first metacarpal bone is an example of aberrant epiphysis, which is a deviation from the norm (and rarely found).

2. c. Trapezium
- ❑ The capitate bone is the largest of the carpal bones in the human hand, and occupies the center of the wrist. It articulates with trapezoid (not trapezium) bone.

3. **a. Epiphysis is at the head**
   - ❑ Epiphysis is present on the heads of all metacarpals, except first metacarpal (epiphysis is at the base).
   - ❑ Epiphysis at the head of the first metacarpal bone is an example of aberrant epiphysis, which is a deviation from the norm (and rarely found).
   - ❑ First metacarpal is shortest and stoutest of all metacarpals, rotated medially through 90 degrees with respect to other metacarpals.
   - ❑ The base of the first metacarpal bone has a convexo-concave articular surface to make a saddle synovial joint with trapezium (first carpometacarpal joint).

4. **c. Major supply from dorsal surface**
   - ❑ Major blood supply (~80%) of scaphoid comes through dorsal surface via dorsal branches of radial artery.
   - ❑ The artery enters just distal to waist area and supply the proximal part in retrograde fashion.

▶ Hand Muscles

- ❑ There are 20 intrinsic muscles in hand: Thenar (3), Hypothenar (3), Adductor pollicis, Lumbricals (4), Interossei (8) and Palmaris brevis.
- ❑ Thenar muscles: Abductor pollicis brevis, Flexor pollicis brevis, Opponens pollicis.
- ❑ Hypothenar muscles: Abductor digiti minimi, Flexor digiti minimi, Opponens digiti minimi.
- ❑ Superficial head of **flexor pollicis brevis** is innervated by the recurrent motor branch of the median nerve, and the deep head by the deep branch of the ulnar nerve.
- ❑ **Abductor pollicis brevis** is innervated by the recurrent motor branch of the median nerve and is the only thenar muscle that is constantly supplied by the median nerve.
- ❑ **Opponens pollicis** is usually mentioned to innervated by the lateral terminal branch of the median nerve (but **Gray's anatomy** mentions that it also receives a branch of the deep terminal branch of the ulnar nerve).

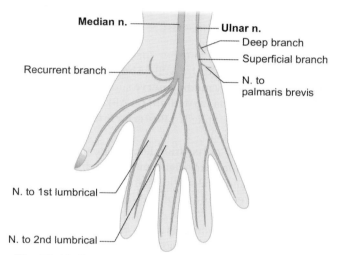

Fig. 54: Median nerve and ulnar nerve distribution in hand

- ❑ **Adductor pollicis, abductor digiti minimi, flexor digiti minimi brevis, opponens digiti minimi and all the interossei are** innervated by the deep branch of the ulnar nerve; the first dorsal interosseous and adductor pollicis are supplied by its most distal portion.
- ❑ **Palmaris brevis** is innervated by the superficial branch of the ulnar nerve.
- ❑ The **first and second lumbricals** are innervated by the median nerve, and the **third and fourth lumbricals** by the deep terminal branch of the ulnar nerve. The third lumbrical frequently receives a supply from the median nerve. The first and second lumbricals are, occasionally, innervated by the deep terminal branch of the ulnar nerve.

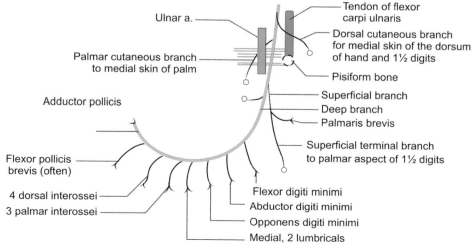

Fig. 55: Ulnar nerve course and distribution in hand

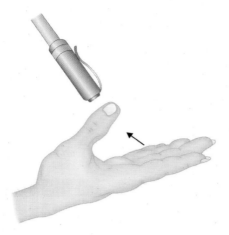

Fig. 56: Pen test

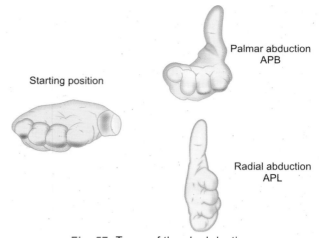

Fig. 57: Types of thumb abduction

- ❏ **Pen test** is to check anterior (palmar) abduction of thumb, carried out by APB (**Abductor pollicis brevis**), supplied by **median nerve** supply.
- ❏ Radial abduction is carried out by APL (**Abductor pollicis longus),** supplied by **Posterior interosseous nerve** (Radial nerve).
- ❏ Lumbricals 1 and 2 arise from lateral side of lateral two tendons of the flexor digitorum profundus.
- ❏ Lumbricals 3 and 4 take origin from adjacent sides of medial three tendons of the flexor digitorum profundus.
- ❏ The tendons of lumbricals cross the lateral side of metacarpophalangeal joints to be inserted into the lateral side of **dorsal digital expansion** of the corresponding digit from second to fifth.
- ❏ The major action of lumbricals is to cause extension at interphalangeal joint. They also cause weak metacarpophalangeal flexion.
- ❏ Pinching the index finger against the thumb without a lumbrical would result in a nail-to-nail contact.

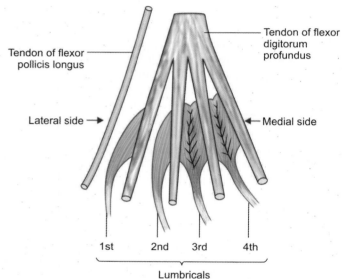

Fig. 58: Lumbricals: Origin—Tendons of flexor digitorum profundus; Insertion—Dorsal digital expansion

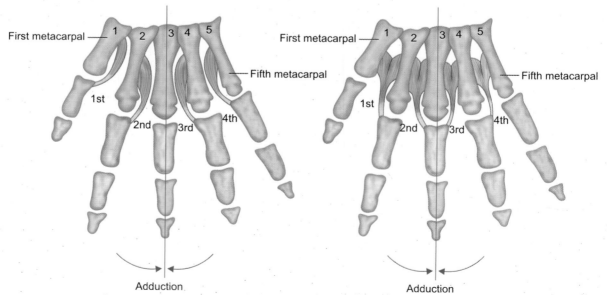

Fig. 59: Palmar and dorsal interossei

❑ **Interossei**

➤ 4 **P**almar interossei adduct ('**PAD**'-Palmar **AD**duct) the fingers towards the longitudinal axis of the middle finger

➤ 4 **D**orsal interossei abduct ('**DAB**'-Dorsal **AB**duction) the fingers away from the longitudinal axis of the middle finger.

➤ The 8 interossei muscles also work along with 4 lumbricals for MCP flexion and IP extension (glass holding position).

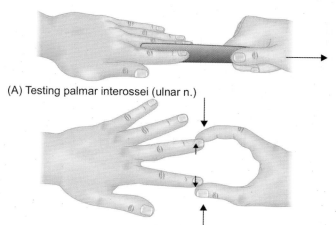

(A) Testing palmar interossei (ulnar n.)

❑ **Card Test** is for palmar interossei (adductors) of the fingers.

➤ Patient is asked to tightly hold a card between the fingers while the examiner tries to pull it out. If **palmar interossei** are weak, patient cannot do palmar **adduction** to grasp. (AIIMS 2015)

(B) Testing dorsal interossei (ulnar n.)

Fig. 60: Clinical testing of interossei muscles

❑ **Egawa's** Test is for dorsal interossei (abductors) of the fingers.

➤ Patient is asked to abduct fingers against examiner's resistance palm facing downward.

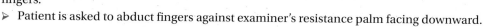

1. **Which muscle does NOT contribute to dorsal digital expansion** *(NEET Pattern 2013)*
   a. Interossei
   b. Lumbricals
   c. Extensor digitorum
   d. Adductor pollicis

2. **Mallet finger is a flexion deformity of the distal phalanx, which occurs due to** *(UPSC)*
   a. Avulsion fracture of middle phalanx
   b. Rupture of collateral slips of extensor expansion
   c. Rupture of central slip of extensor expansion
   d. Dislocation of distal interphalangeal joint

3. **Action of dorsal interossei**
   a. Extension at metacarpophalangeal joint
   b. Adduction at metacarpophalangeal joint
   c. Flexion at metacarpophalangeal joints
   d. Flexion at interphalangeal joints

4. **Flexion of MCP joint and extension of IP joints is the major action of** *(NEET Pattern 2015)*
   a. Palmar interossei
   b. Dorsal interossei
   c. Lumbricals
   d. FDS

5. **FALSE statement regarding adductor pollicis muscle** *(JIPMER 2008)*
   a. Has 2 heads
   b. Supplied by median nerve
   c. Causes adduction of thumb
   d. Arterial supply is from arteria princeps pollicis

6. **A patient cannot hold a sheet of paper between the 2nd and 3rd digits. Nerve damaged is**
   a. Deep branch of ulnar nerve
   b. Deep branch of radial nerve
   c. Superficial branch of ulnar nerve
   d. Median nerve

7. **Compression of a nerve within the carpal tunnel produce inability to** *(AIIMS; NEET Pattern 2014)*
   a. Abduct the thumb
   b. Adduct the thumb
   c. Flex the distal phalanx of the thumb
   d. Oppose the thumb

8. **Power grip of hand is due to** *(NEET Pattern 2014)*
   a. Palmaris
   b. Long flexors
   c. Short flexors
   d. Lumbricals

9. **Identify the structure marked by the arrow** *(JIPMER 2017)*
   a. Palmar branch of median nerve
   b. Recurrent median nerve
   c. Communicating branch of median and ulnar nerve
   d. Deep palmar branch of ulnar nerve

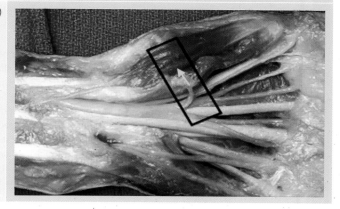

QUESTIONS

10. **Identify the function of the shown muscle in the diagram**
    (NEET Pattern 2018)
    a. Flexion at IP joint
    b. Extension at MCP joint
    c. Flexion at MCP joint
    d. Abduction at MCP joint

11. **De Quervain's disease is tenosynovitis of**
    (NEET Pattern 2018)
    a. Abductor pollicis brevis and extensor pollicis longus
    b. Abductor pollicis longus and extensor carpi radialis brevis
    c. Abductor pollicis longus and extensor pollicis brevis
    d. Abductor pollicis brevis and extensor carpi radialis longus

1. **d. Adductor pollicis**
   - ❑ Dorsal digital expansion is a tendinous modification of extensor digitorum and receives attachment of lumbricals, interossei but not adductor pollicis.

2. **b. Rupture of collateral slips of extensor expansion**
   - ❑ Mallet finger is a flexion deformity of the distal phalanx due to injury to the extensor digitorum at its insertion to the base of the distal phalanx (the collateral slips)

3. **c. Flexion at metacarpophalangeal joints**
   - ❑ Digital abduction is a function of the 4 dorsal interossei ('DAB'-Dorsal ABduction) and digital adduction is a function of
   - ❑ 4 palmar interossei ('PAD'-Palmar ADduct).
   - ❑ The 8 interossei muscles also work along with 4 lumbricals for MCP flexion and IP extension (glass holding position).

4. **c. Lumbricals**
   - ❑ This is a wrong QUESTIONS since it has multiple ANSWERS.
   - ❑ Lumbricals and interossei work together for metacarpophalangeal flexion and interphalangeal extension.
   - ❑ The major action of lumbricals is to cause extension at interphalangeal joint. They also cause weak metacarpophalangeal flexion.
   - ❑ Palmar interossei adduct (PAD) the fingers and dorsal interossei abduct (DAB) the fingers. Interossei also contribute to metacarpophalangeal joint flexion and interphalangeal extension.

5. **b. Supplied by median nerve**
   - ❑ Adductor pollicis muscle has two heads, both supplied by the ulnar nerve.

6. **a. Deep branch of ulnar nerve**
   - ❑ Holding a paper between fingers require adduction, carried out by the palmar interossei (PAD) - Card test. All the interossei are supplied by deep branch of ulnar nerve.

7. **d. Oppose the thumb**
   - ❑ Carpal tunnel syndrome leads to compression of median nerve, paralysing the abductor pollicis brevis, hence loss of thumb opposition.
   - ❑ Thumb opposition has three components:
   - ❑ Anterior abduction of thumb (carried out by abductor pollicis brevis supplied by median nerve)
   - ❑ Medial rotation of thumb (carried out by opponens pollicis supplied by median and ulnar nerve)
   - ❑ Flexion of thumb (carried out by flexor pollicis brevis supplied by median and ulnar nerve)
   - ❑ Paralysis of abductor pollicis brevis leads to loss of the first component of thumb opposition, plus thumb remains in adduction deformity (due to unopposed adductor pollicis supplied by ulnar nerve).
   - ❑ In this patient there is loss of anterior abduction (abductor pollicis brevis; median nerve) but lateral abduction of thumb (abductor pollicis longus supplied by posterior interosseous nerve, radial nerve) is still possible.
   - ❑ Adduction of thumb is carried out by the adductor pollicis (ulnar nerve).
   - ❑ Since the compression of median nerve is within the carpal tunnel (paralysing the distal muscles in hand) the proximal muscles of forearm are still functional. Flexion of distal phalanx (flexor pollicis longus supplied by anterior interosseous nerve, median nerve) is possible.

8. b. Long flexors > d. Lumbricals

- ❑ In power grip while the wrist is fixed in dorsiflexion (by extensor muscles) long finger flexors and intrinsic muscles of hand (like lumbricals) work to grip the object.
- ❑ Power grip is used for carrying heavy bags or for holding on to a handle, the grip is characterised by the flexion of digits 2-5 and flexion and adduction of the thumb around the object but in opposing directions.
- ❑ Three extrinsic hand muscles provide majority of power generated: Flexor Digitorum Superficialis, Flexor Digitorum Profundus and Flexor Pollicis Longus.

9. b. Recurrent median nerve

- ❑ The marker shows recurrent branch of median nerve, which curls upwards to supply thenar muscles (abductor pollicis brevis, flexor pollicis brevis, and opponens pollicis). It usually passes distal to the transverse carpal ligament. It may be affected in carpal tunnel syndrome and can be injured during carpal tunnel surgery.

10. c. Flexion at MCP joint

- ❑ The diagram shows the **palmar interossei** which are involved in adduction of the fingers. 'PAD - Palmar interossei work for Adduction'.
- ❑ Additionally, all the 8 interossei and 4 lumbricals work for **metacarpo-phalangeal flexion** and interphalangeal extension.

11. c. Abductor pollicis longus and extensor pollicis brevis

- ❑ Abductor pollicis longus and extensor pollicis brevis make the **lateral border** of anatomical snuff box and are inflamed in De Quervain's tenosynovitis.

- ❑ **Ape thumb deformity** (median nerve injury) presents with **thenar atrophy** and thumb remains laterally rotated and adducted (**paralysed** abductor pollicis brevis and opponens pollicis; **intact** adductor pollicis).
- ❑ Musician's nerve - Clumsiness of hand occurs due to paralysis of intrinsic muscles of hand like lumbricals & interossei, supplied by ulnar nerve
- ❑ Small hand muscles are supplied by branches of the lower trunk of brachial plexus (C8; T1) via median and ulnar nerve.
- ❑ **Dupuytren's** contracture is a progressive thickening, shortening, and fibrosis of the palmar fascia, especially the **palmar aponeurosis**, producing a fixed flexion deformity of fingers in which the fingers are pulled toward the palm (inability to fully extend fingers), especially the ring and little fingers.

◢ Dorsal Digital Expansion

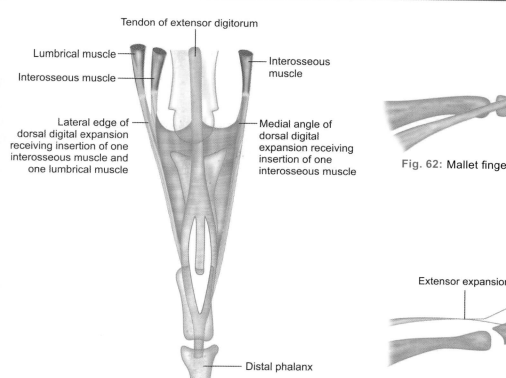

Fig. 61: Dorsal digital expansion

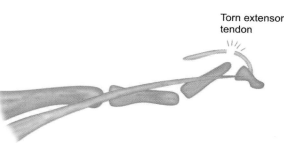

Fig. 62: Mallet finger with swan neck deformity

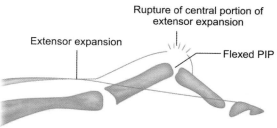

Fig. 63: Boutonniere buttonhole deformity. Proximal interphalangeal (PIP) joint pokes through the extensor expansion

❑ **Dorsal digital expansion** forms a functional unit to coordinate the actions of long extensors, long flexors, lumbricals and interossei on the digit.

❑ Extensor digitorum sends a **single central band** which inserts on the base of the middle phalanx, whereas **two lateral bands** join to form a single terminal band to insert on the base of the distal phalanx.

❑ The tendons of **lumbricals** and **interossei** are inserted into this expansion.

❑ On the index finger and little finger, the expansion is strengthened by extensor indicis and extensor digiti minimi respectively, which blends with it.

❑ **Mallet finger** (hammer or baseball finger) is a finger with **permanent flexion of the distal phalanx** due to an avulsion of the **lateral bands** of the extensor tendon to the distal phalanx. It occurs due to A forceful blow on the tip of the finger causing **sudden and strong flexion** of the phalanx.

❑ **Boutonniere** (button-hole) deformity is characterized by flexion of proximal interphalangeal joint and hyperextension of distal phalanx. It occurs when the flexed PIP joint pokes through the extensor expansion following rupture of its 'central band of dorsal digital expansion due to a direct end on trauma to the finger. It is opposite to mallet finger deformity.

❑ Curves laterally deep to palmar

▶ Arteries in Hand

Artery	Origin	Course
Superficial palmar arch	Direct continuation of ulnar artery; arch is completed on lateral side by superficial branch of radial artery or another of its branches	Curves laterally deep to palmar aponeurosis and superficial to long flexor tendons; curve of arch lies across palm at level of distal border of extended thumb
Deep palmar arch	Direct continuation of radial artery; arch is completed on medial side by deep branch of ulnar artery	Curves medially, deep to long flexor tendons; is in contact with bases of metacarpals
Common palmar digital	Superficial palmar arch	Pass distally on lumbricals to webbing of digits
Proper palmar digital	Common palmar digital arteries	Run along of 2nd–5th digits
Princeps pollicis	Radial artery as it turns into palm	Descends on palmar aspect of 1st metacarpal; divides at base of proximal phalanx into two branches that run along sides of thumb
Radialis indicis	Radial artery but may arise from princeps pollicis artery	Passes along lateral side of index finger to its distal end
Dorsal carpal arch	Radial and ulnar arteries	Arches within fascia on dorsum of hand

Table 18: Palmar arches		
	Superficial palmar arch (SPA)	**Deep palmar arch (DPA)**
Formation	It is the direct continuation of ulnar artery (beyond flexor retinaculum), usually completed laterally by anastomosis with the small superficial palmar branch of the radial artery.*	Is formed by the main termination of the radial artery and is completed medially by the small deep palmar branch of the ulnar artery (at the base of the fifth metacarpal).
Relations	Superficial: ▪ Palmar aponeurosis Deep: ▪ Long flexor tendons ▪ Digital branches of the median and ulnar nerves	Superficial: ▪ Long flexor tendons of the fingers ▪ Lumbricals Deep: ▪ Proximal parts of shafts of the metacarpals ▪ Interosseous muscles
Branches	▪ Three common palmar digital arteries** ▪ One proper digital artery runs along the medial side of the little finger. ▪ Cutaneous branches	▪ Three palmar metacarpal arteries** ▪ Three perforating arteries, which anastomose with dorsal metacarpal arteries ▪ Recurrent branches run proximally in front of carpus to end in the palmar carpal arch
Surface anatomy	It is convex distally and level with a transverse line through the distal border of the fully extended base of the thumb	Lies about 1 cm proximal to the superficial palmar arch. In its concavity, running laterally, is the deep branch of the ulnar nerve.

*As a variation, SPA may be completed by radialis indicis artery or princeps pollicis artery occasionally.

** In the interdigital clefts, the common palmar digital arteries (from SPA). Are joined by the palmar metacarpal arteries (from DPA)

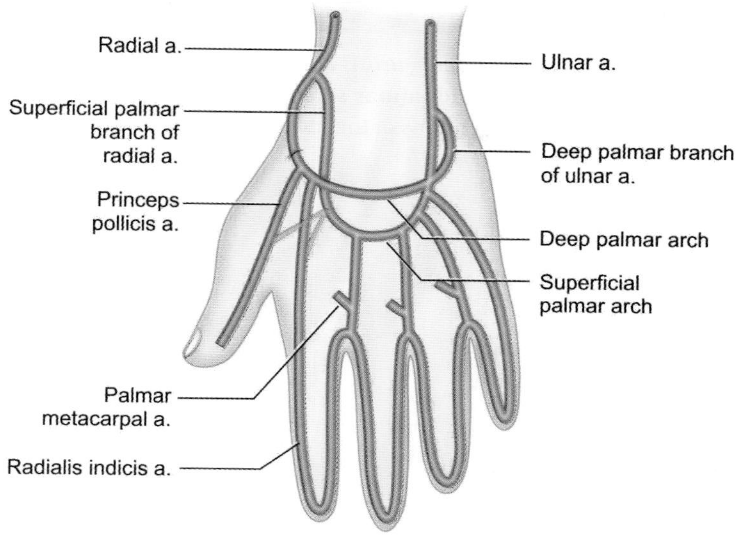

Radial a. ─────

Superficial palmar branch of radial a. ─────

Princeps pollicis a. ─────

───── Ulnar a.

───── Deep palmar branch of ulnar a.

───── Deep palmar arch

───── Superficial palmar arch

Palmar metacarpal a. ─────

Radialis indicis a. ─────

Fig. 64: Palmar arterial arches

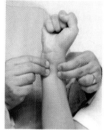

Fig. 65: Patient makes a tight fist and both ulnar and radial arteries compressed

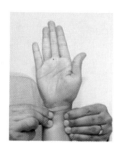

Fig. 66: Patient opens the fist to reveal the pale palm.

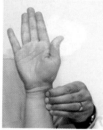

Fig. 67: Ulnar artery compression is removed. Palm turns red, including the thumb zone.

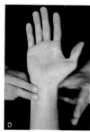

Fig. 68: Reverse Allen test: Compression on the radial artery released

- ❑ **Allen test** is done to check the interconnection (integrity) between the superficial and deep palmar arches and patency of the **radial and ulnar** arteries at the wrist and so determines whether each individual artery is sufficient to maintain the arterial supply to the hand **in isolation.**
- ❑ **Procedure**: The patient **makes a tight fist** so as to express the blood from the skin of the palm and fingers; the examiner **digitally compresses both** the ulnar and radial arteries. Next the patient opens the fist to reveal the **pale palm**. As the ulnar artery compression is removed in next step, the **palm turns red**, including the thumb zone. **If blood fails to return to the thumb zone** it reveals that the anastomosis between the two palmar arches is inadequate and **Allen test is positive**. Radial artery cannulation is **not advisable** in such patient, since it puts the thumb zone at risk of injury.
- ❑ **Anatomical basis:** The hand is normally supplied by blood from the ulnar and radial arteries. The arteries undergo anastomosis in the hand. Thus, if the blood supply from one of the arteries is cut off, the other artery can supply adequate blood to the hand. A **minority** of people lack this dual blood supply.
- ❑ It is performed **prior to radial arterial blood sampling** or cannulation. An uncommon complication of radial arterial blood sampling/cannulation is disruption of the artery (obstruction by clot), placing the hand at risk of ischemia. Those people who lack the dual supply are at much **greater risk of ischemia.**
- ❑ **Reverse Allen test** is done to check the **patency of radial artery**, as the compression on the radial artery is removed the palm should turn red, even if the ulnar artery compression was in place.

QUESTIONS

1. **TRUE about deep palmar arch**   *(NEET Pattern 2015)*
   a. Main contribution is by ulnar artery
   b. Lie superficial to lumbricals
   c. Gives three perforating branches
   d. Gives four palmar metacarpal arteries

2. **Allen's test is done for checking**
   a. Neural disorders
   b. Patency of ulnar artery
   c. Patency of radial artery
   d. Blood flow in cephalic vein

ANSWERS

1. **c. Gives three perforating branches**
   ❑ Deep palmar arch is mainly fed by radial artery, lies deep to lumbricals and gives three perforating and three palmar metacarpal arteries.

2. **b. Patency of ulnar artery > c. Patency of radial artery**
   ❑ Allen test is done to check the patency of both radial and ulnar artery.
   ❑ To check the radial artery, it is named as reverse Allen test.

▶ Spaces in Hand

❑ Fascial spaces of the palm are deep to the *palmar aponeurosis* and divided by a midpalmar (oblique septum attached to third metacarpal) into the **thenar** space and the **midpalmar** space. **Thenar Space** is the lateral space that contains the flexor pollicis longus tendon and the other flexor tendons of the index finger.

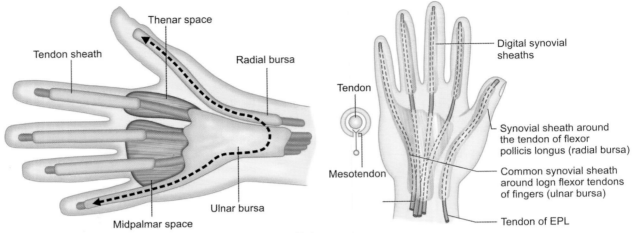

Fig. 69: Palmar spaces

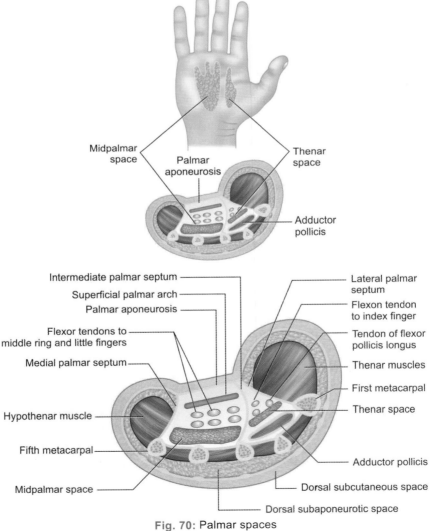

Fig. 70: Palmar spaces

❏ **Midpalmar Space** is the medial space that contains the **flexor tendons of the medial three** digits. The tendons of the second, third, and fourth digits have separate synovial sheaths so that the infection is confined to the infected digit, but *rupture* of the proximal ends of these sheaths allows the infection to spread to the **midpalmar space.**

❏ **First lumbrical space** communicates with **thenar space** whereas, 2, 3 and 4 lumbrical canals are continuous with midpalmar space. Infection from thumb and index finger passes towards the thenar space along the **first lumbrical canal.** Middle, ring finger and little finger drain towards **midpalmar space** along the 2, 3 and 4th lumbrical canals.

❏ **Ulnar bursa** is the common synovial flexor sheath which envelops the tendons of both the flexor digitorum superficialis and profundus muscles. The synovial sheath of the **little finger** is usually continuous with the common synovial sheath (**ulnar bursa**), and thus, tenosynovitis may spread to the common sheath and thus through the palm and carpal tunnel to the forearm

❏ **Radial Bursa** is the synovial flexor sheath for flexor pollicis longus. Tenosynovitis in the **thumb** may spread through the synovial sheath of the flexor pollicis longus (**radial bursa**).

❏ **Forearm space of Parona** lies proximal to the flexor retinaculum and is continuous with the radial and ulnar bursa. Flexor retinaculum separates forearm space of Parona from the thenar and midpalmar space and they are non-continuous.

❏ **Note: Bursa is defined as a potential space lined by synovial membrane.**

QUESTIONS

1. **Content of midpalmar space are all EXCEPT**
   (NEET Pattern 2012)
   a. FDP of 4th finger
   b. FDP of 3rd finger
   c. 2nd lumbrical
   d. 1st lumbrical

2. **Midpalmar space of hand communicates with all EXCEPT**
   a. Forearm space
   b. Fascial sheath of first lumbrical
   c. Fascial sheath of second lumbrical
   d. Fascial sheath of third lumbrical

3. **Infection draining the index finger goes to**
   (NEET Pattern 2014)
   a. Thenar space
   b. Midpalmar space
   c. Ulnar bursa
   d. Radial bursa

4. **Radial bursa is the synovial sheath covering the tendon of**
   (NEET Pattern 2013)
   a. FDS
   b. FDP
   c. FPL
   d. FCR

ANSWERS

1. **d. 1st lumbrical**
   ❏ **First lumbrical** arises from the FDP (flexor digitorum profundus) tendon of index finger and communicates with **the thenar** space.
   ❏ FDP of middle (3), ring (4) and little (5) fingers lies in the **mid-palmar space** and hence the lumbricals 2, 3 and 4 are present in midpalmar space.

2. **b. Fascial sheath of first lumbrical**
   ❏ First lumbrical arises from the FDP (flexor digitorum profundus) tendon of index finger and fascial sheath of first lumbrical is continuous with thenar space.
   ❏ FDP of middle (3), ring (4) and little (5) fingers lies in the mid-palmar space and hence the lumbricals 2,3 and 4 are present in midpalmar space. Midpalmar space is continuous with the medial three web-spaces through medial three lumbrical canals.

3. **a. Thenar space**
   ❏ Ring finger pus drains towards the thenar space

4. **c. FPL**
   ❏ Radial bursa is the synovial sheath covering the tendon of flexor pollicis longus.

- Only muscle that suspends the pectoral girdle from the cranium is **trapezius**
- Widest muscle on the back of the body is **latissimus dorsi**
- **Climbing muscles** are Latissimus dorsi and pectoralis major
- All the rotator cuff muscles are the rotators of the humerus except **supraspinatus**
- Tendon of **supraspinatus** is most commonly torn in **rotator cuff injury.**
- **Largest** synovial bursa in body is **subacromial** (subdeltoid) bursa
- **Strongest** ligament of upper limb is **coracoclavicular** ligament
- Most prominent superficial vein in the body is **median cubital vein**
- Most commonly used vein for venepuncture is **median cubital vein**
- Most preferred vein for cardiac catheterization is **basilic vein**
- Most of the superficial lymph vessels of the upper limb drain into **Lateral group** of the axillary lymph nodes
- Most distal superficial lymph node in the upper limb is **supratrochlear**/epitrochlear node
- Longest superficial vein of the upper limb is **cephalic vein**
- Most lateral bony point of the shoulder region **is greater tubercle** of the humerus
- Most felt arterial pulse for recording blood pressure is **brachial pulse** in the cubital fossa
- Best place to compress the brachial artery to stop hemorrhage in the arm and hand is medial aspect of humerus **near the middle** of arm (site of insertion of coracobrachialis)
- Neurovascular structures jeopardized in **midshaft fracture** of the humerus are **radial nerve and profunda brachii artery**
- Damage of the radial nerve in spiral groove causes only weakness in extension of elbow and **not the total inability to extend elbow**, because branches of the radial nerve supplying **long and lateral heads of triceps** arise in axilla, i.e., above radial groove.

- **Ligament of Struthers** is the fibrous band extending between the supratrochlear spur and medial epicondyle of humerus
- All the flexor muscles of the forearm lie on the front of forearm except **brachioradialis**, which lies on the back of the forearm
- All the superficial flexors of the forearm are supplied by median nerve **except flexor carpi ulnaris**, which is supplied by the ulnar nerve
- All the muscles on the back of the forearm are extensors **except brachioradialis**, which is a flexor of the forearm
- Chief source of blood supply to the forearm is **ulnar artery**
- Deepest artery on the front of the forearm is **anterior interosseous artery**
- **Eye of the hand**/peripheral eye is median nerve in the hand.
- **Biceps brachii** is a *powerful* supinator at the radio-ulnar joint and helps in *screw driving movements*.
- **Common interosseous artery** is a branch of **ulnar artery** near the elbow joint and divides into anterior and posterior interosseous artery.
- There is often an enlargement or **pseudoganglion** on the axillary nerve branch to teres minor. The termination of posterior interosseous nerve also shows a **pseudo-ganglion** Deep fibular nerve in lower limb may also develop a **pseudoganglion** in a branch to extensor digitorum brevis.
- Fracture of the surgical neck may injure the axillary nerve and the posterior humeral circumflex artery as they pass through the quadrangular space.
- **Colles fracture** of the wrist is a distal radius fracture in which the distal fragment is displaced (tilted) **posteriorly**, producing a characteristic bump described as dinner (silver) **fork deformity** because the forearm and wrist resemble the shape of a dinner fork. If the distal fragment is displaced anteriorly, it is called a reverse Colles fracture **(Smith fracture)**. This fracture may show styloid processes of the radius and ulna line-up on a radiograph.
- **Bennett fracture** is a fracture of the **base of the metacarpal** of the thumb. **Boxer's fracture** is a fracture of the necks of the second and third metacarpals, seen in professional boxers, and typically of the fifth metacarpal in unskilled boxers.
- **Tennis elbow** (lateral epicondylitis) is caused by a chronic inflammation or irritation of the origin (tendon) of the extensor muscles of the forearm from the **lateral epicondyle** of the humerus as a result of repetitive strain. It is a painful condition and common in tennis players and violinists.
- **Golfer's elbow** (medial epicondylitis) is a painful condition caused by a small tear or an inflammation or irritation in the origin of the flexor muscles of the forearm from the **medial epicondyle**. Avoidance of repetitive bending (flexing) of the forearm is advised in order to not compress the ulnar nerve.
- **Nursemaid's elbow** or pulled elbow is a radial head subluxation and occurs in toddlers when the child is lifted by the wrist. It is caused by a partial tear (or loose) of the annular ligament and thus the radial head to slip out of position.
- **Volkmann contracture** is an ischemic muscular contracture (flexion deformity) of the fingers and sometimes of the wrist, resulting from ischemic necrosis of the forearm flexor muscles, caused by a pressure injury, such as compartment syndrome, or a tight cast. The muscles are replaced by fibrous tissue, which contracts, producing the flexion deformity.
- **Trigger finger** results from stenosing tenosynovitis or occurs when the flexor tendon develops a nodule or swelling that interferes with its gliding through the pulley, causing an audible clicking or snapping.
- **Jersey finger** (Rugby finger or Sweater finger) is a type of injury due to avulsion of the flexor digitorum profundus (FDP) at the base of the distal interphalangeal joint.

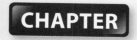
Abdomen

Landmarks

❑ **Murphy's point** lies below the right costal margin at the mid-clavicular line (the approximate location of the fundus of gallbladder).

❑ The point is at the **intersection** of the right linea semilunaris and right costal margin, at the tip of the right 9th costal cartilage.

❑ In **acute cholecystitis**, when the anterior abdominal wall is pressed below this point the patient **winces** (while taking a deep breath) due to pain.

❑ **McBurney's point** lies over the right side of the abdomen, at the junction of the medial 2/3rd and lateral 1/3rd of the line joining the umbilicus with the anterior superior iliac spine.

❑ It corresponds to the most common location of the base of the appendix (where it is attached to the cecum) and is the site of **maximum tenderness** in acute appendicitis.

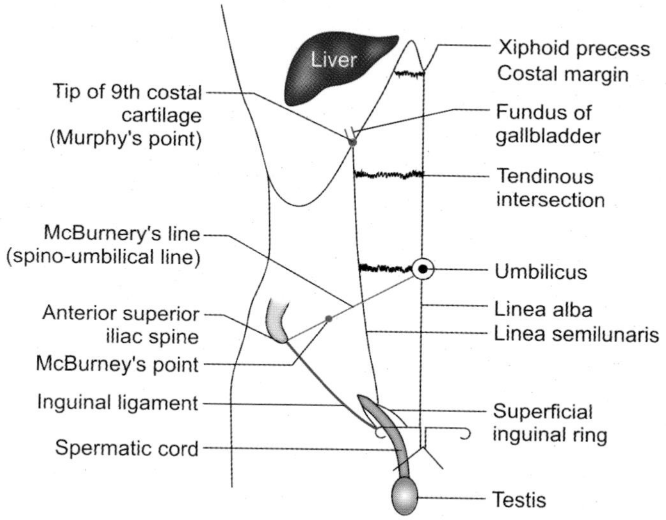

Mid-inguinal Point

❑ The **mid-inguinal point** lies at the midpoint of a line between the pubic symphysis and the anterior superior iliac spine. In adults, it is the approximate surface marking of the **femoral artery** (just below the ligament) and the **deep inguinal ring** (just above the ligament).

❑ The deep inguinal ring is an opening in the transversalis fascia, approximately **midway** between the anterior superior iliac spine and the pubic symphysis, and about 1 cm above the inguinal ligament.

Fig. 1: Various landmarks in the abdomen region in relation with gallbladder, appendix, and spermatic cord

Abdominal Planes

Nine regions of the abdominal cavity are used to describe the location of abdominal organs.

❑ The regions are delineated by **four planes**: two sagittal (**vertical**) and two transverse (**horizontal**) planes.

❑ The two sagittal planes are usually the **midclavicular planes** that pass from the midpoint of the clavicles (approximately 9 cm from the midline) to the **midinguinal points** (midpoints of the lines joining the anterior superior iliac spine and the pubic symphysis on each side).

❑ Most commonly, the transverse planes are the **subcostal plane** (upper border of L3 vertebra), passing through the inferior border of the 10th costal cartilage on each side, and the **transtubercular plane**, passing through the iliac tubercles (approximately 5 cm posterior to the ASIS on each side) and the **upper border of L5 vertebra**.

❑ **Some clinicians** use the **transpyloric** and **interspinous** planes to establish the nine regions.

❑ The **transpyloric plane** lies midway between the **suprasternal notch** of the manubrium and the upper border of the **pubic symphysis,** commonly **transects the pylorus** (the distal, more tubular part of the stomach) when the patient is recumbent (supine or prone).

➤ It is approximately midway between the xiphisternal joint and the umbilicus.

➤ Posteriorly, the plane intersects the **lower border of L1 vertebra** and anteriorly, it intersects the costal at the **ninth costal cartilage**, where the linea semilunaris crosses.

➤ The plane is a **useful landmark** because it also transects many other important structures: the **fundus** of the gallbladder, **neck** of the pancreas, origins of the **superior mesenteric artery** and the **renal arteries**, origin of hepatic **portal vein**, **root** of the transverse mesocolon, duodenojejunal **junction**, and **hila** of both the kidneys, **termination** of adult spinal cord.

Table 1: Abdominal regions and their main contents	
Region	**Contents**
Right hypochondrium	▪ Liver ▪ Gallbladder
Epigastric region	▪ Stomach ▪ Pancreas ▪ Duodenum
Left hypochondrium	▪ Spleen ▪ Left colic flexure
Right lumbar region	▪ Right kidney ▪ Right ureter ▪ Ascending colon
Umbilical region	▪ Loops of small intestine ▪ Aorta ▪ Inferior vena cava
Left lumbar region	▪ Left kidney ▪ Left ureter ▪ Descending colon
Right iliac fossa	▪ Cecum ▪ Appendix
Hypogastric region	▪ Coils of small intestine ▪ Urinary bladder (if distended) ▪ Uterus (in enlarged)
Left iliac fossa	▪ Sigmoid colon

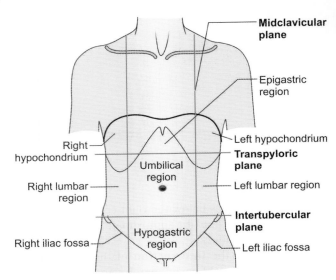

Fig. 2: Nine regions of the abdomen

❑ The **interspinous plane** (upper border of S1 vertebra) passes through the easily palpated ASIS on each side.

❑ For more **general clinical descriptions, four quadrants** of the abdominal cavity (right and left upper and lower quadrants) are defined by two readily defined planes: (1) the **transverse transumbilical** plane, passing through the umbilicus (and the intervertebral disc between the **L3 and L4 vertebrae**), dividing it into upper and lower halves, and (2) the **vertical median plane**, passing longitudinally through the body, dividing it into right and left halves.

❑ **Supracristal plane** is the transverse plane lying at **highest point of iliac crest**. This is usually at the level of the **L4 vertebrae** and passes **through the umbilicus**. It is a landmark for the performance of **lumbar puncture**. The **aorta bifurcates** in this plane.

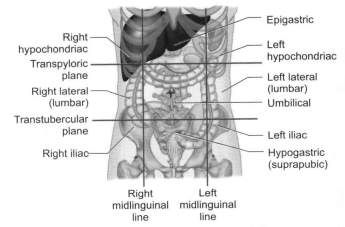

Fig. 3: Planes of subdivision of the abdomen

Kidneys

The posterior aspects of the superior poles of the kidneys lie on the diaphragm and are anterior to the twelfth rib on the right, and to the eleventh and twelfth ribs on the left.

QUESTIONS

1. Transpyloric plane separates: *(NEET Pattern 2015)*
   a. Hypogastrium from lumbar region
   b. Hypochondrium from lumbar region
   c. Iliac fossa from lumbar region
   d. Umbilical region from lumbar region

2. Which of the following structure is NOT present in transpyloric plane?
   a. First lumbar vertebra
   b. Fundus of gallbladder
   c. Hilum of right kidney
   d. Inferior mesenteric vein

ANSWERS

1. **b. Hypochondrium from lumbar region**
   ❑ Transpyloric plane separates **hypochondrium** from **lumbar** region and **epigastrium** from **umbilical** region.

2. **d. Inferior mesenteric vein**
   ❑ Transpyloric plane is present at the **lower border of L1 vertebra** and superior (**not inferior**) mesenteric artery lies here.
   ❑ The **pylorus of stomach** may be found in the transpyloric plane **but is not a constant feature**.
   ❑ **Hila of each kidney** is present at this plane.
   ❑ **Fundus** of gallbladder can be touched at this plane (**Murphy's sign**).

- **Supracristal** plane passes through the lower part of the body of **L4** vertebra *(NEET Pattern 2016)*
- **Supracristal** plane is above **highest point of iliac crest** *(NEET Pattern 2016)*
- **Renal angle** lies between **12th rib** and lateral border of **sacrospinalis** (erector spinae) *(AIIMS 2007; NEET Pattern 2012)*
- **Highest point** of **iliac crest** lies at the level of spine of **L4 vertebra** *(NEET Pattern 2014)*
- **Fundus** of gallbladder is present at **L1 vertebral** level *(NEET Pattern 2015)*
- **Transtubercular** plane lies at **L5 vertebral** level *(NEET Pattern 2013)*

Abdominal Wall

The anterior abdominal wall is firm and elastic. It consists of eight layers. From **superficial to deep**, these are:

Skin → Superficial fascia → External oblique muscle → Internal oblique muscle → Transversus abdominis muscle → Fascia transversalis → Extra peritoneal tissue → Parietal layer of peritoneum.

- ❏ The umbilicus is a fibrous cicatrix that lies a little below the midpoint of the linea alba, and is covered by an adherent area of skin.
- ❏ It consists of skin, a fibrous layer (representing the area of fusion between the **round ligament** of the liver, the **median umbilical** ligament, and two **medial umbilical** ligaments), the transversalis fascia, the umbilical fascia surrounding the urachal remnant, and peritoneum.
- ❏ **Peritoneal folds** are seen in the anterior abdominal wall, raised by various **embryological remnants** (umbilical ligaments).
- ❏ **The ureter** lies on posterior abdominal wall (**retroperitoneally**), crosses **pelvic brim** lying over bifurcation of common iliac arteries, **hook under uterine artery** and enter urinary bladder at **postero lateral angles**.
- ❏ **Vas deferens** passes through the deep inguinal ring (**lying lateral** to inferior epigastric vessels), **pass superior to ureter** and receive secretions of seminal vesicles, and **continue as ejaculatory ducts**, to open into prostatic urethra.

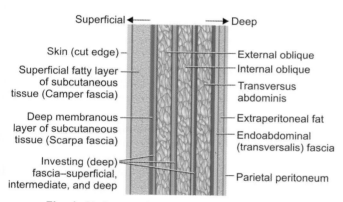

Fig. 4: Six layers of anterior and abdominal wall

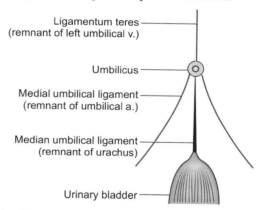

Fig. 5: Four embryological remnant at the umbilicus

Fasciae and Ligaments of the Anterior Abdominal Wall

- ❏ Are organized into superficial (tela subcutanea) and deep fasciae. The superficial fascia has **two layers**: the superficial fatty layer **(Camper fascia)** and the deep membranous layer **(Scarpa fascia)**.
- A. Superficial Fascia
  1. **Superficial** (Fatty) Layer of the Superficial Fascia (Camper Fascia)
     - Continues over the inguinal ligament to merge with the superficial fascia of the thigh.
     - Continues over the pubis and perineum as the superficial layer of the superficial perineal fascia.
  2. **Deep** (Membranous) Layer of the Superficial Fascia (Scarpa Fascia)
     - Is attached to the fascia lata just below the inguinal ligament.^Q
     - Continues over the pubis and perineum as the membranous layer (Coll' fascia) of the superficial perineal fascia.
     - Continues over the penis as the superficial fascia of the penis and over the scrotum as the tunica dartos, which contains smooth muscle.
     - May contain extravasated urine between this fascia and the deep fascia of the abdomen, resulting from rupture of the spongy urethra.

Deep Fascia

- ➤ Covers the muscles and continues over the spermatic cord at the superficial inguinal ring as the **external spermatic fascia**.
- ➤ Continues over the penis as the deep fascia of the penis **(Buck fascia)** and over the pubis and perineum as the deep perineal fascia.

Linea Alba

- ➤ Is a **tendinous median raphe** between the two rectus abdominis muscles, formed by the fusion of the aponeuroses of the external oblique, internal oblique, and transverse abdominal muscles.
- ➤ Extends from the xiphoid process to the pubic symphysis and, at its lower end, the superficial fibers attach to pubic symphysis, and deeper fibers to the pubic crests.
- ➤ In pregnancy, it becomes a pigmented vertical line (linea nigra), probably due to hormone stimulation to produce more melanin.
- ➤ **Epigastric hernia** is a protrusion of extraperitoneal fat or a small piece of greater omentum through a defect in the linea alba above the umbilicus and may contain a small portion of intestine.

Linea Semilunaris

- ➤ Is a curved line along the **lateral border** of the rectus abdominis.

Linea Semicircularis (Arcuate Line)

- ➤ Is a crescent-shaped line marking the **inferior limit** of the posterior layer of the rectus sheath just below the level of the iliac crest.

Transversalis Fascia

- ❑ The transversalis fascia is a thin layer of connective tissue lying between the deep surface of transversus abdominis and the extraperitoneal fat.
- ❑ It is part of the general layer of thin fascia between the peritoneum and the abdominal wall.
- ❑ **Posteriorly**, it fuses with the anterior layer of the thoracolumbar fascia and anteriorly, it forms a continuous sheet.
- ❑ **Superiorly**, it blends with the fascia covering the inferior surface of the diaphragm. **Inferiorly**, it is continuous with the iliac and pelvic parietal fasciae, and is attached to the iliac crest between the origins of transversus abdominis and iliacus, and to the posterior margin of the inguinal ligament between the anterior superior iliac spine and the femoral sheath. Medial to the femoral sheath it is thin and fused to the pubis behind the conjoint tendon.
- ❑ An inferior extension of the transversalis fascia forms the anterior part of the **femoral sheath**.
- ❑ The fascia displays a discrete thickening known as the **iliopubic tract** (also called the deep crural arch), which runs parallel to the inguinal ligament it consists of transverse fibers that fan out laterally towards the anterior superior iliac spine to blend with the iliopsoas fascia and run medially behind the conjoint tendon to the pubic bone.
- ❑ The iliopubic tract is recognized as an **important** structure during open and **laparoscopic inguinal hernia repair**.
- ❑ A further thickening of the transversalis fascia, the **interfoveolar** ligament, runs inferior to the inguinal ligament at the medial margin of the deep inguinal ring; it may contain muscle fibers.
- ❑ The transversalis fascia is prolonged as the **internal spermatic fascia** over the structures that pass through the deep inguinal ring (the testicular vessels and vas (ductus) deferens in the male and the round ligament of the uterus in the female).

Extraperitoneal Connective Tissue

- ❑ The extraperitoneal connective tissue lying between the peritoneum and the fasciae lining the abdominal and pelvic cavities contains a variable amount of fat.
- ❑ The fat is especially abundant on the posterior wall of the abdomen around the kidneys (particularly in obese men) and scanty above the iliac crest and in much of the pelvis.

QUESTION

1. TRUE about Scarpa's fascia   *(NEET Pattern 2015)*
   a. Deep fascia of anterior abdominal wall
   b. Also called Buck's fascia
   c. Attached to Iliotibial tract
   d. Forms suspensory ligament of penis

ANSWER

1. d. Forms suspensory ligament of penis
   ❑ Scarpa's fascia forms the **suspensory ligament** of penis or clitoris in median plane.
   ❑ Scarpa's fascia is the **superficial** fascia of abdomen, it becomes **continuous with Buck's fascia** over the penis and is attached to the **fascia lata of thigh**.

Table 2: Muscles of anterolateral abdominal wall

Muscle	Origin	Insertion	Innervation	Main Action[a]
External oblique (A)	External surfaces of 5th 12th ribs	Linea alba, pubic tubercle, and anterior half of iliac crest	Thoracoabdominal nerves (T7–T11 spinal nerves) and subcostal nerve	Compresses and supports abdominal viscera,[b] flexes and rotates trunk

Muscle	Origin	Insertion	Innervation	Main Action[a]
Internal oblique (B)	Thoracolumbar fascia, anterior two-thirds of iliac crest, and connective tisue deep to lateral third of inguinal ligament	Inferior borders of 10th–12th ribs, linea alba, and pecten pubis via conjoint tendon	Thoracoabdominal nerves (anterior rami or T6–T12 spinal nerves) and first tumbar nerves	
Transversus abdominis (C)	Internal surfaces of 7th–12th costal cartilages, thoracolumbar fasdcia, iliac crest, and connective tissue deep to lateral third of inguinal ligament	Linea alba with aponeurosis of internal oblique, pubic crest, and pecten pubis via conjoint tendon		Compresses and supports abdominal viscera[b]
Rectus abdominis (D)	Pubic symphysis and pubic crest	Xiphoid process and 5th–7th costal cartilages	Thoracoabdominal nerves (anterior rami of T6–T12 spinal nerves)	Flexes trunk (lumbar vertebrae) and compresses abdominal viscera;[b] stabilizes and controls tilt of pelvis (antilordosis)

[a]Approximately 80% of people have an insignificant muscle, the *pyramidalis*, which is located in the rectus sheath anterior to the most inferior part of the rectus abdominis. It extends from the pubic crest of the lip bone to the linea alba. This small muscle draws doen on the linea alba.
[b]In so doing, these muscles act as antagonists of the diaphragm to produce expiration.

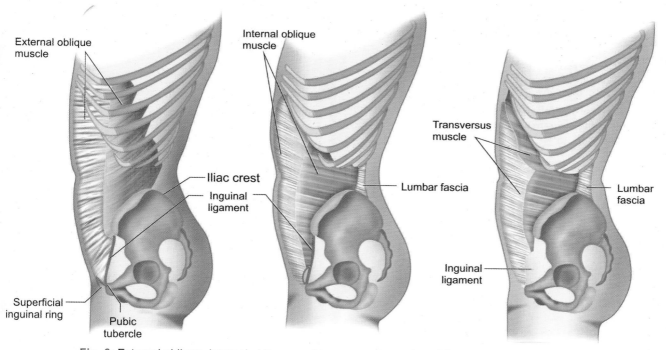

Fig. 6: External oblique, internal oblique, and transversus muscles of the anterior abdominal wall

Muscles

The muscles of the abdominal wall include the **rectus abdominis, transverse abdominis, internal oblique, and external oblique**.

Clinical Procedure

Paracentesis is a procedure whereby a needle is inserted through the layers of the abdominal wall to withdraw excess peritoneal fluid. Knife wounds to the abdomen will also penetrate the layers of the abdominal wall.

Flank Approach

- ❏ The needle or knife will pass through the following structures in succession: **Skin → superficial fascia (Camper and Scarpa) → external oblique muscle → internal oblique muscle → transverse abdominis muscle → transversalis fascia → extraperitoneal fat → parietal peritoneum.**
- ❏ **Pyramidalis** is a small triangular muscle, anterior to the rectus abdominis muscle, and contained in the rectus sheath. It takes **origin** from pubic symphysis and pubic crest and **inserts** into linea alba. It is supplied by **subcostal** nerve (T12) and helps in **tensing the linea alba**.

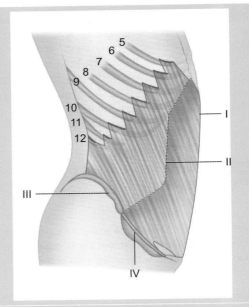

1. **Which of the following is the correct matching, regarding the attachments of external oblique muscle?** *(AIIMS 2016)*
   a. I - Linea alba, II - Linea semilunaris, III - Inner lip of iliac crest, IV - Inguinal ligament
   b. I - Linea alba, II - Linea semilunaris, III - Outer lip of iliac crest, IV - Inguinal ligament
   c. I - Linea semilunaris, II - Linea alba, III - Outer lip of iliac crest, IV - Inguinal ligament
   d. I - Linea semilunaris, II - Arcuate line, III - Inner lip of iliac crest, IV - Inguinal ligament

2. **Function of external oblique muscle:** *(NEET Pattern 2016)*
   a. Anterior flexion of vertebral column
   b. Active expiration
   c. Closure of inguinal ring
   d. All of the above

3. **Rectus abdominis is inserted into:**
   a. Xiphoid process
   b. Median raphe
   c. Linea alba
   d. 1/4 ribs

4. **Which of the following marker is conjoint tendon in the following diagram of transversus abdominis:** *(AIIMS 2017)*
   a. A
   b. B
   c. C
   d. D

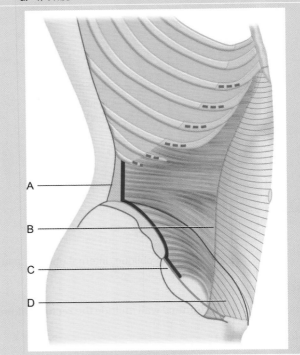

(PGIC 2010)

5. **Flexors of lumbar spine are all EXCEPT:**
   a. Erector spinae
   b. External oblique muscle
   c. Internal oblique muscle
   d. Rectus abdominis
   e. Psoas major

QUESTIONS

ANSWERS

1. **b. I - Linea alba, II - Linea semilunaris, III - Outer lip of iliac crest, IV - Inguinal ligament**
   ❑ External oblique muscle takes origin from the **external surfaces of lower** 8 (5-12th) **ribs**.
   ❑ It inserts into the **linea alba** (marker 'I'), pubic tubercle, and outer lip of the anterior two-thirds of the iliac crest (marker 'III').
   ❑ At **linea semilunaris** (marker 'II') the muscular fibers of muscle become aponeurotic.
   ❑ The free lower border of the aponeurosis is rolled inward on itself to form the **inguinal ligament** (marker 'IV').

2. d. All of the above
- ❑ External oblique contributes to the maintenance of **abdominal tone**, **increasing intra-abdominal pressure** (as in active expiration), and **lateral flexion** of the trunk against resistance. Bilateral contraction flexes the trunk forward.
- ❑ Contraction of external oblique muscle **approximates** the two crura (medial and lateral) of superficial inguinal ring like a **slit valve** to maintain the integrity of inguinal canal.

3. a. Xiphoid process
- ❑ Rectus abdominis takes origin from the **crest of pubis** and Inserts into **costal cartilages** of ribs 5-7 and Xiphisternum.
  Note: Rectus abdominis muscle is **NOT** attached to the median raphe- linea alba.

4. d. D
- ❑ **Conjoint tendon** (marker D) is formed from the lower part of the common aponeurosis of the **internal abdominal oblique** and the **transverse abdominal** as it inserts into the crest of the pubis and pectineal line.
- ❑ **Key**- A: Thoracolumbar fascia; B: Line of demarcation between muscular and aponeurotic parts of muscle; C: Origin from lateral 1/3 of inguinal ligament; D: Conjoint tendon.

5. a. Erector spinae
- ❑ **Forward flexors**: **Rectus abdominis**, **external abdominal oblique**, **internal abdominal obliquus**, transversus abdominis and **iliacus-psoas**.
- ❑ **Lateral flexors**: Ipsilateral contraction of the oblique and transversus abdominal muscles and quadratus lumborum.

- ▪ Pyramidalis is supplied by **Subcostal** nerve (NEET Pattern 2015)

▸ Rectus Sheath

Rectus Sheath

- ❑ Is formed by fusion of the **aponeuroses** of the external oblique, internal oblique, and transverse muscles of the abdomen.
- ❑ Encloses the rectus abdominis and sometimes the pyramidal muscle.
- ❑ Also contains the superior and inferior epigastric vessels and the ventral primary rami of thoracic nerves 7 to 12.
- ❑ Anterior Layer of the Rectus Sheath
  - ➢ **Above** the level of costal margin: Aponeurosis of external oblique only.
  - ➢ **Between** costal margin and above the arcuate line: Aponeuroses of the external and internal oblique muscles.
  - ➢ **Below** the arcuate line: aponeuroses of the external oblique, internal oblique, and transverse muscles.

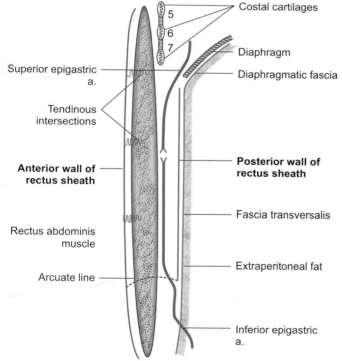

Fig. 7: Sagittal section of rectus sheath showing anterior and posterior wall. Tendinous intersections are attached only to the anterior wall

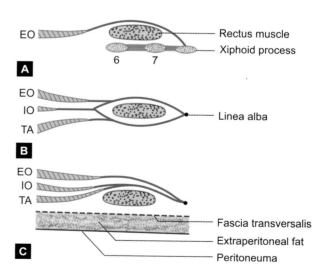

Figs. 8A to C: Formation of the rectus sheath as seen in transverse sections through rectus abdominis and its sheaths at three different levels: A. Above the costal margin; B. Between costal margin and arcuate line; C. Below the arcuate line (EO = external oblique, IO = internal oblique, TA = transversus abdominis)

- ❑ **Posterior Layer** of the Rectus Sheath
  - ➢ Above the level of costal margin: Is deficient and rectus muscle lies directly on the 5th, 6th, and 7th costal cartilages.
  - ➢ Between costal margin and above the arcuate line: Aponeuroses of the internal oblique and transverse muscles.
  - ➢ Below the arcuate line: Is **deficient** and rectus abdominis is in contact with the transversalis fascia.
- ❑ The rectus sheath **contains** the following structures: Muscles: Rectus abdominis and pyramidalis (if present).
- ❑ **Vessels:** Superior epigastric and inferior epigastric artery and veins.
- ❑ **Six nerves:** Terminal parts of lower six thoracic nerves, including lower five intercostal nerves and subcostal nerve. (They are accompanied by terminal parts of posterior intercostal vessels).

Note: Recently some authors mention the aponeuroses of all the three muscles (external, internal, and transversus) are bilaminar thus giving six laminae in all. The three layers form anterior wall and three layers form posterior wall of the rectus sheath. The laminae decussate with other laminae across the midline, i.e., in the region of linea alba and continue as the laminae of contralateral muscles.

- ▪ In rectus sheath superior epigastric artery (branch of internal thoracic artery) anastomose with inferior epigastric artery (branch of external iliac artery). *(PGIC 2008)*

QUESTIONS

1. **Posterior wall of rectus sheath below the level of anterior superior iliac spine is formed by:**
   a. Internal oblique   b. Transversus abdominis
   c. Lacunar ligament   d. Fascia transversalis

2. **Rectus sheath contains all of the following EXCEPT:**
   a. Pyramidalis muscle   b. Genitofemoral nerve
   c. Inferior epigastric vessels   d. Superior epigastric vessels

   (PGIC 2006, 2007)

3. **TRUE statement about lower 1/4 anterior abdominal wall:**
   a. Linea alba is poorly formed
   b. Rectus abdominis is divided by tendinous intersections
   c. Two layers of rectus sheath present
   d. External oblique muscle is poorly formed
   e. External oblique muscle is well developed

ANSWERS

1. **d. Fascia transversalis**
   ❑ Rectus abdominis lies on the transversalis fascia **below the arcuate line**.

2. **b. Genitofemoral nerve**
   ❑ Rectus sheath contains the muscles (rectus abdominis **and pyramidalis**); vessels (**superior** epigastric and **inferior** epigastric artery and veins) and terminal parts of **lower six** thoracic nerves.

3. **a. Linea alba is poorly formed; d) External oblique muscle is poorly formed**
   ❑ Linea alba is wider and more obvious above the umbilicus and is **almost linear and less visible** below this level.
   ❑ External oblique muscle is **aponeurotic** in the lower part.
   ❑ Tendinous intersections divide rectus abdominis muscle, but this is **not a feature in the lower part**.
   ❑ Posterior layer of rectus sheath is **deficient in the lower part**.

▶ Abdominal Wall Hernia

Umbilical Hernia

- ❑ The most extreme variety of umbilical hernia is known as an **omphalocele** or exomphalos, a congenital malformation in which abdominal viscera, covered by a membrane, protrude through a wide umbilical defect.
- ❑ The defect arises from a failure of closure of the umbilical ring after return of the herniated midgut loop in the embryo.
- ❑ The most common variety of umbilical hernia is caused by a weakness of the umbilical scar tissue, and is often seen in babies, especially those of African descent.
- ❑ The vast majority of these will close spontaneously during early childhood.
- ❑ Most umbilical hernias in adults are acquired as a result of stretching of the supporting umbilical fascia and are due to obesity and chronically increased intra-abdominal pressure (e.g. from multiple pregnancies or ascites).

Spigelian Hernia

- ❑ A **spigelian hernia** is a protrusion of preperitoneal fat or a peritoneal sac through a congenital or acquired defect in the abdominal wall

▶ Neurovasculature

- ❑ The ventral rami of the sixth to eleventh intercostal nerves, the subcostal nerve (twelfth thoracic) and first lumbar nerve (iliohypogastric and ilioinguinal nerves) supply the muscles and skin of the anterior abdominal wall.
- ❑ The seventh to the twelfth thoracic ventral rami continue anteriorly from the intercostal and subcostal spaces into the abdominal wall.
- ❑ Approaching the costal margin, the seventh to tenth nerves curve medially across the deep surface of the costal cartilages between the digitations of the diaphragm and transversus abdominis.

❑ The **subcostal nerve** gives a branch to the first lumbar ventral ramus (dorsolumbar nerve) that contributes to the lumbar plexus.

❑ It accompanies the subcostal vessels along the inferior border of the twelfth rib, passing **behind the lateral arcuate ligament** and kidney, and anterior to the upper part of the quadratus lumborum.

❑ All these segmental nerves run anteriorly within a thin layer of fascia in the neurovascular plane between transversus abdominis and internal oblique, where they branch and interconnect with adjacent nerves.

❑ Muscular branches innervate transversus abdominis and internal and external oblique.

❑ Cutaneous branches supply the skin of the lateral and anterior abdominal walls.

❑ The thoracic nerves enter the rectus sheath at its lateral margin and pass posterior to rectus abdominis, where they again intercommunicate.

❑ Each nerve then pierces rectus abdominis from its posterior aspect and gives off muscular branches to this muscle (and a branch to pyramidalis from the subcostal nerve), and cutaneous branches that pierce the anterior rectus sheath to supply overlying skin.

❑ The ninth intercostal nerve supplies skin above the umbilicus, the **tenth** supplies skin that consistently includes the **umbilicus**, and the eleventh supplies skin below the umbilicus.

❑ The subcostal nerve supplies the anterior gluteal skin just below the iliac crest, and the skin of the lower abdomen and inguinal region (overlapping with the L1 dermatome in this region).

❑ The ventral rami of the lower intercostal and subcostal nerves also provide sensory fibers to the costal parts of the diaphragm and parietal peritoneum.

◤ Nerves

Iliohypogastric nerve originates from the superior branch of the **anterior ramus** of spinal nerve **L1** after this nerve receives fibers from **T12** via the subcostal nerve.

❑ It runs in the **neurovascular plane** (i.e., between the internal oblique and transversus abdominis) and pierces the internal oblique about 2.5 cm in front of the anterior superior iliac spine.

❑ It becomes cutaneous by piercing the external oblique aponeurosis about 2.5 cm above the superficial inguinal ring. It is **motor** to the **internal** and **transverse** abdominal muscles and supplies the skin on posterolateral **gluteal** region and **suprapubic** region.

❑ The nerve is occasionally **injured** by a surgical incision in the **right iliac fossa** (e.g. during an inguinal hernia repair, open appendectomy).

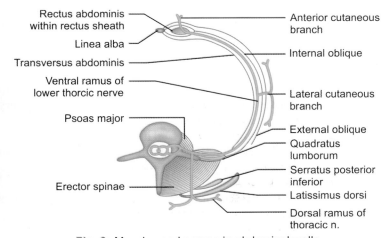

Fig. 9: Muscles and nerves in abdominal walls

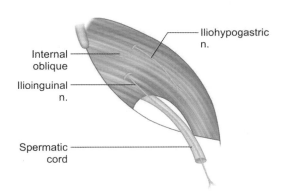

Fig. 10: Iliohypogastric and ilioinguinal nerves

Table 3: Nerves anterolateral abdominal wall			
Nerves	**Origin**	**Course**	**Distribution**
Thoracoabdominal (T7–T11)	Continuation of lower (7th–11th) intercostal nerves distal to costal margin	Run between second and third layer or abdominal muscles; branches enter subcutaneou tissue a lateral cutaneous branches of T10-T11 (in anterior axillary line) and anterior cutaneous branches of T7-T11 (parasternal line)	Muscle of anterolateral abdominal wall and overlying skin

Nerves	Origin	Course	Distribution
7th-9th lateral cutaneous branches	7th-9th intercostal nerves (anterior rami of spinal nerves T7-T9)	Anterior division ion continue across costal margin in subcutaneous tissue	Skin of right and left hypochondriac regions
Subcostal (anteior ramu of T12)	Spinal nerve T12	Run along inferior border of 12th rib: then passes onto subumbilical wall between second and third layer of abdominal muscles	Muscles of anterolateral abdominal wall (including most inferior slip of external oblique) and overlying skin, Superior to iliac crest and inferior to umbilicus

Ilioinguinal Nerve

❏ Originates from the (T12), L1 (L2) and emerges from the lateral border of psoas major, with or just inferior to the iliohypogastric nerve, passes obliquely across quadratus lumborum and the upper part of iliacus.

❏ It enters transversus abdominis about 3 cm medial and 4 cm inferior to the anterior superior iliac spine, where it is readily **blocked by local anesthetic**.

❏ It pierces internal oblique a little lower down, supplies it, and then traverses the inguinal canal superficial to the spermatic cord or round ligament. It emerges with the cord from the **superficial inguinal ring** and divides into terminal sensory branches.

❏ The ilioinguinal and genitofemoral nerves may interconnect within the inguinal canal and, consequently, each innervates the skin of the genitalia to a variable extent.

❏ The ilioinguinal nerve supplies motor nerves to transversus abdominis and internal oblique.

❏ It innervates the skin of the **proximal medial thigh** and the skin over the **root of the penis** and upper part of the scrotum in males, or the skin covering the mons pubis and the adjoining labium majus in females.

❏ The nerve may be injured or entrapped during inguinal **surgery**, particularly for **inguinal hernia**, leading to sensory disturbances and pain over the skin of the genitalia and upper medial thigh.

▼ Arteries

Superior Epigastric Artery and Veins

❏ The superior epigastric artery is a terminal branch of the **internal thoracic artery**.

❏ It arises at the level of the **sixth costal cartilage** and descends between the costal and xiphoid slips of the diaphragm, accompanied by two or more veins that drain to the internal thoracic vein.

❏ The vessels pass anterior to the lower fibers of transversus thoracis and the upper fibers of transversus abdominis before entering the rectus sheath, where they run inferiorly behind rectus abdominis.

Inferior Epigastric Artery and Veins

❏ The inferior epigastric artery (Often referred to as the deep inferior epigastric artery in clinical practice in order to distinguish it from the superficial (inferior) epigastric artery) originates from the medial aspect of the **external iliac artery** just proximal to the inguinal ligament.

❏ Its accompanying veins, usually two, unite to form a single vein that **drains into the external iliac vein**.

❏ It curves forwards in the anterior extraperitoneal tissue and ascends obliquely along the medial margin of the deep inguinal ring.

❏ It lies posterior to the spermatic cord, separated from it by the transversalis fascia.

❏ It pierces the transversalis fascia and enters the rectus sheath by passing anterior to the arcuate line. In this part of its course, it is visible through the parietal peritoneum of the anterior abdominal wall and forms the lateral umbilical fold.

❏ Branches of the inferior epigastric artery **anastomose with branches of the superior epigastric artery** within the rectus sheath posterior to rectus abdominis at a variable level above the umbilicus.

❏ Other branches anastomose with terminal branches of the **lower five** posterior intercostal, subcostal and lumbar arteries at the lateral border of the rectus sheath.

❏ The inferior epigastric artery ascends along the **medial margin** of the deep inguinal ring.

❏ The vas deferens in the male, or the round ligament in the female, passes medially after hooking around the artery at the deep inguinal ring.

❏ The artery forms the **lateral border of Hesselbach's inguinal triangle**, an important landmark in laparoscopic inguinal hernia repair; the inferior border of the triangle is formed by the inguinal ligament, and the medial border is formed by the lateral margin of rectus abdominis.

❏ The inferior epigastric artery also gives off the **cremasteric artery**, a pubic branch, and muscular and cutaneous branches.

- ❑ The cremasteric artery accompanies the spermatic cord in males, supplies cremaster and the other coverings of the cord and anastomoses with the testicular artery.
- ❑ In females, the artery is small and accompanies the round ligament.
- ❑ The superior and inferior epigastric arteries are important sources of collateral blood flow between the internal thoracic artery and the external iliac artery when aortic blood flow is compromised.
- ❑ An enlarged **pubic branch of the inferior epigastric artery** either takes the place of the obturator artery (**replaced obturator artery**), or joins it as an **accessory** obturator artery, in approximately 20% of people
- ❑ This artery runs close to or across the femoral ring to reach the obturator foramen and could be closely related to the **neck of a femoral hernia**. Consequently, this artery **could be involved** in a strangulated femoral hernia.

A collateral circulation between the external and internal iliac system is known as **corona mortis** (circle of death). It refers to the **vascular ring** formed by the anastomosis of **an aberrant artery** with the normal obturator artery arising from a branch of the internal iliac artery. At the time of laparoscopic hernia this vessel is torn both end of vessel can **bleed profusely** because both arise from a major artery.

Posterior intercostal, subcostal and lumbar arteries

- ❑ The tenth and eleventh posterior intercostal arteries, the subcostal artery, and the lumbar arteries pierce the posterior aponeurosis of transversus abdominis to enter the neurovascular plane of the abdominal wall deep to internal oblique.
- ❑ The anterior abdominal wall is also supplied by branches of the femoral artery: namely, the superficial epigastric, superficial circumflex iliac, and superficial external pudendal arteries, and by the deep circumflex iliac artery arising from external iliac artery.

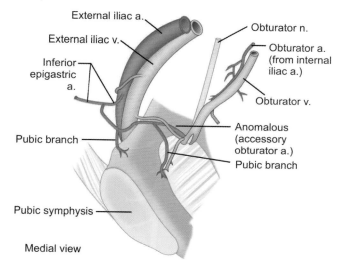

Fig. 11: Accessory obturator artery and corona mortis

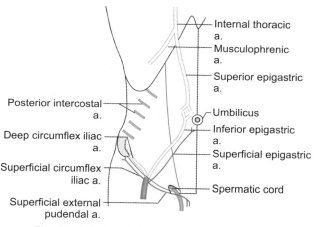

Fig. 12: Arteries of the anterior abdominal wall

Table 4: Arteries of anterolateral abdominal wall			
Artery	**Origin**	**Course**	**Distribution**
Musculophrenic	Internal thoracic artery	Descends along costal margin	Superficial and deep abdominal wall of hypochondriac region; anterolateral diaphragm
Superior epigastric		Descends in rectus sheath deep to rectus adbominis	Rectus abdominis muscle; superificial and deep abdominal wall of epigastric and upper umbilical regions
10th and 11th posterior intercostal arteries	Aorta	Arteries continue beyond ribs to descend in abdominal wall between internal oblique and transversus abdominis muscles	Superficial and deep abdominal wall of lateral (lumbar or flank) region
Subcostal artery			
Deep Inferior epigastric circumflex iliac	External iliac artery	Runs superiorly and enters rectus sheath; runs deep to rectus abdominis	Rectus abdominis muscle; deep abdominal wall of pubic and inferior umbilical regions
		Runs on deep aspect of anterior abdominal wall, parallel to inguinal ligament	Iliacus muscle and deep abdominal wall of inguinal region; iliac fossa
Superficial circumflex iliac	Femoral artery	Runs in subcutaneous tissue along inguinal ligament	Superficial abdominal wall of inguinal region and adjacent anterior thigh
Superificial epigastric		Runs in subcutaneous tissue toward umbilicus	Superficial abdominal wall of pubic and inferior umbilic regions

Veins

Veins accompany the cutaneous arteries and drain as follows:

❏ **Below the umbilicus** they run downward and drain into the great saphenous vein in the groin and thus eventually in the inferior vena cava.

❏ **Above the umbilicus** they run toward the axilla and drain into the axillary vein and thus eventually in the superior vena cava.

❏ **Thoraco-epigastric vein** is formed by the anastomosis of lateral thoracic vein (a tributary of **axillary** vein) with the superficial epigastric vein (a tributary of **great saphenous** vein).

❏ Small tributaries of the inferior epigastric vein draining the skin around the umbilicus anastomose with terminal branches of the umbilical vein draining the umbilical region via the falciform ligament.

❏ These portosystemic anastomoses may open widely in cases of portal hypertension, when portal venous blood may drain into the systemic circulation via the inferior epigastric veins.

❏ The pattern of dilated superficial veins radiating from the umbilicus is referred to as the 'caput medusae'.

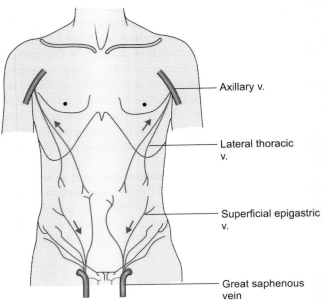

Fig. 13: Superficial veins of the anterior abdominal wall

Lymphatics

❏ Superficial lymphatic vessels accompany the subcutaneous blood vessels immediately below the dermis

❏ Vessels from the lumbar and gluteal regions run with the superficial circumflex iliac vessels, and those from the infra-umbilical skin run with the superficial epigastric vessels.

❏ Both drain into **superficial inguinal nodes**.

❏ The **supraumbilical** region is drained by vessels draining to **axillary** and parasternal nodes.

❏ The deep lymphatic vessels accompany the deeper arteries.

❏ Laterally, they run either with the lumbar arteries to drain into the lateral aortic nodes, or with the intercostal and subcostal arteries to posterior mediastinal nodes.

❏ Lymphatics in the upper anterior abdominal wall run with the superior epigastric vessels to **parasternal** nodes while those in the lower abdominal wall run with the deep circumflex iliac and inferior epigastric arteries to **external iliac nodes**.

Lymphatic drainage of the anterolateral abdominal wall follows the following patterns:

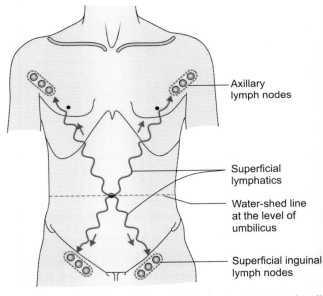

Fig. 14: Superficial lymphatics of the anterior abdominal wall

❏ Superficial lymphatic vessels accompany the subcutaneous veins; those superior to the transumbilical plane drain mainly to the axillary lymph nodes and parasternal lymph nodes. Superficial lymphatic vessels inferior to the transumbilical plane drain to the superficial inguinal lymph nodes.

❏ The deep lymphatic vessels accompany the deeper arteries. Laterally, they run either with the lumbar arteries to drain into the lateral aortic nodes, or with the intercostal and subcostal arteries to posterior mediastinal nodes.

Note: The **water-shed line** for lymphatics lies at the level of the umbilicus.

1. Lymphatic drainage of umbilicus is towards: *(PGIC 2014)*
   a. Axillary lymph nodes only
   b. Inguinal lymph nodes only
   c. Both axillary and inguinal lymph nodes
   d. Celiac lymph nodes
   e. Aortic lymph nodes

2. Corona mortis is: *(NEET Pattern 2016)*
   a. Is a vascular anastomosis
   b. Post-mortem heart and coronary arteries examination
   c. Another term used for rigor mortis
   d. None of the above

QUESTIONS

3. **In rectus sheath which branch of aorta make anastomosis with superior epigastric artery:** *(PGIC 2008)*
   a. Subclavian artery
   b. Axillary artery
   c. External iliac artery
   d. Internal iliac artery
   e. Femoral artery

ANSWERS

1. **c. Both axillary and inguinal lymph nodes; e) Aortic lymph nodes**
   ❑ Umbilicus drains into **both the directions**, supra-umbilically into **axillary** lymph nodes and infra-umbilically into **inguinal** lymph nodes.
   ❑ The deep lymph vessels **follow the arteries** and drain into the internal thoracic, external iliac, posterior mediastinal, and para-aortic (lumbar) nodes.

2. **a. Is a vascular anastomosis**
   ❑ A collateral circulation between the external and internal iliac system is known as **corona mortis**.
   ❑ It is a common variant vascular anastomosis between the **external iliac artery** or **deep inferior epigastric artery** with the **obturator artery**.

3. **c. External iliac artery**
   ❑ In rectus sheath superior epigastric artery (branch of internal thoracic artery) anastomoses with inferior epigastric artery (branch of external iliac artery).

- Nerve supply to the skin around the **umbilicus** is **10th** thoracic ventral ramus.
- **Neurovascular bundle** in anterior abdominal wall lies **between** internal oblique and transverse abdominis *(NEET Pattern 2012)*
- **Inferior epigastric artery** is a branch of **external iliac artery** *(NEET Pattern 2016)*
- **Accessory obturator artery** is a branch of **Inferior epigastric artery** *(NEET Pattern 2016)*
- Usually internal iliac (anterior division) gives the obturator artery.
- **Accessory obturator artery** is related to **lacunar ligament** *(NEET Pattern 2016)*
  – The artery should be protected in **reduction of femoral hernia**, while the lacunar ligament is cut to **enlarge the femoral ring**.

▶ Posterior Abdominal Wall

Fascia on the posterior abdominal wall

Thoracolumbar Fascia

❑ The thoracolumbar fascia is composed of a complex arrangement of multiple fascial layers that is most prominent at the caudal end of the lumbar spine. In the lumbar region, it is often described as having **three layers**.
❑ The **posterior layer** is attached medially to the spines of the lumbar vertebrae and to the supraspinous ligament; it has a superficial lamina (the aponeurosis of latissimus dorsi) and a deep lamina that covers the posterior surface of the paraspinal muscles.
❑ The **middle layer** is attached medially to the tips of the transverse processes of the lumbar vertebrae and extends laterally behind quadratus lumborum; inferiorly, it attaches to the iliac crest, and superiorly to the lower border of the twelfth rib.
❑ The **anterior layer** covers the anterior surface of quadratus lumborum and is attached medially to the transverse processes of the lumbar vertebrae behind psoas major. Laterally, it fuses with the transversalis fascia and the aponeurosis of transversus abdominis.
❑ Inferiorly, it is attached to the **iliolumbar ligament** and adjoining iliac crest.
❑ Superiorly, it is attached to the inferior border of the twelfth rib and extends to the transverse process of the first lumbar vertebra, forming the lateral arcuate ligament of the diaphragm.
❑ The posterior and middle layers of the thoracolumbar fascia fuse at the lateral margin of the paraspinal muscles (the so-called 'lateral raphe'), thereby enclosing the paraspinal muscles in an osteofascial compartment.
❑ Although contained in layers of thoracolumbar fascia, the paraspinal muscles are conceptualized as part of 'the back'.
❑ The aponeurosis of transversus abdominis fuses with both the anterior layer of thoracolumbar fascia at the lateral margin of quadratus lumborum and with the lateral raphe behind quadratus lumborum.

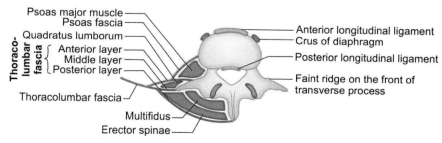

Psoas major muscle
Psoas fascia
Quadratus lumborum
Thoracolumbar fascia { Anterior layer / Middle layer / Posterior layer
Thoracolumbar fascia
Multifidus
Erector spinae

Anterior longitudinal ligament
Crus of diaphragm
Posterior longitudinal ligament
Faint ridge on the front of transverse process

Fig. 15: Attachments of the lumbar vertebra

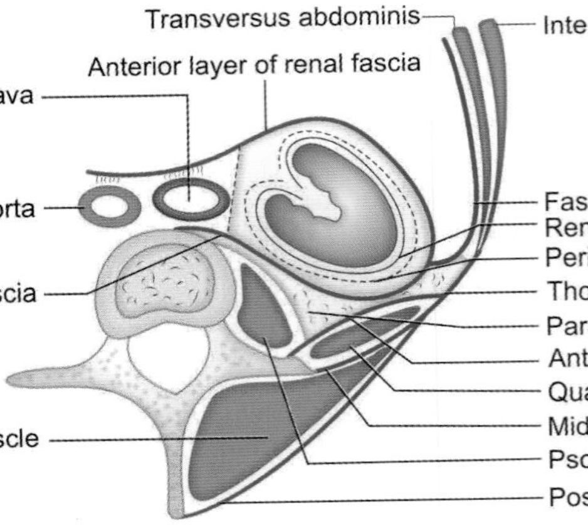

Fig. 16: Transverse section through lumbar region showing transverse disposition of thoracolumbar fasica and coverings of the kidney

QUESTIONS

1. All are true about thoracolumbar facia EXCEPT: *(AIPG 2000)*
   a. Attached to spinous process of lumbar vertebra
   b. Attached to transverse process of lumbar vertebra
   c. The fascia lies posterior to posterior abdominal wall muscles
   d. Gives attachment to Transverse abdominal and internal oblique

2. Which of the following is derived from thoracolumbar fascia? *(NEET Pattern 2016)*
   a. Medial arcuate ligament
   b. Lateral arcuate ligament
   c. Lacunar ligament
   d. Cruciate ligament

ANSWERS

1. **c. The fascia lies posterior to posterior abdominal wall muscles**
   ❏ Thoracolumbar fascia **lies posterior** as well as **anterior** to the posterior abdominal wall.
   ❏ Posterior abdominal wall muscles (e.g., psoas major and minor, iliacus, quadratus lumborum) are **enclosed within** layers of thoracolumbar fascia.

2. **c. Lateral arcuate ligament**
   ❏ Superiorly, thoracolumbar fascia is attached to the inferior border of the **twelfth rib** and extends to the transverse process of the first lumbar vertebra, forming the **lateral arcuate ligament** of the diaphragm.

▼ Muscles

Table 5: Muscles of posterior abdominal wall

Muscle	Supeior attachment	Inferior attachment	Innervation	Main action
Psoas major*	Transverse processes of lumbar vertebrae; sides of bodies of T12–L5 vertebrae and intervening intervertebral discs	By a strong tendon to lesser trochanter of femur	Anterior rami of lumbar nerves **L1, L2, L3**	Acting inferiorly with iliacus, it flexes thigh; acting superiorly it flexes vertebral column laterally; it is used to balance the trunk; when sitting it acts inferiorly with iliacus to flex trunk
Iliacus*	Superior two-thirds of iliac fossa, ala of sacrum, and anterior sacro-iliac ligaments	Lesser trochanter of femur and shaft inferior to it, and to psoas major tendon	Femoral nerve **(L2–L4)**	Flexes thigh and stabilizes hip joint; acts with psoas major
Quadratus lumborum	Medial half of inferior border of 12th ribs and tips of lumbar transverse processes	Iliolumbar ligament and internal lip of iliac crest	Anterior branches of T12 and L1–L4 nerves	Extends and laterally flexes vertebral column; fixes 12th rib during inspiration

*Psoas major and iliacus muscles merge inferiorly; collectively form iliopsoas muscle.

▼ Nerve supply

Genitofemoral Nerve

❏ Originates from the L1 and L2 ventral rami, descends obliquely forwards through the psoas major muscle to emerge on its **anterior surface** nearer the medial border, opposite the third or fourth lumbar vertebra.

❏ It then descends beneath the peritoneum on psoas major, crosses obliquely **behind the ureter**, and divides into genital and femoral.

- ❏ The **genital branch** enters the inguinal canal through the deep ring and accompanies the spermatic cord or round ligament. It exits the superficial inguinal ring, usually dorsal to the spermatic cord or round ligament, and supplies the **cremaster muscle** and skin of the external Genitalia (scrotum, mons pubis, labia majora). Like the ilioinguinal nerve, the genital branch may be injured during inguinal surgery (open and laparoscopic), leading to neuralgic pain.
- ❏ The **femoral branch** pass behind the inguinal ligament (occasionally, through it) and enter the femoral sheath **lateral to the femoral artery**. It pierces the anterior layer of the femoral sheath and fascia lata, and supplies the skin of the upper part of the femoral triangle. It also innervate the anteromedial skin of the thigh via its femoral branch.

Table 6: Autonomic innervation of abdominal viscera (Splanchnic nerves)

Splanchnic nerves	Autonomic fiber Type[a]	System	Origin	Destination
A. Cardiopulmonary (cervical and upper thoracic)	Postsynaptic		Cervical and upper thoracic sympathetic trunk	Thoracic cavity (viscera superior to level of diaphragm)
B. Abdominopelvic 1. Lower thoracic a. Greater b. Lesser c. Least 2. Lumbar 3. Sacral	Presynaptic		Lowre thoracic and abdominopelvic sympathetic trunk: 1. Thoracic sympathetic trunk a. T5–T9 or T10 level b. T10–T11 level c. T12 level 2. Abdominal sympathetic trunk 3. Pelvic (sacral) sympathetic trunk	Abdomiopelvic cavity (prevertebral ganglia serving viscera and suprarenal glands inferior to level of diaphragm) 1. Abdominal prevertebral ganglia: a. Celiac ganglia b. Aorticorenal ganglia c. and 2. Other abdominal prevertebral ganglia (superior and interior mesenteric, and of intermesenteric/hypogastric plexuses) 3. Pelvic prevertebral ganglia
C. Pelvic	Presynaptic	Parasympathetic	Anterior rami of S2–S4 spinal nerves	Intrinsic ganglia of descending and sigmoid colon, rectum, and pelvic viscera

ANS in abdomen

- ❏ Two components:
    1. Sympathetic chains.
    2. Autonomic plexuses on the posterior abdominal wall.

Sympathetic chain in the abdomen

- ❏ It is a ganglionated chain situated on either side of the lumbar vertebrae.
- ❏ It begins deep to the **medial arcuate ligament** of the diaphragm (as the continuation of the thoracic sympathetic chain).
- ❏ It runs vertically downward along the **sides** of bodies of the lumbar vertebrae overlapped on the right side by the IVC and on the left side by the abdominal aorta. The lumbar arteries lie deep to the chain but the lumbar veins may cross superficial to it.
- ❏ The chain enters the pelvis in front of the ala of sacrum beneath the common iliac vessels, where it continues as the sacral sympathetic chain in front of the sacrum.
- ❏ The right and left sympathetic chain converges and unites in front of the coccyx to form the ganglion impar.
- ❏ Each lumbar sympathetic chain possesses four ganglia, the first and second often being fused together.
- ❏ The cell bodies of neurons of the sympathetic supply of the abdomen and pelvis lie in the intermediolateral grey matter of T1-12 and L1-2 spinal segments.
- ❏ **White ramus** communicans: Myelinated axons from these neurons travel in the ventral ramus of the spinal nerve of the same segmental level, leaving it via a white ramus communicans to enter a thoracic or lumbar paravertebral sympathetic ganglion.
- ❏ **Splanchnic nerves**: Visceral branches convey preganglionic motor and visceral sensory (pain) fibers may exit at the same level or ascend or descend several levels in the sympathetic chain before exiting; they leave the ganglia without synapsing and pass medially, giving rise to the paired greater, lesser and least splanchnic nerves, and the lumbar and sacral splanchnic nerves.

Note: **Grey ramus** communicans: Axons destined to supply somatic structures (like skin) synapse in the sympathetic ganglion of the same level, and postganglionic, unmyelinated axons leave the ganglion as one or more grey rami communicantes to enter the spinal nerve of the same segmental level.

Greater Splanchnic Nerve

❑ Root value: T5-9.
❑ It enters the abdomen through the fibers of the ipsilateral crus of the diaphragm, to enter the superior aspect of the Celiac ganglion, where most of the preganglionic fibers synapse (but not those destined for the suprarenal medulla).

Lesser Splanchnic Nerve

❑ Root value: T10-11 (or T9-10).
❑ It enters the abdomen running through the lowermost fibers of the ipsilateral crus of the diaphragm or under the medial arcuate

Ligament

❑ It joins the aorticorenal ganglion and may give branches to the lateral aspect of the Celiac ganglion.

Least splanchnic nerve

❑ Root value: T-11 and/or T-12.
❑ It enters the abdomen medial to the sympathetic chain under the medial arcuate ligament of the diaphragm and runs inferiorly to join the renal plexus.
❑ The trunk of the nerve enters the aorticorenal ganglion and may give branches to the lateral aspect of the Celiac ganglion.

Lumbar splanchnic nerves

❑ They contribute to the **superior and inferior hypogastric plexuses** to innervate the bladder neck, ductus deferens and prostate, among other structures. Damage to these nerves, e.g. during aortoiliac surgery, can result in sexual dysfunction.
❑ Four lumbar splanchnic nerves pass as medial branches from the ganglia to join the Celiac, inferior mesenteric and superior hypogastric plexuses.
❑ The first lumbar splanchnic nerve, from the first ganglion, gives branches to the Celiac, renal and inferior mesenteric plexuses.
❑ The second nerve joins the inferior part of the intermesenteric or inferior mesenteric plexus.
❑ The third nerve arises from the third or fourth ganglion and joins the superior hypogastric plexus.
❑ The fourth lumbar splanchnic nerve from the lowest ganglion passes anterior to the common iliac vessels to join the lower part of the superior hypogastric plexus, or the hypogastric nerves.

Pelvic sympathetic chain

❑ It converges caudally to form a solitary retroperitoneal structure, the ganglion impar (of Walther), which lies at a variable level between the sacrococcygeal joint and the tip of the coccyx.
❑ Ganglion impar conveys sympathetic efferents to and nociceptive afferents from the perineum and terminal urogenital. Regions and it is blocked to treat intractable perineal pain of sympathetic origin in patients with pelvic cancers.

Somatic and vascular branches

❑ Grey rami communicantes containing postganglionic sympathetic nerves pass from the pelvic sympathetic ganglia to the sacral and coccygeal spinal nerves. There are no white rami communicantes at this level.
❑ The postganglionic fibers are distributed via the sacral and coccygeal plexuses.
❑ Thus, sympathetic fibers in the tibial nerve are conveyed to the popliteal artery and its branches in the leg and foot, whilst those in the pudendal and superior and inferior gluteal nerves accompany these arteries to the perineum and buttocks.

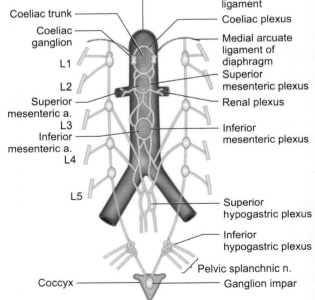

Fig. 17: Lumbar sympathetic chain and autonomic plexuses of the posterior abdominal wall

Sacral splanchnic nerves

- ❑ Sacral splanchnic nerves pass directly from the ganglia to the inferior hypogastric plexus and, from there, to pelvic viscera; they usually arise from the first two sacral sympathetic ganglia.
- ❑ Autonomic plexus on the posterior abdominal wall
- ❑ The preganglionic and postganglionic sympathetic fibers, preganglionic parasympathetic fibers, and visceral afferent fibers form a plexus of nerves around the abdominal aorta.
- ❑ It is constituted by two plexuses: Celiac and superior hypogastric plexuses.

Celiac (solar) plexus

- ❑ The Celiac plexus is located at the level of the T-12 and L1 vertebrae, and is the largest major autonomic plexus.
- ❑ It lies **anterolateral to the aorta** and surrounds the Celiac artery and the root of the superior mesenteric artery.
- ❑ It is posterior to the stomach and lesser sac, and anterior to the crura of the diaphragm and the beginning of the abdominal aorta, and lies medial to the suprarenal glands.
- ❑ The plexus and ganglia receive the **greater** and **lesser splanchnic nerves** and branches from the **vagal** trunks. The plexus is in continuity with small branches along adjacent arteries and is connected to the phrenic, splenic, hepatic, superior mesenteric, suprarenal, renal and gonadal plexuses.
- ❑ Visceral afferents in the Celiac plexus convey pain and other sensations from upper abdominal viscera. Celiac plexus block is undertaken to treat intractable pain from pancreatic disorders.

Celiac and Aorticorenal Ganglia

- ❑ The Celiac ganglia receive greater splanchnic nerve in the upper part and the lesser splanchnic nerve joins the lower part.
- ❑ The lowermost part of each ganglion forms the aorticorenal ganglion, which receives the ipsilateral lesser splanchnic nerve and gives origin to the majority of the renal plexus.

Superior Mesenteric Plexus and Ganglion

- ❑ The superior mesenteric plexus lies in the pre-aortic connective tissue posterior to the pancreas, around the origin of the superior mesenteric artery.
- ❑ It is an inferior continuation of the Celiac plexus, and includes branches from the posterior vagal trunk and Celiac plexus.
- ❑ Its branches accompany the superior mesenteric artery and its divisions.
- ❑ The superior mesenteric ganglion lies superiorly in the plexus, usually above the origin of the superior mesenteric artery.

Intermesenteric Plexus

- ❑ Like other parts of the abdominal aortic autonomic plexus, the intermesenteric plexus is not a discrete structure but is part of a continuous periarterial nerve plexus connected to the gonadal, inferior mesenteric, iliac and superior hypogastric plexuses.
- ❑ It lies on the lateral and anterior aspects of the aorta, between the origins of the superior and inferior mesenteric arteries, and consists of numerous fine, interconnected nerve fibers and a few ganglia continuous superiorly with the superior mesenteric plexus and inferiorly with the superior hypogastric plexus.
- ❑ It is not well characterized but receives parasympathetic and sympathetic branches from the Celiac plexus and additional sympathetic rami from the first and second lumbar splanchnic nerves.

Inferior mesenteric plexus

- ❑ The inferior mesenteric plexus lies around the origin of the inferior mesenteric artery and is distributed along its branches.
- ❑ It is formed predominantly from the aortic plexus, supplemented by sympathetic fibers from the first and second lumbar splanchnic nerves and ascending pelvic parasympathetic fibers from the inferior hypogastric plexus (via the hypogastric nerves and superior hypogastric plexus).
- ❑ Disruption of the inferior mesenteric plexus alone rarely causes clinically significant disturbances of autonomic function.

Superior hypogastric plexus

- ❑ The superior hypogastric plexus lies anterior to the aortic bifurcation.
- ❑ The plexus is formed by branches from three main sources: the aortic plexus (sympathetic and parasympathetic), lumbar splanchnic nerves (sympathetic) and pelvic splanchnic nerves (parasympathetic), which ascend from the inferior hypogastric plexus via the right and left hypogastric nerves.
- ❑ The superior hypogastric plexus conveys branches to the inferior mesenteric plexus and to the ureteric, gonadal and common iliac nerve plexuses; additional small branches turn abruptly forwards into the upper mesorectum to travel with the superior rectal artery.

Inferior Hypogastric Plexus

❑ The inferior hypogastric plexus lies on the pelvic side wall anterolateral to the mesorectum, posterolateral to the base of the urinary bladder.

❑ The inferior hypogastric plexus is formed mainly from pelvic splanchnic (**parasympathetic**) and sacral splanchnic (**sympathetic**) branches; a smaller contribution is derived from sympathetic fibers (from the lower lumbar ganglia), which descend into the plexus from the superior hypogastric plexus via the hypogastric nerves.

❑ It supply the vas deferens, seminal vesicles, prostate, accessory glands and penis in males; the ovary, Fallopian tubes, uterus, uterine cervix and vagina in females; and the urinary bladder and distal ureter in both sexes. The plexus plays a key role in continence and sexual function.

❑ **Hypogastric nerves**: The hypogastric nerves are usually paired nerve bundles but may consist instead of multiple filaments. They contain sympathetic fibers (mostly descending from the superior hypogastric plexus) and parasympathetic fibers (ascending from the inferior hypogastric plexus). The nerves run between the superior and inferior hypogastric plexuses on each side.

Table 7: Pain referral from abdominal viscera

Organ	Referral area	Pathway
Diaphragm:		
Central	C3–C5: neck and shoulder	Phrenic nerve
Marginal	T5–T10: thorax	Intercostal nerves
Foregut:		
Stomach, gallbladder, liver, bile duct, superior duodenum	T5–T9: lower thorax, epigastric region	Celiac plexus to greater splanchnic nerve
Midgut:		
Inferior duodenum, jejunum, ileum, appendix, ascending colon, transverse colon	T10–T11: umbilical region	Superior mesenteric plexus to lesser splanchnic nerve
(Kidney, upper ureters, gonads)	T12–L1: lumbar and ipsilateral inguinal	Aorticorenal plexus to least splanchnic nerve regions
Hindgut:		
Descending colon, sigmoid colon, mid-ureters	L1–L2: suprapubic and inguinal regions, anterior secretum or labia, anterior thigh	Aortic plexus to lumbar splanchnic nerves

Table 8: Pain referral from pelvic viscera

Organ	Referral areas	Pathway
Testes and ovaries	T10–T12: umbilical and pubic regions	Gonadal nerves to aortic plexus and then to lesser and least splanchnic nerves
Middle ureters, urinary bladder, uterine body, uterine tubes	L1–L2: pubic and inguinal regions, anterior scrotum or labia, anterior thigh	Hypogastric plexus to aortic plexus and then to lumbar splanchnic nerves
Rectum, superior anal canal, pelvic ureters, cervix, epididymis, vas deferens, seminal vesicles, prostate gland	S2–S5: perineum and posterior thigh	Pelvic plexus to pelvic splanchnic nerves

Table 9: Pelvic visceral afferent innervation

Organ	Afferent pathway	Level	Referral areas
Kidneys Renal pelvis Upper ureters	Aorticorenal plexus, least splanchnic nerve, white ramus of T12, subcostal nerve	T12	Subcostal and pubic regions
Descending colon Sigmoid colon Mid-ureters Urinary bladder Oviducts Uterine body	Aortic plexus, lumbar splanchnic nerves, white rami of L1–L2, spinal nerves L1–L2	L1–L2	Lumbar and inguinal regions, anterior mons and labia, anterior scrotum, anterior thigh

Organ	Afferent pathway	Level	Referral areas
None	No white rami between L3–S1	L3–S1	No visceral pain refers to dermatomes L3–S1
Cervix Pelvic ureters Epididymis Vas deferens Seminal vesicles Prostate gland Rectum Proximal anal canal	Pelvic plexus, pelvic splanchnic nerves, spinal nerves S2–S4	S2–S4	Perineum, thigh, lateral leg and foot

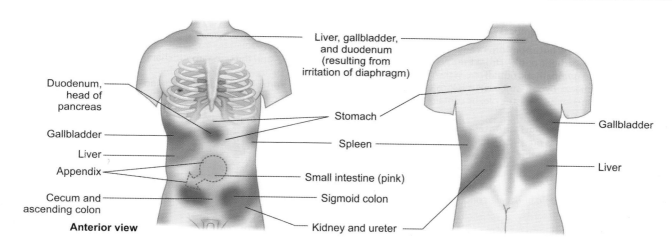

Fig. 18: Referred pain of various on the body surface

Parasympathetic innervation

❑ The parasympathetic neurons innervating the abdomen and pelvis are present in the dorsal motor nucleus of the vagus nerve and in the intermediolateral grey matter of the second, third and fourth sacral spinal segments.

❑ The vagus nerves supply parasympathetic innervation to the abdominal viscera as far as the distal transverse colon, i.e. they supply the foregut and midgut.

❑ The hindgut is supplied by parasympathetic fibers travelling via the pelvic splanchnic nerves.

❑ The vagal trunks are derived from the esophageal plexus and enter the abdomen via the esophageal hiatus.

❑ The anterior vagal trunk is mostly derived from the left vagus and the posterior from the right vagus. The nerves supply the intra-abdominal esophagus and stomach directly.

❑ The anterior trunk gives off a hepatic branch, which innervates the liver parenchyma and vasculature, the biliary tree including the gallbladder, and the structures in the free edge of the lesser omentum.

❑ The posterior trunk supplies branches to the celiac plexus; these fibers frequently constitute the largest portion of the fibers contributing to the plexus. They arise directly from the posterior vagal trunk and from its gastric branch, and run beneath the peritoneum, deep to the posteriorwall of the upper part of the lesser sac, to reach the Celiac plexus. Their synaptic relays with postganglionic neurons are situated in the myenteric (Auerbach's) and submucosal (Meissner's) plexuses in the wall of the gut.

Pelvic splanchnic nerves

❑ They travel in the anterior rami of the second, third and fourth sacral spinal nerves. They leave the nerves as they exit the anterior sacral foramina.

❑ Most pass anterolaterally into the network of nerves that form the inferior hypogastric plexus; from here, they pass to the pelvic viscera. Some join directly with the hypogastric nerves and ascend out of the pelvis, as far as the superior hypogastric plexus; from here, they are distributed with branches of the inferior mesenteric artery.

❑ The pelvic splanchnic nerves are motor to the smooth muscle of the hindgut and bladder wall, supply vasodilator fibers to the erectile tissue of the penis and clitoris, and are secretomotor to the hindgut.

Applied Anatomy:

❑ **Visceral pain:** The viscera are insensitive to cutting, crushing, or burning but visceral pain does occur following excessive distension, spasmodic contraction of smooth muscles, and ischemia of the viscera. The visceral pain is usually referred to the skin supplied by same segmental nerves (referred pain).

❑ **Lumbar sympathectomy:** It is done for vaso-occlusive disease of lower limb (Buerger's disease). Usually the second, third, and fourth lumbar ganglia are excised along with intermediate chain. This causes adequate vasodilation of the lower limb. Consequently the skin of the lower limb Clinical correlation becomes warm, pink, and dry. The first lumbar ganglion is preserved because it plays an important role in ejaculation (keeps the sphincter vesicae closed during ejaculation).

❑ Removal of first lumbar sympathetic ganglion results in **dry coitus**.

QUESTIONS

1. Relation of celiac plexus: *(AIIMS 2010)*
   a. Anterolateral to aorta
   b. Posteromedial to aorta
   c. Anteromedial to lumbar sympathetic chain
   d. Posterolateral to lumbar sympathetic chain

2. Which nerve supplies celiac plexus: *(NEET Pattern 2012)*
   a. Phrenic nerve
   b. Greater splanchnic nerve
   c. Iliohypogastric nerve
   d. Inguinal nerve

3. TRUE about the autonomic nervous system is: *(AIPG 2003)*
   a. The sympathetic outflow from the CNS is through both the cranial nerves and the sympathetic chain
   b. The parasympathetic outflow from the CNS is through cranial nerves only
   c. The superior hypogastric plexus is located at the anterior aspect of the aortic bifurcation and fifth lumbar vertebra
   d. The superior hypogastric plexus contains sympathetic fibers only

ANSWERS

1. a. Anterolateral to aorta > Anteromedial to lumbar sympathetic chain
   ❑ Celiac plexus is present on the **anterior side** of the aorta **around** the beginning of celiac trunk.
   ❑ It lies over the **anterolateral surface of the aorta** at the T12 / L1 vertebral level.

2. b. Greater splanchnic nerve
   ❑ Celiac plexus receives preganglionic sympathetic fibers contributed by the **greater** and **lesser** splanchnic nerves.
   ❑ Parasympathetic fibers are contributed by **vagus** nerve. Postganglionic fibers **accompany the respective blood vessels** to the target organs.

3. c. The superior hypogastric plexus is located at the anterior aspect of the aortic bifurcation and fifth lumbar vertebra
   ❑ Superior hypogastric plexus is **chiefly sympathetic** but some **parasympathetic** fibers from pelvic splanchnic nerves ascend from the inferior hypogastric plexus **via the right and left hypogastric nerves to reach** the superior hypogastric plexus.
   ❑ The sympathetic outflow is thoracolumbar (T1-L2) and **doesn't involve cranial nerves**.
   ❑ Parasympathetic flow is **craniosacral** and involves cranial nerves (3,7,9,10) and sacral nerves (S2,3,4).

▶ Vasculature - Arteries

Table 10: Key anatomical reference points

Structure	Vertebral level
Ductus arteriosus	T4–5
Celiac artery	T12
Superior mesenteric artery	T12–L1
Renal artery	L1
Inferior mesenteric artery	L3
Aortic bifurcation	L4–5

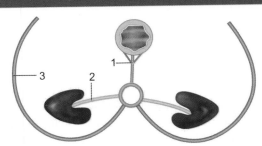

Fig. 19: Arteries of posterior abdominal wall—branches of the aorta

Table 11: Branches of abdominal aorta

Vascular plane	Class	Distribution	Abdominal branches (arteries)	Vertebral level
▪ Anterior midline	Unpaired visceral	Digestive tract	Celiac	T12
			Superior mesenteric	L1
			Inferior mesenteric	L3
▪ Lateral	Paired visceral	Urogenital and endocrine organs	Suprarenal	L1
			Renal	L1
			Gonadal (testicular or ovarian)	L2
Posterolateral	Paired parietal (segmental)	Diaphragm; body wall	Subcostal	L2
			Inferior phrenic	T12
			Lumbar	L1–L4

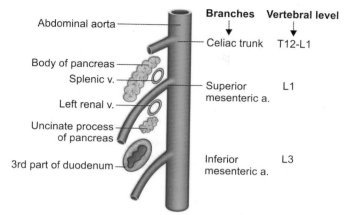

Fig. 20: Three ventral branches of the abdominal aorta as seen in left lateral view of a sagittal section through the abdominal aorta. **Note:** Superior mesenteric artery at its origin is sandwiched between splenic and left renal veins

The abdominal aorta begins at the level of the body of the T-12 vertebra as it passes through aortic hiatus. It descends and bifurcates at L4 vertebra just to the left of the midline.

❑ IVC-L5

Abdominal Aorta

Major Branches

Celiac Trunk is located at **T12** vertebral level and supplies viscera that derive embryologically from the **foregut** (i.e., intra-abdominal portion of esophagus, stomach, upper part of duodenum, liver, gallbladder, and pancreas). The celiac trunk further branches into the following:

a. **Left gastric artery**
b. **Splenic artery**
c. **Common hepatic artery**

❑ **Superior Mesenteric Artery** is located at **L1** vertebral level and supplies viscera that derive embryologically from the **midgut** (i.e., lower part of duodenum, jejunum, ileum, cecum, appendix, ascending colon, and proximal two-thirds of transverse colon)

Renal Arteries supply the kidneys.

Gonadal Arteries supply the testes or ovary.

Inferior Mesenteric Artery is located at **L3** vertebral level and supplies viscera that derive embryologically from the **hindgut** (i.e., distal one-third of transverse colon, descending colon, sigmoid colon, and upper portion of rectum).

Common Iliac Arteries are the terminal branches of the abdominal aorta.

❑ **Collateral Circulation.** The abdominal vasculature has a fairly robust collateral circulation. Any blockage between the superior mesenteric artery at L1 vertebral level and inferior mesenteric artery at L3 vertebral level will cause blood to be diverted along two routes of collateral circulation. The first route uses the middle colic artery (a branch of superior

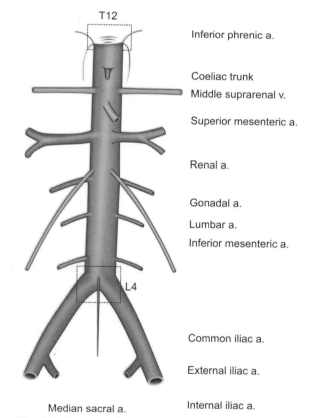

Fig. 21: Course and branches of the abdominal aorta

mesenteric artery) which anastomoses with the left colic artery (a branch of inferior mesenteric artery). The second route uses the marginal artery.

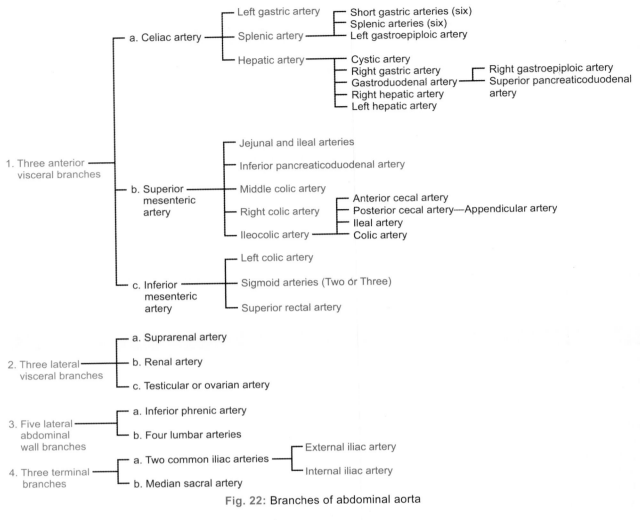

Fig. 22: Branches of abdominal aorta

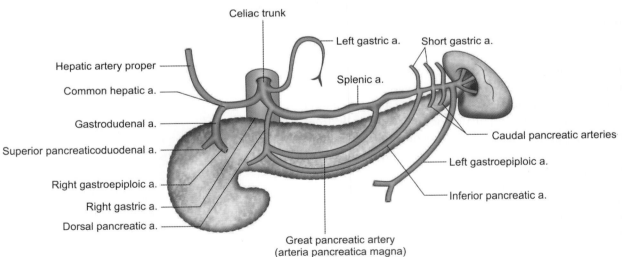

Fig. 23: Celiac trunk

Table 12: Arterial supply to abdominal foregut derivatives: Esophagus, stomach, liver, gallbladder, pancreas, and spleen			
Artery	**Origin**	**Course**	**Distribution**
Celiac trunk	Abdominal aorta (at level of aortic hiatus)	After short anteroinferior course, bifurcates into splenic and common hepatic arteries	Esophagus, stomach proximal duodenum, liver/giving apparatus, pancreas

Artery	Origin	Course	Distribution
Left gastric	Celiac trunk	Ascends retroperitoneally to esophageal hiatus, giving rise to an esophagial branch; then descending along lesser curvature to anastomose with right gastric artery	Distal (mostly abdominal) part of esophagus and lesser curvature of stomach
Splenic		Runs retroperitoneally along superior border of pancreas; traverses splenorenal ligament to hilium of spleen	Body of pancreas, spleen, and greater curvature and posterior stomach body
Posterior gastric	Splenic artery posterior to stomach	Ascends retroperitoneally along posterior wall of lesser omental bursa to enter gastrophrenic ligament	Posterior wall and fundus of stomach
Left gastro-omental (left gastroepiploic)	Splenic artery in hilum spleen	Passes between layers of gastrosplenic ligament to stomach. The along greater curvature in greater omentum to anastomose with right gastro-omental artery	Left portion of greater curvature of stomach
Short gastric (n = 4–5)		Passes between layers of gastrosplenic ligament to fundus of stomach	Fundus of stomach
Hepatic	Celiac trunk	Passes retroperitoneally to reach hepatoduodenal ligament; passing between layers to porta hepatis; bifurcates into right and left hepatic arteries	Liver, gallbladder and biliary ducts, stomach, duodenum, pancreas, and respective lobes of liver
Cystic	Right hepatic artery	Arises within hepatoduodenal ligament (in cystohepatic triangle of Calot)	Gallbladder and cystic duct
Right gastric	Hepatic artery	Runs along lesser curvature of stomach to anastomose with left gastric artery	Right portion of lesser curvature of stomach
Gastroduodenal		Descends retroperitoneally, posterior to gastroduodenal junction	Stomach, pancreas, first part of duodenum, and distal part of bile duct
Right gastro-omental (right gastroepiploic)	Gastroduodenal artery	Passes between layers of greater omentum along greater curvature of stomach to anastomose with left gastro-mental artery	Right portion of greater curvature of stomach
Superior pancreaticoduodenal		Divides into anterior and posterior arteries that descend on each side of pancreatic head, anastomosing with similar branches of inferior pancreaticoduodenal artery	Proximal portion of duodenum and superior part of head of pancreas
Inferior pancreaticoduodenal	Superior mesenteric artery	Divides into anterior and posterior arteries that ascend on each side of pancreatic head, anastomosing with similar branches of superior pancreaticoduodenal artery	Distal portion of duodenum and head of pancreas

For descriptive purposes, the hepatic artery is often divided into the common hepatic artery, from its origin to the origin of the gastroduodenal artery, and hepatic artery proper, made up of the remainder of the vessel.

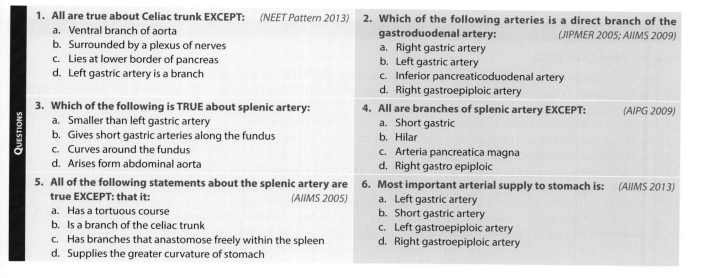

QUESTIONS

1. **All are true about Celiac trunk EXCEPT:** *(NEET Pattern 2013)*
   a. Ventral branch of aorta
   b. Surrounded by a plexus of nerves
   c. Lies at lower border of pancreas
   d. Left gastric artery is a branch

2. **Which of the following arteries is a direct branch of the gastroduodenal artery:** *(JIPMER 2005; AIIMS 2009)*
   a. Right gastric artery
   b. Left gastric artery
   c. Inferior pancreaticoduodenal artery
   d. Right gastroepiploic artery

3. **Which of the following is TRUE about splenic artery:**
   a. Smaller than left gastric artery
   b. Gives short gastric arteries along the fundus
   c. Curves around the fundus
   d. Arises form abdominal aorta

4. **All are branches of splenic artery EXCEPT:** *(AIPG 2009)*
   a. Short gastric
   b. Hilar
   c. Arteria pancreatica magna
   d. Right gastro epiploic

5. **All of the following statements about the splenic artery are true EXCEPT: that it:** *(AIIMS 2005)*
   a. Has a tortuous course
   b. Is a branch of the celiac trunk
   c. Has branches that anastomose freely within the spleen
   d. Supplies the greater curvature of stomach

6. **Most important arterial supply to stomach is:** *(AIIMS 2013)*
   a. Left gastric artery
   b. Short gastric artery
   c. Left gastroepiploic artery
   d. Right gastroepiploic artery

7. **Arterial supply of stomach:**
   a. Right gastric artery
   c. Splenic artery
   e. Superior mesenteric artery

   b. Left gastric artery
   d. Inferior phrenic artery

   (PGIC 2001, 03)

1. **c. Lies at lower border of pancreas**
   - ❑ Celiac trunk lies at the upper aspect of pancreas (**not lower**)
   - ❑ Celiac trunk is a **ventral** branch of abdominal aorta, is surrounded by the nerve plexus called **celiac plexus**.
   - ❑ It gives three branches, including **left gastric artery**.

2. **d. Right gastroepiploic artery**
   - ❑ Right gastroepiploic (gastro-omental artery) artery is one of the two **terminal** branches of the gastroduodenal artery.
   - ❑ It runs from **right to left along** the greater curvature of the stomach, **between** the layers of the greater omentum, **anastomosing with** the left gastroepiploic artery, a branch of the splenic artery.

3. **b. Gives short gastric arteries along the fundus**
   - ❑ Splenic artery is the **largest** branch of Celiac trunk, runs **posterior** to stomach (in stomach bed) and send **short gastric arteries** in gastrosplenic ligament to reach the **fundus** of stomach.

4. **d. Right gastroepiploic**
   - ❑ Right gastroepiploic artery is a branch of **gastroduodenal** artery. Splenic artery gives the **left** gastroepiploic artery.
   - ❑ **Short gastric** arteries are the branches of splenic artery, which travel in the **gastrosplenic ligament** and supply the fundus of stomach.
   - ❑ Splenic artery runs **posterior** to the superior border of pancreas and supplies the organ by giving pancreatic branches) like **arteria pancreatica magna**.
   - ❑ It reaches the hilum of the kidney and gives the **hilar branches**, which enter the spleen as **end arteries**.

5. **c. Has branches that anastomose freely within the spleen**
   - ❑ **Splenic** artery branches **do not anastomose** within the substance of spleen (**end arteries**).
   - ❑ Splenic artery is the **largest** branch of celiac trunk, with a **tortuous** course to allow for movement of spleen.
   - ❑ It supplies body and tail of pancreas via pancreatic branches; **greater curvature** of stomach by giving short gastric and left gastroepiploic branches.

6. **a. Left gastric artery**
   - ❑ The **consistently largest artery** to the stomach is **left gastric artery**.

7. **a. Right gastric artery; b. Left gastric artery; c. Splenic artery**
   - ❑ Inferior **phrenic** artery supplies **diaphragm**. Superior mesenteric artery supplies **mid-gut derivatives**.

- ▪ **Common hepatic artery** is a branch of **Celiac trunk** *(NEET Pattern 2016)*
- ▪ **Gastroduodenal** artery is derived from **hepatic** artery *(AIIMS 2005)*
- ▪ **Arteria pancreatic magna** is a branch of **splenic artery** *(NEET Pattern 2015)*
- ▪ **Short gastric** arteries are branches of **splenic artery** *(NEET Pattern 2013)*
- ▪ **Posterior gastric** artery is a branch of **splenic** artery *(JIPMER 2011; NEET Pattern 2014)*
- ▪ **Superior pancreaticoduodenal** artery is a branch of **gastroduodenal artery**
- ▪ **Left colic** artery is a branch of **inferior mesenteric** artery
- ▪ **Appendicular** artery is a branch of **ileocolic** artery
- ▪ **Caudate process** of liver lies to the **right side** of celiac trunk
- ▪ **Superior mesenteric** artery **does not** supply **stomach** *(NEET Pattern 2014)*

▶ Venous Drainage of Abdomen

Inferior Vena Cava (IVC)

- ❑ The IVC is formed by the union of the **right and left common iliac veins** at vertebral level L5.
- ❑ The IVC drains all the blood from below the diaphragm (even portal blood from the GI tract after it percolates through the liver) to the right atrium.
- ❑ The IVC is in jeopardy during surgical repair of a herniated intervertebral disc.
- ❑ The IVC above the kidneys (suprarenal) should never be ligated (there is a 100% mortality rate).
- ❑ The IVC below the kidneys (infrarenal) may be ligated (there is a 50% mortality rate).
- ❑ The **right gonadal vein** drains directly into the IVC, whereas the **left gonadal vein** drains into the left renal vein.
  - ➢ This is important in females where the appearance of a **right-side hydronephrosis** may indicate thrombosis of the right ovarian vein that constricts the ureter since the right ovarian vein crossed the ureter to drain into the IVC.
  - ➢ This is also important in males where the appearance of a **left-side testicular varicocele** may indicate occlusion of the **left testicular vein** and/or **left renal vein** due to a malignant tumor of the kidney.

❑ **Routes of collateral venous return** exist in case the IVC is blocked by either a malignant retroperitoneal tumor or a large blood clot (thrombus). These include the following:
  ➤ Azygos vein → SVC → right atrium
  ➤ Lumbar veins → external and internal vertebral venous plexuses → cranial dural sinuses → internal jugular vein → right atrium

▶ IVC

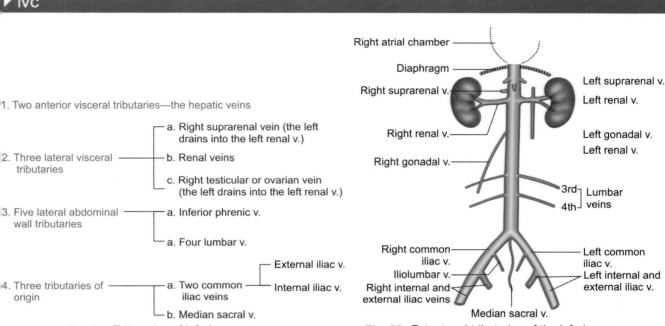

1. Two anterior visceral tributaries—the hepatic veins

2. Three lateral visceral tributaries
  a. Right suprarenal vein (the left drains into the left renal v.)
  b. Renal veins
  c. Right testicular or ovarian vein (the left drains into the left renal v.)

3. Five lateral abdominal wall tributaries
  a. Inferior phrenic v.
  a. Four lumbar v.

4. Three tributaries of origin
  a. Two common iliac veins — External iliac v. / Internal iliac v.
  b. Median sacral v.

Fig. 24: Tributaries of inferior vena cava

Fig. 25: Extent and tributaries of the inferior vena cava

Left inferior phrenic, suprarenal and gonadal veins do not drain into inferior vena cava[Q].

Relations of IVC (from below upwards)

Anterior	Posterior
Root of mesentery ▪ Right gonadal vessels ▪ Third part of duodenum	▪ Right psoas major muscle ▪ Right renal artery ▪ Right Celiac ganglion and sympathetic chain
Head of pancreas with bile duct ▪ First part of duodenum and portal vein (**epiploic foramen**) ▪ Liver	▪ Right suprarenal gland ▪ Right middle suprarenal vein. ▪ Right inferior phrenic artery

Portal vein

❑ The superior mesenteric vein joins splenic vein to form portal vein **behind the neck of the pancreas** at the level of the L1/2 intervertebral disc (at the **transpyloric plane**).

❑ It is approximately **8 cm long** in the adult and ascends obliquely to the right behind the **first part of the duodenum**, the common bile duct and gastroduodenal artery; at this point, it is directly anterior to the inferior vena cava.

❑ It enters the right border of the lesser omentum and ascends anterior to the epiploic foramen to reach the right end of the porta hepatis, where it divides into right and left main branches, which accompany the corresponding branches of the hepatic artery into the liver.

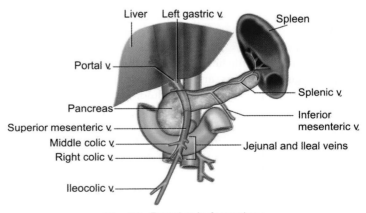

Fig. 26: Portal vein formation

❑ In the lesser omentum, the portal vein lies posterior to both the common bile duct and the hepatic artery.

❑ The main extrahepatic tributaries of the portal vein are the left gastric (coronary) vein and the posterior superior pancreaticoduodenal vein. Within the liver, the left branch receives the obliterated umbilical vein via the ligamentum teres, which connects to its vertical portion.

Hepatic Portal System

❑ In general, the term "portal" refers to a vein interposed between two capillary beds, i.e., capillary bed → vein → capillary bed.

❑ The hepatic portal system consists specifically of the following vascular structures: Capillaries of GI tract → portal vein → hepatic sinusoids.

❑ The **portal vein** is formed posterior to the neck of pancreas by the union of the **splenic vein** and **superior mesenteric vein**. The **inferior mesenteric vein** usually ends by joining the splenic vein.

❑ The blood within the portal vein carries high levels of nutrients from the GI tract and products of red blood cell destruction from the spleen.

❑ **Collateral circulation.** The hepatic portal system has a fairly robust collateral circulation. When blood flow through the liver is severely reduced (e.g., **portal hypertension** due to liver cirrhosis), portal blood will be diverted along three routes of collateral circulation.

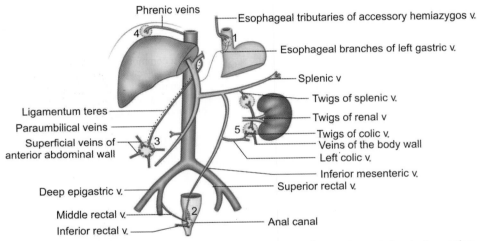

Fig. 27: Site of portocaval anastomosis: 1 = lower end of esophagus; 2 = anal canal; 3 = in the region of umbilicus; 4 = at the bare area of liver; 5 = between the colic veins and the renal veins

➤ The first route at the esophagus uses the left gastric vein (portal system) which anastomoses with the esophageal vein (IVC system) forming **esophageal varices**.

➤ The second route at the umbilicus uses the paraumbilical vein (portal system) which anastomoses with the superficial and inferior epigastric veins (IVC system) forming a **caput medusae**.

➤ The third route at the rectum uses the superior rectal vein (portal system) which anastomoses with middle and inferior rectal veins (IVC system) forming **anorectal varices**.

❑ **Clinical consideration: Portal hypertension.** Portal IVC (caval) anastomosis becomes clinically relevant when **portal hypertension** occurs. Portal hypertension will cause blood within the portal vein to reverse its flow and enter the IVC in order to return to the heart. There are three main sites of portal IVC anastomosis.

❑ **Esophagus, umbilicus,** and **rectum.** Clinical signs of portal hypertension include vomiting copious amounts of blood, enlarged abdomen due to ascites fluid, and splenomegaly. Portal hypertension may be caused by alcoholism, liver cirrhosis, and schistosomiasis. The photograph shows an elderly man with portal hypertension demonstrating caput medusae.

Table 13: Common sites of porto-systemic anastomoses in portal hypertension and associated clinical implications		
Portal vein tributaries	**Systemic veins**	**Clinical presentations**
Left gastric vein	Distal esophageal veins draining into azygos and hemiazygos veins	Esophageal and gastric varices
Superior rectal veins	Middle and inferior rectal veins draining into internal iliac and pudendal veins	Rectal varices

Persistent tributaries of left branch of portal vein in ligamentum teres	Periumbilical branches of epigastric and intercostal veins	Caput medusae
Tributaries of right branch of portal vein overlying 'bare area' of liver	Retroperitoneal veins draining into azygos, hemiazygos, lumbar, intercostal and phrenic veins	Dilated retroperitoneal veins at risk during surgery or interventional procedures
Omental and colonic veins near hepatic and splenic flexures	Retroperitoneal veins near hepatic and splenic flexures	May be problematic during surgery

QUESTIONS

1. **TRUE about inferior vena cava:** *(PGIC 2003)*
   a. Passes through diaphragm at D10 vertebra
   b. Right suprarenal vein drains directly into it
   c. It lies anterior to renal artery
   d. It forms the posterior boundary of epiploic foramen
   e. It is related to psoas muscle

2. **Tributaries of left renal vein are all EXCEPT:** *(NEET Pattern 2014)*
   a. Left adrenal vein
   b. Left lumbar vein
   c. Left testicular vein
   d. Diaphragmatic vein

3. **Vein that doesn't cross the midline is:** *(AI 2007)*
   a. Left brachiocephalic vein
   b. Hemiazygous vein
   c. Left renal vein
   d. Left gonadal vein

4. **FALSE statement about portal vein is:** *(JIPMER 2011)*
   a. It is formed by the union of the superior mesenteric and splenic vein
   b. It ascends posterior to the neck of the pancreas and the superior part of the duodenum
   c. The bile duct and the hepatic artery lie anterior in its upper part
   d. It ends by dividing into the hepatic veins

5. **Which of the following vein (s) is/are part of portal circulation:** *(PGIC 2015)*
   a. Splenic vein
   b. Paraumbilical vein
   c. Superior rectal vein
   d. Left gastric vein
   e. Inferior rectal vein

6. **Which of the following is FALSE about portal vein:**
   a. Formed behind the neck of pancreas
   b. Bile duct lies anterior and right to it
   c. Gastroduodenal artery lies to the left and anterior to it
   d. Ascends behind the 2nd part of duodenum

7. **Which veins drain directly into inferior vena cava:** *(NEET Pattern 2012)*
   a. Superior mesenteric vein
   b. Inferior mesenteric vein
   c. Hepatic vein
   d. Splenic vein

ANSWERS

1. **b. Right suprarenal vein drains directly into it; c. It lies anterior to renal artery; d. It forms the posterior boundary of epiploic foramen; e. It is related to psoas muscle**
   ❑ Inferior vena cava passes through the **central tendon** of diaphragm at D8 (**not D10**) vertebra level.

2. **b. Left lumbar vein**
   ❑ Left inferior **phrenic** (diaphragmatic) vein, left **adrenal** vein and left **gonadal** vein are tributaries of left renal vein (but **not the left lumbar** vein).
   ❑ On the right side the corresponding veins drain directly into IVC (and not into the right renal vein).

3. **d. Left gonadal vein**
   ❑ Left gonadal vein drains into left renal vein and **remains on the left side** of midline (doesn't cross it).
   ❑ Veins **crossing the midline** to join the **drainage structures** lying on **right side of midline** are:
     ■ **Left brachiocephalic** vein crosses the midline to join right counterpart and form **SVC**.
     ■ **Hemiazygous vein** crosses the midline at T8 vertebra level to drain into **azygous vein**.
     ■ **Left renal vein** crosses the midline to enter the **IVC**.
   Note: Left suprarenal, and left inferior phrenic vein enter the left renal vein (**do not cross** the midline).

4. **d. It ends by dividing into the hepatic veins**
   ❑ Portal vein ends at the **right end of porta hepatis** by dividing into a right and a left branch.

5. **a. Splenic vein; b) Paraumbilical vein; c) Superior rectal vein; d) Left gastric vein**
   ❑ The final common pathway for transport of venous blood from spleen, pancreas, gallbladder and the abdominal portion of the gastrointestinal tract (**with the EXCEPT:ion** of the inferior part of the anal canal and sigmoid) is through the **hepatic portal vein**.
   ❑ Inferior rectal vein belongs to **systemic circulation** as it drains eventually into the **inferior vena cava**.

6. **d. Ascends behind the 2nd part of duodenum**
   ❑ Portal vein ascends behind **first part** of duodenum
   ❑ Other options are correct.

7. **c. Hepatic vein**
   ❑ **Hepatic veins** drain the liver into inferior vena cava.
   ❑ Superior mesenteric vein is joined by splenic vein to form the **portal vein**, which itself drains into the liver.
   ❑ **Inferior mesenteric** vein drains into the **splenic** vein, before it drains into **portal** vein.

- **Portal vein** is formed by the union of **splenic** and **superior mesenteric** veins *(NEET Pattern 2013)*
- Structure immediately posterior to pancreatic head is **right renal vein**. *(NEET Pattern 2012)*
- Hepatic veins drain **directly** into IVC (not into mesenteric or splenic veins)
- Portal venous system is **valveless** *(AIIMS 2008)*
- **Portocaval anastomosis** is seen between **superior rectal** vein and **inferior rectal** vein.
- At lower end of esophagus, **porto-caval** anastomosis is in between tributary of **left gastric vein** (portal circulation) and **esophageal vein** (systemic circulation).
- Porto systemic shunt is NOT seen in **spleen** *(AIPG 2007)*
- Inferior epigastric vein drains into external iliac vein *(NEET Pattern 2015)*

◣ Lymphatics

- ☐ Aortic lymph nodes are present on the posterior abdominal wall and divided into – pre, lateral and retro aortic.
- ☐ Preaortic lymph nodes lie anterior to abdominal aorta and is divided into – Celiac, superior mesenteric and inferior mesenteric.
- ☐ They receive afferents from the intermediate nodes. And their efferents are the intestinal trunks which enter the cisterna chyli.
- ☐ Lateral aortic lymph nodes lie on each side of abdominal aorta and receive afferents mainly from the common iliac lymph nodes.
- ☐ The efferents form the lumbar trunks, which enter the cisterna chyli.
- ☐ Few efferents pass to pre-aortic/retroaortic lymph nodes.
- ☐ Retroaortic lymph nodes are considered as an extension of lateral aortic lymph nodes only.
- ☐ Lymph flow from the pelvic region: Sacral/External/Internal iliac → Common iliac → Lateral aortic → Lumbar trunks → Cisterna chyli. Lateral sacral lymph nodes drain into the common iliac group. Para-colic lymph nodes (midgut and hindgut) drain into the superior/inferior mesenteric lymph nodes—preaortic lymph nodes. The efferents are the intestinal trunks towards the cisterna chyli.

◣ Inguinal Region and External Genitalia

Inguinal Region. The inguinal region is an area of weakness of the anterior abdominal wall due to the penetration of the testes and spermatic cord (in males) or the round ligament of the uterus (in females) during embryologic development. **Deep inguinal ring** is an opening in the transversalis fascia, which continues into the inguinal canal as the internal fascia of the structures passing through the inguinal canal. **Superficial inguinal ring** is a defect in the aponeurosis of the **external oblique muscle** located lateral to the pubic tubercle. **Inguinal canal** is an obliquely oriented passageway that begins at the deep inguinal ring (i.e. the entrance) and ends at the superficial inguinal ring (i.e. the exit). The inguinal canal transmits the **spermatic cord** (in males) or **round ligament of the uterus** (in females). The inguinal canal also transmits blood vessels, lymphatic vessels, and the genital branch of the genitofemoral nerve in both sexes.

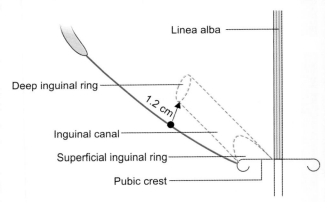

Fig. 28: Surface marking of the inguinal canal

Deep Inguinal Ring

- ☐ It is an oval opening in the **transversalis fascia**, approximately midway between the anterior superior iliac spine and the pubic symphysis, and about 1 cm above the inguinal ligament.
- ☐ It is related above to the arched lower margin of transversus abdominis and medially to the interfoveolar ligament.
- ☐ The inferior epigastric vessels are important medial relations of the deep inguinal ring. They lie on the transversalis fascia as they ascend obliquely behind the conjoint tendon to enter the rectus sheath.
  The length of inguinal canal is 4 cm *(NBEP 2013)*

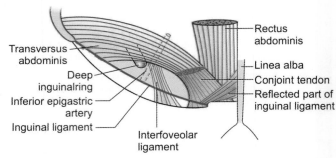

Fig. 29: Interfoveolar ligament

Inguinal Ligament (Poupart Ligament)

❑ Is the coiled lower border of the aponeurosis of the external oblique muscle, extending between the anterior superior iliac spine and the pubic tubercle.
❑ Forms the **floor (inferior wall)** of the inguinal canal.
❑ Modifications of external oblique muscle:
  ➤ Inguinal ligament, lacunar ligament, pectineal (Cooper's) ligament, external spermatic fascia.

Reflected Inguinal Ligament

❑ Is formed by fibers derived from the medial portion of the inguinal ligament and lacunar ligament and runs upward over the conjoint tendon to end at the linea alba.

Falx Inguinalis (Conjoint Tendon)

❑ Is formed by the aponeuroses of the internal oblique and transverse muscles of the abdomen and is inserted into the pubic tubercle and crest.
❑ It descends behind the superficial inguinal ring and strengthens the posterior wall of the medial half of the inguinal canal.

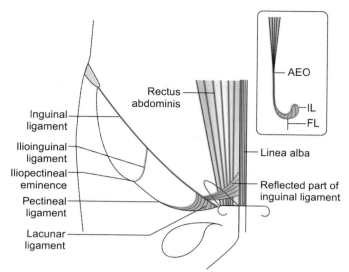

Fig. 30: Inguinal ligament and its extensions. Figure in the inset shows formation of inguinal ligament and its attachment to the fascia lata (AEO = aponeurosis of external bolique, IL = inguinal ligament, FL = fascia lata)

Lacunar Ligament (Gimbernat Ligament)

❑ Represents the medial triangular expansion of the inguinal ligament to the pectineal line of the pubis.
❑ Forms the medial border of the femoral ring and the floor of the inguinal canal.

Pectineal (Cooper) Ligament

❑ Is a strong fibrous band that extends laterally from the lacunar ligament along the pectineal line of the pubis.

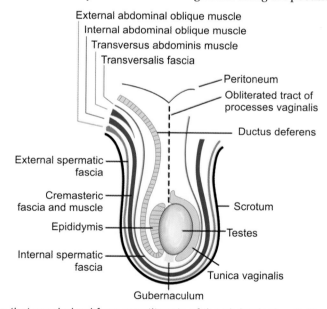

Fig. 31: Coverings of the testes that are derived from constituents of the abdominal wall. These coverings are formed as the testes migrate through the wall in route from their retroperitoneal location in the abdominal cavity to the scrotum

The Scrotum

A. General Features. The scrotum is an outpouching of the lower abdominal wall, whereby layers of the abdominal wall continue into the scrotal area to cover the spermatic cord and testes.

Table 14: Comparison between the layers of the anterior abdominal wall and the scrotum

Layer of anterior abdominal wall	Layer of scrotum
Skin	Skin
Superficial fascia	Dartos muscle
External oblique muscles	External spermatic fascia
Internal oblique muscle	Cremasteric muscle and fascia
Transversus abdominis muscle	No corresponding layer (Note: The transversus abdominis muscle does not continue into the scrotum)
Fascia transversalis	Internal spermatic fascia

❑ **Inguinal canal** is an oblique passage in the lower part of the anterior abdominal wall, situated just above the medial half of the inguinal ligament. It is about **3.75 cm** (1.5 inches) long, and is directed downwards, forwards and medially extending from the deep inguinal ring to the superficial inguinal ring. The deep inguinal ring is an oval opening in the fascia transversalis, situated 1.2 cm above the mid-inguinal point, and immediately lateral to the stem of the inferior epigastric artery. The superficial inguinal ring is a triangular gap in the external oblique aponeurosis. It is shaped like an obtuse angled triangle.

❑ Anterior wall (in its whole extent) is formed by skin; superficial fascia; and external oblique aponeurosis. In its lateral one-third the fleshy fibers of the internal oblique muscle are also present. The posterior wall (in its whole extent) is formed by the fascia transversalis, extraperitoneal tissue, and parietal peritoneum. Additionally in its medial two-thirds is present the **conjoint tendon**; at its medial end the reflected part of the inguinal ligament, and over its lateral one-third the interfoveolar ligament. The roof is formed by the arched fibers of the internal oblique and transversus abdominis muscles and at the floor is the grooved upper surface or the inguinal ligament; and at the medial end by the **lacunar ligament**.

Table 15: Features of the inguinal canal

Features		Formed by
Boundaries	▪ Anterior wall	External oblique aponeurosis (supplemented by internal oblique)
	▪ Posterior wall	Fascia transversalis (supplemented by conjoint tendon in the medial 2/3rd)
	▪ Roof	Internal oblique and transversus abdominis muscles (arched fibers)
	▪ Floor	Inguinal ligament (supplemented by lacunar ligament medially)
Openings	▪ Superficial inguinal ring	Triangular aperture in external oblique aponeurosis above and lateral to the pubic crest
	▪ Deep inguinal ring	Oval aperture in fascia transversalis 1.25 cm above the midinguinal point

Contents of inguinal canal

❑ Spermatic cord in male or round ligament of uterus in female.
❑ Ilioinguinal nerve: It enters through the interval between external and internal oblique muscles.
❑ Genital branch of genitofemoral nerve is a constituent of spermatic cord.

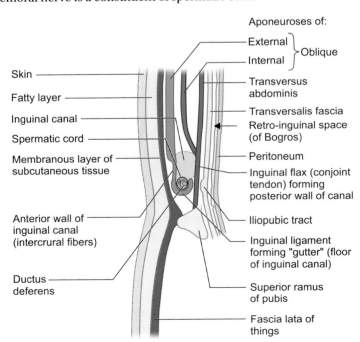

Aponeuroses of:
External ⎫
Internal ⎬ Oblique

Skin
Fatty layer
Inguinal canal
Spermatic cord
Membranous layer of subcutaneous tissue
Anterior wall of inguinal canal (intercrural fibers)
Ductus deferens

Transversus abdominis
Transversalis fascia
Retro-inguinal space (of Bogros)
Peritoneum
Inguinal flax (conjoint tendon) forming posterior wall of canal
Iliopubic tract
Inguinal ligament forming "gutter" (floor of inguinal canal)
Superior ramus of pubis
Fascia lata of things

Fig. 32: Schematic sagittal section of inguinal canal

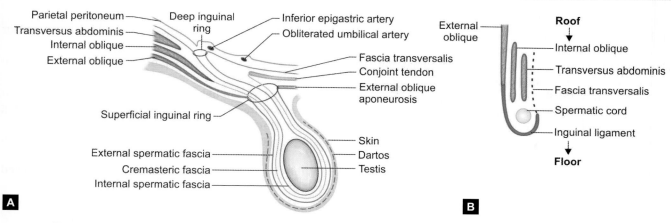

Figs. 33A and B: Boundaries of the inguinal canal: A. Anterior and posterior walls as seen in coronal section; B. Roof and floor as seen in sagittal section

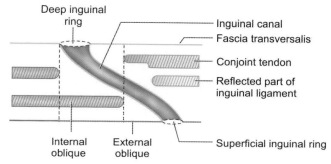

Fig. 34: Structures protecting the anterior and posterior walls of the inguinal canal

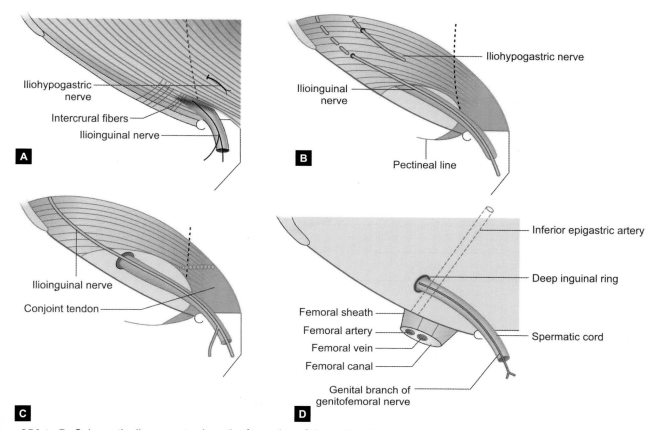

Figs. 35A to D: Schematic diagrams to show the formation of the walls of inguinal canal from outside inwards: A. External oblique; B. Internal oblique; C. Transversus abdominis; D. Fascia transversalis. The formation of anterior and posterior walls and location of inguinal rings can easily be deduced from these figures

Integrity of inguinal canal is maintained by:
- ❑ **Flap-valve Mechanism**: The canal is **oblique** and in occasion of raised intra-abdominal pressure, the anterior and posterior walls of the canal are **approximated** like a flap.
- ❑ **Guarding** of the Inguinal Rings: Deep inguinal ring is guarded **anteriorly by the internal oblique** muscle, and superficial inguinal ring is guarded **posteriorly by the conjoint tendon** and reflected part of the inguinal ligament.
- ❑ **Shutter Mechanism**: Internal oblique surrounds the canal in **front, above, and behind** like a flexible mobile arch, upon it contraction the roof is pulled and **approximated** on the floor like a **shutter**. **Conjoint tendon** is formed by the merging fibers of internal oblique and transversus abdominis muscle on **posterior wall** of inguinal canal.
- ❑ **Slit-valve Mechanism**: Contraction of external oblique muscle approximates the **two crura** (medial and lateral) of superficial inguinal ring like a **slit valve**.
- ❑ **Ball-valve Mechanism**: Contraction of **cremaster muscle** pulls the testis up and the superficial inguinal ring is **plugged** by the spermatic cord.

Table 16: Structures passing through the deep and superficial inguinal rings	
Deep inguinal ring	
In male	**In female**
▪ Ductus deferens and its artery ▪ Testicular artery and the accompanying veins ▪ Obliterated remains of processus vaginalis ▪ Genital branch of genitofemoral nerve ▪ Autonomic nerves and lymphatics	▪ Round ligment of uterus ▪ Obliterated remains of processus vaginalis ▪ Lymphatics from the uterus
Superficial inguinal ring	
In male	**In female**
▪ Spermatic cord ▪ Ilioinguinal nerve*	▪ Round ligament of uterus ▪ Ilioinguinal nerve*

*Ilioinguinal nerve enters the inguinal canal by piercing the wall and not through the deep inguinal ring

Iliopubic tract

It is the thickened inferior margin of the fascia transversalis which appears as a fibrous band running parallel and deep (posterior) to the inguinal ligament. When the inguinal region is viewed from its posterior aspect, the iliopubic tract is seen running posterior to inguinal ligament.

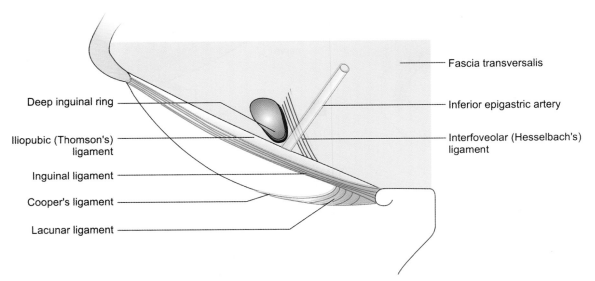

Fig. 36: Iliopubic tract

Iliopectineal arcus or ligament in the pelvi-femoral space

- ❑ Is a fascial partition that separates the muscular (lateral) and vascular (medial) lacunae deep to the inguinal ligament.
  - ➢ The muscular lacuna transmits the iliopsoas muscle.
  - ➢ The vascular lacuna transmits the femoral sheath and its contents, including the femoral vessels, a femoral branch of the genitofemoral nerve, and the femoral canal.

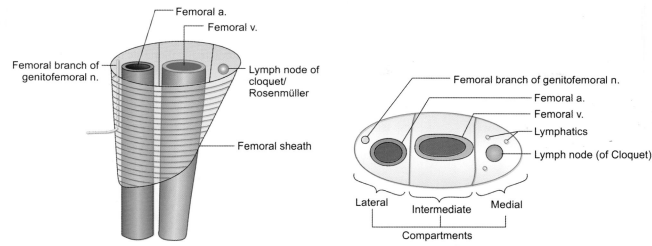

Fig. 37: Walls and contents of the femoral sheath (anterior view)

Fig. 38: Compartment of the femoral sheath

Femoral sheath is a funnel-shaped fascial sheath enclosing the upper 3–4 cm of the femoral vessels. It has three compartments:

- ❏ **Lateral** compartment contains femoral artery and femoral branch of the genitofemoral nerve
- ❏ **Intermediate** compartment contains the femoral vein
- ❏ **Medial** compartment (**femoral canal**) contains deep inguinal lymph node and lymphatics.

▶ Triangles

Inguinal triangle (of Hesselbach)

- ❏ It is bounded inferiorly by the medial third of the inguinal ligament, medially by the lower lateral border of rectus abdominis, and laterally by the inferior epigastric vessels.
- ❏ It is related to the posterior wall of inguinal canal.

Inguinal Triangle (Hesselbach's Triangle)

The inguinal triangle is situated deep to the posterior wall of the inguinal canal; hence, it is seen on the inner aspect of the lower part of the anterior abdominal wall.

Boundaries

- ❏ The boundaries of the inguinal triangle are as follows:
- ❏ Medial: Lower 5 cm of the lateral border of the rectus abdominis muscle.
- ❏ Lateral: Inferior epigastric artery.
- ❏ Inferior: Medial half of the inguinal ligament.
- ❏ The floor of the triangle is covered by the peritoneum, extra-peritoneal tissue, and fascia transversalis.

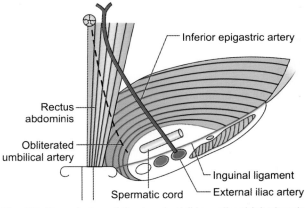

Fig. 39: Boundaries of the inguinal (Hesselbach's) triangle

Note: The medial umbilical ligament (obliterated umbilical artery) crosses the triangle and divides it into medial and lateral parts. The medial part of the floor of the triangle is strengthened by the conjoint tendon.

- ❏ The lateral part of the floor of the triangle is weak, hence direct inguinal hernia usually occurs through this part.

Triangle of Doom is bounded by **testicular vessels** laterally, **vas deferens** medially and **peritoneal fold** covering external iliac vessels at the base.

- ❏ The **apex** is directed towards the deep inguinal ring.
- ❏ **Contents**: External iliac vessels
- ❏ **Applied anatomy**: During laparoscopic repair of inguinal hernia, application of **staples is avoided** in this triangle so as to prevent injury to the contents–external iliac vessels.

Triangle of Pain: A triangular area in the inguinal region, encountered during surgery for inguinal hernias, bounded inferomedially by **gonadal vessels** and superolaterally by the **iliopubic tract**; the lateral femoral cutaneous nerve and the femoral branch of the genitofemoral nerve pass through this area and could be entrapped by staples during surgical procedures.

❑ During laparoscopic inguinal hernia repair, if a tacker is placed below and lateral to the iliopubic tract, the nerve involved is—lateral cutaneous nerve of thigh. It gives features like Meralgia paresthetica.

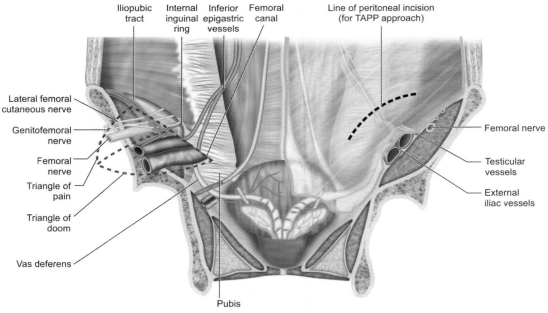

Fig. 40: Antevior abdominal wall (interior view)

1. **Triangle of Doom is bounded by all EXCEPT:** *(AIIMS 2008)*
   a. Vas deferens
   b. Testicular vessels
   c. Cooper ligament
   d. Reflected peritoneal fold

2. **Which structure (s) passes behind the inguinal ligament?** *(PGIC 2010)*
   a. Femoral branch of genitofemoral nerve
   b. Saphenous vein
   c. Superficial epigastric artery
   d. Psoas major
   e. Femoral vein

3. **All are boundaries of inguinal triangle EXCEPT:**
   a. Inguinal ligament
   b. Medial border of pyramidalis
   c. Inferior epigastric vein
   d. Lateral border of rectus abdominis

4. **Content of deep inguinal ring:** *(NEET Pattern 2016)*
   a. Inferior epigastric vessels
   b. Spermatic cord
   c. Ilioinguinal nerve
   d. Femoral branch of genitofemoral nerve

5. **Protective mechanism of inguinal canal:** *(NEET Pattern 2016)*
   a. Obliquity of inguinal canal
   b. Contraction of cremasteric muscle
   c. Contraction of conjoint tendon
   d. All of the above

6. **TRUE about inguinal canal:** *(PGIC 2003)*
   a. It is an intermuscular canal
   b. In male vas deferens passes through it
   c. Superficial inguinal ring is situated superior and lateral to pubic tubercle
   d. Deep inguinal ring is supero-medial to attachment of rectus abdominis
   e. Transmits blood vessels and nerves through it

7. **All of the following are true about inguinal canal EXCEPT:** *(AIPG 2001)*
   a. Conjoint tendon forms part of the posterior wall
   b. Superficial ring is present in external oblique aponeurosis
   c. Deep ring is an opening in transversalis abdominis
   d. Internal oblique forms both roof and anterior wall

8. **TRUE about deep inguinal ring is:** *(AIIMS 2005)*
   a. A defect in fascia transversalis
   b. Lies an inch above the mid-inguinal point
   c. Present medial to inferior epigastric artery
   d. Commonest site of direct hernia

9. **Structures passing through the inguinal canal are all EXCEPT:** *(AIPG 2012; NEET Pattern 2014)*
   a. Genital branch of genitofemoral nerve
   b. Ilio-inguinal nerve
   c. Inferior epigastric artery
   d. Lymphatics from uterus

10. **Which of the following are associated with external oblique muscles:** *(PGIC 2014)*
    a. Poupart's ligament
    b. Lacunar ligament
    c. Superficial inguinal ring
    d. Conjoint tendon
    e. Cremaster muscle

QUESTIONS

QUESTIONS

11. **Roof of inguinal canal is /are formed by:** *(PGIC 2013)*
    a. Internal oblique muscle
    b. Fascia transversalis
    c. Transversus abdominis muscles
    d. External oblique muscle
    e. Conjoint tendon

12. **Which of the following statement is TRUE about conjoint tendon:** *(NEET Pattern 2014)*
    a. Formed by internal oblique and transversus abdominis
    b. Forms the posterior wall of inguinal canal
    c. It is pushed anteriorly by direct inguinal hernia
    d. All of the above

ANSWERS

1. **c. Cooper's ligament**
   - ❑ Cooper's ligament is **not** the boundary for triangle of Doom.
   - ❑ Triangle is bounded by: **Vas deferens** medially, **testicular vessels** laterally and a **peritoneal fold** at the base covering external iliac vessels (these vessels become **content** of the triangle as well).
   - ❑ The **apex** is directed towards the **deep inguinal ring**.

2. **a. Femoral branch of genitofemoral nerve; d. Psoas major; e) Femoral vein**
   - ❑ The muscles (psoas major and iliacus) and neurovascular structures of posterior abdominal wall/pelvis pass into the femoral region of the thigh **through this space**.
   - ❑ This space is called as **pelvi-femoral space**, ilio-pectineal arcus lies here.
   - ❑ Saphenous vein joins femoral vein **below** inguinal ligament.
   - ❑ Superficial epigastric artery passes **anterior** to inguinal ligament.

3. **b. Medial border of pyramidalis**
   - ❑ Hesselbach's inguinal triangle is present on the anteroinferior abdominal wall bounded by the **rectus abdominis** muscle, the **inguinal ligament**, and the **inferior epigastric vessels**.

4. **b. Spermatic cord**
   - ❑ **Spermatic cord** passes through deep inguinal ring. Inferior epigastric vessels **lie medial** to the ring.
   - ❑ Genital (**not femoral**) branch of genitofemoral nerve passes through deep inguinal ring.
   - ❑ Ilioinguinal nerve enters the inguinal canal by piercing the wall and **not through the deep inguinal ring**.

5. **d. All of the above**
   - ❑ Integrity of inguinal canal is maintained by: **Flap-valve** mechanism, **shutter** mechanism, **slit-valve** mechanism, **ball-valve** mechanism.

6. **a. It is an intermuscular canal; b. In male vas deferens passes through it; c. Superficial inguinal ring is situated superior and lateral to pubic tubercle; e. Transmits blood vessels and nerves through it**
   - ❑ Inguinal canal is an **intermuscular** canal surrounded by anterior abdominal wall muscles.
   - ❑ It transmits the **vas deferens** (inside spermatic cord), in males and round ligament of the uterus, in females.
   - ❑ Superficial inguinal ring is an aponeurotic opening in the external oblique muscle, lying **supero-lateral** to pubic tubercle.
   - ❑ Deep inguinal ring is a deficiency in the fascia transversalis.
   - ❑ Inguinal canal transmits **blood vessels**, lymphatic vessels, and the genital branch of the genitofemoral **nerve** in both sexes.

7. **c. Deep ring is an opening in transversalis abdominis**
   - ❑ Deep inguinal ring is an opening in the transversalis fascia (**not the muscle**).
   - ❑ Internal oblique muscle and transversalis muscles **arch over** inguinal canal as roof and reach posterior wall, where together they form **conjoint tendon**.

8. **a. A defect in fascia transversalis**
   - ❑ Deep inguinal ring is present 1/2 inch (1.25cm) above the **mid-inguinal point**.
   - ❑ The ring is present lateral (**not medial**) to Inferior epigastric artery (and vein).
   - ❑ Indirect (**not direct**) inguinal hernia comes through the deep inguinal ring.

9. **c. Inferior epigastric artery**
   - ❑ Inferior epigastric artery is a branch given by external iliac artery, which ascends supero-medially, becomes **medial relation of deep inguinal ring**, and subsequently enters rectus sheath.
   - ❑ It is **not a content** of inguinal canal.
   - ❑ **Lymphatics** from uterus follow the round ligament of uterus through the inguinal canal.

10. **a. Poupart's ligament; b. Lacunar ligament; c. Superficial inguinal ring.**
    - ❑ Poupart's (Inguinal) ligament is the lower in-turned **modification of external oblique** muscle, it further sends **lacunar ligament** posteriorly to attach to pectineal line.
    - ❑ Superficial inguinal **ring** is an aponeurotic opening in **external oblique** muscle.
    - ❑ Conjoint tendon is formed by the converging fibers of **internal oblique** and **transversus abdominis** muscle on the posterior wall of inguinal canal.
    - ❑ Cremaster muscle is an extension of **internal oblique** muscle into the scrotum.

11. **a. Internal oblique muscle; c. Transversus abdominis muscles**
    - ❑ The roof is formed by the **arched fibers** of the internal oblique and transversus abdominis muscles.

12. **d. All of the above**
    - ❑ Conjoint tendon is present in the **posterior wall** of inguinal canal (medial 2/3).
    - ❑ It is formed by the **merging fibers** of internal oblique and transversus abdominis muscles.
    - ❑ It becomes one of the covering of the **medial direct hernia**, coming through the medial part of the **Hesselbach's triangle**.

▶ Inguinal Hernia

Inguinal Hernia

- ❏ Although the inguinal canal is arranged such that the weaknesses in the anterior abdominal wall caused by the deep and superficial inguinal rings are supported, the region is a common site of herniation, particularly in males.
- ❏ An inguinal hernia involves the protrusion of a viscus through the tissues of the inguinal region of the abdominal wall.

Indirect Inguinal Hernia

- ❏ An indirect inguinal hernia arises through the deep inguinal ring lateral to the inferior epigastric vessels.
- ❏ Many indirect hernias are related to the abnormal persistence of a patent processus vaginalis, a tube-like extension of peritoneum through the inguinal canal that is present during normal development and normally becomes occluded after birth.
- ❏ Others are acquired as a result of progressive weakening of the posterior wall of the inguinal canal in the region of the deep inguinal ring.
- ❏ The hernia may pass through the deep ring or may expand the deep ring such that it is no longer a clear entity.
- ❏ Small indirect hernias lie below and lateral to the fibers of the conjoint tendon, but larger hernias often distort and thin the tendon superiorly.
- ❏ Small indirect hernias that do not protrude beyond the inguinal canal are covered by the same inner layers as the spermatic cord: namely, the internal spermatic fascia and cremaster.
- ❏ If the hernia extends through the superficial inguinal ring, it is also covered by external spermatic fascia.
- ❏ In hernias related to a persistent fully patent processus vaginalis, the hernia contents may descend as far as the tunica vaginalis anterior to the testis.
- ❏ In many individuals with a partial or fully patent processus vaginalis, an indirect hernia will manifest in childhood, but in others, an actual hernia into the potential sac may not develop until adult life, often as a consequence of increased intra-abdominal pressure or sudden muscular strain.

Direct Inguinal Hernia

- ❏ A direct inguinal hernia arises **medial** to the inferior epigastric vessels.
- ❏ Direct hernias are always caused by an acquired weakness of the posterior wall of the inguinal canal; as they enlarge, they frequently extend through the anterior wall of the inguinal canal or superficial inguinal ring, becoming covered by external spermatic fascia in the process.
- ❏ A direct inguinal hernia may closely resemble an indirect hernia and can be difficult to distinguish on clinical examination.

Clinical Features of Inguinal Hernias

- ❏ Indirect inguinal hernias often descend from lateral to medial, following the path of the inguinal canal, whereas direct inguinal hernias tend to protrude more directly anteriorly.
- ❏ With the hernia reduced, pressure applied over the region of the deep inguinal ring may prevent the appearance of an indirect hernia on standing or straining, but distinguishing an indirect from a direct inguinal hernia by clinical examination alone is not reliable (Ralphs et al 1980, Tromp et al 2014).
- ❏ Direct hernias are more likely to have a wide neck, making strangulation less likely.

Types of Hernias

1. **Direct Inguinal Hernia**
2. **Indirect Inguinal Hernia**
3. **Femoral Hernia**

Note: Surgical hernia repair may damage the **iliohypogastric nerve,** causing anesthesia of the ipsilateral abdominal wall and inguinal region, and/or the **ilioinguinal nerve,** causing anesthesia of the ipsilateral penis, scrotum, and medial thigh.

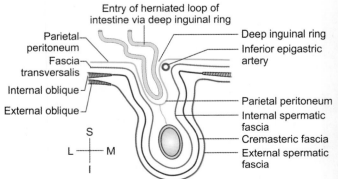

Fig. 41: Coverings of the indirecti inguinal hernia

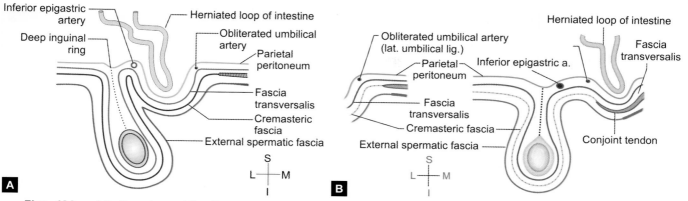

Figs. 42A and B: Coverings of the direct inguinal hernia: A. Lateral direct inguinal hernia; B. Medial direct inguinal hernia

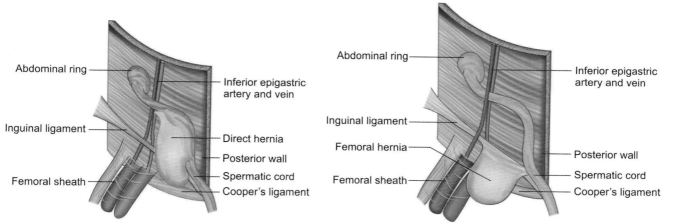

Fig. 43: Direct inguinal hernia. The abdominal ring is intact. A hernia defect is a diffuse bulge in the posterior inguinal wall medial to the inferior epigastric vessels

Fig. 44: Femoral hernia. The defect is through the femoral canal, but otherwise involves similar strucutres and insertions as a direct inguinal hernia

Table 17: Differences between inguinal and femoral hernias		
	Inguinal hernia	**Femoral hernia**
Sex	More common in males	More common in females
Protrusion of hernial sac	Into inguinal canal	Into femoral canal
Neck of protrusion of hernia	Lies above and medial to pubic tubercle	Lies below and lateral to the pubic tubercle

Table 18: Differences between the indirect and direct inguinal hernia		
	Indirect inguinal hernia	**Direct inguinal hernia**
Site of protrusion of hernial sac	Deep inguinal ring	Posterior wall of inguinal canal
Shape	Pear shaped	Globular
Extent	Generally scrotal	Rarely scrotal
Direction	Oblique (directed downward, forward, and medially)	Straight (directed forward)
Neck of hernial sac	Narrow and lies lateral to the inferior epigastric vessels	Wide and lies medial to the inferior epigastric vessels
Reducibility	Sometimes irreducible	Generally always reducible
Age group	Occurs in young age	Occurs in middle and old age
Interanal ring occlusion test*	Positive	Negative

*After reducing the hernia, the pressure is applied over deep inguinal ring and patient is asked to cough. If hernia does not appear, it is indirect (because herniation occurs through the deep inguinal ring), and if hernia appears, it is direct (because herniation occurs through the Hesselbach's triangle).

Femoral Hernia

- **Femoral hernia** passes through the femoral ring into the femoral canal, and **femoral vein** lies lateral to it.
- Femoral hernias occur just below the inguinal ligament, when abdominal contents pass through a naturally occurring weakness called the **femoral canal.**
- The femoral canal is located below the inguinal ligament on the lateral aspect of the pubic tubercle.
- The hernia must pass the **femoral ring** to enter the femoral canal.
- The ring is bounded by the inguinal ligament anteriorly, **pectineal ligament** posteriorly, **lacunar ligament** medially, and the femoral vein laterally.
- The three compartments of the femoral sheath (From lateral to medial): **Femoral artery** and its branches, **Femoral vein** and its tributaries, Femoral canal, which contains lymphatic vessels and deep inguinal lymph nodes.

QUESTIONS

1. TRUE about anatomy of inguinal hernia: *(PGIC 2005)*
   a. Superficial inguinal ring is an opening in external oblique aponeurosis
   b. Indirect inguinal hernia lies just medial to inferior epigastric artery
   c. Posterior wall is formed by transversalis fascia and conjoint tendon
   d. Cremasteric artery is a branch of external iliac artery
   e. Indirect hernia lies anteromedial to spermatic cord

2. Which of the following does NOT form boundary of femoral ring: *(PGIC 2012)*
   a. Femoral artery
   b. Femoral vein
   c. Femoral nerve
   d. Lacunar ligament
   e. Inguinal ligament

3. A 30-year-old lady presented with swelling below inguinal ligament lateral to pubic tubercle, which structure is lateral to this swelling: *(JIPMER 2016)*
   a. Femoral artery
   b. Femoral vein
   c. Obturator vessels
   d. Internal iliac artery

ANSWERS

1. **a. Superficial inguinal ring is an opening in external oblique aponeurosis; c. Posterior wall is formed by transversalis fascia and conjoint tendon; e. Indirect hernia lies anteromedial to spermatic cord**
   - Indirect inguinal hernia lies just lateral (**not medial**) to inferior epigastric artery (and vein).
   - Cremasteric artery is a branch of **inferior epigastric artery** (which itself is a branch of external iliac artery).
   - Indirect inguinal hernia protrudes from peritoneal cavity into **deep inguinal ring**, lies anteromedial to spermatic cord, passes through inguinal canal, exit through superficial inguinal ring to enter the scrotum/labia majus.

2. **a. Femoral artery; c. Femoral nerve**
   - Femoral ring is bounded by the **inguinal ligament** anteriorly, **pectineal ligament** of Cooper posteriorly, **lacunar ligament** medially, and the **femoral vein** laterally.

3. **b. Femoral vein**
   - This is a case of **femoral hernia**, where the sac is **inferolateral** to the pubic tubercle (below the inguinal ligament).
   - The hernia passes through the femoral **ring** into the femoral **canal**, lateral to which lies the femoral vein.

- **Femoral vein** lies **lateral** to sheath of femoral hernia *(AIIMS 2011)*
- Femoral artery **doesn't** lie in the boundary of femoral ring *(AIPG 2005)*
- Femoral nerve lies **outside** the femoral sheath.
- In femoral hernia, the intestine may enter the **femoral ring**, and the **femoral canal** to reach **thigh** region, and lie **inferolateral** to pubic tubercle.
- **Inferior epigastric artery** enters the rectus sheath and is a landmark to **differentiate between** direct and indirect inguinal hernia.
- **Indirect inguinal** hernia: In young adults, intestine may pass through the deep inguinal ring (**lateral** to inferior epigastric artery), enter the inguinal canal and reach the scrotum.
- **Direct** inguinal hernia: In elderly patients, intestine may pass **medial** to inferior epigastric artery and enter the scrotum.

Note: Inguinal hernia (direct or indirect) lies supero-medial to pubic tubercle and enters the scrotum. Whereas, **femoral hernia** lies inferolateral to pubic tubercle and enters the thigh region.

- **Superficial inguinal ring** is a hiatus in the **aponeurosis** of external oblique, just **above and lateral** to the crest of the pubis.
- Deep inguinal ring is a deficiency in **transversalis fascia** *(AIIMS 2005)*

Spermatic Cord

- **Spermatic cord** is formed by the vas deferens and surrounding tissue that runs from the deep inguinal ring down to the testis.
- It has a serosal covering (tunica vaginalis), which is an extension of the peritoneum that passes through the transversalis fascia.
- It is ensheathed in three layers of tissue:
  - External spermatic fascia (derived from aponeurosis of the external oblique muscle)

- ➤ Cremasteric muscle and fascia (continuation of the internal oblique muscle and its fascia)
- ➤ Internal spermatic fascia (continuation of transversalis fascia)
- ❑ Contents:
  - ➤ Ductus deferens
  - ➤ Tunica vaginalis (remains of the processus vaginalis)
  - ➤ Arteries: testicular artery, artery to ductus deferens, cremasteric artery
  - ➤ Nerves: Nerve to cremaster (genital branch of the genitofemoral nerve), sympathetic and parasympathetic nerves (testicular plexus of nerves).

Note: Ilio-inguinal nerve is 'not' located inside the spermatic cord, but runs along the outside of it (in the inguinal canal) on the superficial surface of the external spermatic fascia.

- ➤ Pampiniform venous plexus
- ➤ Lymphatic vessels

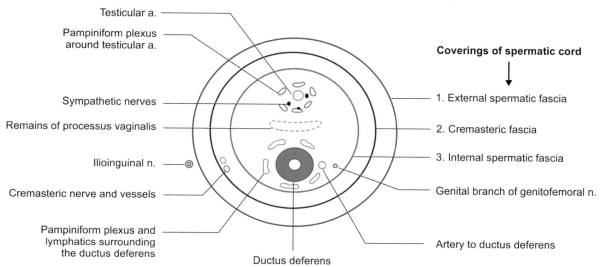

Fig. 45: Transverse section of the spermatic cord showing its covering content

1. All are components of Spermatic cord EXCEPT:
(NEET Pattern 2016)
- a. Genital branch of genitofemoral nerve
- b. Ilioinguinal nerve
- c. Vas deferens
- d. Pampiniform plexus

2. Coverings of spermatic cord are all EXCEPT:
(NEET Pattern 2016)
- a. Internal spermatic fascia
- b. Dartos muscle
- c. Cremasteric fascia
- d. External spermatic fascia

1. b. Ilioinguinal nerve
- ❑ Ilioinguinal nerve is **not** a content of spermatic cord.

2. b. Dartos muscle
- ❑ Dartos is a layer of connective tissue found in the **penile shaft** and **scrotum**.
- ❑ Ilioinguinal nerve is **not** a content of spermatic cord and is **NOT at risk** of injury during vasectomy *(AIIMS 2012)*

◤ Testis, Epididymis and Scrotum

- ❑ **Testis** develops retroperitoneally in the abdomen and descends into the pelvis and eventually reach scrotum.
- ❑ It is surrounded incompletely (medially, laterally, and anteriorly, but not posteriorly) by a sac of peritoneum called the **tunica vaginalis**.
- ❑ Beneath the tunica vaginalis, the testis is surrounded by a thick connective tissue capsule **tunica albuginea** (white).
- ❑ **Tunica vasculosa** is a highly vascular layer of connective tissue beneath the tunica albuginea.
- ❑ Tunica albuginea projects connective tissue septa inward toward the mediastinum and divides the testes into about 250 lobules, each of which contains one to four highly coiled **seminiferous tubules**. These septa converge toward the midline on the posterior surface, where they meet to form a ridge-like thickening known as the **mediastinum**.
- ❑ The testes contain the seminiferous tubules with Leydig (interstitial) cells.
- ❑ In the seminiferous tubules of the testes spermatogonial stem cells adjacent to the inner tubule wall divide in a centripetal direction, beginning at the walls and proceeding towards lumen, to produce sperm.

❑ Spermatogenesis takes **74 days** to complete and about 200 to 300 million spermatozoa are produced daily (about half of these become viable sperm).

❑ Leydig cells secrete **testosterone**, androstenedione and dehydro-epiandrosterone (DHEA), when stimulated by the pituitary hormone luteinizing hormone (LH).

❑ Sequence of sperm movement in testis: Seminiferous tubules → straight tubules → rete testis → efferent ductules in testis

Tunica vaginalis is the pouch of serous membrane that covers the testes. It is derived from the process vaginalis of the peritoneum, which in the fetus precedes the descent of the testes from the abdomen into the scrotum.

❑ It is the serous sac of the peritoneum that covers the front and sides of the testis and epididymis.

❑ It consists of a parietal layer that forms the innermost layer of the scrotum and a visceral layer adherent to the testis and epididymis.

❑ **Processus Vaginalis** is the embryonic diverticulum of the peritoneum that traverses the inguinal canal, accompanying the testis in its descent into the scrotum (or round ligament in the female) and closes forming the tunica vaginalis in the male. Persistent processus vaginalis leads to development of a congenital indirect inguinal hernia, but if its middle portion persists, it develops a congenital hydrocele.

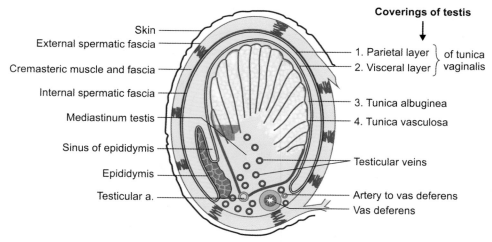

Fig. 46: Transverse section of the left testis and its surrounding structures to show the coverings of the testis

Arterial Supply

❑ **Testicular arteries** (branches of abdominal aorta, just inferior to the renal arteries).

❑ A rich collateral arterial supply comes from the internal iliac artery (via the artery of the ductus deferens), inferior epigastric artery (via the cremasteric artery), and femoral artery (via the external pudendal artery).

❑ The collateral circulation is sufficient to allow ligation of the testicular artery during surgery.

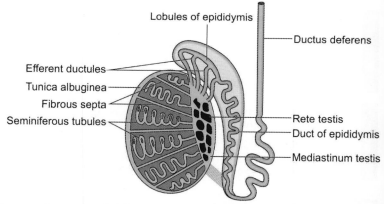

Fig. 47: Longitudinal section of the testis and epididymis showing their structures

Venous Drainage

❑ **Pampiniform plexus** of spermatic veins is present on the surface of the epididymis and run parallel to the spermatic arteries. This provides a countercurrent exchange of heat and testosterone between the two vessels.

❑ **Testicular veins** are formed by the union of the veins of the pampiniform plexus around testis.

❑ Right testicular vein empties into the inferior vena cava and the left testicular vein empties into the left renal vein.

Lymphatic Drainage

❑ Testicular lymphatics drain into the to the para (lateral) and pre (anterior) **aortic lymph nodes**.

Epididymis is a long (6 m) and highly coiled duct for propulsion of the spermatozoa into the ductus deferens.

❑ It has a head, body, and tail (which is continuous with the ductus deferens).

❑ Sperms undergo **maturation**, gain **progressive motility** in epididymis and are **stored there until ejaculation**.

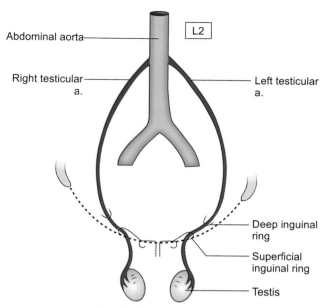

Fig. 48: Testicular arteries

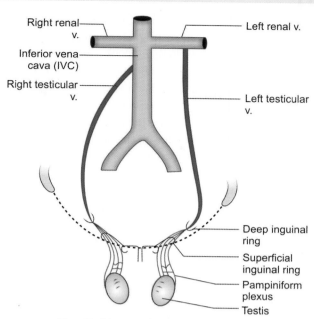

Fig. 49: Venous drainage of the testis

- The principal cells lining the epididymis have the following functions:
  - ➢ Continued resorption of testicular fluid that began in the efferent ductules.
  - ➢ Phagocytosis of degenerating sperm or spermatid residual bodies not phagocytosed by the Sertoli cells
  - ➢ Secretion of glycoproteins, which bind to the surface of the cell membrane of the sperm, sialic acid, and glycero-phospho-choline (which inhibits capacitation, thus preventing sperm from fertilizing a secondary oocyte until the sperm enters the female reproductive tract).
- In the tail region of the epididymis, the muscular coat consists of three layers: Inner longitudinal, middle circular and outer longitudinal layer of smooth muscle. These layers contract to force sperm from the tail of the epididymis to the ductus deferens (sperm emission).
- After the sperm have been in the epididymis for 18 to 24 hours, they develop the capability of motility, even though several inhibitory proteins in the epididymal fluid still prevent final motility until after ejaculation.

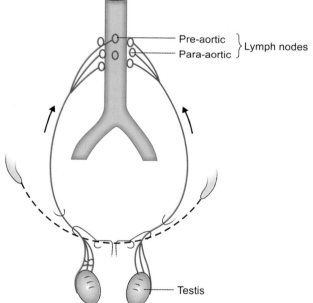

Fig. 50: Lymphatic drainage of the testis

- The transit time of sperm through the epididymis is thought to take up to 12 days, though sperms may be stored in the epididymis for several weeks.
- Once ejaculated into the female, the spermatozoa move up the uterus to the isthmus of the uterine tubes, to undergo **capacitation**.
  - ➢ This further maturation process involves two components: increasing the motility of the spermatozoa and facilitating their preparation for the acrosome reaction.
  - ➢ Capacitation normally lasts for 1 to 10 hours (average 7), during the process sperms gradually lose much of their other **excess cholesterol** and the acrosome membrane becomes much weaker. The membrane of the sperm also becomes much **more permeable to calcium ions**.
  - ➢ From the isthmus, the capacitated spermatozoa move rapidly to the tubal **ampulla**, where **fertilization** takes place.
- After ovulation has occurred, the oocyte (ovum) remains fertilizable for 48 hours, although the chance is mostly lost by **18–24 hours**.

- ❑ Spermatozoa have a life span of 24–48 hours within the female reproductive tract, if hostile mucus is absent.
  - ➢ When there is proper estrogenic cervical mucus, the fertilizing capacity of sperm can last 3–7 days in the periovulatory period (Pallone and Bergus, 2009).
  - ➢ Sperms **usually** do not retain their power of fertilization after **24–48 hours** of coitus.
- ❑ **Scrotum** contains the testis and the epididymis.
  - ➢ It regulates the temperature of the testes and maintains it at 35° Celsius (95° Fahrenheit), i.e. two degrees below the body temperature of 37° Celsius (98.6° Fahrenheit), which is an essential requirement for spermatogenesis.
  - ➢ It has thin skin covered with sparse hairs and no fat.
  - ➢ **Dartos** muscle is subcutaneous (which wrinkles the skin), and is continuous with the superficial penile fascia and superficial perineal fascia.
  - ➢ The **cremaster** muscle covers scrotum and upon contraction elevates the testis.
  - ➢ **Arterial supply**: External pudendal arteries and the posterior scrotal branches of the internal pudendal arteries.
  - ➢ **Nerve supply**: Anterior scrotal branch of the **ilioinguinal nerve**, the genital branch of **genitofemoral nerve**, the posterior scrotal branch of the perineal branch of the **pudendal nerve**, and the perineal branch of the posterior femoral cutaneous nerve.

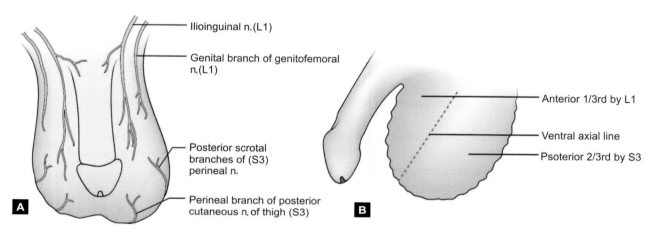

Figs. 51A and B: Nerve supply of the scrotum: A. Cutaneous nerves of the scrotum anterior view; B. Lateral view showing segmental innervation

Dartos is a layer of connective tissue found in the **penile** shaft and **scrotum**.
- ❑ Penile portion is referred to as the **superficial fascia of penis**, which continues as scrotal part as the dartos proper.
- ❑ It is also **continuous with Colles fascia** of the perineum and **Scarpa's fascia** of the abdomen.
- ❑ It lies just below the skin, **just superficial to** the external spermatic fascia in the scrotum and to Buck's fascia in the penile shaft.
- ❑ It has **smooth** muscles, which receive innervation from postganglionic **sympathetic** nerve fibers arriving via the ilioinguinal nerve and the posterior scrotal nerve.

QUESTIONS

1. **Sperm maturation takes place in:** (NEET Pattern 2012)
   a. Vas deferens
   b. Seminiferous tubules
   c. Epididymis
   d. Female genital tract

2. **CORRECT sequence of sperm movements:** (AIPG 2008)
   a. Rete testis → straight tubules → efferent ductules
   b. Straight tubules → efferent ductules → epididymis
   c. Efferent ductules → rete testis → straight tubules
   d. Straight tubules → rete testis → efferent ductules

3. **Injury to which nerve during a herniorrhaphy may cause paraesthesia at the root of scrotum and base of penis:** (AIIMS 2001)
   a. Ilioinguinal
   b. Pudendal
   c. Genitofemoral
   d. Iliohypogastric

ANSWERS

1. **c. Epididymis**
   - ❑ Spermatozoa undergo a **maturation** process and acquire motility and fertility as they migrate from the proximal to the distal end of **epididymis**.
   - ❑ The process of maturation **continues in the female genital tract** as well.

2. **d. Straight tubules → rete testis → efferent ductules**
   - ❑ Sperms form in the **seminiferous tubules** and pass on to the **straight tubules** (tubuli recti).
   - ❑ Next, they enter a network of tubules (**rete testis**) and then reach the **efferent ductules**.
   - ❑ Efferent ductules lead them to the **epididymis** where storage takes place **before ejaculation**.

3. a. **Ilioinguinal**
   - ❑ During herniorrhaphy **ilio-inguinal** nerve is damaged, while working in the **inguinal canal,** whereas, ilio-hypogastric nerve may be damaged while putting the incision for herniorrhaphy at the inguinal region.
   - ❑ Ilioinguinal nerve pierces the obliquus internus, distributing filaments to it, and, accompanying the spermatic cord through the superficial inguinal ring, is distributed to the skin of the **upper and medial part of the thigh**, and to the following locations in the male and female:
     - ▪ In the male (anterior scrotal nerve) to the skin over the **root** of the penis and **anterior** part of the scrotum
     - ▪ In the female (anterior labial nerve) to the skin covering the **mons pubis** and **labium majus**
   - ❑ Ilio-hypogastric nerve supplies skin over the iliac crest, upper inguinal and hypogastric areas. (not the scrotum or penis).

- ▪ **Right** testicular vein drains into **IVC** *(JIPMER 2016)*
- ▪ **Left** testicular vein drains into **Left** renal vein *(NEET Pattern 2015)*
- ▪ Most of the sperms are stored in the **epididymis**, although a small quantity is stored in the **vas deferens.**
- ▪ Lymphatic drainage of testes is **Para-aortic** lymph nodes *(NEET Pattern 2012)*
- ▪ Left testis descent begins early, and it lies slightly at the lower level than the right (**Left - Lower**) *(NEET Pattern 2013)*
- ▪ The intricately and prodigiously looped system of veins and arteries that lie on the surface of the epididymis is known as **pampiniform plexus** of veins *(AIPG 2004)*
- ▪ **Capacitance** of sperm takes place in **isthmus of the uterine tubes.**
- ▪ Sperm acquires motility in **Epididymis** *(NEET Pattern 2014)*
- ▪ Normal volume of adult testis is **15-20 mL** *(NEET Pattern 2016)*
  - – Testis measure 4–5 cm in length, 2–3 cm in breadth and 3–4 cm in anteroposterior diameter; their weight varies between 12 and 20 g.
- ▪ **Corpus spongiosum** get terminally expanded to form **glans penis.**
- ▪ Penile urethra runs in **corpus spongiosum.**
- ▪ **Anterior one third** of scrotum is supplied by **ilioinguinal** nerve (L1) and **genital branch** of the genitofemoral nerve (L1) *(NEET Pattern 2016)*
- ▪ **Posterior two third** of scrotum is supplied by **posterior scrotal nerves** (S3) and perineal branch of **posterior cutaneous nerve** of thigh(S3).
- ▪ **Dartos** muscle and **cremasteric** muscles are supplied by the **genital branch** of the genitofemoral nerve.
- ▪ Cremasteric artery is a branch of inferior epigastric artery *(NEET Pattern 2015)*
  - – It accompanies the spermatic cord and anastomoses with the testicular artery (internal spermatic artery).

◤ Prostate Gland

- ❑ Prostate gland is located between the base of the urinary bladder and the urogenital diaphragm.
- ❑ It consists of glandular tissue in fibromuscular stroma.
- ❑ It has **three surfaces**:
  - ➢ Muscular anterior surface related to the retropubic space
  - ➢ Inferior lateral surfaces related to the levator ani
  - ➢ Posterior surface related to the seminal vesicles and the ampulla of the rectum.

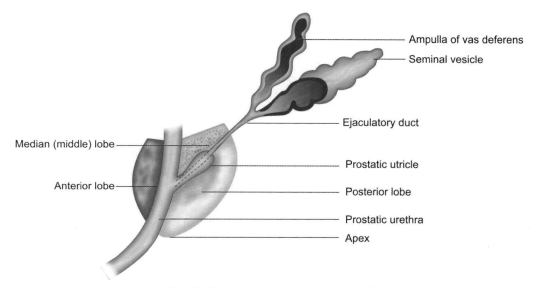

Fig. 52: Prostate gland (sagittal section)

Name	Fraction of gland	Description
Peripheral zone	~70%	The sub-capsular portion of the posterior aspect of the prostate gland that surrounds the distal urethra and is prone to cancer.
Central zone	~25%	It lies posterior to urethra and surrounds the ejaculatory ducts, accounts for ~2.5% of prostate cancers.
Transition zone	~5%	It surrounds the proximal urethra (periurethral zone) and grows throughout life and is responsible for the benign prostatic hypertrophy. ~10–20% of prostate cancers originate in this zone.
Anterior fibromuscular zone	~5%	It has fibromuscular components only (glandular components absent)

- ❑ It has **five lobes** developmentally and are well observed in fetal prostate:
  - ➤ Anterior lobe (or isthmus) lies in front of the urethra and is devoid of glandular substance.
  - ➤ Middle (median) lobe, which lies between the urethra and the ejaculatory ducts and is prone to BPH (benign prostatic hypertrophy) obstructing the internal urethral orifice.
  - ➤ Posterior lobe, which lies behind the urethra and below the ejaculatory ducts., contains glandular tissue, and is prone to carcinomatous transformation.
  - ➤ Lateral lobes (a pair), which are situated on either side of the urethra and form the main mass of the gland.
- ❑ Cut surface of an adult prostate do not resemble to lobes and is described in **four zones**:
- ❑ **Anterior** lobe roughly corresponds to part of **transitional** zone; **posterior** lobe to **peripheral** zone; lateral lobes span all zones and **median** lobe roughly corresponds to part of **central** zone.

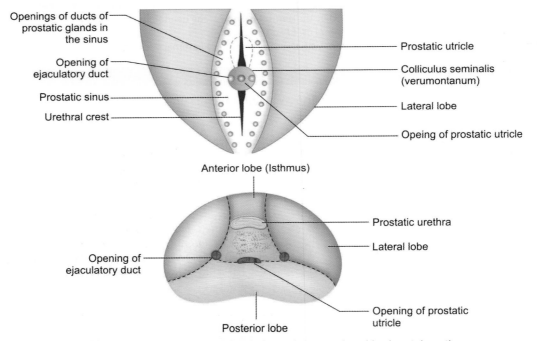

Fig. 53: Lobes of the prostate gland shown in coronal and horizontal sections

- ❑ Prostate has the **urethral crest** located on the posterior wall of the prostatic urethra.
  - ➤ There are numerous openings for the prostatic ducts on either side in **prostatic sinus** — a groove between the urethral crest and the wall of the prostatic urethra.
  - ➤ The crest has a rounded elevation called the **seminal colliculus** (verumontanum), on which the two ejaculatory ducts and the prostatic utricle open.
  - ➤ **Prostatic utricle** is a blind pouch (5 mm deep); it is considered as an analogue to the uterus and vagina in the female.
- ❑ Prostate secretes a fluid that produces the characteristic odor of semen.
- ❑ In the secretions are prostate-specific antigen (PSA), prostaglandins, citric acid and acid phosphatase, and proteolytic enzymes.

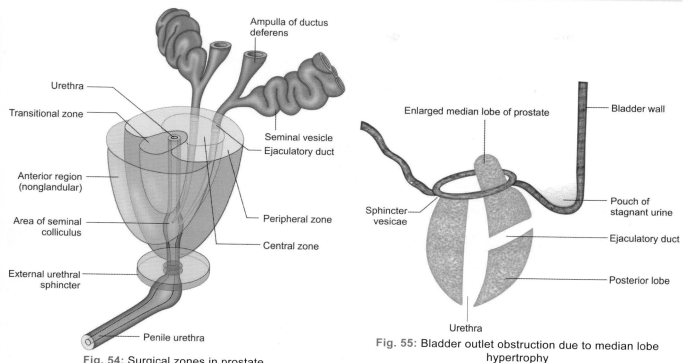

Fig. 54: Surgical zones in prostate

Fig. 55: Bladder outlet obstruction due to median lobe hypertrophy

Arterial Supply

Prostate gland is supplied by the branches of inferior vesical, middle rectal, and internal pudendal arteries (branches of internal iliac artery).

Venous Drainage

Prostate drains by two pathways:

❑ Prostatic venous plexus → internal iliac veins → IVC.
  ➢ Prostatic cancer may metastasize to the heart and lungs, through this channel.
❑ Prostatic venous plexus → vertebral venous plexus → cranial dural venous sinuses.
  ➢ Prostatic cancer may metastasize to the vertebral column and brain, through this channel.
  Benign prostatic hyperplasia (BPH) is seen in the periurethral (transitional) zone, and involves the median lobe.
❑ It leads to compression of the prostatic urethra and causes BOO (bladder outlet obstruction) to the urine flow.
❑ The uvula vesicae is a small rounded elevation just behind the urethral orifice at the apex of the trigone. It is raised by the median lobe of prostate gland, and becomes more prominent in BPH, leading to stagnancy of urine.
❑ TURP (Transurethral resection of the prostate) is the surgical removal of the prostate by means of a cystoscope passed through the urethra. Approximately > 75 % patients develop retrograde ejaculation of semen post TURP, due to injury to internal urethral sphincter during the procedure.

Corpora amylacea, are small hyaline masses (detected microscopically) found in the **prostate gland**, **neuroglia**, and **pulmonary alveoli**. They are derived from degenerate cells or thickened secretions and occur more frequently with advancing age.

QUESTIONS

1. **UNTRUE about prostate is:**
   a. Behind the urethra and between the two ejaculatory ducts lie the median lobe
   b. Colliculus seminalis is an elevation on urethral crest showing three openings
   c. Its urethra is convex anteriorly
   d. Its urethra appears crescentic in transverse section

2. **Most common site of prostatic carcinoma:**
   (NEET Pattern 2015)
   a. Anterior lobe
   b. Median lobe
   c. Posterior lobe
   d. Central zone

3. **A 50-year-old man suffering from carcinoma of prostate showed areas of sclerosis and collapse of T10 and T11 vertebrae in X-ray. The spread of this cancer to the above vertebrae was must probably through:** *(AIIMS 2003)*
   a. Sacral canal
   b. Lymphatic vessels
   c. Internal vertebral plexus of veins
   d. Superior rectal veins

1. **c. Its urethra is convex anteriorly**
   - ❑ Urethra is **concave anteriorly**, as it passes through the prostate gland.
2. **c. Posterior lobe**
   - ❑ **Posterior lobe** roughly corresponds to **peripheral zone**, which is the sub-capsular portion of the posterior aspect of the prostate gland.
   - ❑ 70–80% of prostatic cancers **originate** in this region.
3. **c. Internal vertebral plexus of veins**
   - ❑ Prostatic venous plexus drains into the **internal iliac vein** which connects with the **vertebral venous plexus**, this is thought to be the route of **bone metastasis** of prostate cancer.

- Seminal colliculus is present in **urethra** (NEET Pattern 2016)
- **Prostatic artery** is a branch of Inferior vesical artery (NEET Pattern 2015)
- Zone prone to benign prostatic hypertrophy is **transitional zone**.
- Benign Prostatic hypertrophy is associated with enlargement of **Median lobe** (AIPG 2005; NEET Pattern 2016)
- **Median lobe** of prostate gland raises **uvula vesicae**.

▶ Cowper's Gland

Bulbourethral (BU) Glands of Cowper

A. The BU glands are located in the deep perineal space embedded in the skeletal muscles of the urogenital diaphragm (i.e., deep transverse perineal muscle and sphincter urethrae muscle) and adjacent to the membranous urethrae.
B. The ducts of the BU glands open into the penile urethra.
C. The BU fluid is a clear, mucus-like, slippery fluid that contains galactose, galactosamine, galacturonic acid, sialic acid, and methylpentose.
D. This fluid makes up a major portion of the preseminal fluid (or pre-ejaculate fluid) and probably serves to lubricate the penile urethra.

▶ Seminal Vesicle

Seminal Vesicles

- ❑ Are enclosed by dense endopelvic fascia and are lobulated glandular structures that are diverticula of the ductus deferens.
- ❑ Seminal vesicles produce the alkaline constituent of the seminal fluid, which contains fructose and choline
A. The seminal vesicles are highly coiled tubular diverticula that originate as evaginations of the ductus deferens distal to the ampulla.
B. Contraction of the smooth muscle of the seminal vesicle during emission will discharge seminal fluid into the ejaculatory duct.
C. The seminal fluid is a whitish yellow viscous material that contains **fructose** (the principal metabolic substrate for sperm) and **other sugars, choline, proteins, amino acids, ascorbic acid, citric acid,** and **prostaglandins.**
D. Seminal fluid accounts for 70% of the volume of the ejaculated semen.
E. In **forensic medicine,** the presence of fructose (which is not produced elsewhere in the body) and choline crystals are used to determine the presence of semen.

▶ Ductus Deferens and Ejaculatory Ducts

- ❑ The ductus deferens begins at the inferior pole of the testes, ascends to enter the spermatic cord, transits the inguinal canal, enters the abdominal cavity by passing through the deep inguinal ring, crosses the external iliac artery and vein, and enters the pelvis.
- ❑ The distal end of the ductus deferens enlarges to form the **ampulla,** where it is joined by a short duct from the seminal vesicle to form the **ejaculatory duct**.
- ❑ The smooth muscular coat of the ductus deferens is similar to the tail region of the epididymis (i.e., **inner longitudinal layer, middle circular layer,** and **outer longitudinal layer of smooth muscle**) and contributes to the force of emission.
- ❑ **Arterial Supply.** The arterial supply of the ductus deferens is from the **artery of the ductus deferens,** which arises from the internal iliac artery and anastomoses with the testicular artery.
- ❑ **Venous Drainage.** The venous drainage of the ductus deferens is to the **testicular vein** and the **distal pampiniform plexus**.
- ❑ **Clinical Consideration: Vasectomy.** The scalpel will cut through the following layers in succession to gain access to the ductus deferens: Skin → Colles' fascia and dartos muscle → external spermatic fascia → cremasteric fascia and muscle → internal spermatic fascia → extraperitoneal fat. The tunica vaginalis is not cut.

Ejaculatory Duct

- ❑ The distal end of the ductus deferens enlarges to form the **ampulla,** where it is joined by a short duct from the seminal vesicle to form the **ejaculatory duct.**

- The ejaculatory duct passes through the prostate gland and opens into the prostatic urethra at the **seminal colliculus** of the urethral crest.
- The ejaculatory duct has no smooth muscular coat, so it does not contribute to the force for emission.

QUESTIONS

1. TRUE about seminal vesicle is: *(NEET Pattern 2016)*
   a. Lined by ciliated columnar cells
   b. Has acidic secretion
   c. Contributes to 30% of semen
   d. Secretes secretion rich in fructose

2. All of the following statements regarding vas deferens are true EXCEPT: *(AIPG 2005)*
   a. The terminal part is dilated to form ampulla
   b. It crosses ureter in the region of ischial spine
   c. It passes lateral to inferior epigastric artery at deep inguinal ring
   d. It is separated from the base of bladder by the peritoneum

ANSWERS

1. d. Secretes secretion rich in fructose
   - Seminal vesicle is lined by cuboidal to **pseudostratified columnar** epithelium, secretes fluid that contributes to **two thirds** of the total ejaculate volume.
   - The fluid is rich in **fructose**, coagulation proteins and prostaglandins, with a pH in the neutral to **alkaline** range.

2. d. It is separated from the base of bladder by the peritoneum
   - Vas deferens lies on the posterior wall (base) of the bladder and there is **no peritoneum between them**. So, there is no separation of vas deferens from the base of bladder by the peritoneum.
   - Peritoneum actually lies more posterior to the vas deferens and forms the **recto-vesical pouch**.
   - Below the pouch lies the fascia of Denonvillier's–a pelvic fascia condensation to support the pelvic viscera.
   - Vas deferens hooks around the inferior epigastric artery (**laterally**) at deep inguinal ring and **crosses to the ureter** (superiorly) in the region of ischial spines. It shows a terminal dilatation called as **ampulla**, before it joins the duct of seminal vesicle to form common ejaculatory duct.

▶ Penis

Penis has three masses of vascular erectile tissue: **corpora cavernosa** (paired) and the midline **corpus spongiosum**, which are individually bounded by tunica albuginea.

- Penis has a root, which includes two crura and the bulb of the penis, and the body, which contains the three erectile corpora.
- **Glans penis** is the terminal part of the corpus spongiosum, covered by a fold of skin (**prepuce**). **Frenulum** is a median ventral fold passing from the deep surface of the prepuce.
   ➤ The prominent margin of the glans penis is the **corona**, the median slit near the tip of the glans is the external urethral orifice, and the terminal dilated part of the urethra in the glans is the **fossa navicularis**.
- **Smegma** is secreted by the preputial sebaceous glands of the corona, at the inner surface of the prepuce and neck of the glans penis.
- Deep fascia of the penis (**Buck Fascia**) is a continuation of the deep perineal fascia.
   ➤ It is continuous with the fascia covering the external oblique muscle and the rectus sheath.
- **Tunica Albuginea** is a dense fibrous layer that envelops both the corpora cavernosa and the corpus spongiosum.
   ➤ It is more dense around the corpora cavernosa and more elastic around the corpus spongiosum.

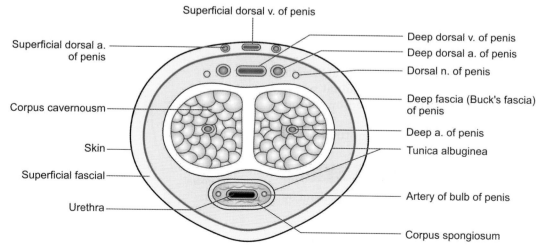

Fig. 56: Transverse section through the body of the penis

▸ Artery Supply

❑ Three arteries arise from internal pudendal arteries, branches of anterior divisions of internal iliac arteries.
- ➤ Arteries to crura of the penis (deep artery of penis).
- ➤ Artery to the bulb of penis (supplies proximal half of corpus spongiosum
- ➤ Dorsal artery of penis which supplies distal part of corpus spongiosum and the glans penis
- ➤ Superficial dorsal arteries of penis.

Note: Deep arteries fill the lacunae of erectile tissue in corpus cavernosum. In the flaccid state of the penis, these vessels appear spiral hence termed **helicine arteries**.

Venous Drainage

❑ Deep dorsal vein of the penis is a midline vein lying deep to the deep (Buck) fascia and superficial to the tunica albuginea.
- ➤ It leaves the perineum through the gap between the arcuate pubic ligament and the transverse perineal ligament and drains into the prostatic and pelvic venous plexuses.

❑ Superficial dorsal vein of the penis runs toward the pubic symphysis between the superficial and deep fasciae and terminates in the external (superficial) pudendal veins, which drain into the greater saphenous vein.

Lymphatic Drainage

❑ The lymphatics from the glans penis drain into the deep inguinal lymph nodes (of Cloquet and Rosenmuller). Rest of penis drain into superficial inguinal lymph nodes.

▸ Cremaster Reflex

Cremasteric Reflex

❑ Stroking of the skin on the front and inner side of the thigh evokes a reflex contraction of cremaster, which retracts the ipsilateral testis.

❑ The afferent limb for cremaster reflex is **femoral branch of genitofemoral nerve** (and by **ilio-inguinal nerve** additionally) and efferent limb is carried by **genital branch of genitofemoral nerve**.

❑ The reflex is usually absent if there is torsion of the testicle.

▸ Erection and Ejaculation

Erection is under parasympathetic system — carried out by pelvic splanchnic nerves.

❑ There occurs dilatation of the arteries supplying the erectile tissue, and thus causes engorgement of the corpora cavernosa and corpus spongiosum, compressing the veins and thus impeding venous return and causing erection.

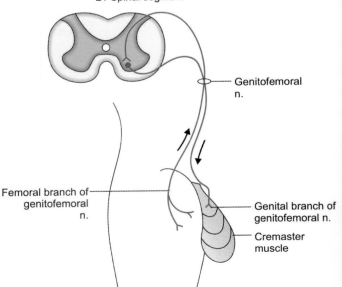

Fig. 57: Neural pathway for cremasteric reflex

- Erection is maintained by contraction of the bulbospongiosus and ischiocavernosus muscles, which compresses the erectile tissues of the bulb and the crus.

Ejaculation is under sympathetic system

- Friction to the glans penis and other sexual stimuli result in excitation of sympathetic fibers.
- There occurs contraction of the smooth muscle of the epididymal ducts, the ductus deferens, the seminal vesicles, and the prostate.
- The contraction of the smooth muscles push spermatozoa and the secretions of both the seminal vesicles and prostate into the prostatic urethra, where they join secretions from the bulbourethral and penile urethral glands.
- Rhythmic contractions of the bulbospongiosus compresses the urethra and pushes and ejects the secretions from the penile urethra.
- Ejaculation is accompanied by contraction of the internal urethral sphincter (of the bladder), which prevents retrograde ejaculation of the semen into the bladder.

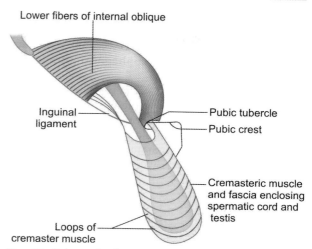

Fig. 58: Schematic diagram to show cremaster muscle

- Root value of cremaster reflex is **L1,2** (AIIMS 2017)

Abdominal Cavity and Peritoneum

In the beginning peritoneum forms **a closed sac**, but when it becomes invaginated by a number of abdominal viscera it is divided into two layers: **outer parietal layer** and **inner visceral layer**.

- The folds of peritoneum by which viscera are suspended are called **mesentery.**
- Peritoneum presents with two layers: **Parietal** peritoneum and **visceral** peritoneum. Parietal peritoneum lines the internal surface of the abdominopelvic walls and visceral peritoneum covers the viscera.

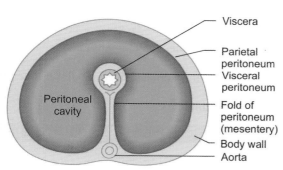

Fig. 59: Schematic transverse section of the abdomen showing arrangement of the peritoneum

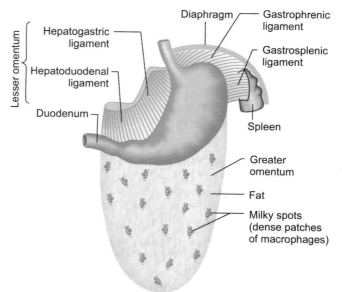

Fig. 60: Peritoneal folds: Omenta and ligaments

The **peritoneal folds** are classified into three types: **Mesentery, omenta,** and **ligaments**. They **carry neurovascular bundles** to the corresponding viscera.

- ❏ **Mesentery**: The **double fold** of visceral peritoneum suspending the gut tube is called **mesentery**. It gets modified into various names: meso-**oesophagus**, meso-**gastrium**, meso-**duodenum**, meso-**colon** according to the structure it is attached.
- ❏ **Omenta** are the double fold of peritoneum that connect the **stomach** with other viscera. It includes **greater omentum**, attaching to greater curvature of stomach and connecting with transverse colon; **lesser omentum**, attaching to lesser curvature of stomach and connecting the stomach with the liver.
- ❏ **Ligaments**: They are double folds of peritoneum that connect organs to the abdominal wall or to each other. **Gastrosplenic** ligament lies between stomach and spleen, **lienorenal** ligamentum lies between kidney and spleen, and **coronary** ligaments lies between liver and diaphragm.

Phrenocolic ligament	Support anterior end of spleen and prevents its downwards displacement.
Lienorenal ligament	Contains splenic vessels and tail of pancreas.
Gastrosplenic ligament	Contains short gastric vessels.

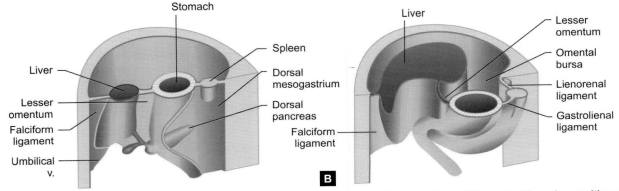

Figs. 61A and B: A. The positions of the spleen, stomach, and pancreas at the end of the fifth week. Note the position of the spleen and pancreas in the dorsal mesogastrium. B. Position of spleen and stomach at the 11th week. Note formation of the omental bursa (lesser peritoneal sac)

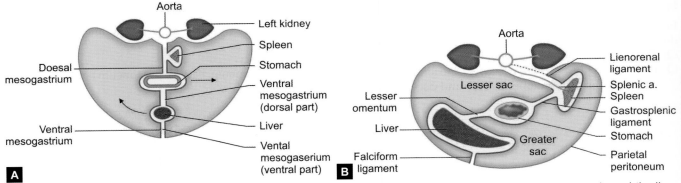

Figs. 62A and B: Transverse section (inferior view) of developing foregut showing ventral and dorsal mesogastria and the ligaments of spleen: A, early stage; B, later stage. As the stomach rotates to right by 90°, a small space (lesser sac) lying behind the stomach, is created in the peritoneal cavity

Peritoneal cavity gets divided into two parts: **Greater** sac and **lesser** sac (omental bursa).

- ❏ **Greater sac** is the larger compartment of the peritoneal cavity and extends across the whole breadth and length of the abdomen.
- ❏ **Lesser sac** is the smaller compartment of the peritoneal cavity, which lies behind the stomach, liver, and lesser omentum as a diverticulum from the greater sac.
- ❏ Greater sac communicates with lesser sac through the **epiploic foramen of Winslow**.

▶ Lesser/Greater Omentum

A. Lesser Omentum
  - ➤ A fold of peritoneum that extends from the porta hepatis of the liver to the lesser curvature of the stomach.
  - ➤ It consists of the hepatoduodenal ligament and hepatogastric ligament.

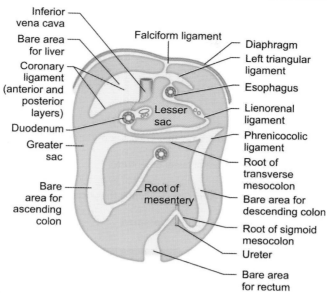

Fig. 63: Attachments of the peritoneum on the posterioir abdominal wall. Note the division of peritoneal cavity into greater sac (orange color) and lesser sac (light blue color)

Contents:

❑ Along the lesser curvature of the stomach the lesser omentum contains: Right and left gastric vessels and associated gastric lymph nodes and branches of the left gastric nerve.

❑ The portal triad lies in the free margin of the hepatoduodenal ligament and consists of the following:
  ➢ Common bile duct (anterior and to the right)
  ➢ Hepatic artery (anterior and to the left)
  ➢ Portal vein (lies posterior)

B. Greater Omentum
  ➢ A fold of peritoneum that hangs down from the greater curvature of the stomach. It is known as the **abdominal policeman** because it adheres to areas of inflammation.

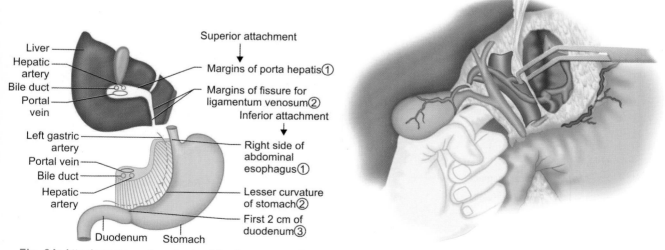

Fig. 64: Attachments and contents of the lesser omenium

Fig. 65: Pringle's maneuver

❑ **Pringle's maneuvre:** A finger is guided through epiploic foramen to put a large atraumatic haemostat and **clamp** the hepatoduodenal ligament (free border of the lesser omentum) interrupting the flow of blood through the **hepatic artery** and the **portal vein** and thus helping to **control bleeding** from the liver.

1. **Structures injured while resecting the free edge of lesser omentum:** *(PGIC 2012)*
   a. Hepatic artery proper
   b. Portal vein
   c. Cystic duct
   d. Hepatic vein
   e. Common bile duct

2. **Free margin of lesser omentum has following contents EXCEPT:** *(NEET Pattern 2015; JIPMER 2016)*
   a. Hepatic vein
   b. Hepatic artery
   c. Portal vein
   d. Bile duct

1. **a. Hepatic artery proper; b) Portal vein; e) Common bile duct.**
   ❏ **Free edge** of lesser omentum contains the structures that enter the porta hepatis **(DAV).** D – Duct (Common bile), A- Artery (proper hepatic), V – Vein (portal).
   ❏ **Cystic duct** and **hepatic vein** are **not** the content of lesser omentum.

2. **a. Hepatic vein**
   ❏ Free edge of lesser omentum contains the 'DAV' structures that enter the porta hepatis. D - Duct (bile), A - Artery (hepatic), V - Vein (portal).
   ❏ These structures form the **anterior boundary of epiploic foramen**.

▶ Greater/Lesser Sac; Morison Pouch

❏ Peritoneal cavity is a potential space between the visceral and parietal peritoneum.
❏ It is divided into the lesser sac and greater sac.

Lesser Peritoneal Sac (Omental Bursa)

❏ A small space behind the stomach that is also called as left posterior intraperitoneal space (LPIS).
❏ Lesser sac forms due to the clockwise rotation of the stomach by 90-degree during embryologic development.
❏ Boundaries
❏ Anterior wall (from above downwards)
   ➢ Caudate lobe of liver

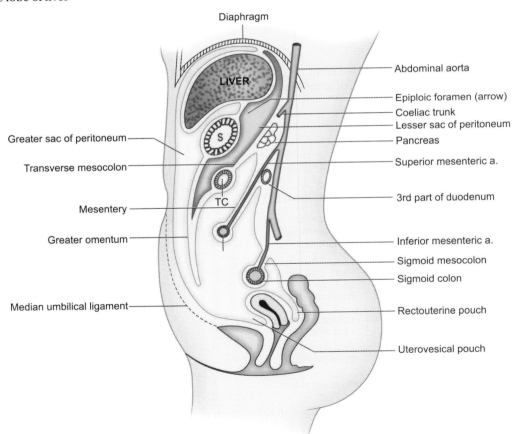

Fig. 66: Sagittal section of the abdominopelvic cavity (female) to show the vertical disposition of peritoneum
(S = stomach, TC = transverse colon, SI = small intestine)

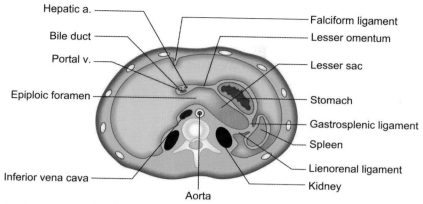

Fig. 67: Peritoneal cavity showing greater and lever sac. Epiploic foramen boundaries are also evident

- ➢ Lesser omentum
- ➢ Stomach (postero-inferior surface)
- ➢ Greater omentum (anterior two layers)
- ❑ Posterior wall (from below upward)
  - ➢ Greater omentum (posterior two layers)
  - ➢ Structures forming the **stomach bed** (EXCEPT: spleen)
    - ▪ Transverse colon.
    - ▪ Transverse mesocolon.
    - ▪ Pancreas.
    - ▪ Upper part of the left kidney and left suprarenal gland
  - ➢ Diaphragm.
- ❑ Right border: Liver
- ❑ Left border: Gastrosplenic and splenorenal ligaments

Applied anatomy: Acute pancreatitis is probably the most common cause of a fluid collection within the lesser sac. Bleeding from trauma or a ruptured splenic artery aneurysm and perforation of a posterior gastric ulcer are other causes of lesser sac collections.

Greater Peritoneal Sac

- ❑ The remainder of the peritoneal cavity and extends from the diaphragm to the pelvis.
- ❑ It contains a number of pouches, recesses, and Paracolic gutters through which peritoneal fluid circulates.
- ❑ Paracolic gutters are channels that run along the ascending and descending colon. Normally, peritoneal fluid flows upward through the paracolic gutters to the subphrenic recess, where it enters the lymphatics associated with the diaphragm.
- ❑ In supine position excess Peritoneal Fluid due to peritonitis or ascites flows upward through the paracolic gutter to the subphrenic recess and the hepatorenal recess (most dependent location).
- ❑ In upright (sitting/standing) position excess Peritoneal Fluid due to peritonitis or ascites flows downward through the paracolic gutters to the rectovesical pouch (in males) or the rectouterine pouch (in females).

Note: Rectouterine pouch of Douglas is the peritoneal space between the rectum and uterus. It is the most dependent part of the peritoneal cavity in upright position. In the supine position it is the most dependent part of the pelvic cavity.

▶ Morison pouch/ Winslow foramen

Hepatorenal pouch of Morrison is the right **subhepatic** space, lies between the inferior surface of the right lobe of the **liver** and the upper pole of the **right kidney**.
- ❑ It is situated between the posteroinferior surface of the liver and front of the right kidney
- ❑ Boundaries
  - ➢ Anterior: Posteroinferior (visceral) surface of the liver.
  - ➢ Posterior: Peritoneum covering the front of the upper pole of the right kidney and the diaphragm.
  - ➢ Above: Posterior (inferior) layer of the coronary ligament.
  - ➢ Below: Transverse colon and mesocolon.
- ❑ Communications
  - ➢ On the left: It communicates through foramen epiploicum with the lesser sac of peritoneum (omental bursa).
  - ➢ Along the sharp inferior border of liver: It communicates with the right anterior intraperitoneal compartment.

Omental (Winslow) Foramen

- ❏ The opening (or connection) between the greater peritoneal sac and lesser peritoneal sac.
- ❏ Boundaries
- ❏ Anterior: Free margin of lesser omentum containing DAV (Duct, Artery, Vein)
- ❏ Posterior: T12 vertebra, with IVC and right adrenal gland
  - ➤ Superior: Liver (1st part, caudate lobe)
  - ➤ Inferior: Duodenum (1st part)

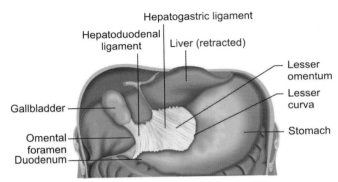

Fig. 68: Epiploic (omental) foramen of Winslow

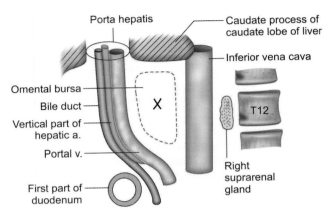

Fig. 69: Boundaries of the foramen epiplocuim

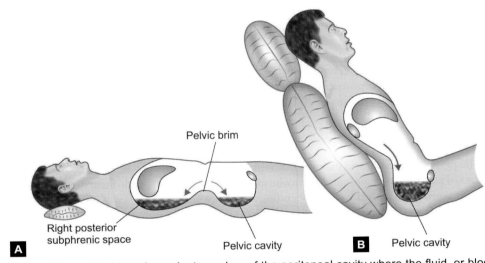

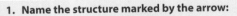

Figs. 70A and B: Most dependent pouches of the peritoneal cavity where the fluid, or blood, or pus collects: (A) when subject is in supine position; (B) when subject is in semi-upright position.

1. Name the structure marked by the arrow: *(AIIMS 2017)*

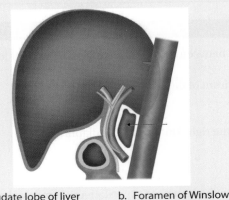

a. Caudate lobe of liver   b. Foramen of Winslow
c. Duodenum   d. Lesser omentum

2. A posteriorly perforating ulcer in the pyloric antrum of the stomach is likely to produce initial localized peritonitis or abscess formation in the: *(AIIMS 2004)*
   a. Greater sac
   b. Right subhepatic/hepatorenal space (pouch of Morison)
   c. Omental bursa
   d. Right subphrenic space

QUESTIONS

3. All are true about boundaries of epiploic foramen EXCEPT:
(NEET Pattern 2015)
a. Anterior: portal vein and hepatic artery
b. Posterior: IVC
c. Inferior: liver
d. Inferior: duodenum

4. Lesser sac of stomach is bounded by:
a. Posterior wall of stomach
b. Visceral surface of spleen
c. Under surface of liver
d. Greater omentum
e. Transverse mesocolon

ANSWERS

1. b. Foramen of Winslow
❑ This diagram shows the boundaries of **foramen of Winslow**.
  ▪ Superior: **Caudate lobe** of liver
  ▪ Inferiorly: **Duodenum** (1st part)
  ▪ Anteriorly: Free margin of **lesser omentum** containing bile duct, hepatic artery and portal vein
  ▪ Posteriorly: Inferior vena cava

2. d. Omental bursa
❑ A posterior perforation of ulcer in the pyloric antrum of the stomach will discharge the contents **behind** the stomach into the **lesser sac** (omental bursa).

3. c. Inferior liver
❑ Liver (caudate lobe) is the superior (**not inferior**) boundary of epiploic foramen.

4. a. Posterior wall of stomach; c) Under surface of liver; d) Greater omentum; e) Transverse mesocolon
❑ Spleen is **separated** from the lesser sac by the **gastrosplenic** and **lienorenal** ligaments.

▪ The **most dependent** part of abdomen in **standing** position is **rectouterine pouch of Douglas**. *(NEET Pattern 2013)*
▪ Rectouterine pouch of Douglas lies between rectum (posteriorly) and uterus and **posterior fornix of vagina** (anteriorly).
▪ A posteriorly **perforating ulcer** in the pyloric antrum of the stomach is likely to produce initial localized peritonitis or abscess formation in the **lesser sac** (omental bursa). *(AIPG 2003, AIIMS 2004)*
▪ **Bile duct** lies **anterior** to epiploic foramen *(NEET Pattern 2014)*
▪ In **Pringle's** manoeuvre the structure clamped is **portal pedicle** (Bile duct, hepatic artery and portal vein).
▪ Caudate (**not quadrate**) lobe lies as the superior border of the epiploic foramen.
▪ **Spleen** projects into the **greater sac** of peritoneal cavity *(AIIMS 2008, 11)*
▪ **Foramen of Winslow** is a communication between greater sac and lesser sac *(NEET Pattern 2016)*
▪ Free edge of lesser omentum contains bile **duct**, hepatic **artery** and portal **vein** *(JIPMER 2016)*
▪ Common bile duct **lies right** to hepatic artery *(JIPMER 2013)*

▶ Root of Mesentery

A. Attached border
  ➤ It is attached to an oblique line across the posterior abdominal wall, extending from the duodenojejunal junction to the ileocecal junction.
  ➤ The duodenojejunal junction lies to the left side of L2 vertebra, whereas the ileocaecal junction lies in right iliac fossa, at the upper part of the right sacroiliac joint.
  ➤ The root of mesentery from above downward crosses in front of:
  ➤ Horizontal (third) part of duodenum
  ➤ Abdominal aorta
  ➤ Inferior vena cava
  ➤ Right gonadal vessels
  ➤ Right ureter
  ➤ Right psoas major muscle

Note: The root of mesentery divides the infracolic compartment into two parts: Right and left. The right one is small and terminates in the right iliac fossa. The left one is larger and passes without interruption into true pelvis.

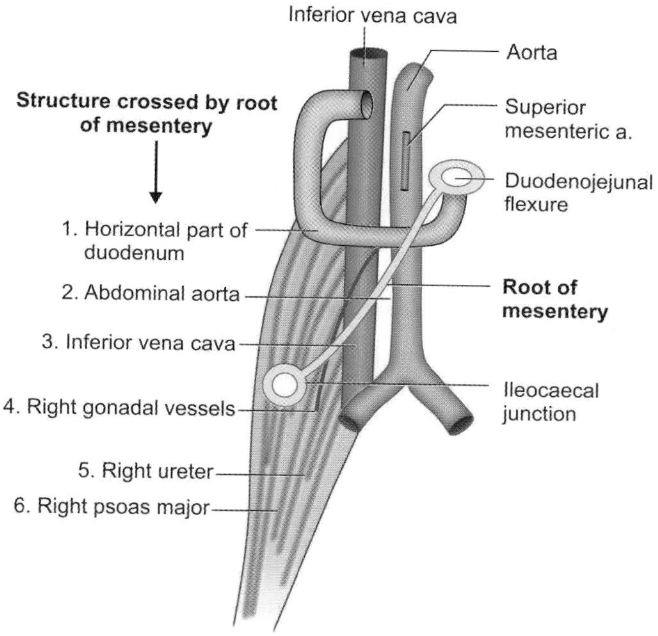

B. Free border (intestinal border)
❑ **It is about 6 m (20 feet) long** and encloses the jejunum and ileum.

❑ The root of mesentery is 6 inches (15 cm) long whereas its periphery (free border) is 6 m long. This accounts for the formation of folds (pleats) in it (a frill-like arrangement).

Structure crossed by root of mesentery

1. Horizontal part of duodenum
2. Abdominal aorta
3. Inferior vena cava
4. Right gonadal vessels
5. Right ureter
6. Right psoas major

Inferior vena cava
Aorta
Superior mesenteric a.
Duodenojejunal flexure
Root of mesentery
Ileocaecal junction

Fig. 71: Structures crossed by the root of the mesentery

❑ It has fat deposition along its root, which diminishes toward the intestinal border. Near the intestinal border it presents fat-free windows (translucent are of peritoneum. The amount of fat is greater in the distal part of the mesentery.

C. Contents of mesentery:
❑ Superior mesenteric artery and vein (in the root) and its jejunal, ileal branches.
❑ Jejunum and ileum (enclosed in the free border)
❑ Lymph nodes (100–200 in number) and lymphatics
❑ Autonomic nerve plexuses
❑ Fat and connective tissue

QUESTION

1. The mesentery of small intestine, along its attachment to the posterior abdominal wall, crosses all or the following structures EXCEPT: *(AIIMS 2004, AIPG 2011)*
   a. Left gonadal vessels
   b. Third part of duodenum
   c. Aorta
   d. Right ureter

ANSWER

1. a. Left gonadal vessels
   ❑ The root of mesentery lies on the **right side** of abdominal cavity and crosses right gonadal vessels (**not left**).
   ❑ The root of the mesentery lies along a line **running diagonally** from the duodenojejunal flexure on the left side of the second lumbar vertebral body to the right sacroiliac joint.
   ❑ It crosses over the **third (horizontal) part** of the duodenum, aorta, inferior vena cava, right ureter and right psoas major.
   ❑ It **does not cross the left ureter**, left gonadal vessels or superior mesenteric artery.
   ❑ Superior mesenteric artery is a **content** of the mesentery.

▶ Spleen: Peritoneal Connections

❑ **Gastrosplenic ligament** extends from the hilum of the spleen to the upper one-third of the greater curvature of the stomach. It contains **short gastric vessels**.
❑ **Lienorenal ligament** extends from the hilum of the spleen to the anterior surface of the left kidney. It contains tail of the pancreas, **splenic vessels**, and lymphatics.
❑ **Phrenico-colic ligament** is a triangular fold of the peritoneum which extends from the **left colic flexure** to the diaphragm opposite to the 10th rib. It passes below the lateral end of the spleen, which it **supports**; hence, it is also termed **sustentaculum lienis**.

▶ Peritoneal Spaces

❑ Peritoneal cavity can be divided into several spaces and pathological processes are often contained within these spaces.
❑ Peritoneal cavity into **two main compartments**, supramesocolic (supracolic) and inframesocolic (or infracolic), which are partially separated by the transverse colon and its mesentery.
❑ Supracolic compartment has a number of spaces: 1. Right subphrenic space; 2. Right subhepatic space (Hepato-renal pouch of Morison); 3. Lesser sac; 4. Left subphrenic space; 5. Left subhepatic space. Infracolic compartment spaces: 1. Right para-colic gutter; 2. Left para-colic gutter.
❑ The right paracolic gutter is continuous with the right supracolic compartment, and hence, bile/pus/blood released from viscera above can reach inferiorly till the pelvic cavity. For example. Tracking of pus in gastric ulcer perforation:
   ➤ Pus of gastric antral perforation moves into lesser sac → Epiploic foramen → Hepatorenal pouch of Morison (supra-colic compartment) → Right paracolic gutter (Infracolic compartment) → Pouch of Douglas (pelvic cavity).

Supramesocolic Compartment

❑ This lies between the diaphragm and the transverse mesocolon.
❑ It can be arbitrarily divided into right and left supramesocolic spaces.
❑ The right supramesocolic space can be subdivided into the right subphrenic space, the right subhepatic space and the lesser sac.
❑ The left supramesocolic space can be divided into two subspaces: the left subphrenic space and the left perihepatic space. These 'spaces' usually communicate but may nevertheless be sites of localized fluid collections.

Paracolic Gutters

❑ The right and left **paracolic gutters** are peritoneal depressions on the posterior abdominal wall alongside the ascending and descending colon, respectively.
❑ The principal paracolic gutter lies **lateral to the colon** on each side.
❑ A less obvious medial paracolic gutter may be present, more often on the right side, if the ascending or descending colon possesses a short mesentery for part of its length.
❑ The **right** (lateral) paracolic gutter runs from the superolateral aspect of the hepatic flexure of the colon, down the lateral aspect of the ascending colon and cecum.

- It is continuous with the peritoneum of the pelvic cavity below.
- Superiorly, it is continuous with the peritoneum that lines the **hepatorenal pouch** and with the lesser sac through the **epiploic foramen**.
- Bile, pus, blood or other fluid may run along the gutter and collect in sites distant to the organ of origin.
- In **supine** patients, infected fluid from the right iliac fossa may **ascend** in the gutter to the right subphrenic space.
- In **erect** or semi-recumbent positions, fluid from the stomach, duodenum or gallbladder may **run down** the gutter to collectin the right iliac fossa (mimicking acute appendicitis) or pelvis to form an abscess.
- The right paracolic gutter is deeper than the left, which, together with the partial barrier provided by the **phrenicocolic** ligament, may explain why subphrenic collections are more common on the right.

Recesses of the Peritoneal Cavity

- Peritoneal fossae or recesses within the peritoneal cavity are occasionally sites of **internal herniation**.
- If a loop of intestine becomes stuck in fossa or recess, the bowel may become obstructed or strangulate from a constriction at the entrance to the recess.
- The contents of the peritoneal fold forming the fossa/recess must be considered when repairing such a hernia.

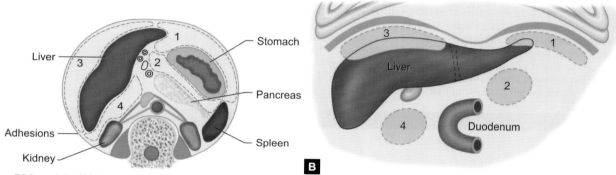

Figs. 72A and B: (A) Intraperitoneal abscesses on transverse section: (1) the left subphrenic space, (2) left subhepatic space/ lesser sac, (3) right subphrenic space, (4) right subhepatic space. (B) Intraperitoneal abscesses on sagittal section: (1) left subphrenic, (2) left subhepatic/lesser sac, (3) right subphrenic, (4) right subhepatic

- **Left subphrenic space** is bounded above by the **diaphragm** and behind by the left triangular ligament and the **left lobe** of the liver, the gastro-hepatic omentum and the anterior surface of the stomach.
  - To the right is the falciform ligament and to the left the spleen, gastrosplenic omentum and diaphragm.
  - The common cause of an abscess here is **an operation** on the stomach, the tail of the pancreas, the spleen or the splenic flexure of the colon.
- **Left subhepatic space** (lesser sac): The most common cause of infection here is complicated **acute pancreatitis**.
  - A **perforated gastric ulcer** rarely causes a collection here because the potential space is obliterated by adhesions.
- **Right subphrenic space** lies between the right lobe of the liver and the diaphragm.
  - It is limited posteriorly by the anterior layer of the coronary and the right triangular ligaments and to the left by the falciform ligament.
  - Common causes of abscess here are perforating cholecystitis, a perforated duodenal ulcer, a duodenal cap 'blow-out' following gastrectomy and appendicitis.
- **Right subhepatic space** lies transversely beneath the right lobe of the liver **in Rutherford Morison's pouch**.
  - It is bounded on the right by the **right lobe of the liver** and the diaphragm. To the left is situated the foramen of Winslow and below this lies the duodenum.
  - In front are the liver and the gall bladder and behind are the upper part of the **right kidney** and the diaphragm.
  - The space is bounded above by the liver and below by the transverse colon and hepatic flexure.
  - It is the **deepest space** of the four and the most common site of a **subphrenic abscess**, which usually arises from appendicitis, cholecystitis, a perforated duodenal ulcer or following upper abdominal surgery.

1. **Which structure lies in the intersigmoid recess**
   a. Left ureter
   b. Left ureter and left common iliac artery
   c. Left ureter and left common iliac vein
   d. Left ureter, left common Iliac artery and left common iliac vein

2. **Sub-diaphragmatic right posterior intraperitoneal space is**
   (JIPMER 2010)
   a. Lesser sac
   b. Morison's pouch
   c. Hepatorenal pouch
   d. Superior part of supracolic compartment

3. **Which of the following is TRUE about location of omental bursa**
   (JIPMER 2004)
   a. Left subhepatic
   b. Left subphrenic
   c. Right subhepatic
   d. Right subphrenic

1. **a. Left ureter**
   - ❑ **Left ureter** crossing the **bifurcation** of left common iliac artery lies **behind intersigmoid recess**, which is a surgical guide for locating left ureter.
   - ❑ Intersigmoid recess is **constantly present** in the foetus and in early infancy but **may disappear with age**.

2. **b. Morrison's pouch**
   - ❑ **Right posterior intraperitoneal space (RPIS)** or **right subhepatic space** is hepatorenal pouch of Morrison.

3. **c. Left subhepatic**
   - ❑ Omental bursa (Lesser sac) is **left posterior intraperitoneal space (LPIS)**, also called **left subhepatic space**.
   - ❑ **Right** subhepatic space is the **hepatorenal pouch** of Morison.

- Morison's pouch is **right subhepatic space** (*NEET Pattern 2015*)
- **Inferior mesenteric** vein is found in relation to the **paraduodenal** fossa (*AIPG 2008*)
- The vessel traversing mesocolon is **middle colic artery** (*NEET Pattern 2016*)
- **Denonvilliers fascia** separates posterior surface of prostate from rectum. It represents the obliterated rectovesical pouch of peritoneum in male.
- Spleen develops in the **dorsal mesentery** and projects into the **greater sac** of peritoneal cavity.
- **Liver** develops in the **ventral mesentery** and also project into the greater sac.
- Lesser sac is the **smaller** part of peritoneal cavity lying **posterior** to the stomach. It is also called as left posterior (sub-hepatic) space.
- Spleen is separated from the lesser sac by the **Gastrosplenic** and **Lienorenal** ligaments.
- Left anterior (subhepatic) space reaches the spleen, but spleen is not projecting into it.
- **Spleen** lies above the level of transverse colon and is in the **supracolic** compartment (not the infracolic).
- Infracolic compartments lie **below the transverse colon** and are having the right and left **paracolic gutters**.
  - This compartment extends till true pelvis. Spleen is separated from the left paracolic gutter by **the phrenocolic ligament**.
- **Phrenocolic ligament** attaches the splenic flexure of transverse colon to the diaphragm and **supports** the anterior end of spleen preventing its projection into the left paracolic gutter.

▶ Gut tube

Stomach

Parts: **Cardia** is the initial segment continuous with esophagus. **Fundus** is formed by the upper curvature of the organ. The **body** is the main central region and **pylorus** is the lower section continuous with duodenum.

Stomach bed: Diaphragm, left kidney, left suprarenal gland, pancreas, transverse mesocolon, left colic flexure (splenic flexure of colon), splenic artery, spleen.

Pancreas (**EXCEPT: tail**) is in the posterior relation of stomach. Splenic artery (**and not vein**) is in the posterior relation of stomach.

Arterial supply

The arterial supply of the stomach is from the following:
- ❑ **Right and left gastric arteries** which supply the lesser curvature (abdominal aorta → celiac trunk → common hepatic artery → right gastric artery; abdominal aorta → celiac trunk → left gastric artery).

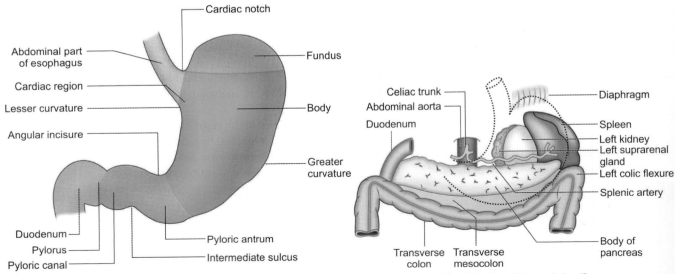

Fig. 73: The parts of the stomach

Fig. 74: The "Stomach bed"

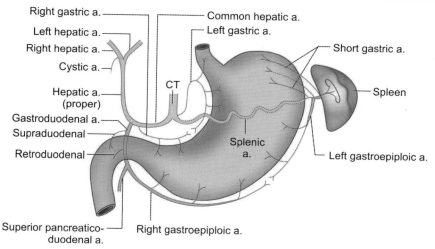

Fig. 75: Arteries of the stomach (CT = Celiac trunk)

- ❑ **Right and left gastroepiploic arteries** which supply the greater curvature (abdominal aorta → celiac trunk → common hepatic artery → gastroduodenal artery → right gastroepiploic artery; abdominal aorta → celiac trunk → splenic artery → left gastroepiploic artery).
- ❑ **Short gastric arteries** which supply the fundus (abdominal aorta → celiac trunk → splenic artery → short gastric arteries).

Venous drainage

- ❑ The venous drainage of the stomach from the following:
- ❑ **Right and left gastric veins** (right and left gastric veins → portal vein → hepatic sinusoids → central veins → hepatic veins → inferior vena cava).
- ❑ **Left gastroepiploic vein** and **short gastric veins** (left gastroepiploic vein and short gastric veins → splenic vein → portal vein → hepatic sinusoids → central veins → hepatic veins → inferior vena cava).
- ❑ **Right gastroepiploic vein** (right gastroepiploic vein → superior mesenteric vein → portal vein → hepatic sinusoids → central veins → hepatic veins → inferior vena cava).

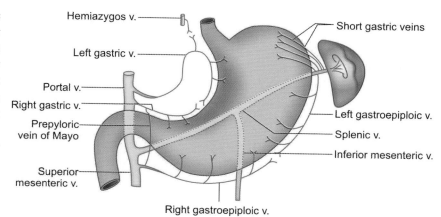

Fig. 76: Venous drainage of the stomach

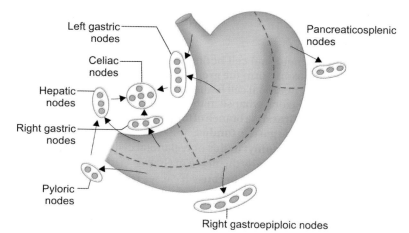

Fig. 77: Lymphatic drainage of the stomach: Lymph node groups drawing the lymphatic territories of the stomach

- ❑ Posterior gastric artery is a branch of splenic artery *(JIPMER 2008)*
- ❑ The left gastric artery usually arises directly from the Celiac trunk. The short gastric arteries, left gastroepiploic artery and when present, the posterior gastric artery are branches of the splenic artery. The right gastric artery and right gastroepiploic artery arise from the hepatic artery and its gastroduodenal branch, respectively.
- ❑ The left gastroepiploic artery is the largest branch of the splenic artery.

  Lymphatic drainage: Territorial lymph nodes → **Celiac nodes** → intestinal lymph trunk → cisterna chyli.

- ❏ **Area 1** drains into **left gastric lymph nodes** along the left gastric artery. These lymph nodes also drain the abdominal part of the esophagus.
- ❏ **Area 2** includes the **pyloric antrum** and **pyloric canal** along the **greater** curvature of the stomach and drain into right gastroepiploic lymph nodes along the right gastroepiploic artery and pyloric nodes.
- ❏ **Area 3** drains into pancreatico-splenic nodes along the splenic artery.
- ❏ **Area 4** includes the **pyloric antrum** and **pyloric canal** along the **lesser** curvature of the stomach. The lymph from this area is drained into **right gastric nodes** along the right gastric artery and **hepatic nodes** along the hepatic artery.

Innervation

- ❏ The innervation of the stomach is by the **enteric nervous system** which is in the stomach consists of the myenteric plexus of Auerbach only. The enteric nervous system is modulated by the parasympathetic and sympathetic nervous systems.
- ❏ **Parasympathetic**
  - ➤ Preganglionic neuronal cell bodies are located in the **dorsal nucleus of the vagus**. Preganglionic axons run in CN X and enter the **anterior and posterior vagal trunks**.
  - ➤ Postganglionic neuronal cell bodies are located in the enteric nervous system, some of which are the 'traditional' postganglionic parasympathetic neurons that release ACh as a neurotransmitter.
  - ➤ The postganglionic axons terminate on mucosal glands and smooth muscle.

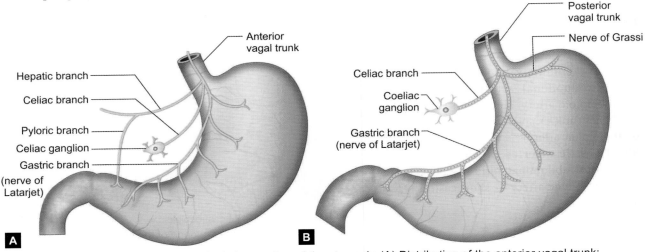

Figs. 78A and B: Parasympathetic innervation of the stomach: (A) Distribution of the anterior vagal trunk; (B) Distribution of the posterior vagal trunk

- ❏ **Sympathetic**
  - ➤ Preganglionic neuronal cell bodies are located in the **intermediolateral cell column** of the spinal cord (T5 to T9). Preganglionic axons form the **greater splanchnic nerve.**
  - ➤ Postganglionic neuronal cell bodies are located in the **celiac ganglion.**
  - ➤ Postganglionic axons synapse in the complex circuitry of the enteric nervous system.

  Criminal nerve of Grassi is a branch of the posterior vagal trunk (**right vagus**) which arises at the level of the gastroesophageal junction and supplies the **gastric fundus.**
- ❏ **Highly selective vagotomy**: In this only parietal cells of the stomach are denervated by cutting the anterior and posterior gastric branches particularly the nerve of Grassi.
- ❏ It is known as criminal nerve **because** it causes recurrence of gastric ulcer even after vagotomy.

  Nerve of Latarjet (posterior nerve of the lesser curvature) is a branch of the **anterior** vagal trunk which supplies the **pylorus**. It is cut in selective vagotomy and preserved in highly selective vagotomy.

  The advantage of **high selective vagotomy** is that nerves of Latarjet and their antral branches are preserved. As a result, the **gastric emptying remains normal**.

Clinical Considerations

- ❏ **Gastric ulcers** are most often occur within the **body of the stomach** along the **lesser curvature** above the **incisura angularis.**
- ❏ **Carcinomas of the stomach** are most commonly found in the **pylorus** of the stomach and may metastasize to **supraclavicular lymph nodes (Virchow nodes)** on the left side which can be palpated within the posterior triangle of the neck. Carcinomas of the stomach may also metastasize to the ovaries where it is called a **Krukenberg tumor.**

1. **Accessory organ which may be found in stomach:**
   (NEET Pattern 2016)
   a. Spleen   b. Liver
   c. Pancreas   d. Kidney

2. **The bed of stomach is NOT formed by:**
   a. Left kidney   b. Left suprarenal vein
   c. Splenic vein   d. Tail of pancreas

3. **Lymphatic drainage of stomach includes all EXCEPT:**
   (NEET Pattern 2012)
   a. Right gastroepiploic nodes b. Pyloric nodes
   c. Preaortic nodes   d. Celiac nodes

4. **Right gastric nodes drain from which part of stomach:**
   (NEET Pattern 2016)
   a. Fundus   b. Greater curvature
   c. Lesser curvature   d. Pylorus

1. **c. Pancreas**
   ❑ Accessory (ectopic) **pancreatic** tissue may be found at various sites usually in the **upper GIT**.

2. **c. Splenic vein and d. Tail of pancreas**
   ❑ Splenic artery (not vein) is present in the stomach bed.
   ❑ Body (not tail) is in relation.

3. **c. Preaortic nodes**
   ❑ Preaortic lymph node term is **not mentioned** in the lymphatic drainage of stomach.

4. **d. Pylorus**
   ❑ Pyloric antrum and pyloric canal along the **lesser** curvature of the stomach drain lymph into **right gastric nodes** (along right gastric artery) and **hepatic nodes** (along hepatic artery).

- **Nerve of Grassi** is a branch of the **right vagus**. *(NEET Pattern 2014)*
  – Failure to divide this nerve may result in **recurrent ulcer.**
- **Nerve of Latarjet** of vagus is seen in the **stomach**. *(NEET Pattern 2014)*
- Stomach do **not** drain into preaortic lymph nodes directly. *(NEET Pattern 2013)*

▶ Intestine - Duodenum, Jejunum, Ileum

Duodenum

A. General Features: The duodenum pursues a C-shaped course around the head of the pancreas.
The duodenum is divided into four parts. Which are as follows:

1. **Superior Part (First Part)**
   ➢ The first 2 cm of the superior part is intraperitoneal and therefore has a mesentery and is mobile; the remaining distal 3 cm of the superior part is retroperitoneal.
   ➢ Radiologists refer to the first 2 cm of the superior part of the duodenum as the **duodenal cap** or **bulb**.
   ➢ The superior part begins at the pylorus of the stomach (**gastroduodenal junction**) which is marked by the **prepyloric vein**.
   ➢ Posterior relationships include the **common bile duct** and **gastroduodenal artery**. The **hepatoduodenal ligament** attaches superiorly and the **greater omentum** attaches inferiorly.
   ➢ Abdominal Viscera

2. **Descending Part (Second Part)**
   ➢ The descending part is retroperitoneal and receives the **common bile duct** and **main pancreatic duct** on its posterior/medial wall at the **hepatopancreatic ampulla (ampulla of Vater).**

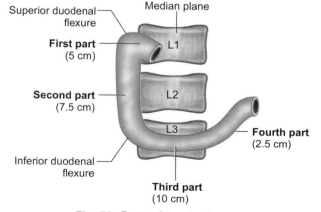

Fig. 79: Parts of the duodenum

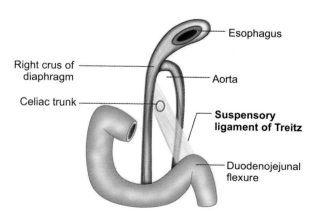

Fig. 80: Suspensory ligament of Treitz

3. **Horizontal Part (Third Part)**
   ➢ The horizontal part is retroperitoneal and runs horizontally across the L3 vertebra between the superior mesenteric artery anteriorly and the aorta and inferior vena cava (IVC) posteriorly.
   ➢ In severe abdominal injuries, this part of the duodenum may be crushed against the L3 vertebra.

4. **Ascending Part (Fourth Part)**
   ➢ The ascending part is intraperitoneal and ascends to meet the jejunum at the **duodenojejunal junction** which occurs approximately at the L2 vertebral level about 2 to 3 cm to the left of the midline.
   ➢ This junction usually forms an acute angle which is called the **duodenojejunal flexure** which is supported by the **ligament of Treitz** (represents the cranial end of the dorsal mesentery).
   ➢ The ligament of Treitz serves as the anatomical landmark for the distinction between **upper and lower gastrointestinal (GI) tract bleeds**.

B. **Arterial Supply:** The arterial supply of the duodenum is from the following:
   ➢ **Supraduodenal artery** which supplies the upper portion of the duodenum (abdominal aorta → celiac trunk → common hepatic artery → gastroduodenal artery → supraduodenal artery).
   ➢ **Anterior and posterior superior pancreaticoduodenal arteries** (abdominal aorta → celiac trunk → common hepatic artery → gastroduodenal artery → anterior and posterior superior pancreaticoduodenal arteries).
   ➢ **Anterior and posterior inferior pancreaticoduodenal arteries** (abdominal aorta → superior mesenteric artery → anterior and posterior inferior pancreaticoduodenal arteries).

C. **Venous Drainage.** The venous drainage of the duodenum is to the following:
   ➢ **Anterior and posterior superior pancreaticoduodenal veins** (anterior and posterior superior pancreaticoduodenal veins → portal vein → hepatic sinusoids → central veins → hepatic veins → inferior vena cava).
   ➢ **Anterior and posterior inferior pancreaticoduodenal veins** (anterior and posterior inferior pancreaticoduodenal veins → superior mesenteric vein → portal vein → hepatic sinusoids → central veins → hepatic veins → inferior vena cava).

D. **Innervation.** See Section VI.

E. **Clinical Considerations**
   ➢ **Duodenal ulcers** most often occur on the anterior wall of the first part of the duodenum (i.e., at the **duodenal cap**) followed by the posterior wall (danger of perforation into the pancreas).
   ➢ **Perforations of the duodenum** occur most often with ulcers on the **anterior wall** of the duodenum. Perforations occur less often with ulcers on the **posterior wall**. However, posterior wall perforations may erode the **gastroduodenal artery** causing severe hemorrhage and extend into the pancreas.

Clinical findings

☐ Air under the diaphragm, pain radiates to the left shoulder.

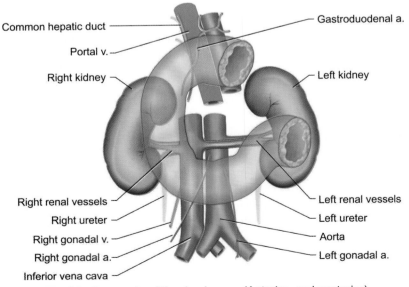

Common hepatic duct
Portal v.
Right kidney
Gastroduodenal a.
Left kidney
Right renal vessels
Right ureter
Right gonadal v.
Right gonadal a.
Inferior vena cava
Left renal vessels
Left ureter
Aorta
Left gonadal a.

Fig. 81: Four parts of the duodenum. (Anterior and posterior)

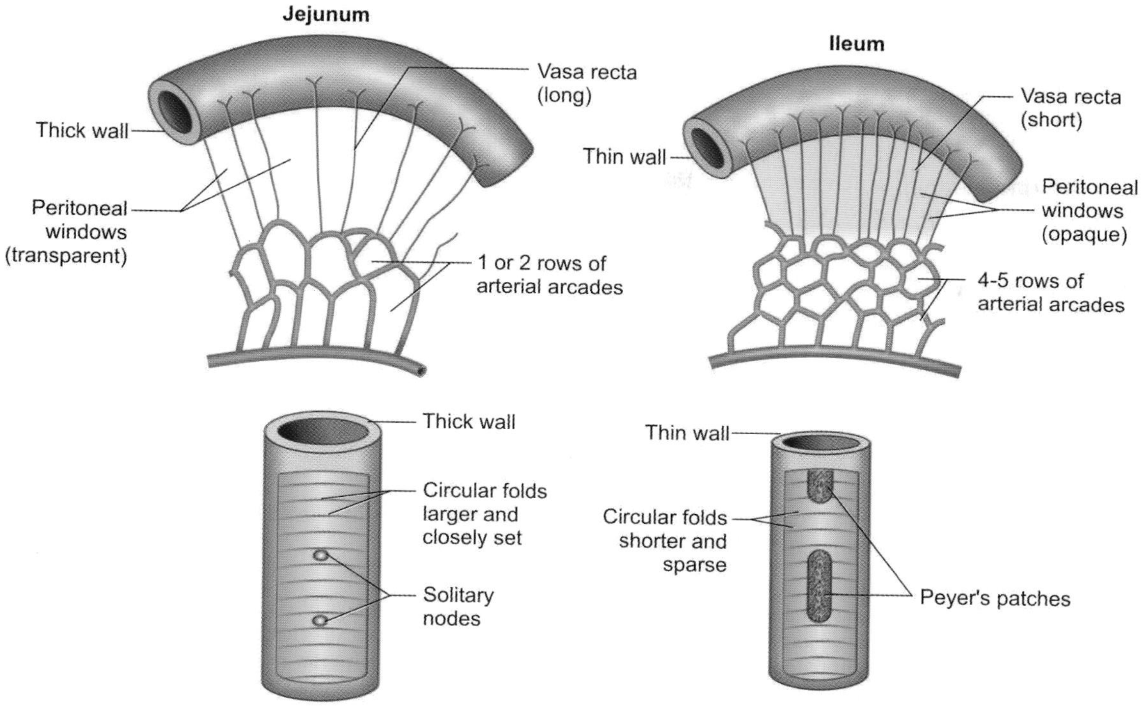

Fig. 82: Differences between the jejunum and ileum

Table 19: Differences between the jejunum and ileum.		
Features	**Jejunum**	**Ileum**
Walls	Thicker and more vascular	Thinner and less vascular
Lumen	Wider and often found empty (diameter = 4 cm)	Narrower and often found full (diameter = 3.5 cm)
Circular folds/plicae circulares (valves of Kerckring)	Longer and closely set	Smaller and sparsely set
Villi	More, larger, thicker, and leaf-like	Less, shorter, thinner, and finger-like
Aggregated lymph follicles (Peyer's patches)	Small, circular, and few in number, and found only in the distal part of the jejunum	Large oval and more in number (± 10 cm × 1.5 cm) and found throughout the extent of ileum being maximum in the distal part
Mesentery	Contains less fat and becomes semitranslucent between the vasa recta called peritoneal windows	Contains more fat and there are no peritoneal windows between the vasa recta
Arterial arcades	One or two rows with long vasa recta	Four or five rows with short vasa recta

Circular folds (valves of Kerckring, plicae circulares, valvulae conniventes) are large valvular flaps (involving both mucosa and submucosa) projecting into the lumen of the small intestine.

❑ Unlike the gastric folds in the stomach, they are **permanent**, and are **not obliterated** when the intestine is distended.
❑ They are **not found** at the commencement of the duodenum but begin to appear about 2.5 or 5 cm beyond the pylorus.
❑ They are **large and numerous** in lower part of the **descending duodenum** and **upper half of the jejunum.**
❑ They gradually **diminish** in size and they almost entirely **disappear** in the lower part of the ileum.
❑ Valvulae conniventes are more prominent in the jejunum giving the '**feathery appearance**' on barium and reduced distally giving a '**featureless**' appearance of **distal ileum**.

1. Which of the following is related to third part of duodenum:
(NEET Pattern 2012)
   a. Portal vein
   b. Head of pancreas
   c. Hepatic artery
   d. Superior mesenteric vein

2. All of these supply the first 2 cm of the duodenum EXCEPT:
(AIIMS 02)
   a. Supraduodenal artery
   b. Common hepatic artery
   c. Gastroduodenal artery
   d. Superior pancreaticoduodenal artery

QUESTIONS

3. **All of the statements are true about ileum EXCEPT:**
   a. Smaller diameter than jejunum
   b. 3-6 arcades in continuation
   c. Large circular mucosal folds
   d. Lymph nodes in mesentery

4. **Valvulae conniventes are seen in:**   (PGIC 2009)
   a. Jejunum   b. Ileum
   c. Stomach   d. Colon
   e. Appendix

5. **On contrast radiography which among the following is FALSE:**   (AIIMS 2011)
   a. Ileum is featureless
   b. Colon has haustrations
   c. Jejunum is feathery
   d. Distal part of duodenum has a cap

6. **WRONG about ileum as compared with jejunum is:**
   a. Short club shaped villi
   b. Long vasa recta
   c. More lymphoid nodules
   d. More fat in mesentery

ANSWERS

1. **d. Superior mesenteric vein > b) Head of pancreas**
   - ❑ Superior mesenteric vein (and artery) cross the **anterior** to the third part of the duodenum to enter the mesentery of small intestine.
   - ❑ Head of pancreas is in **superior** relation.

2. **d. Superior pancreaticoduodenal artery**
   - ❑ Duodenal cap (first 2.5 cm) of duodenum is supplied by branches of various arteries namely, **common hepatic**, right gastric, right gastroepiploic, **gastroduodenal**, **supraduodenal** artery of Wilkie, etc.

3. **c. Large circular mucosal folds**
   - ❑ Circular mucosal folds are **smaller and fewer**
   - ❑ Ileum has **narrower** lumen, as compared with jejunum. There are 3 or 6 arterial arcades with **no windows**.
   - ❑ Lymphatics drain into the lymph nodes in the **mesentery** and finally drain into **superior mesenteric** nodes.

4. **a. Jejunum; b) Ileum**
   - ❑ Valvulae conniventes (Kerckring folds, plicae circulares) are mucosal folds of the small intestine starting from the **second** part of the duodenum, they are **large** and thick at the **jejunum** and considerably decrease in size distally in the ileum.

5. **d. Distal part of duodenum has a cap**
   - ❑ **First part** of the duodenum is visible as a **triangular shadow** on barium studies and is known as **duodenal cap**.
   - ❑ Small intestine contains mucosal folds known as **plicae circulares** that are visible on barium studies and help in the distinction between small intestine and colon.
   - ❑ **Colon** instead can be identified by presence of **haustrations**.
   - ❑ Valvulae conniventes are more prominent in the jejunum giving the '**feathery appearance**' on barium and reduced distally giving a '**featureless**' appearance of **distal ileum**.

6. **b. Long vasa recta**
   - ❑ Ileum has **short vasa recta** with relatively more arcades.

- Circular folds are **absent** in the 1st part of duodenum. (NEET Pattern 2016)
  - The initial 2.5 cm having no folds is seen as the **duodenal cap** in barium meal radiographs.
- **Brunner's glands** are related to **proximal** part of duodenum. (NEET Pattern 2012)
- Length of the intestine is about 8 meter. (NEET Pattern 2015)
  - **Small** intestine is about **6 meters** and the large intestine is about 1.5 meters.
- **Minor** duodenal papilla is opening of **accessory** pancreatic duct. (NEET Pattern 2012)
- Arterial supply of the duodenum is by both **celiac arteries** and **superior mesenteric.**
- Maximum mucosa associated **lymphoid tissue** in small intestine is seen in **Ileum.**
- **Gastroduodenal artery** passes behind the **first part** of duodenum and is prone to **bleeding** in posterior perforation of duodenal ulcer.

◤ Large Intestine

The large intestine is about **1.5 m long** and extends from the cecum in the right iliac fossa to the anus in the perineum. The **shortest** part of the colon is ascending colon (5 inches) and the **longest** is the transverse colon (20 inches).

The three cardinal features of the large intestine are the presence of **taenia coli**, **appendices epiploicae** and **sacculations** (haustrations).

❑ **Taenia coli** are **three ribbon-like bands** of the longitudinal muscle coat. These bands **converge proximally** at the base of the appendix and spread out distally to become **continuous with** the longitudinal muscle coat of the **rectum**.

❑ **Appendices epiploicae** are small pouches of visceral **peritoneum filled with fat** attached to the taenia coli. They are present in the **4 parts** of large intestine (the four parts of colon - ascending, transverse, descending and sigmoid)) and **absent** from the other **4 parts** (cecum, appendix, rectum and anal canal).

❑ **Sacculations** are a series of **pouches** (dilatations) in the wall of cecum and colon between the taenia. They are produced because length of taenia fall short of the length of circular muscle coat.

Arterial supply: Large intestine is supplied by **superior mesenteric artery** (branches: Ileocolic, right colic, middle colic and **inferior mesenteric artery** (branches: Left colic, sigmoidal and superior rectal artery).

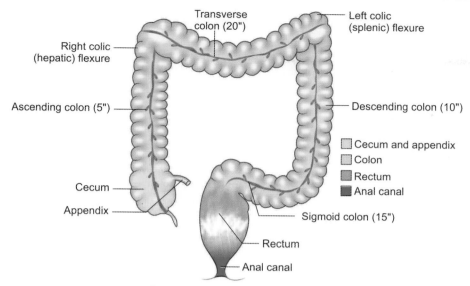

Fig. 83: Parts of the large intestine

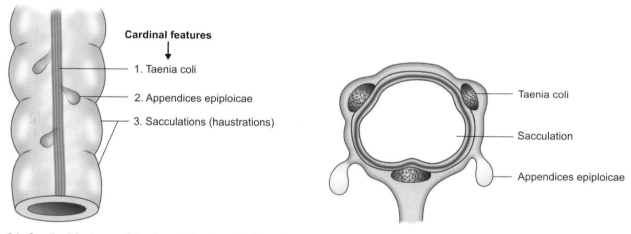

Figs. 84: Cardinal features of the large intestine: Surface view

Fig. 85: Large intestine in cross-sectional view

There are areas of colon with **poor blood supply** resulting from incomplete anastomosis of marginal arteries. These waterhed areas of colon are prone to early ischemia and include:

❑ Splenic flexure (**Griffith** point): Water shed area between superior mesenteric artery and inferior mesenteric artery.

❑ Rectosigmoid junction (**Sudeck's** point): Water shed zone between inferior mesenteric artery and internal iliac artery.

❑ During times of blockage of one of the arteries that supply of the watershed area, such as in atherosclerosis, these regions are **spared** from ischemia by the virtue of their **dual supply**.

❑ However, during times of systemic hypoperfusion such as in DIC or Heart failure, these regions are particularly vulnerable to ischemia by the virtue of the fact that they are supplied by the **most distal branches** of their arteries, and thus the **least likely** to receive sufficient blood.

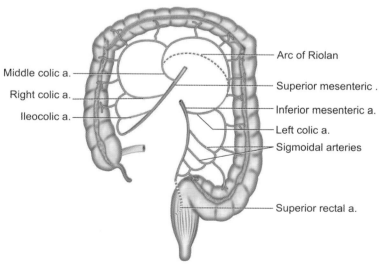

Fig. 86: Arterial supply of the colon. Note the formation of marginal artery of Drummond

▶ Intestine: Vasculature

Table 20: Arterial supply to Intestines.

Artery	Origin	Course	Distribution
Superior mesenteric	Abdominal aorta	Runs in root of mesentery to ileocecal junction	Part of gastrointestinal tract derived from midgut
Intestinal (jejunal and ileal) (n = 15–18)	Superior mesenteric artery	Passes between the two layers of mesentery	Jejunum and ileum
Middle colic		Ascends restroperitoneally and passes between the layers of transverse mesocolon	Transverse colon
Right colic		Passes retroperitoneally to reach the ascending colon	Ascending colon
Ileocolic	Terminal branch of superior mesenteric artery	Runs along root of mesentery and divides into ileal and colic branches	Ileum, cecum, and ascending colon
Appendicular	Ileocolic artery	Passes between layers of meso-appendix	Appendix
Inferior mesenteric	Abdominal aorta	Descends retroperitoneally to left of abdominal aorta	Supplies part of gastrointestinal tract derived from hindgut
Left colic	Inferior mesenteric artery	Passes retroperitoneally towards left to descending colon	Descending colon
Sigmoid (n = 3 – 4)		Passes retroperitoneally towards left to decending colon	Descending and sigmoid colon
Superior rectal	Terminal branch of inferior mesenteric artery	Descends retroperitoneally to rectum	Proximal part of rectum
Middle rectal	Internal iliac	Passes retroperitoneally to rectum	Midparts of rectum
Inferior rectal	Internal pudendal artery	Crosses ischioanal fossa to reach rectum	Distal part of rectum and anal canal

Venous drainage: The veins draining the colon **accompany the arteries**: ileocolic, right colic, and middle colic to join the **superior mesenteric vein**, while the veins, accompanying the branches of inferior mesenteric artery, join the **inferior mesenteric vein**. The superior and inferior mesenteric veins finally drain into the **portal circulation**.

Lymphatic drainage

❑ Lymph nodes related to the colon form **four groups**: epicolic, paracolic, intermediate colic and preterminal colic nodes.

❑ Epicolic nodes are minute whitish nodules on the serosal surface of the colon, sometimes within the appendices epiploicae.

❑ Paracolic nodes lie along the medial borders of the ascending and descending colon and along the mesenteric borders of the transverse and sigmoid colon.

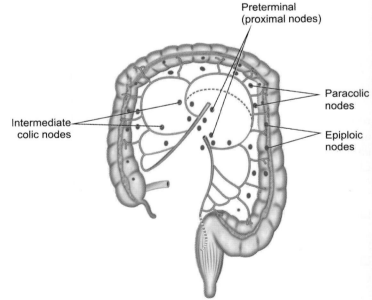

Fig. 87: Lymphatic drainage of the colon.

❑ Intermediate colic nodes lie along the named colic vessels (the ileocolic, right colic, middle colic, left colic, sigmoid and superior rectal arteries).

❑ Preterminal colic nodes lie along the main trunks of the superior and inferior mesenteric arteries and drain into preaortic nodes at the origin of these vessels.

Appendix

A. General Features

- The appendix is an intraperitoneal (**mesoappendix**), narrow, muscular tube attached to the posteromedial surface of the cecum.
- The appendix is located ≈2.5 cm below the ileocecal valve.
- The appendix may lie in the following positions: **Retrocecal (65%), pelvis (32%), subcecal (2%), anterior juxta-ileal (1%), and posterior juxta-ileal (0.5%).**

B. Arterial Supply

- The arterial supply of the appendix is from the **appendicular artery** (abdominal aorta → superior mesenteric artery → ileocolic artery → posterior cecal artery → appendicular artery).

C. Venous Drainage

- The venous drainage of the appendix is to the **posterior cecal vein** (posterior cecal vein → superior mesenteric vein → portal vein → hepatic sinusoids → central veins → hepatic veins → inferior vena cava).

D. Clinical Consideration

Appendicitis begins with the obstruction of the appendix lumen with a fecal concretion (fecalith) and lymphoid hyperplasia followed by distention of the appendix. Clinical findings include initial pain in the umbilical or epigastric region (later pain localizes to the right lumbar region), nausea, vomiting, anorexia, tenderness to palpation, and percussion in the right lumbar region. Complications may include peritonitis due to rupture of the appendix. **McBurney point** is located by drawing a line from the right anterior superior iliac spine to the umbilicus. The midpoint of this line locates the root of the appendix. The appendix is suspended by the **mesoappendix** (i.e., intraperitoneal) and is generally found in the **retrocecal fossa** (although its position is variable).

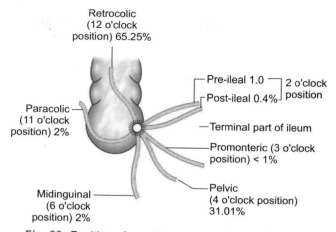

Fig. 88: Position of vermiform appendix (after Treves): Actual position

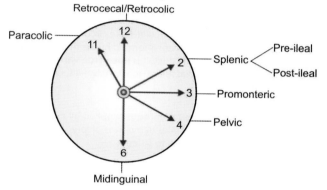

Fig. 89: Positions according to the needle of clock

1. **Which of the following is the terminal group of lymph node for colon:** (AIIMS 2008)
   a. Paracolic
   b. Epicolic
   c. Preaortic
   d. Ileocolic

2. **Arterial supply of sigmoid colon is by:** (PGIC)
   a. Middle colic artery
   b. Marginal artery of Drummond
   c. Left colic artery
   d. Sigmoid artery
   e. Superior hemorrhoidal artery

3. **Structure NOT forming watershed area:** (NEET Pattern 2015)
   a. Splenic flexure
   b. Brain
   c. Duodenum
   d. Spinal cord

4. **Appendix epiploicae present in:** (AIIMS 2010)
   a. Vermiform appendix
   b. Cecum
   c. Sigmoid colon
   d. Rectum

5. **All of the following are the features of large intestine EXCEPT:**
   a. Large intestine secretes acidic mucus which helps in formation of stools
   b. It is a site of mucocutaneous junction
   c. Its epithelium contains goblets cells in large numbers
   d. Absorbs salt and water

6. **TRUE statement about Vermiform appendix:** (PGIC 2006)
   a. Develops from hindgut
   b. Supplied by interior mesenteric artery
   c. Supplied by appendicular branch of ileocolic artery
   d. Does not have mesentery
   e. Has taenia coli

7. **Which fold of GIT is NOT permanent:** (AIIMS 2008)
   a. Ruga
   b. Plicae semilunaris
   c. Spiral Valve of Heister
   d. Transverse rectal

8. **Ligation of the Celiac artery mostly affects all EXCEPT:**
   a. Stomach
   b. Jejunum
   c. Pancreas
   d. Spleen

9. **All are branches of inferior mesenteric artery EXCEPT:** (NEET Pattern 2013)
   a. Left colic
   b. Superior rectal
   c. Middle rectal
   d. Sigmoidal artery

10. **Absence of which amongst the following is the most common variation:** (AIIMS 2014)
    a. Right colic artery
    b. Middle colic artery
    c. Left colic artery
    d. Superior rectal artery

1. **c. Preaortic**
   - ❏ Terminal nodes for colon are superior mesenteric and inferior mesenteric nodes (both are **preaortic** nodes).
   - ❏ Epicolic ⊠ paracolic ⊠ intermediate colic ⊠ preterminal colic ⊠ **preaortic** (direction of lymphatic flow).

2. **b. Marginal artery; d. Sigmoidal artery; e. Superior rectal artery**
   - ❏ Sigmoid colon is supplied by the sigmoidal branches of the **inferior mesenteric** artery and **superior rectal** (hemorrhoidal) artery.
   - ❏ Marginal artery supplies **till rectosigmoid** junction.

3. **c. Duodenum**
   - ❏ Watershed area is supplied by the **small terminal branches** of two or more arteries in an overlapping zone **vulnerable to ischemia**.

4. **c. Sigmoid colon**
   - ❏ Appendices epiploicae are the pouches of peritoneum containing fat present in **all the 4 parts of the colon** (ascending, transverse, descending and sigmoid).
   - ❏ They are absent in the **other 4 parts** of large intestine: At the beginning (cecum and appendix) and at ending (rectum and anal canal).

5. **a. Large intestine secretes acidic mucus which helps in the formation of stools.**
   - ❏ Secretions of large intestine are **alkali** (not acidic).
   - ❏ Mucocutaneous junction is present in the **terminal anal canal**.

6. **c. Supplied by appendicular branch of ileocolic artery**
   - ❏ Vermiform appendix develops from midgut (not hindgut), hence it is supplied by superior (**not inferior**) mesenteric artery.
   - ❏ It has a **mesentery** which carries appendicular branch of ileocolic artery. It **does not** have taenia coli.

7. **a. Ruga**
   - ❏ **Ruga** are the mucosal folds present in the stomach which **disappear** on distension, hence are not permanent.
   - ❏ Plicae semilunaris/circulares are circular folds of mucous membrane and are **permanent** (not obliterated by distension).
   - ❏ Spiral valve of Heister is formed by the mucosal folds at the terminal opening of cystic duct into the common hepatic duct to form the common bile duct. It is **not a true valve** but is permanent and narrows down the lumen of cystic duct at the terminal end.
   - ❏ Transverse **rectal** folds (Houston's valves, plicae transversalis) are **permanent mucosal folds** and are more marked during rectal distension.

8. **c. Jejunum**
   - ❏ Jejunum is a part of **midgut** supplied by the branches of **superior mesenteric** artery (not celiac artery).
   - ❏ Celiac artery supplies derivatives of foregut like stomach, pancreas.
   - ❏ It also gives branch to **spleen**.

9. **c. Middle rectal**
   - ❏ Middle rectal artery is a branch of the **anterior division** of internal iliac artery.
   - ❏ Inferior mesenteric artery supplies **hindgut** derivatives by giving branches like left colic, sigmoidal, superior rectal arteries.

10. **a. Right colic artery**
    - ❏ Right colic artery is a **small** vessel that is **highly variable** in its anatomy and may be absent.

- The **shortest** part of colon is **ascending** colon.
- NOT seen in colon **Peyer's patches**. *(NEET Pattern 2012)*
- Colon is NOT supplied by the Internal iliac artery. *(NEET Pattern 2015)*
- Commonest anatomical position of appendix is **retro-caecal**. *(NEET Pattern 2013)*
- Appendicular artery is a branch of **Ileocolic** artery. *(NEET Pattern 2012)*
- **Valve of Gerlach** is an inconstant fold of mucous membrane resembling a valve at the caecal end of the vermiform appendix. *(NEET Pattern 2016)*
- **Watershed area** between superior mesenteric artery and inferior mesenteric artery prone to early ischemia is **splenic flexure**. *(AIIMS 2007)*
- **Rectum** is devoid of sacculations, appendices epiploicae or mesentery.

◤ Liver and Hepatobiliary Apparatus

Functional anatomy of the liver is based on Couinaud's division of the liver into eight (subsequently nine, then later revised back to eight) functional segments, based on the distribution of portal venous branches in the parenchyma. Further understanding of the intrahepatic biliary anatomy is used as the main guide for division of the liver by few investigators. The liver is divided into four portal sectors by the four main branches of the portal vein. These are right lateral, right medial, left medial and left lateral. The three main hepatic veins lie between these sectors as intersectoral veins. These intersectoral planes are also called portal fissures (or scissures). Each sector is subdivided into segments (usually two), based on their supply by tertiary divisions of the vascular biliary (Glissonian) sheaths.

◤ Liver

General Features

> The liver stroma begins as a thin connective tissue capsule called **Glisson capsule** that extends into the liver around the portal triads, around the periphery of a hepatic lobule, extends into the perisinusoidal space of Disse to surround hepatocytes, and then terminates around the central vein.

The components of the **porta hepatis** are the following: Bile duct, portal vein, hepatic artery, lymphatic vessels, hepatic nerves.

    Historically, the liver was divided into **left** and **right** lobes by the obvious **external** landmark of the **falciform ligament**. Not only was this description **oversimplified**, but it was **anatomically incorrect** in relation to the blood supply to the liver.

- ❏ The **functional anatomy** of the liver is composed of **eight segments**, each supplied by **a single portal triad** (also called a pedicle) composed of a **portal vein**, **hepatic artery**, and **bile duct**.
- ❏ These segments are further organized into **four sectors** separated by **scissura** containing the **three main hepatic veins**.
- ❏ The four sectors are even further organized into the right and left liver. The terms right liver and left **liver** are preferable to the terms right **lobe** and left lobe **because there is no external mark** that allows the identification of the right and left liver.
- ❏ This system was originally described in 1957 by Goldsmith and Woodburne and by **Couinaud**. It defines hepatic anatomy because it is **most relevant to surgery** of the liver.
- ❏ The functional anatomy is **more often** seen as **cross-sectional imaging.**

Lobes of the Liver

- ➢ The liver is classically divided into the **right lobe** and **left lobe** by the **interlobar fissure** (an invisible line running from the gallbladder to the IVC), **quadrate lobe**, and **caudate lobe**.
- ➢ The left lobe contains the **falciform ligament** (a derivative of the ventral mesentery) with the **ligamentum teres** (a remnant of the left umbilical vein) along its inferior border.
- ➢ The **bare area** of the liver is located on the diaphragmatic surface and is devoid of peritoneum.
- ➢ **Liver segmentation**. The right portal fissure, the main portal fissure, and the umbilical fissure divide the liver into four vertical divisions. Three of the four vertical divisions are further divided by the transverse portal plane into eight liver segments (I to VIII) each supplied by a tertiary branch of the portal triad. Liver segments I to VIII each has its own intrasegmental blood supply and biliary drainage.
- ➢ Liver is divided into lobes following two classifications:
  1. Anatomical lobes
  2. Physiological (functional) lobes

Note: Recently these two classification have become more and more overlapping.

Anatomical Lobes

- ❏ **Falciform ligament** (diaphragmatic surface) divides liver into right and left anatomical lobes. On the visceral surface falciform ligament is followed to **fissure for ligamentum venosum** and **fissure for ligamentum teres**, hence demarcating left anatomical lobe from right.
- ❏ Anatomical right lobe is approximately six times larger than the left lobe.
- ❏ Some authors mention four lobes of liver:

Note: Two fissures and two fossa form a H-shaped figure dividing liver into 4 lobes.

1. Right lobe to right of groove for IVC and the fossa for gallbladder.
2. Left lobe to the left of the fissures for ligamentum teres and ligamentum venosum.
3. **Caudate lobe** lying between the groove for ligamentum venosum (on left) and groove for the inferior vena cava (on the right), located above porta hepatis.
4. **Quadrate lobe** bounded by fissure for ligamentum teres (on left) and gallbladder fossa (on right), lying below porta hepatis.

Functional (Physiological) Lobes

- ❏ This division of the liver into **lobes** is based on the intrahepatic distribution of branches of the **bile ducts, hepatic artery, and portal vein**.

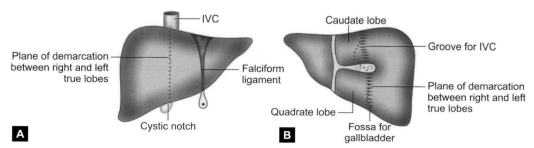

Figs. 90A and B: True/physiological lobes of the liver: (A) Plane of demarcation on anterosuperior surface; (B) Visceral surface is shown by the interrupted redline

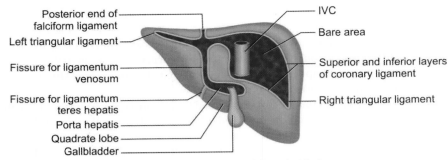

Fig. 91: Liver—viewed from behind

❏ It is further subdivided into four **sectors** (divisions) and then into eight **segments**, each served independently by a secondary or tertiary branch of the portal triad, respectively.

Note: **Cantlie's line** divides liver into right- and left hemiliver and passes through the fossa for gallbladder to the groove for IVC. On the posterior surface it runs from fossa for IVC to the cystic notch.

❏ Each physiological lobe of the liver has its own primary branch of the hepatic artery and portal vein and is drained by its own hepatic duct.
According to Gray's Anatomy (Edition 41) the **functional anatomy** of the liver is based upon.

1. **Portal vein** branches
2. **Biliary duct** distribution
3. **Vascular biliary** (Glissonian) sheath

Note: There is a mention of **hepatic veins** being in the portal **fissures** (scissures) as well.

❏ **Couinaud's division** of the liver into eight (subsequently nine, then later revised back to eight) functional segments based on the distribution of **portal venous branches** in the parenchyma.
❏ The liver is divided into **four portal sectors** by the four main branches of the portal vein. These are right lateral, right medial, left medial and left lateral (sometimes the term posterior is used in place of lateral, and anterior in place of medial).
❏ The three main hepatic veins lie between these sectors as intersectoral veins.
❏ These intersectoral planes are also called portal fissures (or scissures).
❏ Each sector is subdivided into segments (usually two) based on their supply by tertiary divisions of the **vascular biliary (Glissonian) sheaths.**

Note: Glisson's capsule of the liver becomes condensed as Glissonian sheaths around the branches of the portal triad structures as they enter the liver parenchyma and subdivide into segmental branches. Thus, each bile duct, hepatic artery and portal vein is surrounded by a single fibrous sheath which Couinaud called the 'Valoean sheath'.

Couinaud's Classification

❏ Hepatic segments are numbered I to VIII in a clockwise direction.
❏ Segments I to IV belong to left hemiliver and V to VIII are present in the right hemiliver.
❏ Segment I to IV (left lobe) are supplied by the left branch of hepatic artery, left branch of portal vein and drained by left hepatic duct.
❏ Segments V to VIII of right lobe are supplied by the right hepatic artery, right branch of portal vein and drained by right hepatic duct.

Caudate Lobe

❏ **Segment I** corresponds to the anatomical **caudate lobe** and is a boundary line structure (belongs to both right and left hemiliver). It has dual artery, venous and biliary supply.
❏ It lies posterior to segment IV and is subdivided into three parts (caudate process, Spiegel lobe and paracaval portion).
❏ The Glissonian sheaths to segment I arise from both right and left main sheaths; the segment therefore receives vessels from both the left and right branches of the portal vein and hepatic arteries.
❏ Caudate lobe drains bile into both the hepatic ducts and venous drainage is directly into IVC (and not the major hepatic veins).

Fissures of Liver

Three major fissures (main, left and right portal fissures) are not visible on the surface, run through the liver parenchyma and contain the three main hepatic veins.

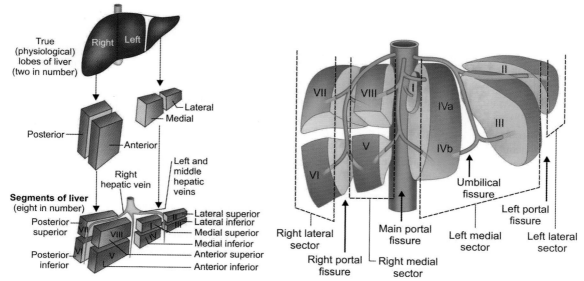

Figs. 92A and B: Segment of the liver

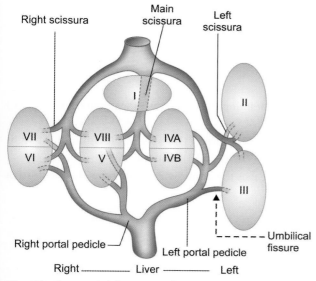

Fig. 93: Segmental Anatomy of the Liver. Each segment receives its own portal pedicle (triad of portal vein, hepatic artery, and bile duct). The eight segments are illustrated, and the four sectors, divided by the three main hepatic veins running in scissura, are shown. The umbilical fissure (not a scissura) is shown to contain the left portal pedicle

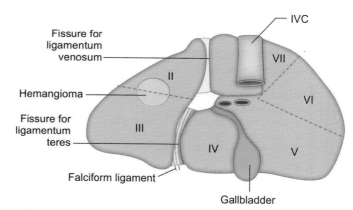

Fig. 94: Posteroinferior view of liver showing hemangioma to the left of falciform ligament

Three minor fissures (umbilical, venous and fissure of Gans) are visible as physical clefts of the liver surface. The fissure of Gans is also known as Rouvière's sulcus or the incisura hepatis dextra.

The liver has two lobes, which can be further subdivided into four sectors/divisions and then into eight surgically resectable hepatic segments, each served independently by a secondary or tertiary branch of the portal triad, respectively.

▼ Liver Lobes, Sectors and Segments

❏ Right lobe:
  ➢ The anterior sector of the right lobe contains superior (VIII) and inferior (V) segments.
  ➢ The posterior sector of the right lobe has superior (VII) and inferior (VI) segments.
❏ Left lobe:
  ➢ The medial sector of the left lobe (quadrate lobe, segment IV) is the part of the left lobe from a surgical perspective but lies to the right of the midline; it is further divided into a superior subsegment (A) and an inferior subsegment (B).
  ➢ The lateral sector of the left lobe contains segments II and III.

Table 21: Terminology for subdivision of liver.

Anatomical term	Right lobe				Left Lobe	Caudate Lobe	
Function/ Surgical term	Right (part of liver [Right portal lobe*])			Left (part of) Liver [Left portal lobe⁺]		Posterior (part of) liver	
	Right lateral division	Right medial division	Left medial division		Left lateral division	[Right caudate lobe⁺]	[Left caudate lobe*]
	Posterior lateral segment **Segment VII** [Posterior superior area]	Posterior lateral segment **Segment VIII** [Anterior superior area]	[Medial superior area] Left medial segment **Segment IV** [Medial inferior area = quadrate lobe]		Lateral segment **Segment II** [Lateral superior area]	Posterior segment **Segment I**	
	Right anterior lateral segment **Segment VI** [Posterior inferior area]	Anterior medial segment **Segment V** [Anterior inferior area]			Left lateral anterior segment **Segment III** [Lateral inferior area]		

The labels in the table and figures above reflect the new **Terminologia Antaomica: International antomical Terminology (1998). Previous terminology is in brackets.
Under the schema of the previous terminology, the caudate lobe was divided into right and left halves, and
*The right half of the caudate lobe was considered a subdivision of the right portal lobe
⁺The left half of the caudate lobe was considered a subdivision of the left portal lobe.
⁺⁺Cantile line and the right sagittal fissure are surface markings defining the main portal fissure.

Liver transplantation: Donor's liver regains its original size in 2 to 3 weeks.

❑ For **pediatric** cases, the left lateral segment (segments II and III) or a total **left hepatic lobectomy** (segments II, III, and IV) is generally enough to provide sufficient liver mass.

❑ For **adult-to-adult** transplantation, **right hepatic lobectomy** is usually required. The surgical technique for right hepatectomy involves separation of the right hepatic lobes (segments V, VI, VII, and VIII) from the left.

❑ Right hepatectomy results in a graft weighing 500 to 1000 grams, which leaves the donor with approximately one third of the original liver mass.

1. **Relation of caudate lobe of liver is:**
   a. Posterior to portal vein
   b. Anterior to right inferior phrenic artery
   c. Posterior to ligamentum teres
   d. Posterior to ligamentum venosum

2. **According to Couinaud's classification, the 4th segment of the liver is:** *(AIIMS 2007)*
   a. Caudate lobe
   b. Quadrate lobe
   c. Left lobe
   d. Right lobe

3. **A hemangioma was found on the left of the attachment of falciform ligament of the liver. Surgeon dissecting Couinaud's segments of liver to the left of attachment of falciform ligament resects which lobes:** *(AIPG 2008, 13)*
   a. 2,3
   b. 1,3
   c. 2,4a
   d. 1,4a

4. **Which among the following about biliary drainage of liver is NOT true:** *(AIIMS 2009,11)*
   a. Caudate lobe drains only left hepatic duct
   b. Right anterior hepatic duct formed by V and VIII segment
   c. Left hepatic duct formed in umbilical fissure
   d. Left hepatic duct crosses IV segment

5. **All of the following segments of liver drains into right hepatic duct EXCEPT:** *(AIIMS 2009)*
   a. I
   b. III
   c. V
   d. VIII

6. **All are true about functional divisions of liver EXCEPT:** *(AIIMS 2015)*
   a. Based upon portal vein and hepatic vein
   b. Divided into 8 segments
   c. Three major and three minor fissures
   d. 4 sectors

7. **Liver is divided into two surgical halves by all EXCEPT:**
   a. Cantlie's line
   b. Right hepatic vein
   c. Portal vein at porta hepatis
   d. Biliary duct at porta hepatis

8. **Liver is divided into right and left lobe by all EXCEPT:** *(NEET Pattern 2016)*
   a. Hepatic vein
   b. Portal vein
   c. Hepatic artery
   d. Hepatic ducts

9. **Liver is divided in 2 halves by all EXCEPT:** *(NEET Pattern 2013)*
   a. Hepatic vein
   b. Portal vein
   c. Hepatic artery
   d. Hepatic duct

1. **b. Anterior to right inferior phrenic artery**
   - ❑ Caudate lobe lies **anterior** to right inferior phrenic artery.
   - ❑ It is **superior** to portal vein and to **right of** fissure for ligament venosum.

2. **b. Quadrate lobe**
   - ❑ Quadrate lobe (4b) of liver is **inferior** part of segment 4, better visualized from the **posterior** aspect of liver.
   - ❑ Caudate (comma-shaped) lobe is the beginning of the segmental nomenclature as is taken as segment-I (posterior segment).
   - ❑ Segments are numbered in a **clockwise** direction when liver is **visualized in anterior view**.
   - ❑ **EXCEPT: for the caudate** lobe (**third liver**), the liver is divided into right and left livers based on the primary (1 degree) division of the **portal triad into right and left branches**.
   - ❑ The plane between the right and left livers being the **main portal fissure** in which the **middle hepatic** vein lies.

3. **a. 2, 3**
   - ❑ Segments **2 and 3 lie to the left of** the falciform ligament and will be resected in this patient.
   - ❑ Couinaud's classification divides liver into various segments based upon the distribution of portal vein and biliary ducts.
   - ❑ Major removal of the liver segments follows the Couinaud's classification for putting the lines of resection.
   - ❑ The **hepatic veins** provide **surgical planes** to dissect the liver, but the surgeon has to bear with the hemorrhage, as they are followed and are a major source of bleeding during dissection.

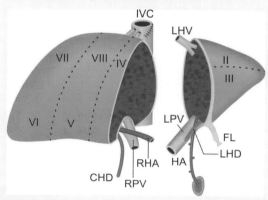

Key: L – Left, R – Right, C - Common; HA – Hepatic Artery, HV – Hepatic Vein; HD – Hepatic Duct; FL – Falciform Ligament

4. **a. Caudate lobe drains only left hepatic duct**
   - ❑ Caudate lobe is a **boundary line** structure and drains bile into **both the hepatic ducts**.
   - ❑ It may in fact be considered a **third** liver; its vascularization is **independent** of the bifurcation of the portal triad (it receives vessels from **both** right and left **bundles**).

5. **b. III**
   - ❑ Segment III belongs to **left liver** and drains bile into left (**not right**) hepatic duct.
   - ❑ Right liver has segment V, VI, VII and VIII which drain into right hepatic duct.
   - ❑ Caudate lobe (segment I) drains into **both** right and left hepatic duct.

6. **c. Three major and three minor fissures**
   - ❑ Gray's Anatomy mentions three major fissures (**not minor**) in the functional division of liver.
   - ❑ **Functional anatomy** of the liver is based on Couinaud's division of the liver into eight functional segments based on the distribution of **portal venous branches** in the parenchyma.
   - ❑ The liver is divided into **four portal sectors** by the four main branches of the **portal vein**. These are right lateral, right medial, left medial and left lateral.
   - ❑ The **three main hepatic veins** lie between these sectors as **intersectoral** veins. These intersectoral planes are also called portal fissures (or scissures) namely: Main, left and right portal fissures.
   - ❑ Each functional segment receives its own primary branch of the hepatic artery and hepatic portal vein and is drained by its own hepatic duct.

7. **b) Right hepatic vein**
   - ❑ Liver is divided into **two surgical halves** by following **middle** hepatic vein (**not the right** hepatic vein).

8. **a. Hepatic vein**
   - ❑ Liver is divided into right and left lobe by DAV (Bile Ducts, hepatic Artery and portal Vein) structures and **not** the **hepatic veins**.

9. **a. Hepatic vein**
   - ❑ Liver is divided into two halves (right and left) and each receives its own primary branch of the hepatic **artery** and hepatic portal **vein** and is drained by its own hepatic **duct**.
   - ❑ From a surgical point of view, the liver is divided into right and left lobes of almost equal (60:40) size by a major fissure (**Cantlie's line**) running from the gallbladder fossa in front to the IVC fossa behind.
   - ❑ This division is based on the right and left branches of the hepatic **artery**, portal **vein**, and tributaries of hepatic **ducts**.
   - ❑ The **middle** hepatic vein (MHV) lies in **Cantlie's line**.

- **Caudate lobe** of liver is segment I. *(NEET Pattern 2013)*
- Liver segment which is **physiologically independent** is segment I. *(NEET Pattern 2015, 16)*
- The **right lobe** of liver consists of segments: V, VI, VII, VIII. *(AIIMS 2004)*

Table 22: Relations of diaphragmatic and visceral surfaces of the liver

Surface		Relations
Diaphragmatic surface (parietal surface)	Superior surface with diaphragm intervening	- Corresponding lung and pleura on either side - Pericardium and heart in the centre
	Anterior surface	- Xiphoid process - Anterior abdominal wall
	Right lateral surface with diaphragm intervening	- Lung and pleura in the upper one-third - Costodiaphragmatic recess in the middle one-third - 10th and 11th ribs in the lower one-third
	Posterior surface: a. With peritoneum intervening b. With peritoneum not intervening	- Abdominal part of the esophagus - Right suprarenal gland - Inferior vena cava
Visceral surface (inferior surface)	a. With peritoneum intervening b. With peritoneum not intervening	- Stomach - Duodenum - Right colic flexure - Right kidney - Gallbladder

Most of the liver is covered by the peritoneum. The areas which are not covered by the peritoneum are:

- ❑ Bare area of the liver: It is a triangular area on the posterior aspect of the right lobe.
- ❑ Fossa for gallbladder, on the inferior surface of the liver between right and quadrate lobes.
- ❑ Groove for IVC, on the posterior surface of the right lobe of the liver.
- ❑ Groove for ligamentum venosum.
- ❑ Porta hepatis.
- ❑ **Arterial Supply**
  - ➤ The arterial supply of the liver is from the **right hepatic artery** and **left hepatic artery** (abdominal aorta → celiac trunk → common hepatic artery → proper hepatic artery → right hepatic artery and left hepatic artery → hepatic sinusoids).
- ❑ **Portal Supply**
  - ➤ The portal supply of the liver is from the **portal vein** (superior mesenteric vein, inferior mesenteric vein, and splenic vein → portal vein → hepatic sinusoids).
  - ➤ The portal vein is formed by the union of the splenic vein and superior mesenteric vein.
  - ➤ The inferior mesenteric vein joins the splenic vein.
  - ➤ The arterial blood and portal blood mix in the hepatic sinusoids.
- ❑ **Venous Drainage**
  - ➤ The venous drainage of the liver is to the **central veins** located at the center of a classic liver lobule (central veins → hepatic veins → inferior vena cava).
- ❑ **Innervation**
  - ➤ The exact function of both the parasympathetic and sympathetic innervations is unclear, EXCEPT: that sympathetics play a role in vasoconstriction.
  - ➤ Pathology involving the diaphragmatic surface of the liver may be referred via the phrenic nerve to the right shoulder region (C3, 4, 5 dermatomes).

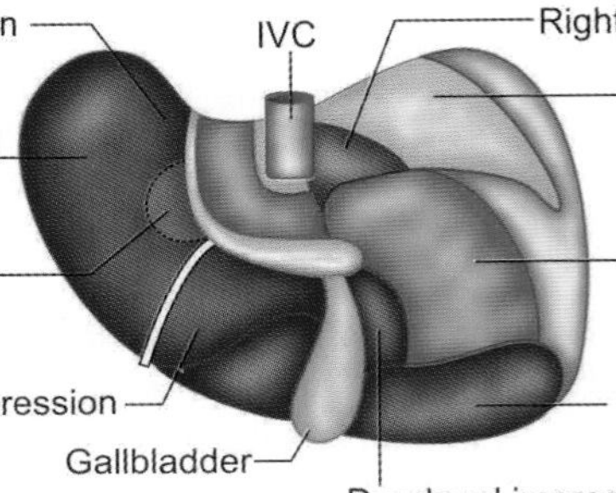

Fig. 95: Visceral relations of the liver (relations of the inferior/visceral surface of the liver)

(labels: Esophageal impression, IVC, Right suprarenal impression, Gastric impression, Bare area of liver, Tuber omentale, Right renal impression, Pyloric impression, Colic impression, Gallbladder, Duodenal impression)

1. **TRUE statement regarding bare area of liver:** *(JIPMER 2008)*
   a. Covered by visceral peritoneum
   b. Supplied by phrenic nerve
   c. Present In the left lobe of liver
   d. Attached to the diaphragm

2. **Blood supply of the liver is:** *(NEET Pattern 2013)*
   a. 80% hepatic artery, 20% portal vein
   b. 20% hepatic artery, 80% portal vein
   c. 50% hepatic artery, 50% portal vein
   d. 100% hepatic artery

3. **Which of the following statement about portal triad is CORRECT:** *(JIPMER 2016)*
   a. Hepatic artery is medial to portal vein
   b. Common bile duct is medial to hepatic artery
   c. Portal vein is posterior to both common bile duct and hepatic duct
   d. Portal vein is anterior to common bile duct but posterior to portal vein

1. **d. Attached to the diaphragm**
   - ❑ Bare area of liver is present in right (**not left**) lobe of liver, in contact with diaphragm and **not** covered by visceral peritoneum is supplied by autonomic nervous system (**not phrenic nerve**).
   - ❑ Areas **not** covered by peritoneum: Fossa for gallbladder, fissure for ligamentum venosum, groove for IVC

2. **b. 20% hepatic artery, 80% portal vein**
   - ❑ Liver receives a **dual** blood supply from the hepatic **portal vein** and **hepatic arteries**.
   - ❑ **Portal vein** delivers approximately 75-80% of the liver's blood supply, and carries **venous blood** drained from the spleen, gastrointestinal tract, and its associated organs.
   - ❑ **Hepatic artery** supplies arterial blood to the liver accounting for the remaining quarter of its blood flow. **Oxygen** is provided from both sources; approximately **half** of the liver's oxygen demand is met by the portal vein, and **half** is met by the hepatic artery.
   - ❑ Blood flows through the liver sinusoids and empties into the **central vein** of each lobule. The central veins coalesce into **hepatic veins**, which leave the liver and drain into the **inferior vena cava**.

3. **c. Portal vein is posterior to both common bile duct and hepatic duct**
   - ❑ The arrangement of structures at the porta hepatis is DAV (in **anterior to posterior order**): Duct (bile duct) → Artery (hepatic) → Vein (portal).
   - ❑ Hepatic artery lies medial to the bile duct, both being anterior to portal vein.

- ▪ **Venous blood** of liver is drained by **hepatic veins**.
- ▪ Liver weights about 1500-1600 g in males and 1200 g-1300 g in females. *(NEET Pattern 2013)*
- ▪ **Bare area of liver** is related to **hepatic veins** draining into inferior vena cava. *(NEET Pattern 2015)*

▼ Gallbladder

A. General Features
- ➢ The gallbladder is divided into the **fundus** (anterior portion), **body,** and the **neck** (posterior portion).
- ➢ A small pouch **(Hartmann pouch)** may extend from the neck as a sequela to pathologic changes and is a common site for gallstones to lodge.
- ➢ **Rokitansky-Aschoff sinuses** occur when the mucosa of the gallbladder penetrates deep into the muscularis externa. They are an early indicator of pathologic changes (e.g. acute cholecystitis or gangrene).

B. Arterial Supply
- ➢ The arterial supply of the gallbladder is from the **cystic artery** (abdominal aorta → celiac trunk → common hepatic artery → proper hepatic artery → right hepatic artery → cystic artery).

C. Venous Drainage
- ➢ The venous drainage of the gallbladder is to the **cystic vein** (cystic vein → portal vein → hepatic sinusoids → central veins → hepatic veins → inferior vena cava).

▼ Extrahepatic Biliary Ducts

A. General Features
- ➢ The **right and left hepatic ducts** join together after leaving the liver to form the **common hepatic duct**.
- ➢ The common hepatic duct is joined at an acute angle by the **cystic duct** to form the **bile duct**.
- ➢ The cystic duct drains bile from the gallbladder. The mucosa of the cystic duct is arranged in a spiral fold with a core of smooth muscle known as the **spiral valve (valve of Heister)**. The spiral valve keeps the cystic duct constantly open so that bile can flow freely in either direction.

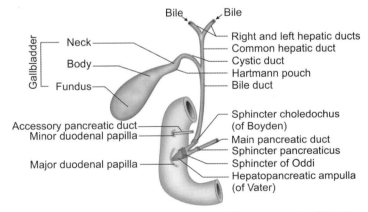

Fig. 96: Components of the extrahepatic biliary apparatus. Note the sphincters around hepatopancreatic ampulla and terminal parts of the bile, and main pancreatic duct

- ❑ The bile duct passes posterior to the pancreas and ends at the **hepatopancreatic ampulla (ampulla of Vater)** where it joins the **pancreatic duct**.
  The **sphincter of Oddi** is an area of thickened smooth muscle that surrounds the bile duct as it traverses the ampulla. The sphincter of Oddi **controls bile flow** (sympathetic innervation causes contraction of the sphincter).
- ❑ Minor duodenal papilla is the opening of accessory pancreatic duct. *(NBEP 2013)*
- ❑ The gallbladder is a blind pouch joined to a single cystic duct in which numerous mucosal folds form the spiral valve (of Heister).
- ❑ The cystic duct joins with the common hepatic duct, and together they form the common bile duct that leads into the duodenum.

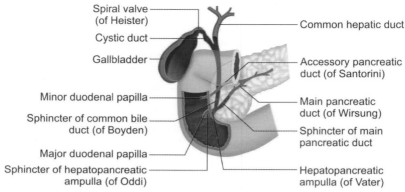

Figs. 97: Relationship of hepatic, pancreatic, and gallbladder duct

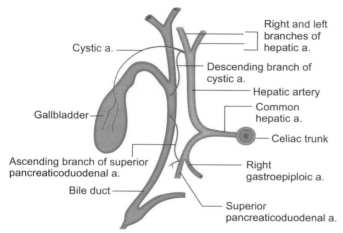

Fig. 98: Blood supply of the gallbladder and bile duct

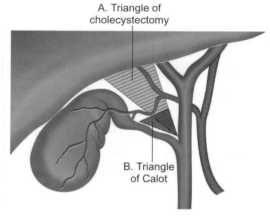

Fig. 99: Blood supply of the gallbladder and bile duct

❏ At the entry to the duodenum, the common bile duct is joined by the main pancreatic duct to form the hepatopancreatic ampulla (of Vater), and together they enter the second part of the duodenum.

❏ Sphincters of the common bile duct (of Boyden), the main pancreatic duct, and the hepatopancreatic ampulla (of Oddi) control the flow of bile and pancreatic secretion into the duodenum.

❏ When the common bile duct sphincter contracts, bile cannot enter the duodenum; it backs up and flows into the gallbladder, where it is concentrated and stored.

Calot's Triangle

❏ Hepatobiliary triangle is a region formed between the cystic duct, the common hepatic duct and the inferior surface of the liver. It is often mistakenly referred to as Calot's triangle, which is an isosceles triangle based on the common hepatic duct, with the cystic artery and cystic duct forming its sides.

1. Sensory nerve supply of gall bladder is through:
(NEET Pattern 2016)
a. Vagus nerve
b. Phrenic nerve
c. Sympathetic nerve
d. Splanchnic nerve

2. Spiral valve of Heister is seen in: (NEET Pattern 2012, 13)
a. Neck of gallbladder
b. Cystic duct
c. Pancreatic duct
d. Pylorus

3. Sphincter of Oddi consists of: (AIIMS 2009,11)
a. 2 sphincters
b. 3 sphincters
c. 4 sphincters
d. 5 sphincters

4. Which is NOT a boundary of Calot's triangle:
(NEET Pattern 2015)
a. Common hepatic duct
b. Cystic duct
c. Right lobe of liver
d. Gallbladder

5. Calot's triangle is bounded by all EXCEPT:
a. Inferior surface of liver
b. Common hepatic duct
c. Cystic duct
d. Cystic artery

6. Which of the following statements is/are TRUE regarding the relation of bile duct: (PGIC 2005)
a. Posteriorly related to 1st part of duodenum
b. Anteriorly related to 1st part of duodenum
c. Related posteriorly to the tunnel of pancreatic head
d. Related to IVC posteriorly
e. Lies left to hepatic artery in the free border of lesser omentum

7. True regarding common bile duct is all EXCEPT: *(AIPG 2000)*
a. Opens 10 cm distal to the pylorus
b. Lies anterior to IVC
c. Portal vein lies posterior to it
d. Usually opens into duodenum separate from the main pancreatic duct

8. Predominant blood supply to the supraduodenal bile duct is derived from: *(AIPG 2012)*
a. Vessels that run upward along the bile duct from the duodenal end of the duct such as the retroduodenal and the gastroduodenal arteries.
b. Vessels that run downward along the bile duct from the hepatic and of the duct such as the right hepatic artery.
c. Vessels that arise from the hepatic artery proper as it runs up along the common bile duct and supplies it with twigs in a non-axial distribution.
d. Vessels that arise from the cystic artery.

1. b. Phrenic nerve
- Innervation of the gallbladder consists of **sympathetic** fibers from the celiac plexus (T7–T9), **parasympathetic** fibers from the vagus (right and left) nerve and **sensory** fibers from the **right phrenic** nerve.

2. b. Cystic duct
- Spiral valve of Heister is formed by the mucosal folds at the terminal opening of **cystic duc**t into the common hepatic duct to form the common bile duct. It narrows down the lumen of cystic duct at the terminal end.
- It is **not a true valve** but is made up of permanent mucosal folds and when the duct is distended, the spaces between the folds get dilated, making the folds more obvious.

3. b. 3 sphincters > c. 4 sphincters > d. 5 sphincters
- The entire sphincter mechanism is actually composed of numerous muscle fiber sphincters and the answer stands **controversial**.
- The latest information points to a total number of **three** (Gray's Anatomy, edition 41), though there have been mention of **four**, **five** and still more higher number in the past.
- The portal for entry of bile and pancreatic juice in humans has been divided into **three** parts: (i) **biliary** (choledochus), (ii) **pancreaticus**, and (iii) **ampulla**.

4. d. Gallbladder
- Calot's triangle is an **isosceles** triangle with the following boundaries (Gray's Anatomy edition 41):
  - Medially (Base): Common hepatic duct
  - Superiorly: Cystic artery
  - Inferiorly: Cystic duct
Note: Some authors consider right lobe of liver as the superior boundary of Calot's triangle.

5. a. Inferior surface of liver
- Calot's triangle lies between three Cs—Common hepatic duct, Cystic duct, and Cystic artery.
- **Inferior** surface of liver forms the boundary for the triangle of cholecystectomy.
- The cystic artery commonly arises from the right hepatic artery is the boundary for the Calot's triangle.
- In the angle between common hepatic duct and cystic duct lies in the **Calot's lymph node of Lund** which gets inflamed in cholecystitis.

6. b. Anteriorly related to 1st part of duodenum; c. Related posteriorly to the tunnel of pancreatic head; d. Related to IVC posteriorly
- Bile duct has four parts:
  - **Supraduodenal** part - Descends in the right free margin of the lesser omentum to the right of the hepatic artery proper and anterior to the portal vein.
  - **Retroduodenal** part - Descends behind the first part of the duodenum with the gastroduodenal artery on its left and IVC on its posterior aspect.
  - **Infraduodenal** (or pancreatic) part - It runs in the groove on the posterior surface of the pancreas. Here it lies in front of the IVC and is accompanied on its left side by the gastroduodenal artery.
  - **Intraduodenal** part

7. d. Usually opens into duodenum separate from the main pancreatic duct
- Common bile duct joins the pancreatic duct to form **hepatopancreatic duct** which opens into 2nd part of duodenum at major **duodenal papilla**.

8. a. Vessels that run upward along the bile duct from the duodenal end of the duct such as the retroduodenal and the gastroduodenal arteries
- Blood supply of supraduodenal bile duct
  - **Axial** blood supply
  - The blood supply to the supraduodenal bile duct is essentially axial (98%)
  - The most important of these vessels run along the lateral borders of the bile duct and are called the '3 o clock' and '9 o' clock arteries.
  - These together with other smaller branches and retroportal vessels from a free anastomosis within the wall of the bile duct.
  - 60% of the blood supply occurs from the duodenal (caudal) end of the duct primarily from branches of the retroduodenal artery (Posterior superior pancreaticoduodenal artery).
  - 38% of the blood supply occurs from the hepatic (cephalic) end of the right hepatic artery.
- **Non-axial** blood supply
  - Non-axial blood supply accounts for only 2% of blood supply to the supraduodenal bile duct.
  - This non-axial blood supply is derived from the branches of the hepatic artery proper as it runs along the common bile duct.

- Cystic artery is usually a branch of which of the **right hepatic artery**. *(NEET Pattern 2012)*
  - As a variation, It may arise from the main trunk of the hepatic artery, from the left hepatic artery, or from the gastroduodenal artery.
- **Medial** boundary of Calot's triangle is formed by common **hepatic duct**. *(NEET Pattern 2016)*
- **In** the angle between common hepatic duct and cystic duct lies the **Calot's lymph node of Lund**. *(NEET Pattern 2012)*
- Pancreatic and bile ducts open into duodenum at **Ampulla**. *(NEET Pattern 2013)*
- **Fibromuscular wall** is seen in the Gallbladder. *(NEET Pattern 2012)*
- **Hartmann pouch** is seen in the Gallbladder. *(NEET Pattern 2015)*
  - Located at the **junction** of the neck of the gallbladder and the cystic duct, may be a site where **gall stone** impacts.

▼ Spleen

General Features

- ❏ The spleen is located in the left hypochondriac region anterior to the 9th, 10th, and 11th ribs which puts the spleen in jeopardy in the case of rib fractures.
- ❏ The spleen does not extend below the costal margin and, therefore, is not palpable unless splenomegaly is present.
- ❏ The spleen is attached to the stomach by the gastrosplenic ligament which contains the short gastric arteries and veins and the left gastroepiploic artery and vein.
- ❏ The spleen is attached to the kidney by the splenorenal ligament which contains the five terminal branches of the splenic artery, tributaries of the splenic vein, and the tail of the pancreas.
- ❏ Accessory spleens occur in 20% of the population and are commonly located near the hilum, tail of the pancreas, or within the gastrosplenic ligament.
- ❏ The functions of the spleen include removal of old or abnormal red blood cells (RBCs), removal of inclusion bodies from RBCs [e.g. Howell-Jolly bodies (nuclear remnants), Pappenheimer bodies (iron granules), Heinz body (denatured hemoglobin)], removal of poorly opsonized pathogens, IgM production by plasma cells, storage of platelets, and protection from infection.

Arterial Supply

- ❏ The arterial supply is from the splenic artery (the largest branch of the celiac trunk) which gives off the following branches: Dorsal pancreatic artery, great pancreatic artery, caudal pancreatic arteries, short gastric arteries, left gastroepiploic artery, and ends with about five terminal branches.
- ❏ The five terminal branches of the splenic artery supply individual segments of the spleen with no anastomosis between them (i.e. end arteries) so that obstruction or ligation of any terminal branch will result in splenic infarction (i.e. the spleen is very prone to infarction).
- ❏ Splenic artery aneurysms show a particularly high incidence of rupture in pregnant women such that these aneurysms should be resected in women of childbearing age.

Venous Drainage

- ❏ The venous drainage is through the splenic vein via tributaries.
- ❏ The splenic vein joins the superior mesenteric vein to form the portal vein.
- ❏ The inferior mesenteric vein usually joins the splenic vein.
- ❏ Splenic vein thrombosis is most commonly associated with pancreatitis and shows the following clinical signs: Gastric varices and upper gastrointestinal bleeding.
- ❏ The spleen (mesodermal) appears about the sixth week as a localized thickening of the coelomic epithelium of the dorsal mesogastrium.
- ❏ Anterior end of the spleen is held up by phrenocolic ligament. *(NBEP 2013)*
- ❏ The Harris' dictum of odd numbers 1, 3, 5, 7, 9, 11 summarizes some splenic statistics, viz., it measures 1 inch in thickness, 3 inches in breadth, 5 inches in length, weighs 7 oz, and lies deep to 9, 10, and 11 ribs.
- ❏ Visceral Relations
- ❏ The visceral surface of the spleen is related to the following viscera:
  - ➢ Fundus of the stomach.
  - ➢ Anterior surface of the left kidney.
  - ➢ Left colic flexure.
  - ➢ Tail of pancreas.
- ❏ These viscera produce impressions on this surface *(for details see visceral surface on page 104)*.
- ❏ The diaphragmatic surface of the spleen is related to the diaphragm, which separates it from the costophrenic recess of the pleura, lung, and 9 to 11 ribs.
- ❏ Accessory Spleens
- ❏ The failure of fusion of splenunculi results in the formation of accessory spleens (splenunculi). These are usually found in the derivatives of the dorsal mesogastrium, viz. (a) in the gastrosplenic ligament, (b) in the lienorenal ligament, and (c) in the greater omentum. Rarely they are formed in the left spermatic cord and in the broad ligament of the uterus (left side).

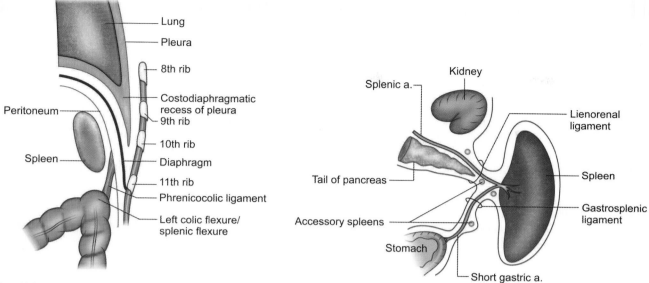

Fig. 100: Longitudinal section through the midaxillary line to show the relations of diaphragmatic surface of the spleen

Fig. 101: Peritoneal relations of the spleen

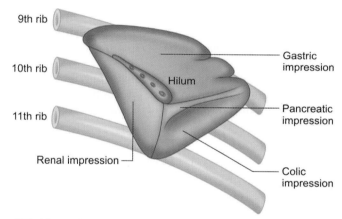

Fig. 102: Visceral surface of the spleen showing different impressions

❏ Rupture of spleen: Although well protected by 9th, 10th, and 11th ribs, the spleen is the most frequently ruptured organ in the abdomen following severe external blow.

The pain is referred to the left shoulder due to irritation of the left dome of diaphragm by the splenic blood. It is called 'Kehr's sign'.

QUESTION

1. All of the following form visceral relations of spleen EXCEPT:
   a. Stomach
   b. Splenic flexure of colon
   c. Kidney
   d. Adrenal gland

ANS

1. d. Adrenal gland
   ❏ Visceral surface of spleen has **gastric**, **renal** and **colic** impressions but **not adrenal.**

- Spleen extends from **9th to 11th rib**. *(NEET Pattern 2012)*
- Downward displacement of enlarged spleen is prevented by **Phrenico-colic ligament**. *(NEET Pattern 2016)*
- Most common location of accessory spleen is **hilum of spleen**. *(NEET Pattern 2015)*
- **Right isomerism** is associated with **asplenia**. *(AIPG 2011)*

▶ Pancreas

A. General Features
  ➤ In the adult, the pancreas is a retroperitoneal organ that measures 15 to 20 cm in length and weighs about 85 to 120 g.
  ➤ The pancreas is both an exocrine gland and an endocrine gland.
  The pancreas consists of four parts which are as follows:

1. Head of the Pancreas
  ❑ The head is the expanded part of the pancreas that lies in the concavity of the C-shaped curve of the duodenum and is firmly attached to the descending and horizontal parts of the duodenum.
  ❑ The uncinate process is a projection from the inferior portion of the pancreatic head.
  ❑ The structures that lie posterior to the head of the pancreas are the IVC, right renal artery, right renal vein, and the left renal vein.

2. Neck of the Pancreas
  ❑ The structures that lie posterior to the neck of the pancreas are the confluence of the superior mesenteric vein and splenic vein to form the portal vein.

3. Body of the Pancreas
  ❑ The structures that lie posterior to the body of the pancreas are the aorta, superior mesenteric artery, left suprarenal gland, left kidney, renal artery, and renal vein.

4. Tail of the Pancreas
  ❑ The tail of the pancreas is related to the splenic hilum and the left colic flexure.

B. Arterial Supply.
  The arterial supply of the pancreas is from the following:
  ➤ Anterior and posterior superior pancreaticoduodenal arteries which supply the head and neck of the pancreas (abdominal aorta → celiac trunk → common hepatic artery → gastroduodenal artery → anterior and posterior superior pancreaticoduodenal arteries).
  ➤ Anterior and posterior inferior pancreaticoduodenal arteries which supply the head and neck of the pancreas (abdominal aorta → superior mesenteric artery → anterior and posterior inferior pancreaticoduodenal arteries).
  ➤ Dorsal pancreatic artery which supplies the body and tail of the pancreas (abdominal aorta → celiac trunk → splenic artery → dorsal pancreatic artery).

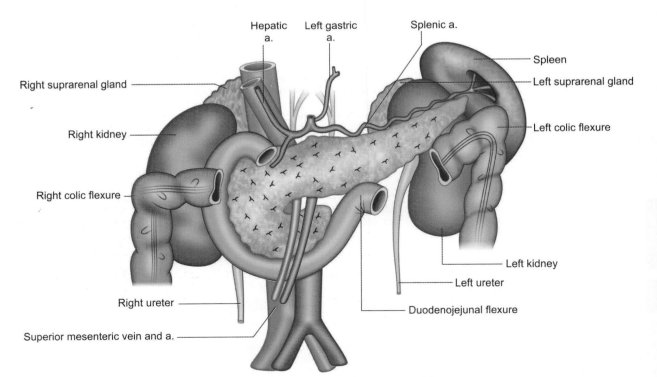

Fig. 103: Visceral relations of the different parts of the pancreas

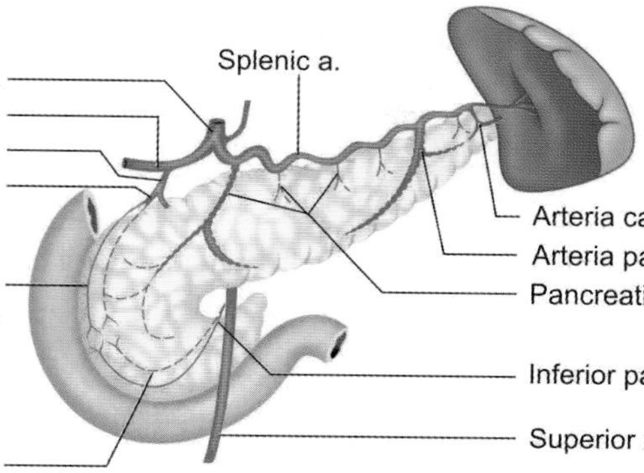

Fig. 104: Arterial supply of the pancreas

> Great pancreatic artery which supplies the body and tail of the pancreas (abdominal aorta → celiac trunk → splenic artery → great pancreatic artery).
> Caudal pancreatic arteries which supply the body and tail of the pancreas (abdominal aorta → celiac trunk → splenic artery → caudal pancreatic arteries).

C. Venous Drainage.

The venous drainage of the pancreas is from the following:

❑ Splenic vein (splenic vein → portal vein → hepatic sinusoids → central veins → hepatic veins → inferior vena cava).
❑ Superior mesenteric vein (superior mesenteric vein → portal vein → hepatic sinusoids → central veins → hepatic veins → inferior vena cava).
❑ Superior mesenteric vein and artery are anterior relations of uncinate process (pancreas).
❑ Abdominal aorta lies posterior to uncinate process (pancreas).
❑ Structure immediately posterior to head of pancreas is right renal vein. *(NBEP 2013)*
❑ Posterior relations of pancreatic head are IVC, terminal parts of right and left renal veins, common bile duct.
❑ Behind the neck of pancreas, superior mesenteric vein joins splenic vein to form portal vein: *(AIIMS 2005)*

1. **Posterior relations of head of pancreas are all EXCEPT:**
   (AIPG 2011)
   a. Common bile duct
   b. Inferior vena cava
   c. First part of duodenum
   d. Aorta

2. **All of the following statements regarding relations of pancreas are true EXCEPT:**
   a. Right renal vein is immediately posterior to the head
   b. Superior mesenteric vein lies anterior to the uncinate process
   c. First part of duodenum is posterior to the head
   d. Superior mesenteric vein lies posterior to the neck

3. **Regarding artery supply of pancreas, which of the following is/are CORRECT:**   *(PGIC)*
   a. Both superior and inferior pancreaticoduodenal arteries are branches of gastroduodenal artery
   b. Posterior superior pancreaticoduodenal artery is a branch of superior mesenteric artery
   c. Anterior inferior pancreaticoduodenal artery is a branch of superior mesenteric artery
   d. Posterior inferior pancreaticoduodenal artery is a branch of gastroduodenal artery
   e. Body and tail are supplied by splenic artery

1. **c. First part of duodenum > d. Aorta**
   ❑ First part of duodenum is **anterior** and **superior** to the head of pancreas.
   ❑ Aorta is posterior to the uncinate process of pancreas (**not the head**)
   ❑ Right and left renal veins drain into IVC behind the head of pancreas (**3 veins lie posterior**).
   ❑ Bile duct passes **behind the head** of pancreas and is joined by pancreatic duct, before opening into second part of duodenum.

2. **c. First part of duodenum is posterior to the head**
   ❑ First part of duodenum is **anterior** and **superior** to the head of pancreas.

3. **c. Anterior inferior pancreaticoduodenal artery is a branch of superior mesenteric artery; e. Body and tail are supplied by splenic artery**
   ❑ Gastroduodenal artery gives **superior** pancreaticoduodenal arteries (anterior and posterior both).
   ❑ Superior mesenteric artery gives **inferior** pancreaticoduodenal arteries (anterior and posterior both).
   ❑ Splenic artery runs on the **superior border** of pancreas and give multiple branches to **body** and **tail** of pancreas.

▪ Structure immediately posterior to pancreatic **head** is right renal vein *(NEET Pattern 2012)*
  – **Right** and **left** renal veins drain into **IVC** behind the head of pancreas.
▪ The **neck** of pancreas is related on its posterior surface to **superior mesenteric vein** *(AIIMS 2005)*

Kidney

❑ Is a retroperitoneal organ lying on posterior abdominal wall at the level of T12 –L3.

Note: Right kidney lies little lower than the left because of the large size of the right lobe of the liver.

❑ 11 cm long, 6 cm wide, and 3 cm thick, and weighs 150 g in men and 135 g in women.
❑ Location:

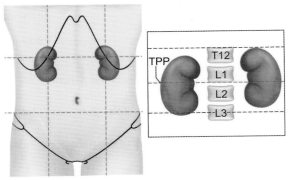

Fig. 105: Surface marking for kidneys

❑ Kidney occupies epigastric, hypochondriac, lumbar and umbilical regions.
❑ Transpyloric plane (TPP) passes through the upper part of the hilum of the right kidney and the lower part of the hilum of the left kidney.

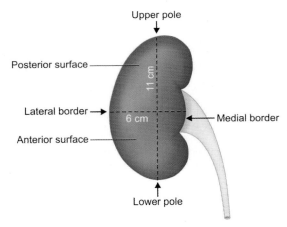

Fig. 106: External features and measurements of the kidney

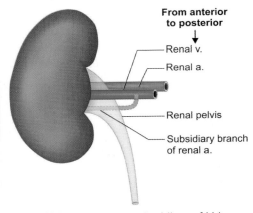

Fig. 107: Structures at the hilum of kidney (also shown are the relations)

❑ Hilus is an indentation on its medial border, through which the ureter, renal vessels, and nerves enter or leave the kidney (Anterior to posterior arrangement of structures is vein artery pelvis (VAP).

Structure

Kidney consists of the medulla and cortex containing 1 to 2 million nephrons (in each kidney) which are the anatomic and functional units of the kidney. Each nephron consists of a renal corpuscle (found only in the cortex), a proximal convoluted tubule, Henle loop, and a distal convoluted tubule.
❑ Renal papilla opens into minor calyx.

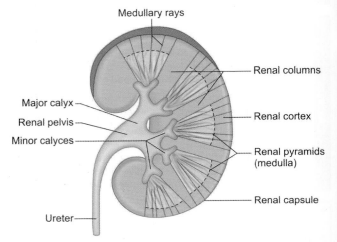

Fig. 108: Location of the uriniferous tubule within the kidney

Cortex

- Forms the outer part of the kidney and also projects into the medullary region between the renal pyramids as renal columns (of Bertini).
- Contains renal corpuscles and proximal and distal convoluted tubules. The renal corpuscle consists of the glomerulus (a tuft of capillaries) surrounded by a glomerular (Bowman) capsule which is the invaginated blind end of the nephron.

Medulla

- Forms the inner part of the kidney and consists of 8 to 12 renal pyramids (of Malpighi) which contain straight tubules (Henle's loops) and collecting tubules.
- **An apex of the renal pyramid, the renal papilla, fits into the cup-shaped minor calyx**^{Q} on which the collecting tubules open (10 to 25 openings).

Note:

➢ A renal pyramid along with its covering cortical tissue forms a **lobe of the kidney.**

➢ **Minor calyces** receive urine from the collecting tubules and empty into two or three **major calyces** which in turn empty into an upper dilated portion of the ureter the **renal pelvis.**

▶ Neurovascular Supply

Renal Arteries

- Arise from the abdominal aorta (at L1 vertebra level) inferior to the origin of the superior mesenteric artery.
- The right artery is longer and a little lower than the left and passes posterior to the IVC; the left artery passes posterior to the left renal vein.
- Give rise to the inferior suprarenal and ureteric arteries.
- At or near the hilum of the kidney, each renal artery divides into anterior and posterior divisions.

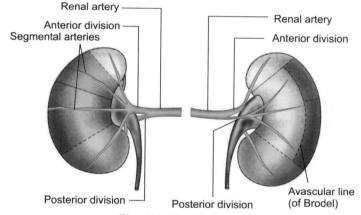

Fig. 109: Renal arteries

Anterior and Posterior Divisions

- The anterior division branches are divided into four **anterior segmental arteries** which supply anterior segments of the kidney called the **apical segmental artery, anterosuperior segmental artery, anteroinferior segmental artery,** and **inferior segmental artery.**
- The posterior division continues as the posterior segmental artery which supplies the posterior segment of the kidney.

Segmental Arteries

- The segmental arteries are end arteries (i.e. they do not anastomose) and are distributed to various segments of the kidney. Segmental arteries have the following clinical importance:
  ➢ Since there is a very little collateral circulation between segmental arteries (i.e. end arteries), an **avascular line (Brodel white line)** is created between anterior and posterior segments such that a longitudinal incision through the kidney will produce minimal bleeding. This approach is useful for surgical removal of renal (staghorn) calculi.
  ➢ Ligation of a segmental artery results in necrosis of the entire segment of the kidney.

Note: Supernumerary renal arteries - In about 30% individuals accessory renal arteries are also found. They commonly arise from the aorta and enter the kidney at the hilus or at one of its poles usually the lower pole.

Vasculature

- The segmental arteries branch into 5 to 11 **interlobar arteries** (run between pyramids) which turn along the base of the pyramid **(arcuate arteries)** and further branch into smaller **interlobular arteries** that supply the cortex.
- In the cortex, the **interlobular artery** gives off the afferent arterioles (one to each glomerulus) which give rise to the capillaries that form the glomerulus. The **glomerular capillaries** reunite to form a single **efferent arteriole** that in turn, gives rise to a second network of capillaries, the **peritubular capillaries.**
- Some of the peritubular capillaries form long loops called the **vasa recta** which accompany the thin segments of the nephrons.

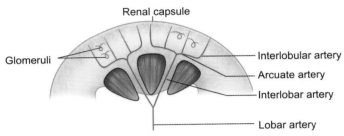

Fig. 110: Arrangement of arteries within the kidney

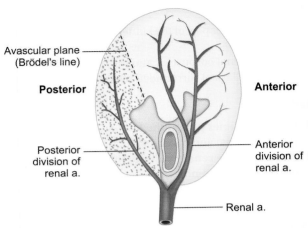

Fig. 111: Schematic diagram showing avascular plane of the kidney (Brödel's line)

The subdivisions of the renal arteries are described sequentially as segmental, lobar, interlobar, arcuate and interlobular arteries, and afferent and efferent glomerular arterioles.

Venous Drainage

❏ Peritubular capillaries drain into the interlobular veins → arcuate veins → interlobar veins → renal vein → IVC.
❏ The left is three times longer[Q] than the right (7.5 cm and 2.5 cm, respectively), and for this reason, **the left kidney is the preferred side for live donor nephrectomy[Q].**
❏ The left renal vein runs from its origin in the renal hilum, posterior to the splenic vein and the body of pancreas, and then across the **anterior aspect of the aorta just below the origin of the superior mesenteric artery[Q].** **Nutcracker syndrome,** characterized by left renal vein hypertension secondary to compression of the vein between the aorta and the superior mesenteric artery has been associated with hematuria and varicocele in children. The left gonadal vein enters the left renal vein from below, and the left suprarenal vein usually receiving one of the left inferior phrenic veins, enters above but nearer the midline.

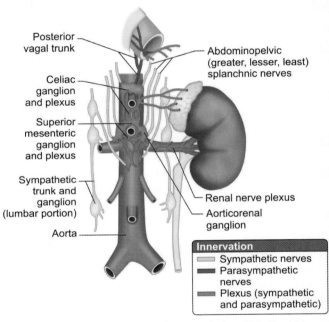

Fig. 112: Location of the uriniferous tubule within the kidney

Lymphatic Drainage

❏ The lymphatics from the kidney drain into the **paraaortic** lymph nodes at the level of origin of the renal arteries.

Nerve Supply (Renal Plexus)

❏ Rami from the **Celiac ganglion and plexus[Q],** aorticorenal ganglion, lowest thoracic splanchnic nerve, first lumbar splanchnic nerve and aortic plexus form a dense plexus of autonomic nerves around the renal artery.
❏ The **sympathetic** fibers are derived from T10-L2 spinal segments, and the **parasympathetic** fibers are derived from vagus nerves.

Renal Pain

❏ Radiates downward and forward from loin into the groin along the T12 (±2) dermatome.
❏ It occurs due to stretching of the renal capsule and spasm of the smooth muscle in the renal pelvis.
❏ The afferent fibers pass successively through the renal plexus, lowest splanchnic nerve, sympathetic trunk, and enter the T12 spinal segment.
❏ The pain is felt in the renal angle and gets referred along the subcostal nerve to the flank and anterior abdominal wall and along the **ilioinguinal nerve (L1)** into the groin.

Note: Renal angle lies between the lower border of the 12th rib and the lateral border of sacrospinalis (erector spinae) muscle.

▶ Relations

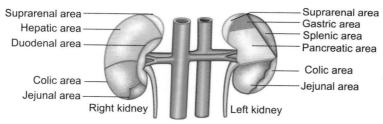

Fig. 113: Anterior relations of the kidneys

Relations of Kidney

Anterior Relations

Right	Left
▪ Right suprarenal gland	▪ Left suprarenal gland
▪ Right lobe of the liver	▪ Spleen
▪ Second part of the duodenum	▪ Stomach
▪ Hepatic (right) colic flexure	▪ Pancreas and splenic vessels
▪ Jejunum	▪ Splenic (left) colic flexure
	▪ Jejunum

Note: Tail of pancreas is not related to the left kidney.

Posterior Relations (both kidneys)

- ▪ Muscles: Diaphragm, quadratus lumborum, psoas major, and transversus abdominis.
- ▪ Nerves: Subcostal (T12), iliohypogastric (L1), and ilioinguinal (L1).
- ▪ Vessels: Subcostal vessels.
- ▪ Ribs: 12th Rib (Left kidney is related to the 11th rib as well).
- ▪ Ligaments: Medial and lateral arcuate ligament.

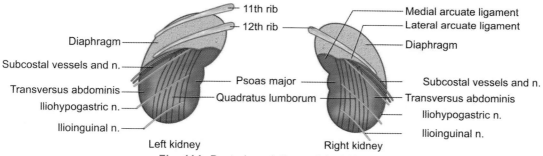

Fig. 114: Posterior relations of the kidneys

Renal transplantation: Left kidney transplantation is preferred (due to longer renal vein). The donor kidney is placed retroperitoneally in the iliac fossa with hilum parallel to the external iliac vessels. The renal artery is anastomosed end to end to the internal iliac artery and renal vein is anastomosed end to side to the external iliac vein. The ureter is implanted into the urinary bladder (ureterocystostomy).

1. All of the following are true regarding blood supply to the kidney EXCEPT: *(AIPG 2002)*
   a. Stellate veins drain the superficial zone
   b. It is a type of portal circulation
   c. Renal artery divides into five segmental arteries before entering the hilum
   d. Its segmental arteries are end arteries

2. Nerve supply to kidney is from: *(NEET Pattern 2012)*
   a. Lumbar plexus
   b. Celiac plexus
   c. Inferior mesenteric nerve
   d. Vagus

3. Right kidney is separated by peritoneum from: *(NEET Pattern 2016)*
   a. Suprarenal gland
   b. Duodenum
   c. Liver
   d. Stomach

4. All of the following are the posterior relations of the kidney EXCEPT: *(NEET Pattern 2014)*
   a. Psoas major
   b. Quadratus lumborum
   c. Sympathetic chain
   d. Ilioinguinal nerve

QUESTIONS

5. All are TRUE about right kidney EXCEPT: *(AIIMS 2001)*
 a. Right renal vein is shorter than left
 b. Related to duodenum
 c. Right kidney is preferred over left for transplantation
 d. Right kidney is placed at the lower level than left

6. Left renal vein crosses the Aorta:
(AIIMS 2007; NEET Pattern 2012)
 a. Anteriorly, above the superior mesenteric artery
 b. Anteriorly, below the superior mesenteric artery
 c. Posteriorly, at the level of superior mesenteric artery
 d. Anteriorly, below the inferior mesenteric artery

(NEET Pattern 2016)

7. NOT true about blood supply of kidney:
 a. Renal artery is a branch of internal iliac artery
 c. Branches of renal artery are end arteries
 b. Right renal artery passes behind IVC
 d. Renal vein drains into IVC

ANSWERS

1. b. It is a type of portal circulation.
 ❑ In the renal glomeruli, the **glomerular capillary bed** lies between afferent and efferent arterioles and **may** be considered as a portal circulation, **but it is not mentioned in Gray's anatomy**.
 ❑ In essence, a **portal system** is a capillary network that **lies between the two veins**. Blood supplying the organ thus passes through **two sets of capillaries before** it returns to the heart.
 ❑ Renal artery divides close to the hilum into **five segmental arteries** that are **end arteries** (i.e. they do not anastomose significantly with other segmental arteries, so that the area supplied by each segmental artery is an **independent, surgically resectable unit** or renal segment).

2. b. Celiac plexus > d. Vagus
 ❑ Rami from the **Celiac ganglion** and **plexus**, aorticorenal ganglion, lowest thoracic splanchnic nerve, first lumbar splanchnic nerve and aortic plexus form a dense plexus of autonomic nerves around the renal artery which supplies the kidney (Gray's Anatomy edition 41).
 ❑ **Vagus** nerve contributes to **celiac plexus** which itself send nerves to kidney **along the renal arteries**.

3. c. Liver
 ❑ Liver is covered by peritoneum in its **anterior relation** with right kidney.
 ❑ Suprarenal gland, duodenum, colon and pancreas are **retroperitoneal** organs, and they are in direct contact with kidney which itself is retroperitoneal.
 Note: Stomach relates with left kidney (**not right kidney**).

4. c. Sympathetic chain
 ❑ Nerves related to kidneys posteriorly are: Subcostal (T12), iliohypogastric (L1), and ilioinguinal (L1).
 ❑ **Four muscles** are in posterior relations of kidney: Diaphragm, quadratus lumborum, psoas major, and transversus abdominis.

5. c. Right kidney is preferred over left for transplantation
 ❑ The **left kidney from a living** related donor is preferred for kidney transplantation because it has a **longer renal vein** and thus is easier to implant in the recipient.
 ❑ Because of the presence of liver, **right kidney is at a lower level** than left. Left kidney relates with 11th and 12 th ribs whereas, **right is related to only 12th rib.**

6. b. Anteriorly, below the superior mesenteric artery
 ❑ Left renal vein **crosses in front of the aorta** from left to right towards the IVC.
 ❑ It lies **below and behind** the superior mesenteric artery.
 ❑ It may be compressed by an aneurysm of the superior mesenteric artery as the vein crosses anterior to the aorta.

7. a. Renal artery is a branch of internal iliac artery
 ❑ Renal artery is a branch of **abdominal aorta** and pass **behind IVC**.
 ❑ Renal arteries are **end arteries**, as they do not anastomose significantly with adjacent branches.
 ❑ Renal veins drain into IVC. **Right** renal vein is **shorter** than left renal vein.
 ❑ Left renal vein is **longer**, passes **in front of aorta**, crosses the midline and **drain into IVC**.

- Pancreas lies **directly anterior** to kidney **without a fold of peritoneum** in between them.
- Kidney is supplied by **renal plexus of nerves** (along renal artery) having sympathetic (T10–L1) and parasympathetic (vagus) contributions.
- **Nutcracker syndrome**: Compression of the left renal vein between the aorta and the superior mesenteric artery, causing hypertension in the kidney with flank pain and sometimes fever and gross hematuria.
- Since inferior vena cava is **not laterally symmetrical**, the left renal vein often receives the following veins: left **inferior phrenic** vein, left **suprarenal** vein, left **gonadal** vein (left testicular vein in males, left ovarian vein in females) and left 2nd lumbar vein.
  – This is in contrast to the right side of the body, where these veins drain **directly into the IVC.**
- The **azygos** vein is connected to the **IVC**, while the **hemiazygos** vein is connected to the **left renal vein**.
- While **exposing the kidney from behind**, nerves are liable to injury are Ilioinguinal nerve, subcostal nerve and Ilio-hypogastric nerve. *(AIPG 2004)*
- **Anterior relations** of the right kidney are liver, hepatic flexure, adrenal gland and 2nd (**not 4th**) part of duodenum. *(NEET Pattern 2013)*
- Most medially located renal structure is **renal pelvis**.
  – Arranged medial to lateral: Renal pelvis → major calyx → minor calyx → renal medulla → renal cortex.
- Renal **papilla** opens into **minor calyx.** *(NEET Pattern 2012)*
  – An apex of the renal pyramid, the renal papilla fits into the cup-shaped minor calyx.
- Kidney hilum contains following structures (**anterior to posterior**): Renal Vein, renal Artery, and Pelvis (VAP).
- Definitive renal artery arises from aorta. *(NEET Pattern 2016)*
- **Posterior relations** of the right kidney are diaphragm, subcostal nerve, ilioinguinal nerve (but not 11th rib). *(NEET Pattern 2016)*

▼ Ureter

Embryology

❑ Develops from the **ureteric bud** given by the **mesonephric duct**.

Ureter

❑ A muscular tube that begins as a continuation of renal pelvis extending from the kidney to the urinary bladder.
❑ Length 25-30 cm (proximal half lies in the abdomen and distal half lies in the pelvic cavity). Lumen = 3 mm.
  ➤ It begins at the **ureteropelvic junction** where the renal pelvis joins the ureter (at the lower end of kidney).
  ➤ Within the abdomen, the ureters descend **retroperitoneal** and anterior to the **psoas major** muscle where they cross the pelvic inlet to enter the minor (or true) pelvis.

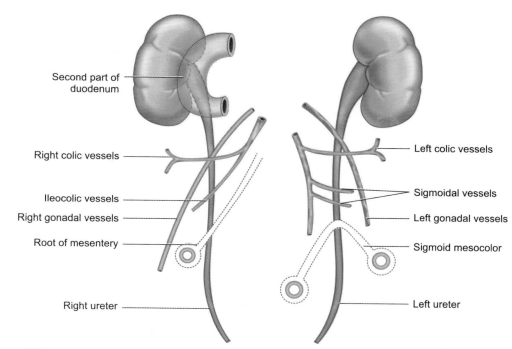

Figs. 115A and B: Anterior relations of the abdominal parts of the ureters: A. Right ureter; B. Left ureter

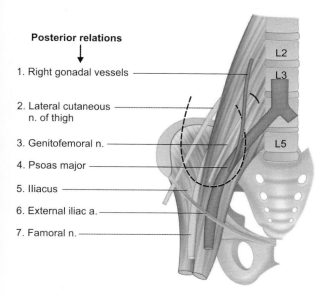

Fig. 116: Posterior relations of the cecum. The position of cecum is outlined by a thick broken black line

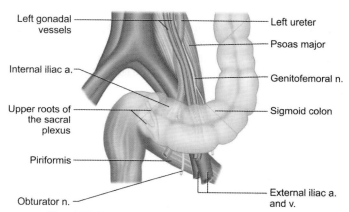

Fig. 117: Posterior relations of the sigmoid colon

- ➤ Within the minor (or true) pelvis, the ureters descend **retroperitoneal** and anterior to the **common iliac artery and vein** where they may be compromised by an aneurysm of the common iliac artery.
- ➤ The ureters end at the **ureterovesical junction** surrounded by the **vesical venous plexus**.
- ➤ The ureters end by traveling obliquely through the wall of the urinary bladder (i.e. the **intramural portion of the ureter**) and define the upper limit of the **urinary bladder trigone**.
- ➤ Ureter is valveless though the intramural portion of the ureter functions as a check valve (**ureterovesical valve of Sampson**) to prevent urine reflux.

Also note the relations of ureter.

- ❑ Sigmoid mesocolon is present **anterior** to ureter in the abdomen.
- ❑ Left gonadal vessels cross the ureter (**anteriorly**), medial to lateral.
- ❑ Ureter lies **anterior** to common iliac artery **bifurcation,** as it crosses the **pelvic brim** to enter pelvic cavity.
- ❑ Ureter lies **anterior** to psoas major and genitofemoral nerve.

Note: Medially the right ureter is related to inferior vena cava and left ureter is related to left gonadal vein and inferior mesenteric vein.

Anterior relations	
Right ureter	▪ Duodenum (2nd part) ▪ Right colic vessels ▪ Ileocolic vessels ▪ Right gonadal vessels ▪ Root of mesentery
Left ureter	▪ Left colic vessels ▪ Sigmoid vessels ▪ Left testicular or ovarian vessels ▪ Sigmoid mesocolon

Posterior relations: Both the ureters run anterior to psoas major muscle and bifurcation of common iliac artery

Note: Respective colic and gonadal vessels run anterior to ureters.

Relations (in pelvis)

- ❑ **In the male,** the ureters pass posterior to the **ductus deferens.**
- ❑ **In the female,** the ureters pass posterior and inferior to the **uterine artery** which lies in the **transverse cervical ligament** (or **cardinal ligament of Mackenrodt**) and lie 1 to 2 cm lateral to the **cervix of the uterus**. During gynecologic operations (e.g. hysterectomy), the ureters may be inadvertently injured. The most common sites of injury are at the pelvic brim where the ureter is close to the ovarian blood vessels and where the uterine artery crosses the ureter along the side of the cervix.

Normal Constrictions in Ureter

- ❑ Ureter may be obstructed by renal calculi (kidney stones) where it joins the renal pelvis (ureteropelvic junction), where it crosses the pelvic brim over the distal end of the common iliac artery, or where it enters the wall of the urinary bladder (ureterovesicular junction).
- ❑ The vesicoureteric junction is the narrowest of these areas and can be responsible for arresting the passage of stones of as little as 2–3 mm.

Note: Surgery books also mention sites of constrictions at juxtaposition of the vas deferens/broad ligament and other at trigonal opening.

- ❑ Radiopaque shadow of ureteric calculus are seen at the following sites:
  - a. Near the tips of the transverse processes of lumbar vertebra.
  - b. Overlying the sacroiliac joint.
  - c. Overlying or slightly medial to the ischial spine.

Vascular Supply

- ❑ Receives arterial supply from:
- ❑ Renal.
- ❑ Gonadal (Testicular/ovarian)
- ❑ Direct branches from abdominal aorta
- ❑ Common and internal iliac (but not external iliac)
- ❑ Vesical (superior and inferior)
- ❑ Middle rectal
- ❑ Uterine.

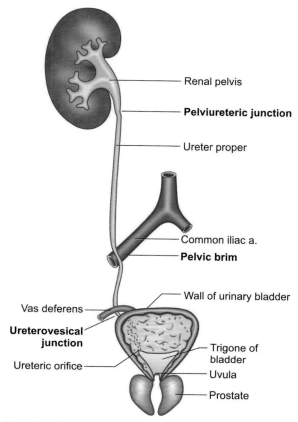

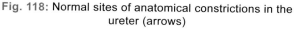

Fig. 118: Normal sites of anatomical constrictions in the ureter (arrows)

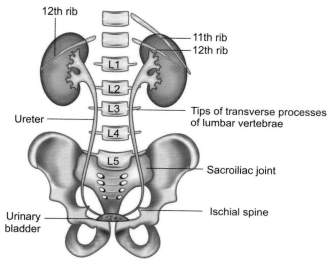

Fig. 119: Drawing from an intravenous pyelogram to show the relationship of the ureters to the bony landmarks

❑ **Venous drainage:** Veins follow the arteries supplying ureter.
❑ **Lymphatic drainage:** The lymph from the ureter is drained into lateral aortic and iliac nodes.

Nerve Supply

❑ T10 - L2 (sympathetic) and S2-4 (parasympathetic) fibers reach ureter by branches from the renal and aortic plexuses, and the superior and inferior hypogastric plexuses.
❑ The nerves are not essential for the initiation and propagation of ureteric contraction waves, they are just modulatory in function.
❑ Peristalsis wave is generated in smooth muscle cells of the minor calyces (**pacemaker**).
❑ Impulse propagation is myogenic conduction mediated by the electrotonic coupling of one muscle cell to its immediate neighbors by the means of intercellular 'gap' junctions.

Referred Pain

❑ Excessive distension of the ureter or spasm of its muscle may be caused by a stone (calculus) and provokes severe pain (ureteric colic, which is commonly, but mistakenly called renal colic).
❑ The spasmodic pain is referred to cutaneous areas innervated from spinal segments that supply the ureter, shoots down and forwards from the **loin to the groin** and scrotum or labium majus.

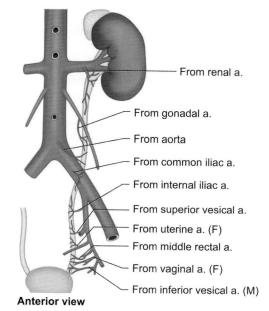

Anterior view

Fig. 120: Normal sites of anatominical constrictions in the ureter (arrows)

❑ Pain from **upper** ureteral obstruction is referred to the lumbar region (T12 and L1) and from middle ureteral obstruction is referred to the inguinal, scrotal or mons pubis and upper medial aspect of the thigh **genitofemoral nerve** (L1, L2). The cremaster which has the same innervation, may reflexly retract the testis.
❑ Calculus at the lower portion of ureter send pain via the **nervi erigentes** (S2, 3, 4) and felt at the posterior thigh converging on to the midline openings of in the perineum (pudendal nerve territory).

QUESTIONS

1. Ureter derives its blood supply from: *(PGIC 2003, 2010)*
   a. Renal artery
   b. Gonadal artery
   c. Common iliac artery
   d. Inferior vesical artery
   e. Superior mesenteric artery

2. About ureter TRUE is: *(PGIC 2005, 2008)*
   a. Begins at hilum
   b. 25 cm
   c. Enters true pelvis after crossing iliac vessels
   d. Totally retroperitoneal
   e. Changes its direction at ischial spine

3. Ureteric constrictions are at all sites EXCEPT: *(NEET Pattern 2013)*
   a. Pelvi-ureteric junction
   b. Lesser pelvis
   c. Ischial spine
   d. Urinary bladder wall

4. The narrowest part of the ureter is at: *(AIIMS 2005)*
   a. Uretero-pelvic junction
   b. Iliac vessel crossing
   c. Pelvic ureter
   d. Ureterovesicle junction

5. Left ureter is related to: *(PGIC 2003)*
   a. Quadratus lumborum
   b. Left gonadal vessels
   c. Superior mesenteric vein
   d. Sigmoid mesocolon
   e. Internal iliac artery

6. Anterior relations of right ureter are all EXCEPT: *(JIPMER 2016)*
   a. Gonadal vessels
   b. Root of mesentery
   c. Ileocolic vessels
   d. Bifurcation of right common iliac artery

7. All are relations of left ureter EXCEPT: *(AIIMS 2016)*
   a. Sigmoid mesentery
   b. Bifurcation of common iliac artery
   c. Quadratus lumborum
   d. Gonadal vessels

8. All structures are posterior relations of cecum EXCEPT: *(NEET Pattern 2016)*
   a. Appendix
   b. Psoas major
   c. Greater omentum
   d. Femoral nerve

ANSWERS

1. a. Renal artery; b. Gonadal artery; c. Common iliac artery; d. Inferior vesical artery
   ❏ Ureter has multiple arteries supplying it, but it is not supplied by **inferior mesenteric artery.**

2. b. 25 cm; c. Enters true pelvis after crossing iliac vessels; d. Totally retroperitoneal; e. Changes its direction at ischial spine
   ❏ Ureter has a total length of 25 cm (12.5 cm abdominal and **12.5 cm pelvic**).
   ❏ Ureter begins as a downward continuation of renal pelvis at the medial margin of the lower end of the kidney (it **does not** begin at hilum)
   ❏ It is a **retroperitoneal** structure and enters true pelvis passing pelvic brim **at the bifurcation of** common iliac artery (It is also the level of beginning of external iliac artery at sacro-iliac joint).
   ❏ In its downward course, **opposite the ischial spine**, ureter **turns antero-medial** and runs towards the base of bladder.

3. b. Lesser pelvis
   ❏ Lesser pelvis is a **vague option** and does not specify a precise location.
   ❏ Ureter has **five constrictions** in its course:
      ■ Pelvi-ureteric junction (tip of transverse process of vertebra, radiologically)
      ■ Pelvic brim (sacro-iliac joint radiologically)
      ■ Juxtaposition of vas deferens/broad ligament
      ■ Ureterovesical junction (ischial spine, radiologically)
      ■ Opening at trigone.

4. d. Uretero-vesicle junction
   ❏ The narrowest lumen is where the ureter enters the bladder wall (**ureterovesicle junction**) and may be responsible for arresting the passage of stones of as little as 2–3 mm.
   Note: Sometime the question may not have the option of ureterovesical junction, in that case the **intramural ureter** (the part inside detrusor) may be taken as the answer.

5. b. Left gonadal vessels; d. Sigmoid mesocolon; e. Internal iliac artery
   ❏ Left gonadal vessels and sigmoid mesocolon are present **anterior** to ureter in the abdomen.
   ❏ Internal iliac artery is present **posterior** to ureter in the pelvic cavity.
   ❏ Inferior mesenteric vein (**not superior mesenteric vein**) is present on medial aspect of left ureter.

6. d. Bifurcation of right common iliac artery
   ❏ Bifurcation of right common iliac artery is **posterior** to the ureter.

7. c. Quadratus lumborum
   ❏ Left ureter is related posteriorly to psoas major muscle (**not quadratus lumborum**).
   ❏ Posterior relations: Both the ureters run anterior to psoas major muscle and bifurcation of common iliac artery.
   ❏ Gonadal vessels cross the ureters anteriorly (**medial to lateral**) and descend down along with them.
   ❏ **Medially** the right ureter is related to **inferior vena cava** and left ureter is related to **inferior mesenteric vein**.

ANSWERS

8. c. Greater omentum
- ❏ Greater omentum may lie in anterior (**not posterior**) relation of cecum.

- Ureter is **not supplied by** external iliac artery.
- Genitofemoral nerve lies on psoas major muscle, and both are posterior (**not anterior**) relations of ureter. *(AIPG 2012)*
- Ureteric peristalsis is due to **pacemaker activity** of the smooth muscle cells in the **renal pelvis**. *(AIIMS 2007)*
- During surgeries ureter can identified by the **peristalsis**.

▶ Adrenal Gland

Suprarenal (Adrenal) Gland

- ❏ Retroperitoneal organ lying on the superomedial aspect of the kidney. It is surrounded by a capsule and renal fascia.
- ❏ Is pyramidal on the right and semilunar on the left.
- ❏ **Cortex** secretes three types of steroid hormones. The outer zona **glomerulosa** produces mineralocorticoids (aldosterone); the middle zona **fasciculata** produces glucocorticoids (cortisol) and the inner zona **reticularis** produces androgens.
- ❏ **Medulla** receives preganglionic sympathetic nerve fibers directly, and secretes epinephrine and norepinephrine.

Vascular Supply

- ❏ Receives arteries from **three** sources: **inferior phrenic** artery, **abdominal aorta**, and the **renal artery**[Q].
- ❏ Is drained via the suprarenal vein, which empties into the IVC on the right and the renal vein on the left .

Nerve Supply

- ❏ Sympathetic preganglionic neuronal cell bodies are located in the intermediolateral cell column of the spinal cord (T10-L1). Preganglionic axons run with the splanchnic nerves.
- ❏ Modified postganglionic neuronal cell bodies called **chromaffin cells** are located in the adrenal medulla.

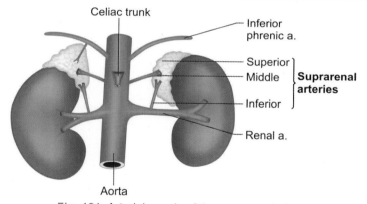

Fig. 121: Arterial supply of the suprarenal gland

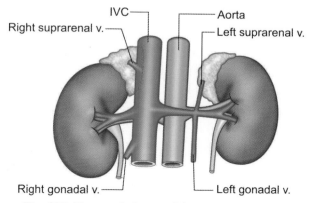

Fig. 122: Venous drainage of the suprarenal gland

1. Suprarenal gland gets its blood supply from all of the following arteries EXCEPT:
   a. Aorta
   b. Renal artery
   c. Inferior phrenic vein
   d. Superior mesenteric artery

2. All of the following statements of adrenal gland are true EXCEPT: *(AIPG)*
   a. Both are supplied by three arteries
   b. Both adrenal glands drain directly into inferior vena cava
   c. Right gland is pyramidal in shape
   d. Average weight is about 5 gms

(NEET Dec. 16 Pattern)

3. True of left suprarenal gland are all EXCEPT:
   a. Semilunar
   b. Drains into renal vein
   c. Related to stomach
   d. Related to bare area of liver

1. d. Superior mesenteric artery
   ❏ Arterial supply of adrenal gland is by three arteries:
   - Superior suprarenal artery (branch of **inferior phrenic** artery).
   - Middle suprarenal artery (branch of **abdominal aorta**).
   - Inferior suprarenal artery (branch of **renal artery**).

2. b. Both adrenal glands drain directly into inferior vena cava
   ❏ Venous drainage is through **suprarenal vein**.
   ❏ Right suprarenal (adrenal) vein drains **into IVC**, and left suprarenal vein drains into **IVC via the left renal vein**.
   ❏ Adrenal gland weighs approximately 5 g (the **medulla** contributes about **one-tenth** of the total weight).

3. d. Related to bare area of liver
   ❏ Right (**not left**) suprarenal gland is related to **bare area of liver.**

- **Right** adrenal vein drains **into inferior vena cava**. *(NEET Pattern 2014)*
- Lymphatics of suprarenal gland drain into **Paraaortic** lymph nodes.
- Left adrenal gland drains into renal vein whereas, right adrenal gland drains into IVC. *(NEET Pattern 2016)*

Pelvis and Perineum

▼ Bones of Pelvis and Perineum

- ❑ **Pelvic diaphragm** separates the pelvic cavity above from the perineal region (including perineum) below.
- ❑ **Perineum** is a part of the pelvic outlet located inferior to the pelvic diaphragm.
- ❑ The pelvic cavity of the true pelvis has the pelvic floor as its inferior border (and the pelvic brim/inlet as its superior border).

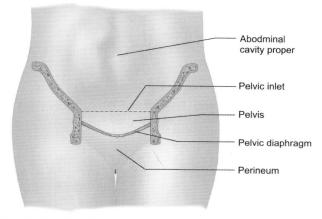

Fig. 1: Relationship between abdomen, pelvis and perineum

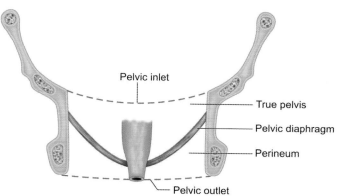

Fig. 2: Relationship between pelvis and perineum

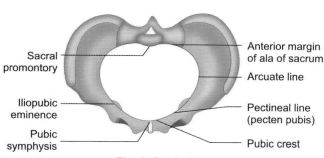

Fig. 3: Pelvic inlet

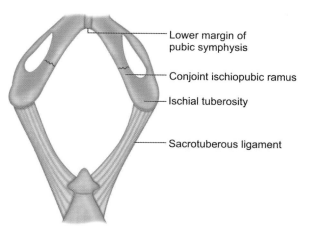

Fig. 4: Pelvic outlet

- ❑ **Pelvic Inlet**/Brim leads into the lesser pelvis and is the superior rim of the pelvic cavity and is bounded posteriorly by the promontory of the sacrum and the anterior border of the ala of the sacrum (sacral part), laterally by the **arcuate or iliopectineal line** of the ilium (iliac part) and anteriorly by the pectineal line, the pubic crest, and the superior margin of the pubic symphysis (pubic part).
- ❑ The **linea terminalis** includes the pubic crest, iliopectineal line, and arcuate line.
- ❑ **Pelvic Outlet** is the diamond-shaped aperture bounded posteriorly by the sacrum and coccyx; laterally by the ischial tuberosities and sacrotuberous ligaments; and anteriorly by the pubic symphysis, arcuate pubic ligament, and rami of the pubis and ischium. It is closed by the pelvic and urogenital diaphragms.

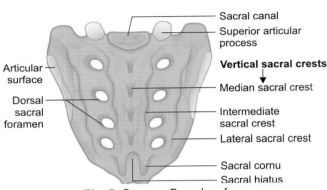

Fig. 5: Sacrum: Dorsal surface

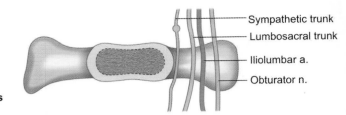

Fig. 6: Structure related to the smooth medial part of the ala of sacrum

- The smooth medial part of the ala of sacrum is related to the following structures (lateral to medial): Obturator nerve, Iliolumbar artery, Lumbosacral trunk, Sympathetic chain (**Mnemonic - OILS**).
- Articular surface of the sacrum extends onto the upper three or **three and a half** sacral vertebrae in adult male.
- In females it extends onto the upper **two or two and a half** of the sacral vertebrae.

QUESTIONS

1. Sacral ala is NOT crossed by   (NEET Pattern 2016)
- a. Ureter
- b. Sympathetic chain
- c. Iliolumbar artery
- d. Obturator nerve

2. Upper border of pubic ramus forms   (NEET Pattern 2014)
- a. Pubic tubercle
- b. Pubic symphysis
- c. Arcuate line
- d. Upper margin of obturator foramen

3. The type of joint between the sacrum and the coccyx is a   (AIPG 2005)
- a. Symphysis
- b. Synostosis
- c. Synchondrosis
- d. Syndesmosis

4. Sacral promontory is the landmark for   (NEET Pattern 2013)
- a. Origin of superior mesenteric artery
- b. Termination of presacral nerve
- c. Origin of inferior mesenteric artery
- d. None of the above

5. Lower limit of sacroiliac joint lies upto which level in females   (NEET Pattern 2015)
- a. 1 to 11/2
- b. 2 to 11/2
- c. 3 to 31/2
- d. 4 to 41/2

ANSWERS

1. a. Ureter
- The smooth medial part of the ala of sacrum is related to the following structures (lateral to medial): Obturator nerve, Iliolumbar artery, lumbosacral trunk, sympathetic chain (OILS).

2. c. Arcuate line
- Upper border of superior pubic ramus is called pectineal line (or pecten pubis). It contributes to arcuate line.
- Upper border of inferior pubic ramus forms lower margin of obturator foramen.

3. a. Symphysis
- Sacrococcygeal joint is a secondary cartilaginous joint – symphysis.
- Symphysis are midline joints and may turn into synostosis with advancing age. For example, symphysis menti becomes a synostosis after the age of 1 year.

4. b. Termination of presacral nerve
- Superior hypogastric plexus (presacral nerve) lies in front of the bifurcation of the abdominal aorta and body of the fifth lumbar vertebra between the two common iliac arteries.
- Origin of superior mesenteric artery lies at L1 and inferior mesenteric artery at L3 vertebral level.

5. b. 2 to 11/2
- Articular surface of the sacrum (lower limit of sacro iliac joint) extends on to upper 2 or 21/2 of the sacral vertebrae in females.
- In males, it extends on to the upper 3 or 31/2 of the sacral vertebrae.

◤ Nerve Supply Pelvis and Perineum

Table 1: Innervation of the female genitalia

	Origin	Proximal course	Distal course	Organ	Function
Parasympathetic	S2–S4	Pelvic splanchnic nerves	Pelvic ganglia	Uterine tube, uterus	Vasodiation
		Cavernous (deep, cavernosal) nerves of clitoris		Vagina, clitoris	Transudation, Erection

	Origin	Proximal course	Distal course	Organ	Function
Sympathetic	T12, L1–L2	Superior mesenteric and renal plexus Superior hypogastric plexus	Ovarian plexus Hypogastric nerve ↓ Inferior hypogastric plexus ↓ Uterovaginal plexus (Frankenhauser ganglion)	Ovary Uterine tube, uterus, upper vagina	Vasoconstriction Contraction
Somatic	S2, 3, 4	Pudendal nerve Pudendal nerve	Dorsal nerve of clitoris Posterior labial nerves	Clitoris Lower vagina Labia majora Ischiocavernosus Bulbospongiosus	 Contraction

- ❏ **Sympathetic** fibers arising from intermediolateral horn cells of lower thoracic and upper lumbar spinal segments (T10-12; L1-2) and carried by the **lumbar splanchnic nerves**.
- ❏ **Parasympathetic** innervation to the pelvic viscera derives from **vagus** nerve and **pelvic splanchnic nerves** (also termed nervi erigentes).
  - ➤ Neurone bodies of vagus nerve are present in the **dorsal nucleus of vagus** (medulla oblongata)
  - ➤ Preganglionic neuronal cell bodies are located in the gray matter (intermediolateral horn cells) of the S2 to S4 spinal cord and form the pelvic splanchnic nerves.
  - ➤ Postganglionic neuronal cell bodies are located near or within the respective viscera.
- ❏ **Superior hypogastric plexus** (also termed the presacral nerve).
  - ➤ It is the downward continuation of the aortic plexus (intermesenteric plexus) from the inferior mesenteric ganglion. It receives the L3 and L4 lumbar splanchnic nerves.
  - ➤ Beginning below the aortic bifurcation and extending downward retroperitoneally, this plexus is formed by sympathetic fibers arising from spinal levels (T10-12; L1-2).
  - ➤ It descends anterior to the L5 vertebra and at the level of the sacral promontory, this superior hypogastric plexus divides into a right and a left **hypogastric nerve** which run downward along the pelvis side walls and lies in the extraperitoneal connective tissue lateral to the rectum.
    - Hypogastric nerves provide branches to the sigmoid colon and the descending colon and is joined by the pelvic splanchnic nerves to form the **inferior hypogastric** (or pelvic plexus).
  - ➤ Superior hypogastric plexus contains preganglionic and postganglionic **sympathetic** fibers, **visceral afferent** fibers, and few, if any, **parasympathetic** fibers which may run a **recurrent** course through the **inferior** hypogastric plexus.
- ❏ **Inferior hypogastric plexus** (also termed the pelvic plexus) is formed by the union of **two hypogastric nerves** (sympathetic), **two pelvic splanchnic nerves** (parasympathetic), and **sacral splanchnic nerves** (L5 and S1 to S3).
  - ➤ It is **retroperitoneal** collection of nerves lying at the S4 and S5 level, against the posterolateral pelvic wall, lateral to the rectum, vagina, and base of the bladder.
  - ➤ It contains pelvic ganglia in which both sympathetic and parasympathetic preganglionic fibers synapse. Fibers of this plexus accompany internal iliac artery branches to their respective pelvic viscera.
  - ➤ It gives rise to **rectal** plexus, **utero-vaginal** plexus, **vesical** plexus, and **prostatic** plexus.
- ❏ **Sacral splanchnic nerves** consist of preganglionic sympathetic fibers that come off the sympathetic chain and synapse in the inferior hypogastric (pelvic) plexus.
- ❏ **Pelvic splanchnic nerves (Nervi Erigentes)** arise from the sacral segment of the spinal cord (S2–S4) and are the only splanchnic nerves that carry parasympathetic fibers. (All other splanchnic nerves are sympathetic).
  - ➤ They contribute to the formation of the pelvic (or inferior hypogastric) plexus, and supply the descending colon, sigmoid colon, and other viscera in the pelvis and perineum.
- ❏ **Sacral sympathetic trunk** is a continuation of the paravertebral sympathetic chain ganglia in the pelvis. The sacral trunks descend on the inner surface of the sacrum medial to the sacral foramina and converge to form the small median **ganglion impar** anterior to the coccyx.
- ❏ **Coccygeal plexus** is formed by the anterior primary rami of S4 and S5 spinal nerves and the coccygeal nerve. **Coccygeal nerve** innervates the coccygeus muscle, part of the levator ani muscles, and the sacrococcygeal joint.
- ❏ **Anococcygeal nerve** arise from coccygeal plexus and innervate the skin between the tip of the coccyx and the anus.

Table 2: Nerves of perineum - I			
Nerve	Origin	Course	Distribution
Anterior labial nerves (♀); Anterior scrotal nerves (♂)	Terminal part of ilioinguinal nerve (L1)	Arise as ilioinguinal exits superficial inguinal ring; pass anteriorly and inferiorly	*In females*, sensory to mons pubis and anterior part of labium jajus; *in males*, sensory to pubic region, skin of proximal penis, and anterior aspect of scrotum, and adjacent thigh

Nerve	Origin	Course	Distribution
Genital branch of genitofemoral nerve	Genitofemoral nerve (L1 and L2)	Emerges through or near superficial inguinal ring	*In females,* sensory to anterior labia majora; *in males,* motor to cremaster muscle, sensory to anterior aspect of scrotum and adjacent thigh
Perineal branch of posterior cutaneous nerve of thigh	Posterior cutaneous nerve of thigh (S1–S3)	Arises deep to interior border of gluteus maximus; passes medially over sacrotuberous ligament to parallel ischiopubic ramus	Sensory to lateral perineum (labia majora in ♀, scrotum in ♂), genitofemoral sulcus, and superior most medial thigh; may overlap lateral parts of perineum supplied by pudendal nerve
Inferior clunial nerves	Posterior cutaneous nerve of thigh (S1–S3)	Arises deep to and emerge from inferior border of gluteus maximus, ascending in subcutaneous tissue	Skin of inferior gluteal region (buttocks)—gluteal fold and area superior to it

Table 3: Nerves of perineum - II

Nerve	Origin	Course	Distribution
Pudendal nerve (S2–S4)	Sacral plexus (anterior rami of S2–S4)	Exits pelvis via infrapiriform part of greater sciatic foramen; passes posterior to sacrospinous ligament; enters perineum via lesser sciatic foramen, immediately dividing into branches as it enters pudendal canal	Motor to muscles of perineum and sensory to majority of perineal region via its branches, the inferior rectal and perineal nerves, and the dorsal nerve of clitoris or penis
Inferior anal (rectal) nerve	Pudendal nerve (S3–4)	Passes medially from area of ischial spine (entrance to pudendal canal), traversing ischio-anal fat body	External and sphincter; participates in innervation of inferior and medial-most part of levator ani (puborectalis); sensory to anal canal inferior to pectinate line and circumanal skin
Perineal nerve	Pudendal nerve	Arises near entrance to pudendal canal, paralleling parent nerve to and of canal, then passes medially	Divides into superficial and deep branches, the posterior labial or scrotal nerve and the deep perineal nerve
Posterior labial nerve (♂), posterior scrotal nerves (♀)	Superficial terminal branch of perineal nerve	Arise in anterior (terminal) end of pudendal canal, passing medially and superficially	Motor to muscles of superficial perineal pouch (ischiocavernosus, bulbospongiosus, and superficial perineal muscles); in females, sensory to vestibule of vagina and inferior part of vagina
Deep perineal nerve	Deep terminal branch of perineal nerve	Arise in anterior (terminal) end of pudendal canal, passing medially and superficialy	Motor to muscles of superficial perineal pouch (ischiocavernosus, bulbospongiosus, and superficial perineal muscles); in females, sensory to vestibule of vagina and inferior part of vagina

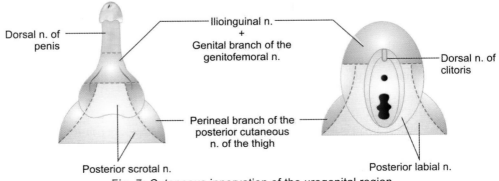

Fig. 7: Cutaneous innervation of the urogenital region

Pudendal Nerve

Pudendal nerve is formed by the anterior primary rami of S2–4 in the pelvic cavity.

- ❑ It leaves the **pelvic cavity** by passing through the **greater sciatic foramen** (between the piriformis and coccygeus muscles).
- ❑ It crosses the **ischial spine** posteriorly and enters the perineum with the internal pudendal artery through the **lesser sciatic foramen**.
- ❑ Next it enters the **pudendal canal** gives rise to the inferior rectal nerve and the perineal nerve, and **terminates** as the dorsal nerve of the penis (or clitoris).
- ❑ **Inferior rectal nerve** is a branch of pudendal nerve given within the pudendal canal divides into several branches, **crosses the ischiorectal fossa**, and innervates the sphincter ani externus and the skin around the anus.
- ❑ **Perineal nerve** divides into a deep branch which supplies all of the perineal muscles, and a superficial (posterior scrotal or labial) branch, which supplies the scrotum or labia majora.
- ❑ **Dorsal nerve** of the penis (or clitoris) is the terminal branch, pierces the perineal membrane, runs between the two layers of the suspensory ligament of the penis (or clitoris), and runs deep to the deep fascia on the dorsum of the penis (or clitoris) to innervate the skin, prepuce, and glans.

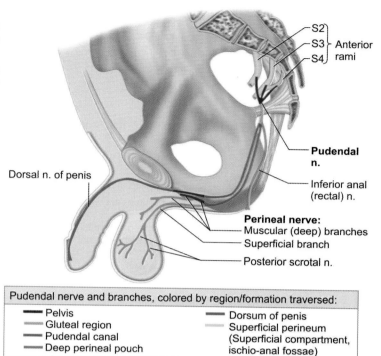

Fig. 8: Pudendal nerve: Formation, course and branches

- ❑ **Alcock's pudendal canal** is present in the lateral wall of ischiorectal fossa, **within layers of obturator fascia**. It has a length of 2.5 cm and lies above the ischial tuberosity. It extends from the lesser sciatic foramen to the posterior limit of the deep perineal pouch.
- ❑ It contains pudendal nerve, internal pudendal artery and vein and send inferior rectal nerve and vessels medially through the fossa towards the anal canal.

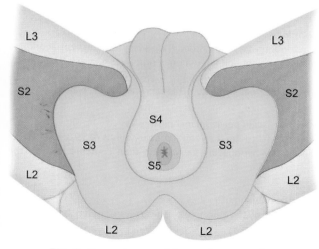

Fig. 9: Dermatomes of the perineum region

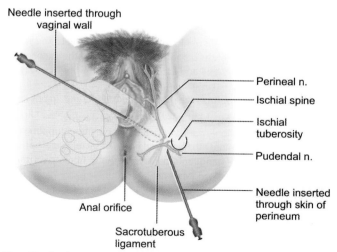

Fig. 10: Pudendal nerve block: Needle is directed at the ischial spine

- ❑ **Pudendal nerve block**: Ischial spine is the landmark and is palpated through the vagina. A needle is guided by the finger to the **ischial spine**. A 1% lignocaine solution is injected transvaginally or just lateral to the labia majora around the tip of the ischial spine and through the sacrospinous ligament.
- ❑ Pudendal block paralyses the skeletal muscles of perineum and anesthetizes the skin of perineum. It also leads to the loss of sensation at the openings of urethra, vagina and anal canal.

❑ Pudendal block leads to urinary and fecal **incontinence**, hence urine and fecal matter needs to be evacuated prior to the procedure (Rectal enema and Foley's catheterization).

❑ For a complete anesthesia of the perineal region, the **ilioinguinal** nerve (which branches into the anterior labial nerves), **genitofemoral** nerve, and perineal branch of the posterior **femoral** cutaneous nerve are also anesthetized.

QUESTIONS

1. Pelvic splanchnic nerves supply all EXCEPT (AIIMS 2009,10)
a. Vermiform appendix
b. Urinary bladder
c. Uterus
d. Rectum

2. All of the following are true regarding the pudendal nerve EXCEPT (AIPG)
a. Both sensory and motor
b. Derived from S2, 3, 4 spinal nerve roots
c. Leaves pelvis through the lesser sciatic foramen
d. Only somatic nerve to innervate the pelvic organ

3. Pelvic pain is mediated by (NEET Pattern 2013)
a. Pudendal nerve
b. Sciatic nerve
c. Autonomic nerves
d. None of the above

4. True about nervi erigentes are all EXCEPT (NEET Pattern 2015)
a. Autonomic nerves
b. Parasympathetic outflow
c. Arise from ventral rami of S2, 3, 4
d. Joins superior hypogastric plexus

5. Preganglionic parasympathetic nerve fibers which supply pelvic viscera is/are (PGIC 2003)
a. Ventral rami of S2,3,4   b. Hypogastric plexus
c. Pudendal nerve   d. Splanchnic nerve
e. Inferior mesenteric plexus

6. Pudendal nerve block abolishes pain from (JIPMER 2016)
a. Upper cervix
b. Superior part of vagina
c. Lower cervix
d. Inferior part of vagina

ANSWERS

1. a. Vermiform appendix
❑ Vermiform appendix is a part of mid-gut under the supply of vagus nerve (not pelvic splanchnic nerves).
❑ Pelvic splanchnic nerves are the parasympathetic nerves to supply the pelvic viscera like urinary bladder, uterus and rectum.

2. c. Leaves pelvis through the lesser sciatic foramen
❑ Pudendal nerve (S2–S4) passes out of the pelvic cavity through the greater sciatic foramen (not the lesser sciatic foramen) and enters the gluteal region.
❑ It travels around the posterior surface of the ischial spine, and re-enters the pelvic cavity through the lesser sciatic foramen.
❑ Next the pudendal nerve travels within the fascia of the obturator internus muscle (called the pudendal canal of Alcock) and gives rise to the inferior rectal and perineal nerves, and terminates as the dorsal nerve of the penis (or clitoris).
❑ It is a somatic and mixed (sensory and motor) nerve supplying skin and skeletal muscles of perineum.
❑ It is the only somatic nerve that supplies the terminal portions of the pelvic organs (urethra, vagina and anal canal).

3. c. Autonomic nerves
❑ Pelvic pain is carried by the autonomic nervous system: Sympathetic component is carried by lumbar splanchnic nerves (T-12, L1,2) and parasympathetic component is nervi erigentes (S 2,3,4).

4. d. Joins superior hypogastric plexus
❑ There is no answer in this question, because all the statements are true.
❑ Nervi erigentes belong to the parasympathetic component of autonomic nervous system. They arise from the ventral primary ramus of S2,3,4 and ascend from the inferior hypogastric plexus via the right and left hypogastric nerves to reach the superior hypogastric plexus.
Note: Some authors are of the opinion that they do not join the superior hypogastric plexus. This explains the given answer.

5. a. Ventral rami of S2,3,4; d. Splanchnic nerve
❑ Preganglionic parasympathetic nerve fibers suppling pelvic viscera are called pelvic splanchnic nerves.
❑ They originate in the lateral horns of sacral spinal cord (S 2,3,4) and pass through the ventral primary ramus of S 2,3,4.
❑ These preganglionic parasympathetic fibers pass through the inferior hypogastric plexus, and then continue towards the respective pelvic viscera.

6. d. Inferior part of vagina
❑ Pudendal nerve supplies the structures in the perineum including the opening of vagina.
❑ Pelvic viscera (including cervix and major portion of vagina) are supplied by the autonomic nervous system: Lumbar splanchnic nerves (sympathetic) and nervi erigentes (parasympathetic).

▼ Muscles of Pelvis and Perineum

❑ **Pelvic floor** is composed of several overlapping sheets of muscles and connective tissues.
➤ It closes the pelvic and abdominal cavities and bear the load of the visceral organs.
➤ It controls the openings of the gastrointestinal and urogenital tubes that pierce through it.
➤ It has two hiatuses: Anteriorly urogenital hiatus through which urethra and vagina pass through and posteriorly anal hiatus through which anal canal passes.

- ❑ Pelvic diaphragm = Levator ani + Ischiococcygeus
- ❑ Levator ani = Pubococcygeus + Iliococcygeus
- ❑ Pubococcygeus (male) = Puborectalis + Puboprostaticus
- ❑ Pubococcygeus (female) = Puborectalis + Pubovaginalis
- ❑ **Pelvic diaphragm** separates the pelvic cavity above from the perineal region below.
  - ➤ It lies posterior and deep to the urogenital diaphragm and medial and deep to the ischiorectal fossa.
  - ➤ It is composed of muscle fibers of the **levator ani** and the **coccygeus** muscle (covered by the parietal pelvic fascia on their upper and lower aspects), and associated connective tissue which span the area underneath the pelvis.

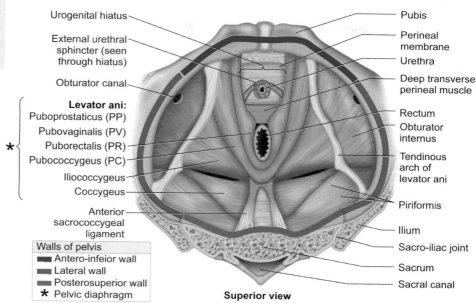

Fig. 11: Floor and walls of pelvis

- ➤ These muscles arise between the symphysis and the ischial spine and converge on the coccyx and the anococcygeal ligament which spans between the tip of the coccyx and the anal hiatus.
- ➤ Right and left levator ani lie almost horizontally in the floor of the pelvis separated by a narrow gap that transmits the urethra, vagina, and anal canal.
- ➤ The levator ani muscle has two parts: **pubococcygeus** (anterior) and **iliococcygeus** (posterior).
  1. **Pubococcygeus** runs backward from the body of the pubis toward the coccyx. Some fibers are inserted into the prostate, urethra, vagina and anorectal junction and named accordingly: Puboprostaticus, pubourethralis, pubovaginalis, puborectalis, respectively.
  2. **Iliococcygeus** attaches to the ilium part of the hip bone and coccyx bone lies posteriorly and is not well developed.
- ➤ Ischiococcygeus (simply called coccygeus) is situated behind the levator ani and frequently tendinous as much as muscular, extends from the ischial spine to the lateral margin of the sacrum and coccyx.

Note: Some sources do not consider 'pelvic floor' and 'pelvic diaphragm' to be identical. It is mentioned that diaphragm consists of only the levator ani and coccygeus, while the 'floor' should also include the perineal membrane and deep perineal pouch.

Functions of Pelvic Diaphragm

- ❑ Excellent support of pelvic viscera (urinary bladder, uterus, rectum, etc.). On contraction, raises the entire pelvic floor.
- ❑ Help in maintenance of continence as a part of the urinary, vaginal and anal sphincters.
- ❑ Facilitates birth by resisting the descent of the presenting part causing the fetus to rotate forwards to navigate through the pelvic girdle.
- ❑ Helps to maintain optimal intra-abdominal pressure.
- ❑ Damaged pelvic diaphragm leads to prolapse of pelvic viscera and incontinence. Pelvic floor muscles can be strengthened with Kegel exercises.

Table 4: Muscles of pelvic walls and floor					
Boundary	**Muscle**	**Proximal Attachment**	**Distal Attachment**	**Innervation**	**Main Action**
Lateral wall	Obturator internus	Pelvic surfaces of ilium and ischium; obturator membrane	Greater trochanter of femur	Nerve to obturator internus (L5, S1, S2)	Rotates thigh laterally; assits in holding head of femur in acetabulum
Posterosuperior wall	Piriformis	Pelvic surface of S2–S4 segments; superior margin of greater sciatic notch and sacrotuber-ous ligament	Greater trochanter of femur	Anterior rami of S1 and S2	Rotates thigh laterally; abducts thigh; assists in holding head of femur in acetabulum

Boundary	Muscle	Proximal Attachment	Distal Attachment	Innervation	Main Action
Floor	Coccygeus (ischiococcygeus)	Ischial spine	Inferior end of sacrum and coccyx	Branches of S4 and S5 spinal nerves	Forms small part of pelvic diaphragm that supports pelvic viscera; flexes coccyx
	Levator ani (puborectalis, pubococcygeus, and iliococcygeus	Body of pubis; tendinous arch of obturator fascia; ischial spine	Perineal body; coccyx; anococcygeal ligament; walls of prostate or vagina, rectum, and canal	Nerve to levator ani (branches of S4), inferior and (rectal) nerve, and coccygeal plexus	Forms most of pelvic diaphragm that helps support pelvic viscera and resists increases in intra-abdominal pressure

Table 5: Muscles of perineum - I

Muscle	Origin	Course and distribution	Innervation	Main action
External sphincter	Skin and fascia surrounding anus; coccyx via anococcygeal ligament	Passes around lateral aspects of anal canal, insertion into perineal body	Inferior anal (rectal) nerve, a branch of pudendal nerve (S2–S4)	Constricts anal canal during peristalsis, resisting defecation; supports and flexes perineal body and pelvic floor
Bulbospongiosus	*Male:* Median rapheon ventral surface of bulb of penis; perineal body	*Male:* Surrounds lateral aspects of bulb of penis and most proximal part of body of penis, inserting into perineal membrane, dorsal aspect of corpus spongiosum and corpora cavernosa, and fascia of bulb of penis	Muscular (deep) branch of perineal nerve, a branch of pudendal nerve (S2–S4)	*Male:* Supports and fixes perineal body/pelvic floor; compresses bulb of penis to expel last drops of urine/semen; assists erection by compressing outflow via deep perineal vein and by pushing blood from bulb into body of penis
	Female: Perineal body	*Female:* Passes on each side of lower vagina, enclosing bulb and greater vestibular gland; inserts into pubic arch and fascia of corpora cavernosa of clitoris		*Female:* Supports and flexes perineal body/pelvic floor; 'sphincter' of vagina; assists in erection of clitoris (and perhaps bulb of vestibule); compresses greater vestibular gland

- ❏ **Bulbospongiosus** muscle compress the bulb in the male, impeding venous return from the penis and thereby maintaining erection.
- ❏ Contraction (along with contraction of the ischiocavernosus) constricts the corpus spongiosum, thereby **expelling the last drops** of urine (or semen in ejaculation).
- ❏ Compress the erectile tissue of the vestibular bulbs in the female and constrict the vaginal orifice (vaginal sphincter).

Table 6: Muscles of perineum - II

Muscle	Origin	Course and distribution	Innervation	Main action
Ischiocavernosus	Internal surface of ischiopubic ramus and ischial tuberosity	Embraces crus of penis of clitoris, inserting onto inferior and medial aspects of crus and to perineal membrane medial to crus	Muscular (deep) branch of perineal nerve, a branch of pudendal nerve (S2–S4)	Maintains erection of penis or clitoris by compressing outflow veins and pushing blood from the root of penis or clitoris into the body of penis or clitoris
Superficial transverse perineal muscle		Passes along inferior aspect of posterior border of perineal membrane to perineal body		Supports and flex perineal body/pelvic floor to support abdominopelvic viscera and resist increased intra-abdominal pressure
Deep transverse perineal muscle		Passes along superior aspect of posterior border of perineal membrane to perineal body and external anal sphincter		

Muscle	Origin	Course and distribution	Innervation	Main action
External urethral sphincter	(Compressor urethra portion only)	Surrounds urethra superior to perineal membrane; in males, it also ascends anterior aspect of prostate; in females, some fibers also enclose vagina (urethrovaginal sphincter)	Dorsal nerve of penis or clitoris, the terminal branch of the pudendal nerve (S2–S4)	Compresses urethra to maintain urinary continence; in females, urethrovaginal sphincter portion also compresses vagina

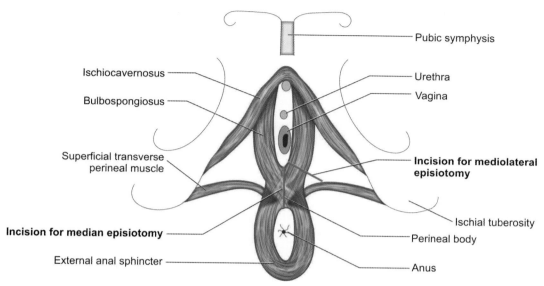

Fig. 12: Perineal body

- **Perineal body** (central perineal tendon) is the fibromuscular tissue located in the midline at the junction between the anal and urogenital triangles, just anterior to the anal sphincter.
- In males, it is found between the bulb of penis and the anus and in females, it is present between the vagina and anal canal, and about 1.25 cm in front of the anus.
- **Structures attaching to perineal body**: External anal sphincter; Bulbospongiosus muscle; Superficial and deep transverse perineal muscle; Anterior fibers of the levator ani (including puborectalis or pubovaginalis, etc.); Fibers from external urinary sphincter; Conjoint longitudinal coat (of rectum).
- Perineal body is an important support of pelvic viscera and is essential for the integrity of the pelvic floor.
  - **Perineal body tear** during vaginal delivery leads to widening of the gap between the anterior free borders of levator ani muscle of both sides, thus predisposing the woman to prolapse of pelvic viscera (urinary bladder, uterus, rectum, etc.)
  - **Episiotomy** is a surgical incision of the perineum (and the posterior vaginal wall) to enlarge the vaginal opening during childbirth. It is done during second stage of labor to quickly enlarge the opening for the baby to pass through.
- The right and left puborectalis unite behind the anorectal junction to form a muscular sling. Some regard them as a part of the sphincter ani externus.
- **Sacrospinous ligament** may represent either a degenerate part or an aponeurosis of the muscle *Ischiococcygeus*.

QUESTIONS

1. **Muscle(s), which form the Pelvic floor** (PGIC 2016)
   a. Obturator internus   b. Puborectalis
   c. Ischiococcygeus   d. Piriformis
   e. Pubococcygeus

2. **Name the muscle forming pelvic diaphragm**
   a. Deep transverse perinei   b. Sphincter urethrae
   c. Levator ani   d. Piriformis

3. **Levator ani muscle include all EXCEPT** (NEET Pattern 2016)
   a. Puborectalis
   b. Pubococcygeus
   c. Iliococcygeus
   d. Ischiococcygeus

4. **Pudendal nerve supplying motor part to external sphincter is derived from** (NEET Pattern 2013)
   a. L5-S1 roots
   b. S1- S2 roots
   c. L2-L3 roots
   d. S2-S3 roots

ANSWERS

1. **b. Puborectalis; c. Ischiococcygeus; e. Pubococcygeus**
   - Pelvic floor is formed by pelvic diaphragm which is contributed by **ischiococcygeus** muscle and levator ani muscle (**Puborectalis, pubococcygeus**, iliococcygeus).
   - **Obturator internus** is present in the lateral wall of the pelvic floor and **Piriformis** forms the postero-superior wall.

2. **c. Levator ani**
  ❑ Pelvic diaphragm is contributed by **levator ani** (pubococcygeus and Iliococcygeus) and ischiococcygeus muscles.
  ❑ Parts of pubococcygeus: Pubourethralis, puboprostaticus, pubovaginalis, puborectalis are the components of the diaphragm.
  ❑ **Deep transverse perinei** and **sphincter urethrae** are the together components of urogenital diaphragm.
  ❑ **Piriformis** forms the postero-superior wall of the pelvic cavity.

3. **d. Ischiococcygeus**
  ❑ **Ischiococcygeus** muscle is a component of pelvic diaphragm, but is **not** included under levator ani muscle.
  ❑ Levator ani muscle is subdivided into named portions according to their attachments and the pelvic viscera to which they are related (**pubococcygeus, iliococcygeus** and **puborectalis**).
  ❑ Pubococcygeus is often subdivided into separate parts according to the pelvic viscera to which each part relates (puboperinealis, puboprostaticus or pubovaginalis, puboanalis, puborectalis).
  Note: Ischiococcygeus (coccygeus) is not a part of levator ani muscle, lies immediately cranial and contiguous with it. Together with levator ani muscle it forms the pelvic diaphragm.

4. **d. S2-S3 roots**
  ❑ Pudendal nerve is contributed by the anterior primary ramus of S 2, 3, 4 in the sacral plexus and supply external sphincters of urethra, vagina and anal canal. External anal sphincter is supplied by inferior rectal nerve branch of pudendal nerve (S 2,3,4).

▶ Arteries of Pelvis and Perineum

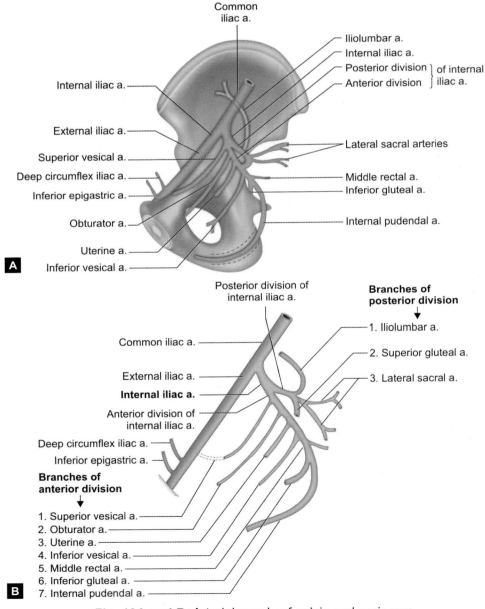

Fig. 13A and B: Arterial supply of pelvis and perineum

Table 7: Arteries of Pelvis - I

Artery	Origin	Course	Distribution	Anastomosis
Gonadal	Abdominal aorta	Descends retroperitoneally;		
Testicular (♂)		Traverses inguinal canal and enter scrotum	Abdominal and/or pelvic ureter, ovary, and ampullary end of uterine tube	Cremasteric artery, artery of ductus deferens
Ovarian (♀)		Crosses pelvic brim, descends in suspensory ligament of ovary	Abdominal and/or pelvic ureter, ovary, and ampulary end of uterine tube	Uterine artery via tubal and ovarian branches
Superior rectal	Continuation of inferior mesenteric artery	Crosses left common iliac vessels and descends into pelvis between layers of sigmoid mesocolon	Superior part of rectum	Middle rectal artery; inferior rectal (internal pudendal) artery
Median sacral	Posterior aspect of abdominal aorta	Descends close to midline over L4 and L5 vertebrae, sacrum, and coccyx	Inferior lumbar vertebrae, sacrum, and coccyx	Lateral sacral artery (via medial sacral branches)
Internal iliac	Common iliac artery	Passes medially over pelvic brim and descends into pelvic cavity; often forms anterior and posterior divisions	Main blood supply to pelvic organs, gluteal muscles, and perineum	
Anterior division of internal iliac	Internal iliac artery	Passes medially over pelvic brim and descends into pelvic cavity; often forms anterior and posterior divisions	Main blood supply to pelvic organs, gluteal muscles, and perineum	
Umbilical	Anterior division of internal iliac artery	Runs a short pelvic course, gives off superior vesical arteries, then obliterates, becoming medial umbilical ligament	Superior aspect of urinary bladder and, in some males, ductus deferens (via superior vesical arteries and artery to ductus deferens)	(Occasionally the patent part of the umbilical artery)
Superior vesical	(Patent proximal umbilical artery)	Usually multiple; pass to superior aspect of urinary bladder	Superior aspect of urinary bladder; in some males, ductus deferens (via artery to ductus deferens)	Inferior vesical (♂); Vaginal artery (♀)
Obturator		Runs anterio-inferiorly on obturator fascia of lateral pelvic wall, exiting pelvis via obturator canal	Pelvic muscles, nutrient artery to ilium, head of femur, and muscles of medial compartment of thigh	Inferior epigastric (via pubic branch); umbilical artery
Inferior vesical (♂)		Passes subperitoneally in lateral ligament of bladder, giving rise to prostatic artery (♂) and occasionally the artery to the ductus deferens	Inferior aspect of male urinary bladder, pelvic part of urete; prostate, and seminal glands; occasionally ductus deferens	Superior vesical artery
Artery to ductus deferens (♂)	(Superior or inferior vesical artery)	Runs subperitoneally to ductus deferens	Ductus deferens	Testicular artery; cremasteric artery
Prostatic branches (♂)	(Inferior vesical artery)	Descends on posterolateral aspects of prostate	Prostate and prostatic urethra	Deep perineal (internal pudendal)
Uterine (♀)		Runs anatomically in base of broad ligament/superior cardinal ligament, gives rise to vaginal branch, then crosses ureter superiorly to reach lateral aspect of uterine cervix	Uterus, ligaments of uterus, medial parts of uterine tube and ovary, and superior vagina	Ovarian artery (via tubal and ovarian branches); vaginal artery
Vaginal (♀)	(Uterine artery)	Divides into vaginal and inferior vesical branches, the former descending on the vagina, the latter passing to the urinary bladder	Vaginal branch: Lower vagina, vestibular bulb, and adjacent rectum; inferior vesical branch: fundus of urinary bladder	Vaginal branch of uterine artery, superior vesical artery

Artery	Origin	Course	Distribution	Anastomoses
Internal pudendal	Anterior division of internal iliac artery	Exits pelvis via infrapiriform part of greater sciatic foramen, enters perineum (ischio-anal fossa) via lesser sciatic foramen, passes via pudendal canal to crogenital UG triangle	Main artery of perineum, including muscles and skin of anal and urogenital triangles, erectile bodies	(Umbilical artery; prostatic branches of inferior vesical artery in males)
Middle rectal		Descends in pelvis to inferior part of rectum	Inferior part of rectum, seminal glands, prostate (vagina)	Superior and inferior rectal arteries
Inferior gluteal		Exits pelvis via infrapiriform part of greater sciatic foramen	Pelvic diaphragm (coccygeus and levator ani), piriformis, quadratus femoris, superiormost hamstrings, gluteus maximus, and sciatic nerve	Profunda femoris artery (via medial and lateral circumflex femoral arteries)

Table 8: Arteries of Pelvis - II			
Artery	Origin	Course	Distribution in perineum
Internal pudendal	Anterior division of internal iliac artery	Leaves pelvis through greater sciatic foramen; hooks around ischial spine to enter perineum via lesser sciatic foramen; enters pudendal canal	Primary artery of perineum and external genital organs
Inferior rectal	Internal pudendal artery	Arises at entrance to pudendal canal; traverses ischio-anal fossa to anal canal	Anal canal inferior to pectinate line; anal sphincters; peri-anal skin
Perineal		Arises within pudendal canal; passes to superficial pouch (space) on exit	Supplies superficial perineal muscles and scrotum of male/vestibule of female
Posterior scrotal (♂) or labial (♀)		Runs in superficial fascia of posterior scrotum or labia majora	Skin of scrotum or labia majora and minora
Artery of bulb of penis (♂) or vestibule (♀)	Terminal branch of perineal artery	Pierces perineal membrane to reach bulb of penis or vestibule of vagina	Supplies bulb of penis (including bulbar urethra) and bulbo-urethral gland (male) or bulb of vestibule and greater vestibular gland (female)
Deep artery of penis (♂) or clitoris (♀)	Terminal branch of internal pudendal artery	Pierces perineal membrane to enter crura of corpora cavernosa of penis or clitoris; branches run proximally and distally	Supplies most erectile tissue of corpora cavernosa of penis or clitoris via helicine arteries
Dorsal artery of penis (♂) or clitoris (♀)		Passes to deep pouch; pierces perineal membrane and traverses suspensory ligament of penis or clitoris to run on dorsum of penis or clitoris to glans	Deep perineal pouch; skin of penis; fascia of penis or clitoris; distal corpus spongiosum of penis, including spongy urethra; glans penis or clitoris
External pudendal, superficial, and deep branches	Femoral artery	Pass medially from thigh to reach anterior aspect of the urogenital triangle or perineum	Anterior aspect of scrotum and skin at root of penis of male; mons pubis and anterior aspect of labia of female

Internal Pudendal Artery is a branch from the anterior division of internal iliac artery.

❑ It leaves the pelvis by way of the greater sciatic foramen between the piriformis and coccygeus and immediately enters the perineum through the lesser sciatic foramen by hooking around the ischial spine, accompanied by the pudendal nerve during its course.

❑ It passes along the lateral wall of the ischiorectal fossa in the **pudendal canal**.

QUESTIONS

1. **Branch of internal iliac artery is/are**   (PGIC 2014)
   a. Inferior vesical artery
   b. Inferior epigastric artery
   c. Iliolumbar artery
   d. Internal pudendal artery
   e. Obturator artery

2. **Internal pudendal artery is a branch of**   (NEET Pattern 2015)
   a. Anterior division of internal iliac
   b. Posterior division of internal iliac
   c. Anterior division of external iliac
   d. Posterior division of external iliac

3. **All are branches of the internal iliac artery EXCEPT**   (NEET Pattern 2012)
   a. Ovarian artery   b. Superior vesical artery
   c. Middle rectal artery   d. Inferior vesical artery

4. **Artery to ductus deferens is a branch of**   (NEET Pattern 2016)
   a. Superior vesical artery   b. Inferior vesical artery
   c. Internal pudendal artery   d. Middle rectal artery

1. **a. Inferior vesical artery; c. Iliolumbar artery; d. Internal pudendal artery; e. Obturator artery**
   - ❏ Inferior epigastric artery is a branch of external (not internal) iliac artery.

2. **a. Anterior division of internal iliac**
   - ❏ Anterior division of internal iliac artery gives the internal pudendal artery which accompanies pudendal nerve in the pudendal canal and supply the perineum region.

3. **a. Ovarian artery**
   - ❏ Ovarian artery is a branch of the abdominal aorta.
   - ❏ Gonads develop in the abdomen region and gonadal arteries are branches of abdominal aorta.
   - ❏ As the gonads descend down to pelvic cavity, gonadal arteries become longer (Testicular > Ovarian in length).

4. **a. Superior vesical artery > b. Inferior vesical artery > d. Middle rectal artery**
   - ❏ Vas deferens is usually derived from the superior vesical artery, and occasionally from the inferior vesical artery, both branches of the internal iliac artery.
   - **Note:** It may also arise from middle rectal artery.

Venous and Lymphatic drainage of Pelvis and Perineum

Pelvic Venous Plexus

It lies within the minor (true) pelvic cavity and is formed by intercommunicating veins surrounding the pelvic viscera and include the rectal venous plexus, vesical venous plexus, prostatic venous plexus, uterine venous plexus, and vaginal venous plexus.

Components

- ❏ Pelvic venous plexuses → internal iliac veins which join the external iliac veins to form the common iliac veins → common iliac veins, which join to form the inferior vena cava (IVC). This is the major pathway.
- ❏ Pelvic venous plexuses → median sacral vein → common iliac vein → IVC
- ❏ Pelvic venous plexuses → ovarian veins → IVC
- ❏ Pelvic venous plexuses → superior rectal vein → inferior mesenteric vein → portal vein
- ❏ Pelvic venous plexuses → lateral sacral veins → internal vertebral venous plexus → cranial dural sinuses

Lymphatics

Lymphatic drainage of the **Pelvis**

- ❏ The lymphatics follow the internal iliac vessels to the internal iliac nodes to the common iliac nodes and subsequently to the lumbar (aortic) nodes.
- ❏ Internal iliac nodes receive lymph from the upper part of vagina and other pelvic organs, and they drain into the common iliac and then to the lumbar (aortic) nodes.
- ❏ Lymph from the uppermost part of the rectum drains along the superior rectal vessels, inferior mesenteric nodes, and then aortic nodes.
- ❏ Lymph from the testis and epididymis or ovary drains along the gonadal vessels directly into the aortic nodes.
- ❏ Lymph vessels from the prostate drain into the internal iliac nodes.
- ❏ Lymph vessels from the ovary, uterine tube, and fundus follow the ovarian artery and drain into the para-aortic nodes. Lymph vessels from the uterine body and cervix and bladder drain into the internal and external iliac nodes.

Lymphatic drainage of the **Perineum**

- ❏ Lymphatics drain via the superficial inguinal lymph nodes which receive lymph from the lower abdominal wall, buttocks, penis, scrotum, labium majus, and lower parts of the vagina and anal canal.
- ❏ These lymph nodes have efferent vessels that drain primarily into the external iliac nodes and ultimately to the lumbar (aortic) nodes.
- ❏ Lymphatics from the glans penis (or clitoris) and labium minus pass to the deep inguinal and external iliac nodes.

Table 9: Lymphatic drainage of pelvis and perineum			
Lymph node group		**Structures typically drainage to lymph node group**	
Lumbar	*Female:* Along ovarian vessels	Gonads and associated structures; common iliac nodes	*Female:* Ovary; uterine tube (except isthmus and intrauterine parts); fundus of uterus
	Male: Along testicular vessels		*Male urethra:* Testis; epididymis

Lymph node group	Structures typically drainage to lymph node group	
Inferior mesenteric	Superiormost rectum; sigmoid colon; descending colon; pararectal nodes	
Common iliac	External and internal iliac lymph nodes	
Internal iliac	Inferior pelvic structures; deep perineal structures; sacral nodes	*Female:* Base of bladder; inferior pelvic ureter; anal canal (above pectinate line); inferior rectum; middle and upper vagina; cervix; body of uterus
		Male: Prostatic urethra; prostate; base of bladder; inferior pelvic ureter; inferior seminal glands; cavernous bodies; anal canal (above pectinate line); inferior rectum
External iliac	Anterosuperior pelvic structures; deep inguinal nodes	*Female:* Superior bladder: superior pelvic ureter; upper vagina; cervix; lower body of uterus
		Male: Superior bladder; superior pelvic ureter; upper seminal gland; pelvic part of ductus deferens; intermediate and spongy urethra (secondary)
Superficial inguinal	Lower limb: Superficial drainage of inferolateral quadrant of trunk including anterior abdominal wall inferior to umbilicus, gluteal region, and superficial perineal structures	*Female:* Superolateral uterus (near attachment of round ligament); skin of perineum including vulva; ostium of vagina (inferior to hymen); prepuce of clitoris; peri-anal skin; anal canal inferior to pectinate line
		Male: Skin of perineum including skin and prepuce of penis; scrotum; peri-anal skin; anal canal inferior to pectinate line
Deep inguinal	Clitoris glans or penis; superficial inguinal nodes	*Female:* Clitoris glans
Sacral	Postero-inferior pelvic strucutres; inferior rectum; inferior vagina	
Pararectal	Superior rectum	

QUESTIONS

1. **Superficial inguinal lymphatics drain all of the following EXCEPT:** *(NEET Pattern 2015)*
   a. Anal canal below pectinate line
   b. Glans penis
   c. Urethra
   d. Perineum

2. **Infection/inflammation of all of the following causes enlarged superficial inguinal lymph nodes EXCEPT:** *(AIPG 2004)*
   a. Isthmus of uterine tube
   b. Inferior part of anal canal
   c. Big toe
   d. Penile urethra

ANSWERS

1. **b. Glans penis**
   - Glans penis drains into deep inguinal lymph nodes (Cloquet).
   - Anal canal below pectinate line drains into superficial inguinal lymph nodes, and above the pectinate line into internal iliac lymph nodes.
   - Proximal urethra drains into iliac and distal urethra into inguinal lymph nodes.
   - Perineum majorly drains into superficial inguinal lymph nodes.

2. **d. Penile urethra**
   - Lymphatics from the penile urethra (and glans penis) mainly run towards deep inguinal lymph nodes.
   - Though few lymphatics may end up in the superficial inguinal lymph nodes.
   - Isthmus of uterine tube, inferior part of anal canal and big toe all drain towards the superficial group of lymph nodes. Lymphatics from the isthmus follow the round ligament of uterus and lymphatics from the great toe follow the great saphenous vein, both reaching the superficial inguinal lymph nodes.

▶ Female Reproductive System

Ovaries are the female gonads located in the pelvic cavity, posterior to the broad ligament, in the **ovarian fossa of Waldeyer**, between the divergent external and internal iliac vessels.

- They are attached to the lateral pelvic wall by the **suspensory ligament of the ovary** (a region of the broad ligament) which contains the ovarian artery, vein, and nerve.
- The blood vessels, lymphatics, and nerves pass over the pelvic inlet, cross the external iliac vessels, and then enter the suspensory ligament of the ovary (lateral end of broad ligament) and finally enter the hilum of ovary via the **mesovarium**.
- The ovary consists of a **cortex** and **medulla**. In young women, the outermost portion of the cortex is smooth, has a dull white surface (**tunica albuginea**).
- The surface of the ovaries is not covered by mesothelium, but instead by a simple cuboidal epithelium called the **germinal epithelium of Waldeyer**.
- Beneath this epithelium, the **cortex** contains oocytes and developing follicles. The **medulla** is the central portion which is composed of loose connective tissue.
- There are a large number of arteries and veins in the medulla and a small number of smooth muscle fibers.

   Ovarian fossa of Waldeyer: Ovarian fossa is a shallow depression in the peritoneal lining of lateral wall of the pelvis, where in the ovary (in nulliparous) lies.

- It lies below the pelvic brim.
- Behind the ovarian fossa are retroperitoneal structures including the **ureter**, internal iliac vessels, obturator vessels and nerve, and the **origin of the uterine artery**.
- Posterior border of ovary is free and faces the peritoneum which overlies the upper part of the internal iliac artery and vein, and the ureter.
- Ovarian fossa is bounded anteriorly (and superiorly) by the external iliac vessels and inferiorly by the uterine tubes (in the free margin of broad ligament).
- Obliterated umbilical artery (medial umbilical ligament) crosses anteriorly.
- The obturator nerve and vessels cross the floor of the fossa (inferiorly).

Peritoneal Relations

- Ovarian ligament is a fibromuscular cord that extends from the ovary to the uterus below the uterine tube, running within the layers of the broad ligament.

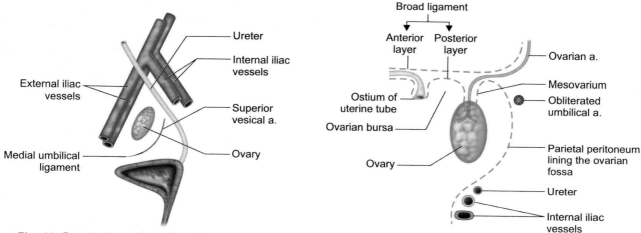

Fig. 14: Boundaries and relation of ovarian fossa

Fig. 15: Peritoneal relations of the ovary

- Suspensory ligament of the ovary is a band of peritoneum that extends upward from the ovary to the pelvic wall and transmits the ovarian vessels, nerves, and lymphatics.

Arterial Supply

- Ovarian arteries (branch of abdominal aorta) and ascending branches of the uterine arteries (branch of internal iliac artery).

Venous Drainage

- Ovaries drain into ovarian veins, right ovaries veins empties into the inferior vena cava and the left ovarian vein empties into the left renal vein.

Lymphatic Drainage

- Lymphatics drain into the para (lateral) and pre (anterior) aortic lymph nodes.

Nerve Supply

- Sympathetic nerves are derived from spinal segment T10, 11.
- Parasympathetic nerves are vagus (laterally) and nervi erigentes (medially) nerve.
- Sensory (general visceral afferent) fibers follow the ovarian artery and enter at T10,11, spinal cord level.
  - Ovarian pain is referred in the umbilical region (T10).
  - The intractable ovarian pain can be alleviated by transecting the suspensory ligament, which contain the afferent fibers.

1. Ureter is present in which wall of ovarian fossa
(NEET Pattern 2016)
- a. Anterior
- b. Posterior
- c. Medial
- d. Lateral

2. Ovarian fossa is formed by all EXCEPT   (NEET Pattern 2015)
- a. Obliterated umbilical artery
- b. Internal iliac artery
- c. Ureter
- d. Round ligament of ovary

3. Ovarian pathology is referred to
(AIIMS 2010)
- a. Gluteal region
- b. Anterior thigh
- c. Medial part of thigh
- d. Back of thigh

QUESTIONS

1. b. Posterior
- ❑ Behind the ovarian fossa are retroperitoneal structures including the ureter, internal iliac vessels, obturator vessels and nerve, and the origin of the uterine artery.

2. d. Round ligament of ovary
- ❑ Round ligament of ovary is inferomedial to the ovary.

3. c. Medial part of thigh
- ❑ Ovarian pathology may irritate the obturator nerve lying in the vicinity which leads to a referred pain in the medial thigh (Dermatome: L2).
- ❑ Obturator nerve (L2, 3 and 4) is the nerve of medial thigh and supplies the skin on the medial thigh. This type of pain is a somatic referred pain.
- ❑ Another example is the pain felt in the knee joint in a case of Perthes' disease which is pathology of hip joint but referred somatic pain is felt in the knee joint, since, both the joints are supplied by a common nerve – the obturator nerve.
- ❑ The visceral pain of the ovary is carried by the visceral nerves having root value T-10, 11. Hence, visceral referred pain from the ovarian pathology which will be felt in the skin bearing (dermatome T-10, 11).
- ❑ Pain in the medial thigh could be a referred pain from viscera like ureter, hind gut, uterus, urinary bladder. Or it could be a somatic referred pain irritating obturator nerve as in a case of appendicitis, pelvic abscess or ovarian pathology as in the present case.

▶ Uterus

- ❑ **Cervix** is the lower part of the uterus that measures about 2.5 to 3 cm in length. The external os in a nulliparous woman is **round** and **transverse** in a parous woman.
- ❑ Cervix is divided into a supravaginal portion (**endocervix**) and a vaginal portion (**ectocervix**) which protrudes into the vagina.
- ❑ At puberty, the **simple columnar epithelium** of the endocervical canal extends onto the ectocervix and its exposure to the acidic (pH = 3) of the vagina induces a transformation from columnar to stratified **squamous epithelium** (i.e., squamous metaplasia) and the formation of a transformation zone.

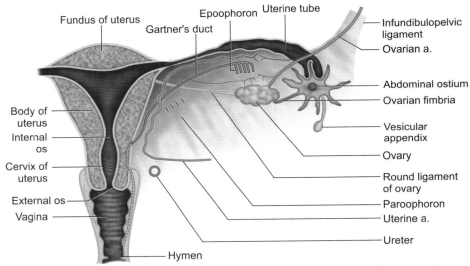

Fig. 16: Contents of the broad ligament (posterior aspect of the right broad ligament) of the uterus

- ❑ **Broad ligament** consists of double layer of parietal peritoneum, extending from the uterus to the lateral pelvic wall and functions to hold the uterus in position.
  - ➤ It does not contain the ovary but is attached to the ovary through the mesovarium.
  - ➤ It has a posterior layer that curves from the isthmus of the uterus (the rectouterine fold) to the posterior wall of the pelvis alongside of the rectum.
  - ➤ It has four regions:
    1. Mesovarium connects the posterior layer of the broad ligament with anterior surface of the ovary.
    2. Mesosalpinx is the fold of the broad ligament that suspends the uterine tube.
    3. Mesometrium is the part of the broad ligament below the mesosalpinx and mesovarium.
    4. Suspensory ligament of the ovary.

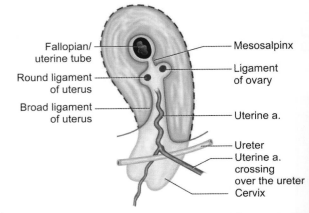

Fig. 17: Sagittal section through the broad ligament of the uterus showing structures that lie within the broad ligament

❑ **Contents**: Ovarian NVB (artery, vein, and nerves), ovarian ligament of the uterus (which is a remnant of the gubernaculum in the embryo), Uterine tubes and NVB (Uterine artery, vein, and nerves - which lie at the base of the broad ligament within the transverse cervical ligament), Round ligament of the uterus (which is a remnant of the gubernaculum in the embryo), Epoophoron and paroophoron (which are remnants of the mesonephric tubules in the embryo), Gartner's duct (which is a remnant of the mesonephric duct in the embryo), Ureter (which lies at the base of the broad ligament posterior and inferior to the uterine artery), nerve plexus, and lymphatic vessels.

Position of the Uterus

❑ Uterus is normally in an anteverted and anteflexed position which places the uterus in a nearly horizontal position lying on the superior wall of the urinary bladder.

❑ **Anteversion**: The long axis of the uterus is bent forward on the long axis of the vagina against the urinary bladder. It is the anterior bend of the uterus at the angle between the cervix and vagina.

❑ **Anteflexion**: It refers to the anterior bend of the uterus at the angle between the cervix and body of the uterus.

Arterial supply: The uterus is supplied by uterine arteries and partly by the ovarian arteries.

❑ Uterine artery is a branch of anterior division of internal iliac artery runs medially across the pelvic floor in the base of the broad ligament towards the uterine cervix.

❑ It passes superior to the ureter, superolateral to the fornix of the vagina.

❑ Then it ascends along the side of the uterus. At the superolateral angle of uterus it turns laterally, runs along the uterine tube and anastomose with the ovarian artery.

❑ Uterine artery supplies vagina, uterus, medial two-third of the uterine tube, ovary, ureter, and structures within the broad ligament.

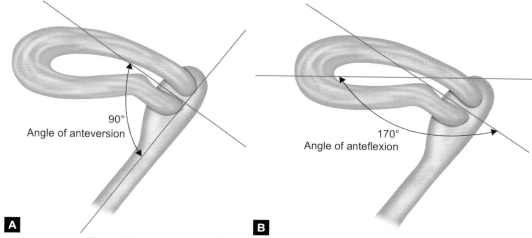

Figs. 18A and B: A. Position of anteversion B. Position of anteflexion

❑ **Branches**: Near the cervix after crossing the ureter, it gives ureteric, vaginal, and cervical branches.
  ➤ The cervical branches form circular anastomosis around the isthmus.
  ➤ Along the side of body of the uterus it gives off arcuate branches which run transversely on the anterior and posterior surfaces of the body of uterus and anastomoses with their counter parts along the midline.

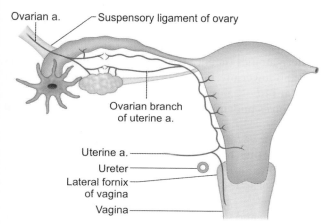

Fig. 19: Uterus: Arterial supply

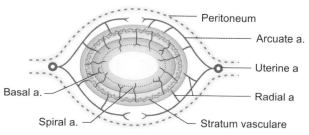

Fig. 20: Intrinsic arterial circulation of the uterus

  ➤ Along the fallopian tube it gives off tubal and ovarian branches.

❑ Sequence of arterial branches (peripheral to deeper): Arcuate → Radial → Basal & Spiral (**ARBS**)

Intrinsic uterine circulation

❑ Uterine artery gives **arcuate** (coronary) arteries which anastomose on the anterior and posterior surfaces of the body of the uterus in the midline.
  ➢ **Radial** arteries arise from the arcuate arteries and pierce the myometrium centripetally, anastomose with each other and form stratum vasculare in the middle layer of myometrium.
  ➢ From stratum vasculare **basal** and **spiral** are given to supply the endometrium.
  ➢ Spiral arteries supply the functional zone of the endometrium (which is cast off during menstruation) and basal arteries supply the basal zone of the endometrium (which helps in the regeneration of the denuded endometrium).
❑ **Venous Drainage** of the uterus is to the internal iliac veins (which empties into the IVC).
❑ **Fundus** and upper part of the body: Pre-and para-aortic lymph nodes along the ovarian vessels.
  ➢ Few lymphatics from the lateral angles of the uterus travel along the round ligaments of the uterus and drain into the superficial inguinal lymph nodes.
❑ **Middle part of the body**: External iliac nodes via broad ligament.
❑ From **cervix**, on each side the lymph vessels drain in three directions:
  1. Laterally: External iliac and obturator nodes
  2. Posterolaterally: Internal iliac nodes (major drainage)
  3. Posteriorly: Sacral nodes.

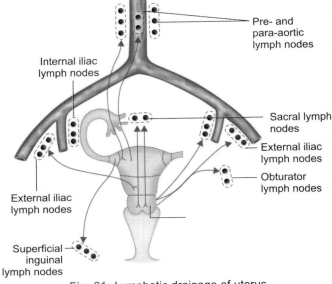

Fig. 21: Lymphatic drainage of uterus

Nerve supply

The nerve supply to the uterus is predominantly from the **inferior hypogastric plexus** and branches are carried by arteries (**uterine** and **ovarian**).

❑ Nerves ascend with uterine arteries in the broad ligament and connect with tubal nerves with the ovarian plexus.
❑ Nerves to the cervix form a plexus that contains small paracervical ganglia.
❑ Sympathetic preganglionic efferent fibers are derived from neurones in the last thoracic and first lumbar spinal segments (T10-12; L1-2) which synapse on the postganglionic neurones in the superior and inferior hypogastric plexuses. These fibers produce uterine contraction (in non-pregnant uterus) and vasoconstriction. Uterine contraction in pregnant uterus is under oxytocin hormone.
❑ Parasympathetic preganglionic fibers arise from neurones in the second to fourth sacral spinal segments (S 2,3,4) and relay in the paracervical ganglia, and cause uterine inhibition and vasodilation, but these activities are complicated by hormonal control of uterine functions.
❑ Most afferent sensory fibers from the **uterus** ascend through the **inferior hypogastric plexus** and enter the spinal cord via **lumbar splanchnic** (T10-12; L1-2) and corresponding spinal nerves. The sensory nerves from the **cervix** and upper part of the **birth canal** pass through the pelvic splanchnic nerves (**nervi erigentes**) to the S 2,3,4 nerves.
❑ Those from the **lower portion** of the birth canal pass primarily through the **pudendal nerve**.

Labor pain

❑ Pain during **first stage of labor** is initially confined to T11 – T12 dermatomes (latent phase), but eventually labor enters active phase and much of the pain is due to dilatation of cervix and lower uterine segment and pain passes through hypogastric plexus and aortic plexus before entering the spinal cord at T10 – L1 nerve roots.
❑ Stretching and compression of the pelvic and perineal structures involves pudendal nerve (S2-4), so pain during **second stage of labor** involves T10 – S4 dermatomes.
❑ **Spinal anesthesia** upto spinal nerve T10 is necessary to block pain for vaginal delivery and upto spinal nerve T4 for cesarean section (due to the sympathetic fiber levels being at higher level than motor or sensory blockade).
❑ **Lumbar spinal anesthesia** (spinal block), in which the anesthetic agent is introduced with a needle into the spinal subarachnoid space and it anesthetizes the intraperitoneal, subperitoneal and somatic structures.
  ➢ It produces complete aesthesia inferior to approximately the waist level.
  ➢ The perineum, pelvic floor, and birth canal are anesthetized, and motor and sensory functions of the entire lower limbs, as well as sensation of uterine contractions, are temporarily eliminated.

- ❑ **Caudal epidural block**, in which the anesthetic agent is administered using an in-dwelling catheter in the sacral canal, and it anesthetizes the subperitoneal and somatic structures.
- ❑ The entire birth canal, pelvic floor, and most of the perineum are anesthetized, but the lower limbs are not usually affected, and the mother is aware of uterine contractions.
- ❑ **Pudendal nerve block** provides local anesthesia over the perineum (S2–S4 dermatomes) and the inferior quarter of the vagina.
  - ➢ It does not block pain from the superior birth canal (uterine cervix and superior vagina), so the mother is able to feel uterine contractions.

QUESTIONS

1. CORRECT sequence of arterial blood flow in uterus is:
    (NEET Pattern 2016)
   a. Uterine → Arcuate → Radial → Spiral
   b. Uterine → Radial → Arcuate → Spiral
   c. Uterine → Spiral → Radial → Arcuate
   d. Uterine → Arcuate → Spiral → Radial

2. Uterine lymphatics drain into all EXCEPT: *(AIPG 2005)*
   a. External iliac
   b. Internal iliac
   c. Superficial inguinal
   d. Deep inguinal

3. Lymphatic drainage of uterine cervix is all EXCEPT:
   a. Obturator
   b. Sacral
   c. External iliac
   d. Internal iliac

4. Uterine cervix drains lymphatics into all EXCEPT:
   a. Parametrial lymph nodes *(AIPG 2006)*
   b. Deep inguinal lymph nodes
   c. Obturator lymph nodes
   d. External iliac lymph nodes

5. All the following pairs are correct concerning the lymphatics of uterus EXCEPT
   a. Fundus: Para-aortic
   b. Mid-uterus: External iliac
   c. Cervix: Superficial inguinal lymph nodes
   d. Cervix: Sacral

6. Labor pain in uterus is carried by *(NEET Pattern 2016)*
   a. Parasympathetic nerves
   b. Sympathetic nerves
   c. Pudendal nerve
   d. Splanchnic nerve

7. In first stage of labor the referred pain from uterus is carried to the dermatome *(AIIMS)*
   a. T10, 11
   b. T12; L1
   c. L1, 2
   d. S2, 3

8. To provide pain relief during first stage of labor which sensory level should be blocked
   a. T8 to L1
   b. T9 to L2
   c. T10 to L1
   d. T11 to L2

9. All are true regarding uterus EXCEPT
    (PGIC 2014)
   a. Lymph vessels from fundus drain to para-aortic lymph nodes
   b. Broad ligament provides primary support to uterus
   c. Mainly supplied by uterine artery
   d. Supplied by ovarian artery
   e. Posterior surface is related to intestine

ANSWERS

1. a. Uterine → Arcuate → Radial → Spiral
   ❑ ARBS: Arcuate → Radial → Basal and Spiral

2. d. Deep inguinal
   ❑ Lymphatics from the uterus reach the superficial inguinal lymph nodes but not the deep inguinal.
   ❑ The lymphatics follow the round ligament of uterus to reach the superficial inguinal lymph nodes.
   ❑ Upper part of the uterus like fundus, drain mainly into the para-aortic lymph nodes.
   ❑ Lymphatics from cervix region spread towards external iliac as well as internal iliac group of lymph nodes.

3. a. Sacral
   ❑ Uterus drains into all the lymphatic destinations mentioned in the choices, hence this appears to be a wrong question, though some standard textbooks do not mention sacral lymph nodes in the lymphatic drainage.

4. b. Deep inguinal lymph nodes
   ❑ Lymphatic drainage from the cervix does not drain into the deep inguinal lymph nodes.
   ❑ Obturator lymph nodes receive a minor component of lymphatic drainage from the cervix.
   ❑ The lymphatics of cervix mainly move towards the internal iliac lymph nodes. Additionally, it drains towards external iliac; rectal and the sacral lymph nodes as well. Parametrial lymph nodes receive the lymphatics of cervix and direct them towards their further destination.

5. c. Cervix: Superficial inguinal lymph nodes
   ❑ Uterine cervix does not drain into the inguinal lymph nodes (superficial or deep).
   ❑ Fundus and upper part of the body: Pre- and para-aortic lymph nodes along the ovarian vessels (few lymphatics from the lateral angles of the uterus travel along the round ligaments of the uterus and drain into superficial inguinal lymph nodes)
   ❑ Middle part of the body: External iliac nodes via broad ligament.
   ❑ From cervix, on each side the lymph vessels drain in three directions:
     ■ Laterally: External iliac and obturator nodes
     ■ Posterolaterally: Internal iliac nodes
     ■ Posteriorly: Sacral nodes.

6. b. Sympathetic nerves > a. Parasympathetic nerves
- ❑ The pain of labor in the first stage is mediated by sympathetic fibers reaching T10 to L1 spinal segments.
- ❑ In the second stage pain is carried by sympathetic fibers to T12 to L1 spinal segments.
- ❑ Visceral afferent fibers conducting pain from subperitoneal structures, such as the cervix and vagina (i.e. the birth canal), travel with parasympathetic fibers to the S2–S4 spinal ganglia.
- ❑ Somatic sensation from the opening of the vagina also passes to the S2–S4 spinal ganglia via the pudendal nerve.

7. b. T12; L1
- ❑ Pain during first stage of labor is due to uterine contraction and cervical dilatation.
- ❑ Initially pain is confined to T11-T12 dermatomes (upper uterine contractions), but eventually dilatation of cervix and lower uterine segment pain passes through hypogastric plexus and aortic plexus before entering the spinal cord at T10-L1 nerve roots.

8. c. T10 to L1
- ❑ Pain during labor is due to uterine contraction and cervical dilatation, initially confined to T11-T12 dermatomes (upper uterine contractions), but eventually dilatation of cervix and lower uterine segment pain reach the spinal cord at T10-L1 nerve roots.

9. b. Broad ligament provides primary support to uterus
- ❑ Broad ligament is a fold of peritoneum and poor support of uterus. Primary supports of uterus are muscular supports.
- ❑ Lymphatics from the uterine fundus drain towards the para-aortic lymph nodes.
- ❑ Uterus is supplied by uterine (mainly) and ovarian arteries.
- ❑ Posterior surface of uterus is related to coils of the terminal ileum and to the sigmoid colon. It is covered with peritoneum and forms the anterior wall of the rectouterine pouch.

▶ Supports of Pelvic Viscera

Pelvic viscera (like urinary bladder, uterus, rectum, etc.) are supported by numerous structures. Supports of uterus has been discussed in great detail.

Supports of uterus
- ❑ Muscular (dynamic supports) - provide excellent support
  - ➤ Pelvic diaphragm (levator ani and coccygeus)
  - ➤ Urogenital diaphragm (urethral sphincter and deep transverse perinei)
  - ➤ Perineal body (common perineal tendon for the attachment of numerous perineal muscles)
- ❑ **Pelvic fascia condensations** (passive supports) – provide good support
  - ➤ Transverse cervical ligaments (of Mackenrodt).
  - ➤ Pubocervical ligaments.
  - ➤ Uterosacral (sacrocervical) ligaments
- ❑ Peritoneal folds - provide **poor support**
  - ➤ Broad ligaments
  - ➤ Round ligament of uterus (remnant of the gubernaculum in the embryo)
  - ➤ Uterovesical fold of peritoneum
  - ➤ Rectovaginal fold of peritoneum
- ❑ Uterine position and axis (anteflexed and anteverted)

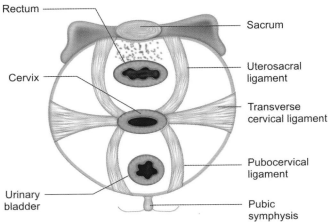

Fig. 22: Ligamentous (fibromuscular) supports of the uterus (Superior view)

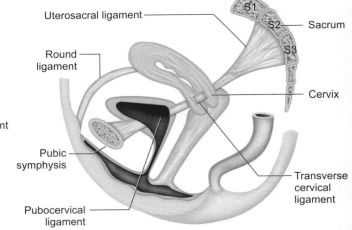

Fig. 23: Lateral view: All these ligaments (except round ligaments) are formed by the pelvic fascia condensations (visceral layer)

- ❑ **Transverse cervical ligaments** of Mackenrodt are the most important ligaments of the uterus, hence often called cardinal ligaments.

- They are the fibromuscular condensation of pelvic fascia around the uterine vessels, at the base of broad ligament.
- They are fan-shaped fibromuscular bands extending from the lateral aspect of cervix and upper vaginal wall to the lateral pelvic wall.
- They form a hammock which supports the uterus and prevent its downward displacement.
- **Pubocervical ligaments** are a pair of fibrous bands which extend from the cervix to the posterior aspects of the pubic bones.
- **Uterosacral ligaments** are a pair of fibrous bands which extend from the cervix to the second and third sacral vertebrae, and pass on each side of the rectum.
  - These ligaments pull the cervix backward against the forward pull of the round ligaments and help in the maintenance of anteflexed and anteverted positions of the uterus.
- **Round ligaments** of the uterus are a pair of fibromuscular bands which lie between the two layers of broad ligament.

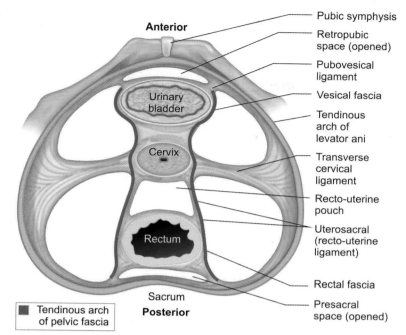

Fig. 24: Ligamentous supports of pelvic viscera

- It begins at the **lateral angle of the uterus**, passes forward and laterally **between the two layers of broad ligament**, enters the **deep inguinal ring** after winding around the **lateral side** of the inferior epigastric artery.
- It traverses the **inguinal canal**, emerges through the superficial inguinal ring, and splits into numerous thread-like fibrous bands which merge with the fibroareolar tissue of the **labium majus**.
- These ligaments pull the fundus forward and help to maintain the **anteversion** and **anteflexion** of the uterus.
- **Sacrocervical** ligaments extend from the lower end of the sacrum to the cervix and the upper end of the vagina.
- **Rectouterine** (Sacrouterine) Ligaments hold the cervix back and upward and sometimes elevate a shelf-like fold of peritoneum (rectouterine fold), which passes from the isthmus of the uterus to the posterior wall of the pelvis lateral to the rectum.
  - It corresponds to the sacrogenital (rectoprostatic) fold in the male.

Prolapse of uterus may occur if the supports are weakened.

- During parturition the muscular supports undergo lot of stretching and may give up, leading to uterus being pushed inside vagina and come out into the perineum.
- Surgical support: The cardinal ligaments have enough fibrous content to provide anchor for the wide loops of sutures during several surgical procedures.
- Endopelvic fascia lies between, and is continuous with, both visceral and parietal layers of pelvic fascia.
- **Hypogastric sheath** is a condensation of pelvic fascia which lies along the postero-lateral pelvic walls and carries the neuro-vascular bundles towards the pelvic viscera. It also provides pelvic viscera support and has three lamina:
  - **Anterolateral** ligament of urinary bladder which carries superior vesical arteries and veins.
  - **Posterolateral** ligaments of rectum which carries middle rectal arteries and veins.
  - **Middle** lamina which in male forms recto-vesical septum (between urinary bladder and rectum) and in female forms cardinal ligament of uterus which carries uterine artery in its superior-most portion at the base of broad ligament of uterus.

Pelvic fascia

Parietal pelvic fascia covering the obturator internus and levator ani muscles and the visceral pelvic fascia surrounding the pelvic organs are continuous where the organs penetrate the pelvic floor, forming a tendinous arch of pelvic fascia bilaterally.

Additional ligaments

- Pubovesical (Female) or puboprostatic (Male) ligaments are condensations of the pelvic fascia that extend from the neck of the bladder (or the prostate gland in the male) to the pelvic bone.
- Inferior pubic (Arcuate pubic) ligament arches across the inferior aspect of the pubic symphysis and attaches to the medial borders of the inferior pubic rami.

1. **Which is NOT a part of the hypogastric sheath**
   a. Transverse cervical ligament b. Broad ligament
   c. Lateral ligament of bladder d. Uterosacral ligament

2. **Support of prostate is** *(NEET Pattern 2013)*
   a. Pubococcygeus b. Ischiococcygeus
   c. Iliococcygeus d. None of the above

3. **Supports of the uterus are all EXCEPT** *(AIIMS 2006)*
   a. Uterosacral ligament b. Broad ligament
   c. Mackenrodt ligament d. Levator ani

4. **Which of the following does not prevent prolapse of uterus**
   a. Perineal body b. Pubocervical ligament
   c. Broad ligament d. Transverse cervical ligament

5. **Anteversion of uterus is maintained by** *(NEET Pattern 2018)*
   a. Cardinal ligaments
   b. Uterosacral ligaments
   c. Pubocervical ligaments
   d. Round ligaments

1. **b. Broad ligament**
   ❑ Hypogastric sheath is a condensation of the pelvic fascia which transmits vessels and nerves along the lateral pelvic wall towards the pelvic viscera.
   ❑ Broad ligament of uterus is not a part of the hypogastric sheath. It is a peritoneal fold.
   ❑ Parts of the hypogastric sheath:
   ▪ Anterior lamina: Lateral ligament of bladder.
   ▪ Middle lamina: Transverse cervical ligament, rectovesical septum in males.
   ▪ Posterior lamina: Presacral fascia, uterosacral ligament (containing middle rectal vessels).
   Note: The endopelvic fascia lies between, and is continuous with, both visceral and parietal layers of pelvic fascia.

2. **a. Pubococcygeus**
   ❑ Anterior fibers of pubococcygeus surround the prostate to form levator prostatae muscle, which supports the prostate.
   ❑ Pubovaginalis in the female is the equivalent of levator prostate in the male.
   ❑ Both originate from the posterior pelvic surface of the body of the pubis bone. Fibers pass inferiorly, medially and posteriorly to insert into a midline raphe, the central perineal tendon.

3. **b. Broad ligament**
   ❑ Broad ligament is a double fold of peritoneum and is a weak support of uterus, its function as uterine support is comparatively insignificant.
   ❑ The best supports of pelvic viscera are the muscular supports like Levator ani.
   ❑ The pelvic fascia condensations like uterosacral- and Mackenrodt ligaments are considered as good supports of uterus.

4. **c. Broad ligament**
   ❑ Broad ligament is a peritoneal fold and poor support of uterus.
   ❑ Perineal body is a central perineal tendon which receives attachment of perineal muscles which support the pelvic viscera.
   ❑ Pubocervical and transverse cervical ligaments are the pelvic fascia condensations which are good supports of pelvic viscera.

5. **Ans. d. Round ligaments**
   ❑ *Round ligaments pull the fundus forward and help to maintain the anteversion and anteflexion of the uterus.
   ❑ Angle of anteversion is the forward angle between the long axis of the vagina and the long axis of the cervix.

▶ Uterine Tube

Uterine tubes (oviducts) extend 8 to 14 cm from the uterine cornua and anatomically classified along their length as an **interstitial** (1 cm) portion, **isthmus** (3 cm), **ampulla** (5 cm), and **infundibulum** (1 cm).

❑ **Interstitial** (intramural) portion is embodied within the uterine muscular wall.

❑ **Isthmus** has narrow lumen (2—3 mm) and widens gradually into the (5—8 mm) more laterally.

❑ **Ampulla** is the longest and has the widest lumen, and fertilization takes place here.

❑ **Infundibulum** is the funnel-shaped fimbriated distal extremity which opens into the peritoneal cavity.

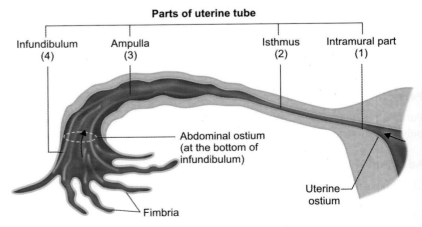

Parts of uterine tube

Infundibulum (4) Ampulla (3) Isthmus (2) Intramural part (1)

Abdominal ostium (at the bottom of infundibulum)

Uterine ostium

Fimbria

Fig. 25: Parts of the uterine tube

The mucosa is thrown into longitudinal folds which are the **most pronounced distally at the infundibulum** and decrease to shallow bulges in the intrauterine (intramural) portion.

In cross section, the extrauterine fallopian tube contains a mesosalpinx, myosalpinx, and endosalpinx.

❑ Mesosalpinx which is a region of the broad ligament, has a single-cell mesothelial layer functioning as visceral peritoneum.
❑ Myosalpinx has smooth muscle arranged in an inner circular and an outer longitudinal layer.
❑ Endosalpinx is the tubal mucosa having columnar epithelium composed of **ciliated** and secretory (peg) cells resting on a sparse lamina propria. The ciliated cells are most abundant at the fimbriated end.

Arterial Supply

❑ Ovarian arteries (branches of abdominal aorta) and the ascending branches of the uterine arteries (branches of internal iliac artery).

Venous Drainage

❑ Uterine tubes drain into ovarian veins and the uterine veins.

Nerve Supply

❑ Preganglionic parasympathetic fibers are derived from the vagus for the lateral half of the tube, and pelvic splanchnic nerves for the medial half.
❑ Preganglionic sympathetic supply is derived from neurones in the intermediolateral column of the T10—L2 spinal segments; postganglionic sympathetic fibers are most likely derived from the superior hypogastric plexus via the superior hypogastric and hypogastric nerves.
❑ Visceral afferent fibers travel with the sympathetic nerves and enter the cord through corresponding dorsal roots to reach spinal segment T10; they may also travel with parasympathetic fibers.

QUESTIONS

1. **Which part of the uterine tube acts as anatomical sphincter**
   a. Intramural part
   b. Isthmus
   c. Ampulla
   d. Infundibulum

2. **The sensory supply of the fallopian tube and ovary is from**
   a. T6 to T8
   b. T8 to T10
   c. T10 to T12
   d. L2 to L4

ANSWERS

1. **b. Isthmus > a. Intramural part**
   ❑ The arrangement of the muscles at the isthmus is such that it can work like a sphincter, preventing the oocyte from entering the uterine cavity.
   ❑ Some authors mention the location of sphincter at the junction of uterus and uterine tube (intramural part).

2. **c. T10 to T12**
   ❑ Visceral afferent fibers travel with the sympathetic nerves and enter the cord through corresponding dorsal roots (T12 ±2).

▸ Female External Genitalia

❑ Female external genitalia (or vulva/pudendum) consists of a vestibule of vagina and its surrounding structures such as mons pubis, labia majora, labia minora, clitoris, vestibular bulb and pair of greater vestibular glands.
❑ Bartholin gland is located at the junction of middle 1/3 and posterior 1/3 of labia majora.

Vestibule of the Vagina represents the embryologic urogenital sinus.

❑ It is the space between the labia minora which contains the urethral orifice, paraurethral glands (of Skene), vaginal introitus (incompletely covered by the hymen), greater vestibular glands (of Bartholin), and lesser vestibular glands.

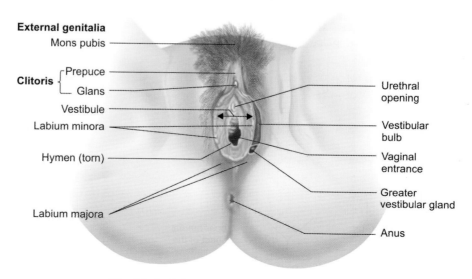

External genitalia
- Mons pubis
- Clitoris { Prepuce / Glans }
- Vestibule
- Labium minora
- Hymen (torn)
- Labium majora
- Urethral opening
- Vestibular bulb
- Vaginal entrance
- Greater vestibular gland
- Anus

Fig. 26: An inferior view of the female perineum

Greater Vestibular (Bartholin) Glands lie in the **superficial perineal pouch** deep to the vestibular bulbs in the female.

- ❑ They are homologous to the **bulbourethral glands** in the male.
- ❑ They consist of two small oval bodies that flank the vaginal orifice in contact with, and often overlapped by the posterior end of the vestibular bulb.
- ❑ They are compressed during coitus and secrete mucus that lubricates the vagina.
- ❑ They are located **slightly posterior** and on each side of the opening of the vagina. Each open into the vestibule by a 2 cm duct situated in the groove between the hymen and the labium minora.
- ❑ The glands are composed of tubuloacinar type with columnar cells. The epithelium of the Bartholin duct is **cuboidal** near the gland but becomes transitional and finally **stratified squamous** near the opening of the duct.

QUESTIONS

1. **All are parts of vulva EXCEPT:**   *(NEET Pattern 2012)*
   a. Labia minora
   b. Labia majora
   c. Perineal body
   d. Clitoris

2. **All is true about Bartholin gland EXCEPT:**
   a. Homologous of male bulbourethral gland
   b. Present in the superficial perineal pouch
   c. Located at the junction of anterior 1/3 and middle 1/3 of labia majora
   d. Opens into the vestibule between hymen and labia minora

   (PGIC 2016)

3. **TRUE about anatomy of vagina**
   a. Anterior wall is longer than posterior wall
   b. Covered by columnar epithelium
   c. Covered by nonkeratinized stratified squamous epithelium
   d. Vaginal secretion is from transudation of vaginal epithelium
   e. Supplied by cervico-vaginal branch of the uterine artery

ANSWERS

1. **c. Perineal body**
   - ❑ The female external genitalia (or vulva/pudendum) consists of a vestibule of vagina and its surrounding structures such as mons pubis, labia majora, labia minora, clitoris, vestibular bulb and pair of greater vestibular glands.

2. **c. Located at the junction of anterior 1/3 and middle 1/3 of labia majora**
   - ❑ Bartholin gland is located at the junction of middle 1/3 and posterior 1/3 of labia majora.
   - ❑ The duct opens in the posterolateral wall of vagina (vestibule).
   - ❑ The epithelium of the Bartholin duct is cuboidal near the gland, but becomes transitional and finally stratified squamous near the opening of the duct.

3. **c. Covered by non-keratinized stratified squamous epithelium; d. Vaginal secretion is from transudation of vaginal epithelium; e. Supplied by cervico-vaginal branch of the uterine artery**
   - ❑ The vaginal mucosa is attached to the uterine cervix higher on the posterior cervical wall than on the anterior; the anterior wall is approximately 7.5 cm long and the posterior wall is approximately 9 cm long.
   - ❑ The epithelium of vagina is non-keratinized stratified squamous similar to, and continuous with that of the ectocervix.
   - ❑ Superior portion of the vagina is supplied by the vaginal branches of uterine artery (branch of internal iliac artery).
   - ❑ Middle and lower portions of the vagina are supplied by the internal pudendal artery which arises from the internal iliac artery.

▶ **Perineum**

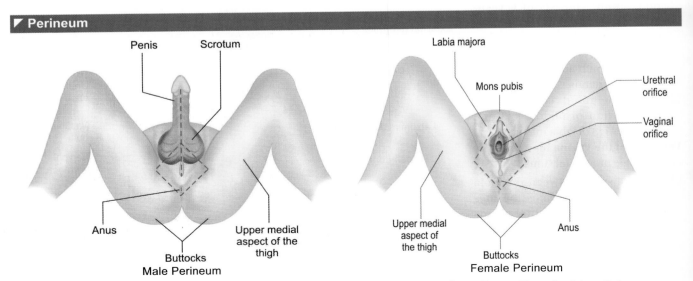

Fig. 27: Perineum as seen in lithotomy position. Interrupted red lines indicate the position of pelvic outlet

Perineum is the diamond-shaped region between the thighs which corresponds to the outlet of the pelvis and presents with openings of urethra, vagina and anal canal.

- ❏ It includes **perineal pouches** (superficial and deep); **ischiorectal fossa**; pudendal canal and anal canal.
- ❏ **Boundaries**: Anterior: Pubic symphysis, arch and the arcuate ligament
    - ➤ Anterolateral: Ischiopubic rami
    - ➤ Lateral: Ischial tuberosities
    - ➤ Postero-lateral: Sacrotuberous ligaments
    - ➤ Posterior: Tip of the coccyx
    - ➤ Floor: Skin and fascia
    - ➤ Roof: Pelvic diaphragm and associated fascia
- ❏ It is divided into an anterior **urogenital triangle** and a posterior **anal triangle** by a line drawn across the surface connecting the ischial tuberosities.

Urogenital triangle contains the superficial and deep perineal pouches (spaces):

Superficial Perineal Pouch

- ❏ It lies between the perineal membrane (inferior fascia of the urogenital diaphragm) and the Colles fascia (membranous layer of superficial perineal fascia).
- ❏ It is an open compartment due to the fact that anteriorly the space communicates freely with the potential space lying between the superficial fascia of the anterior abdominal wall and the anterior abdominal muscles.

Deep perineal pouch is enclosed in part by the perineum, and located superior to the perineal membrane (inferior fascia of urogenital diaphragm).

- ❏ It lies between the superior and inferior fascia of the urogenital diaphragm.
- ❏ Recently the deep pouch is being described as the region between the perineal membrane and pelvic diaphragm.

Urogenital diaphragm (triangular ligament) is the term used **occasionally** to describe the muscular components of the deep perineal pouch.

- ❏ Urethra and the vagina pass through the urogenital diaphragm.
- ❏ The term urogenital diaphragm should not be confused with the pelvic diaphragm (pelvic floor) which is a true diaphragm supporting the pelvic viscera.

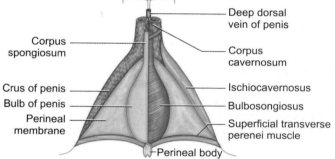

Fig. 28: Root of the penis and superficial perineal muscles. The superficial perineal muscles are removed in the left of the figure to show crus and bulb of the penis

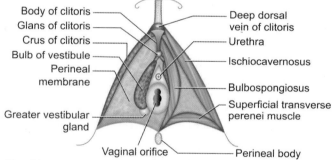

Fig. 29: Root of clitoris and superficial perineal muscles. Superficial perineal muscles have been removed in the left half of the figure to show the bulb of the vestibule and greater vestibular gland

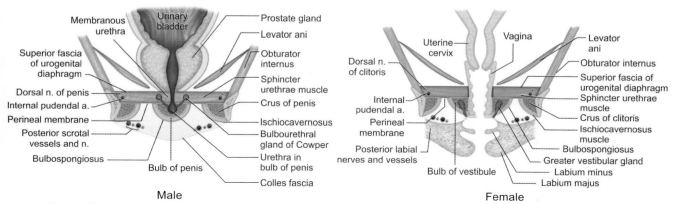

Fig. 30: Coronal sections of the urogenital region showing contents of the superficial and deep perineal pouches

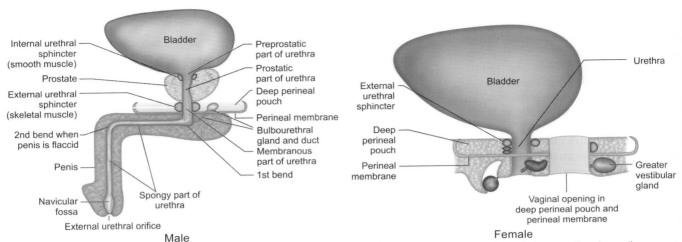

Fig. 31: Sagittal sections of the urogenital region showing the contents of the superficial and deep perineal pouches

- ❏ Traditionally, a trilaminar, triangular musculo-fascial diaphragm, in the anterior part of perineum has been described as making up the deep perineal pouch.
- ❏ It consisted of the perineal membrane (inferior fascia of the UG diaphragm) inferiorly, a superior fascia of the UG diaphragm superiorly, and deep perineal muscles in between.
- ❏ The deep pouch was the space between the two fascial membranes occupied by two muscles: a disc-like 'sphincter urethra' anterior to transversely oriented 'deep transverse perineal' muscle.
- ❏ In males, the bulbourethral glands are also considered occupants of the pouch.

Current Concept

- ❏ In the female, the posterior edge of the perineal membrane is typically occupied by a mass of smooth muscle in the place of the deep transverse perineal muscles.
- ❏ Immediately superior to the posterior half of the perineal membrane, the flat, sheet-like, deep transverse perineal muscle, when developed (typically only in males) offers dynamic support for the pelvic viscera.
- ❏ The only 'superior fascia' is the intrinsic fascia of the external urethral sphincter muscle. Though some authors consider the inferior fascia of the pelvic diaphragm to be the superior boundary of the deep pouch.

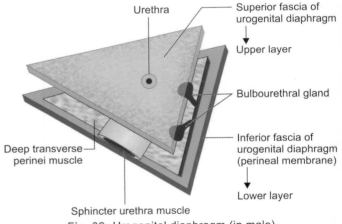

Fig. 32: Urogenital diaphragm (in male)

Note: In both views, the strong perineal membrane is the inferior boundary (floor) of the deep pouch, separating it from the superficial pouch. The perineal membrane is indeed with the perineal body the final passive support of the pelvic viscera.

- ❏ **Bulbourethral** (Cowper) Glands lie among the fibers of the sphincter urethra in the deep perineal pouch in the male, on the posterolateral sides of the membranous urethra.
- ❏ The ducts pass through the perineal membrane to reach superficial perineal pouch and open into the bulbous portion of the spongy (penile) urethra.

Table 10: Structure within the deep and superficial perineal spaces	
Male	**Female**
Structures within the deep perineal space	
Membranous urethra	Urethra, Vagina
Urogenital (UG) diaphragm Deep transverse perineal muscle Sphincter urethra muscle	UG diaphragm Deep transverse perineal muscle Sphincter urethra muscle

Male	Female
Branches of internal pudendal artery Artery of the penis	Branches of internal pudendal artery Artery of the clitoris
Branches of pudendal nerve Dorsal nerve of the penis	Branches of pudendal nerve Dorsal nerve of the clitoris
Bulbourethral glands (Cowper)	No glands
Structures within the superficial perineal space	
Penile (spongly) urethra	Urethra, Vestibule of the vagina
Bulbospongiosus muscle Ischiocavernosus muscle Superficial transverse perineal muscle	Bulbospongiosus muscle Ischiocavernosus muscle Superficial transverse perineal muscle
Branches of internal pudendal artery Perineal artery → posterior scrotal arteries Dorsal artery of the penis Deep artery of the penis	Branches of internal pudendal artery Perineal artery → posterior labial arteries Dorsal artery of the clitoris Deep artery of the clitoris
Branches of pudendal nerve Perineal nerve → posterior scrotal nerves Dorsal nerve of the penis	Branches of pudendal nerve Perineal nerve → posterior labial nerves Dorsal nerve of the clitoris
Bulb of the penis Crus of the penis	Vestibular bulb Crus of the clitoris
Perineal body	Perineal body Round ligament of the uterus
Duct of the bulbourethral gland	Greater vestibular glands (of Bartholin)

▼ Perineal fascia

Perineal fascia has two parts (superficial and deep) and each of these can be subdivided into superficial and deep parts.
- ❑ Superficial perineal fascia
  - ➢ Fatty layer
  - ➢ Deeper membranous layer (Colles' fascia)
- ❑ Deep perineal fascia
  - ➢ Perineal membrane (inferior fascia of urogenital diaphragm)
  - ➢ Superior fascia of urogenital diaphragm (Considered hypothetical)
- ❑ During dissection in the perineum, the arrangement of layers (from superficial to deep) is:

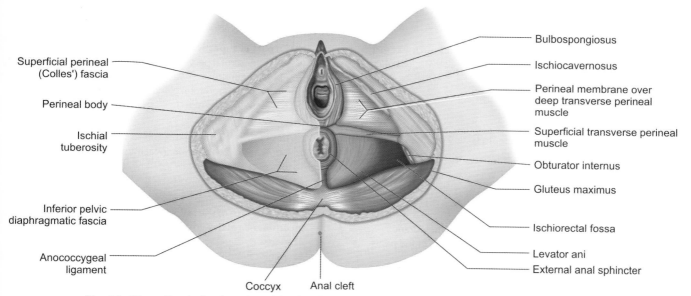

Fig. 33: Dissection in the female pelvis showing relations of superficial and deep perineal pouches

Skin → superficial perineal fascia (fatty layer) → superficial perineal fascia (deeper membranous layer - Colles' fascia) → superficial perineal pouch → perineal membrane (inferior fascia of urogenital diaphragm) → Deep perineal pouch → superior fascia of urogenital diaphragm (hypothetical) → fascia and muscles of pelvic floor (levator ani, coccygeus) → pelvic viscera.

Note: The location of perineal body and ischiorectal fossa

Colles' fascia is the deep membranous layer (of the superficial perineal fascia) and forms the floor (inferior boundary) of the superficial perineal pouch.

➢ On either side it is firmly attached to the margins of the rami of the pubis and ischium, lateral to the crus of penis and as far back as the tuberosity of the ischium.
➢ Posteriorly, it curves around the superficial transverse perineal muscle to join the lower margin of the perineal membrane.
➢ It emerges from the inferior side of the perineal membrane and continues along the ventral (inferior) penis without covering the scrotum.
➢ It separates the skin and subcutaneous fat from the superficial perineal pouch and covers the muscles in the pouch.
➢ It becomes **continuous with the dartos tunic of the scrotum** with the superficial fascia of the penis, and with the **Scarpa fascia** of the anterior abdominal wall.
➢ **Straddle injuries** may rupture of the **bulbous spongy urethra** below the perineal membrane leading to extravasation of urine into the superficial perineal pouch which may spread inferiorly into the scrotum, anteriorly around the penis, and superiorly into the lower part of the abdominal wall.

Perineal membrane is the inferior fascia of urogenital diaphragm.

❑ Location: It is the roof (superior boundary) of the superficial perineal pouch, and the floor (inferior boundary) of the deep perineal pouch.
➢ It is thickened anteriorly to form the **transverse ligament of the perineum** which spans the subpubic angle just behind the deep dorsal vein of the penis (or clitoris).
❑ Shape: It is triangular in shape and about 4 cm in depth.
➢ Apex is directed forward, and is separated from the arcuate pubic ligament by an oval opening for the transmission of the deep dorsal vein of the penis (or clitoris).
➢ Lateral margins are attached on either side to the inferior rami of the pubis and ischium above the crus penis.
➢ Base is directed toward the rectum, and connected to the perineal body posteriorly. The base is fused with both the pelvic fascia and Colles' fascia.
❑ Relations: It is continuous with the deep layer of the superficial fascia behind the superficial transverse perineal muscle, and with the inferior layer of the diaphragmatic part of the pelvic fascia.

QUESTIONS

1. **Superficial perineal muscles include**   *(PGIC 2002)*
   a. Superficial transverse perineal muscle
   b. Bulbospongiosus
   c. Ischiocavernosus
   d. Iliococcygeus
   e. Pubococcygeus

2. **Urogenital diaphragm is contributed by all EXCEPT**
   (NEET Pattern 2012)
   a. Sphincter urethra
   b. Perineal body
   c. Colles' fascia
   d. Perineal membrane

3. **All are the contents of deep perineal pouch EXCEPT**
   (AIIMS 2008; AIPG 2009)
   a. Bulb/Root of penis
   b. Dorsal nerve of penis
   c. Sphincter urethra
   d. Bulbourethral glands

4. **NOT a part of superficial perineal pouch**   *(AIIMS 2011)*
   a. Posterior scrotal nerves
   b. Sphincter urethra
   c. Ducts of bulbourethral glands
   d. Bulbospongiosus muscle

5. **Nerve supply to the perineum is**   *(NEET Pattern 2012)*
   a. Pudendal nerve
   b. Inferior rectal nerve
   c. Pelvic splanchnic nerves
   d. Hypogastric plexus

6. **All of the following are attached to perineal body EXCEPT:**
   a. Superficial transverse perineal muscle   *(NBE 2013)*
   b. Iliococcygeus
   c. Bulbospongiosus
   d. Ischiocavernosus

7. **The deep perineal space**
   a. Is formed superiorly by the perineal membrane
   b. Contains a segment of the dorsal nerve of the penis
   c. Is formed inferiorly by Colles' fascia
   d. Contains the greater vestibular glands

8. **Injury to which of the following muscle may lead to urinary incontinence along with cystocele, rectocele and prolapse of uterus**   *(AIIMS 2017)*
   a. Ischiocavernosus
   b. Pubococcygeus
   c. Bulbospongiosus
   d. Urethral and anal sphincter

9. Which of the following marked structure in the figure given below forms the pelvic diaphragm *(AIIMS 2017)*
   a. A
   b. B
   c. C
   d. D

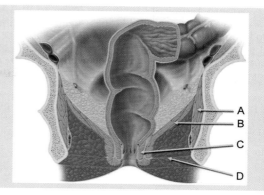

1. **a. Superficial transverse perineal muscle; b. Bulbospongiosus; c. Ischiocavernosus**
   - ❑ Muscles in the superficial perineal pouch are ischiocavernosus, bulbospongiosus and superficial transverse perineal muscle.
   - ❑ Iliococcygeus and pubococcygeus are components of pelvic diaphragm.

2. **c. Colles' fascia**
   - ❑ Urogenital diaphragm contains the deep perineal pouch and is lined inferiorly by the perineal membrane and not Colles' fascia.
   - ❑ Colles' fascia lies at the floor (inferior lining) of superficial perineal pouch.

3. **a. Bulb/Root of penis**
   - ❑ Bulb/root of penis lies in the superficial perineal pouch and not the deep perineal pouch.
   - ❑ Bulb of vagina/root of clitoris also lie in the superficial perineal pouch.

4. **b. Sphincter urethra**
   - ❑ Sphincter urethra (external urethral sphincter) is present in the wall of membranous urethra in the deep perineal pouch, it also extends vertically, around the anterior aspect of the prostatic urethra.

5. **a. Pudendal nerve**
   - ❑ Pudendal nerve is the nerve of perineum. It is a mixed (sensory and motor) nerve to supply skin and skeletal muscles of perineum.

6. **d. Ischiocavernosus**
   - ❑ Ischiocavernosus is not a midline muscle and is not attached to the central perineal tendon (perineal body).
   - ❑ Superficial and deep transverse perineal muscles both attach to the perineal body.
   - ❑ Iliococcygeus (pelvic diaphragm) has attachment to the perineal body
   - ❑ Bulbospongiosus is a muscle in the superficial perineal pouch which covers the bulb of penis (or vagina) and attaches to perineal body.

7. **b. Contains a segment of the dorsal nerve of penis.**
   - ❑ Dorsal nerve of penis is a content of both superficial and deep perineal pouch. Other choices are applicable to superficial perineal pouch.

8. **b. Pubococcygeus**
   - ❑ Pubococcygeus is a component of pelvic diaphragm (a pelvic viscera support). Injury to this muscle leads to loss of support to the pelvic viscera (urinary bladder, uterus, rectum, etc.) leading to their prolapse.

9. **b. B**
   - ❑ This is a coronal section of the pelvic region showing the relations of ischiorectal fossa.
   - ❑ Pelvic diaphragm is majorly contributed by the levator ani muscle (Marker B).
   - ❑ Key: Marker A: Obturator internus muscle; C: Internal anal sphincter; D: Perianal fascia

▶ Anal triangle

Anal triangle has two components: Muscles and Ischiorectal fossa.
- ❑ Muscles of the anal triangle: External anal sphincter, obturator internus, levator ani and coccygeus muscles.
- ❑ Ischiorectal Fossa (IRF) is present on either side of the anorectum and is separated from the pelvic cavity by the levator ani muscle (and fascia).
  - ➤ **Boundaries**:
    - ▪ Anterior: Urogenital diaphragm (with perineal membrane)
    - ▪ Posterior: Gluteus maximus (and sacrotuberous ligament)

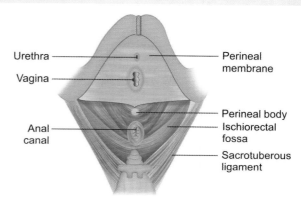

Fig. 34: Surface view of the ischiorectal fossa and perineal membrane

- Superomedial: Sphincter ani externus and levator ani
- Lateral: Obturator internus muscle (with obturator fascia) on ischial tuberosity
- Floor: Skin
- Roof: Meeting point of obturator fascia (covering obturator internus) and inferior fascia of the pelvic diaphragm (covering levator ani muscle).

➤ **Contents**: Inferior rectal neurovascular bundle (nerve, artery and vein); fat; perineal branches of the posterior femoral cutaneous nerve, and the pudendal canal (with pudendal nerve, internal pudendal artery and vein).

❑ A communication (horse shoe shaped) is present between the two IRF passing behind the anal canal.

Note: Pudendal canal is formed either by the splitting of the obturator fascia (or by separation between the fascia lunata and the obturator fascia).

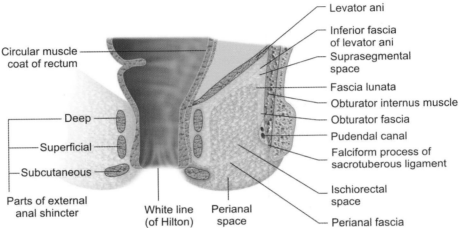

Fig. 35: Boundaries of the ischiorectal fossa as seen in coronal section through the anal triangle

1. Boundaries of ischiorectal fossa are *(NEET Pattern 2014)*
a. Posterior: Perineal membrane
b. Anterior: Sacrotuberous ligament
c. Lateral: Obturator internus
d. Medial: Gluteus maximus

2. During incision and drainage of ischiorectal abscess, which nerve is/are injured *(PGIC 2012)*
a. Superior rectal nerve
b. Inferior rectal nerve
c. Superior gluteal nerve
d. Inferior gluteal nerve
e. Posterior labial nerve

3. Pudendal canal is a part of *(NEET Pattern 2014)*
a. Colles' fascia
b. Obturator fascia
c. Scarpa's fascia
d. None

4. UNTRUE about ischiorectal fossa
a. Obturator fascia meets anal fascia at the apex
b. A communication is present between the two IRF in front of anal canal
c. Alcock's canal is located at the lateral wall
d. Inferior rectal nerve and vessels pass through it

1. c. Lateral: Obturator internus
❑ Lateral boundaries of ischiorectal fossa is the ischial bone with obturator internus muscle covered by obturator fascia.
❑ Perineal membrane lies anterior and sacrotuberous ligament and gluteus maximus are posterior. Medial boundary is levator ani muscle.

2. b. Inferior rectal nerve; e. Posterior labial nerve
❑ Dissection of ischiorectal fossa, may involve injury to inferior rectal, pudendal, posterior scrotal (or labial) nerve and vessels along with perforating branches of S2-S3 and perineal branches of S4 nerve.

3. b. Obturator fascia
❑ Pudendal canal is formed in the obturator fascia in the lateral wall of the ischiorectal fossa.

4. b. A communication is present between the two IRF in front of anal canal
❑ A communication is present between the two IRF is behind the anal canal.
❑ Apex (roof): Meeting point of obturator fascia (covering obturator internus) and inferior fascia of the pelvic diaphragm (covering levator ani muscle)
❑ Alcock's pudendal canal is present in the lateral wall of ischiorectal fossa and send inferior rectal nerve and vessels medially through the fossa towards the anal canal.

Urinary Bladder and Urethra

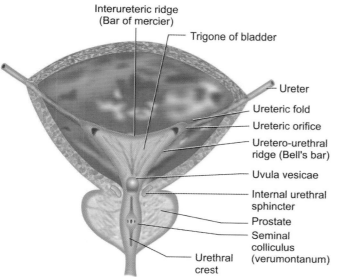

Fig. 36: Interior of the urinary bladder as seen in the coronal section

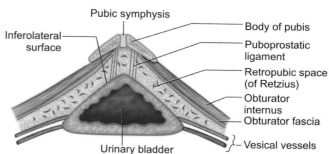

Fig. 37: Relations of the inferolateral surfaces of the urinary bladder

Trigone of the bladder is located on the posterior surface of the bladder (fundus or base).

❑ Its limits are defined superiorly by the openings of the ureters and inferiorly by the internal urethral orifice, around which is a thick circular layer called the internal urethral sphincter (sphincter vesicae).

❑ It is always **smooth-surfaced** because the mucosa is tightly adherent to the detrusor muscle.

❑ Ureter enters the urinary bladder at the lateral angle has an oblique course through it and is valveless. The intramural portion of the ureter functions as a check valve (ureterovesical valve of Sampson) to prevent urine reflux.

❑ Internal urethral orifice lies at the apex of urinary bladder.

❑ **Urethral crest** is a longitudinal fold on the posterior wall of the prostatic urethra extending from the uvula of the bladder. In both sexes, the superficial trigone muscle becomes continuous with the smooth muscle of the proximal urethra, and extends in the male along the urethral crest as far as the openings of the ejaculatory ducts.

❑ **Uvula vesicae** which is a small eminence at the apex of its trigone, projecting into the orifice of the urethra.

Arterial Supply

❑ Superior and inferior vesical arteries (branches of internal iliac artery), obturator artery, and inferior gluteal artery.

❑ In females, branches of the uterine artery and vaginal artery additionally supply the bladder.

Venous Drainage

❑ Urinary bladder drains into the prostatic (or vesical) plexus of veins which empties into the internal iliac vein.

Nerve supply

Urinary bladder is innervated by the **vesical plexus** which receives the input from the **inferior hypogastric plexus**.

❑ The vesical plexus contains both parasympathetic and sympathetic components.
  ➤ Parasympathetic (for urine evacuation)
    ▪ Preganglionic neuronal cell bodies are located in the intermediolateral cell column of the S2 to S4 spinal cord segments and the axons travel to the vesical plexus as the pelvic splanchnic nerves.
    ▪ Postganglionic neuronal cell bodies are located in the vesical plexus and the bladder wall and axons are distributed to the detrusor muscle of the bladder where they cause contraction of the detrusor muscle and relaxation of the internal urethral sphincter.
  ➤ Sympathetic (for storage of urine)
    ▪ Preganglionic neuronal cell bodies are located in the intermediolateral cell column of **T10-L2 spinal cord segments**.
    ▪ Preganglionic axons pass through the paravertebral ganglia (do not synapse) to become the lesser thoracic splanchnic nerve, least thoracic splanchnic nerve, first lumbar splanchnic nerve, and second lumbar splanchnic nerve and travel to the inferior hypogastric plexus by way of the superior hypogastric plexus.
    ▪ Postganglionic neuronal cell bodies are located in the **inferior hypogastric plexus** and the axons enter the vesical plexus and are distributed to the detrusor muscle of the bladder.
    ▪ They lead to **relaxation** of the **detrusor muscle** and **contraction** of the **internal urethral sphincter** (although some investigators claim their action is strictly on the smooth muscle of blood vessels).

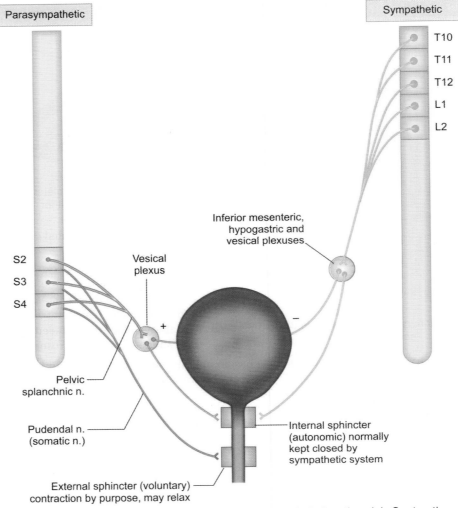

Fig. 38: Motor innervation of the urinary bladder. (+): Contraction, (−): Relaxation, (±): Contraction and relaxation

➢ Sensory innervation: Sensory information from the bladder is carried by both parasympathetic (mainly) and sympathetic fibers.
  ▪ Parasympathetic afferent (sensory) neurons whose cell bodies are located in the dorsal root ganglion run with **the pelvic splanchnic nerves** and relay pain and stretch information from the bladder to S2 to S4 spinal segments within the CNS.
    – The pain associated with bladder pathology may be referred over the S2 to S4 dermatomes (i.e. perineum and posterior thigh).
    – The stretch information associated with bladder fullness from stretch receptors in the bladder wall runs with the pelvic splanchnic nerves and serves as the afferent limb in the micturition reflex.
  ▪ Sympathetic afferent (sensory) neurons whose cell bodies are located in the dorsal root ganglion run with the lesser thoracic splanchnic nerve, least thoracic splanchnic nerve, first lumbar splanchnic nerve, and second lumbar splanchnic nerve, and relay pain information from the bladder to the T10-L2 spinal cord segments with the CNS.
    – The pain associated with bladder pathology may be referred over the T10-L2 dermatomes (i.e. lumbar region, inguinal region, and anterosuperior thigh).
  Micturition (Urination) is the release of urine from the urinary bladder through the urethra to the exterior.
❑ It is initiated by stimulating **stretch receptors** in the detrusor muscle in the bladder wall due to increasing volume (approximately 300 mL for adults) of urine.
❑ It is assisted by contraction of the abdominal muscles which increases the intra-abdominal and pelvic pressures.
❑ It involves the following processes:
  ➢ The **sympathetic** nervous system (general visceral efferent) works for **storage** of urine in urinary bladder.
  ➢ It relaxes the detrusor muscle and constrict the internal sphincter, inhibiting emptying.
  ➢ General visceral afferent impulses arise from stretch receptors in the bladder wall and enter the spinal cord (S2–S4) via the nervi erigentes.

➢ **Parasympathetic** preganglionic (GVE) fibers help in urine **evacuation** by contraction of the detrusor muscle and relaxation of the internal urethral sphincter. It is brought about by nervi erigentes which synapse in the pelvic (inferior hypogastric) plexus.

➢ General somatic efferent fibers in the pudendal nerve can contract the external urethral sphincter (skeletal muscle) to hold the urine at our own will.

➢ At the end of micturition, the external urethral sphincter contracts, and bulbospongiosus muscles in the male expel the last few drops of urine from the urethra.

QUESTIONS

1. TRUE about ureter's entry into bladder *(PGIC 2009)*
   a. At medial angle of trigone
   b. At lateral angle of trigone
   c. Make an angle
   d. Is straight
   e. Valveless

2. All are true about the trigone of the urinary bladder EXCEPT: *(AIIMS 2006)*
   a. Mucosa is loosely associated to the underlying musculature
   b. Mucosa is smooth
   c. It is lined by transitional epithelium
   d. It is derived from the absorbed part of the mesonephric duct

3. FALSE regarding trigone of bladder *(NEET Pattern 2015)*
   a. Lined by transitional epithelium
   b. Mucosa smooth and firmly adherent
   c. Internal urethral orifice lies at lateral angle of base
   d. Developed from mesonephric duct

4. All are true about urinary bladder EXCEPT: *(NEET Pattern 2016)*
   a. Trigone is lined by transitional epithelium
   b. Trigone mucosa is thrown into rugae
   c. There is no submucosal coat in trigone
   d. All are true

5. Urethral crest is due to *(AIIMS 2013)*
   a. Opening of prostatic glands
   b. Puboprostatic spread
   c. Insertion of detrusor
   d. Insertion of trigone

6. Where is the cave of Retzius present *(NEET Pattern 2012)*
   a. Between urinary bladder and rectum
   b. Between urinary bladder and cervix
   c. In front of the bladder
   d. Between the cervix and the rectum

7. All are related to posterior surface of urinary bladder EXCEPT *(JIPMER 2001)*
   a. Ureter
   b. Rectum through rectovesical pouch
   c. Seminal vesicles
   d. Vas deferens

8. In bladder injury pain is referred to all EXCEPT *(NEET Pattern 2012)*
   a. Upper part of thigh
   b. Lower abdominal wall
   c. Flank
   d. Penis

9. If a missile enters the body just above the pubic ramus through the anterior abdominal wall it will most likely pierce which of the following structures *(AIIMS 2000)*
   a. Abdominal aorta   b. Left renal vein
   c. Urinary bladder   d. Spinal cord

10. Nerve supply to musculature of urinary bladder is *(NEET Pattern 2015)*
   a. Sympathetic   b. Parasympathetic
   c. Both   d. None

11. TRUE about nerve supply of urinary bladder *(NEET Pattern 2016)*
   a. Sympathetic supply is via pelvic splanchnic nerves   b. Parasympathetic segmental supply is T11- L2
   c. Micturition reflex is mediated by pelvic splanchnic nerve d. All are correct

ANSWERS

1. b. At lateral angle of trigone; c. Make an angle; e. Valveless
   ❑ Ureter enters the urinary bladder at the lateral angle has an oblique course through it and is valveless.
   ❑ The intramural portion of the ureter functions as a check valve (ureterovesical valve of Sampson) to prevent urine reflux.

2. a. Mucosa is loosely associated to the underlying musculature
   ❑ Mucosa is tightly adherent to the underlying musculature in the trigone of urinary bladder.
   ❑ The mucosa appears smooth at the trigone because of this tight adherence, since folding is not possible in the mucosa.
   ❑ In other places the mucosa is highly folded in storage (may stretched in distension).
   ❑ Trigone of bladder is derived by the absorption of the mesonephric duct into the bladder wall.
   ❑ Transitional epithelium lines the urinary bladder throughout its extent including the trigone.

3. c. Internal urethral orifice lies at lateral angle of base
   ❑ Internal urethral orifice lies at the apex (no the lateral angle of base) of urinary bladder.
   ❑ It's the ureters that open at lateral angles.

4. b. Trigone mucosa is thrown into ruga
   ❑ At the trigone of urinary bladder, the mucous membrane is firmly bound to the muscular coat (no submucosa) and therefore, is smooth (no rugae).

5. d. Insertion of trigone
   ❑ Urethral crest is a longitudinal fold on the posterior wall of the urethra extending from the uvula of the bladder.
   ❑ In both sexes, the superficial trigone muscle becomes continuous with the smooth muscle of the proximal urethra, and extends in the male along the urethral crest as far as the openings of the ejaculatory ducts.

6. c. In front of the bladder
   ❑ Cave of Retzius (retropubic space) is the extraperitoneal space between the pubic symphysis and urinary bladder.
   ❑ It is basically a preperitoneal space behind the transversalis fascia and in front of peritoneum.

7. **a. Ureter**
   - ❏ Ureters join the superolateral angles of urinary bladder (not related to the posterior surface).
   - ❏ Relations of posterior surface of urinary bladder:
     - ■ Upper part is separated from rectum by the rectovesical pouch containing coils of the small intestine.
     - ■ Lower part is separated from rectum by the terminal parts of vas deferens and seminal vesicles.
     - ■ The triangular area between the vas deferens is separated from the rectum by rectovesical fascia (of Denonvillier).

8. **c. Flank**
   - ❏ This is a wrong question with no appropriate answer. The best possible option is flank region, as little is known about the functional significance of thoracolumbar afferents.
   - ❏ Pain fibers of urinary bladder are carried by both sympathetic and parasympathetic fibers.
   - ❏ Parasympathetic fibers (nervi erigentes) are derived from S2, S3, S4 segments of the spinal cord and the referred pain is felt in the corresponding dermatomes in perineum and posterior thigh.
   - ❏ Sympathetic fibers are derived from T11, 12 and L1, 2 segments of the spinal cord and the pain is referred to the lumbar region, inguinal region, and anterosuperior thigh.s

9. **c. Urinary bladder**
   - ❏ A distended urinary bladder may be ruptured by the injuries of lower abdominal wall as mentioned in the question.
   - ❏ Spinal cord terminates at L1 vertebral level; left renal vein is given at L1-2 level and abdominal aorta bifurcates at L4. None of the mentioned structures reach the level of pubic ramus.

10. **c. Both**
    - ❏ Sympathetic nervous system (T12 ± 2) leads to storage of urine by relaxing the detrusor muscle and contracting the internal urethral sphincter.
    - ❏ Parasympathetic nervous system works for evacuation of urine (S2,3,4) by stimulating contraction of detrusor and relaxing the internal urethral sphincter.

11. **c. Micturition reflex is mediated by pelvic splanchnic nerve**
    - ❏ Parasympathetic nervous system works for evacuation of urine acting through pelvic splanchnic nerves (S2,3,4) which stimulate contraction of detrusor and relax the internal urethral sphincter.
    - ❏ Sympathetic nervous system (T12 ± 2) leads to storage of urine by relaxing the detrusor muscle and contracting the internal urethral sphincter.

▶ Urethra

Male urethra serves as a passage for urine (and semen) to the exterior and has a **length of about 20 cm.**

- ❏ It begins at the internal urethral orifice of the bladder where the detrusor muscle extends longitudinally into the prostatic urethra and forms a complete collar around the neck of the bladder called the **internal urethral sphincter.**
- ❏ Male urethra consists of three parts: prostatic, membranous, and spongy **Prostatic** urethra courses through and is surrounded by the prostate gland.
- ❏ **Membranous** urethra courses through the urogenital diaphragm (deep perineal pouch) where it becomes related to the deep transverse perineal muscle and sphincter urethra muscle (external urethral sphincter), both of which are skeletal muscles innervated by the pudendal nerve.

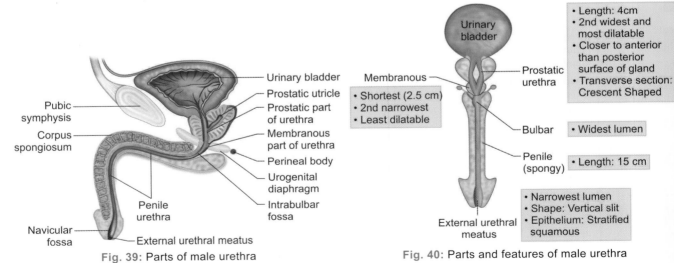

Fig. 39: Parts of male urethra   Fig. 40: Parts and features of male urethra

- ❏ **Spongy** urethra has two parts; Bulbous and penile.
- ❏ **Bulbous spongy urethra** courses through the bulb of the penis and develops endodermal outgrowths into the surrounding mesoderm to form the bulbourethral glands of Cowper.

Note: The glands are present in males in relation with membranous urethra (in the deep perineal pouch), whereas the duct opens into the bulbous spongy urethra (in superficial perineal pouch).

❏ **Penile spongy** (cavernous) urethra courses through and is surrounded by the **corpus spongiosum**. Distal part of the penile urethra courses through the glans penis and terminates as the navicular fossa at the external urethral orifice.

❏ **Prostatic urethra** and the membranous urethra together are considered as the **posterior urethra** and bulbous urethra plus the penile urethra are called the **anterior urethra**.

❏ The **narrowest** lumen is present at the external urethral meatus and the **second narrowest** is in the membranous urethra.

❏ The **widest** lumen is present in the bulbous part of penile urethra, **second widest** is the prostatic urethra.

Table 11: Parts of Male urethra

Part	Length	Location/Disposition	Features
Intramural (preprostatic) part	0.5–1.5 cm	Extends almost vertically through the neck of bladder	Surrounded by internal urethral sphincter: Diameter and length vary depending on whether bladder is filling or emptying
Prostatic urethra	3.0–4.0 cm	Descends through anterior prostate, forming a gentle, anteriorly concave curve; is bounded anteriorly by a vertical trough-like part (rhabdosphincter) of external urethral sphincter	Widest and most dilatable part; features urethral crest with seminal colliculus, flanked by prostatic sinuses into which prostatic ducts open; ejaculatory ducts open onto colliculus, hence urinary and reproductive tracts merge in this part
Intermediate (membranous) part	1.0–1.5 cm	Passes through deep perineal pouch, surrounded by circular fibers of external urethral sphincter; penetrates perineal membrane	Narrowest and least distensible part (except for external urethral orifice)
Spongy urethra	~15 cm	Courses through corpus spongiosum; initial widening occurs in the blub of penis; widens again distally as navicular fossa (in glans penis)	Longest and most mobile part; bulbourethral glands open into bulbous part; distally, urethral glands open into small urethral lacuna entering lumen of this part

Note: Prostatic urethra is considered as the widest and most dilatable part though recent literature mentions that bulbous part of spongy urethra has the widest lumen.

Table 12: Urethra (Lymphatics)

Region	Lymph nodes
Posterior urethra	Internal iliac, external iliac (few)
Membranous urethra	Internal iliac
Anterior urethra (with glans penis)	Deep inguinal, superficial inguinal (few), external iliac

Table 13: Urethra (Epithelium)

Region	Epithelium
Proximal part of prostatic urethra	Transitional (urothelium)
Distal part of prostatic urethra, membranous urethra, major part of penile urethra	Pseudostratified or stratified columnar
Distal penile urethra	Stratified squamous

❏ Female urethra is approximately **4 cm long** begins at the internal urethral orifice of the bladder where the detrusor muscle extends longitudinally into the urethra but does **not** form a significant **internal urethral sphincter**.

➤ It courses through the **urogenital diaphragm** (deep perineal pouch) where it becomes related to the deep transverse perineal muscle and sphincter urethra muscle.

➤ Posterior surface of the female urethra fuses with the anterior wall of the vagina such that the external urethral sphincter does not completely surround the female urethra.

➤ Female urethra drains into both the internal and external iliac lymph nodes.

Urethra Sphincter System

Urethra has two sphincter muscles: external urethral sphincter and internal urethral sphincter.

External urethral sphincter muscle is derived from **sphincter urethra** of urethra which surrounds the whole length of the membranous portion of the urethra and is enclosed in the fascia of the urogenital diaphragm.

❏ Its external fibers arise from the junction of the inferior rami of the pubis and ischium and from the neighboring fascia.

❏ They arch across the front of the urethra and bulbourethral glands, pass around the urethra, and behind it unite with the muscle of the opposite side by means of a tendinous raphe. It is also inserted into the perineal body.

❏ Its innermost fibers form a continuous circular investment for the membranous urethra.

❏ It is **innervated by somatic fibers (S2,3,4).**

❏ **Male** external urethral sphincter is formed by two muscles: sphincter urethra and compressor urethra muscles both in the deep perineal space.

❑ **Female** external urethral sphincter is formed by three muscles: sphincter urethra, compressor urethrae and urethrovaginalis muscles.

➢ **Urethro-vaginalis sphincter** is attached to the anterolateral wall of the vagina that compresses both the urethra and vagina.

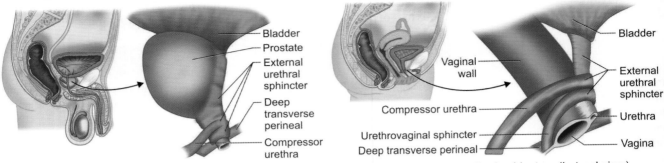

Male external urethral sphincters (Lateral view)   Female external urethral sphincters (Lateral view)

Fig. 41: Superior external urethral sphincter ascends to the neck of the bladder. Inferior sphincter includes cylindrical and loop-like portions (compressor urethra)

Internal urethral sphincter

❑ Male:
➢ It is the (pre-prostatic) sphincter at the junction of the urethra with the urinary bladder, surrounding the internal urethral orifice and constricts it.
➢ It is derived from the bladder musculature of trigonal region.
➢ It is a **smooth** muscle, kept tonically contracted by lumbar plexus of the sympathetic nervous system.
➢ During urination it is relaxed via branches from the inferior hypogastric plexus (S2-S4) parasympathetic nervous system.
➢ It is the primary muscle for maintenance of **continence of urine**.
➢ During ejaculation, it contracts to **prevent reflux of semen** into the urinary bladder (retrograde ejaculation). It is innervated by the L1 sympathetic fibers. L1 fibers should not be cut while performing lumbar sympathectomy otherwise, would result in **retrograde ejaculation** of semen.

❑ Female:
➢ Unlike male anatomy, in which the bladder neck and prostate comprise the internal urinary sphincter, the internal sphincter in females is **functional rather than anatomic**.
➢ The bladder neck and proximal urethra constitute the female internal sphincter.
➢ Urinary continence in females is maintained by the following muscles: Sphincter urethra, Compressor urethra, sphincter urethrovaginalis, pubourethralis (part of Levator ani muscle).

---

1. Prostatic urethra is characterized by all of the following features EXCEPT: *(AIPG)*
   a. Is the widest and most dilatable part
   b. Presents a concavity posteriorly
   c. Lies closer to anterior surface of prostate
   d. Receives prostatic ductules along its posterior wall

2. NOT true about prostatic urethra: *(AIIMS 2009,10)*
   a. Trapezoid shape in cross section
   b. Presence of verumontanum
   c. Opening of prostatic ducts
   d. Urethral crest on posterior wall

3. Bulbourethral glands open into which part of the urethra *(NEET Pattern 2012)*
   a. Membranous   b. Spongy
   c. Prostatic   d. Intramural

4. WRONG statement about male urethra is
   a. Length of male urethra is 20 cm
   b. Membranous urethra has shortest length
   c. Narrowest lumen is at the external urethral meatus
   d. Prostatic urethra has the widest lumen

5. Which of the following combination is/are TRUE regarding epithelial fining of urinary system: *(PGIC 2015)*
   a. Urinary bladder: Transitional
   b. Pre-prostatic urethra: Stratified columnar
   c. Membranous urethra: Transitional epithelium
   d. Distal part of penile urethra: Non-keratinized stratified squamous epithelium
   e. Urethral meatus: Keratinized stratified squamous epithelium

6. Distal part of spongy male urethra drains via which lymph nodes: *(AIPG 2009)*
   a. Superficial inguinal
   b. External Iliac
   c. Deep inguinal
   d. Aortic

7. All of the following statements are true about sphincter urethra EXCEPT: *(AIIMS 2014)*
   a. Located at the bladder neck
   b. Originate from ischiopubic ramus
   c. Is a voluntary muscle
   d. Supplied by pudendal nerve

8. Vaginal sphincter is formed by all EXCEPT: *(AIIMS 2009, 10)*
   a. Internal urethral sphincter
   b. External urethral sphincter
   c. Pubovaginalis
   d. Bulbospongiosus

1. b. Presents a concavity posteriorly

- ❏ Prostatic urethra presents an anterior (and not posterior) concavity which becomes more prominent in the membranous part. It runs downwards and forward to exit prostate slightly anterior to its apex.
- ❏ Prostatic urethra passes more anteriorly through the prostate and is at the junction of anterior 1/3 and posterior 2/3 rd of prostate. Hence, it lies closer to the anterior surface of the prostate. It receives multiple openings of prostatic ductules at its posterior wall.

2. a. Trapezoid shape in cross section

- ❏ Transverse section of prostate shows crescent (semilunar) shaped lumen of urethra (and not trapezoid).
- ❏ Verumontanum (seminal colliculus) is a rounded elevation on the posterior wall of prostatic urethra showing three openings.
- ❏ Prostatic urethra has a midline elevation on the posterior wall of prostatic urethra called urethral crest.
- ❏ There are multiple openings found on the sides of urethral crest for the glandular secretions of prostate.

3. b. Spongy

- ❏ Bulbourethral glands are present in males in relation with membranous urethra (in the deep perineal pouch), whereas the duct opens into the bulbous spongy urethra (in superficial perineal pouch).

4. d. Prostatic urethra has the widest lumen

- ❏ Male urethra has a total length of 20 cm and is divided mainly into 4 parts.
- ❏ Membranous urethra has the shortest length - 1.5 cm.
- ❏ The narrowest lumen is present at the external urethral meatus and the second narrowest is in the membranous urethra.
- ❏ The widest lumen is present in the bulbous part of penile urethra, second widest is the prostatic urethra.

5. a. Urinary bladder: Transitional; d. Distal part of penile urethra: Non-keratinized stratified squamous epithelium;

- ❏ e) Urethral meatus: Keratinized stratified squamous epithelium
- ❏ Urothelium (transitional epithelium) extends from the ends of the collecting ducts through the ureters and bladder to the pre-prostatic urethra and the proximal portion of the prostatic urethra (as far as the ejaculatory ducts). In females, it extends as far as the urogenital membrane.
- ❏ The epithelium changes below the openings of the ejaculatory ducts to a pseudostratified or stratified columnar type which lines the membranous urethra and the major part of the penile urethra. Towards the distal end of the penile urethra, the epithelium changes to stratified squamous, also lines the navicular fossa and becomes keratinized at the external meatus.

6. c. Deep inguinal

- ❏ Distal spongy urethra and the glans penis drain into the deep inguinal lymph nodes of Cloquet or Rosenmuller.

7. a. Located at the bladder neck

- ❏ Sphincter urethra (external urethral sphincter) is a content of deep perineal pouch (not the bladder neck).
- ❏ It is a skeletal (voluntary) muscle supplied by somatic pudendal nerve (S2,3,4) and works for urinary continence.
- ❏ It takes its origin from the ischiopubic ramus on each side and unite with the muscle of the opposite side by means of a tendinous raphe.
- ❏ Internal urethral sphincter (sphincter vesicae) is located at the bladder neck is a smooth (involuntary) muscle engaged in preventing retrograde ejaculation of semen supplied by L1 sympathetic fibers.

8. a. Internal urethral sphincter

- ❏ Internal urethral sphincter does not function as vaginal sphincter. The internal sphincter in females is functional rather than anatomic.
- ❏ Muscles that compress the vagina and act as sphincters include the pubovaginalis, external urethral sphincter (especially its urethrovaginal sphincter part), and bulbospongiosus.
- ❏ The external urethral sphincter surrounds the vagina also and works as urethro-vaginal sphincter. It is innervated by the nerve fibers of Onuf's nucleus (S2, 3, 4) via the pudendal nerve.
- ❏ Pubovaginalis is a part of pubococcygeus (Levator ani) and functions as genital tract sphincter. Levator ani muscle forms the pelvic diaphragm.
- ❏ Bulbospongiosus is a muscle of superficial perineal pouch and is a constrictor of genital tract.

▶ Extravasation of Urine

- ❏ Attachments of Scarpa's- and Colles' fascia are such that they prevent the passage of extravasated urine due to urethral rupture backward into the ischiorectal fossa and downward into the thighs.
- ❏ The line of fusion of Scarpa's fascia passes over Holden's line, body of pubis, margins of pubic arch, and posterior border of the perineal membrane/ posterior edge of the urogenital diaphragm.

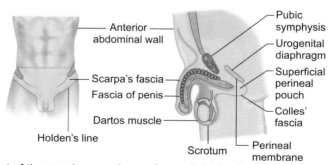

Fig. 42: Extent of the membranous layer of superficial fascia of the abdomen (Scarpa's fascia): Anterior view and Sagittal section. Rupture urethra in the perineum, lets the extravasated urine collects first in the superficial pouch and then on to the anterior abdominal wall inferior to the umbilicus in the superficial inguinal space

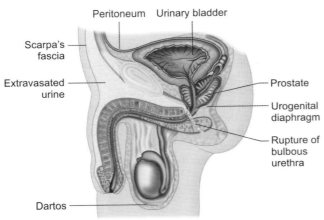

Fig. 43: Rupture of the bulbous urethra above the urogenital diaphragm leading extravasation

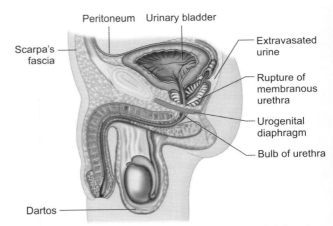

Fig. 44: Rupture of the urethra leading to superficial to deep extravasation

- ❑ In a case of **fundal rupture of urinary bladder** (as may occur in bomb explosions), the peritoneum covering the fundus is also ruptured leading to extravasation of urine into the peritoneal cavity (**ascites**).
- ❑ Pelvic fractures may result in pulling of pubo-prostatic ligaments and rupture of the **membranous part of the urethra**. In this case urine escapes into the deep perineal pouch and can extravasate upward into the peri-vesical space (around the prostate and bladder) or downward into the superficial perineal space (if there is associated rupture of perineal membrane).
- ❑ In a case of straddle injury, there is rupture of the **bulbous portion of the spongy urethra** below the urogenital diaphragm and the extravasated urine may pass into the **superficial perineal space** and spread inferiorly into the **scrotum**, anteriorly around the **penis**, and superiorly into the lower part of the **abdominal wall**.
- ❑ The urine cannot spread laterally into the thigh because the inferior fascia of the urogenital diaphragm (the perineal membrane) and the superficial fascia of the perineum are firmly attached to the ischiopubic rami and are connected with the deep fascia of the thigh (fascia lata).
- ❑ It cannot spread posteriorly into the anal region (ischiorectal fossa) because the perineal membrane and **Colles' fascia** are continuous with each other around the superficial transverse perineal muscles.
- ❑ It cannot enter the deep perineal pouch because **perineal membrane** prevents that.
- ❑ **Penile fracture:** Diagnosis of albugineal rupture is usually made from a characteristic history of severe pain with a cracking or popping sound during acute bending of the erect penis followed by immediate detumescence, penile swelling, and deformity.
- ❑ **Albugineal rupture** is associated with urethral injury in 10–20% of cases.
- ❑ **Penile hematoma is confined to the shaft when the Buck's fascia is intact**.
- ❑ If the Buck fascia has been violated, the swelling and ecchymosis are contained within the Colles' fascia. In this instance, a 'butterfly-pattern' ecchymosis may be observed over the perineum, scrotum, and lower abdominal wall.

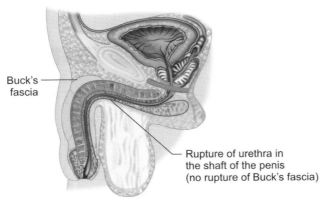

Fig. 45: Extravasation of urine: Urine is confined to penile shaft (if Buck's fascia is intact)

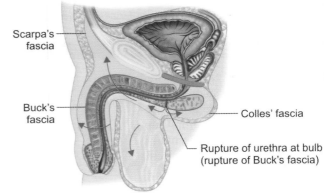

Fig. 46: Urine extravasation is into the penile and scrotal layers and along the anterior abdominal wall (if Buck's fascia is ruptured)

QUESTIONS

1. **Scarpa's fascia gets attached to** *(JIPMER 2010)*
   a. Inguinal ligament
   b. Fascia lata of thigh
   c. Conjoint tendon
   d. Pubic crest

2. **In bulbous urethra, extravasated urine from this injury can spread into which of the following structures**
   a. Scrotum
   b. Ischiorectal fossa
   c. Deep perineal space
   d. Thigh

3. **Injury to the male urethra above the perineal membrane due to a pelvic fracture causes urine to accumulate in all of the following EXCEPT**
   a. Space of Retzius   b. Deep perineal pouch
   c. Superficial perineal pouch   d. Peritoneal cavity

4. **Injury to the male urethra below the perineal membrane causes urine to accumulate in**   *(AIPG 2007)*
   a. Superficial perineal pouch   b. Deep perineal pouch
   c. Space of Retzius   d. Pouch of Douglas

5. **A patient exposed to bomb explosion injury presents with rupture of the fundus of urinary bladder. The extravasated urine reaches**
   a. Space of Retzius
   b. Deep perineal pouch
   c. Superficial perineal pouch
   d. Peritoneal cavity

6. **After fracture of the penis (injury to the tunica albuginea with intact Buck's fascia, there occurs hematoma**
   a. The penis and scrotum
   b. At the perineum in a butterfly shape
   c. Penis, scrotum, perineum and lower part of anterior abdominal wall
   d. Shaft of the penis only

1. **b. Fascia lata of thigh**
   ❑ Scarpa's fascia is the deep membranous layer of superficial fascia of anterior abdominal wall.
   ❑ It crosses the inguinal ligament and gets attached to the fascia lata of thigh along Holden's line below and parallel to inguinal ligament.

2. **a. Scrotum**
   ❑ Extravasation of urine may result from the rupture of the bulbous spongy urethra below the perineal membrane; the urine may pass into the superficial perineal pouch and spread inferiorly into the scrotum, anteriorly around the penis, and superiorly into the lower part of the abdominal wall.
   ❑ The urine cannot spread laterally into the thigh because the perineal membrane and the superficial fascia of the perineum are firmly attached to the ischiopubic rami and are connected with the deep fascia of the thigh (fascia lata).
   ❑ It cannot spread posteriorly into the anal region (ischiorectal fossa) because the perineal membrane and Colless' fascia are continuous with each other around the superficial transverse perineal muscles.

3. **d. Peritoneal cavity > c. Superficial perineal pouch**
   ❑ Rupture of membranous part of the urethra may lead to urine escaping into the space around the prostate and bladder and extraperitoneal space (but not the peritoneal cavity).
   ❑ If the urogenital diaphragm is also disrupted urine leaks into the deep perineal space and into the superficial perineal space (as the perineal membrane is also ruptured).
   ❑ The most common type of urethral injury is at the junction of posterior and anterior (bulbous) urethra. Radiologists consider a type III urethral injury as a combined anterior/posterior urethral injury.

4. **a. Superficial perineal pouch**
   ❑ Superficial perineal pouch lies below the perineal membrane and has the spongy part of urethra lying in it. Any injury to the spongy urethra like the bulbous rupture of urethra leads to the extravasation of urine into the superficial perineal pouch.
   ❑ The urine can track from the superficial pouch towards the anterior abdominal wall and reach just anterior to the external oblique aponeurosis.
   ❑ Perineal membrane separates the deep perineal pouch from the superficial and prevents urine from entering the deep perineal pouch from superficial.
   ❑ Space of Retzius is an extraperitoneal space lying between the pubic bones and the urinary bladder.
   ❑ Membranous rupture of urethra (above the perineal membrane) may cause accumulation of blood and urine in this space.
   ❑ Pouch of Douglas is the recto-vesical (or rectouterine) pouch of peritoneum. Douglas pouch is intraperitoneal and also well separated from the superficial pouch. Neither of the two varieties of urethral rupture the urine can reach into this space.

5. **d. Peritoneal cavity**
   ❑ Rupture of the dome (superior wall) of the urinary bladder leads to rupture of peritoneum and results in an intraperitoneal extravasation of urine within the peritoneal cavity (ascites).
   ❑ It is caused by a compressive force on a full bladder.

6. **d. Shaft of the penis only**
   ❑ Penile Fracture - Diagnosis of albugineal rupture is usually made from a characteristic history of severe pain with a cracking or popping sound during acute bending of the erect penis followed by immediate detumescence, penile swelling, and deformity.
   ❑ Albugineal rupture is associated with urethral injury in 10–20% of cases.
   ❑ Penile hematoma is confined to the shaft when the Buck's fascia is intact.
   ❑ If the Buck fascia has been violated, the swelling and ecchymosis are contained within the Colles' fascia. In this instance, a 'butterfly pattern' ecchymosis may be observed over the perineum, scrotum, and lower abdominal wall.

⬛ Rectum

Rectum is the part of the large intestine which lies between the sigmoid colon and the anal canal.

❑ It begins at vertebral level S3 and ends at the tip of the coccyx (i.e., the **anorectal junction**) where the **puborectalis muscle** forms a U-shaped sling causing an 80° **perineal flexure**.
❑ **Ampulla of the rectum** is a dilated portion of the rectum that lies just above the pelvic diaphragm.
❑ Rectum is normally empty of fecal matter.
❑ Unlike the sigmoid colon, rectum has no sacculations, appendices epiploicae or taenia coli.

- ❑ Rectum has three **lateral curvatures**: the upper and lower are convex to the right, and the middle (most prominent) is convex to the left.
- ❑ On the luminal aspect, these three curves are marked by semi-circular folds (Houston's valves).

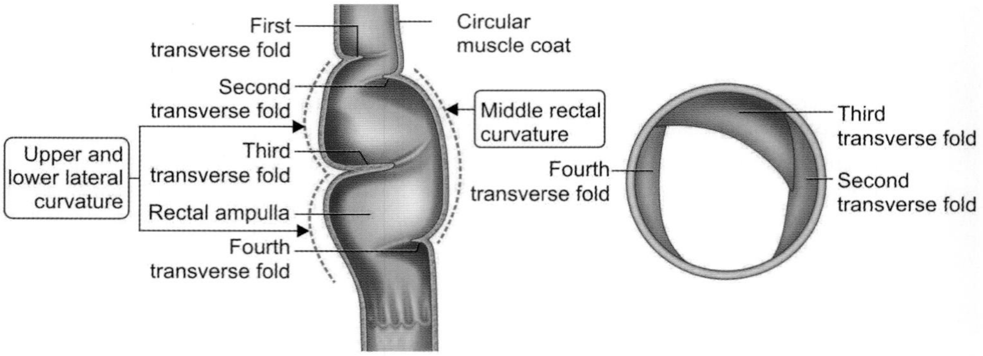

There are two types of **mucosal folds** in rectum: temporary and permanent.

1. When the rectum is empty, the mucosa has several longitudinal folds in its lower part which are temporary and disappear during distension.

2. **Permanent folds**, also called Houston' valves are crescentic (semilunar) **transverse** folds situated against the concavities of the lateral curvatures of the rectum.
   - ➤ They are formed by the mucosa, submucosa and inner circular layer of smooth muscle that permanently extend into the lumen of the rectum to support the fecal mass.
   - ➤ They are **permanent** and become more prominent when the rectum is distended.
   - ➤ They are usually three in number;

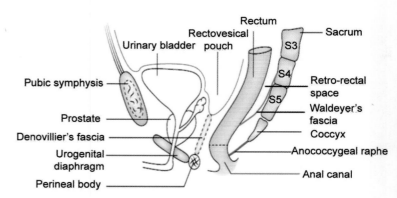

Fig. 47: Rectum in Coronal view and Transverse view

Fig. 48: Fascia related to rectum

sometimes a fourth is found, and occasionally only two are present, and numbered from above downward are as follows:
   - ▪ First fold (or superior fold) is at the commencement of the rectum, distal to the rectosigmoid junction. It projects from the right (or left wall) and may occasionally encircles the rectal lumen (Not mentioned in most of the books).
   - ▪ Second fold projects from the left rectal wall along the concavity of upper lateral curvature. It lies opposite the middle of rectum.
   - ▪ Third fold is the **largest and most constant** lies immediately above the rectal ampulla. It projects from the anterior and right wall just below the level of the anterior peritoneal reflection, along the concavity of middle lateral curvature. It has prominent circular muscle.
   - ▪ Fourth (inferior) fold is the most variable and projects from the left wall of the rectum along the concavity of lower lateral curvature. It lies about 2.5 cm above the anus.
   - ➤ These transverse folds of the rectum (rectal valves) provide support to hold the feces and prevent its urging toward the anus which would produce a strong urge to defecate. They are visible per anum with the aid of a speculum.
- ❑ **Denonvilliers' fascia** is a membranous partition separating the rectum from the prostate and urinary bladder.
   - ➤ This structure in the male corresponds to the fascia rectovaginalis in female.
- ❑ **Waldeyer's fascia** is the presacral fascia present between rectum and sacrum.
   - ➤ It lies in the anterior aspect of the sacrum, enclosing the sacral vessels and nerves.
   - ➤ It lies at the floor of the retro-rectal space.
   - ➤ It continues anteriorly as the pelvic parietal fascia covering the entire pelvic cavity.
- ❑ Lower third of rectum is below the peritoneum which is reflected anteriorly on to the urinary bladder in males to form the **rectovesical pouch**, or on to the posterior vaginal fornix in females to form the **recto-uterine pouch (of Douglas).**
   - ➤ It contains peritoneal fluid and some of the small intestine.
   - ➤ The level of this reflection is higher in males; the rectovesical pouch is approximately 7.5 cm above the anorectal junction in males, while the recto-uterine pouch is approximately 5.5 cm above the anorectal junction in females.
- ❑ **Waldeyer's fascia** is the **presacral fascia** present between rectum and sacrum.
   - ➤ It lies, the anterior aspect of the sacrum, enclosing the sacral vessels and nerves.
   - ➤ It continues anteriorly as the pelvic parietal fascia, covering the entire pelvic cavity.
   - ➤ It is limited posteroinferiorly, as it fuses with the mesorectal fascia lying above the levator ani muscle at the level of the anorectal junction.
   - ➤ It has been mistakenly described as the posterior aspect of the mesorectal fascia. These two fascia are separate entities.
- ❑ During rectal surgery and mesorectum excision, dissection along the **avascular alveolar plane** between these two fascia, facilitates a straightforward dissection and preserves the sacral vessels and hypogastric nerves.

QUESTIONS

1. Pelvic fascia between rectum and sacrum is
(NEET Pattern 2012,15)
- a. Denonvilliers' fascia
- b. Colles' fascia
- c. Waldeyer's fascia
- d. Scarpa's fascia

2. Fascia of Waldeyer belongs to *(JIPMER 2012)*
- a. Fascia of the pelvic wall to anorectal junction
- b. Fascia of the pelvic floor
- c. Fascia of the pelvic viscera
- d. None of the above

3. Anterior relation to the upper part of rectum in male is
(NEET Pattern 2016)
- a. Sacrum
- b. Rectovesical pouch
- c. Seminal vesicle
- d. Ductus deferens

4. Which of the following statements about Valves of Houston is TRUE *(AIPG 2012)*
- a. Middle valve corresponds to the middle convex fold to the right
- b. Upper valve corresponds to peritoneal reflections
- c. Valves contain all three layers of muscle wall
- d. Valves disappear after the mobilization of rectum

ANSWERS

1. c. Waldeyer's fascia
- ❑ Waldeyer's fascia (presacral fascia) lies in the anterior aspect of the sacrum, enclosing the sacral vessels and nerves.
- ❑ It is limited posteroinferiorly, as it fuses with the mesorectal fascia lying above the levator ani muscle.
- ❑ Identification and preservation of the Waldeyer's fascia is of fundamental importance in preventing complications and reducing local recurrences of rectal cancer.
- ❑ Denonvillier's fascia is a membranous partition separating the rectum from the prostate and urinary bladder; this structure in the male corresponds to the fascia rectovaginalis in the female.

2. a. Fascia of the pelvic wall to anorectal junction
- ❑ Presacral fascia of Waldeyer, lies the anterior aspect of the sacrum, enclosing the sacral vessels and nerves. It continues anteriorly as the pelvic parietal fascia covering the entire pelvic cavity and is limited posteroinferiorly, as it fuses with the mesorectal fascia, lying above the levator ani muscle at the level of the anorectal junction.

3. b. Rectovesical pouch
- ❑ Upper two-third of rectum is related to rectovesical pouch and coils of the small intestine and sigmoid colon within it.

4. d. Valves disappear after the mobilization of rectum
- ❑ Valves of Houston are lost after full mobilization of the rectum. The middle valve is located on the right wall but correspond to the middle convex fold to the left. The middle (not upper) valve corresponds to the level of peritoneal reflection. These valves do not contain all three layers of the muscle wall.

▶ Anal Canal

Anal canal is the terminal portion of the large intestine having a length of ~ 4 cm long and extends from the rectum at the anorectal junction to the surface of the body at the anus.

- ❑ It divides into an upper two-third (visceral portion) which belongs to the intestine, and a lower one-third (somatic portion) which belongs to the perineum.
- ❑ A point of demarcation between visceral and somatic portions is called the **pectinate** (dentate) line which is a serrated line following the anal valves.
- ❑ Pectinate line is the water-shed line having different neurovascular bundle above and below it.

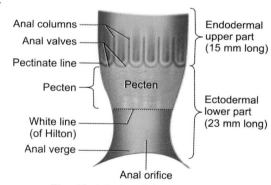

Fig. 49: Interior of the anal canal

Upper Anal Canal

- ❑ Mucosa of the upper anal canal is thrown into longitudinal folds called the **anal columns** (of Morgagni). The base of the anal columns marks the **pectinate line**.
- ❑ At the base of the anal columns are folds of tissue called the **anal valves**. Behind the anal valves are small, blind pouches called the **anal sinuses** into which anal glands open.
- ❑ Upper anal canal is surrounded by the internal anal sphincter which is a continuation of smooth muscle from the rectum with involuntary control via autonomic innervation.
- ❑ It is lined by **simple columnar epithelium**.

Lower Anal Canal

- ❑ It extends from the pectinate line to the anal verge (the point at which perianal skin begins).
- ❑ It is surrounded by external anal sphincter which is a skeletal muscle under voluntary control via the pudendal nerve.
- ❑ It is lined by **stratified squamous epithelium** (non-keratinized) till Hilton's line. Below that it becomes keratinized.
- ❑ **Hilton's white line** is the intermuscular (intersphincteric groove) between the lower border of the internal anal sphincter and the subcutaneous part of the external anal sphincter. It indicates the junction between keratinized stratified squamous epithelium and non-keratinized stratified squamous epithelium.

- ❑ **Anal transition zone** (ATZ) is interposed between uninterrupted colorectal-type mucosa above and uninterrupted squamous epithelium below, irrespective of the type of epithelium present in the zone itself.
  - ➢ It lies above the dentate (pectinate line) and reaches upto 2 cm.
  - ➢ It is composed of 5-9 cells layers. The surface cells can be columnar, cuboidal or somewhat more flattened
- ❑ **Pecten** is the zone in the lower half of the anal canal between the pectinate line and the anal verge.
- ❑ **Anal verge** is the distal end of the anal canal forming a transitional zone between the epithelium of the anal canal and the perianal skin.

Table 14: Comparison between upper and lower anal canal

Features	Upper anal canal	Lower anal canal
Arterial supply	Superior rectal artery (branch of inferior mesenteric artery)	Inferior rectal artery (branch of internal pudendal artery)
Venous drainage	Superior rectal vein → inferior mesenteric vein → hepatic portal system	Inferior rectal vein → internal pudendal vein → internal iliac vein → IVC
Lymphatic drainage	Deep nodes	Superficial inguinal nodes
Innervation	Motor: Autonomic innervation of internal anal sphincter (smooth muscle) Sensory: Stretch sensation; no pain sensation	Motor: Somatic innervation (pudendal nerve) of external anal sphincter (striated muscle sensory: Pain, temperature, touch sensation)
Embryologic derivation	Endoderm (hindgut)	Ectoderm (proctodeum)
Epithelium	Simple columnar	Stratified squamous non-keratinized
Tumors	Palphable enlarged superficial nodes will NOT be found. Patients do NOT complain of pain	Palpable enlarged superficial nodes will be found. Patients do complain of pain
Hemorrhoids	Internal hemorrhoids (varicosities of superior rectal veins) Covered by rectal mucosa. Patients do NOT complain of pain	External hemorrhoids (varicosities of inferior rectal veins). Covered by skin. Patients do complain of pain

- ❑ Transitions occurring at pectinate line:
  - ➢ Vessels and nerves superior to the pectinate line are visceral; those inferior to the pectinate line are parietal or somatic.
  - ➢ This orientation reflects the embryological development of the anorectum.

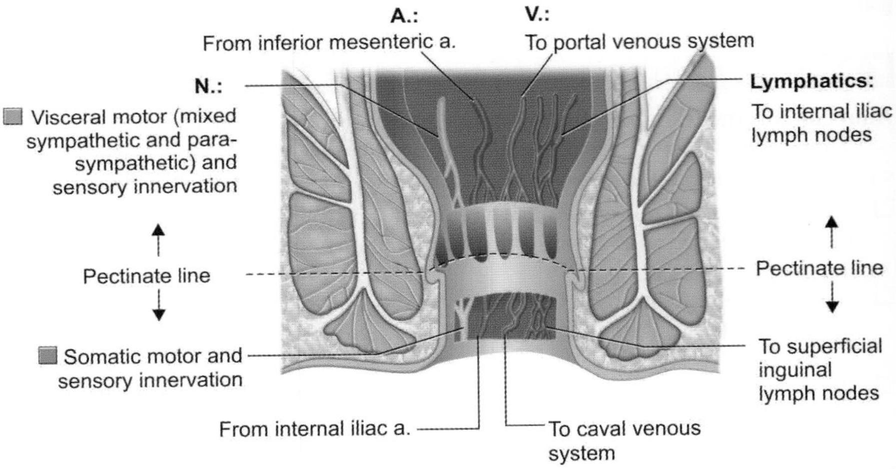

Fig. 50: Separation of 'visceral' and 'parietal' at the pectinate line

Arterial supply

- ❑ Rectum
  - ➢ **Superior rectal artery** (continuation of the inferior mesentery artery) is the chief supply.
  - ➢ **Middle rectal artery** (branch of anterior division of the internal iliac artery).
  - ➢ **Inferior rectal artery** (branch of internal pudendal artery)
  - ➢ **Median sacral artery** (branch of the abdominal aorta)
- ❑ Anal canal
  - ➢ It is supplied by terminal branches of the **superior rectal artery** and the **inferior rectal artery** together with a small contribution from the **median sacral artery**.
  - ➢ Middle rectal artery does not supply the anal canal.

Venous drainage

- ❑ Venous drainage of the rectum and anal canal parallels the arterial supply.
- ❑ Upper portions are drained predominantly by the **superior rectal veins**, tributaries portal mesenteric venous system; some blood returns to the systemic circulation via the **middle rectal veins**.
  - ➢ **Superior rectal vein** → inferior mesenteric vein → portal vein → hepatic sinusoids → central veins → hepatic veins → inferior vena cava
  - ➢ **Middle rectal vein** → internal iliac vein → common iliac vein → inferior vena cava

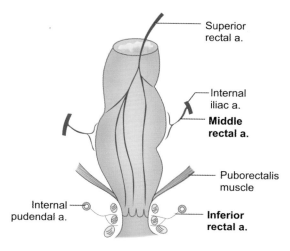

Fig. 51: Arterial supply of rectum and anal canal

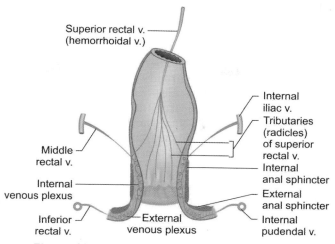

Fig. 52: Venous drainage of rectum and anal canal

❑ Lower portions drain via the **inferior rectal** branches of the internal pudendal vein into systemic circulation.
  ➢ **Inferior rectal vein** → internal pudendal vein → internal iliac vein → common iliac vein → inferior vena cava

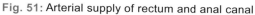

Note: Portosystemic anastomosis: Superior rectal vein (tributary of **portal vein**) forms anastomosis with middle and inferior rectal veins (tributaries of **inferior vena cava**).

❑ Rectum
  ➢ Upper half lymphatics accompany the superior rectal vessels and drain into the **inferior mesenteric nodes**. Few of these vessels drain into the pararectal lymph nodes (on each side of the rectosigmoid junction).
  ➢ Lower half lymphatics accompany the middle rectal vessels and drain into the **internal iliac nodes**.
❑ **Anal canal** Pectinate line forms the 'water shed line' of the anal canal
  ➢ **Upper** half lymphatics drain into the **internal iliac lymph nodes**
  ➢ **Lower** half lymphatics drain into the **superficial inguinal** lymph nodes (horizontal group).

Nerve Supply

❑ Rectum
  ➢ Lumbar splanchnic nerves are the sympathetic component derived from L1, L2 segments of the spinal cord.
  ➢ Nervi erigentes are the parasympathetic nerves from S2, S3, S4 segments of the spinal cord.
❑ Anal canal
  ➢ **Upper** anal canal is supplied by autonomic nervous system (parasympathetic and sympathetic nerves)
    ▪ Internal anal sphincter is a smooth muscle under involuntary control
    ▪ Sensations are limited to stretch and ischemia .
  ➢ **Lower** anal canal is supplied by the somatic pudendal nerve.
    ▪ External anal sphincter is a skeletal muscle under voluntary control
    ▪ It is sensitive to somatic sensations like touch, pain, temperature, etc.
  Anorectal ring (or flexure) is the demarcation between the rectum and the anal canal where the puborectalis muscle forms a sling around the posterior aspect of the anorectal junction kinking it anteriorly.
❑ It is **formed by fusion** of fibers of:
  ➢ Puborectalis
  ➢ Uppermost fibers of external anal sphincter
  ➢ Internal anal sphincter.

At rest

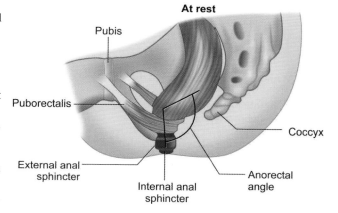

During straining

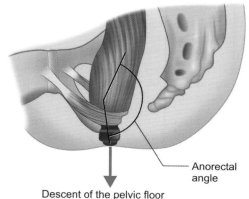

Fig. 53: Anorectal ring and angle

Anorectal Angle

❑ Fecal continence is maintained by normal rectal sensation and tonic contraction of the internal anal sphincter and the puborectalis muscle which wraps around the anorectum maintaining an anorectal angle **between 80° and 110°.**

❑ The angle is 2–3 cm anterior to and slightly below the tip of the coccyx level with the apex of the prostate in males.

Rectal or digital (finger) examination is performed for palpating enlargements, tissue hardening, hemorrhoids, rectal carcinoma, prostate cancer, seminal vesicle, ampulla of the ductus deferens, bladder, uterus, cervix, ovaries, anorectal abscesses, perineal body, etc.

❑ During defecation, the pelvic floor muscles (including the puborectalis) relax, allowing the anorectal angle to straighten by atleast 15°, and the perineum descends by 1-3.5 cm.

❑ Damage to the anorectal ring results in **rectal incontinence**.

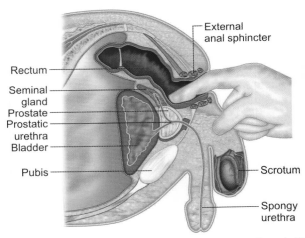

Fig. 54: Rectal digital examination-Medial view (from left)

QUESTIONS

1. **Internal anal sphincter is a part of** *(JIPMER 2012)*
   a. Internal longitudinal fibers of rectum
   b. Internal circular muscle fibers of rectum
   c. Puborectalis muscle
   d. Deep perineal muscles

2. **TRUE statement about anatomy of anal canal** *(PGIC 2010)*
   a. Puborectalis is essential to maintain continence
   b. Internal sphincter is skeletal muscle
   c. Internal sphincter remains in the state of tonic contraction
   d. External sphincter is supplied by gluteal nerve
   e. Pectinate line forms 'water shed line'

3. **TRUE about pectinate line** *(NEET Pattern 2015)*
   a. Part above pectinate line develops from proctodeum
   b. Arterial supply above pectinate line is through superior rectal artery
   c. Lymphatic drainage above pectinate line is through superficial inguinal nodes
   d. Part above pectinate line is supplied by somatic nerves

4. **Anal valves are found in which part of anal canal** *(NEET Pattern 2015)*
   a. Upper
   b. Middle
   c. Lower
   d. Anal verge

5. **Anal canal is NOT supplied by** *(AIIMS 2015)*
   a. Superior rectal artery
   b. Inferior rectal artery
   c. Median sacral artery
   d. Middle rectal artery

6. **All form of anorectal ring EXCEPT** *(AIIMS 2013)*
   a. External anal sphincter
   b. Internal anal sphincter
   c. Puborectalis
   d. Anococcygeal raphe

7. **Anorectal angle is formed due to action of** *(NEET Pattern 2016)*
   a. Internal anal sphincter
   b. Puborectalis
   c. Circular layer of smooth muscles
   d. Longitudinal layer of smooth muscle

8. **True about internal anal sphincter are all EXCEPT** *(NEET Pattern 2016)*
   a. Contributed by puborectalis
   b. Involuntary
   c. Usually remains contracted
   d. Supplied by superior hypogastric plexus

9. **Internal rectal venous plexus drains into** *(NEET Pattern 2016)*
   a. Superior rectal vein
   b. Middle rectal vein
   c. Inferior rectal vein
   d. All the above

10. **The nerve mediating pain of external hemorrhoids** *(AIPG 2002; NEET Pattern 2014)*
   a. Hypogastric nerve
   b. Inferior rectal nerve
   c. Pelvic splanchnic nerve
   d. Sympathetic plexus

ANSWERS

1. **b. Internal circular muscle fibers of rectum**
   ❑ Internal and sphincter is formed by thickened circular muscle coat of the anal canal (which is continuous with rectum) and surrounds the upper two-third of the canal.

2. **a. Puborectalis is essential to maintain continence; c. Internal sphincter remains in the state of tonic contraction; e. Pectinate line forms 'water shed line'**
   ❑ Puborectalis is essential to maintain continence by making a sling to increase anorectal angle.
   ❑ Internal anal sphincter is a smooth muscle under autonomic control and remains in tonically contracted state.
   ❑ External anal sphincter is a skeletal muscle supplied by the somatic nerve- inferior rectal nerve and perineal branch of 4th sacral nerve.

3. **b. Arterial supply above pectinate line is through superior rectal artery**
   ❑ Part below (not above) pectinate line develops from proctodeum drain into superficial inguinal nodes and is supplied by somatic nerves.

4. **a. Upper**
   ❑ Anal valves are crescentic folds of the mucous membrane located in the upper part of the anal canal.

5. **d. Middle rectal artery**
   - ❏ Middle rectal artery supplies the rectum, but 'not' the anal canal.
   - ❏ The anal canal is supplied by terminal branches of the superior rectal artery and the inferior rectal artery branch of the internal pudendal artery together with a small contribution from the median sacral artery.
   - ❏ The arterial supply to the epithelium of the lower anal canal in the midline particularly posteriorly is relatively deficient and is thought to predispose to the occurrence of acute and chronic anal fissures which are most commonly found in the midline especially posteriorly.

6. **d. Anococcygeal raphe**
   - ❏ Anorectal ring is a muscular present at the junction of rectum and anus. It is formed by fusion of fibers of puborectalis, uppermost fibers of external anal sphincter and internal anal sphincter.
   - ❏ Anococcygeal raphe is a fibrous median raphe in the floor of the pelvis which extends between the coccyx and the margin of the anus and is not a component of anorectal ring.
   - ❏ Damage to the anorectal ring results in rectal incontinence.

7. **b. Puborectalis**
   - ❏ Anorectal angle is formed due to action of puborectalis muscle.

8. **a. Contributed by puborectalis**
   - ❏ Internal anal sphincter is an involuntary (smooth muscle) sphincter which remains in the state of contraction usually. It is supplied by sympathetic fibers through superior hypogastric plexus and by parasympathetic fibers from nervi erigentes.

9. **a. Superior rectal vein**
   - ❏ The tributaries of superior rectal vein begin in the anal canal from the internal rectal venous plexus.
   - ❏ The internal venous plexus is present in the submucous coat and surrounds the anal canal above Hilton's line.

10. **b. Inferior rectal nerve**
    - ❏ External hemorrhoids lie below the pectinate line and pain is carried by inferior rectal nerve (branch of pudendal nerve).

- Pelvic organ with **thickest** muscular walls **is uterus.**
- Bulk of semen is formed by the secretion of **seminal vesicles.**
- **Sacred bone** is sacrum and **tail bone** is coccyx.
- Largest branch of the anterior division of the internal iliac artery is **inferior gluteal artery.**
- **Inferior rectal artery** is a branch of internal pudendal artery.
- **Superior rectal vein** drains the upper regions of rectum and anal canal into vein of hindgut - inferior mesenteric vein.
- Most fixed part of the urinary bladder is **neck** of the urinary bladder.
- Uterus and vagina in the male is represented by **Prostatic utricle.**
- Prostate gland in the females is represented by **Paraurethral glands** (of Skene).
- **Least movable** part of the uterus is cervix.
- Most common site of fertilization is **ampulla** of the uterine tube.
- Most important ligaments of the uterus is **transverse cervical ligaments** (of Mackenrodt).
- Most important surgical relation of the uterine artery where it **crosses the ureter** anterosuperiorly (from lateral to medial side) – Water below the bridge.
- Most prominent lateral curvature of the rectum is **middle lateral curvature** (being convex to the left).
- Most important is **Houston valve** is the third transverse rectal fold of the mucous membrane.
- Chief artery of the rectum is **superior rectal artery** and vein is **superior rectal vein.**
- Location of **primary internal piles** in lithotomy position are 3, 7, and 11 o'clock positions

▶ Embryology

❏ Lower limb is first recognizable as a laterally projecting thickening in the body wall opposite somites at **day 28**. The core of mesenchymal cells is derived from both **somatopleuric** (bones and connective tissue) and **paraxial** (muscles) mesenchyme.

❏ Lower limb rotates in utero **medially 90°**, while the upper limb rotates laterally 90°. Thus, the limbs are **180° out of phase** with one another (knee anterior and **big toe medial** versus elbow posterior and thumb lateral).

❏ The **extensor** compartment in lower limb comes **anterior** and the flexor compartment becomes posterior.

❏ The blood supply to the lower limb is derived from the lateral branch of the **fifth lumbar intersegmental artery**, which continues into the limb bud as the axial artery.

❏ The **preaxial** vein becomes the long **saphenous** vein, which drains into the femoral vein at the saphenous opening and **postaxial vein** becomes the short saphenous vein, which passes deep and joins the popliteal vein.

▶ Hip Bone

❏ **Ischial tuberosity** gives attachment to the posterior thigh (hamstring) muscles. The upper area of the tuberosity is subdivided by an **oblique line** into a superolateral part for **semimembranosus** and an inferomedial part for the **long head of biceps femoris** and **semitendinosus**.

❏ The lower area is subdivided by an irregular **vertical ridge** into lateral and medial areas. **Hamstring part of adductor magnus** originates from the inferolateral aspect of the ischial tuberosity. Infero-medial aspect of gluteal tuberosity has no muscle; is covered by **fibrofatty tissue**; has the sciatic bursa of gluteus maximus and supports the body in sitting.

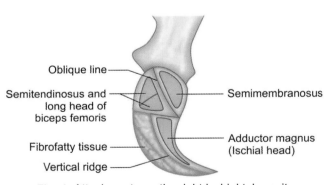

Fig. 1: Attachments on the right ischial tuberosity (posterior aspect)

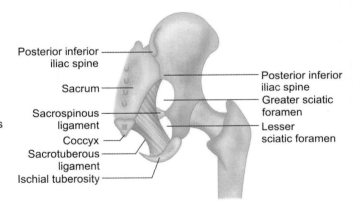

Fig. 2: Sacrotuberous & sacrospinous ligaments and the related greater and lesser sciatic foramina

❏ **Sacrotuberous ligament** (runs from the sacrum to the ischial tuberosity) and **sacrospinous ligaments** (runs from the sacrum to the ischial spine) convert the **greater** and **lesser sciatic notches** of the hip bone into greater and lesser sciatic foramina, the two important exits from the pelvis.

❏ Sacrotuberous ligament **is pierced by** the coccygeal branches of the inferior gluteal artery, the perforating cutaneous nerve (S2,3) and filaments of the coccygeal plexus (formed by S4,5 & **coccygeal nerve**).

❏ Sacrospinous ligament is regarded as a degenerate part of **coccygeus** muscle.

QUESTIONS

1. The ischial tuberosity provides attachment to:
(NEET Pattern 2015)

a. Obturator internus
b. Quadratus femoris
c. Gluteus maximum
d. Adductor magnus

2. TRUE about attachment at ischial tuberosity
(NEET Pattern 2015)

a. Origin of semitendinosus from superolateral area
b. Origin of semimembranosus from superolateral area
c. Origin of long head of biceps from inferolateral area
d. Origin of adductor magnus from inferomedial area

ANSWERS

1. d. Adductor magnus
Posterior (hamstring) part of adductor magnus takes origin from the ischial tuberosity.

2. b. Origin of semimembranosus from superolateral area
Semimembranosus arises by a long, flat tendon from a superolateral impression on the ischial tuberosity.

❏ Greater sciatic foramen: **Piriformis** muscle pass through it, above which the **superior gluteal** vessels and nerve leave the pelvis.

❏ Below piriformis, the inferior gluteal vessels and nerve, **sciatic nerve** and posterior femoral cutaneous nerves, nerve to quadratus femoris and **PIN structures** (Pudendal nerve, Internal pudendal vessels and Nerve to obturator internus) leave the pelvis.

❏ The tendon (**not muscle**) of obturator internus passes through the lesser sciatic notch.

❏ Injury **to superior gluteal nerve**, which passes superior to piriformis and winds around greater sciatic notch, paralyzes **gluteus medius** muscle *(NEET Pattern 2012)*

  ➤ **PIN** (Pudendal nerve, Internal pudendal vessels and Nerve to obturator internus) structures come from pelvic cavity, pass through the **greater sciatic notch**, hook behind the ischial spine (in gluteal region) and move into the **lesser sciatic notch**.

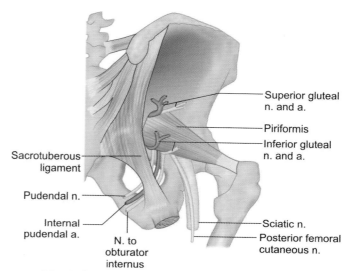

Fig. 3: Structures passing through the greater and lesser sciatic foramina

❏ All the structures enter the gluteal region through greater sciatic foramen except **tendon of obturator internus** which enters the gluteal region through lesser sciatic foramen.

❏ Both superior and inferior gluteal nerves pass through greater sciatic foramen.

QUESTIONS

1. All the following structures pass through lesser sciatic foramen EXCEPT: *(NEET Pattern 2013)*
a. Pudendal nerve
b. Obturator internus muscle
c. Internal pudendal vessels
d. Nerve to obturator internus

2. Structure passing through both greater and lesser sciatic foramen are all EXCEPT: *(NEET Pattern 2015)*
a. Pudendal nerve
b. Internal pudendal vein
c. Nerve to obturator internus
d. Tendon of obturator internus

3. Sacrotuberous ligament is pierced by: *(NEET Pattern 2015)*
a. S1 Nerve
b. L5 Nerve
c. Coccygeal nerve
d. None

4. Structures passing through obturator foramen are all EXCEPT: *(NEET Pattern 2016)*
a. Internal pudendal vessels
b. Obturator nerve
c. Obturator artery
d. Obturator vein

ANSWERS

1. b. Obturator internus muscle
❏ It is the tendon (not muscle) of obturator internus, which passes through lesser sciatic notch.

2. d. Tendon of obturator internus
❏ PIN (Pudendal nerve, Internal pudendal vessels and Nerve to obturator internus) structures come from pelvic cavity, pass through the greater sciatic notch, hook behind the ischial spine (in gluteal region) and move into the lesser sciatic notch.
❏ The tendon (and not muscle) of obturator internus passes through the lesser sciatic notch.

3. c. Coccygeal nerve
❏ The sacrotuberous ligament is pierced by the coccygeal branches of the inferior gluteal artery, the perforating cutaneous nerve (S2,3) and filaments of the coccygeal plexus (formed by S4,5 & coccygeal nerve).

4. a. Internal pudendal vessels
❏ Internal pudendal vessels pass through greater and lesser sciatic foramina (not through obturator foramen).

▶ Femur

- ❑ **Linea aspera** is a prominent longitudinal ridge or crest, on the middle third of the bone, presenting a medial and a lateral lip. It is an important insertion point for the adductors and the intermuscular septa that divides the thigh into three compartments.
- ❑ Superiorly the medial lip becomes continuous with the **spiral line** and the outer (lateral) lip becomes continuous with the **gluteal tuberosity**, which extends up to the root of greater trochanter.

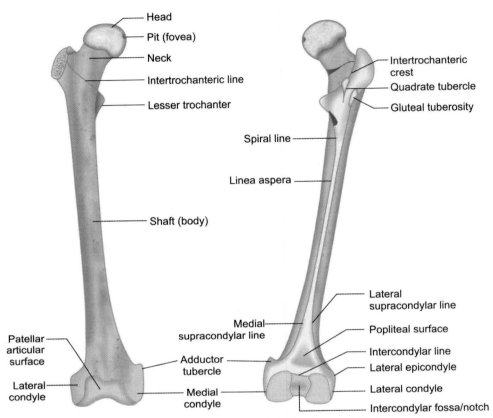

Fig. 4: General features of the femur: Anterior view and Posterior view

- ❑ Linea aspera is perforated a little below its center by the **nutrient canal**, which is directed obliquely upward.

    The main nutrient artery to femur is usually derived from **the second perforating artery** (branch of profunda femoris artery).

- ❑ Lower end of femur has **one secondary centre of ossification**, which appears near the birth (9 months of intrauterine life) and fuses by 20th year.
- ❑ Lower end of femur and upper end of tibia, ossification centres are unique in the sense that they **appear just before birth** (ninth month of IUL). It is of **medicolegal importance** because their presence in radiograph indicates maturity of the fetus (foul play can be detected).

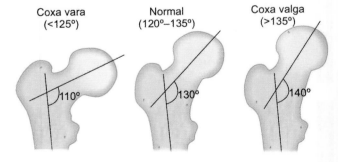

Fig. 5: Femur - Neck shaft angle

The angle formed by axis of femoral shaft and line drawn along axis of femoral neck is about 127° (125–140°)

In normal adult it is about 125° and 135° in a child at age 3 years.

It is widest at birth and diminishes gradually until the age of 10 years; it is smaller in females.

if < 125 (coxa varus) and if > 135 (coxa valgus) deformity.

Note: Angle of torsion is between the axis of head and neck of the femur and transverse axis of femoral condyles (7° to 12°).

Attachments on linea aspera:

❏ From the **medial** lip of the linea aspera vastus **medialis** originates.

❏ From the **lateral** lip the vastus **lateralis** and short head of biceps femoris takes origin.

❏ The **adductor magnus** is inserted into the linea aspera, and to its lateral prolongation above, and its medial prolongation below.

❏ Between the vastus lateralis and the adductor magnus **two muscles** are attached: the gluteus maximus inserted above, and the short head of the biceps femoris originating below.

❏ Between the adductor magnus and the vastus medialis muscles **two muscles** inserted are: the adductor brevis and adductor longus.

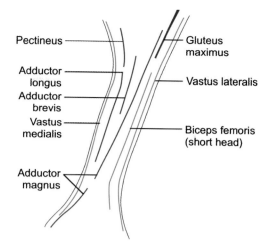

Fig. 6: Structures attached to the lines aspera (magnified view)

1. TRUE about linea aspera: (NEET Pattern 2013)
   a. Forms lateral border of femur
   b. Forms medial border of femur
   c. Continues as gluteal tuberosity
   d. Present on the posterior surface of femur

2. Muscle attached to medial lip of linea aspera of femur: (NEET Pattern 2015)
   a. Short lead of biceps femoris b. Vastus lateralis
   c. Vastus intermedius
   d. Vastus medialis

3. Lower end of femur is ossified from how many ossification centers: (NEET Pattern 2013)
   a. 1   b. 2
   c. 3   d. 4

4. Angle of the neck of femur to shaft is: (JIPMER 2007; NEET Pattern 2013)
   a. 110°   b. 125°
   c. 135°   d. 100°

1. c. Continues as gluteal tuberosity
   ❏ Linea aspera is present on the middle third of the posterior border (not surface) of femur.
   ❏ Superiorly the medial lip becomes continuous with the spiral line and the outer (lateral) lip becomes continuous with the gluteal tuberosity.

2. d. Vastus medialis
   ❏ From the medial lip of the linea aspera vastus medialis originates.

3. a. 1
   ❏ Lower end of femur has **one secondary centre** of ossification, which appears near the birth (9 months of intrauterine life) and fuses by 20th year.

4. b. 125°
   ❏ The angle formed by axis of femoral shaft and line drawn along axis of femoral neck is about 127° (125–140°)

▶ Tibia

Tibia is a **pre-axial** bone. It has no articulation with patella.

Secondary centre for the upper end is present at birth and fuses with the shaft by 16 years in females and 18 in males.

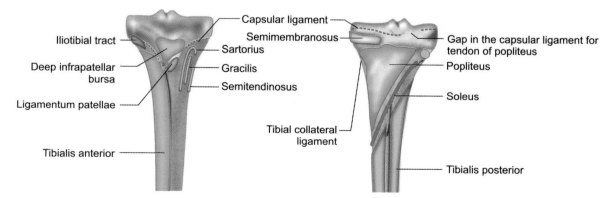

Fig. 7: Upper end of tibia

❏ **Nutrient artery** is a branch of the posterior tibial artery (may also be a branch from the anterior tibial artery)

❏ Nutrient foramen is present on shaft, **directed away** from the upper growing end.

- **Largest nutrient artery** in the body is nutrient artery of tibia.
- **Semi-membranosus** is attached to the medial condyle (posteriorly)
- Intercondylar area provides attachments to various structures (anterior to posterior). (**Mnemonic**: Medical College Lucknow, Lucknow Medical College)
- ACL and PCL are intracapsular and extrasynovial ligaments, lined by synovial membrane almost entirely.

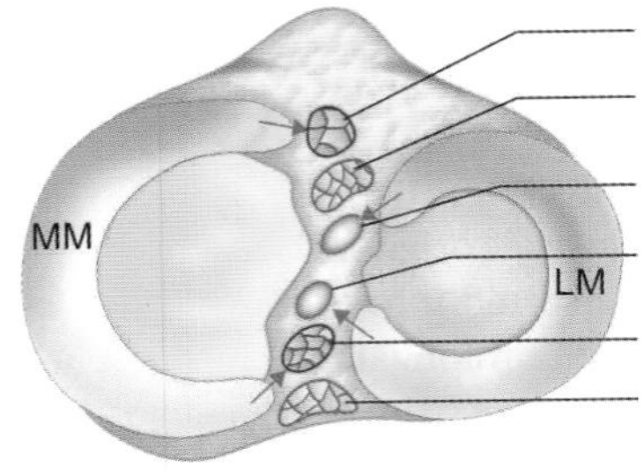

Medial meniscus (anterior end)
Cruciate ligament (anterior)
Lateral meniscus (anterior end)
Lateral meniscus (posterior end)
Medial meniscus (posterior end)
Cruciate ligament (posterior)

Fig. 8: Structures attached in intercondylar area on the superior aspect of the tibia (MM - Medial meniscus, LM – Lateral meniscus)

QUESTIONS

1. **All the following are true about upper end of tibia EXCEPT:**
   (AIPG 2000)
   a. Ossification centre for the upper end fuses by 18 years
   b. Meniscal cartilage is attached to the intercondylar area
   c. Gives attachment to semimembranosus
   d. Posterior aspect of patella articulates with upper end of tibia laterally

2. **Most anterior structure on tibial plateau Transverse ligament:**
   (PGIC 2017)
   a. Anterior horn of lateral meniscus
   b. Anterior horn of medial meniscus
   c. Anterior cruciate ligament
   d. Ligamentum patella

3. **Nutrient artery to tibia arises from which of the following arteries?**
   (JIPMER 2008)
   a. Popliteal artery
   b. Anterior tibial artery
   c. Posterior tibial artery
   d. Peroneal artery

4. **FALSE about tibia fibula is:**
   (NEET Pattern 2015)
   a. Nutrient artery of tibia is from posterior tibial artery
   b. Nutrient artery of fibula is from peroneal artery
   c. Proximal end of tibia is related to common peroneal nerve
   d. Tibia is the most common site of osteomyelitis

ANSWERS

1. **d. Posterior aspect of patella articulates with upper end of tibia laterally**
   - Patella has no articulation with tibia; it is articulated to femur only.
   - Ossification: Secondary centre for the upper end is present at birth and fuses with the shaft by 16 years in females and 18 in males.
   - Both medial and lateral menisci are attached to the intercondylar area on tibia.
   - Semi-membranosus muscle is attached to the medial condyle of tibia, posteriorly.

2. **b. Anterior horn of medial meniscus**
   - Anterior horn of medial meniscus is the most anterior structure attached on the intercondylar area on the superior surface of tibia.

3. **c. Posterior tibial artery**
   - Nutrient artery is a branch of the posterior tibial artery; it may also arise at the level of the popliteal bifurcation or as a branch from the anterior tibial artery.

4. **c. Proximal end of tibia is related to common peroneal nerve**
   - Proximal end of fibula (not tibia) is related to common peroneal nerve.
   - Primary hematogenous osteomyelitis is more common in infants and children, usually occurring in the long bone metaphysis, upper end of tibia being the commonest site of acute osteomyelitis

Tibio-femoral condyles are involved in weight transmission (**pressure epiphysis**) and are intracapsular.
- Styloid process of fibula bone gives attachment to fibular collateral ligament (knee joint) and biceps femoris.

◤ Joints

Table 1: Type of joints in lower limb

Joint	Type
Sacroiliac joint	Plane synovial
Pubis symphysis	Symphysis (secondary cartilaginous)
Hip	Ball and socket synovial
Knee	Bicondylar (>Modified hinge) synovial
Superior tibiofibular joint	Plane synovial
Middle radioulnar	Fibrous (Syndesmosis)
Inferior tibiofibular	Fibrous (Syndesmosis)
Ankle	Hinge synovial
Talocalcaneonavicular	Ball and socket synovial
Subtalar (talocalcaneal)	Plane synovial

Joint	Type
Calcaneocuboid	Saddle synovial
Other Intercarpal and midcarpal	Plane synovial
Metatarsophalangeal	Ellipsoid (> Condylar) synovial
Interphalangeal	Hinge

❑ The strongest flexor of hip joint is **iliopsoas** muscle.
❑ Hip flexion is done by sartorius, pectineus, rectus femoris (but not gluteus maximus).
❑ The **iliofemoral ligament of Bigelow** (that forms an inverted Y shape) is the strongest ligament of the hip joint and limits hyperextension.
❑ **Langenbeck triangle** has its apex at the anterior superior spine of the ilium, base along the anatomical neck of the femur, and its external side by the external face of the greater trochanter of the femur *(JIPMER 2015)*.

▶ Hip Joint

Hip joint is a synovial ball-and-socket joint and exhibits a very effective compromise between mobility and stability that allows movement in all three orthogonal planes.

Ligaments of hip joint

❑ **Capsule** attaches to acetabular margin of hip bone, labrum and transverse acetabular ligament.
  ➢ On the femur, it is attached anteriorly to the intertrochanteric line and posteriorly 1 cm in front of (medial to) the intertrochanteric crest.
  ➢ It has two types of fibres—inner circular (zona orbicularis) fibres and outer longitudinal fibres (which are reflected along the neck toward the head to form the retinacula).

Note: The synovial membrane lines inner aspect of the fibrous capsule, the intracapsular portion of the femoral neck, glenoid labrum (both surfaces), transverse acetabular ligament, ligamentum teres, and fat in the acetabular fossa.

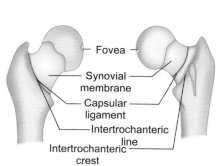

Fig. 9: Attachment of the capsular ligament of hip joint on the femur

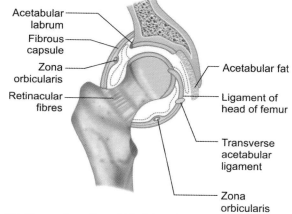

Fig. 10: Coronal section of hip joint showing the fibrous capsule and the lining of synovial membrane

❑ **Iliofemoral** ligament (of Bigelow) lies anteriorly and blends with the capsule.
  ➢ It has **inverted Y-shaped**, whose apex is attached to the lower half of the anterior inferior iliac spine and acetabular margin and the base to the intertrochanteric line.
  ➢ It has **three parts**: A lateral thick band of oblique fibres, a medial thick band of vertical fibres, and a large central thin portion.
  ➢ It is the **strongest ligament of body** and prevents the trunk from falling backward in the standing posture.
  ➢ It also **prevents hyperextension** of hip joint during standing.
❑ **Pubofemoral ligament** reinforces the fibrous capsule inferiorly, extends from the pubis bone to the femoral neck, and **limits abduction** and extension.

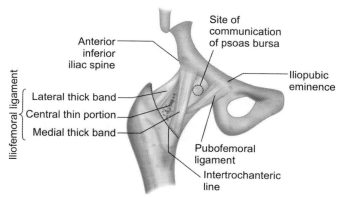

Fig. 11: Iliofemoral and pubofemoral ligaments

❏ **Ischiofemoral ligament** supports the capsule posteriorly. Its fibres attach to ischium bone, spiral behind the femoral neck to be attached into the greater trochanter deep to the iliofemoral ligament.

❏ **Ligamentum teres** (round) of the head of femur is actually a flat triangular ligament with apex attached to the fovea of the head, and its base to the transverse acetabular ligament.
  ➤ It carries acetabular branches of the obturator and medial circumflex femoral arteries.

❏ **Acetabular labrum** is a fibrocartilaginous rim attached to the acetabular margin to deepen it. It's transverse acetabular part bridges the acetabular notch.

Movements	Muscles producing movements
Flexion	▪ Psoas major and iliacus (chief flexor) ▪ Sartorius, rectus femoris, and pectineus
Extension	▪ Gluteus maximum (chief extensor) ▪ Hamstring muscles
Abduction	▪ Gluteus medius and minimus (chief abductors) ▪ Tensor fasciae latae and sartorius
Adduction	▪ Adductor longus, adductor brevis, and adductor magnus (chief adductors) ▪ Pectineus and gracilis
Medial rotation	▪ Anterior fibres of gluteus minimus and medius (chief medial rotators) ▪ Tensor fasciae latae
Lateral rotation	▪ Piriformis, obturator externus, obturator internus and associated gemelli, quadratus femoris (These muscles are generally termed short rotators)

QUESTIONS

1. **Regarding hip joint, which of the following statements is TRUE?** *(NEET pattern 2014)*
   a. Retinaculum attaches femur to hip bone
   b. Inferior gluteal nerve supplies the hip abductors
   c. Capsule is attached to the intertrochanteric line
   d. Iliopsoas causes hip abduction

2. **Iliofemoral ligament arise from Ischial tuberosity:** *(PGIC 2008;14)*
   a. Ischial tuberosity
   b. Anterior superior iliac spine
   c. Iliopubic rami
   d. Anterior inferior iliac spine
   e. Iliac crest

3. **Abduction of the thigh is limited by:**
   a. Tension in the adductors
   b. Tension in the adductors and iliofemoral ligament
   c. Tension in the adductors and pubofemoral ligament
   d. Tension in the adductors and ischiofemoral ligament

4. **Gluteo-femoral bursa is in between gluteus maximus and:** *(NEET Pattern 2014)*
   a. Greater trochanter
   b. Lesser trochanter
   c. Ischial tuberosity
   d. Vastus lateralis

ANSWERS

1. **c. Capsule is attached to the intertrochanteric line**
   ❏ Capsule of the hip joint is attached to the intertrochanteric line.
   ❏ Retinacular fibres are reflected capsular fibres running on the neck of femur and carry arterial supply to neck and head of femur. They are not attached to hip bone.
   ❏ Inferior gluteal nerve supplies gluteus maximus muscle, which is the chief extensor at hip joint. Hip abductors are supplied by superior gluteal nerve.
   ❏ Iliopsoas muscle is the chief muscle for hip flexion.

2. **d. Anterior inferior iliac spine**
   ❏ Iliofemoral ligament (of Bigelow) is Y shaped, arising from the anterior inferior iliac spine and the rim of the acetabulum, it spreads obliquely downwards and lateral to attach to the intertrochanteric line on the anterior side of the femoral head.

3. **c. Tension in the adductors and pubofemoral ligament**
   ❏ Pubofemoral (adductor) muscles and pubofemoral ligaments pull the femur back towards pubis bone (midline), hence limiting abduction.

4. **d. Vastus lateralis**
   ❏ Gluteofemoral bursa is present between gluteus maximus and vastus lateralis.

❏ **Weaver's bottom** Inflamed and enlarged synovial bursa between the gluteus maximus and ischial tuberosity.

► Knee Joint

❏ Anterior cruciate ligament is **taut during knee extension** and posterior cruciate ligament during knee flexion.
❏ When the knee is flexed, PCL resists the forces pushing tibia posteriorly in relation to femur.
❏ **Anterior cruciate ligament** is attached to the anterior intercondylar area of the tibia and posterior cruciate ligament posteriorly. Note: Naming as anterior and posterior is with reference to their tibial attachments *(NEET Pattern 2015)*

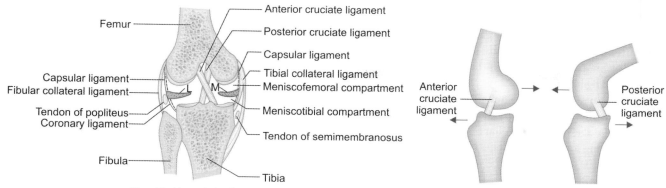

Fig. 12: Knee joint ligaments

Fig. 13: Cruciate ligaments in Knee joint

- ❑ **Coronary ligament** is that part of the capsule which lies between the periphery of menisci and the tibial condyle. It attaches the lower border of both the menisci to the tibia (also called as tibio-meniscal ligament) *(AIIMS 2012)*
- ❑ Morphologically, the **medial collateral ligament** represents the degenerated tendon of insertion of the ischial head of the adductor magnus, & fibular ligament represents the degenerated tendon of the peroneus longus *(NEET Pattern 2016)*.
- ❑ **Largest** synovial cavity in the body is with knee joint.

Table 2: Meniscal ligaments in knee joint	
Medial meniscus	**Lateral meniscus**
▪ C-shaped/semilunar in shape	▪ "O"-shaped/circular in shape
▪ Attached to the medial collateral ligament	▪ Attached to the tendon popliteus muscle
▪ More prone to injury	▪ Less prone to injury

Table 3: Movements at knee joint		
	Muscles producing movements	
Movements	**Chief muscles**	**Accessory muscles**
Flexion	▪ Semimembranosus ▪ Semitendinosus ▪ Biceps femoris	▪ Popliteus (initiates flexion) ▪ Sartorius ▪ Gracilis ▪ Gastrocnemius ▪ Plantaris
Extension	Quadriceps femoris	Tensor fasciae latae
Medial rotation	▪ Semitendinosus ▪ Semimembranosus ▪ Popliteus	▪ Sartorius ▪ Gracilis
Lateral rotation	▪ Biceps femoris	▪ Gluteus maximum ▪ Tensor faciae latae

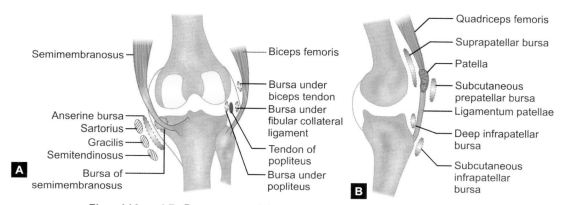

Figs. 14A and B: Bursae around the knee joint: (A) Bursae on the medial and lateral aspects of the knee; (B) Bursae on the front of the knee

- ❑ **'Donoghue's triad'** may occur when a football player's cleated shoe is planted firmly in the turf and the knee is struck from the lateral side.
  - ➤ It is characterized by the (a) rupture of the **tibial collateral ligament**, as a result of excessive abduction; (b) tearing of the **anterior cruciate ligament**, as a result of forward displacement of the tibia; and (c) injury to the **medial meniscus**, as a result of the tibial collateral ligament attachment.

Anserine Bursa

❑ Tendons of one muscle from each of the **three compartments** of the thigh: **sartorius** (anterior), **gracilis** (medial), and **semitendinosus** (posterior) are inserted into the upper part of the **medial surface of the tibia**.

❑ There is an **anserine bursa** at their tibial attachment separating each other near their insertion and also from the tibial collateral ligament.

❑ **Clergyman's** knee (infrapatellar bursitis), indicates that it is due to a position where the patient kneels down in church while praying, may develop bursitis after repeated friction between the skin and the patella.

❑ **Housemaid's** knee (prepatellar bursitis) commonly occurs among individuals whose professions require frequent kneeling and bending forwards – as required in mopping the floor.

Arterial Supply

❑ **Arterial anastomosis** around the knee contributed by: Five genicular branches of popliteal artery, descending genicular branch of femoral artery, descending branch of the lateral circumflex femoral artery, two recurrent branches of the anterior tibial artery, and circumflex fibular branch of the posterior tibial artery.

❑ Superior medial genicular artery **anastomosis** with the descending genicular branch of the femoral artery and inferior medial genicular artery

❑ Inferior medial genicular artery **anastomosis** with the superior medial genicular artery and saphenous artery—a branch of the descending genicular artery (a branch of femoral artery).

❑ Superior lateral genicular artery **anastomosis** with the descending branch of the lateral circumflex femoral artery and inferior lateral genicular artery.

❑ Inferior lateral genicular artery **anastomosis** with the superior lateral genicular artery, anterior and posterior recurrent branches of the anterior tibial artery, and circumflex fibular branch of posterior tibial artery.

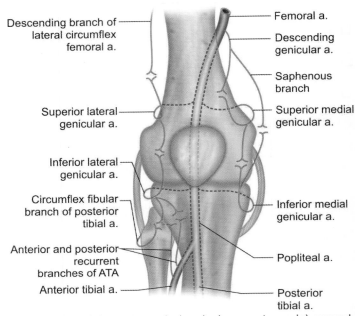

Fig. 15: Arterial anastomosis (genicular anastomosis) around the knee joint (ATA = anterior tibial artery)

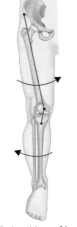

Fig. 16: Locking of knee joint

Table 4: Locking and unlocking of knee joint	
Locking of the knee joint	**Unlocking of the knee joint**
Medial rotation of the femur on tibia during terminal phase of extension	Lateral rotation of the femur on tibia during initial phase of flexion
It is brought about by quadriceps femoris	It is brought about by the popliteus muscle
Locked knee becomes absolutely rigid	Unlocked knee can be further flexed
All ligaments are taut	All ligaments are relaxed

❑ Locking may involve **medial rotation** of femur or **lateral rotation** of tibia, at the last stages of knee extension.

❑ **Tibial tuberosity** moves towards the **lateral border** of patella.

QUESTIONS

1. **A healthy young athlete sitting at table with knee at 90° flexion. What will happen when he fully extends the knee?**
   (AIIMS 2010)
   a. Movement of tibial tuberosity towards medial border of patella
   b. Movement of tibial tuberosity towards lateral border of patella
   c. Movement of tibial tuberosity towards centre of patella
   d. No change in relationship

2. **Physiological locking involves:**
   (AIPG 2008; NEET Pattern 2012)
   a. Internal rotation of femur over stabilized tibia
   b. Internal rotation of tibia over stabilized femur
   c. External rotation of tibia over stabilized femur
   d. External rotation of femur over stabilized tibia

3. **ACL prevents:** *(NEET Pattern 2014; JIPMER 2016)*
   a. Anterior dislocation of tibia
   b. Posterior dislocation of tibia
   c. Anterior dislocation of femur
   d. Posterior dislocation of femur

4. **WRONG statement about posterior cruciate ligament is:**
   a. Extrasynovial *(AIIMS 2017)*
   b. Attach to lateral surface of medial femoral condyle
   c. Prevents posterior displacement of tibia on femur
   d. Primary restrain for internal rotation at knee joint

5. **About posterior cruciate ligament, TRUE statement is:**
   (AIPG 2007; AIIMS 2007)
   a. Inserted on medial side of medial femoral condyle
   b. Intrasynovial
   c. Prevent posterior displacement of tibia
   d. Relaxed in full flexion

6. **Oblique popliteal ligament is pierced by:**
   (NEET Pattern 2013)
   a. Anterior branch of popliteal artery
   b. Medial inferior genicular branch of popliteal artery
   c. Medial superior genicular branch of popliteal artery
   d. Middle genicular branch of popliteal artery

7. **Medial rotation of tibia in flexed leg is brought about by:**
   (JIPMER 2007)
   a. Popliteus
   b. Vastus medialis
   c. Quadriceps femoris
   d. Adductor magnus

8. **TRUE about medial meniscus:** *(PGIC 2014)*
   a. Made up of hyaline cartilage
   b. Injury of lateral meniscus is more frequent than medial meniscus
   c. C-shaped
   d. Fixed to medial collateral ligament
   e. Inner part is more avascular

9. **A boy playing football received a blow to the lateral aspect of the knee and suffered a twisting fall, has been diagnosed as having O'Donoghue's triad, which comprises of:**
   a. Anterior cruciate ligament tear *(PGIC 2015)*
   b. Posterior cruciate ligament tear
   c. Medial meniscus
   d. Lateral meniscus
   e. Medial collateral ligament

10. **Patellar anastomosis is formed by which artery?**
    (NEET Pattern 2014)
    a. Descending genicular
    b. Anterior tibial recurrent
    c. Posterior tibial recurrent
    d. All of the above

11. **The blood supply of anterior cruciate ligament is primarily derived from:**
    (AIPG 2008)
    a. Superior medial genicular artery
    b. Descending genicular artery
    c. Middle genicular artery
    d. Circumflex fibular artery

12. **Pes anserinus includes following three muscles EXCEPT:**
    (NEET Pattern 2015)
    a. Semitendinosus
    b. Semimembranosus
    c. Gracilis
    d. Sartorius

ANSWERS

1. **b. Movement of tibial tuberosity towards lateral border of patella**
   ❑ In sitting posture (when foot is off the ground), full extension leads to knee locking (by lateral rotation of tibia). Hence, tibial tuberosity moves laterally towards the lateral border of patella.

2. **a. Internal rotation of femur over stabilized tibia > c. External rotation of tibia over stabilized femur**
   ❑ When the foot is fixed to the ground and tibia stabilized, during the last stages of knee extension, femur rotates internally (medially) to lock the knee joint.
   ❑ If the foot is off the ground (as sitting on a table) then tibia rotates opposite (externally/laterally) to lock the knee joint.

3. **a. Anterior dislocation of tibia > d. Posterior dislocation of femur**
   ❑ Anterior cruciate ligament (ACL) prevents the anterior displacement of tibia on the bone femur, and posterior displacement of femur on tibia as well.
   ❑ In ACL injury anterior drawer test becomes positive, i.e., tibia becomes loose and can pulled anteriorly on the bone femur.

4. **d. Primary restrain for internal rotation at knee joint**
   ❑ Posterior cruciate ligament is intracapsular and extrasynovial membrane. It is attached to the posterior intercondylar area of the tibia and runs antero-medially to attach to lateral
   ❑ Surface of the medial femoral condyle. It prevents posterior displacement of tibia on femur.

ANSWERS

5. c. Prevent posterior displacement of tibia
- ❑ Posterior cruciate ligament (PCL) prevents posterior displacement of tibia on femur.
- ❑ PCL attaches to the lateral surface of the medial femoral condyle.
- ❑ It is intracapsular and extrasynovial, lined by synovial membrane almost entirely.
- ❑ When the knee is flexed, it resists the forces pushing tibia posteriorly in relation to femur.

6. d. Middle genicular branch of popliteal artery
- ❑ Oblique popliteal ligament is an expansion from the tendon of semimembranosus muscle, running upward and laterally superficial to the capsule to be attached to the intercondylar line of the femur, strengthens the capsule of knee joint posteriorly.
- ❑ It is intimately related to the popliteal artery and pierced by: Middle genicular nerve, middle genicular vessels, and posterior division of the obturator nerve.

7. a. Popliteus
- ❑ Medial rotation of the flexed leg (knee unlocking) is carried out by popliteus, semimembranosus and semitendinosus, assisted by sartorius and gracilis.

8. c. C-shaped; d. Fixed to medial collateral ligament
- ❑ Menisci are crescentic C shape fibrocartilaginous structures.
- ❑ The peripheries are vascularized by capillary loops from the fibrous capsule and synovial membrane, while their inner regions are avascular.
- ❑ Meniscal tears mostly occur in inner zone and seldom heal spontaneously (poor vascularity).
- ❑ Peripheral zone has the potential to heal spontaneously, due to good vascular supply.
- ❑ Medial meniscus is more vulnerable to injury than lateral because of its fixity to the tibial collateral ligament and greater excursion during rotatory movement.
- ❑ Lateral meniscus is pulled and protected by popliteus muscle.

9. a. Anterior cruciate ligament tear; c. Medial meniscus; e. Medial collateral ligament
- ❑ O'Donoghue's triad may occur when a football player's cleated shoe is planted firmly in the turf and the knee is struck from the lateral side. It is characterized by the injured three ligaments: ACL, medial meniscus and tibial collateral ligament.

10. d. All of the above
- ❑ A network of vessels is present around and above the patella and on the contiguous ends of the femur and tibia, forming a superficial and a deep plexus.

11. c. Middle genicular artery
- ❑ Middle genicular artery (branch of popliteal artery) pierces the oblique popliteal ligament and supplies the cruciate ligaments & synovial membrane of knee joint.

12. b. Semimembranosus
- ❑ Tendons of one muscle from each of the three compartments of the thigh: sartorius (anterior), gracilis (medial), and semitendinosus (posterior) are inserted into the upper part of the medial surface of the tibia. Anserine bursa is at their tibial attachment separating each other near their insertion and also from the tibial collateral ligament.

▶ Ankle Joint

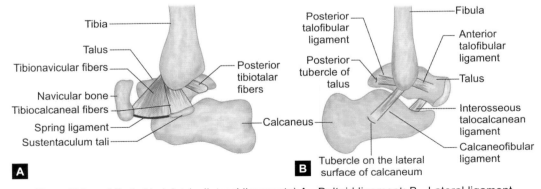

Figs. 17A and B: Ankle joint (collateral ligaments) A - Deltoid ligament; B - Lateral ligament

- ❑ **Spring** (plantar calcaneonavicular) ligament **supports the head of the talus** and the medial longitudinal arch.
- ❑ If this ligament fails, the navicular and calcaneus separate, allowing the talar head, which is the highest point of the medial arch, to descend, leading to a flat-foot deformity *(NEET Pattern 2014)*

Note: Spring ligament is **not attached** to head of talus *(NEET Pattern 2013)*

QUESTIONS

1. Plantar flexion is brought about by which of these muscles? *(PGIC)*
  a. Plantaris
  b. FHL
  c. Tibialis anterior
  d. Peroneus brevis
  e. Soleus

ANSWERS

1. a. Plantaris, b. FHL e. Soleus
  ❑ Calf muscles carry out the movement of plantar flexion.

Table 5: Movements at ankle joint		
Movements	**Muscles producing movements**	
	Principal muscles	**Accessory muscles**
Dorsiflexion	Tibialis anterior	▪ Extensor digitorum longus ▪ Extensor hallucis longus ▪ Peroneus tertius
Plantar flexion	▪ Gastrocnemius ▪ Soleus	▪ Plantaris ▪ Tibialis posterior ▪ Flexor hallucis longus ▪ Flexor digitorum longus

QUESTIONS

1. The stability of the ankle joint is maintained by all of the following EXCEPT: *(AIIMS 2003)*
  a. Plantar calcaneonavicular (spring) ligament
  b. Deltoid ligament
  c. Lateral ligament
  d. Shape of the superior talar articular surface

2. Stability of ankle joint is maintained by all EXCEPT: *(AIIMS 2009)*
  a. Collateral ligaments
  b. Cruciate ligaments
  c. Tendons of muscles crossing the joint
  d. Close apposition of articular surfaces of bones

3. Deltoid ligament is NOT attached to: *(AIIMS 2009)*
  a. Medial cuneiform
  b. Medial malleolus
  c. Sustentaculum tali
  d. Spring ligament

4. Spring ligament consists of all EXCEPT: *(JIPMER 2011; NEET Pattern 2015)*
  a. Plantar calcaneocuboid ligament
  b. Plantar calcaneonavicular ligament
  c. Medial calcaneonavicular ligament
  d. Lateral calcaneonavicular ligament

ANSWERS

1. a. Plantar calcaneonavicular (spring) ligament
  ❑ Spring ligament works for the maintenance of medial longitudinal arch.

2. b. Cruciate ligaments
  ❑ Cruciate ligaments are present in the knee (and not ankle) joint.

3. a. Medial cuneiform
  ❑ Deltoid ligament is a triangular (delta shaped) ligament on the medial side of the ankle attached to tibia (Medial malleolus).
  ❑ Deltoid ligament has four parts attaching to medial malleolus of tibia. It doesn't include calcaneonavicular (spring) ligament.

4. a. Plantar calcaneocuboid ligament
  ❑ Spring (calcaneo-navicular) ligament attaches calcaneum to navicular bone (and not cuboid).
  ❑ It is made up of two distinct structures: the superomedial calcaneonavicular portion and the inferolateral calcaneonavicular portion.

▶ Nerves of Lower Limb

Nerves of the lower limb are derived from the **ventral primary rami** of the lumbar and sacral nerves forming the **lumbar plexus (L1-L4)** in the posterior abdominal wall and the **sacral** plexus (L4–S4) in the pelvis.

Branches	Root value
1. Iliohypogastric nerve	L1
2. Ilioinguinal nerve	L1
3. Genitofemoral nerve	L1, L2 (ventral division)
4. Lateral cutaneous nerve of the thigh	L2, L3 (dorsal divisions)
5. Femoral nerve	L2, L3, L4 (dorsal divisions)
6. Obturator nerve	L2, L3, L4 (ventral divisions)
7. Accessory obturator nerve (occasional)	L3, L4 (ventral divisions)

Branches of the lumbar plexus

❑ **Subcostal nerve** is the anterior division of the twelfth thoracic nerve. Some authors describe it as the first branch of the lumbar plexus.
❑ Femoral nerve is formed by the dorsal divisions of L2,3,4; whereas, obturator nerve is from ventral division of same L2,3,4.

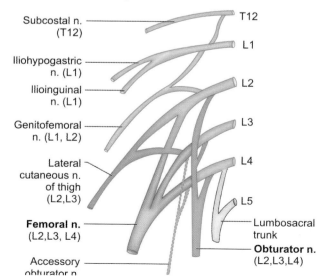

Fig. 18: Lumbar plexus (Dorsal divisions- green colour and Ventral divisions- blue)

1. **All are branches of lumbar plexus EXCEPT:**
   (NEET Pattern 2015)
   a. Iliohypogastric nerve
   b. Ilioinguinal nerve
   c. Obturator nerve
   d. Subcostal nerve

2. **Root value of lumbosacral trunk:** *(NEET Pattern 2015)*
   a. L4,5
   b. L4,5; S1
   c. L4,5; S1,2,3
   d. S1,2,3

1. **d. Subcostal nerve**
   ❑ Subcostal nerve is the anterior division of the twelfth thoracic nerve, is larger than the other intercostal nerves. It runs along the lower border of the twelfth rib.
   ❑ It may give off a communicating branch to the first lumbar nerve and the iliohypogastric nerve.
   ❑ Some authors describe it as the first branch of the lumbar plexus.

2. **a. L4,5**
   ❑ Lumbosacral trunk arises from the anterior rami of the L4 and L5 nerve roots in lumbar plexus. It contributes to the sacral plexus.

Table 6: Branches of sacral plexus			
From root	**Terminal**	**From pelvic surface**	**From dorsal surface**
Muscular branches	Sciatic (L4, L5; S1, S2, S3)	Nerve to quadratus femoris (L4, L; S1)	Superior gluteal nerve (L4, L5; S1)
Pelvic splanchnic nerves	Pedendal (S2, S3, S4)	Nerve to obturator internus (L5, S1; S2)	▪ Inferiogluteal nerve (L5; S1, S2) ▪ Posterior cutaneous nerve of the thigh (S1, S2, S3) ▪ Perforating cutaneous nerve (S2, S3) ▪ Perineal branch of 4th sacral nerve (S4)

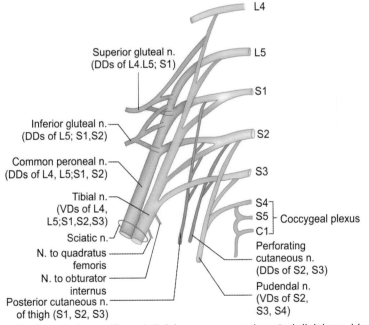

Fig. 19: Sacral plexus (Dorsal divisions- green and ventral divisions- blue)

Obturator internus is supplied by the nerve to obturator internus (L5; S1, S2) and not obturator nerve.

Posterior cutaneous nerve of thigh arises from the sacral plexus with root value S-1,2,3 *(NEET Pattern 2012)*

Sciatic nerve arises from the ventral divisions of L-4,5 and S-1,2,3 *(NEET Pattern 2012)*

Pudendal nerve arises from the ventral primary rami of S-2,3,4 *(NEET Pattern 2014)*

❑ **Medial cutaneous nerve** of the thigh (L2, L3) is a branch of the anterior division of the femoral nerve. It supplies most of the medial aspect of the thigh. Middle part of the medial thigh is supplied by obturator nerve.

❑ In **meralgia paresthetica**, the nerve involved is **lateral cutaneous nerve** of thigh. It presents with constant pain and abnormal perception in the outer side of the thigh, occasionally extending to the knee.

❑ **Saphenous nerve** (branch of femoral nerve) accompanying the great saphenous vein should be identified and secured, during venesection.

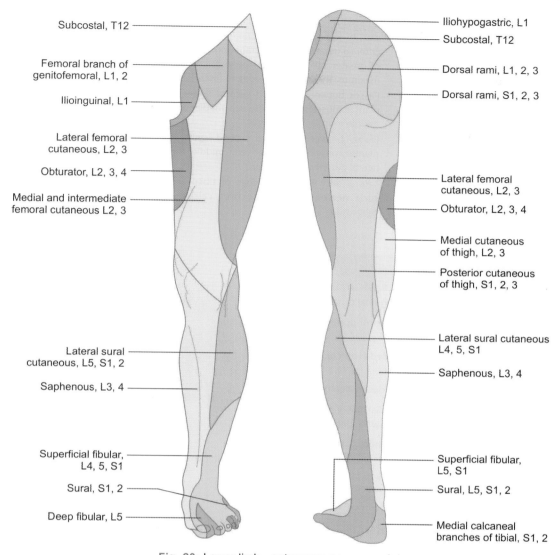

Fig. 20: Lower limb—cutaneous nerve supply

Table 7: Lower limb—Cutaneous nerve supply			
Nerve	**Origin (contributing spinal nerve)**	**Course**	**Distribution in lower limb**
Subcostal	T12 anterior ramus	Courses along inferior border of 12th rib; lateral cutaneous branch descends over iliac crest	Lateral cutaneous branch supplies skin of hip region inferior to anterior part of iliac crest and anterior to greater trochanter
Iliohypogastric	Lumbar plexus (L1: occsionally T12)	Parallels iliac crest; divides into lateral and anterior cutaneous branches	Lateral cutaneous branch supplies superolateral quadrant of buttocks
Ilioinguinal	Lumbar plexus (L1: occasionally T12)	Passes through inguinal canal; divides into fermoral and scrotal or labial branches	Femoral branch supplies skin over medial femoral triangle
Genitofemoral	Lumbar plexus (L1–L2)	Descends anterior surface of psoas major; divides into genital and femoral branches	Femoral branch supplies skin over lateral part of femoral triangle; genital branch supplies anterior scrotum or labia majora
Lateral cutaneous nerve of thigh	Lumbar plexus (L2–L3)	Passes deep to inguinal ligament 2–3 cm medial to anterior superior iliac spine	Supplies skin on anterior and lateral aspects of thigh
Anterior cutaneous branches	Lumbar plexus via fermoral nerve (L2–L4)	Arise in femoral triangle; pierce fascia lata along path of sartorius muscle	Supply skin of anterior and medial aspects of thigh
Cutaneous branch of obturator nerve	Lumbar plexus via obturator nerve, anterior branch (L2–L4)	Following its descent between adductors longus and brevis, anterior division of obturator nerve pierce fascia lata to reach skin of thigh	Skin of middle part of medial thigh

Nerve	Oringin (contributing spinal Nerve)	Course	Distribution in lower limb
Posterior cutaneous nerve of thigh	Sacral plexus (S1–S3)	Enters gluteal region via infrapiriform portion of greater sciatic foramen deep to gluteus maximus; then descends deep to fascia lata	Terminal branches pierce fascia lata to supply skin of posterior thigh and popliteal fossa
Medial plantar nerve	Tibial nerve (L4–L5)	Passes between first and second layers of plantar muscles, then between medial and middle muscles of first layer	Skin of medial side of sole, and plantar aspect, sides, and nailbeds of medial 3½ toes
Lateral plantar nerve	Tibial nerve (S1–S2)	Passes between first and second layers of plantar muscles, then between middle and lateral muscles of first layer	Skin of lateral sole, and plantar aspect, sides, and nailbeds of lateral 1½ toes
Calcaneal nerves	Tibial and sural nerves (S1–S2)	Lateral and medial branches of tibial and sural nerves, respectively, over calcaneal tuberosity	Skin of heel

Table 8: Dermatomes of lower limb	
Dermatome	**Area supplied**
L1	Inguinal area (over inguinal canal)
L2	Anterior and lateral part of upper 2/3rd of thigh.
L3	Anterior, Lateral and Medial part of lower 1/3rd of thigh and knee
L4	Medial side of leg, medial malleolus
L5	Lateral side of leg. Medial half of dorsum of foot, dorsum of first web space
S1	Posterior surface of ankle, and lateral half of dorsum of foot
S2	Posterior of thigh and leg
S3	Gluteal area around perianal region, Groin
S4	Perianal skin and Groin

- Dermatomal supply just **below inguinal ligament** is L1 *(NEET Pattern 2016)*
- **Perianal skin** is supplied by S4 (and S5) root value *(NEET Pattern 2012)*
- Slip disc at L5–S1 vertebrae; involves S-1 root value, leading to involvement of corresponding dermatome on lateral side of the foot and little toe (**sural nerve territory**).
- Great toe has **L5 dermatome**; little toe and heel- S1; S2 lies on the posterior aspect of lower limb.
- The dorsal and ventral **axial lines** both reach the **ankle joint**, ventral reaches the medial aspect
- **Meralgia paresthetica** is due to involvement of lateral cutaneous nerve of thigh. There is constant pain and abnormal perception in the outer side of the thigh, occasionally extending to the knee. *(AIIMS 2015)*
- Root value of **medial cutaneous nerve of thigh** is L2, L3. It is a branch of the anterior division of the femoral nerve. (NEET Pattern 2014)
- Most commonly used nerve in the body for **grafting** is sural nerve.
- **Longest** cutaneous nerve in the body is saphenous nerve.

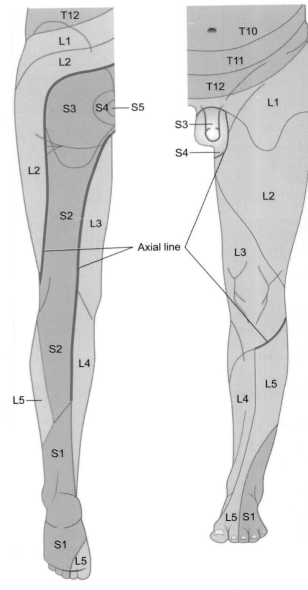

Fig. 21: Dermatomes of lower limb.

1. **Sensory supply of medial side of thigh is:** *(NEET Pattern 2016)*
   - a. Sciatic nerve
   - b. Femoral nerve
   - c. Obturator nerve
   - d. Saphenous nerve

2. **Posterior thigh dermatome is:** *(NEET Pattern 2013)*
   - a. L–4
   - b. L–5
   - c. S–1
   - d. S–2

3. **Posterior cutaneous nerve of thigh supplies skin overlying:** *(PGIC-2012)*
   - a. Lateral aspect of thigh
   - b. Posterior inferior aspect of buttock
   - c. Scrotum
   - d. Back of thigh
   - e. Popliteal fossa

4. **During laparoscopic hernia repair a tack was accidently placed below and lateral to the iliopubic tract. Post-operatively the patient complained of pain in the thigh. This is due to the involvement of:** *(AIIMS-2015)*
   - a. Lateral cutaneous nerve of thigh
   - b. Ilio-inguinal nerve
   - c. Genito-femoral nerve
   - d. Obturator nerve

5. **An altered sensation over the area of great saphenous vein in leg, where a venesection was made, is seen due to injury to which of the following nerve?** *(AIPG 2008)*
   - a. Femoral nerve
   - b. Sural nerve
   - c. Tibial nerve
   - d. Superficial peroneal nerve

6. **S1 nerve root irritation will result in pain located along the:** *(AIIMS 2004)*
   - a. Anterior aspect of the thigh
   - b. Medial aspect of the thigh
   - c. Anteromedial aspect of the leg
   - d. Lateral side of the foot

1. **b. Femoral nerve**
   - ❑ The medial cutaneous nerves from the femoral nerve supply most of the medial aspect of the thigh. Middle part of the medial thigh is supplied by obturator nerve.

2. **d. S-2**
   - ❑ Posterior calf and thigh region has S2 dermatome.

3. **b. Posterior inferior aspect of buttock, c. Scrotum, d. Back of thigh, e. Popliteal fossa**
   - ❑ The root value of posterior cutaneous nerve of thigh is S – 1, 2, 3.
   - ❑ It supplies the cutaneous region of posterior thigh and popliteal fossa.
   - ❑ It also covers the cutaneous region on posterior inferior aspect of buttock region and scrotum.

4. **a. Lateral cutaneous nerve of thigh**
   - ❑ Iliopubic tract runs parallel and deeper to inguinal ligament. The nerve damaged in this scenario is lateral cutaneous nerve of thigh.
   - ❑ Lateral femoral cutaneous nerve arises from the lumbar plexus (L2–L3), passes under the inguinal ligament near the anterior superior iliac spine and supply skin on the anterolateral aspect of thigh.
   - ❑ This is a case of nerve injury in triangle of pain (details in abdomen region).

5. **a. Femoral nerve**
   - ❑ The nerve injured is saphenous nerve (branch of femoral nerve).
   - ❑ Great saphenous vein anterior to medial malleolus is the most preferred site of venesection (cut-down) in emergency.
   - ❑ The saphenous nerve accompanying the vein should be identified and secured, during the procedure.

6. **d. Lateral side of the foot**
   - ❑ Sural nerve supplies the skin over little toe and lateral margin of foot, bearing the dermatome S1.

Table 9: Segmental innervation of the muscles of the lower limb	
Segment	Muscles supplied
L1	Psoas major, psoas minor
L2	Psoas major, iliacus, sartorius, gracilis, pectineus, adductor longus, adductor brevis
L3	Psoas major, quadriceps femoris, adductors (magnus, longus, brevis)
L4	Psoas major, quadriceps femoris, tensor fasciae latae, adductor magnus, obturator externus, tibialis anterior, tibialis posterior
L5	Gluteus medius, gluteus minimus, obturator internus, semimembranosus, semitendinosus, extensor hallucis longus, extensor digitorum longus, fibularis tertius, popliteus
S1	Gluteus maximus, obturator internus, piriformis, biceps femoris, semitendinosus, popliteus, gastrocnemius, soleus, fibularis longus and fibularis brevis, extensor digitorum brevis
S2	Piriformis, biceps femoris, gastrocnemius, soleus, flexor digitorum longus, flexor hallucis longus, some intrinsic foot muscles
S3	Some intrinsic foot muscles (except abductor hallucis, flexor hallucis brevis, flexor digitorum brevis, extensor digitorum brevis)

Table 10: Segmental innervation of joint movements of the lower limb		
Region	Muscles supplied	Segment
Hip	Flexors, adductors, medial rotators	L1–3
	Extensors, abductors, lateral rotators	L5, S1
Knee	Extensors	L3, 4
	Flexors	L5, S1
Ankle	Dorsiflexors	L4, 5
	Plantar flexors	S1, 2
Foot	Invertors	L4, 5
	Evertors	L5, S1
	Intrinsic muscles	S2, 3

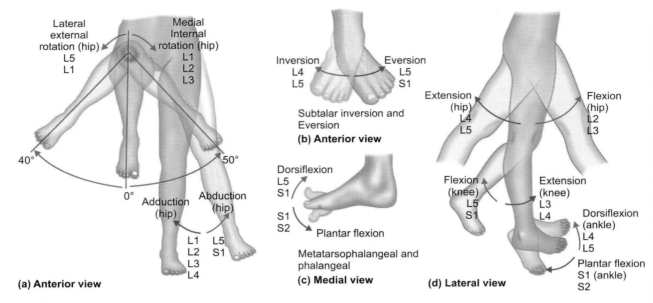

Figs. 22A to D: Myotomes: Segmental innervation of muscle groups and movements of lower limb. The level of spinal cord injury may be determined by the strength and ability to perform particular movements.

Table 11: Nerves of gluteal and posterior thigh region			
Nerve	**Origin**	**Course**	**Distribution**
Sciatic	Sacral plexus (anterior and posterior divisions of anterior rami of L4–S3 spinal nerves)	Enters gluteal region via greater sciatic foramen inferior to piriformis and deep to gluteus maximus; descends in posterior thigh deep to biceps femoris; bifurcates into tibial and common fibular nerves at apex of popliteal fossa	Supplies no muscles in gluteal regions; supplies all muscles of posterior compartment of thigh (tibial division supplies all but short head of biceps, which is supplied by common fibular divison).
Posterior cutaneous nerve of thigh	Sacral plexus (anterior and posterior divisions of anterior rami of S1–S3 spinal nerves)	Enter gluteal region via greater sciatic foramen inferior to piriformis and deep to gluteus maximus, emrging from interior border of latter; descends in posterior thigh deep to fascia lata.	Supplies skin of inferior half of buttocks (through inferior clunial nerves). Skin over posterior thigh and popliteal fossa, and skin of lateral perineum and upper medial thigh (via its perineal branch)
Superior gluteal	Sacral plexus (posterior divisions of anterior rami of L4–S1 spinal nerves)	Enters gluteal region via greater sciatic foramen superior to piriformis; courses laterally between gluteus medius and minimus as far as tensor fasciae latae	Innvervates gluteus medius, gluteus minimus, and tensor fasciae latae muscles
Inferior gluteal	Sacral plexus (posterior divisions of anterior rami of L5-S2 spinal nerves)	Enters gluteal region via greater sciatic foramen superior to piriformis; courses laterally between gluteus medius and minimus as far as tensor fasciae latae	Innvervates gluteus medius, gluteus minimus, and tensor fasciae latae muscles
Nerve to quadratus femoris	Sacral plexus (anterior divisions of anterior rami of L4–S1 spinal nerves)	Enters gluteal region via greater sciatic foramen inferior to piriformis, deep (anterior) to sciatic nerve	Innervates hip joint, inferior gemellus, and quadratus femoris.
Pudendal	Sacral plexus (anterior divisions of anterior rami of S2–S4 spinal nerves)	Exits pelvis via greater sciatic foramen inferior to piriformis; descends posterior to sacrospinous ligament; enters perineum through lesser sciatic foramen	Supplies no structures in gluteal region or posterior thigh (principal nerve to perineum)
Nerve to obturator internus	Sacral plexus (Posterior divisions of anterior rami of L5–S2 spinal nerves)	Exist pelvis via greater sciatic foramen inferior to piriformis; descends posterior to sacrospinous ligament; enters perineum through lesser sciatic foramen	Supplies superior gemellus and obturator internus

QUESTIONS

1. **Which nerve does NOT supply gluteal region?** *(AIIMS 2012)*
   a. Superior gluteal nerve   b. Sciatic nerve
   c. Nerve to quadrates femoris   d. Nerve to obturator internus

2. **Superior gluteal nerve supplies all EXCEPT:** *(AIIMS 2010)*
   a. Gluteus minimus   b. Gluteus medius
   c. Tensor fascia lata   d. Gluteus maximus

ANSWERS

1. **b. Sciatic nerve**
   - Sciatic nerve supplies back of thigh, the leg and foot region.
   - It passes through the gluteal region, but doesn't supply the area.

2. **d. Gluteus maximus**
   - Gluteus maximus is supplied by the inferior gluteal nerve.
   - Superior gluteal nerve supplies the trio – Gluteus medius, Gluteus minimus and Tensor fascia latae.

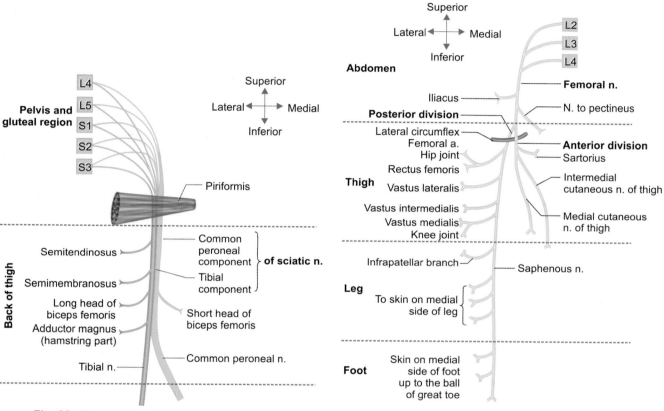

Fig. 23: Sciatic nerve - Origin, course, branches

Fig. 24: Femoral nerve - Origin, course, branches

Sciatic nerve

- All the muscles on the back of thigh are supplied by tibial component of sciatic nerve except **short head of biceps femoris** which is supplied by its common peroneal component of sciatic nerve.
- **Thickest** nerve in the body is sciatic nerve.

QUESTIONS

1. **WRONG statement about femoral nerve is:** *(NEET Pattern 2016)*
   a. Arises from ventral division of ventral rami
   b. Root value is L2,3,4
   c. Largest branch of lumbar plexus
   d. Supplies quadriceps femoris

2. **The patient presented with loss of extension at knee joint with decreased sensation over anterior aspect of thigh. The nerve damaged is:** *(NEET Pattern 2016)*
   a. Obturator   b. Femoral
   c. Common peroneal   d. Tibial

ANSWERS

1. **a. Arises from ventral division of ventral rami**
   - Femoral nerve arises from the dorsal (not ventral) division of ventral rami of L2,3,4.

2. **a. Arises from ventral division of ventral rami**
   - Femoral nerve supplies the extensors at knee joint and skin over the anterior aspect of thigh as well.

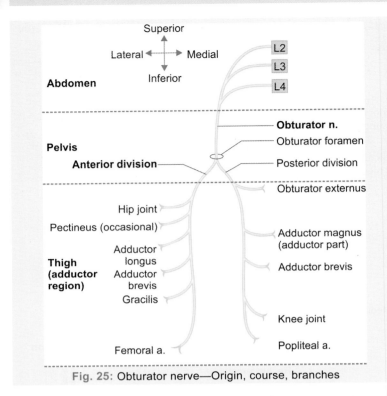

Fig. 25: Obturator nerve—Origin, course, branches

Obturator nerve - Origin, course, branches

❑ Obturator Nerve Enters Thigh Through Obturator Foramen *(NEET Pattern 2014)*
❑ It is the nerve of **hip adduction**.
❑ Obturator nerve doesn't supply obturator internus (which is supplied by a branch from sacral plexus). *(NEET Pattern 2014)*
❑ Obturator nerve gives articular branch to hip as well the knee joint, and may present with pain at knee joint in a lesion of hip joint *(NEET Pattern 2016)*

▶ Nerves of leg region

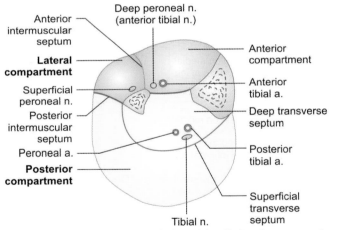

Fig. 26: Transverse section through the mid-calf showing compartments of leg (muscles and neurovascular bundle)

❑ Anterior compartment of leg (Deep Peroneal nerve territory): Dorsiflexor (Extensor) muscles
❑ Posterior compartment of leg (Posterior Tibial nerve territory): Plantar flexor muscles
❑ Lateral compartment of leg (Superficial Peroneal nerve): Evertors of foot

Table 12: Nerves of leg region			
Nerve	**Origin**	**Course**	**Distribution in Leg**
Saphenous	Femoral nerve	Descends with femoral vessels through femoral triangle and adductor canal and then descends with great saphenous veins	Supplies skin on medial side of ankle and foot
Sural	Usually arises from branches of both tibial and common fibular nerves	Descends between heads of a gastrocnemius and becomes superficial at middle of leg; descends with small saphenous vein and passes inferior to lateral malleolus to lateral side of foot	Supplies skin on posterior and lateral aspects of leg and lateral side of foot
Tibial	Sciatic nerve	Forms as sciatic bifurcates at apex of popliteal fossa; descends through popliteal fossa and lies on popliteal; runs inferiorly on tibialis posterior with posterior tibial vessels; terminates beneath flexor retinaculum by dividing into medial and lateral plantar nerves	Supplies posterior muscles of leg and knee joint

Nerve	Origin	Course	Distribution in Leg
Common fibular (peroneal)	Sciatic nerve	Forms as sciatic bifurcates at apex of popliteal fossa and follows medial border of biceps femoris and its tendon; passes over posterior aspect of head of fibula and then winds around neck of fibula deep to fibularis longus.where it divides into deep and superficial fibular nerves	Supplies skin on lateral part of posterior aspect of leg via the lateral sural cutaneous nerve; also supplies knee joint via its articular branch
Superficial fibular (peroneal)	Common fibular nerve	Arises between fibularis longus and neck of fibula and descends in lateral compartment of leg; pierces deep fascia at distal third of leg to become subcutaneous	Supplies fibularis longus and brevis and skin on distal third of anterior surface of leg and dorsum of foot
Deep fibular (peroneal)	Common fibular nerve	Arises between fibularis longus and neck of fibula; passes through extensor digitorum longus and descends on interosseous membrane crosses distal end of tibia and enters dorsum of foot.	Supplies anterior muscles of leg, dorsum of foot and skin of first interdigital cleft; sends articular branches to joints it crosses.

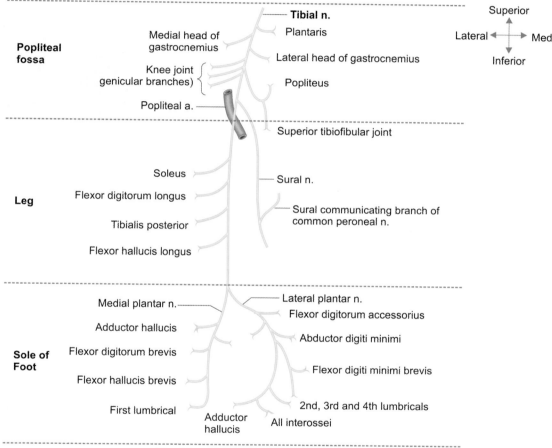

Fig. 27: Tibial nerve - Origin, course, branches

1. Tibial nerve injury causes: *(PGIC 2012)*
a. Dorsiflexion of foot at ankle joint
b. Plantar flexion of the foot at ankle joint
c. Loss of sensation of dorsum of foot
d. Paralysis of muscles of anterior compartment of leg
e. Loss of sensation over the medial border of foot

2. 3rd and 4th lumbrical of foot are supplied by:
(NEET Pattern 2015)
a. Medial planter nerve
b. Lateral plantar nerve
c. Peroneal nerve
d. Posterior tibial nerve

1. a. Dorsiflexion of foot at ankle joint
☐ In tibial nerve injury posterior leg (calf) muscles and sole muscle are paralysed and there is sensory loss on the posterior calf region, lateral foot and sole skin.
☐ The patient is unable to do plantar flexion and the foot remains in dorsiflexion (due to unopposed anterior leg muscles).

2. b. Lateral plantar nerve
☐ First lumbrical of foot is supplied by medial plantar nerve and the lateral three are supplied by the lateral plantar nerve.

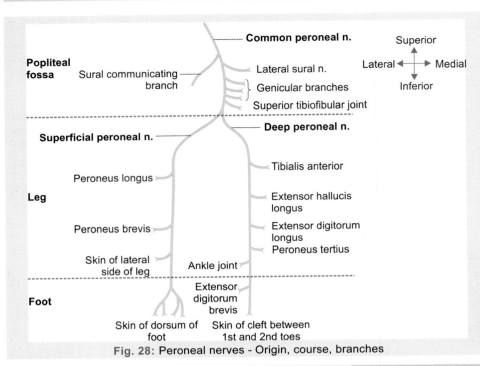

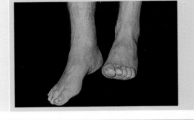

Deep peroneal nerve supplies the skin at the **dorsum of first web space**. A lesion leads to loss of sensation of adjacent sides of 1st and 2nd toe *(AIIMS 2009)*

Fracture neck of fibula results in common peroneal nerve injury, leading to **loss of dorsiflexion** at the ankle (foot drop) and toes, alongwith inability of **foot eversion**.

Fig. 28: Peroneal nerves - Origin, course, branches

1. A person is unable to dorsiflex the foot and there is loss of sensations on dorsal foot. Possible nerve injury is: *(PGIC 2013)*
a. Damage to common peroneal nerve at neck of fibula
b. Damage to common peroneal at medial malleolus
c. Compression of anterior tibial nerve at ankle
d. Damage to superficial peroneal nerve
e. Damage of deep peroneal nerve

2. Which of the following may occur in common peroneal nerve injury? *(PGIC 2015)*
a. Loss of dorsiflexion of toe
b. Foot drop
c. High stepping of foot
d. Eversion of foot affected
e. Loss of sensation over sole

1. c. Compression of anterior tibial nerve at ankle, e. Damage of deep peroneal nerve
❑ Isolated injury to the deep fibular nerve may result from compartment syndrome, from an intraneural ganglion cyst etc.
❑ Individuals with lesions of the deep fibular nerve have weakness of ankle dorsiflexion and extension of all toes but normal foot eversion.
❑ Sensory impairment is confined to the dorsum of first interdigital web space.

2. a. Loss of dorsiflexion of toe; b. Foot drop; c. High stepping of foot; d. Eversion of foot affected
❑ Common peroneal nerve injury leads to loss of dorsiflexion at the ankle (foot drop) and toes, alongwith inability of foot eversion.
❑ There is loss of sensation on the dorsum of the foot (and not sole).

❑ Deep peroneal nerve is called nervus hesitans.
❑ Most commonly injured nerve in the lower limb is **Common peroneal nerve.**

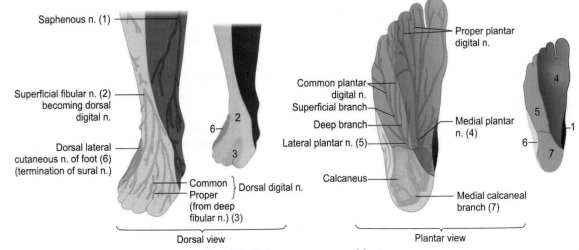

Fig. 29: Cutaneous nerves of foot.

Cutaneous Nerve of Foot

- Most of the dorsum of foot is supplied by **superficial peroneal nerve**, including **medial side of great toe**.
- **Saphenous** nerve supplies the medial side of the dorsum of foot, **only till the ball of great toe**.
- Lateral side of the great toe is supplied by the **deep peroneal nerve**. It supplies the 1st web space on the dorsum of foot.
- **Sural nerve** supplies the little toe and lateral margin of foot.

QUESTIONS

1. In L5 root involvement, which among the following is NOT affected?   *(AIPG 2011)*
   a. Thigh abduction
   b. Knee flexion
   c. Knee extension
   d. Toe extension

2. Clinical features observed in a case of L5-S1 disc prolapse is/are: *(PGIC 2017)*
   a. Radiating pain on the lateral leg
   b. Loss of sensation on lateral aspect of sole and foot
   c. Loss of ankle reflex
   d. Weakness of extensor hallucis longus
   e. Hypertonic reflexes on contralateral side

ANSWERS

1. **c. Knee extension**
   - Knee extension is carried out by L-2, 3 and 4 (Femoral nerve). Lesion at the level of L-5, doesn't affect knee extension.
   - Knee flexion is carried out by the root value: L-5 and S-1 (Tibial nerve).
   - Toe extension requires L-5 (deep peroneal nerve).

2. **b. Loss of sensation on lateral aspect of sole and foot; c. Loss of ankle reflex**
   - In a case of L5-S1 disc prolapse, nerve root compressed is S1, leading to pain and loss of sensation on lateral aspect of sole and foot (sural nerve). Posterior leg muscles are weakened, with loss of ankle reflex (S1 root value).
   - In a case of slip disc at L4-5, L5 root will be compromised leading to sensory problems in lateral leg and anterior leg muscles (like extensor hallucis longus) will be weakened.

Reflexes

Knee Reflex (L2–4)

- With the patient sitting and the knee supported and partially flexed, the patellar ligament is struck with a knee hammer, resulting in a sudden contraction of the quadriceps femoris (extension of the knee joint).
- Its afferent and efferent impulses are transmitted in the femoral nerve (L2–L4).

Ankle-jerk (Achilles) reflex (S1, 2)

- With the patient sitting and the lower limb laterally rotated and partially flexed at the hip and knee, the foot is dorsiflexed by the examiner and the calcaneal tendon struck with a knee hammer.
- A reflex twitch of the triceps surae is induced which causes plantar flexion of the foot.
- Both afferent and efferent limbs of the reflex arc are carried in the tibial nerve.
- This results in plantar flexion of the foot.

Plantar reflex

- With the foot relaxed, the outer edge of the sole is stroked longitudinally with a blunt object such as the tip of the handle of a knee hammer.
- Normally, this action elicits flexion of the toes.
- However, in patients with upper motor neurone lesions, the response includes extension of the great toe (Babinski's sign).

IM Injections

- IM injections are given on the upper outer (superolateral) quadrant of gluteal region, to prevent iatrogenic damage to the sciatic nerve.
- The needle should reach into the gluteus medius (rather than into gluteus maximus).
- A safe alternative is to inject into the lateral aspect of the thigh (vastus lateralis).
- Commonest site of **intramuscular injection** in the thigh is anterolateral aspect of the thigh into the **vastus lateralis** muscle.

Muscles (Anterior thigh)

Muscles of thigh

- Anterior compartment (femoral nerve territory): Flexors of hip, Extensors of knee
- Posterior compartment (Tibial part of sciatic nerve territory): Extensors of hip, Flexors of knee
- Medial compartment (obturator nerve territory): Adductors of thigh

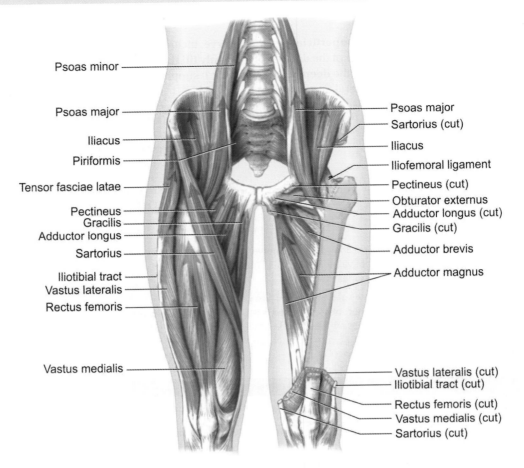

Fig. 30: Muscle of anterior-medial thigh and iliac region

Table 13: Muscles of anterior thigh (hip flexors)				
Muscle	**Proximal attachment[a]**	**Distal attachment**	**Innervation[b]**	**Main action(s)**
Pectineus	Superior ramus of pubis	Pectineal line of femur, just inferior to lesser trochanter	Femoral nerve (**L2**–L3); may receive a branch from obturation nerve	Adducts and flexes thigh; assists with medial rotation of thigh
Iliopsoas	Sides of T12–L5 vertebrae and discs between them; transverse processes of all lumbar vertebrae	Lesser trochanter of femur	Anterior rami of lumbar nerves (**L1**, **L2**, L3)	Act conjointly in flexing thigh at hip joint and in stabilizing this joint
Psoas minor	Sides of T12–L1 vertebrae and intervertebral discs	Pectineal line, iliopectineal eminence via iliopectineal arch	Anterior rami of lumbar nerves (L1, L2)	
Iliacus	Iliac crest, iliac fossa, ala of sacrum, and anterior sacro-ligaments	Tendon of psoas major lesser trochanter, and femur distal to it	Femoral nerve (L2, L3)	
Sartorius	Anterior superior iliac spine and superior part of notch interior to it	Superior part of medial surface of tibia	Femoral nerve (L2, L3)	Flexes abducts, and laterally rotates thigh at hip jonit; flexes leg at knee joint. (medially rotating leg when knee is flexed)[d]

[a]The latin word insertio means attachment. The terms insertion and origin (L. origo) have not been used here (or elsewhere) since they change with function.
[b]The spinal cord segmental innervation is indicated (e.g. L1, L2, L3 means that the nerves supplying the psoas major are derived from the first three lumbar segments of the spinal cord). Numbers in boldface (**L1**, **L2**) indicate the main segmental innervation. Damage to one or more of the listed spinal cord segments or to the moto nerve roots arising from them results in parelysis of the muscles concerned.
[c]The psoas major is also a postural muscle that helps control the deviation of the trunks and is active during standing.
[d]The four actions of the sartorus (L. sartor, tailor) produce the once common cross legged sitting positon used by tailors, hence the name.

Table 14: Muscles of anterior thigh (knee extensors)

Muscle	Proximal attachment	Distal attachment	Innervation[a]	Main action
Quardriceps femoris				
Rectus femoris	Anterior inferior illiac spine and ilium superior to acetabulum	Via common tendinous (quadri-ceps tendon) and independent attachment to base of patella; indirectly via patellar ligament or tibial tuberosity; medial and lateral vasti also attach to tibia and patella via aponeuroses (medial and lateral patellar retinacula)	Femoral nerve (L2, **L3**, **L4**)	Extend leg at knee joint; rectus femoris also steadies hip joint and helps illiopsoas flex thigh
Vastus lateralis	Greater trochanter and lateral lip of linea aspera of femur			
Vastus medialis	Inter-trochanteric line and medial lip of linea aspera of femur			
Vastus intermedius	Anterior and lateral surfaces of shaft of femur			

[a]The spinal cord segmental innervation is indicated (e.g., "L1, L2, L3") means that the nerves supplying the quadriceps femoris are derived from the first three lumbar segments of the spinal cord. Number in boldface **(L3, L4)** indicate the main segmental innervation. Damage to one or more of the listed spinal cord segments or to the motor nerve roots arising from them results in paralysis of the muscles concerned.

Action of rectus femoris at hip and knee joints

❑ **Rectus femoris**, a part of quadriceps femoris pulls the tibia anterior for knee extension.

❑ Rectus femoris also act at the hip joint along with iliopsoas for **hip flexion**.

Note: Rectus femoris arises by two tendons : one attached to anterior inferior iliac spine; the other to the brim of the acetabulum and the capsule of hip joint.

❑ Rectus femoris is called as **Kicking muscle**.

❑ All the parts of quadriceps act on the knee joint only **except** Rectus femoris which acts on both hip joint and knee joint

Sartor (tailor posture) attained by the activity of sartorius muscle.

❑ It causes flexion at both the hip and knee joints.

❑ It also causes abduction and lateral rotation at hip joint.

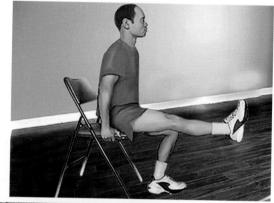

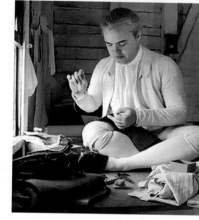

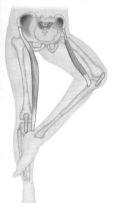

1. Strongest flexor of the hip joint is: *(NEET Pattern 2012)*
a. Sartorius
b. Gluteus maximus
c. Iliopsoas
d. Pectineus

2. Hip flexion is done by all EXCEPT:
a. Ilio-psoas
b. Pectineus
c. Sartorius
d. Semitendinosus

3. Lateral dislocation of patella is prevented by: *(NEET Pattern 2015)*
a. Rectus femoris
b. Vastus intermedius
c. Vastus lateralis
d. Vastus medialis

4. Action of sartorius muscles includes all EXCEPT: *(NEET Pattern 2015)*
a. Flexion of thigh
b. Flexion of leg
c. Extension of leg
d. Lateral rotator of thigh

1. **c. Iliopsoas**
   - ❑ Iliopsoas is the chief flexor at hip joint, assisted by sartorius and pectineus as the accessory muscles.
   - ❑ Gluteus maximus is the chief extensor at hip joint, assisted by hamstrings as the accessory muscles.

2. **d. Semitendinosus**
   - ❑ Hip flexion is chiefly carried out by iliopsoas muscle and assisted by muscles like pectineus, sartorius etc.
   - ❑ Semitendinosus is a hamstring muscle for hip extension along with the gluteus maximus.

3. **d. Vastus medialis**
   - ❑ Vastus medialis stabilizes patella bone and prevents its lateral dislocation on femur.
   - ❑ Restraining action of the medial patellofemoral ligament help in preventing lateral displacement of patella.

4. **c. Extension of leg**
   - ❑ Sartorius muscle help to attain the sartor (tailor) posture.
   - ❑ It causes flexion at both the hip and knee joints.
   - ❑ It also causes abduction and lateral rotation at hip joint.

▶ Muscles (Medial Thigh)

Table 15: Muscles of medial thigh

Muscle[a]	Proximal attachment	Distal attachment	Innervation[b]	Main action
Adductor longus	Body of pubis inferior to pubic crest	Middle third of linea aspera of femur	Obturator nerve, branch of, anterior division (L2, **L3**, L4)	Adducts thigh
Adductor brevis	Body and inferior ramus of pubis	Pectineal lines and proximal part of linea aspera of femur		Adducts thigh; to some extent flexes it
Adductor magnus	Adductor part: inferior ramus of pubis, ramus of ischium Hamstrings part: ischial tuberosity	Adductor part: gluteal tuberosity, linea aspera, medial supracondylar lines Hamstring part: aductor tubercle of femur	Adductor part: obturator nerve (L2, **L3**, L4), branches of posterior division Hamstring part: tibial part of sciatic nerve (L4)	Adducts thigh Adductor part: flexes thigh Hamstrings part: extends thigh
Gracilis	Body and inferior ramus of pubis	Superior part of medial surface of tibia.	Obturator nerve (**L2**, L3)	Adducts thigh; flexes leg; helps rotate leg medially
Obturator externus	Margins of obturator foramen and obturator membrane	Trochanteric fossa of femur	Obturator nerve (L3, **L4**)	Laterally rotates thigh; steadies head of femur in acetabulum

[a]Collectively, the five muscles listed are the adductors of the thigh, but their actions are more complex (e.g., they act as flexors of the hip joint during flexion of the knee joint and are active during walking).
[b]The spinal cord segmental innervation is indicated (e.g., "L2, L3, L4" means that the nerves supplying the adductor longus are derived from the second to fourth lumbar segments of the spinal cord). Numbers in boldface (**L3**) indicated the main segmental innervation. Damage to one or more of the listed spinal cord segments or to the motor nerve roots arising from them results in paralysis of the muscles concerned.

1. **What is TRUE about adductors of thigh**   *(NEET Pattern 2015)*
   - a. Ischial head of adductor magnus is an adductor
   - b. Profunda femoris artery is the main blood supply
   - c. Ischial head of adductor magnus originates from adductor tubercle
   - d. Adductor magnus is the largest muscle

1. **d. Adductor magnus is the largest muscle > b. Profunda femoris artery is the main blood supply**
   - ❑ Adductor magnus is the largest muscle and is a hybrid muscle having two parts.
   - ❑ Posterior ischial head of adductor magnus, takes origin from ischial tuberosity and is a hamstring part (not adductor).
   - ❑ Adductor tubercle receives the insertion (not origin) of adductor magnus.
   - ❑ Profunda femoris artery provides major supply to all the three compartments of thigh including medial (adductor) compartment.

❑ All the muscles of the adductor compartment of thigh are inserted into the femur **except gracilis** (which is inserted into the tibia).

❑ **Rider's bone** is calcified tendon of adductor longus/sesamoid bone in the tendon of adductor longus.

Muscles (Posterior Thigh)

Table 16: Muscles of posterior thigh				
Muscle[a]	Proximal attachment	Distal attachment	Innervation[b]	Main action
Semitendinosus	Ischial tuberosity	Medial surface of superior part of tibia	Tibial division of sciatic nerve part of tibia (L5, S1, S2)	Extend thigh; flex leg and rotate it medially when knee is flexed; when thigh and leg are flexed, these muscles can extend trunk
Semimembranosus		Posterior part of medial condyle of tibia; reflected attachment forms oblique popliteal ligament (to lateral femoral condyle)		
Biceps femoris	Long head: ischial tuberosity Short head: linea aspera and lateral supracondylar line of femur	Lateral side of head of fibula; tendon is split at this site by fibular collateral ligament of knee	Long head: tibial division of sciatic nerve (L5, S1, S2) Short head: common fibular division of sciatic nerve (L5, S1, S2)	Flexes leg and rotates it laterally when knee is flexed; extends thigh (e.g., accelerating mass during first step of gait).

[a]Collectively these three muscles are known as hamstrings
[b]The spinal cord segmental innervation is indicated (e.g., "LS, S1, S2" means that the nerves supplying the semitendinosus are derived from the fifth lumbar segment and first two sacral segments of the spinal cord). Numbers in boldface (L5, S1) indicate the main segmental innervation. Damage to one or more of the listed spinal cord segments or to the motor nerve roots arising from them results in paralysis of the muscles concerned.

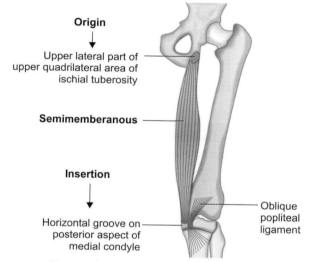

Origin

Upper lateral part of upper quadrilateral area of ischial tuberosity

Semimemberanous

Insertion

Horizontal groove on posterior aspect of medial condyle

Oblique popliteal ligament

Fig. 31: Semimembranosus attachments

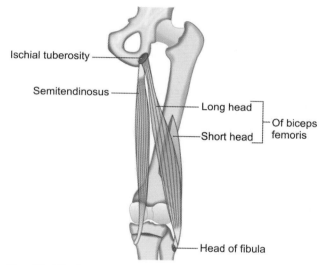

Ischial tuberosity

Semitendinosus

Long head
Short head
} Of biceps femoris

Head of fibula

Fig. 32: Attachments of semitendinosus and biceps femoris

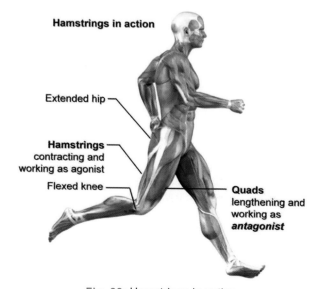

Hamstrings in action

Extended hip

Hamstrings contracting and working as agonist

Flexed knee

Quads lengthening and working as *antagonist*

Fig. 33: Hamstrings in action

- ❑ Hamstrings in action
- ❑ Hamstrings are: Semitendinosus, semimembranosus, long head of biceps femoris and posterior part of adductor magnus
- ❑ They extend the thigh at the hip and flex the leg at the knee and work antagonistically to quadriceps femoris.
- ❑ Main extensors of the hip **during walking** are Hamstring muscles.

1. **The following are part of hamstrings:**   *(PGIC 2014,15)*
   a. Semitendinosus   b. Semimembranosus
   c. Gracilis
   d. Short head of biceps femoris
   e. Sartorius

2. **TRUE regarding semitendinosus:**   *(NEET Pattern 2015)*
   a. Supplied by common peroneal part of sciatic nerve
   b. Proximal fleshy distal thin
   c. Distal fleshy proximal thin
   d. Proximal and distal thin middle fleshy

3. **Biceps femoris, a hamstring muscle causes:**
   a. Hip flexion and knee extension
   b. Hip and knee flexion
   c. Hip and knee extension
   d. Hip extension and knee flexion

4. **Oblique popliteal ligament attaches to:**   *(JIPMER 2006)*
   a. Semimembranosus
   b. Semitendinosus
   c. Adductor magnus
   d. Sartorius

1. **a. Semitendinosus; b. Semimembranosus**
   ❑ Hamstrings are: Semitendinosus, semimembranosus, long head of biceps femoris and posterior part of adductor magnus.

2. **b. Proximal fleshy distal thin**
   ❑ Semitendinosus is fleshy in the upper part and forms a cord-like tendon in the lower part, which lies posterior to semimembranosus muscle.
   ❑ It is a hamstring muscle supplied by the tibial part of sciatic nerve.

3. **d. Hip extension and knee flexion**
   ❑ Biceps femoris is one of the hamstring muscles along with semitendinosus, semimembranosus, and ischial head of the adductor magnus, which extend the thigh at the hip and flex the leg at the knee.

4. **a. Semimembranosus**
   ❑ Oblique popliteal ligament is an expansion from the tendon of semimembranosus muscle, runs upward and laterally superficial to the capsule to be attached to the intercondylar line of the femur.

❑ Some authors equate **sacrotuberous ligament** with the degenerated developmental remnant of the tendon of the **long head of the biceps femoris**.

▶ Muscles (Gluteal region)

Table 17: Muscles of gluteal region (abductors and rotators of thigh)

Muscle	Proximal attachment	Distal attachment	Innervation[a]	Main action
Gluteus maximus	Ilium posterior to posterior gluteal line; dorsal surface of sacrum and coccyx; sacrotuberous ligament	Most fibers end in iliotibial tract, which inserts into lateral condyle of tibia; some fibers insert on gluteal tuberosity	Inferior gluteal nerve (L5, **S1, S2**)	Extends thigh (especially from flexed position) and assists in its lateral rotation; steadies thigh and assists in rising from sitting position
Gluteus medius	External surface of ilium between anterior and posterior gluteal lines	Lateral surface of greater trochanter of femur	Superior gluteal nerve (**LS, S1**)	Abduct and medially rotate thigh; keep pelvis level when ipsilateral limb is weight-bearing and advance opposite
Gluteus minimus	External surface of ilium between anterior and inferior gluteal lines	Anterior surface of greater trochanter of femur		(unsupported) side during its swing phase
Tensor fasciae	Anterior superior iliac spine; anterior part of iliac crest	Iliotibial tract, which attaches to lateral condyle of tibia		
Piriformis	Anterior surface of sacrum; sacrotuberous ligament	Superior border of greater trochanter of femur	Branches of anterior rami of **S1**, S2	Laterally rotate extended thigh and abduct flexed thigh; steady femoral head in acetabulum
Obturator internus	Pelvic surface of obturator membrane and surrounding bones	Medial surface of greater trochanter (trochanteric fossa) of femur[c]	Nerve to obturator internus (LS, **S1**)	Laterally rotate extended thigh and abduct flexed thigh; steady femoral head in acetabulum
Superior and inferior gemelli	Superior: ischial spine Inferior: ischial tuberosity	Medial surface of greater trochanter (trochanteric fossa) of femur[b]	Superior gemellus : same nerve supply as obturator internus Inferior gemellus: same nerve supply as quadratus femoris	

Muscle	Proximal attachment	Distal attachment	Innervation[a]	Main action
Quadratus femoris	Lateral border of ischial tuberosity	Quadrate tubercle on inter-trochanteric crest of femur and area inferior to it	Nerve to quadratus femoris (L5, S1)	Laterally rotates thigh; steadies femoral head in acetabulum

[a]The spinal cord segmental innervation is indicated (e.g., "S1.S2"s means that the nerves supplying the piriformis are derived from the first two sacral segments of the spinal cord). Numbers in boldface (S1) indicate the main segmental innervation. Damage to one or more of the listed spinalcord segments or to the motor nerve roots arising from them. Results in paralysis of the muscles concerned.
[b]The gemelli muscles blend with and share the tendon to the obturator internus as it attaches to the greater trochanter of the femur, collectively forming the triceps coxae.
[c]There are six lateral rotators of the thigh: piriformis, obturator internus, superior and interior gemelli, quadratus temoris, and obturator externus. These muscles also stabilize the hip joint.

❑ Gluteus maximus helps in sitting to standing position: It works as an extensor of trunk on thigh, when **raising the trunk from sitting**, acting from the pelvis, it an extend the flexed thigh and bring it in line with the trunk.
❑ Superior gemellus and obturator internus are supplied by **nerve to obturator internus** (L5, S12)
❑ Inferior gemellus and quadratus femoris are supplied by **nerve to quadratus femoris** (L4,5; S1).

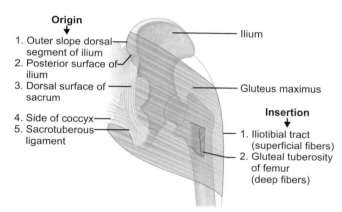

Fig. 34: Attachments of gluteus maximus

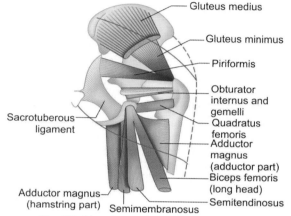

Fig. 35: Muscles under gluteus maximus

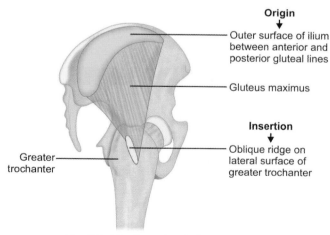

Fig. 36: Attachments of gluteus medius

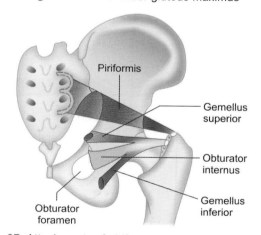

Fig. 37: Attachments of piriformis, obturator internus and gamelli muscles.

❑ **Piriformis** muscle (key muscle of gluteal region) takes its origin from anterior surface of sacrum, gluteal surface of ilium and sacrotuberous ligament. Its round tendon inserts on the tip of the greater trochanter after passing through greater sciatic foramen.
❑ **Largest muscle** of the body is gluteus maximus.

1. **Gluteus maximus is inserted on:** *(NEET Pattern 2014)*
   a. Lesser trochanter
   b. Greater trochanter
   c. Spiral line
   d. Iliotibial tract

2. **TRUE regarding origin and insertion of piriformis:**
   (NEET Pattern 2015)
   a. Origin from sacrum and ilium and insertion on lesser trochanter
   b. Origin from sacrum and ilium and insertion on greater trochanter
   c. Origin from Ischial tuberosity and insertion on lesser trochanter
   d. Origin from ischial tuberosity and insertion on greater trochanter

3. **Muscle attached to lateral surface of greater trochanter:** *(NEET Pattern 2014)*
   - a. Gluteus maximus
   - b. Gluteus medius
   - c. Gluteus minimus
   - d. Piriformis

4. **Lateral rotators of thigh are all EXCEPT:** *(NEET Pattern 2016)*
   - a. Piriformis
   - b. Gluteus medius
   - c. Quadratus femoris
   - d. Obturator internus

5. **Identify the marked muscle in the gluteal region:**
   - a. Obturator externus
   - b. Obturator internus
   - c. Quadratus femoris
   - d. Piriformis

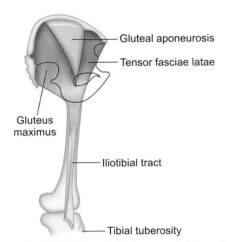

6. **Which of the following muscle is involved in movement from sitting to standing position:** *(NEET Pattern 2014)*
   - a. Gluteus maximus
   - b. Obturator internus
   - c. Gluteus medius
   - d. Gluteus minimus

1. **d. Iliotibial tract**
   - ❑ Most of the fibers of gluteus maximus insert into iliotibial tract and some fibers insert on gluteal tuberosity.

2. **b. Origin from sacrum and ilium and insertion on greater trochanter**
   - ❑ Piriformis muscle takes its origin from anterior surface of sacrum, gluteal surface of ilium and sacrotuberous ligament.
   - ❑ Its round tendon inserts on the tip of the greater trochanter.

3. **b. Gluteus medius**
   - ❑ Gluteus medius attaches to the lateral surface of greater trochanter.
   - ❑ Gluteus minimus attaches to the anterior surface of greater trochanter.
   - ❑ Gluteus maximus attaches on posterior aspect of femur bone at gluteal tuberosity.

4. **b. Gluteus medius**
   - ❑ The pull of gluteus medius muscle passes anterior to hip joint, hence it is a medial rotator at the joint.

5. **c. Quadratus femoris**
   - ❑ Under cover of gluteus maximus, a quadrangular muscle, attached to bone femur is called quadratus femoris.

6. **a. Gluteus maximus**
   - ❑ Gluteus maximus works as an extensor of trunk on thigh, when raising the trunk from sitting, acting from the pelvis, it an extend the flexed thigh and bring it in line with the trunk.

◤ Iliotibial Tract

Ilio-tibial tract

❑ It is a modification of deep fascia (lata) of the lateral aspect of thigh.

Gluteal aponeurosis

Tensor fasciae latae

Gluteus maximus

Iliotibial tract

Tibial tuberosity

Fig. 38: Attachment of the iliotibial tract. Note superficial portion of gluteus maximus and tensor fasciae latae insert into the iliotibial tract from opposite directions

❑ It receives insertion of superficial portion of **gluteus maximus** and **tensor fasciae latae**. It is inserted on the **Gerdy's tubercle** on anterolateral surface of the lateral tibial condyle.

❑ It is not inserted on tibial tuberosity *(NEET Pattern 2015)*

❑ It stabilizes the knee both in semiflexed and extended position; hence it is used constantly during walking and running.

❑ Iliotibial Band Syndrome (pain), may occur in a long-distance runner or cyclist.

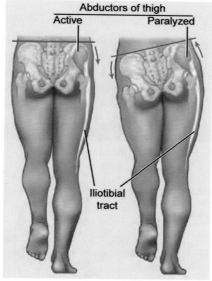

Fig. 29: Trendelenburg test

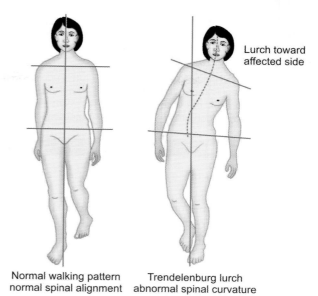

Fig. 40: Lurching gait

Trendelenburg Test

- In a case of left **superior gluteal nerve** injury (left gluteus medius palsy). Patient's right lower limb keep falling down during swing phase of walking cycle (limb length becomes more) and is unable to clear the foot from the ground leading to a lurch to clear it from ground.
- Injury to superior gluteal nerve results in a characteristic motor loss, resulting in a disabling gluteus medius limp, to compensate for weakened abduction of the thigh by the **gluteus medius and minimus**.
- When a standing person is asked to lift one foot off the ground and stand on one foot, the gluteus medius and minimus normally contract as soon as the contralateral foot leaves the floor, preventing the fall of the pelvis to the unsupported side.
- In a **superior gluteal nerve lesion**, when the patient is asked to stand on one leg, the pelvis on the unsupported side descends, indicating that the gluteus medius and minimus on the supported side are non-functional (positive Trendelenburg test).
- When the pelvis descends on the unsupported side, the lower limb becomes, in effect, too long and does not clear the ground when the foot is brought forward in the swing phase of walking. To compensate, the individual leans away from the unsupported side, raising the pelvis to allow adequate room for the foot to clear the ground as it swings forward. This results in a characteristic **lurching gait**. (In bilateral lesion it becomes **waddling gait**).
- Trendelenburg test may also be present in fracture of the greater trochanter (the distal attachment of gluteus medius) and dislocation of the hip joint.

QUESTIONS

1. Inability to maintain pelvis position while standing on one leg, nerve paralysed: *(JIPMER 2016)*
   a. Superior gluteal nerve   b. Inferior gluteal nerve
   c. Tibial part of sciatic nerve   d. Common peroneal nerve

2. Trendelenburg test is positive due to injury to the nerve: *(AIIMS 2008)*
   a. Inferior gluteal   b. Superior gluteal
   c. Obturator   d. Tibial

3. In walking, gravity tends to tilt pelvis and trunk to the unsupported side, major factor in preventing this unwanted movement is:
   a. Adductor muscles   b. Quadriceps
   c. Gluteus maximus
   d. Gluteus medius and minimus

4. An old man has trouble walking. At his physician›s office, he is asked to stand on his right foot and his left hip drops. Which of the following nerves is most likely damaged, causing his problem:
   a. Left inferior gluteal   b. Left superior gluteal
   c. Right inferior gluteal   d. Right superior gluteal

ANSWERS

1. **a. Superior gluteal nerve**
   - When a person who has suffered a lesion of the superior gluteal nerve is asked to stand on one leg, the pelvis on the unsupported side descends, indicating that the gluteus medius and minimus on the supported side are weak or non-functional. This sign is referred to clinically as a positive Trendelenburg test.

2. **b. Superior gluteal**
   - Superior gluteal nerve, if injured, paralyses the 3 muscles: gluteus medius, gluteus minimus and tensor fascia latae and hence lead to Trendelenberg test positive.
   - These 3 muscles, especially the gluteus medius raises the unsupported hip during walking, which otherwise will be pulled down by the gravity.
   - In Trendelenberg test this action of gluteus medius (superior pelvic tilt of contralateral hip) is absent and we actually observe that there is a downward drop of the unsupported hip -due to unopposed action of gravity. This leads to Lurching gait in the patient.

3. d. Gluteus medius and minimus
- ❏ During walking, gravity tends to tilt pelvis and trunk to the unsupported side, these muscles prevent this unwanted movement, by counteracting gravity from the opposite side.

4. d. Right superior gluteal
- ❏ In this patient, the right superior gluteal nerve is damaged, leading to failure of abductor mechanism of gluteus medius.
- ❏ There is also the failure of muscle to cause an upward lift of left hip, when the patient is asked to stand on his right foot.
- ❏ Normally the superior gluteal nerve leads to pelvic stability while a person stands on a single foot, by elevating the opposite hip- the job being performed by gluteus medius.

▼ Hybrid Muscles

Anterior compartment (Femoral nerve territory)	Flexors of hip, Extensors of knee
Posterior compartment (Tibial part of sciatic nerve territory)	Extensors of hip, Flexors of knee
Medial compartment (Obturator nerve territory)	Adductors of thigh

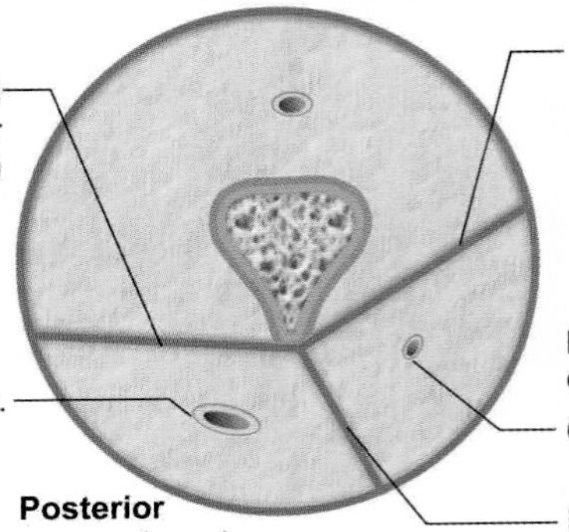

Hybrid muscles

Pectineus: Femoral + Obturator nerve

Adductor magnus: Obturator nerve + Tibial part of sciatic nerve

Biceps femoris: Tibial part of sciatic nerve + Common peroneal nerve

- ❏ **Longest** muscle in the body is **sartorius**.
- ❏ Gluteus maximus is the strongest extensor of the thigh at the hip and especially important when walking uphill, climbing stairs, or rising from a sitting position.
- ❏ **Iliopsoas** muscle is a **powerful flexor** of the thigh and attaches to the lesser trochanter.
- ❏ The tensor fascia lata and rectus femoris muscles can flex the thigh at the hip joint and extend the leg at the knee.
- ❏ In lower limb, **gracilis** is the most common muscle used for **surgical grafting**.

Fig. 41: Transverse section through the middle thigh showing compartments of thigh (with corresponding nerves)

▼ Anterior and Lateral Leg Muscles

Table 18: Muscles of anterior and lateral leg region

Muscle	Proximal attachment	Distal attachment	Innervation[a]	Main action
Anterior compartment Tibialis anterior (1)	Lateral condyle and superior half of lateral surface of tibia and interosseous membrane	Medial and inferior surfaces of medial cuneiform and base of 1st metatarsal	Deep fibular nerve (**L4**, L5)	Dorsiflexes ankle and inverts foot
Extensor digitorum longus (2)	Lateral condyle of tibia and superior three quarters of medial surface of fibula and interosseous membrane	Middle and distal phalanges of lateral four digits		Extends lateral four digits and dorsiflexes ankle
Extensor hallucis longus (3)	Middle part of anterior surface of fibula and interosseous membrane	Dorsal aspect of base of distal phalanx of great toe (hallux)		Extends great toe and dorsiflexes ankle
Fibularis tertius (4)	Inferior third of anterior surface of fibula and interosseous membrane	Dorsum of base of 5th metatarsal		Dorsiflexes ankle and aids in eversion of foot
Lateral compartment Fibularis longus (5)	Head and superior two thirds of lateral surface of fibula	Base of 1st metatarsal and medial cuneiform	Superficial fibular nerve (**L5**, **S1**, S2)	Everts foot and weakly plantarflexes ankle
Fibularis brevis (6)	Inferior two thirds of lateral surface of fibula	Dorsal surface of tuberosity on lateral side of base of 5th metatarsal		

[a]The spinal cord segmental innervation is indicated (e.g., "L4, L5" means that the nerves supplying the tibialis anterior are derived from the fourth and fifth lumbar at the spinal cord). Numbers in boldface (L4) indicate the main segmental innervation. Damage to one or more at the listed spinal cord segments or to the motor nerve roots arising from them results in paralysis of the muscles concerned.

Muscles of anterior and lateral leg region

Extensor TDH (Tom, Dick and Harry): T - Tibialis anterior, D- Extensor digitorum longus, H - Extensor hallucis longus) → Cause extension at ankle and toe joints.

Peroneus (fibularis) tertius is present in anterior leg compartment with extensors *(NEET Pattern 2012)*

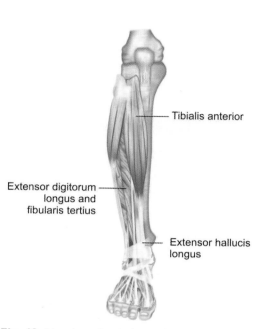

Fig. 42: Muscles of anterior and lateral by region

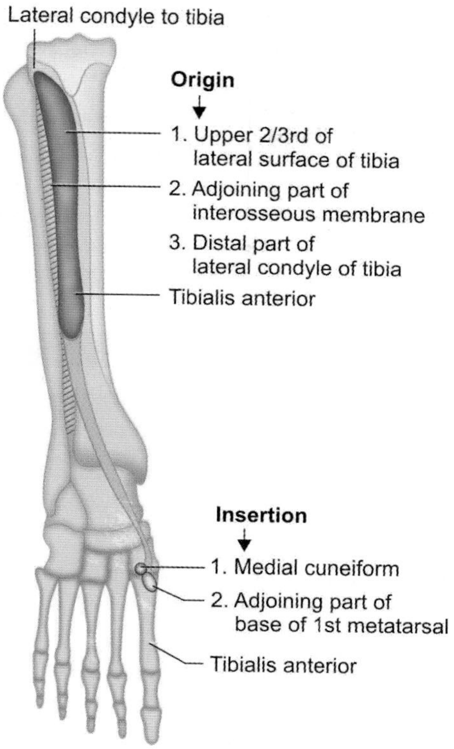

Tibialis anterior

Extensor digitorum longus and fibularis tertius

Extensor hallucis longus

Lateral condyle to tibia

Origin

1. Upper 2/3rd of lateral surface of tibia
2. Adjoining part of interosseous membrane
3. Distal part of lateral condyle of tibia

Tibialis anterior

Insertion

1. Medial cuneiform
2. Adjoining part of base of 1st metatarsal

Tibialis anterior

Fig. 43: Attachments of tibialis anterior

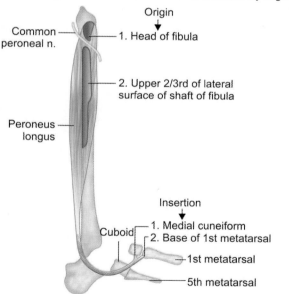

Common peroneal n.

Origin

1. Head of fibula
2. Upper 2/3rd of lateral surface of shaft of fibula

Peroneus longus

Insertion

Cuboid

1. Medial cuneiform
2. Base of 1st metatarsal

1st metatarsal

5th metatarsal

Fig. 44: Attachments of peroneus longus

- Tibialis anterior works for dorsiflexion (extension) and inversion *(NEET Pattern 2015)*; Nerve supply: Deep peroneal (anterior tibial) nerve.
- It is active in both stance and swing phases of walking cycle
- Action of peroneus longus is: Eversion (turn the sole lateral). It also maintains transverse (and lateral longitudinal) plantar arch.
- Nerve supply: Superficial peroneal nerve (branch of common peroneal nerve).
- Violent inversion of the foot will lead to avulsion of tendon of the **peroneus brevis** attached to the tuberosity of the 5th metatarsal *(AIIMS 2007)*
- Peroneus longus and brevis cause **eversion** of foot at **subtalar joint**.
- **Tibialis** anterior and posterior, both cause **inversion** of foot at subtalar joint.

1. **All are true about anterior compartment of leg EXCEPT:**
   (NEET Pattern 2015)
   a. Tibialis anterior causes dorsiflexion of foot
   b. Extensor hallucis longus causes extension of metatarso-phalangeal joint of big toe
   c. Peroneus longus causes eversion of foot
   d. Nerve supply is through deep peroneal nerve

2. **Peroneus longus:**   *(NEET Pattern 2015)*
   a. Invertor of foot
   b. Supplied by deep peroneal nerve
   c. Maintains arches of foot
   d. Arises from tibia

3. **Muscle(s) of anterior compartment of leg is/are:**
   (PGIC 2016)
   a. Peroneus longus
   b. Peroneus brevis
   c. Peroneus tertius
   d. Flexor digitorum longus
   e. Flexor hallucis longus

1. **c. Peroneus longus causes eversion of foot**
   - ❏ Peroneus longus is a muscle of lateral (not anterior) leg compartment.

2. **c. Maintains arches of foot**
   - ❏ Peroneus longus causes foot eversion and maintains lateral longitudinal and transverse arches of foot.
   - ❏ It takes its origin from fibula and is supplied by superficial peroneal nerve.

3. **c. Peroneus tertius**
   - ❏ Peroneus tertius is a muscle of anterior compartment of leg.
   - ❏ Peroneus longus and peroneus brevis belong to lateral leg compartment.
   - ❏ Flexor digitorum longus and Flexor hallucis longus belong to flexor compartment (calf) of leg.

▶ Posterior Leg Muscles

Table 19: Superficial muscles of posterior leg region

Muscle	Proximal attachment	Distal attachment	Innervation[a]	Main action
Gastrocnemius (1)	Lateral head: lateral aspect of lateral condyle of femur	Posterior surface of calcaneus via calcaneal tendon	Tibial nerve (S1, S2)	Plantarflexes ankle when knee is extended; raises heel during walking; flexes leg at knee joint
	Medial head: popliteal surface of femur; superior to medial condyle			
Soleus (2)	Posterior aspect of head and superior quarter of posterior surface of fibula; soleal line and middle third of medial border of tibia; and tendinous arch extending between the bony attachments			Plantarflexes ankle independent of position of knee steadies leg on foot
Plantaris (3)	Inferior end of lateral supracondylar line of femur; oblique popliteal ligament			Weakly assists gastrocnemius in plantarflexing ankle

[a]The spinal cord segmental innervation is Indicated (e.g., "S1, S2' means that the nerves supplying these muscles are derived from the first and second sacral segments of the spinal cord). Damage to one or more of the listed spinal cord segments or to the motor nerve roots arising from them results in paralysis of the muscles concerned.

Table 20: Deep muscles of posterior leg region

Muscle	Proximal attachment	Distal attachment	Innervation[a]	Main action
Popliteus	Lateral surface of lateral condyle of femur and lateral meniscus	Posterior surface of tibia, superior to soleal line	Tibial nerve (L4, LS, S1)	Weakly flexes knee and unlocks it by rotating femur 5° on fixed tibia; medially rotates tibia of unplanted limb
Flexor hallucis longus (4)	Inferior two thirds of posterior surface of fibula; inferior part of interosseous membrane	Base of distal phalanx of great toe (hallux)	Tibial nerve (S2, S3)	Flexes great toe at all joints; weakly plantarflexes ankle: supports medial longitudinal arch of fool
Flexor digitorum longus (5)	Medial part of posterior surface of tibia inferior to soleal line; by a broad tendon to fibula	Bases of distal phalanges of lateral four digits		Flexes lateral four digits; plantarflexes ankle; supports longitudinal arches of foot
Tibialis posterior (6)	Interosseous membrane: posterior surface of tibia inferior to sole-al line: posterior surf ace of fibula	Tuberosity of navicular. cuneiform. cuboid, and sustentaculum tali of calcaneus; bases of 2nd, 3rd, and 4th metatarsals	Tibial nerve (L4, LS)	Plantarflexes ankle: inverts foot

[a]The spinal cord segmental innervation is indicated (e.g. 'S2, S3' means that the nerves supplying the flexor hallucis longus are derived from the second and third sacral segments of the spinal cord). Damage to one or more of the listed spinal cord segments or to the motor nerve roots arising from them results in paralysis of the muscles concerned.

Posterior leg (calf) muscles: Superficial and Deeper group

- ❏ **Superficial (GPS):** Triceps surae -Gastrocnemius, plantaris and soleus.
- ❏ **Deep:** Flexor TDH (Tom, Dick and Harry): Tibialis posterior, flexor digitorum longus, flexor hallucis longus → Cause flexion at ankle and toe joints.

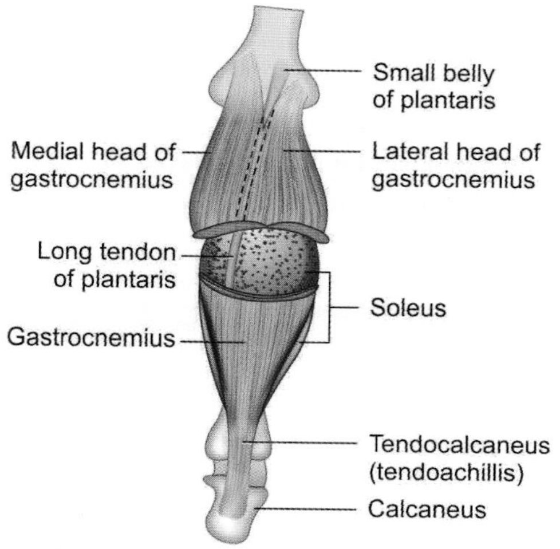

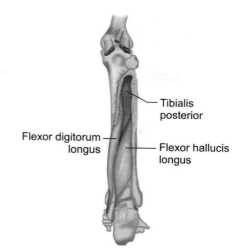

Fig. 45: Posterior leg (calf) muscles: Superficial group

Fig. 46: Posterior leg (calf) muscles: Superficial group

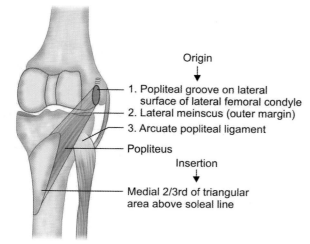

Fig. 47: Attachments of popliteus muscle

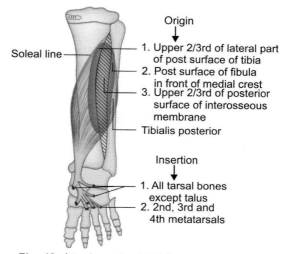

Fig. 48: Attachments of tibialis posterior muscle

❑ Popliteus has **intracapsular** origin from the lateral condyle of femur, has attachment with the lateral lemniscus (not medial) and inserts into the posterior surface of tibia (floor of popliteal fossa).

❑ It is supplied by tibial nerve and unlocks the knee joint by **medial rotation of tibia** (in un-planted foot). It also works with hamstring muscles for knee flexion.

❑ **Tibialis posterior** takes origin from inner posterior borders of both tibia & fibula and also the interosseous membrane *(NEET Pattern 2014)*. It has extensive attachments on the foot bones but is **not attached to talus** bone.

1. Muscle acting both at knee and ankle joint is/are:
   a. Gastrocnemius   b. Soleus   *(PGIC 2014,15)*
   c. Plantaris   d. Tibialis posterior
   e. Flexor hallucis longus

2. All are true about popliteus EXCEPT: *(NEET Pattern 2013)*
   a. Flexes the knee   b. Unlocks the knee
   c. Inserted on medial meniscus d. Is intracapsular

1. a. Gastrocnemius, c. Plantaris
   ❑ The only muscles which cross the knee joint as well as ankle joint are gastrocnemius and plantaris.
   ❑ They both cause flexion at knee joint and plantar flexion at ankle joint.

2. c. Inserted on medial meniscus
   ❑ It has intracapsular origin from the lateral condyle of femur, has attachment with the lateral lemniscus (not medial) and inserts into the posterior surface of tibia (floor of popliteal fossa).
   ❑ It is supplied by tibial nerve and unlocks the knee joint by medial rotation of tibia (in un-planted foot). It also works with hamstring muscles for knee flexion.

❑ Plantaris has a long slender tendon giving the appearance of a nerve (hence termed **freshman's nerve**). It is a vestigial muscle (absent in 5–10% population), tendon is used for grafting.

- Muscle of the leg having maximum concentration of muscle spindles is **plantaris**.
- Muscle functioning as organ of proprioception in the leg is plantaris.
- Soleus is called **peripheral heart**, as it helps pumping the blood in the circulatory system.
- In posterior compartment syndrome, patient keeps the foot in a position of plantar-flexion to maximally relax the fascia/muscles. And there occurs pain on dorsiflexion, due to passive stretching of posterior leg muscles *(AIIMS 2008)*
- Plantaris has a thin tendon, which get stretched and ruptured in **violent dorsiflexion** *(NEET Pattern 2013)*
- "Workhorse" of plantar flexion of the foot soleus.

▶ Arteries of Lower Limb

- Profunda femoris artery is the major artery to all the three compartments of thigh, including posterior thigh.

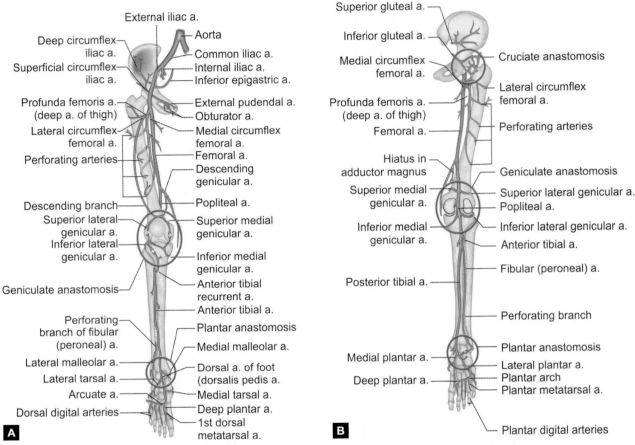

Figs. 49A and B: Arterial supply of lower limb; A. Anterior view; B. Posterior view

- Anterior compartment additionally has femoral artery and medial thigh has additional obturator artery.
- **Five genicular** arteries are given by popliteal artery (including **middle genicular artery**) to supply knee joint. There are two superior (medial & lateral) and two inferior (medial & lateral) as well.
- Most difficult peripheral pulse to feel **Popliteal pulse.**
- Artery most prone to aneurysm in the body Popliteal artery

Table 21: Arteries of anterior and medial thigh			
Artery	**Origin**	**Course**	**Distribution**
Femoral	Continuation of external iliac artery distal to inguinal ligament	Descends through femoral triangle bisecting it; then courses through adductor canal; terminates as it traverses adductor hiatus, where its name becomes popliteal artery	Branches supply anterior and anteromedial aspects of thigh

Artery	Origin	Course	Distribution
Profunda femoris artery (deep artery of thigh)	Femoral artery 1-5 cm inferior to inguinal ligament	Passes deeply between pectineus and adductor longus; descending posterior to latter on medial side of femur	Three to four perforating arteries pass through adductor magnus muscle, winding around femur to supply muscles in medial. posterior, and lateral part of anterior compartments
Medial circumflex femoral	Profunda femoris artery: may arise from femoral artery	Passes medially and posteriorly between pectineus and iliopsoas; enters gluteal region and gives rise to posterior retinacular arteries; then terminates by dividing into transverse and ascending branches	Supplies most of blood to head and neck of femur: transverse branch takes part in cruciate anastomosis of thigh; ascending branch joins inferior gluteal artery
Lateral circumflex femoral		Passes laterally deep to sartorius and rectus femoris, dividing into ascending, transverse, and descending arteries	Ascending branch supplies anterior part of gluteal region; transverse branch winds around femur; descending branch joins genicular periarticular anastomosis
Obturator	Internal iliac artery or (in ~20%) as an accessory or replaced obturator artery from the inferior epigastric artery	Passes through obturator foramen; enters medial compartment of thigh and divides into anterior and posterior branches, which pass on respective sides of adductor brevis	Anterior branch supplies obturator externus, pectineus, adductors of thigh, and gracilis; posterior branch supplies muscles attached to ischial tuberosity

Table 22: Arteries of leg region			
Artery[a]	Origin	Course	Distribution in leg
Popliteal	Continuation of femoral aretery at adductor hiatus in adductor magnus	Passes through popliteal fossa to leg: ends at lower border popliteus muscle by dividing into anterior and posterior tibial arteries	Superior, middle, and inferior genicular arteries to both lateral and medial aspects of knee
Anterior tibial	Popliteal	Passes between tibia and fibula into anterior compartment through gap in superior part of interosseous membrane and descends this membrane between tibialis anterior and extensor digitorum longus	Anterior compartment of leg
Dorsalis pedis (Dorsal artery of foot)	Continuation of anterior tibial artery distal to inferior extensor retinaculum	Descends anteromedially to first interosseous space and divides into plantar and arcuate arteries	Muscles on dorsum of foot; pierces first dorsal interosseous muscles as deep plantar artery to contribute to formation of plantar arch
Posterior tibial	Popliteal	Passes through posterior compartment of leg and terminates distal to flexor retinaculum by diving into medial and lateral plantar arteries	Posterior and lateral compartments of leg: circumflex fibular branch joins anastomoses around knee: nutrient artery passes to tibia
Fibular	Posterior tibial	Descends in posterior compartment adjacent to posterior intermuscular septum	Posterior compartment of leg: perforating branches supply lateral compartment of leg

Thigh positioned in slight flexion, abduction and lateral rotation, femoral artery is represented by the upper two-third of a line, drawn from the midinguinal point to the adductor tubercle *(NEET Pattern 2013)*

Femoral artery and branches

Superficial external pudendal artery is a branch of femoral artery *(NEET Pattern 2015)*

Superficial epigastric artery is a branch of femoral artery *(NEET Pattern 2015)*

❑ Halfway between the anterior superior iliac spine and the pubic symphysis lies the **midinguinal point** (MIP). **Femoral artery pulse** is felt at the midinguinal point ± 1 cm either side *(NEET Pattern 2012)*.

Note: It is mid-inguinal point and not the mid-point of inguinal ligament.

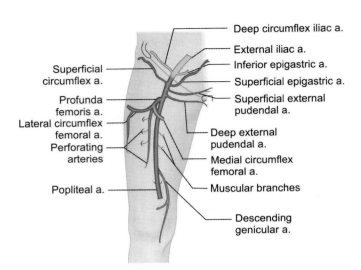

Fig. 50: Branches of the femoral artery

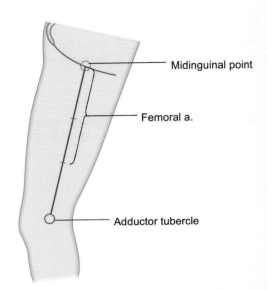

Fig. 51: Surface marking of the femoral artery

❏ Since the **femoral artery** is quite superficial in the femoral triangle, it is the preferred artery for cannulation and injecting dye to perform procedures like angiography. It is also the preferred vessel for performing the coronary angiography and angioplasty.

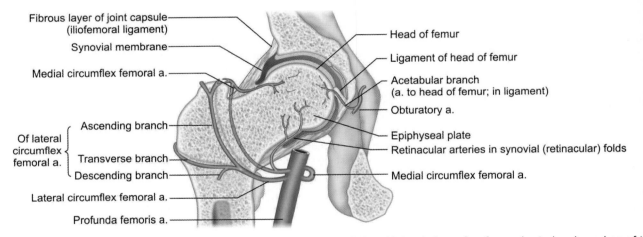

Fig. 52: Blood supply of head and neck of femur. Branches of the medial and lateral circumflex femoral arteries, branches of the profunda femoris artery, and the artery to the femoral head (a branch of the obturator artery) supply the head and neck of the femur. In the adult, the medial circumflex femoral artery is the most important source of blood to the femoral head and adjacent (proximal) neck

Most important source of blood supply to the head of the femur are **retinacular arteries**.

❏ The **lateral epiphyseal artery** (the terminal branch of the medial circumflex femoral artery) is the **primary** blood supply and runs along the postero-superior aspect of the femoral neck before terminating into 2-4 retinacular arteries that enter the femoral head.

❏ The femoral head receives blood supply mostly from the **MFCA** (medial circumflex femoral artery).

❏ Also from the anastomoses that contribute to the blood supply of the femoral head, the **most** important is the anastomosis with the IGA (**inferior gluteal artery**) via the piriformis branch, which can also be a dominant vessel supplying the femoral head.

❏ The anterior nutrient artery of the femoral neck—originating from the **lateral circumflex artery**—and the **obturator artery**, via the artery of the ligamentum teres, constitute a minor component of the blood supply to the femoral head

❏ In **intracapsular fracture**, the retinacular vessels—the chief source of blood supply to the head—are injured. This leads to delayed healing or non-union of fracture, or even **avascular necrosis** of the head of femur.

❏ **Chief artery** for the muscles of thigh is **Profunda femoris artery**.

❏ Largest branch of the profunda femoris artery **Lateral circumflex femoral artery.**

QUESTIONS

1. **Popliteal artery is difficult to palpate because:** *(AIPG 2009)*
   a. It is not superficial
   b. Does not pass over prominent bony structure
   c. Superficial but does not pass over prominent bony structure
   d. Not superficial and does not pass over prominent bony structure

2. **Which nerve passes behind the femoral artery:**
   (NEET Pattern 2016)
   a. Femoral nerve
   b. Saphenous nerve
   c. Lateral cutaneous nerve of thigh
   d. Nerve to pectineus

3. **The blood supply to femoral head is mostly by:**
   (NEET Pattern 2013)
   a. Lateral epiphyseal artery
   b. Medial epiphyseal artery
   c. Ligamentum teres artery
   d. Profunda femoris

4. **The blood supply to femoral head is:** *(PGIC 2014, 2003)*
   a. Obturator artery
   b. Internal pudendal artery
   c. Lateral circumflex femoral artery
   d. Femoral artery
   e. Profunda femoral artery

ANSWERS

1. **d. Not superficial and does not pass over prominent bony structure**
   ❑ Popliteal artery is the most difficult of the peripheral pulses to feel because it lies deep in the popliteal fossa and does not pass over prominent bony structure.

2. **d. Nerve to pectineus**
   ❑ Nerve to the pectineus arises immediately below the inguinal ligament, and passes behind the femoral sheath (and femoral artery) to enter the anterior surface of the muscle.

3. **a. Lateral epiphyseal artery**
   ❑ The lateral epiphyseal artery (the terminal branch of the medial circumflex femoral artery) is the primary blood supply and runs along the postero-superior aspect of the femoral neck before terminating into 2-4 retinacular arteries that enter the femoral head.

4. **a. Obturator artery, c. Lateral circumflex femoral artery, d. Femoral artery, e. Profunda femoral artery**
   ❑ Femoral head is supplied by branch of obturator artery, medial & lateral circumflex arteries and inferior & superior gluteal arteries.
   ❑ Medial circumflex artery may be a direct branch of femoral artery occasionally.
   ❑ It is also supplied by 1st perforating branch of profunda femoral artery.

❑ Unique feature of the **lateral compartment** of the leg is that it does not have its own artery.
❑ **Largest nutrient artery** in the body is nutrient artery to tibia (a branch of the posterior tibial artery).
❑ Largest and most important branch of the posterior tibial artery is **peroneal artery**.

▼ Veins of lower limb

❑ **Femoral vein** is the upward continuation of the **popliteal vein** beginning at the adductor opening and ending posterior to the inguinal ligament as the external iliac vein. It is posterolateral to the femoral artery in the distal adductor canal.

❑ More proximally in the canal, and in the distal femoral triangle (i.e. at its apex), the vein lies posterior to the artery and proximally, at the base of the triangle, the vein lies medial to the artery.

❑ **Tributaries**: Veins accompanying the superficial epigastric, superficial circumflex iliac and external pudendal arteries join the long saphenous vein before it enters the saphenous opening.

❑ Other tributaries are profunda femoris vein, lateral and medial circumflex femoral veins, deep external pudendal vein.

❑ There are usually **four or five valves** in the femoral vein; the two most constant are just distal to the entry of profunda femoris and near the inguinal ligament.

❑ **Great saphenous vein** starts as a continuation of medial marginal vein, ascends 2.5 cm in front (not behind) of the medial malleolus. In the thigh, it is in relation with medial cutaneous nerve of thigh and pass through saphenous opening to end in femoral vein 2.5 cm below the inguinal ligament.

❑ The saphenous opening (fossa ovalis) is an **opening in fascia lata**, closed by a membrane of areolar tissue—the **cribriform fascia** which is pierced by great saphenous vein. The centre of the opening is about **4 cm inferolateral** to the pubic tubercle.

❑ The vein has 10 to 12 valves, which are more numerous in the leg than in relation to the thigh and are usually located just below the perforated vein; there are 4 on average, located below the knee.

❑ **Small (Short) Saphenous Vein** is formed by the union of dorsal vein from the fifth digit (smallest toe) merge with the lateral end of dorsal venous arch of the foot to form the short saphenous vein. Next it runs superiorly behind the lateral malleolus, along the **lateral edge of tendocalcaneus**, and is accompanied by the sural nerve on its lateral side. It keeps ascending in the middle of the back of the leg (not lateral leg), eventually terminates into popliteal vein.

❑ The vein contains 7–13 valves, one of those near termination.

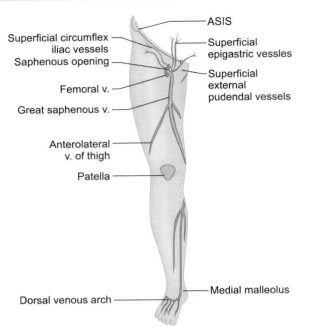

Fig. 53: Great saphenous vein - Formation, course, termination, tributaries and perforators

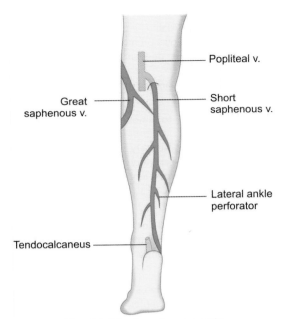

Fig. 54: Short saphenous vein

QUESTIONS

1. **TRUE regarding saphenous vein:** *(PGIC 2014)*
   Long saphenous vein formed as continuation of medial side of deep venous arch
   a. Long saphenous vein — situated posterior to medial malleolus
   b. Long saphenous vein— closely related to saphenous nerve
   c. Short saphenous vein— open into great saphenous vein
   d. Short saphenous vein associated with sural nerve

2. **TRUE about saphenous opening:** *(NEET Pattern 2014)*
   a. Transmits saphenous nerve
   b. Lies 4 cm lateral and superior to pubic tubercle
   c. Covered by cribriform fascia
   d. Opening in cribriform fascia

3. **All are true about short saphenous vein EXCEPT:** *(NEET Pattern 2015)*
   a. Runs behind lateral malleolus
   b. Runs on lateral side of leg
   c. Accompanied by sural nerve
   d. Achilles tendon is medial to vein

ANSWERS

1. **a. Long saphenous vein formed as continuation of medial side of deep venous arch; c. Long saphenous vein- closely related to saphenous nerve; e. Short saphenous vein associated with sural nerve**
   ❑ Long saphenous vein is formed by the union of the medial end of dorsal venous arch with the medial marginal vein which drains the medial side of great toe. It passes upwards anterior (not posterior) to the medial malleolus.
   ❑ The saphenous nerve has a course along with the long saphenous vein.
   ❑ Short saphenous vein is accompanied by the sural nerve and opens into the popliteal vein (not great saphenous vein).

2. **c. Covered by cribriform fascia**
   ❑ Saphenous opening is an oval defect in the fascia lata in front of the thigh, for the passage of great saphenous vein into the femora vein.
   ❑ The centre of the opening is about 4 cm inferolateral to the pubic tubercle.
   ❑ The saphenous opening is closed by a membrane of areolar tissue—the cribriform fascia which is pierced by great saphenous vein, superficial epigastric and superficial external pudendal vessels and lymph vessels connecting superficial and deep inguinal lymph nodes.

3. **b. Runs on lateral side of leg**
   ❑ Short saphenous vein begins at the lateral end of dorsal venous arch, runs superiorly behind the lateral malleolus, along the lateral edge of tendocalcaneus, and is accompanied by the sural nerve on its lateral side.
   ❑ It keeps ascending in the middle of the back of the leg (not lateral leg), eventually terminates into popliteal vein.

❑ There are **no perforator** veins below the inguinal ligament *(AIIMS 2007)*
❑ **Hunterian perforator** is present in mid-thigh at the lower part of adductor (Hunterian) canal. It connects great saphenous vein with the femoral vein *(NEET Pattern 2013)*
❑ **Dodd's perforator** is present in distal thigh and connect great saphenous vein with femoral vein *(NEET Pattern 2016)*
❑ Incompetent valves affecting perforating veins of lower limb makes the blood flow from **deep to superficial** direction.
❑ This makes the superficial veins overfilled with blood and they become dilated, elongated and tortuous – **varicose veins** *(AIIMS 2005)*

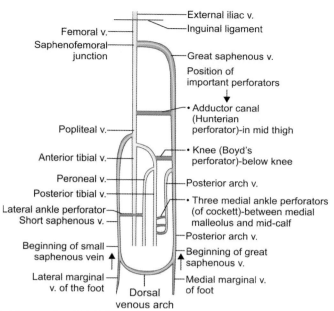

Fig. 55: Veins of the lower limb (deep vein - light blue color, superficial veins - deep blue color, perforating vein - violet color

Perforators	Location	Connection
1. Mid-thigh (Hunterian perforator)	Just above knee (lower part of adductor canal)	Great saphenous with femoral vein
2. Knee (Boyd's perforator)	Just below knee	Great saphenous with posterior tibial vein
3. Leg (lateral ankle)	At the junction of middle of lower third of leg	Short saphenous with peroneal vein
4. 4, 5, 6. Leg (three medial ankle; Cockett's perforator)	a. Upper medial: junction of middle and lower third of leg b. Middle medial: 4 cm above the medial malleolus c. Lower medial: posteroinferior to medial malleolus	Posterior arch vein to posterior tibial vein

❑ **Great saphenous vein** in front of medial malleolus at ankle is the most preferred site of **venesection** (cut-down).
❑ Femoral vein is the preferred vein for intravenous infusions in infants and children and in patients with peripheral circulatory failure.
❑ **Longest** vein in the body is great saphenous vein.

▶ Lymphatics

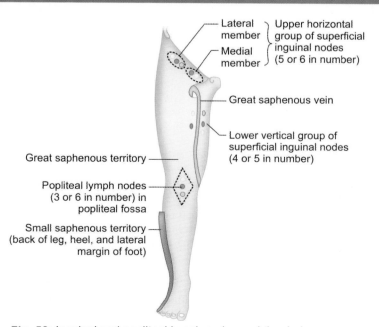

Fig. 56: Inguinal and popliteal lymph nodes and the drainage areas

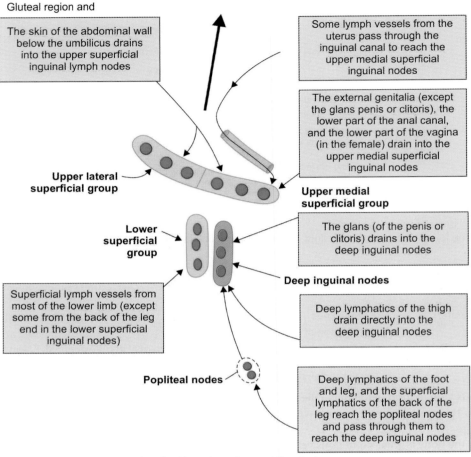

Fig. 57: Inguinal lymph nodes and the drainage areas

1. Skin and facia covering the ball of the big toe drain the lymphatics into: *(NEET Pattern 2015)*
 a. Vertical group of superficial inguinal lymph nodes
 b. Horizontal group of superficial inguinal lymph nodes
 c. Popliteal lymph nodes
 d. Deep inguinal lymph nodes

2. Medial superficial inguinal lymph node drains: *(NEET Pattern 2016)*
 a. Skin of abdominal wall below umbilicus
 b. Lymphatics of thigh
 c. Penis or clitoris
 d. All of the above

1. a. Vertical group of superficial inguinal lymph nodes
 ❑ Lymphatics from skin and superficial fascia of great toe accompany great saphenous vein and drain into superficial inguinal lymph nodes (vertical group).

2. c. Penis or clitoris
 ❑ The lymphatic vessels of the superficial tissue of the penis or clitoris run along with the superficial external pudendal blood vessels, and mainly drain into the superficial inguinal lymph nodes, just like the lymphatic vessels of the scrotum or labia majora. The glans penis, glans clitoris, labia minora, and the terminal inferior end of the vagina, all drain into the deep inguinal and external iliac lymph nodes.

❑ Lymph node of **Cloquet or Rosenmüller** are the deep inguinal lymph node present in the femoral canal.
❑ Most of the lymph from the lower limb is drained into **lower vertical** group of **superficial** inguinal lymph nodes.
❑ **Vein of Leonardo da Vinci** is the posterior arch vein, a tributary of great saphenous vein.

Femoral triangle

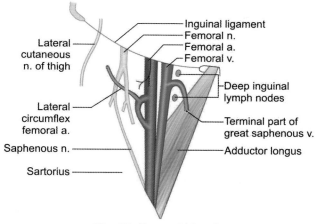

Fig. 58: Femoral triangle

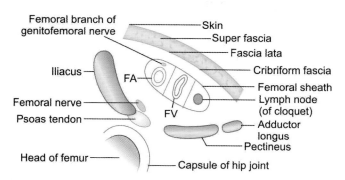

Fig. 59: Relations of femoral triangle

1. The floor of the femoral triangle is formed by all EXCEPT:
(NEET Pattern 2016)
a. Adductor longus   b. Sartorius
c. Psoas major   d. Pectineus

2. What is most medial in the femoral triangle: *(AIIMS 2009)*
a. Lymphatics   b. Nerve
c. Vein   d. Artery

3. All are contents of femoral triangle EXCEPT:
a. Femoral artery   *(NEET Pattern 2015)*
b. Femoral vein
c. Superficial inguinal lymph nodes
d. Nerve to pectineus

4. All are contents of femoral sheath EXCEPT:
a. Femoral artery   *(JIPMER 2001,4; NEET Pattern 2012)*
b. Femoral nerve
c. Femoral vein
d. Genitofemoral nerve

1. b. Sartorius
- Medial margin of sartorius forms the boundary of femoral triangle, thus sartorius muscle lies outside the triangle.

2. a. Lymphatics
- Femoral triangle has the deep inguinal lymph nodes in the medial most region.
- Femoral triangle is present in the anterior thigh and is bounded by superior - inguinal ligament; medial - medial margin of the adductor longus muscle and lateral - medial margin of the sartorius muscle.
- The contents (lateral to medial) are: Lateral cutaneous nerve of thigh; terminal part of the femoral nerve and its branches; the femoral branch of genitofemoral nerve; femoral sheath having three compartments with contents (lateral to medial): Femoral artery and its branches; femoral vein and its tributaries and femoral canal, which contains lymphatic vessels and deep inguinal lymph nodes.

3. c. Superficial inguinal lymph nodes
- The superficial inguinal lymph nodes are found deep to Camper's fascia and superficial to fascia lata.
- Since femoral triangle is a sub-fascial space (fascia lata being the roof), it is only the deep inguinal lymph nodes, which are contents of femoral triangle.

4. b. Femoral nerve
- Femoral nerve is a content of femoral triangle, but is not covered by femoral sheath.

Adductor Canal

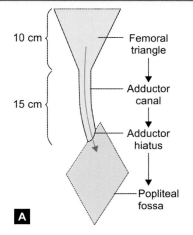

A

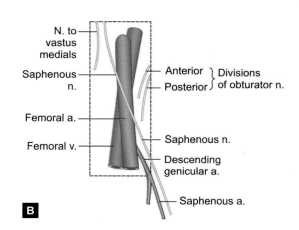

B

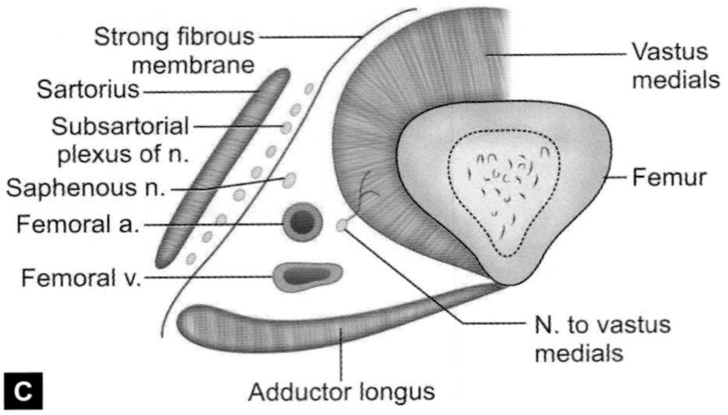

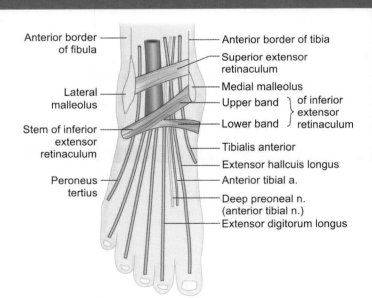

Strong fibrous membrane
Sartorius
Subsartorial plexus of n.
Saphenous n.
Femoral a.
Femoral v.
Vastus medials
Femur
N. to vastus medials
Adductor longus

C

Figs. 60A to C: Adductor canal

❑ **Adductor canal** (Sub-sartorial/Hunter's canal) passes from the apex of the femoral triangle to the popliteal fossa.

QUESTIONS

1. All of the following pairs regarding adductor canal are true EXCEPT: *(JIPMER 2010)*
   a. Roof: Sartorius muscle
   b. Contents: Femoral nerve
   c. Floor: Adductor longus and magnus
   d. Antero-lateral boundary: Vastus medialis

2. Which of the following structure(s) pass through adductor magnus: *(PGIC 2015)*
   a. Femoral vessels   b. Femoral nerve
   c. Femoral sheath   d. Saphenous nerve
   e. Tibial nerve

ANSWERS

1. b. Contents: Femoral nerve
   ❑ Femoral nerve is not a content of adductor canal.
   ❑ Saphenous nerve, a branch of femoral nerve is present in the canal and passes anterior to femoral artery.

2. a. Femoral vessels
   ❑ Adductor magnus has a hiatus through which pass the femoral artery and vein from the **adductor canal** to enter the popliteal fossa.
   ❑ Femoral artery, vein and nerve are present in femoral triangle, artery and vein inside the femoral sheath (nerve being outside the sheath).
   ❑ Saphenous nerve is a branch of femoral nerve in femoral triangle, enters the adductor canal, but does not leave through the adductor hiatus instead penetrates superficially halfway through the adductor canal.
   ❑ Tibial nerve is located in the posterior thigh and descend inferiorly to become a content of popliteal fossa.

▸ Ankle Region Retinacula

QUESTION

1. NOT true about inferior extensor retinaculum: *(NEET Pattern 2015)*
   a. Y shaped
   b. Superior slip attached to lower end of fibula
   c. Inferior slip attached to deep fascia of sole
   d. Laterally attached to calcaneum

ANSWER

1. b. Superior slip attached to lower end of fibula:
   ❑ Superior lip of inferior extensor retinacula attaches to the medial malleolus of tibia.
   ❑ Inferior extensor retinaculum is Y shaped structure, whose stem is attached laterally to superior surface of calcaneum and the inferior lip of Y fuses with the deep fascia of the sole.

Anterior border of fibula
Lateral malleolus
Stem of inferior extensor retinaculum
Peroneus tertius
Anterior border of tibia
Superior extensor retinaculum
Medial malleolus
Upper band ⎫ of inferior
Lower band ⎬ extensor retinaculum
Tibialis anterior
Extensor hallcuis longus
Anterior tibial a.
Deep preoneal n. (anterior tibial n.)
Extensor digitorum longus

Fig. 61: Extensor retinacula

QUESTIONS

1. Structure passing deep to flexor retinaculum is:
                                                  (NEET Pattern 2015)
   a. Posterior tibial artery   b. Long saphenous vein
   c. Tibialis anterior   d. Peroneus tertius

ANSWERS

1. **a. Posterior tibial artery**
   - ❑ Flexor retinaculum is present on the medial side of ankle and let pass the long tendons of calf region towards the foot, along with the **posterior tibial neurovascular bundle**.
   - ❑ Tibialis anterior and peroneus tertius passes under anterior (**extensor retinacula**).

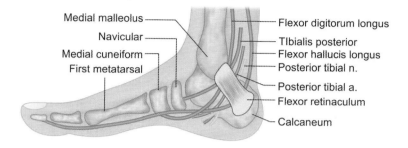

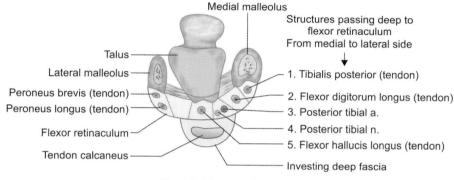

Fig. 62: Flexor retinaculum

QUESTIONS

1. **All of the following pass under the flexor retinaculum EXCEPT:** (PGIC 2000)
   a. Tibialis anterior
   b. Tibialis posterior
   c. Posterior tibial artery
   d. Deep peroneal nerve
   e. Anterior tibial nerve

2. **Neurovascular bundle of anterior compartment of leg passes between the tendons of:** (NEET Pattern 2013)
   a. Tibialis anterior and extensor hallucis longus
   b. Extensor hallucis longus and extensor digitorum longus
   c. Extensor hallucis longus and peroneus tertius
   d. Extensor digitorum longus and peroneus tertius

ANSWERS

1. **a. Tibialis anterior; d. Deep peroneal nerve; e. Anterior tibial nerve**
   - ❑ Tibialis anterior and deep peroneal (anterior tibial) nerve pass under the anteriorly placed extensor retinaculum.

2. **b. Extensor hallucis longus and extensor digitorum longus**
   - ❑ Arrangement of structures (medial to lateral) in front of ankle joint: Tibialis anterior, extensor hallucis longus, anterior tibial artery, deep peroneal nerve, extensor digitorum longus, peroneus tertius.

▶ Foot

Joint	Type (synovial)	Movement
Subtalar (talocalcaneal)	Plane	Inversion and eversion
Talocalcaneonavicular	Ball and socket	Inversion and eversion
Calcaneo-cuboid	Saddle	Inversion and eversion Circumduction
Transverse tarsal (midtarsal) Talonavicular + calcaneocuboid		Inversion and eversion
Tarsometatarsal	Plane	Abduction and adduction
Metatarso-phalangeal	Ellipsoid	Dorsiflexion and plantar flexion Adduction and abduction circumduction
Interphalangeal	Hinge	Dorsiflexion and plantar flexion

Movement	Joints involved
Plantar flexion and dorsiflexion	Ankle Metatarsophalangeal Interphalangeal
Inversion and eversion*	Subtalar (talo-calcaneal) Talocalcaneonavicular Transverse tarsal (midtarsal)
Adduction and abduction**	Transverse tarsal First tarsometatarsal Metatarsophalangeal
Supination (adduction, inversion and plantar flexion) and Pronation (abduction, eversion and dorsiflexion):	Ankle (dorsiflexion and plantar flexion) Talocalcaneonavicular and subtalar (Inversion and eversion) Transverse tarsal First tarsometatarsal Metatarsophalangeal

*Inversion: Medial border of foot is raised so that the sole faces medially and
eversion: Lateral border of the foot is raised so that the sole faces laterally

**Adduction: Movement of the foot towards the midline (in the transverse plane) and abduction: Movement away from the midline

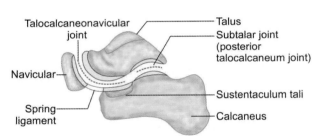

Fig. 63: Subtalar and talocalcaneonavicular joints

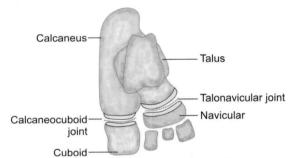

Fig. 64: Transverse tarsal (midtarsal) joint

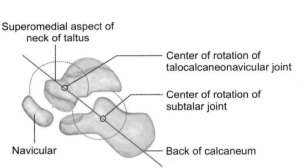

Fig. 65: Axis of inversion and eversion (red line)

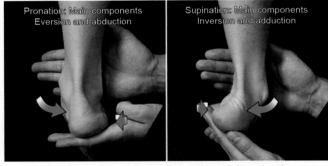

Fig. 66: Foot movements: Pronation and supination

❑ Inversion and eversion occurs mainly at **sub-talar joint**. Major movements occur at talocalcaneonavicular joint.
❑ Other involved joints are transverse tarsal/midtarsal joints (calcaneocuboid & talonavicular).

Table 23: Movements of inversion and eversion		
	Muscles	
Movements	**Principal muscles**	**Accessory muscles**
Inversion (ROM = 30°)	▪ Tibialis anterior ▪ Tibialis posterior	▪ Flexor hallucis longus ▪ Flexor digitorum longus
Eversion (ROM = 20°)	▪ Peroneus longus ▪ Peroneus brevis	▪ Peroneus tertius

QUESTIONS

1. Abduction and adduction of foot occurs at which joints
(NEET Pattern 2016)
- a. Ankle
- b. Subtalar
- c. Tarso-metatarsal
- d. Transverse tarsal

2. In foot pronation, the axis of which two joints become parallel
(AIIMS 2014)
- a. Talo-calcaneal and talonavicular
- b. Talo-calcaneal and calcaneocuboid
- c. Subtalar and Lisfranc
- d. Talo-navicular and calcaneo-cuboid

ANSWERS

1. d. Transverse tarsal
- ❑ Adduction is movement of the foot towards the midline in the transverse plane; abduction is movement away from the midline. This movement occurs at the transverse tarsal joints (a compound joint consisting of calcaneocuboid and talonavicular joints) and, to a limited degree, the first tarsometatarsal and metatarsophalangeal joints.

2. d. Talo-navicular and calcaneo-cuboid.
- ❑ Transverse tarsal (Midtarsal) joint is a collective term for the talonavicular (TN) part of the talocalcaneonavicular joint and the calcaneocuboid (CC) joint.
- ❑ The two joints are separated anatomically but act together functionally.
- ❑ During supination of foot, the soles face each other and there occurs inversion, whereas, in pronation, soles move outwards and is accompanied by eversion (TN and CC joint become parallel)

❑ Talo-calcaneonavicular joint is a Ball & Socket type of synovial joint (AIIMS 2017)
❑ Tarsometatarsal Joint (**Lisfranc Joint**) is the articulation of the tarsal bones with the metatarsals.

◤ Muscles of Sole

- ❑ **Dorsal interossei** abduct (DAB) toes, whereas the **plantar interossei** adduct (PAD) toes. All the interossei (along with lumbricals) flex MTP joints and extend IP joints. Paralysis of lumbrical and interossei leads to claw foot.
- ❑ Dorsal interossei abduct the toes relative to the longitudinal axis of the **second metatarsal**.
  Plantar interossei adduct the third, fourth and fifth toes.
- ❑ Diagrams for foot muscles - Layer 1 and 2 are missing !I have put them on a blank page, next to this one.

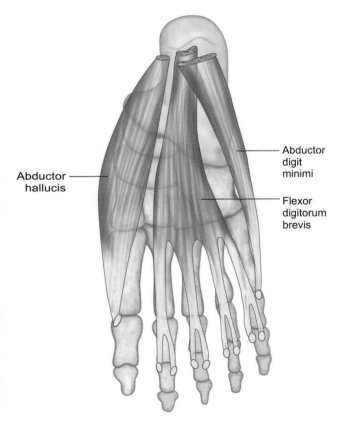

Fig. 67: Muscles of foot (layer 1)

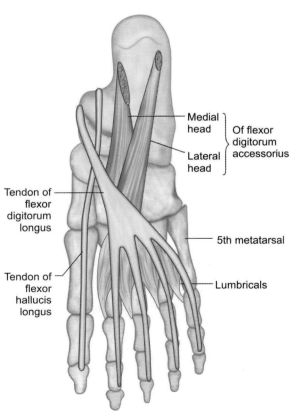

Fig. 68: Muscles of foot (layer 2)

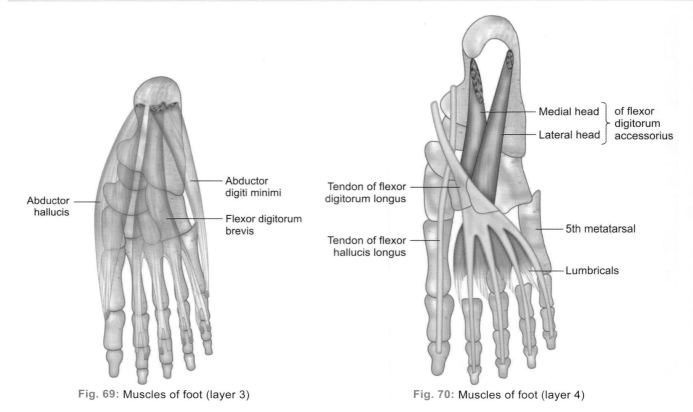

Fig. 69: Muscles of foot (layer 3)

Fig. 70: Muscles of foot (layer 4)

QUESTIONS

1. **First layer of sole has:**   *(NEET Pattern 2014)*
   a. Abductor hallucis   b. Flexor hallucis longus
   c. Flexor hallucis brevis   d. Adductor hallucis

2. **All of the following pairs concerning layers of sole muscles are correct EXCEPT:**
   a. First layer: Adductor hallucis   b. Second layer: Lumbricals
   c. Third layer: Flexor hallucis   d. Fourth layer: Interossei

ANSWERS

1. **a. Abductor hallucis**
   ❑ Abductor hallucis muscle belongs to first layer of sole.
   ❑ Tendon of flexor hallucis longus is found in second layer.
   ❑ Flexor hallucis brevis and adductor hallucis belong to the third layer.

2. **a. First layer: Adductor hallucis**
   ❑ Adductor hallucis belongs to third layer of sole.

All the interossei of sole are supplied by the deep branch of the lateral plantar nerve **except** those in the fourth intermetatarsal space, which are supplied by the superficial branch of the lateral plantar nerve.

▶ Plantar Arches

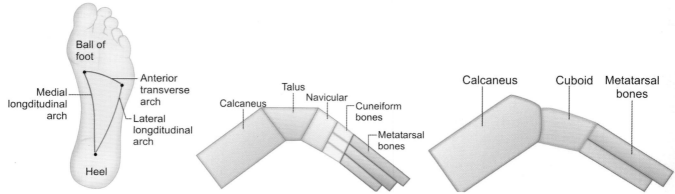

Fig. 71: Plantar arches

Fig. 72: Medial longitudinal arch

Fig. 73: Lateral longitudinal arch

Table 24: Differences between the medial and lateral longitudinal arches	
Medial longitudinal arch	**Lateral longitudinal arch**
▪ Formed by more bones and more joints	▪ Formed by less bones and less joints
▪ Characteristic features is resiliency	▪ Characteristic feature is rigidity
▪ Higher and more mobile	▪ Lower and less mobile
▪ Involved in propulsion during locomotion (i.e., initiating the next step during walking)	▪ Involved in receiving and supporting the body weight
▪ Summit is formed by the talus	▪ Summit is formed by the calcaneum
▪ Main joint is talocalcaneonavicular joint (the most vulnerable part of the arch)	▪ Main joint is calcaneocuboid (the most vulnerable part of the arch)

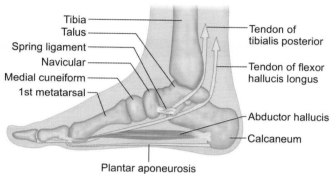

Fig. 74: Factors maintaining the medial longitudinal arch: Supports of the head of talus

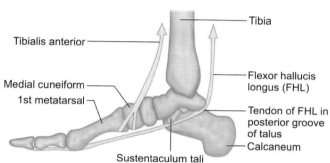

Fig. 75: Factors maintaining the medial longitudinal arch: Slings

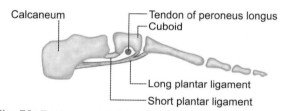

Fig. 76: Factors maintaining the lateral longitudinal arch: Short and long plantar ligaments

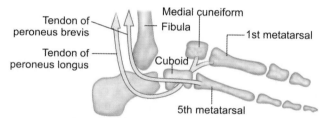

Fig. 77: Factors maintaining the lateral longitudinal arch: Tendons of the peroneus brevis and peroneus longus

❑ The bones involved in the **transverse arch** are the bases of the five metatarsals, the cuboid and the cuneiforms. The intermediate and lateral cuneiforms are wedge-shaped and thus adapted to maintenance of the transverse arch.

❑ The transverse arches are strengthened by the interosseous, plantar, and dorsal ligaments, by the short muscles of the first and fifth toes (especially the **transverse head of the Adductor hallucis**), and by the Peroneus longus, whose tendon stretches across between the piers of the arches.

❑ Most important factors in maintaining the **transverse arch** of the foot ate tendons of peroneus longus and tibialis posterior.

❑ **Keystone** of medial longitudinal arch is talus and for lateral longitudinal arch is cuboid.

❑ Most **vulnerable** part of the medial longitudinal arch is talocalcaneonavicular joint.

❑ Most **vulnerable** part of the lateral longitudinal arch is calcaneocuboid joint.

❑ Most important ligament for maintaining the arches of the foot is **spring ligament.**

❑ Commonest deformity of the foot **Talipes equinovarus**

QUESTIONS

1. **Medial longitudinal arch of the foot is maintained by all EXCEPT:** *(NEET Pattern 2015)*
   a. Peroneus longus
   b. Tibialis posterior
   c. Flexor digitorum longus
   d. Plantar aponeurosis

2. **Which is NOT a part of medial longitudinal arch of foot:**
   a. Third metatarsal
   b. Cuboid
   c. Calcaneum
   d. Talus

3. **Which tendon passes below sustentacula tali:** *(AIPG 2010)*
   a. Tibialis anterior
   b. Tibialis posterior
   c. Flexor hallucis longus
   d. Flexor digitorum longus

4. **Which of the following tendons has attachment on sustentaculum tali:** *(AIPG 2010)*
   a. Tibialis anterior
   b. Tibialis posterior
   c. Flexor digitorum longus
   d. Flexor hallucis longus

1. **a. Peroneus longus**
   - ❑ Peroneus longus and brevis support the lateral longitudinal arch.

2. **b. Cuboid**
   - ❑ Cuboid bone is present at the lateral aspect of the foot, articulates with calcaneum (CC joint is saddle synovial) and both bones contributes to lateral longitudinal arch. Cuboid bone is the keystone bone for the arch.

3. **c. Flexor hallucis longus**
   - ❑ The tendon of flexor hallucis longus passes in a groove between the two tubercles of the posterior talus and then lower surface of the sustentaculum tali. It uses sustentaculum tali as a pulley to pull and flex the great toe (flexor/hallux). This tendon also passes deep to the flexor retinaculum along with the other long tendons of the posterior leg.

4. **b. Tibialis posterior**
   - ❑ Tibialis posterior attaches to the medial margin on sustentaculum tali.

❑ Only intrinsic muscle on the dorsum of the foot is **extensor digitorum brevis.**
❑ Plantar fasciitis is **Policeman's heel**.

▶ Gait Cycle

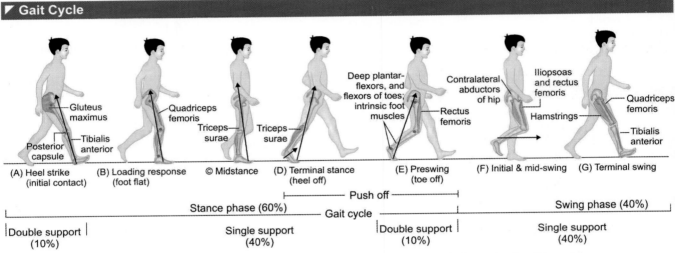

Fig. 78: Gait cycle. The activity of one limb between two repeated events of walking

❑ The kinetic energy of body is least in mid-stance phase of walking cycle, while the body is in single support phase (one foot on ground and the other foot being in air). **Kinetic energy is maximum in double support** (both the feet on ground).
❑ **Tibialis anterior** is active in both swing and stance phase of walking cycle *(AIIMS 2003)*.

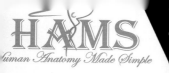

Human Anatomy Made Simple
by Dr. Rajesh K. Kaushal

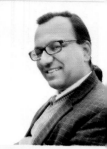

Anatomy Revision Programme
(AIIMS, PGI, JIPMER, NEET, DNB EXAMS)

ARP (Anatomy Revision Programme) is a 4 day (44 hours) concept based Anatomy lecture conducted throughout India and abroad in environment for the PG aspirants preparing for AIIMS, PGIMER, JIPMEr, NEET and DNB Exams.

Dr. Rajesh K Kaushal has been teaching Anatomy to PG Aspirants for past 16 years and actively engaged in taking interactive live classes in different cities across India. His approach towards the subject goes by the slogan **'HAMS-Human Anatomy Made Simple'** which is throughout in his classes.

ARP (Anatomy Revision Programme) Salient Features :

❖ Maximizes confidence and scoring in basic & advanced concepts in Anatomy & related subjects in PG Entrance Examinations.

❖ Coverage of Anatomy based questions in other subjects like Physiology, Pathology, Forensic, Pharmacology, ENT, Ophthalmology, Orhthopaedics, Dermatology, Medicine, Surgery, Obstetrics & Gynaecology, Paediatrics, Radiology, Anaesthesia

❖ High yield topics discussed in simplified language.

❖ Excellent handling of controversial questions with standard textbook references.

❖ Maximum possible content mastered in shortest possible time.

❖ **Study Material :** Anatomy Book (Self Assessment and Review of Anatomy-) is provided to each student registered for the class.

First Ever Comprehensive Anatomy Book by Subject Specialist

SECOND EDITION

Self Assessment and Review of
ANATOMY

Rajesh K Kaushal

Based on facts and concepts of the latest editions of standard books

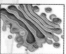

Highlights
- Comprehensive theory and latest pattern questions in all sub-sections of Anatomy—Embryology, Histology, Neuroanatomy and Gross Anatomy (including Surface and Radiological Anatomy)
- Previous years' questions with explanatory answers from the Entrance Examinations conducted by AIIMS, PGIC, JIPMER, NEET, and DNB
- Reference books include Gray's Anatomy (41st Ed), Keith L Moore (7th Ed), Langman's Embryology (13th Ed), Ross Histology (7th Ed), Barr's Neuroanatomy (10th Ed), Dorland's Medical Dictionary (32nd Ed).

Explained Referenced Answers
All Recent Questions 2018–2001
All India (2012–2001)
AIIMS (Nov 2017–2001)
DNB (2012–2001)
JIPMER (2017–2000)
UPSC (2017–2000)
NEET PG (2018–2012)
Image-based questions

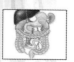

A must-buy book for All India, AIIMS, PGI, JIPMER, DNB, FMGE & State entrance exams

Day wise Schedule

Day-1
○ General Embryology
○ Histology, Osteology and Arthrology
○ NeuroAnatomy-I

Day-2
○ NeuroAnatomy-II
○ Head and Neck
○ Back

Day-3
○ Thorax
○ Upper Limb
○ Abdomen-I

Day-4
○ Abdomen-II
○ Pelvis and Perineum
○ Lower Limb

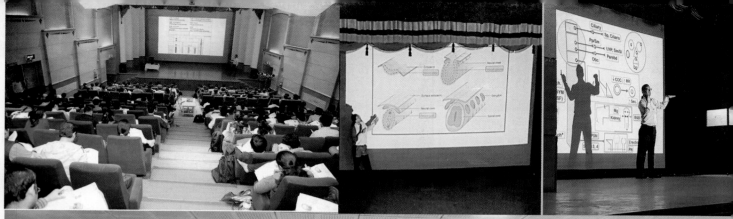

Glimpses of Anatomy Revision Programme

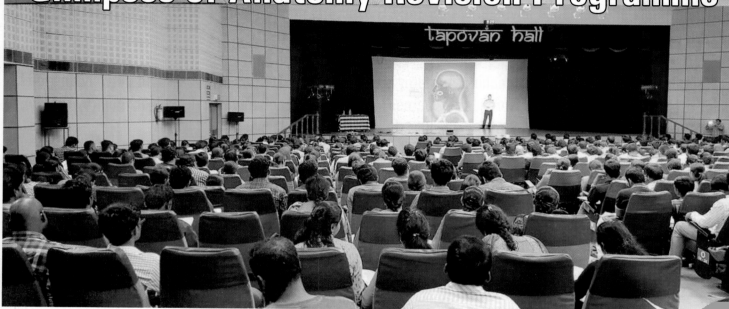

tapovan hall